ATHERO— SCLEROSIS V

Proceedings of the
Fifth International Symposium

Edited by
Antonio M. Gotto, Jr.   Louis C. Smith   Barbara Allen

With 250 illustrations

 Springer-Verlag
New York   Heidelberg   Berlin

Proceedings of the Fifth International Symposium
on Atherosclerosis

Held in Houston, November 6−9, 1979

Sponsored by Baylor College of Medicine and The
Methodist Hospital, Houston, Texas

Printed in the United States of America

9 8 7 6 5 4 3 2 1

ISBN 0-387-90473-5 Springer-Verlag New York Heidelberg Berlin
ISBN 3-540-90473-5 Springer-Verlag Berlin Heidelberg New York

INTERNATIONAL PROGRAM COMMITTEE

Jean-Louis Beaumont
Henry Buchwald
Lars A. Carlson
William E. Connor
Alan J. Day
Frederick H. Epstein
Yuichiro Goto
Antonio M. Gotto, Jr.
M. Daria Haust
William L. Holmes
Anatoli N. Klimov

David Kritchevsky
K.T. Lee
Kare R. Norum
Michael F. Oliver
Rodolfo Paoletti
Gotthard Schettler
Gunther Schlierf
Yechezkiel Stein
Daniel Steinberg
Jack P. Strong

ORGANIZING COMMITTEE

Chairman: Antonio M. Gotto, Jr.
Co-Chairman: Yuichiro Goto
General Secretary: Louis C. Smith
Symposium Coordinator: Jean King
Scientific Editor: Barbara Allen

ACKNOWLEDGEMENTS

We gratefully acknowledge the following individuals, institutions, organizations and companies whose generosity and support made this meeting possible.

William L. Holmes
Lars A. Carlson
Yuichiro Goto
M. Daria Haust
David Kritchevsky
Henry C. McGill
Paul J. Nestel
Michael F. Oliver
Rodolfo Paoletti
Gotthard Schettler
Yechezkiel Stein
Daniel Steinberg
Robert W. Wissler
Baylor College of Medicine
The Methodist Hospital
Council on Arteriosclerosis of the
    American Heart Association

Abbott Laboratories
American Cyanamid Company
Ayerst
Best Foods
Burroughs Wellcome Company
Ciba Geigy Corporation
Dow Chemical Company, USA
Hoffman-LaRoche, Inc.
Eli Lilly and Company
McNeil Laboratories
Mead Johnson Pharmaceutical Division
Merck Sharp and Dohme Research
    Laboratories
Miles Laboratories, Inc.
Norwich Eaton
Ortho Pharmaceutical Corporation
The Proctor and Gamble Corporation

William H. Rorer, Inc.
Sandoz, Inc.
Schering Corporation
G.D. Searle and Company
Smith, Kline and French Laboratories

Standard Brands, Inc.
Sun Company
Syntex Research
The Upjohn Company
Wyeth Laboratories, Inc.

PREFACE

The objective of the program committee of the Fifth International Symposium on Atherosclerosis was to bring together experts in many disciplines to broaden the scope of the attack on this disease and to foster interaction. Our hope was that such interaction would accelerate the eradication of the disease. The symposium achieved that objective and continued the tradition of the previous symposia in providing a forum for summaries of recent research developments in the study, treatment and prevention of atherosclerosis. The leading authorities and researchers in this field and in the related areas of interest have presented the newest information, concepts and ideas that have evolved in the past three years since the previous meeting in Tokyo. The most promising fields for future investigation are clearly identified, as are the nature of the controversies that persist in some highly important aspects of treatment of this disease. The appearance of these proceedings so soon after the meeting will greatly enhance the impact of the symposium on current research in atherosclerosis.

The program committee is particularly indebted to the excellent response of the investigators for their willingness to participate in the symposium and for their successful efforts in bringing high quality to their presentations. Their cooperation in the expeditious delivery of manuscripts for this volume has been particularly gratifying. The efforts of Ms. Barbara Allen in preparing this volume bear special note. The Chairman and the General Secretary gratefully acknowledge their debt of gratitude to Ms. Jean King, whose extraordinary skill and effort provided a pleasant, superbly organized and well-managed context for this symposium.

Antonio M. Gotto, Jr.
Chairman

Louis C. Smith
General Secretary

November 23, 1979
Houston, Texas

INTRODUCTION

Baylor College of Medicine and The Methodist Hospital hosted the Fifth International Symposium on Atherosclerosis in Houston, Texas, November 6−9, 1979. The honorary co-sponsors of the Symposium were Mrs. Mary Lasker of New York and Princesse Lilian of Belgium, two distinguished supporters of biomedical research. Because of their long interest in programs for the treatment and prevention of cardiovascular disease, the Fifth International Symposium conferred distinguished service awards on Mrs. Lasker and Princesse Lilian. Distinguished service awards were also given to Dr. Michael DeBakey, President and Chancellor of Baylor College of Medicine, for his contributions to the surgical treatment of atherosclerosis; to Mr. Ted Bowen, the President of The Methodist Hospital, for his vision, foresight, and administrative leadership in providing the facilities for a comprehensive cardiovascular center; and to Professors Gotthard Schettler of Heidelberg and Yuichiro Goto of Tokyo for their long and dedicated work in the field of atherosclerosis. At the meeting, Professor Schettler announced the establishment of a new organization called the International Atherosclerosis Society. The Fifth International Symposium on Atherosclerosis was the first to be held under the auspices of the new International Atherosclerosis Society.

The Symposium demonstrated the dynamic growth of the field, the progress that has been made since the previous symposium in Tokyo, and the fact that atherosclerosis has become a remarkably interdisciplinary activity. One of the most gratifying aspects of the Symposium was the degree of interchange between basic and clinical scientists, epidemiologists, biochemists, nutritionists, cardiologists and cardiovascular surgeons.

The opening session of the Houston Symposium honored Dr. DeBakey's contributions to the surgical treatment of atherosclerosis. As it presents to the surgeon atherosclerosis may follow a number of different patterns. One is the primary distribution of the lesions, for example, whether the coronary, the carotid or the peripheral arteries are involved, or a combination thereof. Another characteristic feature is whether the disease involves primarily distal or proximal blockage. A third characteristic relates to the rate of progression of the disease: rapid, slow or intermediate. It has not yet been possible to establish correlations between several of the patterns and any known constellation of risk factors. Another type of pattern, of which the frequency is unknown, are those individuals who may have coronary artery spasm, usually superimposed on underlying coronary artery obstruction, but in some instances without significant underlying coronary atherosclerotic lesions.

A workshop was devoted to the topic of coronary bypass surgery. Both the cardiologists and cardiovascular surgeons exhibited a considerable degree of enthusiasm for the procedure. There was even some note of optimism that the procedure may prolong life. Regardless of this last point, which remains a controversial one, the overall consensus of the participants in the workshop was one of enthusiasm for coronary artery bypass surgery as a treatment for obstructive disease of the coronary arteries. The relatively new procedure of coronary angioplasty may also prove to be beneficial to patients with certain types of coronary artery obstruction. This subject was to be extensively discussed at the annual meeting of the American Heart Association and one under intensive investigation.

The question of treatment of hyperlipidemia continues to be spiced with controversy. A number of different methods of reducing blood lipids discussed at the Symposium included diet, the subject of the second plenary session, drugs, ileal bypass surgery, portacaval shunt and plasma exchange procedures. Some preliminary evidence from human studies suggests that atherosclerosis may be reversible in man. The majority of individuals in intervention trials for relatively short periods of time will probably show failure of progression rather than clear-cut evidence of regression. What is needed is a way of achieving more than a marginal reduction of cholesterol or low density lipoproteins (LDL). For example, if it were possible to lower the cholesterol to less than about 150 mg/dl with a concomitant reduction in LDL, then extensive long-term intervention trials might not be required in order to show a clear-cut effect on morbidity and mortality. Some promising new drugs described at the Symposium include a new inhibitor of HMG CoA reductase.

A distinguished group of scientists could not agree on what information should be conveyed to the general public about diet. The fields of nutrition, platelet biochemistry, thrombosis prostaglandin chemistry, and cardiovascular disease are merging, as was illustrated by the plenary sessions on diet and on the vessel wall in which prostaglandin metabolism was discussed. In the platelet membranes from the Eskimo, an increased proportion of phospholipids containing unsaturated C-20:5 eicosopentanoic acid has been found. This most likely occurs as a consequence of ingesting the preformed fatty acids from fish in the Eskimo's diet. The Eskimo has been found to have a prolonged bleeding time. Several reviews claim that the Eskimo has a decreased incidence of coronary artery disease. Firm evidence for this latter point appears to be lacking, and it should be more intensively examined by epidemiologic studies. There is no evidence that consuming larger amounts of the C-20:3 fatty acid homo-γ-linolenic acid would increase the arachidonic acid content of platelets since administration of lipid emulsions containing homo-linolenic acid results in a replacement of arachidonic acid by the homo-linolenic acid. Thus, the role of polyunsaturated fats continues to be a controversial one. Depending upon the polyunsaturated fatty acid composition of the diet, the cholesterol and LDL concentrations may be lowered and bleeding time may be prolonged. It seems likely that the fluidity of the platelet and other cellular membranes may be altered by the specific fatty acid composition and this in turn may affect associated membrane properties.

One of the most encouraging reports at the meeting was that of a positive beneficial effect upon morbidity and mortality from treatment of mild hypertension in Australia. There continues to be much less controversy associated with efficacy of the treatment of hypertension than that of hyperlipidemia. Among the information concerning hypertension presented at the meeting was the report of a possible new marker for essential hypertension, the measurement of an abnormality in the mechanism of potassium transport across the erythrocyte. The use of drugs to affect the renin angiotensin axis also holds promise as providing new avenues for the treatment of hypertension.

The importance of cell biology in atherosclerosis was again emphasized by the presentation of important fundamental work at plenary sessions and at the workshops and oral sessions. The roles of the platelet growth factor of collagen and of glycosaminoglycans were discussed along with a number of other important topics. The study of the arterial wall has focused on the crucial cellular elements, viz., the endothelium, the smooth muscle cell and macrophage. No longer is atherosclerosis viewed as a disease of degeneration but rather one of proliferation. The role of hyperlipidemia in the proliferation of the cellular elements of the arterial wall is an important subject but remains to be defined.

A panel of expert epidemiologists, cardiologists and internists could not agree on an explanation for the declining death rate for cardiovascular disease in the United States, although there was agreement that such a decrease has occurred. The overall decline in the death rate for cardiovascular disease for the past 15 years has been approximately 30% as compared to 17% for noncardiovascular disease. A number of potential contributing factors have been suggested, including more effective detection and treatment of hypertension, a decline in the consumption of tobacco, a decrease in the use of saturated fats with a concomitant increase in consumption of polyunsaturated or vegetable fats, an apparent decline in the concentration of serum cholesterol and a national enthusiasm for exercise. Other countries, particularly European ones, have not shown a decline in death rate, although favorable trends may now be occurring. Despite these encouraging results, cardiovascular disease remains the number one cause of death and disability in Western society, accounting for over one-half the deaths in the United States each year. Approximately one million die each year in the United States from cardiovascular disease, of which about two-thirds are from myocardial infarctions. Thus, there is an enormous challenge yet awaiting physicians and researchers in the field of atherosclerosis and the end of this problem is far from visible at the present.

The results of the World Health Organization study on clofibrate have been reported since the last symposium. These results have been variously interpreted. For those who want to interpret the study in a favorable way, the group receiving clofibrate experienced a 20% lower rate of nonfatal myocardial infarctions, which accompanied a 10% reduction in the concentration of serum cholesterol. For those who wish to interpret the study in a different light, the group taking the clofibrate had a higher mortality as compared to the placebo control group. It is hoped that the results of the Multiple Risk Factor Intervention Trial in the United States and of the Lipid Research Clinics intervention with cholestyramine will give a more clear-cut resolution of the lipid hypothesis.

Regardless of the difficulties in proving or disproving the lipid hypothesis, interest in hyperlipidemia has lead to an explosion of research and knowledge concerning the structure and metabolism of plasma lipoproteins. This subject was extensively discussed in plenary sessions, workshops and in the oral sessions of the Symposium. An awareness of the complexity of the plasma lipoproteins has developed as more knowledge has evolved. Subclasses and subgroups have been identified, some of which may have important metabolic implications. For example, do HDL_2 and HDL_3 differ in their ability to protect against atherosclerosis? A causal relationship between concentrations of HDL and coronary artery disease has not been established, although a strong negative correlation exists. Different subgroups of LDL may exist due to differences in carbohydrate composition or other chemical properties. Work presented at the Symposium showed that some patients treated with drugs such as clofibrate responded with a reduction in LDL, while others exhibited an increase. Such findings illustrate the importance of performing careful metabolic studies of lipoprotein subclasses and apoproteins. Knowledge from such studies may form the basis of clinical tests that can be applied to patients and that can provide a more precise indication of who is likely to respond to a given hypolipidemic drug.

Knowledge of the chemistry of the lipoproteins has greatly expanded with the identification of apoprotein groups extending from A through E. The primary amino acid sequence of five of the apoproteins is known. In addition to binding lipids, certain of the apoproteins have been shown to have other specific functions, for example, the activation of lecithin:cholesterol acyltransferase by apoA-I and apoC-I and lipoprotein lipase by apoC-II. ApoD, also called the thin-line peptide and apoA-III, may be identical to the cholesteryl ester transfer protein. Specific regions of the apoC-II have been identified which activate lipoprotein lipase and which are involved in lipid binding. Extensive evidence now exists to support the role of hydrophobic surfaces in the binding of apoproteins to phospholipids in the plasma lipoproteins. The specific lipid binding sites are located in certain regions of the apoprotein called amphipathic helices.

Often a great deal of valuable information concerning lipoprotein metabolism can be gained by the study of mutants, as was illustrated at the Symposium by work on abetalipoproteinemia, LCAT deficiency, hypobetalipoproteinemia, Tangier disease, a form of type I hyperlipoproteinemia which is due to the complete absence of apoC-II, and familial hyper-cholesterolemia. An outstanding example is the knowledge gained about LDL and choles-terol metabolism from the discovery of the LDL receptor; these investigators rested heavily on the use of patients with familial hypercholesterolemia, who either have a deficiency or a complete absence of the receptor. Evidence was presented at the Symposium to support the occurrence of the receptor in vivo employing chemically modified LDL. Just how much LDL under normal conditions goes through the non-LDL receptor pathway has not been estab-lished. While a deficiency of the LDL receptor can explain the elevation in levels of LDL, additional factors are required to explain why elevation of LDL produces atherosclerosis. If the receptor were working normally in the endothelial cell or smooth muscle cell, the system should be self-regulating. Evidence was reviewed that chemical modification of LDL can enhance its uptake by cells. Whether such mechanisms operate in vivo is not known.

The purpose of my summary is not to list the most important or most significant work discussed at the Symposium, but rather to give a flavor of a few of the subjects discussed in order to indicate the interdisciplinary nature of the research and the great amount of progress that has been made since the last Symposium three years ago. The Symposium highlighted the hope that this progress will one day lead to the elucidation of the basic cause or causes of atherosclerosis and will point the way towards the development of solutions for the problem.

Antonio M. Gotto, Jr., M.D.
Houston, Texas
November 23, 1979

CONTENTS

Workshop: The Arterial Wall—I (Co-Chairpersons: M.D. Haust, K.W. Walton)

Workshop: Lipid, Apoprotein and Lipoprotein Origin and Synthesis (Co-Chairpersons: R.J. Havel, B. Lewis)

Workshop: Lipoprotein Structure (Co-Chairpersons: H.B. Brewer, Jr., W. Stoffel)

xiv

Workshop: Regression (Co-Chairpersons: D.H. Blankenhorn, J.P. Strong)

Workshop: The Interrelationship Between Lipid and Prostaglandin Metabolism
(Co-Chairpersons: S. Bergstrom, G.S. Boyd)

Workshop: Cellular Metabolism of Lipoproteins (Co-Chairpersons: E.L. Bierman,
N. Myant)

CONTRIBUTORS

C.W.M. Adams, M.D., D.Sc., F.R.C.P., F.R.C. Path., Head, Department of Pathology, Guy's Hospital Medical School, London SE1 9RT, England

Edward H. Ahrens, Jr., M.D., The Rockefeller University, 1230 York Avenue, New York, New York 10021, U.S.A.

Kazuo Aihara, M.D., Department of Medicine, Keio University, School of Medicine, 35 Shinano-machi, Shinjuku, Tokyo 160, Japan

Petar Alaupovic, Ph.D., Head, Lipoprotein Laboratory, Oklahoma Medical Research Foundation, 825 Northeast 13th Street, Oklahoma City, Oklahoma 73104, U.S.A.

John J. Albers, Ph.D., Division of Metabolism and Endocrinology, Department of Medicine, Harborview Medical Center, University of Washington School of Medicine, 326 Ninth Avenue, Seattle, Washington 98104, U.S.A.

Mark L. Armstrong, M.D., Cardiovascular Division, Department of Internal Medicine, University of Iowa College of Medicine, Iowa City, Iowa 52242, U.S.A.

Gerd Assmann, M.D., Westfalische Wilhelms-Universität, Medizinische Einrichtungen Zentrallaboratorium, 44 Münster, Westring 3, Federal Republic of Germany

Alan D. Attie, Division of Metabolic Disease, School of Medicine, University of California at San Diego, La Jolla, California 92093, U.S.A.

W. Auerswald, M.D., Atherosclerosis Research Group at the Department of Medical Physiology, University of Vienna, Vienna, Austria

Josef Augustin, M.D., Klinisches Institut für Herzinfarktforschung an der Medizinisches, Universitätsklink Heidelberg, Bergheimer Strasse 58, D 6900 Heidelberg, Federal Republic of Germany

J.M. Augustyn, Ph.D., Laboratory Service, Veterans Administration Medical Center, Albany, New York 12208, U.S.A.

Pietro Avogaro, M.D., Ph.D., Regional General Hospital, Unit for Atherosclerosis, National Council for Research, 30100 Venice, Italy

Giovannella Baggio, M.D., Department of Internal Medicine, Division of Gerentology and Metabolic Diseases, University of Padua, Policlinico, Via Giustiniani 2, 35100 Padua, Italy

Margret Bartholomé, Ph.D., Lehrstuhl für Klinischen Chemie der Medizinischen Einrichtungen der Universität Göttingen, Robert-Koch-Strasse 40, 3400 Göttingen, Federal Republic of Germany

M.F. Baudet, Ph.D., INSERM U 32, Créteil Faculty of Medicine, Henri-Mondor Hospital, Paris XII University, 9400 Créteil, France

Hans R. Baumgartner, M.D., F. Hoffman-La Roche and Company, Department of Pharmacology Research, CH 4002 Basel, Switzerland

Linda L. Bausserman, Ph.D., Brown University Program in Medicine, The Miriam Hospital, 164 Summit Avenue, Providence, Rhode Island 02906

O.B. Bayliss-High, Ph.D., M. Phil., Department of Pathology, Guy's Hospital Medical School, London SE1 9RT, England

J.L. Beaumont, M.D., INSERM U 32, Créteil Faculty of Medicine, Henri-Mondor Hospital, Paris XII University, 9400 Créteil, France

V. Beaumont, M.D., INSERM U 32, Créteil Faculty of Medicine, Henri-Mondor Hospital, Paris XII University, 9400 Créteil, France

Isolde Becht, Kliniches Institut für Herzinfarktforschung an der Medizinischen, Universitätsklinik Heidelberg, Bergheimer Strasse 58, D 6900 Heidelberg, Federal Republic of Germany

Carl Becker, M.D., Department of Pathology, The New York Hospital, Cornell Medical Center, 525 East 68th Street, New York, New York 10021, U.S.A.

Fabrizio Bellini, Ph.D., Departments of Physiology and Biochemistry, The Medical College of Pennsylvania Hospital, 3300 Henry Avenue, Philadelphia, Pennsylvania 19129, U.S.A.

Fabio Belussi, M.D., Regional General Hospital, Unit for Atherosclerosis, National Council for Research, 30100 Venice, Italy

Gunilla Bengtsson, Ph.D., Department of Medical Chemistry, University of Umea, S901 87 Umea, Sweden

Gerald S. Berenson, M.D., Head, Section of Cardiology, Department of Medicine, Director, Specialized Center of Research—Atherosclerosis, Louisiana State University Medical Center, 1542 Tulane Avenue, New Orleans, Louisiana 70112, U.S.A.

G. Michael B. Berger, M.B., Ch.B., Ph.D., Department of Pathology and Lipid Clinic, Red Cross War Memorial Children's Hospital, Randelbosch 7700, Cape Town, Republic of South Africa

Leonard Bickman, Ph.D., Westinghouse National Issues Center, Chicago, Illinois, U.S.A.

Edwin L. Bierman, M.D., Head, Division of Metabolism and Endocrinology, University of Washington School of Medicine, RG Royal Gorge 20, Seattle, Washington 98195, U.S.A.

David W. Bilheimer, M.D., Department of Internal Medicine, The University of Texas Health Science Center at Dallas, 5323 Harry Hines Boulevard, Dallas, Texas 75235, U.S.A.

Sören Bjökerud, M.D., Ph.D., Department of Pathology, University of Goteborg, Sahlgrens Hospital, S-41345 Goteborg, Sweden

Henry W. Blackburn, M.D., Director, Laboratory of Physiological Hygiene, School of Public Health, University of Minnesota School of Medicine, 611 Beacon Street SE, Minneapolis, Minnesota 55455, U.S.A.

Ralph Blackett, M.D., Chairman, Department of Medicine, Prince Henry and Prince of Wales Hospitals, University of New South Wales, Sydney, New South Wales, Australia

David H. Blankenhorn, M.D., Director, Cardiology Division, Department of Medicine, University of Southern California School of Medicine, 2025 Zonal Avenue, Los Angeles, California 90033, U.S.A.

Donna Boggs, R.D., Lipid Research and General Clinical Research Centers, University of Cincinnati College of Medicine, Cincinnati, Ohio 45229, U.S.A.

Gabriele Bittolo Bon, M.D., Regional General Hospital, Unit for Atherosclerosis, National Council for Research, 30100 Venice, Italy

M. Gene Bond, Ph.D., Arteriosclerosis Research Center, Bowman Gray School of Medicine of Wake Forest University, Winston-Salem, North Carolina 27103, U.S.A.

Francois Bonnici, M.B., Ch.B., M.Med., F.C.P., Department of Pediatrics and Lipid Clinic, Red Cross War Memorial Children's Hospital, Cape Town, Republic of South Africa

G.V.R. Born, F.R.C.P., F.R.S., Department of Pharmacology, University of London King's College, Strand, London WC2R 2LS, England

Fred Brand, M.D., Department of Medicine, Boston University School of Medicine, 80 East Concord Street, Boston, Massachusetts 02118, U.S.A.

W. Carl Breckenridge, Ph.D., Lipid Research Clinic, Departments of Medicine and Clinical Biochemistry, University of Toronto, 1 Spadina Crescent, Toronto M5S 2J5, Ontario, Canada

P.J. Brennan, M.B., F.R.A.C.P., Staff Physician, Prince Henry and Prince of Wales Hospitals, Sydney, New South Wales, Australia

H. Bryan Brewer, Jr., M.D., Chief, Molecular Disease Branch, National Heart, Lung and Blood Institute, National Institutes of Health, Building 10, Room 7N117, 9000 Rockville Pike, Bethesda, Maryland 20205, U.S.A.

T.J. Bronzert, Molecular Disease Branch, National Heart, Lung and Blood Institute, National Institutes of Health, Bethesda, Maryland 20205, U.S.A.

Virgil Brown, M.D., Chief, Division of Arteriosclerosis and Metabolism, Department of Medicine, Mount Sinai Medical Center, 1 Gustav Levy Place, New York, New York 10029, U.S.A.

Henry Buchwald, M.D., Ph.D., Department of Surgery, Medical School, University of Minnesota, 516 Delaware Street SE, Minneapolis, Minnesota 55455, U.S.A.

Bill C. Bullock, D.V.M., Arteriosclerosis Research Center, Bowman Gray School of Medicine of Wake Forest University, Winston-Salem, North Carolina 27103, U.S.A.

Kathryn Burton, R.D., Lipid Research and General Clinical Research Center, University of Cincinnati College of Medicine, Cincinnati, Ohio 45229, U.S.A.

Germán Camejo, Ph.D., Head, Laboratorio de Lipoproteínas, Centro de Biofísica y Bioquímica, Instituto Venezolano de Investigaciones Cientificas, Apartado 1827, Caracas-101, Venezuela

Alan D. Cardin, Ph.D., Department of Pharmacology and Biophysics, University of Cincinnati College of Medicine, 231 Bethesda Avenue, Cincinnati, Ohio 45267, U.S.A.

Thomas E. Carew, Ph.D., Division of Metabolic Disease, School of Medicine, University of California, San Diego, La Jolla, California 92093, U.S.A.

William P. Castelli, M.D., Medical Director, Heart Disease Epidemiology Study, National Heart, Lung and Blood Institute, National Institutes of Health, 118 Lincoln Street, Framingham, Massachusetts 01701, U.S.A.

Alberico L. Catapano, Ph.D., Center Enrica Grossi Paoletti, Istituto di Farmacologia e di Farmacognosia, Universita di Milano, Via A. Del Sarto 21, 20129 Milano, Italy

Giuseppe Cazzolato, Ph.D., Regional General Hospital, Unit for Atherosclerosis, National Council for Research, 30100 Venice, Italy

Marian Cheung, Ph.D., Division of Metabolism and Endocrinology, Department of Medicine, University of Washington School of Medicine, Harborview Medical Center, 732 Harborview Hall ZA-36, 326 Ninth Avenue, Seattle, Washington 98104, U.S.A.

G.G. Chetchinachvili, M.D., Institute of Experimental Medicine, Academy of Medical Science USSR, Kirovsky 69/71, Leningrad 197022, U.S.S.R.

John S. Child, M.D., Division of Cardiology, Department of Medicine, University of California Center for the Health Sciences, Los Angeles, California 90024, U.S.A.

Francis V. Chisari, M.D., Department of Molecular Immunology, Scripps Clinic and Research Foundation, 10666 North Torry Pines Road, La Jolla, California 92037, U.S.A.

Aram V. Chobanian,)M.D., Director, Cardiovascular Institute, Department of Medicine, Boston University School of Medicine, 80 East Concord Street, Boston, Massachusetts 02118, U.S.A.

William R. Clarke, Ph.D., Department of Preventive Medicine, Division of Biostatistics, University of Iowa, Iowa City, Iowa 52242, U.S.A.

Thomas B. Clarkson, D.V.M., Department of Comparative Medicine, Director,

Atherosclerosis Research Center, Bowman Gray School of Medicine of Wake Forest University, 300 South Hawthorne Road, Winston-Salem, North Carolina 27103, U.S.A.

Diane Wilson Cox, Ph.D., F.C.C.M.G., Departments of Pediatrics and Genetics, Hospital for Sick Children, Departments of Medical Genetics and Medical Biophysics, University of Toronto, 555 University Avenue, Toronto, Ontario, Canada

Gaetano Crepaldi, M.D., Director, Department of Internal Medicine, Division of Gerentology and Metabolic Diseases, University of Padua, Policlinico, Via Giustiniani 2, 35100 Padua, Italy

Linda K. Curtiss, Ph.D., The Research Institute of Scripps Clinic, Department of Molecular Immunology, 10666 North Torrey Pines Road, La Jolla, California 92037, U.S.A.

Georges Dagher, M.S., INSERM U 7 Research Unit, Hôpital Necker, 161 rue de Sèvres, 74015 Paris, France

E.R. Dalferes, Jr., B.S., Department of Medicine, Louisiana State University Medical Center, 1542 Tulane Avenue, New Orleans, Louisiana 70112, U.S.A.

Assaad S. Daoud, M.D., Chief, Laboratory Service, Veterans Administration Medical Center, Department of Pathology, Albany Medical College, 113 Holland Avenue, Albany, New York 12208, U.S.A.

Jean Davignon, M.D., M.Sc., F.R.C.P., F.A.C.P., Director, Department of Lipid Metabolism and Atherosclerosis Research, Clinical Research Institute of Montreal, Department of Medicine, University of Montreal, 110 Avenue des Pins Ouest, Montreal, Quebec H2W 1R7, Canada

Roger A. Davis, Ph.D., Division of Metabolic Disease, Department of Medicine, University of California at San Diego, La Jolla, California 92093, U.S.A.

Michael E. DeBakey, M.D., Olga Keith Wiess Professor of Surgery, Chairman, Department of Surgery, Baylor College of Medicine and The Methodist Hospital, 6565 Fannin, Houston, Texas 77030, U.S.A.

Ralph B. Dell, M.D., Arteriosclerosis Research Center and the Department of Medicine, Columbia University College of Physicians and Surgeons, 630 West 168th Street, New York, New York 10032, U.S.A.

A.D. Denisenko, M.D., Institute for Experimental Medicine, Academy of Medical Science U.S.S.R., Kirovsky 69/71, Leningrad 197022, U.S.S.R.

Theodore Dubin, D.V.M., Department of Pathology, The New York Hospital, Cornell University Medical Center, New York, New York 10021, U.S.A.

Charles Dubost, M.D., Clinique Chirurgicale Cardiovasculaire, Hospital Broussais, 96 Rue Didot, 75674 Paris, Cedex 14, France

Daniel W. Dubovsky, M.B., Ch.B., F.C.P., Department of Hematology, University of Cape Town Medical School, Cape Town, Republic of South Africa

Thomas S. Edgington, M.D., Department of Molecular Immunology, The Research Institute of Scripps Clinic, 10666 North Torrey Pines Road, La Jolla, California 92037, U.S.A.

Peter A. Edwards, Ph.D., Division of Cardiology, Department of Medicine, University of California for the Health Sciences, Los Angeles, California 90024, U.S.A.

Douglas A. Eggen, Ph.D., Department of Pathology, Louisiana State University Medical Center, 1542 Tulane Avenue, New Orleans, Louisiana 70112, U.S.A.

Shlomo Eisenberg, M.D., Lipid Research Laboratory, Department of Medicine B, Hadassah University Hospital, Jerusalem, Israel

Jean-Luc Elghozi, M.D., INSERM U 7 Research Unit, Hôpital Necker, 161 rue de Sèvres, 75015 Paris, France

Akira Endo, M.D., Fermentation Laboratory, Tokyo, Noko University, 3-5-8 Saiwaicho, Fuchu-shi, Tokyo, 183 Japan

Sven Chr. Enger, M.D., Department of Pathology, Ullevaal Hospital, Oslo, Norway

Sheldon G. Englehorn, Division of Metabolic Disease, Department of Medicine, University of California at San Diego, La Jolla, California 92093, U.S.A.

Frederick H. Epstein, M.D., Institut fur Sozial- und Präventivmedizin, Universität Zürich, Gloriastrasse 32, 8006 Zürich, Switzerland

Domenick J. Falcone, B.A., Department of Pathology, The New York Hospital—Cornell Medical Center, 625 East 68th Street, New York, New York 10021, U.S.A.

Renato Fellin, M.D., Department of Internal Medicine, Division of Gerentology and Metabolic Diseases, University of Padua, Policlinico, Via Giustiniani 2, 35100 Padua, Italy

James Fesmire, B.S., Laboratory of Lipid Research and Lipoprotein Studies, Oklahoma Medical Research Foundation, Oklahoma City, Oklahoma 73104, U.S.A.

Noel H. Fidge, Ph.D., Cardiovascular Metabolism and Nutrition Research Unit, Baker Medical Research Institute, Commercial Road, Prahran, Victoria, Australia 3181

Christopher J. Fielding, Ph.D., Cardiovascular Research Institute, University of California, San Francisco, California 94143, U.S.A.

Phoebe E. Fielding, Ph.D., Cardiovascular Research Institute, University of California, San Francisco, California 94143, U.S.A.

Katti Fischer-Dzoga, M.D., Department of Pathology, The University of Chicago and The Pritzker School of Medicine, 950 East 59th Street, Chicago, Illinois 60637, U.S.A.

Gunther M. Fless, Ph.D., Department of Medicine, The University of Chicago and The Pritzker School of Medicine, 950 East 59th Street, Chicago, Illinois 60637, U.S.A.

C.-H. Florén, M.D., Division of Metabolism and Endocrinology, Department of Medicine, University of Washington School of Medicine, Harborview Medical Center, Seattle, Washington 98104, U.S.A.

R.A. Florentin, M.D., Department of Pathology, Albany Medical College of Union University, 47 New Scotland Avenue, Albany, New York 12208, U.S.A.

Alan Marcus Fogelman, M.D., Division of Cardiology, Department of Medicine, University of California Center for the Health Sciences, Los Angeles, California 90024, U.S.A.

G. Franceschini, Ph.D., Center Enrica Grossi Paoletti, Istituto di Farmacologia e di Farmacognosia, Università di Milano, Via A. Del Sarto 21, 20129 Milano, Italy

Ivan D. Frantz, M.D., Department of Medicine and Biochemistry, University of Minnesota Medical School, Minneapolis, Minnesota 55455, U.S.A.

K.E. Fritz, Ph.D., Atherosclerosis Research, Veterans Administration Medical Center, Albany, New York 12208, U.S.A.

Dennis K. Fujii, Ph.D., Department of Molecular Immunology, The Research Institute of Scripps Clinic, 10666 North Torrey Pines Road, La Jolla, California 92037, U.S.A.

Ricardo P. Garay, M.D., INSERM U 7 Research Unit, Hôpital Necker, 161 rue de Sèvres, 75015 Paris, France

Ruth T. Gardner, Harvard Medical School and Beth Israel Hospital, Boston, Massachusetts 02215, U.S.A.

Peter S. Gartside, Ph.D., Lipid Research and General Clinical Research Centers, University of Cincinnati College of Medicine, Cincinnati, Ohio 45229, U.S.A.

Antoine Gattereau, M.D., M.Sc., F.R.C.P., F.A.C.P., Department of Medicine, University of Montreal, Department of Lipid Metabolism and Atherosclerosis Research, Clinical Research Institute of Montreal, Montreal, Quebec, Canada

John W. Gaubatz, M.S., Department of Medicine, Baylor College of Medicine, 1200 Moursund, Houston, Texas 77030, U.S.A.

Ross G. Gerrity, Ph.D., Cleveland Clinic Foundation, 9500 Euclid, Cleveland, Ohio 44106, U.S.A.

Godfrey S. Getz, M.B., B.Ch. D. Phil., Departments of Pathology and Biochemistry and Specialized Center of Research in Atherosclerosis, University of Chicago and The Pritzker School of Medicine, 950 East 59th Street, Chicago, Illinois 60637, U.S.A.

G.J. Gherardi, M.D., Department of Pathology, Framingham Union Hospital, Framingham, Massachusetts, U.S.A.

G. Gianfranceschi, Ph.D., Center Enrica Grossi Paoletti, Istituto di Farmacologia e di Farmacognosia, Università di Milano, Via A. Del Sarto 21, 20129 Milano, Italy

Peter Giles, Ph.D., D.I.C., M.I. Biol., Department of Child Health, Institute of Child Health, 30 Guilford Street, London WC1N 1EN, England

Dr. Michael A. Gimbrone, Jr., Department of Pathology, Harvard Medical School and the Peter Bent Brigham Hospital, 721 Huntington Avenue, Boston, Massachusetts 02115, U.S.A.

S. Glagov, M.D., Department of Pathology, University of Chicago and The Pritzker School of Medicine, 950 East 59th Street, Chicago, Illinois 60637, U.S.A.

Leonora Glatfelter, R.D., Lipid Research and General Clinical Research Centers, University of Cincinnati, College of Medicine, Cincinnati, Ohio 45229, U.S.A.

Robert M. Glickman, M.D., Department of Medicine, Chief of Gastroenterology, Columbia University College of Physicians and Surgeons, 630 West 168th Street, New York, New York 10032, U.S.A.

Charles J. Glueck, M.D., Director, Lipid Research and General Clinical Research Centers, University of Cincinnati, College of Medicine, 234 Goodman Street, Cincinnati, Ohio 45229, U.S.A.

Itzhak Goldberg, M.D., Harvard Medical School and Beth Israel Hospital, 330 Brookline Avenue, Boston, Massachusetts 02215, U.S.A.

DeWitt S. Goodman, M.D., Tilden-Weger-Bieler Professor, Arteriosclerosis Research Center and the Department of Medicine, Columbia University College of Physicians and Surgeons, 630 West 168th Street, New York, New York 10032, U.S.A.

John F. Goodwin, M.D., F.R.C.P., F.A.C.C., Department of Clinical Cardiology, University of London, Royal Postgraduate Medical School, Hammersmith Hospital, Ducane Road, London W12 OHS, England

Tavia Gordon, 12901 Blue Hill Road, Silver Springs, Maryland 20906, U.S.A.

Yuichiro Goto, M.D., Department of Medicine, Keio University, School of Medicine, 35 Shinano-machi, Shinjuku, Tokyo 160, Japan

Antonio M. Gotto, Jr., M.D., The J.S. Abercrombie Professor of Atherosclerosis and Lipoprotein Research, Chairman, Department of Medicine, Baylor College of Medicine, The Bob and Vivian Smith Professor and Chairman, Department of Internal Medicine, The Methodist Hospital, 6565 Fannin, Houston, Texas 77030, U.S.A.

Peter H.R. Green, F.R.A.C.P., Department of Medicine, Division of Gastroenterology, Columbia University College of Physicians and Surgeons, 630 West 168th Street, New York, New York 10032, U.S.A.

Heiner Greten, M.D., Klinisches Institut für Herzinfarktforschung an der Medizinischen, Universitätsklinik Heidelberg, Bergheimer Strasse 58, D 6900 Heidelberg, Federal Republic of Germany

Jochen Grosser, M.D., Klinisches Institut für Herzinfarktforschung an der Medizinischen, Universitätsklinik Heidelberg, Bergheimer Strasse 58, D 6900 Heidelberg, Federal Republic of Germany

Scott M. Grundy, M.D., Ph.D., Department of Medicine, Veterans Administration Medical Center and The University of California, San Diego, California 92161, U.S.A.

Ryszard J. Gryglewski, M.D., Chairman, Department of Pharmacology, N. Copernicus Medical Academy, 31-531 Cracow, Grzegórzecka 16 Poland

Daniel L. Guerrero, B.A., Department of Pathology, The University of Texas Health Science Center, San Antonio, 7703 Floyd Curl Drive, San Antonio, Texas 78284, U.S.A.

M. Robin Hagens, B.S., Department of Pathology, The University of Texas Health Science Center, San Antonio, 7703 Floyd Curl Drive, San Antonio, Texas 78284, U.S.A.

David P. Hajjar, Ph.D., Department of Pathology, The New York Hospital−Cornell Medical Center, 625 East 68th Street, New York, New York 10021, U.S.A.

Robert L. Hamilton, Ph.D., Cardiovascular Research Institute, University of California, San Francisco, California 94122, U.S.A.

Laurence A. Harker, M.D., Division of Hematology, Department of Medicine, University of Washington School of Medicine, Harborview Medical Center, 325 Ninth Avenue, Seattle, Washington 98105, U.S.A.

Kari Harno, M.D., Third Department of Medicine, University of Helsinki Central Hospital, 00290 Helsinki 29, Finland

Yoshiya Hata, M.D., Department of Medicine, Keio University, School of Medicine, 35 Shinano-machi, Shinjuku, Tokyo 160, Japan

Christian C. Haudenschild, M.D., Department of Pathology, Boston University School of Medicine, 80 East Concord Street, Boston, Massachusetts 02118, U.S.A.

Helmut Hauser, Ph.D., Institut fur Biochemie ETH, Zurich, Switzerland

M. Daria Haust, M.D., Departments of Pathology and Pediatrics, University of Western Ontario and University Hospital Health Sciences Center, London N6A 5C1, Ontario, Canada

Richard J. Havel, M.D., Cardiovascular Research Institute, University of California, San Francisco, California 94143, U.S.A.

Rick Hay, M.D., Ph.D., Department of Pathology, The University of Chicago Hospitals and Clinics and The Pritzker School of Medicine, Chicago, Illinois 60637, U.S.A.

T. Hayashi, M.D., Honolulu Heart Study, Kuakini Medical Center, 347 North Kuakini Street, Honolulu, Hawaii 96817, U.S.A.

William R. Hazzard, M.D., Chief, Division of Gerontology and Geriatric Medicine, Northwest Lipid Research Clinic, University of Washington School of Medicine, 326 Ninth Avenue, Seattle, Washington 98104, U.S.A.

Carol L. Heideman, M.S., Department of Medicine, Baylor College of Medicine, 1200 Moursund, Houston, Texas 77030, U.S.A.

Robert J. Heinen, M.D., Brown University Program in Medicine, The Miriam Hospital, l64 Summit Avenue, Providence, Rhode Island 02906, U.S.A.

G. Heiss, M.D., Ph.D., Lipid Research Clinic Program, Central Patient Registry and Coordinating Centers, Department of Biostatistics, School of Public Health, University of North Carolina, Chapel Hill, North Carolina, U.S.A.

Anders Helgeland, M.D., Department of Pathology, Ullevaal Hospital, Oslo, Norway

L. Omar Henderson, Ph.D., Brown University Program in Medicine, The Miriam Hospital, 164 Summit Avenue, Providence, Rhode Island, 02906, U.S.A.

Peter N. Herbert, M.D., Brown University Program in Medicine, The Miriam Hospital, 164 Summit Avenue, Providence, Rhode Island 02906, U.S.A.

C.C. Heuck, M.D., Ph.D., Department of Medicine, University of Heidelberg, Bergheimer Strasse 58, D6900 Heidelberg, Federal Republic of Germany

Ingvar Hjermann, M.D., Department of Pathology, Ullevaal Hospital, Oslo, Norway

Henry F. Hoff, Ph.D., Department of Medicine, Baylor College of Medicine, 1200 Moursund, Houston, Texas 77030, U.S.A.

Martha Hokom, B.S., Division of Cardiology, Department of Medicine, University of California Center for the Health Sciences, Los Angeles, California 90024, U.S.A.

Ingar Holme, M.D., Department of Pathology, Ullevaal Hospital, Oslo, Norway

William L. Holmes, Ph.D., Chairman, Department of Research, Lankenau Hospital, Lancaster Avenue West of City Line, Philadelphia, Pennsylvania 19151, U.S.A.

Murray W. Huff, Ph.D., Cardiovascular Metabolism and Nutrition Research Unit, Baker Medical Research Institute, Commercial Road, Prahran, Victoria, Australia 3181

Donald B. Hunninghake, M.D., Departments of Medicine and Pharmacology, University of Minnesota, 3-260 Millard Hall, 435 Delaware Street SE, Minneapolis, Minnesota 55455, U.S.A.

Toshitsugu Ishikawa, M.D., Department of Medicine, Jikei University, Aoto Hospital, 6-41-2 Aoto, Katsushika, Tokyo, Japan

Richard L. Jackson, Ph.D., Department of Pharmacology and Cell Biophysics, University of Cincinnati College of Medicine, 231 Bethesda Avenue, Cincinnati, Ohio 45267, U.S.A.

Eric A. Jaffe, M.D., Division of Hematology-Oncology, Department of Medicine, The New York Hospital−Cornell Medical Center, 625 East 68th Street, New York, New York 10021, U.S.A.

J. Jarmolych, M.D., Chief, Anatomical Pathology, Laboratory Service, Veterans Administration Medical Center, Albany, New York 12208, U.S.A.

Mary Jane Jesse, M.D., Vice-Chairman, Department of Pediatrics, University of Miami School of Medicine, Miami, Florida, U.S.A.

Hymie S. Joffe, M.B., Ch.B., M. Med., Department of Pediatrics, Red Cross War Memorial Children's Hospital, Cape Town, Republic of South Africa

J. David Johnson, Ph.D., Department of Pharmacology and Cell Biophysics, University of Cincinnati College of Medicine, 231 Bethesda Avenue, Cincinnati, Ohio 45267, U.S.A.

W.D. Johnson, M.S., Department of Biometry, Louisiana State University Medical Center, 1542 Tulane Avenue, New Orleans, Louisiana 70112, U.S.A.

John P. Kane, M.D., Ph.D., Department of Medicine, Associate Director, Specialized Center of Research on Atherosclerosis, University of California, San Francisco, California 94143, U.S.A.

William B. Kannel, M.D., M.P.H., Chief, Section of Preventive Medicine and Epidemiology, Department of Medicine, Boston University School of Medicine, 80 East Concord Street, Boston, Massachusetts 02118, U.S.A.

Beverly Kariya, Department of Pathology, University of Washington School of Medicine, Seattle, Washington 98195, U.S.A.

Kathe A. Kelly, M.Sc., Lipid Research and General Clinical Research Centers, University of Cincinnati College of Medicine, Cincinnati, Ohio 45229, U.S.A.

Phil Khoury, M.S., Lipid Research and General Clinical Research Centers, University of Cincinnati College of Medicine, Cincinnati, Ohio 45229, U.S.A.

Paavo K.J. Kinnunen, M.D., Third Department of Medicine, University of Helsinki Central Hospital, Helsinki 29, Finland

Tomas Kirchhausen, Ph.D., Department of Medicine, The University of Chicago and The Pritzker School of Medicine, 950 East 59th Street, Chicago, Illinois 60637, U.S.A.

Anatoli N. Klimov, M.D., Head, The Anitchkov Department of Atherosclerosis and Laboratory of Lipid Metabolism, Institute for Experimental Medicine, Academy of Medical Science USSR, Kirovsky 69/71, Leningrad, 197022, U.S.S.R.

Gerald Klose, M.D., Klinisches Institut für Herzinfarktforschung an der Medizinischen, Universitätsklinik Heidelberg, Bergheimer Strasse 58, D 6900 Heidelberg, Federal Republic of Germany

Roger D. Knapp, Ph.D., Department of Medicine, Baylor College of Medicine and The

Methodist Hospital, 6565 Fannin, Houston, Texas 77030, U.S.A.

Robert H. Knopp, M.D., Director, Northwest Lipid Research Clinic, Department of Medicine, University of Washington School of Medicine, 325 Ninth Avenue, Seattle, Washington 98104, U.S.A.

Lawrence Koep, M.D., Department of Surgery, University of Colorado Health Sciences Center, 4200 East Ninth Avenue, Denver, Colorado 80262, U.S.A.

M. Kohlmeier, M.D., Department of Medicine, University of Heidelberg, Bergheimer Strasse 58, D6900 Heidelberg, Federal Republic of Germany

M.G. Kokatnur, Ph.D., Department of Pathology, Louisiana State University Medical Center, 1542 Tulane Avenue, New Orleans, Louisiana 70112, U.S.A.

Gerhard M. Kostner, Ph.D., Institute of Medical Biochemistry, University of Graz, A-8010 Graz, Austria

David Kritchevsky, Ph.D., Associate Director, The Wistar Institute of Anatomy and Biology, University of Pennsylvania, 36th Street At Spruce, Philadelphia, Pennsylvania 19104, U.S.A.

Joan Kruc, M.S., Chicago Heart Association, Chicago, Illinois, U.S.A.

Timo Kuusi, M.D., Third Department of Medicine, University of Helsinki Central Hospital, 00290 Helsinki 29, Finland

Peter O. Kwiterovitch, Jr., M.D., Departments of Pediatrics and Medicine, Johns Hopkins University School of Medicine, Baltimore, Maryland 21205, U.S.A.

Peter Laggner, Ph.D., Institut für Röntgenstrukturanalyse, Steyrergasse 17, Graz, Austria

John M. Laragh, M.D., Master Professor of Surgery, Director, Cardiovascular Center, The New York Hospital–Cornell Medical Center, 525 East 68th Street, New York City, 10021, U.S.A.

Rhea Larsen, R.D., Lipid Research and General Clinical Research Centers, University of Cincinnati College of Medicine, Cincinnati, Ohio 45229, U.S.A.

J. LaRosa, M.D., Director, Lipid Research Clinic, George Washington University Hospital Medical Center, Washington, D.C., U.S.A.

Ronald M. Lauer, M.D., Director, Division of Pediatric Cardiology, Department of Pediatrics, University of Iowa, Iowa City, Iowa 52242, U.S.A.

Peter Laskarzewski, Ph.D., Lipid Research and General Clinical Research Centers, University of Cincinnati College of Medicine, Cincinnati, Ohio 45229, U.S.A.

Gerald M. Lawrie, M.D., M.B.B.S., F.R.C.S., F.R.A.C.S., F.R.C.S., Department of Surgery, Baylor College of Medicine and The Methodist Hospital, 6565 Fannin, Houston, Texas 77030, U.S.A.

K.T. Lee, M.D., Ph.D., Department of Pathology, Albany Medical College of Union University, 47 New Scotland Avenue, Albany, New York 12208, U.S.A.

B. Leelarthaepin, Ph.D., Department of Medicine, Prince Henry Hospital, Sydney, New South Wales, Australia

Robert I. Levy, M.D., Director, National Heart, Lung and Blood Institute, National Institutes of Health, Building 31, Room 5A-52, Bethesda, Maryland 20205, U.S.A.

Paul Leren, M.D., Department of Pathology, Ullevaal Hospital, Oslo, Norway

Barry Lewis, M.D., Department of Chemical Pathology and Metabolic Disorders, St. Thomas's Hospital, London SE1 7EH, England

J. Alick Little, M.D., F.R.C.P., Lipid Research Clinic, Department of Medicine, St. Michael's Hospital, University of Toronto, 1 Spadina Crescent, Toronto M55 2J5, Ontario, Canada

June K. Lloyd, M.D., F.R.C.P., Department of Child Health, St. George's Hospital Medical School, London SW17 ORE, England

Madeleine Lou, M.Sc., Centre de Recherches sur les Maladies Lipidiques, Centre Hospitalier de l'Université Laval, 2705 boulevard Laurier, Ste-Foy, Québec G1V 4G2, Canada

Richard Lovell, A.O., Department of Medicine, University of Melbourne, Royal Melbourne Hospital, Victoria 3050, Australia

Karen M. Lynch, M.S., Brown University Program in Medicine, The Miriam Hospital, 164 Summit Avenue, Providence, Rhode Island 02906, U.S.A.

Paul J. Lupien, M.D., Ph.D., Director, Centre de Recherche sur les Maladies Lipidiques, Centre Hospitalier de l'Université Laval, 2705 Boulevard Laurier, Ste-Foy, Québec G1V 4G2, Canada

Suzanne Lussier-Cacan, Ph.D., Department of Medicine, University of Montreal, Department of Lipid Metabolism and Atherosclerosis Research, Clinical Research Institute of Montreal, Montreal, Quebec, Canada

Robert W. Mahley, M.D, Ph.D., Director, Gladstone Research Foundation, Laboratories for Cardiovascular Disease, University of California, San Francisco, California 94110, U.S.A.

G. T. Malcom, Ph.D., Departments of Pathology and Medical Technology, Louisiana State University Medical Center, 1542 Tulane Avenue, New Orleans, Louisiana 70122, U.S.A.

Kafait U. Malik, D.Sc., Ph.D., Department of Pharmacology, College of Medicine, Center for the Health Sciences, University of Tennessee, 800 Madison Avenue, Memphis, Tennessee 38163, U.S.A.

M.J. Malloy, M.D., Cardiovascular Research Institute, University of California, San Francisco, California 94143, U.S.A.

Carol A. Marzetta, B.S., Arteriosclerosis Research Center, Bowman Gray School of Medicine of Wake Forest University, Winston-Salem, North Carolina 27103, U.S.A.

John Mathews, M.D., Ph.D., F.R.A.C.P., Department of Medicine, University of Melbourne, Royal Melbourne Hospital, Victoria 3050, Australia

Nobuo Matsuoka, M.D., Ph.D., Department of Pharmacology and Cell Biophysics, University of Cincinnati College of Medicine, 231 Bethesda Avenue, Cincinnati, Ohio 45267, U.S.A.

Walter McConathy, Ph.D., Laboratory of Lipid Research and Lipoprotein Studies, Oklahoma Medical Research Foundation, 825 Northeast 13th Street, Oklahoma, City, Oklahoma 73104, U.S.A.

C.A. McGilchrist, Ph.D., School of Mathematics, University of New South Wales, Kensington, New South Wales, Australia

V.M. McGuire, B.S., R.P.Dt., Department of Dietetics, St. Michael's Hospital, 30 Bond Street, Toronto M5B 1W8, Canada

Henry D. McIntosh, M.D., Watson Clinic, P.O. Box 1429, Lakeland, Florida 33802, U.S.A.

P.M. McNamara, B.S., Framingham Study, National Heart, Lung and Blood Institute, National Institutes of Health, Bethesda, Maryland 20205, U.S.A.

Marjorie B. Megan, Department of Medicine, University of Iowa College of Medicine, Iowa City, Iowa 52242, U.S.A.

Margot J. Mellies, M.D., Lipid Research and General Clinical Research Centers, University of Cincinnati College of Medicine, Cincinnati, Ohio 45229, U.S.A.

Soaira Mendoza, M.D., Lipid Research and General Clinical Research Centers, University of Cincinnati College of Medicine, Cincinnati, Ohio 45229, U.S.A.

Philippe Meyer, M.D., Departments of Physiology and Pharmacology, INSERM U 7 Research Unit, Hôpital Necker, 161 rue de Sèvres, 75015 Paris, France

Tatu Miettinen, M.D., Second Department of Medicine, University of Helsinki, 00290 Helsinki 29, Finland

Norman E. Miller, M.D., M.Sc., Ph.D., Department of Chemical Pathology and Metabolic Disorders, 5th Floor, North Wing, St. Thomas's Hospital Medical School, London SE1 7EH, England

Richard R. Miller, M.D., Department of Medicine, Chief of Cardiology, Baylor College of Medicine and The Methodist Hospital, 6565 Fannin, Houston, Texas 77030, U.S.A.

C. Richard Minick, M.D., Department of Pathology, The New York Hospital–Cornell Medical Center, 625 East 68th Street, New York, New York 10021, U.S.A.

Patricia P. Moll, Ph.D., Department of Human Genetics, The University of Michigan Medical School, 1137 E. Catherine Street, Ann Arbor, Michigan 48109, U.S.A.

Salvador Moncada, M.D., Ph.D., The Wellcome Research Laboratories, Department of Prostaglandin Research, Langley Court, Beckenham, Kent, BR3 3BS, England

Richard B. Moore, M.D., Department of Surgery, Medical School, University of Minnesota, 516 Delaware Street S.E., Minneapolis, Minnesota 55455, U.S.A.

Sital Moorjani, Ph.D., Centre de Recherches sur les Maladies Lipidiques, Centre Hospitalier de l'Université Laval, 2705 boulevard Laurier, Ste-Foy, Québec G1V 4G2, Canada

Joel D. Morrisett, Ph.D., Department of Medicine, Baylor College of Medicine and The Methodist Hospital, 6565 Fannin, Houston, Texas 77030, U.S.A.

John A. Morrison, Ph.D., Lipid Research and General Clinical Research Centers, University of Cincinnati College of Medicine, Cincinnati, Ohio 45229, U.S.A.

Howard G. Muntz, Department of Pharmacology and Cell Biophysics, University of Cincinnati College of Medicine, 231 Bethesda Avenue, Cincinnati, Ohio 45267, U.S.A.

Thomas A. Musliner, M.D., Brown University Program in Medicine, The Miriam Hospital, 164 Summit Avenue, Providence, Rhode Island 02906, U.S.A.

James Fraser Mustard, M.D., Ph.D., Faculty of Health Sciences, McMaster University, 1200 Main Street West, Hamilton, Ontario L8S 4J9, Canada

Nicolas Myant, M.D., F.R.C.P, MRC Lipid Metabolism Unit, Hammersmith Hospital, Ducane Road, London W12 OHS, England

Haruo Nakamura, M.D., Department of Medicine, Jikei University, Aoto Hospital, 6-41-2 Aoto Katsushika, Tokyo, Japan

Alberto Nasjletti, M.D., Department of Pharmacology, College of Medicine, The University of Tennessee Center for the Health Sciences, 800 Madison Avenue, Memphis, Tennessee 38163

E.K. Neely, Department of Pharmacology and Cell Biophysics, University of Cincinnati College of Medicine, 231 Bethesda Avenue, Cincinnati, Ohio 45267, U.S.A.

Paul J. Nestel, M.D., F.R.A.C.P., Head, Cardiovascular Metabolism and Nutrition Research Unit, Baker Medical Research Institute, Commercial Road, Prahran, Victoria, Australia 3181

W.P. Newman, III, M.D., Department of Pathology, Louisiana State University Medical Center, 1542 Tulane Avenue, New Orleans, Lousiana 70112, U.S.A.

Esko A. Nikkilä, M.D., Third Department of Medicine, University of Helsinki Central Hospital, 00290 Helsinki 29, Finland

Fujio Numano, M.D., Department of Internal Medicine, Tokyo Medical and Dental University, 5-45, Yushima 1-Chome, Bunkyo-Ku, Tokyo 113, Japan

Celia Oakley, M.D., F.R.C.P., Clinical Cardiology, Hammersmith Hospital, Ducane Road, London W12 OHS, England

M.C. Oalman, D.P.H., Departments of Pathology, Public Health and Preventive Medicine, Louisiana State University Medical Center, 1542 Tulane Avenue, New Orleans, Louisiana 70112, U.S.A.

Takamitsu Oikawa, M.D., Department of Medicine, Keio University, School of Medicine, 35 Shinano-machi, Shinjuku, Tokyo 160, Japan

Thomas Olivecrona, M.D., Department of Medical Chemistry, University of Umea, S 901 87 Umea, Sweden

Michael F. Oliver, M.D., The Duke of Edinburgh Professor of Cardiology, Department of Cardiology, University of Edinburgh Medical School, Royal Infirmary, Edinburgh EH 39YW, Scotland

Anders G. Olsson M.D., King Gustaf V Research Institute, Karolinska Hospital, S 104 01 Stockholm, Sweden

P. Oster, M.D., Department of Medicine, University of Heidelberg, Bergheimer Strasse 58, D6900 Heidelberg, Federal Republic of Germany

Christopher J. Packard, B.Sc., Ph.D., University Department of Biochemistry, Royal Infirmary, Glasgow G4 OSF, Scotland

A. Jean Palmer, M.B., F.R.A.C.P., Division of Preventive Cardiology, Prince Henry and Prince of Wales Hospitals, Sydney, New South Wales, Austr!lia

Sharon Pangburn, Division of Metabolic Disease, School of Medicine, University of California at San Diego, La Jolla, California 92093, U.S.A.

Rodolfo Paoletti, M.D., Centre Enrica Grossi Paoletti, Direttore, Istituto di Farmacologia e di Farmacognosia, Università di Milano, Via A. Del Sarto, 21, 20129 Milano, Italy

L.G. Petrova-Maslakova, M.D., Institute for Experimental Medicine, Academy of Medical Science U.S.S.R., Kirovsky 69/71, Leningrad 197022, U.S.S.R.

Ray C. Pittman, Ph.D., Division of Metabolic Disease, School of Medicine, University of California at San Diego, La Jolla, California 92093, U.S.A.

A. Poli, M.D., Center Enrica Grossi Paoletti, Istituto di Farmacologia e di Farmacognosia, Università di Milano, Via A. Del Sarto 21, 20129 Milano, Italy

Craig M. Pratt, M.D., Department of Medicine, Baylor College of Medicine, Director, Exercise Laboratory, and Co-Director, Coronary Care Unit, The Methodist Hospital, 6565 Fannin, Houston, Texas 77030, U.S.A.

Michael Preece, M.Sc., M.D., M.R.C.P., Department of Growth and Development, Institute of Child Health, 30 Guilford Street, London WC1N 1EN, England

Klaus Preissner, Klinisches Institute für Herzinfarktforschung an der Medizinischen, Universitätsklinik Heidelberg, Bergheimer Strasse 58, D 6900 Heidelberg, Federal Republic of Germany

Margaret Forney Prescott, Ph.D., Department of Pathology, Boston University School of Medicine, 80 East Concord Street, Boston, Massachusetts 02118, U.S.A.

Giobatta Quinci, D.Chem., Regional General Hospital, Unit for Atherosclerosis, National Council for Research 30100 Venice, Italy

B. Radharkrishnamurthy, Ph.D., Departments of Medicine and Biochemistry, Louisiana State University Medical Center, 1542 Tulane Avenue, New Orleans, Louisiana 70112, U.S.A.

Elaine Raines, Department of Pathology, University of Washington School of Medicine, Seattle, Washington 98195, U.S.A.

Rajasekhar Ramakrishnan, Ph.D., Arteriosclerosis Research Center and Department of Pediatrics, Columbia University College of Physicians and Surgeons, 630 West 168th Street, New York, New York 10032, U.S.A.

Eva Ray, Ph.D., Department of Physiology and Biochemistry, The Medical College of Pennsylvania and Hospital, 3300 Henry Avenue, Philadelphia, Pennsylvania 19129, U.S.A.

Catherine Reardon, B.S., Department of Biochemistry, The University of Chicago, Chicago, Illinois 60637, U.S.A.

Carol T. Reed, B.A., M.S., Department of Pathology, The University of Texas Health

Science Center, San Antonio, 7703 Floyd Curl Drive, San Antonio, Texas 78284, U.S.A.

J.M. Reiner, Ph.D., Department of Pathology, Albany Medical College of Union University, 47 New Scotland Avenue, Albany, New York 12208, U.S.A.

G.G. Rhoads, M.D., M.P.H., Honolulu Heart Study, Kuakini Medical Center, 347 North Kuakini Street, Honolulu, Hawaii 96817, U.S.A.

Basil H. Rifkind, M.D., F.R.C.P., Project Officer, Lipid Research Clinic Program, Lipid Metabolism Branch, Division of Heart and Vascular Diseases, National Heart, Lung and Blood Institute, National Institutes of Health, Building 31, Room 4A-19, Bethesda, Maryland 20205, U.S.A.

Ladislas Robert, M.D., Ph.D., Directeur de Recherche au CNRS, Laboratoire de Biochimie du Tissu Conjunctif, Institut de Recherches Universitaire sur les Maladies Vasculaires, Faculté de Medicine, Université Paris—Val de Marne, 6, Rue du General Sarrail, 94010 Créteil, France

Abel Robertson, M.D., Ph.D., Institute of Pathology, School of Medicine, Case Western Reserve University, 2085 Adelbert Road, Cleveland, Ohio 44106, U.S.A.

W.A. Rock, M.D., Department of Pathology, Louisiana State University Medical Center, 1542 Tulane Avenue, New Orleans, Louisiana 70112, U.S.A.

Russell Ross, Ph.D., Department of Pathology, SM-30, University of Washington School of Medicine, Seattle, Washington 98195, U.S.A.

George Rothblat, Ph.D., Departments of Physiology and Biochemistry, The Medical College of Pennsylvania and Hospital, 3300 Henry Avenue, Philadelphia, Pennsylvania 19129, U.S.A.

Richard D. Rucker, M.D., Department of Surgery, School of Medicine, University of Minnesota, 516 Delaware Street, S.E., Minneapolis, Minnesota 55455, U.S.A.

David C. Sabiston, Jr., M.D., James Buchanan Duke Professor of Surgery and Chairman, Department of Surgery, Duke University Medical School, Durham, North Carolina 27710, U.S.A.

Bengt Samuelsson, M.D., Department of Chemistry, Karolinska Institute, S-104 01 Stockholm, Sweden

Ralph Sapsford, F.R.C.S., Department of Surgery, Hammersmith Hospital, Ducane Road, London W12 OHS, England

Angelo M. Scanu, M.D., Department of Medicine, The University of Chicago and The Pritzker School of Medicine, 950 East 59th Street, Chicago, Illinois 60637, U.S.A.

E.J. Schaefer, M.D., Molecular Disease Branch, National Heart, Lung and Blood Institute, National Institutes of Health, Bethesda, Maryland 20205, U.S.A.

Hans-Eckart Schaefer, M.D., Universität zu Köln, Abteilung für Feinstrukturelle Pathologie, Pathologisches Institut, Josef-Stelzmannstrasse 9, D-5 Köln 41, Federal Republic of Germany

T.J. Schaffner, M.D., Department of Pathology, University of Chicago and The Pritzker School of Medicine, 950 East 59th Street, Chicago, Illinois 60637, U.S.A.

G. Schellenberg, M.D., Department of Medicine, University of Heidelberg, Bergheimer Strasse 58, D6900 Heidelberg, Federal Republic of Germany

Gotthard Schettler, M.D., Direktor, Medizinische Universitatis Klinik, University of Heidelberg, Bergheimer Strasse 58, D 6900 Heidelberg, Federal Republic of Germany

Gunther Schlierf, M.D., Department of Medicine, University of Heidelberg, Bergheimer Strasse 58, D 6900 Heidelberg, Federal Republic of Germany

James A. Schoenberger, M.D., Chairman, Department of Preventive Medicine, Rush-Presbyterian-St. Lukes Medical Center, 316 Service Building, 1753 West Congress Parkway, Chicago, Illinois 60612, U.S.A.

Gustav Schonfeld, M.D., Lipid Research Center, Departments of Preventive Medicine and

Medicine, Washington University School of Medicine, Box 8046, 4566 Scott Avenue, St. Louis, Missouri 63110, U.S.A.

Otto Schrecker, M.D., Klinisches Institut für Herzinfarktforschung an der Medizinischen, Universitätsklinik Heidelberg, Bergheimer Strasse 58, D 6900 Heidelberg, Federal Republic of Germany

Colin J. Schwartz, M.D., B.S., F.R.A.C.P., Department of Pathology, The University of Texas Health Science Center, San Antonio, 7703 Floyd Curl Drive, San Antonio, Texas 78284, U.S.A.

R.F. Scott, M.D., Department of Pathology, Albany Medical College of Union University, 47 New Scotland Avenue, Albany, New York 12208, U.S.A.

Janet Seager, M.A., Division of Cardiology, Department of Medicine, University of California Center for the Health Sciences, Los Angeles, California 90024, U.S.A.

Dietrich Seidel, M.D., Department of Clinical Chemistry, Lehrstuhl für Klinische Chemie der Medizinischen Einrichtungen der Universität Göttingen, Robert-Koch-Strasse 40, 3400 Göttingen, Federal Republic of Germany

Alan H. Seplowitz, M.D., Arteriosclerosis Research Center and the Department of Medicine, Columbia University College of Physicians and Surgeons, 630 West 168th Street, New York, New York 10032, U.S.A.

Ishaiahu Schechter, Ph.D., Division of Cardiology, Department of Medicine, University of California Center for the Health Sciences, Los Angeles, California 90024, U.S.A.

James Shepherd, B.Sc., M.B., Ph.D., University Department of Biochemistry, Royal Infirmary, Glasgow G4 OSF, Scotland

Hiroshi Shigematsu, M.D., Department of Medicine, Keio University, School of Medicine, 35 Shinano-machi, Shinjuku, Tokyo 160, Japan

Harris B. Shumacker, Jr., M.D., Distinguished Professor of Surgery Emeritus, Indiana University Medical Center, and Senior Surgical Consultant, St. Vincent Hospital and Health Care Center, 8402 Harcourt Road, Indianapolis, Indiana 46260, U.S.A.

K. Silberbauer, M.D., Atherosclerosis Research Groups at the Department of Medical Physiology, University of Vienna, Vienna, Austria

Judy M. Simpson, B.Sc, Department of Statistics, School of Mathematics, University of New South Wales, Kensington, New South Wales, Australia

Charles F. Sing, Ph.D., Department of Human Genetics, The University of Michigan Medical School, 1137 E. Catherine Street, Ann Arbor, Michigan 48109, U.S.A.

H. Sinzinger, M.D., Atherosclerosis Research Group at the Department of Medical Physiology, University of Vienna, Vienna, Austria

Cesare R. Sirtori, M.D., Ph.D., Center Enrica Grossi Paoletti, Istituto di Farmacologia e di Farmacognosia, Università di Milano, Via A. Del Sarto 21, 20129 Milano, Italy

M. Sirtori, M.D., Center Enrica Grossi Paoletti, Istituto di Farmacologia e di Farmacognosia, Università di Milano, Via A. Del Sarto 21, 20129 Milano, Italy

Joan Slack, D.M., F.R.C.P., MRC Clinical Genetics Unit, Institute of Child Health, 30 Guilford Street, London WC1N 1EN, England

Donald M. Small, M.D., Chief, Biophysics Institute, Departments of Medicine and Biochemistry, Boston University School of Medicine, 80 East Concord Street, Boston, Massachusetts 02118, U.S.A.

Charlene Smith, R.D., Lipid Research and General Clinical Research Centers, University of Cincinnati College of Medicine, Cincinnati, Ohio 45229, U.S.A.

Elspeth B. Smith, Ph.D., B.A., University of Aberdeen, Department of Chemical Pathology, University Medical Buildings, Foresterhill, Aberdeen AB9 2ZD, Scotland

Frank R. Smith, M.D., Arteriosclerosis Research Center and Department of Medicine, Columbia University College of Physicians and Surgeons, 630 West 168th Street, New York, New York 10032, U.S.A.

Louis C. Smith, Ph.D., Department of Medicine, Baylor College of Medicine and The Methodist Hospital, 6565 Fannin, Houston, Texas 77030, U.S.A.

Allen Sniderman, M.D., Edwards Professor of Cardiology, Cardiovascular Research Unit, McGill University, Royal Victoria Hospital, Montreal H3A 1A1, Quebec, Canada

Lilian Socorro, Ms.Sc., Laboratorio de Lipoproteínas, Centro de Biofisica y Bioquímica, Instituto Venezolano de Investigaciones Cientificas, Apartado 1827, Caracas-101, Venezuela

Lars A. Solberg, M.D., Department of Pathology, Ullevaal Hospital, Oslo 1, Norway

Paul Sorlie, B.S., Biometric Section, National Heart, Lung and Blood Institute, National Institutes of Health, Bethesda, Maryland 20205, U.S.A.

James T. Sparrow, Ph.D., Department of Medicine, Baylor College of Medicine and The Methodist Hospital, 6565 Fannin, Houston, Texas 77030, U.S.A.

F. Spengel, M.D., Department of Medicine, Medizinische Poliklink der Universität München, Pettenkoferstrasse 8A, D-8000 München 2, Federal Republic of Germany

Eugene A. Sprague, Ph.D., Department of Pathology, The University of Texas Health Science Center, San Antonio, 7703 Floyd Curl Drive, San Antonio, Texas 78284, U.S.A.

Sathanur R. Srinivasan, Ph.D., Department of Medicine, Louisiana State University Medical Center, 1542 Tulane Avenue, New Orleans, Louisiana 70112, U.S.A.

Richard W. St. Clair, Ph.D., Department of Pathology and the Arteriosclerosis Research Center, Bowman Gray School of Medicine of Wake Forest University, 300 South Hawthorne Road, Winston-Salem, North Carolina, 27103, U.S.A.

Herbert C. Stary, M.D., Department of Pathology, Louisiana State University Medical Center, 1542 Tulane Avenue, New Orleans, Louisiana 70112, U.S.A.

Thomas E. Starzl, M.D., Ph.D., Chairman, Department of Surgery, University of Colorado Health Sciences Center, Denver, Colorado 80262, U.S.A.

A. Stiehl, M.D., Department of Medicine, University of Heidelberg, Bergheimer Strasse 58, D6900 Heidelberg, Federal Republic of Germany

Evan A. Stein, M.D., Department of Medicine, Lipid Research, University of Cincinnati Medical Center, Cincinnati General Hospital, 231 Bethesda Avenue, Cincinnati, Ohio 45267, U.S.A.

Olga Stein, M.D., Department of Experimental Medicine and Cancer Research, Hebrew University, Hadassah Medical School, Jerusalem, Israel

Yechezkiel Stein, M.D., Chairman, Department of Medicine B, Lipid Research Laboratory, Hadassah Medical School, Jerusalem, Israel

Daniel Steinberg, M.D., Head, Division of Metabolic Disease, Department of Medicine, School of Medicine, University of California, San Diego, La Jolla, California 92093, U.S.A.

Robert Steiner, F.F.R., F.R.C.P., Department of Diagnostic Radiology, Hammersmith Hospital, Ducane Road, London W12 OHS, England

Michael B. Stemerman, M.D., Head, Thrombosis and Hemostasis Unit, Department of Medicine and The Thorndike Laboratory, Beth Israel Hospital, 330 Brookline Avenue, Boston, Massachusetts 02215, U.S.A.

Grant N. Stemmermann, M.D., Director of Laboratories, Honolulu Heart Study, Kuakini Medical Center, 347 North Kuakini Street, Honolulu, Hawaii 96817, U.S.A.

Nils H. Sternby, M.D., Chairman, Department of Pathology, University of Lund, Malmo General Hospital, S214 01 Malmo, Sweden

Richard K. Stockton, Department of Medicine, Baylor College of Medicine and The Methodist Hospital, Houston, Texas 77030, U.S.A.

Wilhelm Stoffel, M.D., Ph.D., Department of Biochemistry, Institut für Physiolgische

Chemie, Universität zu Köln, Joseph-Stelzmann-Str. 52, 5000 Köln 41, Federal Republic of Germany

Jack P. Strong, M.D., Chairman, Department of Pathology, Louisiana State University Medical Center, 1542 Tulane Avenue, New Orleans, Louisiana 70112, U.S.A.

Albert J. Sunseri, Ph.D., Chicago Heart Association, Chicago, Illinois, U.S.A.

Naoki Suzuki, M.D., Department of Medicine, Jikei University, Aoto Hospital, 6-41-2 Aoto, Katsushika, Tokyo, Japan

Marja-Riitta Taskinen, M.D., Department of Pharmacology and Cell Biophysics, University of Cincinnati College of Medicine, 231 Bethesda Avenue, Cincinnati, Ohio 45267, U.S.A.

L.M. Tchichatarashvili, M.D., Institute for Experimental Medicine, Academy of Medical Science USSR, Kirovsky 69/71, Leningrad 197022 U.S.S.R.

Babie Teng, M.Sc., Cardiovascular Research Unit, Royal Victoria Hospital, McGill University, Montreal H3A 1A1, Quebec, Canada

Gilbert Thompson, M.D., F.R.C.P., MRC Lipid Metabolism Unit, Hammersmith Hospital, Ducane Road, London W12 OHS, England

Wilbur A. Thomas, M.D., Cyrus Strong Merrill Professor and Chairman, Department of Pathology, Albany Medical College of Union University, 47 New Scotland Avenue, Albany, New York 12208, U.S.A.

Matti Tikkanen, M.D., Third Department of Medicine, University of Helsinki Central Hospital, 00290 Helsinki 29, Finland

Jack L. Titus, M.D., Ph.D., The Moody Chairman, Department of Pathology, Baylor College of Medicine and The Methodist Hospital, 6565 Fannin, Houston, Texas 77030, U.S.A.

V. Toca, M.S., Department of Pathology, Louisiana State University Medical Center, 1542 Tulane Avenue, New Orleans, Louisiana 70112, U.S.A.

R.E. Tracy, M.D., Ph.D., Department of Pathology, Louisiana State University Medical Center, 1542 Tulane Avenue, New Orleans, Louisiana 70112, U.S.A.

Elena Tremoli, Ph.D., Center Enrica Grossi Paoletti, Istituto di Farmacologia e di Farmacognosia, Università di Milano, Via A. Del Sarto 21, 20120 Milano, Italy

V.F. Tryufanov, M.D., Institute of Experimental Medicine, Academy of Medical Science USSR, Kirovsky 69/71, Leningrad 197022, U.S.S.R.

Thomas B. Tschopp, M.D., Department of Pharmacology Research, F. Hoffman-LaRoche and Company, 4002 Basel, Switzerland

P. Tun, M.D., Cardiovascular Research Institute, University of California, San Francisco, California 94143, U.S.A.

Gerd Utermann, M.D., Institute für Humangenetik und Genetische Poliklinik, Der Philipps Universität Marburg, Bahnhofstrasse 7A, 3550 Marburg an der Lahn, Federal Republic of Germany

Richard L. Varco, M.D., Ph.D., Department of Surgery, School of Medicine, University of Minnesota, 516 Delaware Street SE, Minneapolis, Minnesota 55455, U.S.A.

Draga Vesselinovitch, D.V.M., M.Sc., Specialized Center of Research in Atherosclerosis, Department of Pathology, University of Chicago and The Pritzker School of Medicine, 950 East 59th Street, Chicago, Illinois 60637, U.S.A.

Ismo Virtanen, M.D., Third Department of Medicine, University of Helsinki Central Hospital, Helsinki 29, Finland

Arthur Vogel, M.D., Ph.D., Department of Pathology, University of Washington School of Medicine, Seattle, Washington 98195, U.S.A.

John C. Voyta, B.S., Department of Medicine, Baylor College of Medicine and The Methodist Hospital, 6565 Fannin, Houston, Texas 77030, U.S.A.

A.W. Voors, M.D., Dr.P.H., Departments of Public Health and Preventive Medicine and

Medicine, Louisiana State University Medical Center, 1542 Tulane Avenue, New Orleans, Louisiana 70112, U.S.A.

Kenneth W. Walton, M.D., D.Sc., Ph.D., F.R.C.Path., Department of Investigative Pathology, The Medical School, The University of Birmingham, Birmingham B15 2TJ, England

Patsy Wang-Iverson, Ph.D., Division of Arteriosclerosis and Metabolism, Department of Medicine, Mount Sinai Medical Center, 1 Gustav Levy Place, New York, New York 10029, U.S.A.

Emory D. Warner, M.D., Department of Pathology, University of Iowa College of Medicine, Iowa City, Iowa 52242, U.S.A.

G. Russell Warnick, M.S., Division of Metabolism and Endocrinology, Northwest Lipid Research Clinic, Harborview Medical Center, University of Washington School of Medicine, Seattle, Washington 98104, U.S.A.

L.S. Webber, Ph.D., Departments of Medicine and Biometry, Louisiana State University Medical Center, 1542 Tulane Avenue, New Orleans, Louisiana 70112, U.S.A.

Philip Weech, Ph.D., Laboratory of Lipid and Lipoprotein Studies, Oklahoma Medical Research Foundation, 825 Northeast 13th Street, Oklahoma City, Oklahoma 73104, U.S.A.

Richard Weil, III, M.D., Department of Surgery, University of Colorado Health Sciences Center, 4200 East Ninth Avenue, Denver, Colorado 80262, U.S.A.

Donald G. Weilbaecher, M.D., Department of Pathology, Baylor College of Medicine and The Methodist Hospital, 6565 Fannin, Houston, Texas 77030, U.S.A.

N. Weinstock, Ph.D., Lehrstuhl für Klinische Chemie der Medizinischen Einrichtungen der Universität Göttingen, Robert-Koch-Strasse 40, 3400 Göttingen, Federal Republic of Germany

David B. Weinstein, Ph.D., Department of Medicine, M-013D, Division of Metabolic Disease, School of Medicine, University of California at San Diego, La Jolla, California 92093, U.S.A.

Richard J. West, M.D., F.R.C.P., Department of Child Health, St. George's Hospital Medical School, London, SW17 ORE, England

Robert W. Wissler, M.D., Ph.D., Department of Pathology and the Specialized Center of Research in Atherosclerosis, The University of Chicago and The Pritzker School of Medicine, 950 East 59th Street, Chicago, Illinois 60637, U.S.A.

G. Wolfram, M.D., Department of Medicine, Medizinische Poliklinik, Universität München, Pettenkoferstrasse 8A, D-8000 München 2, Federal Republic of Germany

Joan M. Woodhill, D.Sc., Head, Division of Nutrition and Dietetics, Prince Henry and Prince of Wales Hospitals, Sydney, New South Wales, Australia

Minoru Yamamoto, M.D., Department of Medicine, Keio University, School of Medicine, 35 Shinano-machi, Shinjuku, Tokyo 160, Japan

Yoshio Yamauchi, M.D., Department of Medicine, Keio University, School of Medicine, 35 Shinano-machi, Shinjuku, Tokyo 160, Japan

L.A. Zeech, M.D., Molecular Diseases Branch, National Heart, Lung and Blood Institute, National Institutes of Health, Bethesda, Maryland 20205, U.S.A.

Donald B. Zilversmit, M.D., Division of Nutritional Sciences and Section of Biochemistry, Molecular and Cell Biology, Division of Biological Sciences, Cornell University, Ithaca, New York 14853, U.S.A.

Nepomuk Zöllner, M.D., Department of Medicine, Chief, Medizinische Poliklinik, Universität München, Pettenkoferstrasse 8A, D-8000 München 2, Federal Republic of Germany

Yu N. Zubzhitsky, M.D., Institute of Experimental Medicine, Academy of Medical Science U.S.S.R., Kirovsky 69/71, Leningrad 197022, U.S.S.R.

Contributions of Invited Speakers

Plenary Session: Cardiovascular Surgery
Chairperson: David S. Sabiston, Jr.
Speakers: Michael E. DeBakey
                     Harris B. Shumacker, Jr.
                     Charles Dubost

Workshop: Coronary Bypass Surgery
Speakers: John F. Goodwin
                     Gerald M. Lawrie
                     Henry D. McIntosh
                     Richard R. Miller

Workshop: Epidemiology of Atherosclerotic Lesions
Co-Chairpersons: Yuichiro Goto and Jack P. Strong
Speakers: William B. Kannel
                     Lars A. Solberg
                     Grant Stemmermann
                     Nils Sternby

Workshop: Drug Treatment of Hyperlipidemia
Chairperson: David Kritchevsky
Speakers: Donald B. Hunninghake
                     John P. Kane
                     Anatoli N. Klimov
                     Anders G. Olsson
                     Cesare R. Sirtori

Workshop: The Arterial Wall—I
Co-Chairpersons: M. Daria Haust and Kenneth M. Walton
Speakers: Abel Lazzarini Robertson
                     Colin J. Schwartz
                     Elspeth B. Smith
                     Jack L. Titus
Discussants: Colin W.M. Adams
                     Sören Björkerud
                     Ladislas Robert
                     H. Sinzinger

Workshop: Lipid, Apoprotein and Lipoprotein Origin and Synthesis

Co-Chairpersons: Richard J. Havel and Barry Lewis
Speakers: Shlomo Eisenberg
    Akira Endo
    Godfrey S. Getz
    Robert M. Glickman
    Robert L. Hamilton
    David B. Weinstein

Workshop: Lipoprotein Structure

Chairperson: Wilhelm Stoffel
Speakers: Germán Camejo
    Richard L. Jackson
    Gerhard M. Kostner
    Joel D. Morrisett

Atherosclerosis: Patterns and Rates of Progression[1]

Michael E. DeBakey

Despite considerable progress during the past several decades in the acquisition of knowledge about the anatomicopathologic changes that occur in the arterial wall, the exact cause of atherosclerosis is unknown. Our experience with more than 15,000 patients treated over a period of more than two decades has provided highly informative observations about the various patterns of arterial atherosclerotic occlusion as well as the natural course of the disease. For one thing, arteriosclerosis or atherosclerosis tends to assume certain characteristic anatomic, pathologic, and clinical patterns. Moreover, the disease is often segmental, with relatively normal proximal and distal arterial beds, although other forms may show a more generalized distribution. Recognition of the different clinical patterns of atherosclerosis made institution of successful surgical procedures possible.

Distribution According to Sex and Age

In general, atherosclerosis occurs predominately in male patients except after the menopause, when the sex distribution becomes almost equal. The disease becomes clinically manifested usually in persons in the fifth to seventh decades of life.

Patterns of Atherosclerosis

The patterns of the disease may be classified into four major categories in accordance with the anatomic sites of involvement: 1) the coronary arterial bed; 2) the major branches of the aortic arch; 3) the major branches of the upper abdominal aorta; and 4) the lower abdominal aorta and its major branches. In each of these categories this disease tends to assume one of three patterns of anatomic locations in the arterial bed: 1) involvement of the proximal or midportions of the arterial bed, with little or no disease in the distal bed; 2) predominant involvement of the distal arterial bed, with little or no involvement of the proximal portion; and 3) diffuse or generalized disease involving both the proximal and distal portions of the arterial bed.

The first category, namely the coronary arterial bed, is the most serious and disabling. The atherosclerotic lesions may be well localized to a small segment producing complete or incomplete occlusion. Such lesions usually involve the proximal or midportions of the arterial bed, with little or no involvement of the distal arterial bed and are therefore amenable to surgical treatment, consisting, in most cases, in aorto-coronary bypass. In most patients the disease affects both the right and left coronary arteries. In those patients with predominant involvement of the distal portion of the arterial bed and little or no involvement of the proximal portion, surgical treatment is not

[1] Supported in part by U. S. Public Health Service, National Heart and Blood Institute grant HL-17269, The National Heart and Blood Vessel Research and Demonstration Center, Baylor College of Medicine, Houston, Texas.

possible. Similarly, in those patterns characterized by diffuse involvement of the entire arterial bed, surgical treatment is not advisable.

The next pattern affects the innominate, carotid, and subclavian arteries, and their major branches. Several patterns also occur in this region. In one, the proximal segments of these vessels as they arise from the aortic arch are affected; occlusion may be complete or incomplete, and in about 50 per cent of patients more than one of these major arteries is diseased. The disease is almost always well-localized, with a relatively normal distal arterial bed; it is therefore amenable to surgical treatment. Another pattern occurs at the bifurcation of the carotid arteries and the origin of the internal carotid arteries, and at the origin of the vertebral arteries. The arteries both proximal and distal to these well-localized atherosclerotic lesions tend to be relatively normal, so that this pattern is also amenable to surgical treatment. In still another pattern the disease affects the distal arterial bed or intracranial portion, with relatively little or no disease of the proximal segments. It unfortunately is not amenable to surgical treatment.

In most of these patterns the atheroma causes localized stenosis, but in some the lesion is ulcerative, with little or no stenosis. On the surface of the ulcer, fibrin and thrombi develop, portions of which may break off and be swept up by the blood stream producing emboli; when this occurs, the patients may have repeated episodes of transient ischemic attacks.

These anatomic patterns of occlusive atherosclerotic disease tend to produce characteristic cerebrovascular manifestations and neurologic disturbances. The symptoms of a number of patients, unfortunately, do not reflect the exact site and extent of disease because of the high incidence of multiple arterial involvement and the development of collateral circulation. Thus, in some patients with characteristic ischemia due to occlusive lesions of the internal carotid arteries, arteriography may disclose the responsible, and surgically correctable, lesion to be in the proximal segment of the innominate, common carotid, or vertebral arteries. In other patients with characteristic manifestations of basilar arterial insufficiency, the responsible, and surgically correctable, lesion may be in the internal carotid arteries or in the proximal segments of the innominate, common carotid, or subclavian artery.

The third pattern of anatomic distribution of occlusive atherosclerotic disease involves the celiac axis, the superior mesenteric, and the renal arteries. The disease is characteristically well-localized at or near the origin of these arteries from the aorta, with relatively normal distal arterial beds, and hence this pattern is surgically correctable. Ischemia resulting from these occlusive patterns produces 1) abdominal or intestinal angina caused by occlusion of the celiac and superior mesenteric arteries, and 2) renovascular hypertension caused by occlusion of the renal arteries.

The final category of anatomic distribution of atherosclerotic occlusive disease affects the terminal abdominal aorta and its major branches. It, too, has several distinctive patterns. Disease localized to the aorto-iliac segment is one of the most common. Usually beginning at or near the origin of the common iliac arteries, the incomplete occlusion of one or the other common iliac artery gradually enlarges to complete occlusion of both. Later, thrombosis of the abdominal aorta spreads up to the origin of the renal arteries and produces intermittent claudication and sexual impotence. Since the distal arterial bed beyond the aorto-iliac segment is usually fairly normal, this pattern is also surgically correctable.

The next most common pattern in this category consists in disease of the superficial femoral artery in the region of the adductor canal. Usually well-localized, with a relatively patent distal segment in the popliteal artery and its major branches, it too is surgically correctable. Depending on its stage of development, the disease may cause incomplete or complete occlusion. Combined aorto-iliac and superficial femoral arterial occlusion, with some variations as to side of involvement, is also fairly common.

A rather unusual pattern, seen most often in women between 30 and 50 years of age, is one in which the atheroma is localized in the abdominal aorta a few centimeters above the bifurcation, usually on the posterior wall. Often only 2 to 4 cm long, it affects most of the posterior half of the aortic circumference. At endarterectomy, it may be easily separated from the remainder of the aortic wall by a cleavage plane at the site of attachment.

The final pattern in this category affects the popliteal artery and its major branches, with relatively little or no disease of the proximal arterial bed. This pattern is usually seen in patients with diabetes. It is unfortunately not amenable to surgical correction.

Extensive clinical experience suggests some selectivity in the occurrence, in different categories of patients, of the patterns of anatomic distribution of atherosclerotic occlusive disease that have been described. Thus, some patients are prone to cerebrovascular occlusive disease and have little or no evidence of involvement of other major arterial beds. Even in this group, patients with proximal disease of the major arteries arising from the aortic arch tend to be younger than those with disease of the carotid arteries at their bifurcation and of the vertebral arteries. The sex ratio is about 3 to 2. In Negroes distal occlusive patterns are prevalent, and proximal patterns uncommon. Still other patients are prone to coronary arterial occlusion, with little or no evidence of disease elsewhere. In this group the disease develops in both sexes at an earlier age than in those with carotid arterial occlusion. Similarly, patients with predominant aorto-iliac occlusion tend to be younger than those with the femoro-popliteal pattern, but the sex ratio here is about 10 male patients to 1 female patient. The various patterns of anatomic distribution of the disease may also develop simultaneously in some patients, whereas in others this may take place over a period of several years to as much as 20 years.

Rates of Progression

Atherosclerosis has been observed to develop at three different rates. Group I is characterized by rapid development, usually within one to three years. At first, the atheroma appears insignificant, clinically and arteriographically, but in a few years it produces clinical manifestations, and arteriography shows severe stenosis or complete occlusion of the lumen. These atherosclerotic plaques may be localized to a small segment of the artery, or they may be more extensive. Although they have been observed at most anatomic sites previously described, there is some evidence of more frequent occurrence in the carotid, coronary, and femoral arteries. Patients of both sexes in this group appear to be younger than in other groups.

In Group II the rate of progression is moderate, usually over a period of five to eight years. Both clinically and arteriographically, the atheroma proceeds from relative insignificance to severe encroachment on the lumen with consequent ischemic changes. Here again the disease occurs at most anatomic sites previously described. There is no particularly significant sex or age difference in this group. A higher proportion of patients falls into this group than in the others.

In Group III the disease develops slowly, usually over a period of ten years or more. Some patients in this group show no evidence of further progression of the disease up to twenty years after operation. This group also shows no particularly significant sex or age difference. In other patients, the disease at the original site in the artery may not progress, but later, disease appears at another site in the same artery. Thus, ten years after surgical correction of aorto-iliac occlusive disease, significant atherosclerotic occlusive disease may be found in the superficial femoral arteries. In still other patients, the disease may progress in different arteries, as exemplified by the appearance of disease first in the carotid artery, later in the aorto-iliac or femoral arteries, and still later, in the coronary arteries, but with little or no progression in the original diseased artery.

Clinical Significance

Based on more than twenty-five years' experience with over 15,000 patients, including arteriographic documentation, we concluded that arteriosclerosis or atherosclerosis represents several or more different entities, each having distinctive anatomicopathologic and clinical characteristics. Although atheromas have long been known to develop insidiously, enlarge continuously, and produce clinical manifestations when they encroach sufficiently on the lumen to impede circulation, their anatomicopathologic characteristics vary considerably, and they assume well-defined patterns of anatomic distribution as well as rates of progression.

These patterns fall into four major categories according to the anatomic site of disease, with a distinctive tendency to assume predominantly proximal or distal involvement or to be highly segmental or more diffuse with multiple sites of involvement. Patients usually have clinical manifestations reflecting one of these categories, but some patients may have various combinations of these categories simultaneously or sequentially.

The different rates of progression are also of considerable clinical significance. After surgical correction of the original well-localized process, some patients show no evidence of further progression of the disease in other parts of that arterial bed. At least in some patients, the disease appears to progress slowly up to a certain point, beyond which its progression is greatly retarded or even arrested. Moreover, atherosclerosis in some patients may be self-limited.

Although the disease may not progress in the artery in which it was originally manifested, for as long as twenty years, it may develop in another artery many years later, and the pattern of the atheromatous process often assumes similar characteristics in the new arterial site.

Both patterns of disease and rates of progression have prognostic and therapeutic significance. The main therapeutic objective is restoration of normal circulation in the diseased segment. The surgical procedures designed for this purpose include thromboendarterectomy, excision with graft replacement, the bypass graft, and patch-graft angioplasty. Both the feasibility of surgical treatment and selection of the appropriate procedure depend on the pattern of the disease. In general, well-localized or segmental disease with a relatively normal distal artery is amenable to surgical correction, whereas diffuse disease throughout most of the artery or affecting predominantly the distal portion is not amenable to effective surgical treatment.

Perhaps the most important prognostic factor is the rate of progression of atherosclerotic occlusive disease, irrespective of the pattern as originally manifested. Although well-localized disease in the more proximal segments of the arterial bed appear to progress more slowly than more diffuse disease, especially in the distal artery, a certain proportion of the well-localized form will show a rapid rate of progression. Indeed, recurrence of ischemic disturbances and failure within a few years after surgical treatment are usually caused by the rapid progression of the disease distal to the site of surgical correction, whether this be by endarterectomy or the bypass graft. This is well exemplified by a number of our patients in whom long-term excellent results followed operation, with arteriographic evidence of little or no progression of the disease, whereas other patients with recurrence of manifestations within a few years after operation showed progression of the atheromatous process.

In our present state of knowledge, it is not possible to determine the susceptibility of the individual patient to the various patterns and rates of progression at the onset of the disease or before. Certain risk factors, including particularly hypercholesterolemia, hypertension, and cigarette smoking as primary factors, and heredity, sex, age, hypertriglyceridemia, obesity, diabetes mellitus, physical activity, stress, and personality types as secondary factors, have been emphasized by some. I have not been able to establish a strong correlation between individual risk factors and the various patterns and rates of progression of atherosclerosis, or even between risk factors and individual susceptibility. Perhaps one-fourth or more of our patients had no identifiable risk factor.

Finally, I believe that the symptom complex referred to as arteriosclerosis or atherosclerosis represents a number of distinctively different clinical and anatomicopathologic patterns with various rates of progression. Much of the confusion about etiology, diagnosis, treatment, and prevention probably stems from failure to recognize these widely different patterns, which may indeed represent different entities. Certain epidemiologic studies, for example, include all forms of arteriosclerosis or atherosclerosis as a single entity without regard to their distinctly different patterns or rates of progression. Results of such studies, in the absence of precise definition of the patterns involved or their relative incidence in the sample population being studied, can only lead to further confusion. When the exact cause is ultimately found, each of the several or more different patterns conceivably will have a specific etiologic agent or set of etiologic factors.

Surgery for Coronary Artery Disease

David C. Sabiston, Jr.

Coronary artery bypass grafts (CABG) represent the most common cardiac surgical procedure performed today, and advances in this field have greatly altered the management of a number of patients with coronary artery disease. Following much laboratory experience in the direct anastomosis of coronary arteries in experimental animals (Sabiston and Blalock 1958), the first saphenous vein bypass graft to a coronary artery was performed in 1962 (Sabiston). A severe stenosis of the left main coronary artery was successfully corrected by a CABG in 1964 (Garrett et al. 1973). Several years later the procedure became widely used when it was demonstrated that it could be performed with a very low operative mortality (Favaloro 1968; Johnson et al. 1969).

In the majority of patients with angina pectoris, the primary objective of CABG is the relief of anginal pain and success is achieved in approximately 90%. Moreover, 60 to 70% of these patients have complete disappearance of all anginal symptoms and require no subsequent medication. A second objective, and one which has been recently emphasized, is extending the length of life. Although it is difficult to construct an ideal study to evaluate this factor, a frequently quoted series concerning the natural history of coronary artery disease and angina pectoris treated by nonsurgical means is a group of 601 patients with angina pectoris thoroughly evaluated by coronary arteriography and carefully followed over a ten year period with medical management (Bruschke 1978). When these patients were divided into those with single, double, triple vessel, and left main coronary disease, a clear relationship became apparent in comparing the subsequent risk of death with the number of coronary arteries involved (Fig. 1).

In reviewing these data, it becomes apparent that medical therapy alone is often inadequate in the treatment of symptomatic coronary artery disease, both from point of view of relief of symptoms and for life expectancy. Although there is general agreement that relief of pain in the vast majority of patients following CABG has been achieved, the issue of the extension of the length of life has been a controversial issue. In a number of published series, the conclusion has been drawn that CABG clearly increases longevity, and this is most clearly substantiated in those patients with significant stenosis of the left main coronary artery. This condition is well recognized to be associated with a high mortality in patients managed solely by medical means and death rates range up to 50% in the first two years following diagnosis by coronary arteriography (Cohen et al. 1972; Lavine et al. 1972).

One of the most conclusive studies of medical versus surgical management of patients with left main coronary lesions is that reported from a group of Veterans Administration Hospitals. In this study, 113 patients with left main lesions were divided into those managed surgically (65 patients) and those managed medically (48 patients) (Takaro et al. 1976). At the end of three years, 83% of the surgical patients had survived, whereas only 61% of those managed medically were still alive as seen in Figure 2. This series provided indisputable evidence that CABG extended the length of life in this group of patients with coronary artery disease. Moreover, the same conclusion was drawn from other similar studies in patients with double and triple vessel disease (Hurst et al. 1978). In the Veterans Administration Hospital cooperative study, patients with three vessel disease had a longer survival than those managed medically as shown in Figure 3 (Read et al. 1978).

Although criticisms of that study were made by Kaiser (1975), the data from this randomized study nevertheless are quite useful and have been helpful in the assessment of medical versus surgical therapy. In another series of patients with three vessel disease undergoing CABG reported by Cohn and associates (1975), the five year postoperative survival was 97%. While not strictly comparable, a contrast was drawn between these results and those from the series managed nonoperatively from the Cleveland Clinic. The latter group also had three vessel disease and the four year survival was 56% as seen in Figure 4.

The effect of CABG on long term survival of patients with double vessel disease is more controversial, although it has been concluded that the five year survival of surgically managed patients in this group was definitely better than would have been expected from medical management as shown in Figure 5 (Greene et al. 1977; Hurst et al. 1978).

Most believe that there is no convincing evidence thus far that the length of life is significantly increased following CABG for patients with single vessel disease. The primary indication for operation in this group is the relief of angina pectoris. At present, a consensus of available data re lating longevity to CABG is most appropriately summarized by Hurst (1978) who states, "Compared with modern medical therapy, properly performed coronary bypass surgery appears to prolong the life of patients who have obstruction of the left main coronary artery or triple or double vessel disease."

LESIONS OF 1, 2 AND 3 ARTERIES AND LEFT MAIN

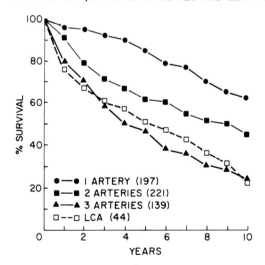

FIG. 1 Graphic illustration of a 10 year follow-up of 601 patients managed medically prior to the availability of coronary artery bypass grafts Bruschke AVG (1978).

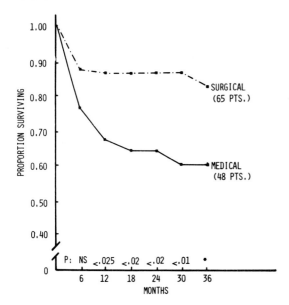

FIG. 2 Results of the prospective randomized
clinical trial of patients with severe obstruction of the left main coronary artery in the Veterans Administration study (Takaro et al. 1976).

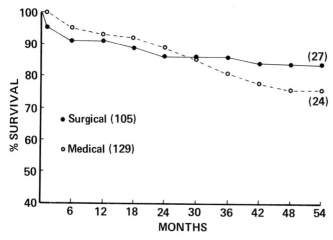

FIG. 3 Survival data among 129 medically treated
and 105 surgically treated patients with triple
vessel disease in the VA randomized study of left
main lesions. (Read et al. 1978).

Selection of Patients for Surgical Management

Although it is difficult to state precisely the number of patients who are
appropriate candidates for myocardial revascularization, it is generally
estimated that at least 20 to 25% of those with angina fail to obtain satisfactory pain relief with medication alone. In some patients, drug intolerance becomes a significant problem, and in others the anginal pain is
refractory to all forms of medical management. In addition to refractory
pain, CABG is also indicated for other specific complications of coronary
artery disease including preinfarction angina, refractory dysrhythmias
which are due to myocardial ischemia, and coronary lesions coexisting with
ventricular aneurysms.

All agree that selective coronary arteriography is essential in choosing
patients for myocardial revascularization. The diseased vessels undergoing consideration for grafting should have a reasonable lumen (1 mm or
more) and the distal coronary bed should be patent. In most series, 80 to
90% of patients with symptomatic coronary artery disease have coronary arterial anatomy appropriate for direct aortocoronary grafts. The majority
of surgical candidates have several significant lesions in the proximal
portions of the major coronary arteries which are potentially correctable
by a graft. In those patients with complete occlusion of a proximal coronary artery, the collateral circulation at the time of coronary arteriography may be inadequate to opacify the distal vessels despite the fact that
a patent lumen may be present. There are a number of studies which have
convincingly demonstrated patent distal vessels which did not previously
opacify at the time of coronary arteriography.

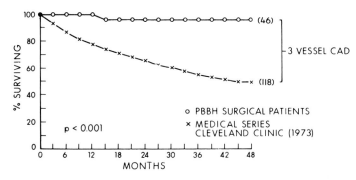

FIG. 4 Survival curves of patients with triple
vessel coronary artery disease (CAD) treated
with bypass surgery at the Peter Bent Brigham
Hospital (PBBH) and treated medically at the
Cleveland Clinic (lower curve); p = probability (Cohn et al. 1975).

While selective coronary arteriography is essential, cardiac catheterization frequently adds much data of importance in the understanding of the total hemodynamic profile. These studies reveal the status of left ventricular wall motion and provide an assessment of the function of the aortic and mitral valves. Characteristic features associated with an increased surgical risk include cardiomegaly, a low ejection fraction (below 25%), and an increased left ventricular volume. Nevertheless, the presence of these abnormalities does not necessarily represent a contraindication to operation or preclude a successful long term result.

The recent introduction of noninvasive radionuclide angiography has simplified an objective assessment of coronary artery disease since this technique makes it possible to obtain reliable values for ventricular volume, ejection fraction, cardiac output, and left ventricular wall motion both at rest and more importantly during exercise. In the normal heart, exercise not only produces an increase in cardiac output but also an increase in the ejection fraction of the left ventricle.

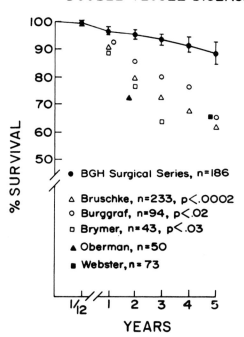

FIG. 5 Survival curves of patients with double vessel obstruction treated with bypass surgery at the Buffalo General Hospital (BGH) (upper curve) and treated medically in five series. n = number of patients; p = probability (Hurst et al. 1978).

In patients with myocardial ischemia due to coronary artery disease, exercise often results in a <u>decrease</u> in the ejection fraction as depicted in Figure 6 (Jones et al. 1978). The response to exercise in 20 patients with more than one vessel coronary artery disease including change in heart rate, cardiac output, pulmonary transit time, and pulmonary blood volume is shown in Figure 7 (Rerych et al. 1978). Such data provide very helpful information in the total assessment of myocardial function and of the likelihood of successful revascularization. Moreover, it provides a mean and comparative postoperative follow-up after CABG.

The surgical mortality of CABG has continued to diminish, and for patients undergoing uncomplicated coronary arterial bypass grafts, the mortality is in the range of 1 to 2%. These improved results have been due to a number of factors including advances in surgical technique, improved pre and postoperative management, and the use of the intra-aortic balloon assist device for diastolic augmentation in patients with extensive coronary disease. It is quite likely that one of the most significant factors in the reduction of perioperative mortality has been the more frequent use of hypothermic potassium cardioplegia, a technique originally developed by Melrose and associates (1955). The motionless heart aids greatly in the technical performance of coronary arterial anastomoses. Interest in clinical cardiople-

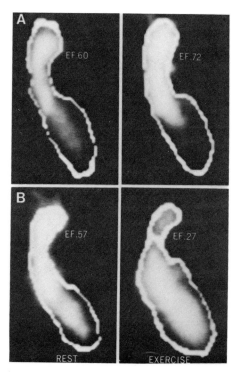

FIG. 6 End-diastolic outlines and end-systolic images demonstrating wall motion at rest and at exercise in a normal subject (A) and a patient with coronary artery disease (B). Patients with myocardial ischemia show marked cardiac dilatation and global hypokinesia with acute exercise (Jones et al. 1978).

gia was reintroduced by the experimental work of Bretschneider and associates in Germany (1975), Hearse et al. in England (1976), and Gay and Ebert
in the United States (1973). Two primary features are mandatory if the
myocardium is to be maximally protected while maintained in a motionless
and nonperfused state: (1) a marked reduction in cardiac temperature, and
(2) diastolic cardiac arrest. These two principles combine to greatly reduce the level of cardiac metabolism and are achieved by the direct administration of cold potassium solution (4° C) into the coronary circulation
where it is allowed to remain and is replenished at intervals in order to
maintain low temperature and an adequate concentration of potassium to
maintain diastolic arrest. In addition, the myocardium is maintained at a
low temperature by continuous bathing of the myocardium with cold saline
or ice slush. Under this combination of circumstances, the oxygen uptake
of the myocardium is reduced to extremely low levels (Chitwood et al. 1979).

RESPONSE TO EXERCISE IN 20 PATIENTS WITH
MORE THAN ONE VESSEL CORONARY ARTERY DISEASE
MEAN AGE 53 YEARS

	Rest	Exercise	P
Heart Rate (beats/min)	75±15	119±26	$<10^{-5}$
Cardiac Output (L/min)	5.7±1.5	11.3±4.3	$<10^{-5}$
Pulmonary Transit Time (sec)	7.7±1.8	5.4±1.7	$<10^{-5}$
Pulmonary Blood Volume (ml)	727±269	953±367	$<.02$

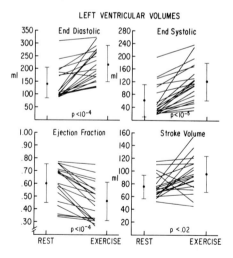

FIG. 7 Hemodynamic response of 20 patients (mean
age, 53 years) with significant stenosis of 2 or
more coronary arteries demonstrating the marked
hemodynamic changes that occur during exercise in
these patients (Rerych et al. 1978).

In summary, for patients who fail to achieve relief of anginal pain despite adequate medical therapy, CABG is indicated and can be performed with a very low mortality and with expectation of excellent clinical results. Randomized studies now indicate that, in certain groups of patients with coronary artery disease, life expectancy is significantly improved following myocardial revascularization. Advances in the proper selection of candidates for operative therapy, improvements in many aspects of surgical technique, the widespread use of hypothermic potassium cardioplegia, and advances in postoperative therapy have each been responsible for the diminishing surgical mortality to a current level of 1 to 2% in most centers.

References

Bretschneider HJ, Hubner G, Knoll D, Lohr B, Nordbeck H, Spieckermann PG (1975) Myocardial resistance and tolerance to ischemia: physiological and biochemical basis. J Cardiovasc Surg 16: 241

Bruschke AVG (1978) Ten-year follow-up of 601 nonsurgical cases of angiographically documented coronary disease. Angiographic correlations. In: The first decade of bypass graft surgery for coronary artery disease. An international symposium. Cleveland Clin Qtly 45: 143

Chitwood WR Jr, Sink JD, Hill RC, Wechsler AS, Sabiston DC Jr (1979) The effects of hypothermia on myocardial oxygen consumption and transmural coronary blood flow in the potassium-arrested heart. Ann Surg 190: 106

Cohen MV, Cohn PF, Herman MV, Gorlin R (1972) Diagnosis and prognosis of main left coronary obstruction. Circulation I-45 and 46: 57

Cohn LH, Boyden CM, Collins JJ Jr (1975) Improved long-term survival after aortocoronary bypass for advanced coronary artery disease. Am J Surg 129: 380

Favaloro RG (1968) Saphenous vein autograft replacement of severe segmental coronary artery occlusion: operative technique. Ann Thorac Surg 5: 334

Garrett HE, Dennis EW, DeBakey ME (1973) Aortocoronary bypass with saphenous vein graft: seven-year follow-up. JAMA 223: 792

Gay WA Jr, Ebert PA (1973) Functional, metabolic, and morphologic effects of potassium-induced cardioplegia. Surgery 74: 284

Greene DG, Bunnell IL, Arani DT (1977) Long-term survival after coronary bypass surgery. Buffalo General Hospital, State University of New York, brochure for exhibit at American Heart Association meeting, Miami

Hearse DJ, Stewart DA, Braimbridge MV (1976) Cellular protection during myocardial ischemia. The development and characterization of a procedure for the induction of reversible ischemic arrest. Circulation 54: 193

Hurst JW, King SB III, Logue RB, Hatcher CR Jr, Jones EL, Craver JM, Douglas JS Jr, Franch RH, Dorney ER, Cobbs BW Jr, Robinson PH, Clements SD Jr, Kaplan JA, Bradford JM (1978) Value of coronary bypass surgery. Controversies in cardiology: part 1. Am J Cardiol 42: 308

Johnson, WD, Flemma RJ, Lepley D Jr, Ellison EH (1969) Extended treatment of severe coronary artery disease. A total surgical approach. Ann Surg 170: 460

Jones RH, Rerych SK, Newman GE, Scholz PM, Howe WR, Oldham HN, Goodrich JK, Sabiston DC Jr (1978) Noninvasive radionuclide procedures for diagnosis and management of myocardial ischemia. World J Surg 2: 811

Kaiser GC, Barner HB, Tyras DH, Codd JE, Mudd JG, Willman VL (1978) Myocardial revascularization: a rebuttal of the cooperative study. Ann Surg 188: 331

Lavine P, Kimbiris D, Segal BL, Linhart JW (1972) Left main coronary artery disease. Clinical, arteriographic and hemodynamic appraisal. Am J Cardiol 30: 791

Melrose DG, Dreyer B, Bentall HH, Baker JBE (1955) Elective cardiac arrest. Lancet 2: 21

Read RC, Murphy ML, Hultgren HN, Takaro T (1978) Survival of men treated for chronic stable angina pectoris. A cooperative randomized study. J Thorac Cardiovasc Surg 75: 1

Rerych SK, Scholz PM, Newman GE, Sabiston DC Jr, Jones RH (1978) Cardiac function at rest and during exercise in normals and in patients with coronary heart disease: evaluation by radionuclide angiocardiography. Ann Surg 187: 449

Sabiston DC Jr (1974) The coronary circulation. The William F. Rienhoff, Jr. Lecture. Johns Hopkins Med J 134: 314

Sabiston DC Jr, Blalock A (1958) Physiologic and anatomic determinants of coronary blood flow and their relationship to myocardial revascularization. Surgery 44: 406

Takaro T, Hultgren HN, Lipton MJ, Detre KM, Participants in the Study Group (1976) The VA cooperative randomized study of surgery for coronary arterial occlusive disease. II. Subgroup with significant left main lesions. Circulation III-54: 107

Review of 30 Years of Surgery of the Heart and the Great Vessels

Ch. Dubost

A review of heart surgery and a discussion of its future perspectives constitute two interesting topics, although retrospection - necessary for the evaluation of our knowledge - may create a non-merited self-satisfaction and projections based on our hopes for the 21st century may create a sophisticated delerium worthy of the best science fiction works.

Rather than composing a catalogue, whose entries would rapidly become fastidious, I will raise several questions and try to offer responses dictated by the experience of 30 years of cardiac and vascular surgery.

Radical Cure or Complete Repair of Congenital Heart Disease?

It is currently possible to evaluate the results of various congenital heart diseases operated during the last 25 years.

In children, teenagers and adults, there are hardly any contraindications for surgery of the ostium secundum, the sinus venosus, the endocardial cushion defect in its partial or intermediate forms and the ventricular septal defect with low pulmonary resistance.

These various cardiopathies consistently indicate surgery even in the 5th, 6th or 7th decade of life; the same is true of ruptured aneurysms of the sinus of Valsalva or of corono-cardiac fistulae. It is possible to speak here of complete repair without the risk of being accused of megalomania by supercilious cardiologists. The same is not true, however, for complete A-V canals and for the truncus arteriosus: a better interpretation of anatomical lesions and more elaborate means of investigation, as well as more sophisticated techniques, have led to greater success in operations which nonetheless remain risky and which often yield only approximate results.

The continuous progress in cyanotic heart diseases has primarily involved the tetralogy of Fallot and, to a lesser extent, the transposition of the great vessels.

Surgical repair of tetralogy of Fallot today represents one of the most important activities in many cardiac surgery centers. It is not rare that several teams have performed hundreds of these operations. Our group at the Hôpital Broussais in Paris has performed 900 radical operations of tetralogy of Fallot during the last 25 years and almost 500 Blalock's operations in the same period, mainly between 1947 and 1955.

The surgical risk of the classical form of tetralogy of Fallot in children and teenagers has progressively decreased and is currently situated at about 5%. The longterm results are excellent and remain so: this was verified by a systematic study of the survivors of 900 operated patients in our group who underwent control catheterization and angiography. The long-term results are less satisfactory, however, for operations in which the infundibulo-pulmonary tract had to be enlarged by a large patch: the resulting pulmonary insufficiency diminished the quality of the functional result. In

17

certain cases, this complication may become sufficiently serious so that certain teams have proposed to avoid it, implanting a Hancock tube armed with a heterograft in order to by-pass the hypoplastic area. We have recently begun to acquire results of hemodynamic studies after the orthotopic implantation of an aortic heterograft at the level of the pulmonary ring in cases of hypoplastic pulmonary annulus in children weighing 8 to 10 kg (18 to 22 lbs.); we implanted heterologous valves as large as No. 21 or 23 with good immediate results.

Optimum patient age for the operation remains to be discussed. The current tendency is to advocate complete repair within the first several months of life for serious cases, which in the past would have undergone a palliating anastomosis. This will be discussed later, in the section on infantile surgery.

Current post-operatory results concerning the tetralogy of Fallot are more than satisfactory, in that a considerable fraction of the patients may be considered as cured. For exacting cardiologists, this cure is not complete, however, since it is often accompanied by an increased cardiac volume which tends to increase with time, by a complete block of the right branch and by ventriculo-pulmonary dynamics which, although near normal, may not be completely so. We thus share to a certain extent the limitation of cardiologists who prefer the term "radical cure" to "complete repair".

The complete transposition of the great vessels poses more difficult problems. The radical cure of this complex lesion may use several different techniques, in view of the varieties of the disease which may be encountered. Mustard's procedure of venous inversion represents the simple and elegant solution to the most common forms of transposition. Radical cure is also possible in the form combining ventricular septal defect with a pulmonary stenosis. The long-term results of these operations are not consistently excellent, however, and the old Senning operation is gradually regaining the place it lost in the cure of transposition.

In addition to the two major groups of cyanotic cardiopathies, other less frequent malformations have fed the inventive fires of surgeons: Fontan treated atresia of the tricuspid valve by an ingeneous derivation between the right auricle and the pulmonary artery; there are other examples, fortunately rare (Ebstein's anomaly of the tricuspid valve, single ventricle), for which palliative measures have been successfully performed. The double outlet right ventricle and auriculo-ventricular discordances with ventricular septal defect and pulmonary stenosis both offer possibilities of radical cure with relatively low surgical risk.

Neo-natal Surgery?

During the last several years, work inspired by Japanese surgeons and continued primarily in the United States, then in Europe, has led to the indication of surgery of certain congenital heart diseases in new-borns or infants.

Certain improved techniques, such as deep hypothermia and membrane oxygenator, have been applied to infants with heart diseases which were heretofore fatal within several weeks or months. The most frequently encountered examples are ventricular septal defect with pulmonary hypertension, poorly tolerated, complete transposition of the great vessels and complete A-V canals. Even certain poorly tolerated forms of tetralogy of Fallot have been proposed for radical cure in the first weeks or months of life. This is clearly an interesting technical acquisition, but for certain forms, the risk of incomplete or only palliative operations eventually yields a high percentage of

failure. Our own belief is that this type of surgery within the first few
days or weeks of life has led to abuses, particularly in radical cure of
tetralogy of Fallot. As for us, we remain faithful to a right or left Blalock procedure, depending on the position of the aortic arch, in those infants threatened by a severe anoxhemia. Radical surgery is undertaken later,
when the infant reaches a size of 10 to 12 kg (22 to 26 lbs.), at a time when
an improvement, both functional and at the level of vessel size, will have
been attained by a prior anastomosis.

Does the Ideal Artificial Valve Exist?

The therapeutic approach to acquired heart disease was revolutionized with
the use of artificial valves in the United States in 1960. I will only
stress that in addition to mechanical valves, ball valves or disk valves,
there also exist biological valves, primarily heterografts. In a number of
cases these biological valves are the response to a particular problem. As
a result of the work of J.P. Binet and A. Carpentier in 1966 and of the improvements introduced by Carpentier in 1968 concerning the glutaraldehyde
preservation technique, a number of teams throughout the world have used
porcine valves, primarily for the replacement of the mitral valve, but also
for the tricuspid and aortic valves. The treated valvular graft is sutured
to the interior of a frame in order to insure an insertion and thus a perfect
functioning, and also to protect the graft from any cellular and lymphatic
penetration from the receiver's aorta. These prepared and chemically treated valves are no longer similar to grafts: in contrast to true grafts, their
permanence does not depend on a regeneration from receiver cells, but rather
on tolerance, stability and resistance of valve tissue.

These valves have been extensively used for the last ten years for the mitral apparatus and less frequently for the tricuspid and aortic apparatus.
The long-term results are excellent and it is entirely valid to believe that
valve replacement by heterograft today represents the best choice, at least
at the level of the mitral apparatus.

During this time in my department, Carpentier attempted to improve the procedures of conservative mitral valvuloplasty by the use of a metal ring surrounded by tissue. The ring was so shaped as to maintain the totality of
the aortic leaflet of the mitral valve spreading while puckering the commissures and shortening this dilated portion of the mitral ring, which is
that of the implantation of the small valve. As far as I am concerned, I
have always been somewhat reticent in the use of the conservative technique
of the mitral valve and have applied it only in the forms of rupture of the
chordae of the small valve in which it was possible to conserve an otherwise
nearly intact mitral apparatus. This is not true for the tricuspid and we
have learned to recognize the danger of a prosthetic replacement which,
regardless of the material used, often led to failure after a short time.
It is for this reason that we remain partial to the conservation of the
tricuspid, whether it be related to a functional dilation of the orifice or
to an anatomical lesion in which a commissurotomy of two commissures
associated with a valvuloplasty can be performed. We prefer partial antero-
posterior valvuloplasty, which enables us to reduce the diameter of the preferentially dilated portion of the tricuspid ring without involving the
region of the septal valve, which retains a normal size. In addition, by
not using circumferential annuloplasty, regardless of the technique utilized,
the risk of post-operative auriculo-ventricular block is suppressed. Finally,
although aortic heterografts have not been used as widely as those of the
mitral apparatus, this is because the aortic diameter often admits only
prostheses of relatively small size; we now know that these small prostheses undergo secondary alteration and calcifications. For this reason,
the aortic heterografts we use in our department are only large sizes,

beginning with caliber 29 or 31, our routine replacement prosthesis being the Smeloff-Cutter valve. We have already implanted more than 1,000 of these valves: it has not been modified since its creation and we have never observed any case of ball variance after its use. It is also interesting to note that certain of these patients, in spite of their physician's advice, are against anticoagulant treatment and that a number of them lead a normal life in the absence of anticoagulation.

Our experience in valve surgery has led us to encounter a disease of mysterious origins, Loëffler's constrictive fibrous endocarditis, manifested by an internal constriction of one or both ventricles. I proposed an operation, and performed it for the first time in 1971, which consists of the resection of the ventricular fibrosis with the involved mitral and tricuspid apparatus and the replacement of the orifices with heterografts. This new technique may be applied to a group of patients otherwise condemned. My personal experience today involves 20 operated cases.

Does Closed Heart Surgery Deserve to Retain a Place?

This question is validly posed only by mitral stenosis. The uncertainties of closed intra-cardiac surgery and the advances in open heart surgery have resulted in the majority of surgeons choosing to operate under visual control, regardless of the circumstances.

We believe, however, that closed mitral commissurotomy performed with a dilator must be retained. In the case of a young woman presenting with a pure mitral stenosis, non-calcified, small heart and sinusal rhythm, I chose a closed heart commissurotomy with dilator (I have remained faithful to the technique of trans-atrial dilatation, which I have used for 25 years) because of its simplicity, its effectiveness and the absence of associated risk. Today we reoperate patients having had commissurotomies 25 years ago and who have lived normally for a quarter of a century. Clearly, in cases of doubt concerning the anatomical nature of the lesion visual control is imposed. I believe, on the other hand, that open heart surgery for all cases of mitral stenosis, in addition to increased risk, also leads to the danger of a too perfect commissurotomy and its corollary, an iatrogenic mitral insufficiency; in addition, this open approach leads to an overestimation of lesions which may result in a certain percentage of unwarranted mitral replacements.

The diagnostic means at our disposal today, including phonomechanograms, image intensifier analyses and echocardiography, enable us to precisely recognize the state of the mitral valve and to preview the true possibilities of conservation.

Is the Aorto-coronary By-pass Capable of Modifying the Course of Coronary Disease?

In the field of acquired heart disease, coronary disease has attained premier importance since 1968, when Favaloro proposed the revascularization of the myocardium by aorto-coronary venous by-pass. This operation soon became very popular and the number of operated cases is spiraling, especially in the United States. It was generally admitted from the beginning that the operation prolonged patient longevity and that under these circumstances it was recommended to treat not only patients suffering from symptomatic coronary disease, but also those in whom routine coronarography exhibited significant lesions of one or several coronary arteries, even in the absence of clinical signs.

Today, ten years after the advent of this technique, it appears that indications are not as clear-cut as they were thought. Evaluations of operations in some American centers prove that patient longevity is not obviously improved after by-pass. The current belief of cardiology teams, at least in France, is that aorto-coronary by-pass should not be as widely used until it has been proven that longevity is significantly increased. This is the reason why we think that this operation should be reserved for intractable anginal pains, as well as for patients with unstable angina, where the coronary by-pass is to be performed as an emergency operation.

Does Palliative Surgery Still Have a Place in Certain Types of Aortic Aneurysms?

Valve surgery and coronary surgery do not represent the totality of surgical possibilities in acquired heart disease: aortic aneurysms represent a large group in which surgery has realized considerable progress. Aneurysm of the thoracic aorta and aneurysm of the abdominal aorta are frequently encountered and it is primarily the latter that benefits from a graft inclusion technique which has been successfully used for a long time.

a) One of the most frequent locations in the thoracic aorta is the ascending aorta. It develops at the level of the sinus of Valsalva and the aneurysm is most often due to a dystrophy of the aortic wall, related to Marfan's syndrome or to an elastorrhexia. Surgery consists of the graft inclusion technique associated with the replacement of the aortic valve with or without the repositioning of the coronary arteries.

b) A privileged localization is represented by the aneurysms of the descending post-subclavian thoracic aorta. Whether it is a traumatic aneurysm or an atheromatous aneurysm, involving only one part of the descending aorta, the technique is simple graft inclusion. This localization is nonetheless accompanied by the risk of post-operative paraplegia resulting from the duration of aortic clamping. For this reason, several techniques have been proposed to avoid this danger: inert shunt and femoro-femoral veno-arterial or left auricle-femoral artery pulsed derivations.

We know today that simple distal and proximal normothermic clamping has a risk factor which is no greater than that associated with methods preserving distal vascularization. This leads us to think that the change in spinal vascularization is not only directly related to the duration of the ischemia, but also to an arterial distribution such that blood supply to the spinal cord is reduced anatomically and cannot be protected by any means. This is the principal reason explaining why most surgical teams today perform surgical cures of moderate size aneurysms of the descending thoracic aorta by simple clamping and graft inclusion.

c) Thoraco-abdominal aneurysms, on the other hand, raise more problems, especially lesions which involve the entire descending thoracic aorta and all or a part of the abdominal aorta; this condition creates higher operatory risks.

Here again, after having performed a retrograde revascularization inspired by the technique of Hou-Yu-Lin, involving neither shunt nor pulsed derivation, our current preferences are for Crawford's technique. This method involves the simplest and most rapid method of graft inclusion with successive cephalo-caudal reimplantation of the visceral branches of the sub-diaphragmatic aorta and the implantation of an aortic fragment with the origins of the pairs of inter-costal and lumbar arteries destined for spinal supply: paraplegia thus decreases from 38% to 14% in this series of cases.

In the eventuality of these voluminous thoraco-abdominal aneurysms, however, the operation is dangerous, with a combined vital and spinal risk of 30%. In spite of the relative rapidity of the operation, a double incision is required: high thoracotomy and a long thoraco-abdominal incision. Aneurysmal dissection time is reduced but it remains necessary to uncover the proximal aorta, to free the diaphragmatic passage and to open the peritoneum in order to clamp the abdominal aorta. Aortic clamping results in an enormous overload for the heart, which proves to be too great for certain poor myocardia. Furthermore, the resulting cerebral hypertension may cause certain neurological complications. Delicate problems are also raised by the control of collateral arteries within the aneurysm.

All these considerations have led us to believe that a palliative operation involving exclusion of the aneurysm is valid in this type of eventuality, especially in patients with other associated vascular or visceral troubles.

We performed this type of operation with R. Soyer in 1975. An aneurysm which extended from the left subclavian artery to the origin of the superior mesenteric artery was operated by left thoracotomy. We realized that a graft inclusion would create undue risk in this patient as a result of per-operative hemorrhage which we were not prepared to control and also because the patient had a poor myocardium and bad kidney function. We thus decided to install a definitive by-pass between the ascending aorta and the abdominal aorta proximal to the iliac bifurcation, then to sever the aorta distal to the origin of the subclavian artery and to suture the two extremities, to reimplant the coeliac trunk on the prosthesis and, finally, to sever the aorta above the renal arteries and to suture the two extremities.

The aneurysm was thus excluded from the aortic stream and only the intercostal and lumbar arteries continued to supply the sac in counter-current circulation. A progressive thrombosis will undoubtedly develop in the pocket, leaving time for the spinal cord arteries to be relieved by collateral circulation. This first case was a success and the results remain perfect four years later.

The anastomosis between the ascending aorta and the graft when performed by left thoracic approach nevertheless is difficult, even if the sternum is incised horizontally. This is primarily because of the location of the trunk of the pulmonary artery, which blocks access. This is the principal reason why we preferred, with Carpentier, to perform the same protocol using a long median sterno-pubic incision. A No. 26 or 29 Dacron tube is sutured to the right flank of the ascending aorta, then pulled across the pericardium and the diaphragm behind the left lobe of the liver; then an end-to-side anastomosis is performed between the Dacron tube and the abdominal aorta above its bifurcation. The aorta is then clamped definitively after the origin of the left subclavian artery with a special metal clamp which is left in place. It is also possible to use a pistol screw-clamp to occlude the aorta: the aorta is first protected by a double thickness of Teflon felt and the plastic ring placed around the aorta is then progressively tightened until the aorta is completely occluded. If one or several visceral branches are included in the aneurysm they are reimplanted on the side of the graft. If the aneurysm does not involve the abdominal visceral branches, it is not necessary to interrupt the aorta at the lower pole of the ectasia. This superior unipolar exclusion of the aneurysm is the simplest solution, leading to the depulsation of the aneurysmal sac, avoiding evolution toward rupture and avoiding the necessity for reimplanting the visceral branches. This is a low risk operation and is well tolerated in patients considered poor risk cases as a result of associated vascular or visceral lesions.

We also believe that it is justified to apply this technique to certain aneurysms of the aortic arch in cases where current techniques do not offer an ideal solution. The operation we recommend above may be performed with less risk.

Once the aorto-aortic shunt is installed, a trifurcating graft is sutured to the by-pass and each of its branches is termino-laterally anastomosed to the innominate trunk, the left carotid and the subclavian. Finally, the aorta is definitively interrupted immediately prior to the innominate trunk and the origins of each of the large branches of the aortic arch are tied. The aneurysm of the arch is thus depulsed and will evolve towards thrombosis while the new aorta will assure the supply of the descending aorta and abdominal visceral branches.

Will Heart Transplantation One Day Enter the Therapeutic Arsenal?

The several teams which continue to perform heart transplants on the clinical level answer in the positive. In his recent publications, Shumway affirmed that heart transplants have left the experimental stage and have become a therapeutic technique. Our belief, however, is that this attitude does not have solid bases which could influence a large number of heart surgery teams. Several factors are responsible. There has recently been a decreased demand for this procedure which can be explained by the advent of new medical or surgical therapies, particularly for coronary heart disease. In addition, the several teams performing this research have limited indications to a group of young patients, less than 40 years of age. It was noted that results in this group were more satisfactory than in those patients already having been operated with cardio-pulmonary by-pass. On the other hand, certain patients whose cardiac disorder has a possible auto-immune nature would be less satisfactory candidates for a transplant. Thus, if we currently note improved results of heart transplantation, this is the consequence not of scientific progress, but rather of the inclusion of several simplifications: at the level of the recipient group and at the level of immunological requirements. Shumway, who today has acquired the widest experience in this field, restricts his choice to the ABO system, ignoring the HLA system and choosing the youngest and healthiest heart whose volume is best adapted to the size of the recipient. Another simplification is at the level of post-operative treatment, where cortisone is used almost exclusively. The last simplification is at the level of heart transplantation itself, where C. Barnard advocates abandoning orthotopic transplants as a result of unacceptably high failures, in favor of heterotopic transplants, i.e. the implantation of a "spare" heart in parallel with the patient's heart, even though the latter will also be exposed to risks of rejection. We thus observe that claimed progress is not obvious, since it is based on restrictive criteria related solely to observation and lacking true scientific bases.

This type of human experimentation has not yet reached the therapeutic stage. Even if application on a larger scale becomes possible, it will be faced with a lack of donors; this lack would become intensified compared with that already existent in renal transplants.

Conclusions

The last 30 years have enabled this new branch of surgery to greatly expand. It has addressed itself to many types of cardiac and aortic diseases and there are tens of thousands of patients throughout the world today who have reaped its benefits.

Considered in the light of a reconstructive technique, cardio-aortic surgery has attained its goal, even if it was only able to offer palliative support to a large number of congenital or complex acquired diseases.

This means that much remains to be done in this field; in the domain of acquired cardiopathies, the ideal valve remains to be found.

The aorto-coronary by-pass is a decisive tool in the fight against certain forms of coronary heart disease and offers relief to the patient which cannot be offered by medical treatment alone. Its future, however, is fraught with uncertainties, especially since no formal proof yet exists that it indeed increases the longevity of operated patients.

We have thus reached a certain plateau today, but I will invoke an optimistic note to conclude this rapid overview of a field of surgery I was involved in at its infancy. With the enthousiastic help of a number of colleagues, I aided in its development and today it has reached an apogee. It is now in a phase of reflection, waiting to make a new leap forward.

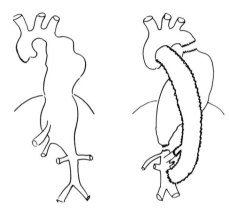

Figure 1a. Thoraco-abdominal aneurysm treated by left thoracic aorto-aortic by-pass, bipolar exclusion and reimplantation of coeliac axis.

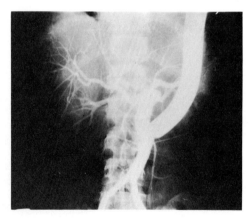

Figure 1b. Control aortography taken 1 year later shows perfect filling of aorto-abdominal branches of iliac axis.

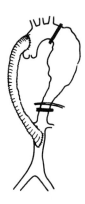

Figure 2. Aorto-aortic by-pass conducted through median sternotomy and xipho-pubic incision and bipolar exclusion by two left-in-place metal clamps.

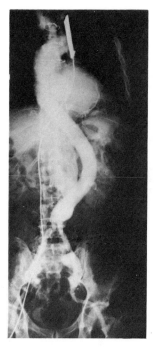

Figure 3. Control aortography of a unipolar exclusion of a thoraco-abdominal aneurysm.

Mechanism of Progress. Page from the History of Cardiovascular Surgery

Harris B. Shumacker, Jr.

Nothing could please me more than to have the privilege and honor of taking part, together with my close friends and distinguished colleagues, Stanley Crawford, Charles Dubost, and David Sabiston, in this important International Symposium's opening Plenary Session which honors one of our hosts and participants, Michael E. DeBakey, upon his retirement from the Presidency of the Baylor College of Medicine. This high post he has held with true eminence through periods of smooth sailing and rough seas, those of rapid, easy progress and of difficult times as well, always maintaining a forward course, so that this institution, which we consider his "Center of Medical Advancement", has become a Mecca for thousands who have sought and gained inspiration and instruction from it. He has helped it grow and acquire the best hospital, library and laboratory aids, but has always kept clearly in mind that great institutions are not made with bricks and mortar, nor even with books and manuscripts, but with people – people who can perform their professional obligations with real skill and who, at the same time, can think critically, receptively, and with originality. He has adhered to the basic philosophy that the primary functions of a medical center must include, in addition to the best possible teaching and post-doctoral training and the most effective clinical care of the patients who come to it for help, an ongoing, vigorous and productive research program. He has realized full well that investigative work is invaluable, not only because of the new knowledge it may yield, but also because it is essential for creating the ideal environment in which young men and women may reach their full potential development. In addition to his local duties, he has given freely of his time to our and other governments, commissions, committees, and societies. Anyone who has had the opportunity of serving with him can recall his apparently placid arrival just in the nick of time after a long day's work in Houston and his hurried farewell once the conference was over in order to return for an early start the next morning following a long night's flight back to Texas.

I must say to my old and dear friend, Mike, that I shall not devote the period which has been allotted to me in citing the contributions he has made, nor those of his associates who have done so much under his inspiring leadership, nor the many high honors he has received from here and abroad – all so well earned and so richly merited. To do so would take all the time I have at my disposal, and possibly more, and would, I fear, only prove embarrassing to him. I know my colleagues, Charles, David, and Stanley will forgive me for omitting reference to the many most important innovations for which we are all deeply indebted to them.

It seems to me appropriate to the occasion that I speak briefly about the mechanisms of progress and illustrate the concepts I have reached by a page from our cardiovascular surgical past. It is clear to all who have paused to ask themselves, "How have we gotten to where we are?" that ideas constitute the fundamental basis of our forward march. They are the treasured seeds of discovery and inventions from which new knowledge evolves, new observations are made, new techniques are developed. Those of merit, properly cultivated, are the glory of our past, the stepping-stones of the present, and the promise of the future. Those which have died unexplored and undeveloped, on the other hand, constitute the sackcloth and ashes we wear in humiliation. Let us take a look at them, examining factors which have killed some before their fertilization, slowed down the evolution of others, and, fortunately, permitted still others to blossom into full maturity almost overnight - factors which account for delays, persistence of erroneous beliefs and practices, as well as for periods of steady forging ahead.

What a pity it is that civilization tends from the beginning to smother, rather than to encourage, the imagination and curiosity inborn in most of us - the constant questioning of the very young "who, what, when, where, why?". What a tragedy it is that one can help students in all stages of self-development relatively easily acquire factual knowledge, that it is possible, though more exacting, to assist them to think critically, yet without prejudice or rigidity, but extremely difficult, if not virtually impossible, to give them a sense of wonder and creativity.

Though, in substantiating my views, I shall use other historical examples, I shall select them primarily from the field of arterial surgery. This is done for two reasons: In the first place, among the many contributions of Mike DeBakey and his colleagues, those in this particular area probably include the most significant - innumerable innovations which have proven of enormous importance in extending the scope of applicable surgery. In the second place, atherosclerosis is the topic of this International Symposium and the majority of the operatively treatable arterial lesions throughout the body, aneurysmal, stenotic, and obstructive, have this disease process as their etiologic basis.

How can I better begin than by referring to the thought-provoking Presidential Address before the American Surgical Association of Alfred Blalock (1956), my former beloved Chief, and David Sabiston's? It deals with the nature of discovery and begins by pointing out that discovery is considered to mean learning what already existed but was not previously known, while invention refers to the development of something not existent before. I should like to make it evident that, unlike Blalock, who limited his remarks to discovery, I shall deal here with discovery, invention, and innovations of all sorts which assist in improving our understanding and bringing about better treatment. He very aptly divided discoveries into those which occur by chance or accident, those which result from intention or design, those which are the consequence of imagination or "hunch", and those which arise from some combination of the others. I have the feeling that there might well be added the concept that some discoveries may well be classified as having come about by necessity. In his first category he mentioned as one example Rudolph Matas's development of the new technique of endoaneurysmorrhaphy which entails the intrasaccular suture of vessels arising from, or entering, an aneurysm. When Matas first encountered back-bleeding from such branches after the main stem artery had been ligated proximally and distally, his new and important contribution resulted not by chance alone, for it was a matter of absolute necessity that he stop the loss of blood or the patient would not have survived. His extensive operative background and his capacity to think with ingenuity led him to conceive at once of closing the orifices by suture from within the aneurysmal sac. I am confident that many of the innovations from this clinic have arisen similarly when DeBakey and his staff, confronted with situations which required treatment and for which there was no good precedent, have, either beforehand, or during the midst of an operation, conceived a worthwhile plan which turned out to constitute a valuable and original method of management. I remember well an occasion some years ago when he and I were serving on a Board of Advisors to a certain university. One important member of our group became utterly annoyed and upset because I expressed the opinion that as persons with the originality and experience of DeBakey went about their daily chores, seeing patients on the wards and in the clinics and carrying out operative procedures, they were, in a sense, performing research just as surely as if they were in the laboratory pursuing a carefully designed program of investigation - that they were always on the verge of something new and useful. What they have accomplished in this way proves, I believe, the correctness of this assumption. I am reminded of Wangensteen's (1978) wise comments following a discussion of Semmelweis' epoch-making observations and the unfortunate view of some that the highest recognition was due only those whose work is "characterized by the use of acceptable scientific methods". He wrote: "Are the methods of current day science so perfected and restricted that the greatest benefits conferred upon mankind do not qualify as being scientific in nature? That great accomplishment is of no moment? ..... We see daily too many examples of application of scientific methods to the resolution of sterile ideas, that at best produce only barren results".

Another means of discovery not listed by Blalock as a separate category, but one he must have had in mind, is that of serendipity - the unexpected side-benefits of a project - the valuable additional gains over and beyond the primary objective sought. Undoubtedly, countless innovations have come about in this manner. Mentioned by him, but not so classified, was the delayed recognition that the wearing of rubber gloves was a most important measure in reducing the incidence of operatively induced infection - something far from Halsted's thoughts when he introduced their use in order to protect from mercuric chloride dermatitis the hands of a beautiful young scrub nurse who was to become his wife and life-long companion.

Thus far the mechanisms which move us ahead have been considered. Let us now examine some of the factors which either impede or assist the conversion of the spark of imagination into new knowledge, better understanding, and more effectual treatment. The ligature, without the utilization of which operative surgery as we currently understand it could never have been developed, serves as an appropriate topic with which to begin. Celsus is said to have employed it and certainly Antylus in the second century not only did so, but operated upon aneurysms by proximal and distal ligation of the main stem artery, following which he opened and packed the sac.[1] Why did we have to wait fourteen long centuries before the ligature was "rediscovered" in 1537 by Paré? It was, of course, due to the mental attitude of the Dark Ages when in medicine, as in other disciplines, it was felt inappropriate, almost sacrilegious, to challenge so-called "authority" - when man was satisfied to go along accepting what he had inherited without question, never taking exception, never thinking of possible new and better understanding nor of improved methods of management. These are, of course, among our cardinal sins - the mistaken notion that authority is synonymous with correctness and our failure to be continuously inquiring, seeking, questioning. One might ask further why another couple of hundred years elapsed before the ligature, proved so effective by Paré, took hold, so to speak, and became the primary method for the control of bleeding. As Samuel Harvey has pointed out in his delightful little book "The History of Hemostasis", for a long while the method of Paré did not clearly win out, for even though the actual cautery now ranked a poor third, the chemical styptic still occupied the top place, the ligature somewhere in between, being used almost exclusively for controlling bleeding from large vessels during amputations through the thigh and arm. It must be remembered, too, that he was referring to an age by no means devoid of great surgeons, but of men such as Petit, Desault, Chopart, Cheselden, Pott, and Heister. The difficulty was clearly much the same, fear of innovation and satisfaction with the status quo.

As far as one can learn, it was in 1759 that the first crude arterial repair was carried out. It was then, 220 years ago, that Hallowell, at the sugges-

---

1 References to which I allude are not included in the appended brief list unless they are not mentioned in the more general review publications which are cited.

tion of his physician friend Lambert, closed a small opening in the brachial artery from which an aneurysm arose by passing a pin through its edges and tying a thread about the pin in the manner of the cobbler's stitch until the arterial luminal integrity was secure. Though this was still in the age of "laudable pus", the repair remained intact and the circulation excellent. This event is historically and educationally important far beyond being a "first". We probably would know nothing of it had it not been for John Hunter who heard about it and persuaded Lambert to publish this observation. Good ideas must be shared and the best method of doing this is by publication. Publication alone, however, is without value unless what is published is read and read with open receptiveness rather than preconceived rigidity as well as with proper critical analysis. The failure to do this has recurred time and again, always slowing progress.

Not long after the Lambert-Hallowell operation the studies of Asman were described in his inaugural dissertation. They indicated that the method was a failure. Few who became familiar with this work appreciated the fact that the crude method which Lambert himself recognized as almost surely applicable only to large arteries was doomed to end in obliteration when applied to the small arteries of experimental animals, and that such observations in no way indicated that the successful repair of arteries was an impossibility. Animal experiments have been of vital importance in the advances which have been made and many of us assembled here have spent a considerable part of our time building suitable experimental laboratories, financing them, and working in them. Yet, animal studies must be examined critically. Not all of them are well done. What proves true in one species may yield entirely different results in others. As an example, decapsulation of the dog's kidneys is followed within a few months by the laying down about it of a dense, heavy, constricting envelope of scar tissue and resultant arterial hypertension (Bounous and Shumacker 1961), but these alterations apparently do not follow removal of the renal capsule of the Macacus Rhesus or of the human (Stone and Fulenwider 1977). Without doubt, not all animal experiments are directly applicable to man. Certain vascular and sympathetic nerve studies fall into this category since, as far as is known, no animal species has a vasomotor apparatus as labile and responsive as man's – nor the variability in reactivity noted even among healthy persons. There is food for thought in Francis Moore's (1979) statement in his recent commentary on the study of trauma: "Research could well start by asking embarrassing questions rather than burrowing deeper into the perfect animal model". Some laboratory studies have, indeed, tended to slow down the clinical application of an excellent idea. If we had waited for the "entirely perfect" animal experiments with the heart-lung machine before applying it in patient usage, we might well be performing only closed and very time-limited, simple open cardiac procedures.

Nevertheless, everyone would agree that if an idea potentially applicable to man can be shown to hold promise, or to be of limited value, or worthless, by carefully planned and executed animal experimentation, this is not only desirable but imperative. A single example will be sufficient. One of the least effectual operative procedures carried out at the time Mike DeBakey and I were young surgeons was the "homeopathic" approach to chronic constrictive pericarditis. With limited exposure through a right or left thoracotomy or an upper abdominal transdiaphragmatic approach all too often only small segments of the encasing pericardium were excised. Naturally, the patients were not often cured and many were subjected to multiple operations of this sort. To be sure, there were some successes, including the initial case treated in this country by Churchill, a hemipericardiectomy. To be sure, too, the total picture of chronic cardiac constriction had been produced in experimental animals by inducing widespread pericarditis. This did not, however, help settle the question argued by our leading thoracic surgeons whether one should decompress the right or the left side of the heart. The evolution of a method for producing in dogs selective and limited, as well as diffuse, cardiac compression in the early 1950s by Parsons and Holman (1950) and by Isaacs and his associates (1952) brought about not only better understanding of the precise hemodynamics of right-sided, left-sided and complete pericardial constriction, but made clear that the proper operative management was radical subtotal resection.

Lack of such considerations of the limitations and value of animal studies led surgeons of great prominence time and again to condemn the idea of arterial repair on the basis of Asman's report. Among them were such men as Velpeau who did so in his treatise published nearly seventy-five years after the Lambert-Hallowell operation and Broca who did the same in his monograph on aneurysms almost twenty-five years later. Animal experimentation, despite its enormous value in contributing important new knowledge, must no more be elevated to the position of a godhead than should a mathematical formula or a computer read-out. All are subject to error.

People who are in positions of unusual respect must realize that their statements and opinions are apt to bear undue weight upon those of lesser stature, that the heavy hand of "authority" may be erroneously interpreted as always representing the truth. Dozens of illustrations to the contrary could be cited. I shall mention only two. When Elliott Cutler's medical associate, Sam Levine, sent to Sir James MacKenzie a reprint of the first operative efforts to treat mitral stenosis at the Brigham Hospital in the 1920s, the reply from the world-renowned cardiologist was to the effect that they had done a very foolish thing in Boston, that patients with rheumatic valvular disease were not ill because of the constriction or incompetence of the valve, but primarily because of the sick state of the heart muscle. The thousands upon thousands of patients treated successfully by valvular repair or replacement attest to the error of his assessment. Sir William Osler, certainly one of the preeminent physicians of his day, and likely the single most highly regarded one, a person long interested in the problems associated with arteriovenous fistulas, in one of his last publications when referring to one such case stated that it "illustrates the wisdom of non-intervention" and subsequently remarked "twice he narrowly escaped operation". This should suffice to establish the point.

Furthermore, simply because the time is not quite right for the application of a new concept, it should not be buried by harsh, unjustified criticism. When Sir Lauder Brunton published a paper entitled, "Surgical Operation for Mitral Stenosis", in Lancet in 1902, the editors waited only until the next week's issue to take him thoroughly to task for making such a preposterous proposal, a suggestion which Brunton himself had simply offered in the hope that further work might be done by others in order to prove or disprove his thesis more promptly and not with the idea that it was ready to be applied in clinical cases. We must also keep in mind the fact that the young should be encouraged and not dissuaded by their elders. All too often they are right, and their seniors are wrong. When I asked Elliott Cutler why he had utilized the transventricular rather than the atrial approach in his early efforts to open the stenotic mitral valve, he told me that his chief, loved and respected Harvey Cushing, had advised him to do so, fearing that the thin-walled atrium would prove more difficult to close by suture than the thick-walled ventricle - certainly a mistaken notion. When Jack Gibbon, working as a Fellow in Churchill's laboratory, proposed to embark upon the difficult project of developing a temporary extracorporeal substitute for the heart and lungs, Churchill told him that he might go ahead but certainly did not lend him real encouragement and Walter Bauer advised him to tackle simpler problems, ones more sure of suitability for publication, in order to forward his academic career. It was only Gene Landis who really encouraged him to proceed and give it a try.

There is another lesson from the Lambert-Hallowell operation, simple and perfectly obvious, but, at the same time, most important. Ideas may readily spill over from one branch of medical practice or medical science to another. It was a physician, Lambert, who, discouraged with the results which followed his surgical colleagues' treatment of peripheral aneurysms by ligating the main arterial stem, conceived the notion of a better method, that is, of preserving the continuity of the parent artery. Similarly, it was another physician, Samways, who first suggested that mitral stenosis might prove amenable to operative treatment, actually fifty years before this operation was demonstrated to be effective. Furthermore, a new concept or innovation in one branch of medicine may spread across many areas of special interest, as weeds may spread across a lawn or, to put it in a prettier way, wild flowers may spread across a barren field. No better example could be cited than the development of new knowledge, techniques and ancillary aids which were brought about by the birth of modern cardiac surgery. The early successful operations of Robert Gross, Clarence Crafoord, Alfred Blalock, and others, and, especially Jack Gibbon's heart-lung machine did much more than stimulate dozens of surgeons around the world, including Mike DeBakey and his colleagues here in Houston, to conceive of operative manipulations for the palliation or cure of most of the acquired and congenital anomalies of the heart. They also made evident the need for better diagnostic methods, improved understanding of the basic anatomical, physiological, physical, and biochemical problems which came to the forefront as the consequence of these new operative advances. How far we have come in solving them by the brilliant hard work of physicians, pediatricians, radiologists, anesthesiologists, basic scientists - indeed, all members of our profession - is truly remarkable. Furthermore, their efforts have resulted in new instrumentation which has facilitated the measurement and monitoring of vital functions and rendered our management more appropriate and safe. In addition, the proper care of patients undergoing complex cardiovascular operative procedures has done more perhaps than anything else to stimulate the institution of badly needed specialized recovery rooms and intensive care units, the working together as a team of physicians and surgeons with diverse special fields of interest, and improved physician-patient relationships. It became clearly evident that patients and their families needed to know precisely what was proposed, why it was suggested, what the alternatives were, what risks were involved, what the prospects for the future would be, since, for one reason or another, patients have a peculiarly intimate concern about their hearts and about cardiac operations.

Let us return for a moment to the ultimate fate of Lambert's idea that the continuity of affected arteries might be operatively maintained or restored. Sadly enough, as the consequence of factors which have been discussed, no other reported closure of an arterial wound was recorded in the literature until Glück did so with small ivory clamps and Postempski by direct suture approximately 125 years after the Hallowell operation. Another decade passed by before our own J. B. Murphy did the first end-to-end suture by his now long-abandoned invagination method. It was in 1906 that Goyanes first bridged an arterial defect in man with an autogenous segment of vein and a year later that Lexer reported the utilization of a free, transplanted autogenous vein graft as an arterial substitute. In the meantime, during the last part of the nineteenth century and the early years of the present one, various workers throughout the world had laid down the fundamentals of the operative repair of blood vessels and the utilization of vascular substitutes. They included Burci, Jassinowsky, Napalkow, Silberberg, Dörfler, Heidenhain, Jaboulay and Briau, Clermont, Dorrance, Frouin, Clementi, Höpfner, Glück, Exner, Carrel and Guthrie. Indeed, with the notable exception of the introduction of various plastic substitutes, we know relatively little more concerning these matters today than they knew from their own work over seventy years ago. They had studied the utilization of veins and arteries, autogenous and homologous, fresh, preserved, and fixed. They knew that they were all capable of functioning as a suitable conduit when introduced into a defect of a host blood vessel, but they also knew that there was evidence of complete survival as a living structure only in the case of autogenous blood vessel grafts.

How tragic it is that this rich inheritance was largely forgotten and the era of vascular suture and blood vessel substitution, with some sporadic and notable exceptions, had to await the stimulus of World War II and the rapidly growing field of operative surgery of the heart, the aorta and its branches. Though this hiatus is difficult to comprehend, some of the delaying factors are known such as the general failure to recognize that the rather poor results obtained in the comparatively few procedures attempted during World War I were related to their having been done under the most unfavorable circumstances - in contaminated or potentially contaminated wounds, often by surgeons untrained in the techniques they were using, without the proper equipment for atraumatic interruption of flow through vessels and fine suture materials and needles known to be necessary from the basic principles laid down by our predecessors. There were, however, exceptions, persons who understood clearly the difficulties which greatly diminished the likelihood of success. Sir George Makins, for example, in reporting upon over 1200 cases of vascular injury incurred in the British Army stated, "I regret not being able to give any information regarding the treatment of gunshot wounds of the arteries by direct suture. In the cases I myself have seen, the nature of the defect in the arterial wall, the condition of the surrounding tissues, or the fact that the septic condition of the primary tract afforded small hope of performing an aseptic operation, mitigated against the choice of this method". Bernheim, who was much interested in blood vessel repair and who was, as far as is known, the first in this country successfully to interpolate an autogenous vein graft in an arterial defect made these remarks about the situation in World War I: "Opportunities for carrying out more modern procedures for the repair or reconstruction of damaged vessels were conspicuous by their absence..... Not that ..... gaping arteries and veins could not be sutured, but it would have been foolhearty to have tried to suture arteries or veins in the presence of such infections as were the rule in practically all the battle wounded. Certain isolated successes will be reported without a doubt, but the teachings of Carrel, together with the laboratory experiences of his followers, have so effectually demonstrated the futility of attempted blood vessel suturing in any but a non-infected field, that it needed but a glance at the type of wound to be dealt with to realize from the onset the hopelessness of finer blood vessel surgery. Excision and ligation were the rule..... It required a high order of self restraint to forego some of these cases." After the war, during civilian life when conditions were more ideal, disappointingly few blood vessels were managed by suture or grafting techniques even up to and almost through World War II. In trying to understand the reluctance to accept these methods which had been placed on a firm basis long beforehand, one has to consider matters such as satisfaction with the existent methods of management, the lack of urge to utilize promising techniques not yet placed on a firm basis by a large body of clinical experience, the failure to have read properly and understood well the literature, the rigidity of professional thinking which often prevailed. Even Daniel Elkin, certainly one of our foremost cardiovascular surgeons and winner of the highly prized Matas Award, throughout World War II failed to take advantage of his unparalleled opportunity as Head of the Vascular Center at the Ashford General Hospital to look into these possibilities and continued to treat aneurysms and arteriovenous fistulas by ligating the main arterial stem rather than by making any effort to maintain or restore the continuity of the affected artery. Only a few military surgeons explored the merits of the latter approach and I am gratified that I was fortunately among the dissidents.

There is another matter which, though a touchy one, deserves serious consideration. I refer to the clinical utilization of new operative techniques. Certainly no one would condone any operative effort which is ill-conceived, potentially or obviously hazardous, and which offers little or no promise of benefit of sufficient degree and durability to justify the risk involved. On the other hand, we must, on occasions, be willing to try new ideas, the worth of which cannot be evaluated in experimental animals, provided that they appear to be rational, that they seemingly can be carried out with relative safety, with the likelihood of yielding good results of satisfactory duration, and also provided that the condition cannot be managed in any other effective way. When John Munro proposed the ligation of the ductus arteriosus in 1907, he said, "At various times I have tried to inspire the pediatric specialists with my views, but in vain". To be sure, Munro's brilliant suggestion was undoubtedly a few years early, but just a few, for it was not long before the basic principles of blood grouping and transfusion had been established, adequate endotracheal anesthesia for procedures within the open thorax was being used, and the techniques of thoracotomy were well understood. To have waited thirty years before John Streeter ligated the first patent ductus - a procedure which might have had a successful outcome had not the patient had subacute bacterial endarteritis - and still yet another year before Robert Gross operated upon the first patient with survival and cure is too long a delay We do know that in 1932 that forward-looking physician, William Sydney Thayer, upon the stimulation of his intern, DeWitt Wilcox, went to Professor Dean Lewis to see whether he would approve of an operative attempt to shut off the ductus in a patient who was in unmanageable heart failure, but was turned down. We know, too, that the idea was considered by George Humphreys who had no opportunity, and by Elliott Cutler in conjunction with Fahr and Wangensteen (O Wangensteen 1979, personal communication) whose patient rejected the proposition.

If there is no logical reason that three decades had to pass before Munro's idea was acted upon, certainly there is none to explain why Souttar's digital approach to the stenotic mitral valve in 1925 should not have brought about satisfactory mitral valvulotomies long before Dwight Harken and Charles Bailey demonstrated that the procedure could be done successfully in 1948. When Harken asked Souttar, then in his ninety-third year of life, why he had not continued with his effort, he responded in this tragically informative manner: "I did not repeat the operation because I could not get another case. Although my patient made an uninterrupted recovery, the physicians declared it was all nonsense and, in fact, that the operation was unjustifiable. In fact, it is of no use to be ahead of one's time!". How all too true!

Finally, I must mention the recognition by Robert Gross, responsible for so many innovations of tremendous value, while he was still an intern, of the probable operative curability of the disabling and often fatal congenital vascular rings. He let his idea be known to his colleagues at the Children's Medical Center, but waited fourteen years before the first case was referred to him for treatment. That is too long a wait.

It is hardly necessary for me to say that the tedious, forward march, - centuries long - broken by starts and stops, characterized by long periods of sterile inactivity and by sudden bursts of productive, innovative work finally reached fruition during the later war years and those that followed. A veritable explosion of cardiovascular surgical advances then occurred on an almost daily basis until most of the cardiac and vascular lesions came into the realm of operative curability or palliation. Neither is it necessary for me to state that the participants in this Plenary Session, Stanley Crawford, Charles Dubost, David Sabiston, and, last but certainly not least, Michael DeBakey and his colleagues were among the leaders and made many of the most significant contributions.

The limitations of time prevent me from pursuing further the ways in which the history of cardiovascular surgery has taught us valuable lessons, and I must terminate my remarks. I am confident that we have profited a great deal from the past and that our future will always be brighter if we heed the good and the bad which has been bequeathed to us.

President DeBakey, you have now been in Houston over thirty-one years. If, in the future, in our field of work there are more men and women with your imagination, critical judgment, open-mindedness, sense of responsibility, energy and drive, the next chapter in cardiovascular surgery will be even brighter than the most resplendent one in the past. As Chancellor and Departmental Chairman, your hard and productive work will continue unabated. You have long been, and will continue to be, our American Cardiovascular Surgical Ambassador-at-Large.

References

Blalock A (1956) Presidential address. The nature of discovery. Ann Surg 144:289-303
Bounous G, Shumacker HB Jr. (1961) Further studies on renal decapsulation. Surg Gynec & Obst 113:567-572
Elkin DC, DeBakey ME (eds) (1955) Vascular surgery. Medical department, United States army. Surgery in world war II. US Government Printing Office, Washington
Guthrie GC, Harbison SP, Fisher B (1959) The contributions of Dr CC Guthrie to vascular surgery. Blood vessel surgery and its applications (a reprint). University of Pittsburgh Press, Pittsburgh
Isaacs JP, Carter BN II, Heller JH Jr. (1952) Experimental pericarditis. Pathologic physiology of constrictive pericarditis. Bull Johns Hopkins Hosp 90:259-300
Matas R (1920) Surgery of the vascular system. In: Keen's surgery. Its principles and practice. (7th printing) WB Saunders, Philadelphia and London. Vol 5 pp 17-350
Meade RH (1961) A history of thoracic surgery. Charles C Thomas, Springfield
Moore FD (1979) The study of trauma. Can we encourage new federal directions? JAMA 241:2269-2271
Parsons HG, Holman E (1950) Experimental ascites. Surgical Forum 1:251-258
Shumacker HB Jr. (1968) Authority, research and publication: Reflections based upon some historical aspects of vascular surgery. Ann Surg 168: 169-182
Shumacker HB Jr., Muhm, HY (1969) Arterial suture techniques and grafts: Past, present, and future. Surgery 66:419-433
Stone HH, Fulenwider JT (1977) Renal decapsulation in the prevention of post-ischemic oliguria. Ann Surg 186:343-355
Wangensteen OH (1978) Surgery and travel groups. Surg Gynec & Obst 147:246-254
Wangensteen OH, Wangensteen, SD (1978) The rise of surgery from empiric craft to scientific discipline University of Minnesota Press, Minneapolis

My Current Views Regarding Coronary Bypass Surgery

J.F. Goodwin

There is ample evidence to indicate that coronary bypass surgery relieves or improves stable angina in 80% or more of patients. My overall view therefore is that it is an operation mainly for symptoms. The impact of the operation upon survival is still being debated.

The Veterans Administration Randomised Multicentre Study (Murphy et al. 1977) on stable angina pectoris has caused great controversy. Initially welcomed by Braunwald (1977) as a timely antedote to excessive enthusiasm for the operation, the report concluded that surgical treatment offered improvement in survival at three years only in patients with left main coronary artery stenosis. This conclusion called down vials of wrath from many quarters. The criticisms of the trial were summed up by Favoloro (1979). They were: only low risk patients were included; only 50% angiographic coronary artery stenosis was required; the initial operative mortality was high; and the patency rate of grafts was low.

Numerous studies have now been published which claim better survival for surgical than medical treatment in various degrees of occlusive coronary artery disease. Many of these trials have been retrospective and therefore are of questionable value (Braunwald 1977; Cohn et al. 1975). Prospective trials have also been reported in the United States (Vismara et al. 1977) to favor surgery but Hurst et al. (1978) have pointed out the difficulties involved, one of the problems being the apparently inexplicably worse prognosis of medically treated patients in trials as compared with those not included in trials.

In Europe the enthusiasm for coronary bypass grafting has been somewhat less explosive than in the United States. A Multicentre European Trial (European Coronary Artery Surgery Study Group 1979) was set up to study the effect of medical and surgical treatment on death and recurrent myocardial infarction in September 1973. The results at two years have now been reported. This trial was a prospective study of matched patients with chronic stable angina: 768 men under the age of 65 years with at least 50% obstruction in two or more major coronary arteries and left ventricular ejection fraction of, or more than 50%, took part. Three hundred seventy-three patients were allocated medical and 395, surgical treatment. Twenty-six "surgical" patients did not undergo operation; six died before operation, 19 refused operation and one was lost to follow-up. Fifty "medical" patients underwent surgery because of symptoms that did not respond to medical treatment so that continued inclusion in the "medical" group was not felt to be justified.

At two years there was no significant difference in mortality between the two groups but in the group of patients with three vessel disease the survival was significantly better for surgical patients. This was also true for patients with stenosis of the left main coronary artery but the numbers were insufficient for conclusions to be firmly drawn.

The surgical hospital mortality was 3.6% for all patients and 1.5% in the last third of patients. Graft patency was 90% within nine months and 77%

between nine and 18 months following operation. Symptomatic improvement was distinctly better in the operative group.

These results suggest a definite improvement in survival for patients with three vessel disease who are treated surgically but recent reports have suggested the same conclusions for patients with two vessel disease (Cohn et al. 1975; Hurst et al. 1978) or even single vessel disease (Lawrie et al. 1978). Lawrie et al. (1978) have emphasized the importance of ventricular function and claim that survival at five years was better in surgically treated patients with single vessel disease than that of the normal population if left ventricular function was good. If patients with both good and poor left ventricular function were included, the survival was the same as the normal population, which seems difficult to understand but, of course, some of the "normal" population contributing to the general U.S. population will have died of unsuspected coronary artery disease.

The general weight of opinion inclines to the view that surgery in single vessel disease will not improve prognosis, except possibly when the artery involved is the left anterior descending.

But there are many unknown factors and unresolved problems. Left ventricular function is a crucial matter and may even be more important, in my opinion, than the site of the coronary artery lesions. Favoloro (1979) has shown in a prospective study that the overall mortality at 40 months was 66% for patients treated medically and 25% for those treated surgically in a group with poor left ventricular function. On the other hand, poor left ventricular function tends to increase the risks of the operation.

As Favoloro has also pointed out, the classification of coronary artery lesions by angiography requires further refinement. The terms "left main," "single," "double" or "triple" disease are much too crude and give little idea of the site of the lesions and their numbers which may be of crucial importance. It is likely that a severe lesion of the left anterior descending artery proximal to the first septal branch would carry a greater risk to life than lesions occurring distally.

A major problem in deciding who should be operated on is presented by the patient who has three vessel disease but no symptoms. This problem will not occur of course if coronary arteriography is performed only on patients with symptoms but Favoloro (1979) has reported a significant number of patients who were symptomless after a myocardial infarction and who had three vessel disease.

Should coronary artery bypass grafting be advised for such patients, the major reason would be to prevent sudden death. Vismara et al. (1977), showed that sudden death was one third as frequent in patients with two or three vessel disease treated surgically as in a medical group in a prospective study. The patients were matched angiographically and followed for 39 months. Hammermeister et al. (1977) reported a prospective study over a period of four years. The rate of sudden death for medically treated patients was 1.8 – 10.9 times higher than the rate for patients who were comparable as regards ejection fraction and extent of coronary artery disease but who were treated surgically. If these figures are representative then every patient with coronary artery disease should have coronary artery bypass grafting. This is not at the present time a feasible or reasonable suggestion and much more information is needed on the prognosis of silent coronary artery disease of various degrees of severity. Comparison of results of medical and surgical treatment on survival are also affected by improvements in medical methods of treatment which may turn out to be superior to surgical methods. The effect of, for example, longterm beta-adrenergic blockade and anti-platelet drugs needs to be evaluated as a method of improving prognosis. Coronary artery bypass grafting should not be considered as an alternative to medical treatment but as an adjunct. As Hurst et al. (1978) have pointed out, bypass grafting improves blood supply to the myocardium while beta-adrenergic blackade diminishes the work of the heart. In addition, the effect of anti-platelet drugs in discouraging thrombosis may be crucial.

As far as stable angina is concerned, before or after infarction, I believe that coronary bypass grafting offers an excellent prospect of significantly relieving the pain at a low risk in the patient with a suitable type of disease. Symptoms need not be "intolerable" nor angina uncontrollable before surgery is indicated.

If there is disease only of the right coronary artery with good left ventricular function, the prognosis will not be influenced and there is a very small chance of deterioration as a result of a peri-operative infarction, as with any coronary artery bypass operation. If there is three vessel disease, especially if this is proximal and associated with impaired left ventricular function, prognosis will be improved as well as pain relieved.

If there is two vessel disease, the effect of operation on prognosis is still uncertain in my view. Proximal disease involving the left coronary artery would certainly increase the likelihood of surgery improving left ventricular function if this is impaired.

The Symptomless Patient

I confess that I find this decision the hardest of all. In general, I doubt if surgery will improve prognosis for the reasons I have mentioned. However, the occasional patient with significant left main stem stenosis who is without symptoms ought to benefit from the operation in terms of survival but the influence of left ventricular function is not fully understood. How much does good left ventricular function improve prognosis irrespective of operation?

All survival curves and life tables in coronary artery disease suffer from the disability that they give no idea of how long the lesions have been present before they were detected. The prognosis of patients who have severe disease but are asymptomatic is not really known, while every "control normal" population must contain a number of people who will feature in the statistics of sudden unexpected death.

After myocardial infarction, and especially after repeated attacks, if left ventricular function is impaired and significant three vessel disease exists, operation is likely to improve prognosis. The Framingham Study (Kannel 1973) has shown that the prognosis for patients with silent myocardial infarction on the electrocardiogram and left ventricular hypertrophy is similar to that in those with clear-cut symptomatic myocardial infarction.

Coronary artery bypass grafting for acute myocardial infarction is not advisable during the period of 12 hours to 14 days after the attack (Scanlon et al. 1977) although Scanlon et al. (1977) consider that there may be circumstances which indicate surgery.

Unstable Angina

Unstable angina is only an indication for operation if pain fails to respond to full medical treatment. Conti (1977) has shown that the incidence of myocardial infarction is greater with surgery than with medical treatment. No difference in mortality rate was noted in his series but persistent angina was more common with medical than surgical treatment. The indicators for surgery for unstable angina therefore tend to be the same as those for stable angina.

Mortality of Surgical Treatment

Mortality for surgery must be taken into account in assessing the need for coronary bypass grafting. In the ideal patient who is under the age of 60, is not hypertensive, does not smoke cigarettes, has no evidence of arterial disease elsewhere, and good left ventricular function, the mortality is now in the region of 2% or less. Mortality may be related to impaired left ventricular function, peri-operative infarction and such other factors as widespread vascular disease elsewhere, diabetes, chronic lung disease and perhaps advanced age. The five year survival should be around 90% (Hurst et al. 1978).

Conclusions

To sum up, coronary bypass grafting is indicated for angina that does not respond fully to medical treatment. This indication does not exclude single vessel disease, even of the right coronary artery, if this is responsible for the symptoms. Bypass grafting is therefore principally a symptomatic operation but will improve prognosis in certain subsets; stenosis of the left main coronary artery, severe three vessel disease with impaired left ventricular function, appear on present evidence to be situation in which prognosis is improved by surgical treatment. The position of two vessel disease is still uncertain. If the disease is proximal and involves the left aterior descending coronary artery, and if left ventricular function is impaired, then probably prognosis will be improved. Much more information is necessary to decide on the effect of surgical treatment on prognosis in patients with two vessel disease, single vessel disease and patients who are symptomless, even with more severe disease.

In general, the operation is well worthwhile for the patient with significant symptoms within the good risk group. It may well be justifiable on symptomatic grounds alone in patients who are less favorable if the symptoms are sufficiently severe. It must be remembered that the results will be less good and the risk higher for the patient with severe generalized vascular disease, poor left ventricular function or diabetes or impaired lung function, particularly over the age of 60.

Further studies are needed regarding the natural history of coronary artery disease and better analyses of comparability of patients is needed with more prospective studies of such comparable patients (Conti 1978).

References

Braunwald E (1977) Coronary artery surgery at the crossroads. N Engl J Med 297:661-663

Cohn LH, Boyden CM, Collins JJ Jr (1975) Improved long-term survival after aorto-coronary bypass for advanced coronary artery disease. Am J Surg 129:380-385

Conti CR (1977) Unstable angina pectoris. In: Yu PN, Goodwin JF (eds) Progress in Cardiology. Lea and Febiger, Philadelphia, Vol 6, pp 51-66

Conti CR (1978) Influence of myocardial infarction on survival. Controversies in cardiology: Part II. Am J Cardiol 42:330-332

European Coronary Artery Surgery Study Group (1979) Coronary artery bypass surgery in stable angina pectoris. Survival at two years. Lancet 1: 890-893

Favoloro RG (1979) Direct myocardial revascularization: A 10 year journey. Myths and realities. Am J Cardiol 43:109

Hammermeister KE, De Rouen TA, Murray JA, et al. (1977) Effect of aorto-coronary bypass grafting on death and sudden death; comparison of non-randomized medical surgically treated cohorts with comparable coronary disease and left ventricular function. Am J Cardiol 39:925-934

Hurst JW, King SB III, Logue RB, et al. (1978) Value of coronary artery bypass surgery. Controversies in cardiology, part 1. Am J Cardiol 42: 308-329

Kannel WB (1973) The natural history of myocardial infarction: The Framingham Study. Leiden University Press, pp 14-15

Lawrie GM, Morris GC Jr, Howell JF, et al. (1978) Improved survival after five years in 1144 patients after coronary bypass surgery. Am J Cardiol 42:709-715

Murphy ML, Hultgren HN, Detre K, et al. (1977) Treatment of chronic stable angina. A preliminary report of survival data of the randomized Veterans Administration Co-operative Study. N Engl J Med 297:621-627

Scanlon PJ, Johnson SA, Loeb HS, et al. (1977) Coronary artery bypass grafts in acute myocardial infarction. In: Yu PN, Goodwin JF (eds) Progress in Cardiology. Lea and Febiger, Philadelphia, Vol 6, pp 113-135

Vismara LA, Miller RR, Price JE, et al. (1977) Improved longevity due to reduction of sudden death by aorta-coronary bypass in coronary atherosclerosis. Prospective evaluation of medical versus surgical therapy in matched patients with multivessel disease. Am J Cardiol 39:919-924

Results of Coronary Bypass: A Long-Term Perspective

Gerald M. Lawrie

The coronary bypass procedure has gained widespread acceptance as a highly effective form of treatment for angina pectoris. There is also evidence that it prolongs life in patients with three vessel or left main coronary stenosis. We have been particularly interested in the late results of coro-nary bypass in regard to relief of symptoms and prolongation of life and have therefore determined the fate of 1578 consecutive patients after coro-nary bypass with followup beyond 5 years in all cases. An initial study was made of clinical, treadmill and angiographic results in 434 patients operated upon between 1968 and 1971. (Lawrie et al. 1977). All patients were followed up for more than 60 months after operation (mean 70.7 months). Of the initial 434 patients, 98 died 0 to 74 (mean 31.1 months) post-oper-atively. Of the 336 survivors, 152 reentered the hospital and underwent standardized clinical assessment. Angina was lessened in 93.4 percent (255 of 273) and absent in 51.3 percent (140 of 273) of these patients. Of pat-ients under 65 years of age, 79.2 percent (152 of 192) were still working. Treadmill exercise tests performed in 107 patients showed an ischemic re-sponse in 44.9 percent (48 of 107) and an indeterminate response in 9.3 per-cent (10 of 107). The duration of the exercise, maximal pulse rate and double product all correlated well with the completeness of revasculariza-tion.

The patency rate in 131 patients with 193 grafts studied 60 to 88 (mean 69.7) months post-operatively was 90.7 percent. In the overall group of 176 pat-ients with 256 grafts studied 12 to 88 (mean 26.2) months post-operatively, the patency rate was 86.3 percent. Overall, 137 patients (78.1 percent) had all grafts patent, and 166 (94.3 percent) had one or more patent grafts. In the group of 131 patients studied after 5 years, 126 (96.2) percent had at least one patent graft. Vein graft morphology was excellent. The complete-ness of revascularization could be assessed in detail in 116 patients. In 37 (31.9 percent), no residual lesion was present; in 56 (48.3 percent) one significant lesion was not bypassed and in 21 (18.1 percent) two signifi-cant lesions remained untreated. Only two patients (1.7 percent) had three significant lesions without functioning bypasses. Histologic examinations of 122 graft specimens obtained up to 7 years after operation indicated that intimal proliferation occurred in all grafts but rarely caused occlu-sion. Atherosclerosis was observed in only 17 grafts and, in our experi-ence, the annual incidence of atherosclerosis up to 7 years after operation has been only 0.5 - 1%. Furthermore, atherosclerosis occurred mainly in patients with severe hyperlipidemia. Thus, in our experience, graft func-tion has remained excellent beyond 5 years. (Lawrie et al. 1976, Lie et al. 1977).

In our patients, left ventricular function, as assessed by end-diastolic pressure and left ventriculography, has been stable over a 5-year interval. Furthermore, because our patients have continued to have good treadmill per-formance beyond 5 years, we believe that the operation is effective in the long-term relief of myocardial ischemia.

In 75 patients, the pre- and post-operative cineangiograms were available and of sufficiently good quality for detailed comparison of changes in the native coronary circulation. The mean interval between studies was 69.7 months (range 60 to 83). The cineangiograms were reviewed by two cardiologists. To minimize the effects of observer variability only progression of a lesion by more than 25 percent or progression to total occlusion was considered significant in this study.

Completely new lesions of more than 70 percent stenosis at previously angiographically normal sites were found in 24 (10.7 percent) of all 225 vessels, 20 (20 percent) of 105 ungrafted vessels and 4 (3.3 percent) of 120 grafted vessels. In the 105 ungrafted vessels, old lesions had progressed by more than 25 percent or had become totally occluded in 19 cases (18.0 percent); however, in 9 of these 19 (47.4 percent) the stenosis was greater than 70 percent initially and in only 5 (26.3 percent) had the lesion progressed from less than 70 to greater than 70 percent stenosis. Thus, the development of a completely new lesion with greater than 70 percent stenosis occurred twice as often as progression of mild lesion (less than 70 percent stenosis) to a significant lesion (more than 70 percent stenosis) (24 of 225 versus 5 of 105).

In 114 patients with 171 grafts, the influence of the graft on the native circulation was examined. In 81 (47.4 percent) of the 171 arteries, the graft was patent and no change had occurred in the recipient artery. In 60 arteries (35.1 percent) the proximal lesion had undergone localized closure but the graft and artery were otherwise patent. However, 62 (87.3 percent) of these lesions were greater than 90 percent initially. Occlusion of the segment between a patent graft and the stenotic lesion was observed in only seven grafts (4 percent). Occlusion of 16 grafts (9.3 percent) was associated with no change in the native circulation, but in 4 (2.3 percent) it was associated with occlusion of the underlying artery. Development of new distal lesions was quite rare, occurring in only three vessels (1.8 percent).

To determine the influence of coronary bypass surgery on late survival, the next 1144 consecutive patients were contacted 60 to 76 months after operation. (Lawrie et al. 1978).There were 1000 men (87.4 percent). The mean age was 50.1 years (range 24 to 75). Operation was performed for angina pectoris with coronary lesions of more than 70 percent reduction in luminal diameter in 1,101 patients (96.2 percent). Forty-three patients (3.8 percent) had congestive heart failure without angina and 240 (21.0 percent) had both heart failure and angina. Unstable angina was present in 149 patients (13 percent). Previous myocardial infarction had occurred in 675 patients (59 percent). Single vessel disease was present in 226 patients (19.8 percent), double vessel disease in 442 (38.6 percent), triple vessel disease in 376 patients (32.9 percent) and greater than 50 percent stenosis of the left main coronary artery in 100 patients (8.7 percent). The overall operative mortality rate was 4.6 percent (52 patients). With exclusion of patients with left main coronary artery disease, this rate was 3.8 percent (40 of 1044) and the overall crude 5 year survival rate was 89.1 percent (930 of 1044). The survival rates of men and women were comparable. Left ventricular function was classified as good if end-diastolic pressure was less than 15 mm Hg and the left ventriculogram revealed no aneurysmal or akinetic area. Among men, the respective survival rates for each subgroup and for those with good left ventricular function within that subgroup were as follows: one vessel disease, 92.9 percent (169 of 182) and 94.9 percent (130 of 137); two vessel disease, 90.3 percent (352 of 390) and 94.3 percent (248 of 263); three vessel disease, 85.7 percent (293 of 342) and 90.9 percent (189 of 208); left main coronary artery disease, 81.4 percent (70 of 86) and 90.6 percent (48 of 53). The graft patency rate in 157 patients was 86.4 percent (247 of 286 grafts), and 149 patients (94.9 percent) had at least one patent graft.

Late survival of all patients with reasonably good pre-operative left
ventricular function was normal compared with the expected number of survivors based on the general U.S. population experience of 1973. Thus, the
survival rates of surgically treated patients with reasonable pre-operative
left ventricular function, regardless of the number of coronary lesions,
were restored to survival rates comparable with those of the general population. With poor ventricular function, survival is impaired but is still
superior to that reported with medical treatment only. We feel that this
data further supports the view that the coronary bypass procedure is effective in the long-term relief of angina and that it favorably influences
late survival in patients with symptomatic multivessel coronary disease.

Our current approach is to offer operation to all operable symptomatic patients unresponsive to medical therapy. We feel patients with three vessel
or left main coronary stenosis should have surgical treatment regardless of
the presence or absence of symptoms or their response to medical treatment.
Exercise thallium scanning has been useful in assessing the severity of
myocardial ischemia in "asymptomatic" patients. We are influenced to operate on "asymptomatic" patients with even single or double vessel disease
if marked myocardial ischemia is demonstrated.

At present we continue to operate on symptomatic patients with marked impairment of left ventricular function in the hope of improving left ventricular performance and long-term survival. We are investigating this
group of patients by means of radionuclide ventriculography and long-term
followup to more clearly define their prognosis with and without operation.

In summary, the coronary bypass procedure has been shown to have a high
success rate in the long-term relief of the adverse sequelae of coronary
artery disease. We feel many points of controversy are now resolved and
that data which is accumulating rapidly will answer many of the remaining
questions.

References

Lawrie GM, Lie JT, Morris GC, Beazley HL (1976) Vein graft patency and
    intimal proliferation after aortocoronary bypass: early and long-term
    angiopathologic correlations. Am J Cardiol 38:856-862

Lawrie GM, Morris GC, Howell JF, Ogura JW, Spencer WH, Cashion WR, Winters
    WL, Beazley HL, Chapman DW, Peterson PK, Lie JT (1977) Results of coro-
    nary bypass more than 5 years after operation in 434 patients:clinical,
    treadmill exercise and angiographic correlations. Am J Cardiol 40:
    665-671

Lawrie GM, Morris GC, Howell JF, Tredici TD, Chapman DW (1978) Improved
    survival after 5 years in 1,144 patients after coronary bypass surgery.
    Am J Cardiol 42: 709-715

Lie JT, Lawrie GM, Morris GC (1977) Aortocoronary bypass saphenous vein
    graft atherosclerosis:anatomic study of 99 vein grafts from normal
    and hyperlipoproteinemic patients up to 75 months post-operatively.
    Am J Cardiol 40: 906-914

Current Views Regarding Coronary Bypass Surgery

Henry D. McIntosh

Coronary heart disease is the most common cause of death in this country. But
the pessimism attached to this fact a decade ago is gradually being replaced
by cautious optimism. Rather than the incidence of death from this cause continuing to increase, as it did during the first half of the century and still
is in many developed and developing countries throughout the world, in the
United States the incidence of death is declining. During the last decade the
decline in mortality has occurred at an accelerated rate. These observations
indicate that coronary heart disease is not an inevitable result of aging,
rather it is an epidemic disease; as such the morbidity and mortality is related, at least in part, to the prevalence of certain behavioral characteristics
of society . . . cigarette smoking, hypertension, elevated cholesterol obesity
and sedentary living. Although a cause and effect relationship has not been
unequivocally established, the decline in the mortality from coronary heart
disease has paralleled the attenuation of the frequency of these risk factors
in this country (Havlik and Feinleib 1979).

Data recently reported by the Metropolitan Life Insurance Company (1979) indicates that the decline in mortality has been greater among urban, predominantly
white middle class males than among persons in the lower socioeconomic nonwhite
strata of society. From 1969 to 1977 age-adjusted death rates from cardiovascular disease among white men in the general population declined from 459 to
367 per 100,000 (19%); among insured men the decline was 387 to 296 per 100,000
(31%). In 1969, the mortality among insured men was 18% lower than among
white males in the general population but by 1977, the death rate among insured
men was 37% lower then the rate among men in the general population. During
the same period the decline in the death rate among white women in the general
population and insured white women was 24 and 26% respectively. (See Figure 1)

This report by Metropolitan supports our concerns about the selection of control populations for the purpose of determining if coronary bypass surgery
postpones premature death (1978). The striking decline in mortality over the
last decade, especially in middle class white males, further emphasizes the
fallacy of comparing the results of patients operated during this decade with
patients treated medically during the last decade. The demonstration that the
rate of decline in mortality is different for different socioeconomic strata
is particularly pertinent. Most reports of the results of surgery have come
from university centers and private clinics. A large percent of operated
patients embraced by such studies are from the same socioeconomic strata as
represented by Metropolitan's male insurees. Lawrie, Morris, Howell et al.
(1977) reported that the survival of a large series of consecutively operated
patients exceeded the survival of the "population at large without heart disease". The report by the Metropolitan supports our previous conclusions that
Lawrie, Morris, Howell et al. (1977) observations were not surprising and in
our judgment the prolonged survival of the operated group might not in any way
be related to the potential or real benefits of surgery (1979). The use of

Age-Adjusted Death Rates From Cardiovascular Diseases

Metropolitan Life Insurance Company, Standard Ordinary Policyholders and United States White Population, 1969-1977

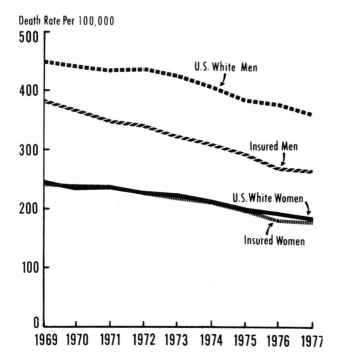

Figure 1. Metropolitan Life Insurance Company Statistical Bulletin, New York, New York, Vol. 60 (2) 1979, Page 2 (Published by permission)

the general population, or a major part thereof, as a control population is fraught with many biases. For example, McMichael (1976) has indicated that a subset of the population may enjoy, when compared to the total population, the "healthy worker effect". Brenner (1976) reported that a 1% increase in the unemployed rate in the U.S. sustained over a six year period was associated with an increase of approximately 36,887 total deaths.

Both DeBakey and Lawrie (1979) and Hurst and his colleagues (1978) have indicated that they are satisfied with the data that indicates that life is prolonged by coronary bypass grafting. They state or imply that further studies are not needed. Hurst et al. (1978) concluded that "we must make up our minds using the data we now have". In our judgment, however, studies such as the Metropolitan's which demonstrate striking changes in the natural history of the disease indicate the need for caution and the need to keep an open mind and avoid premature judgments. As Lewis Thomas (1974), cautioned "it is medicine's oldest dilemma, not to be settled by candor or by any kind of rhetoric; what it needs is a lot of time and patience, waiting for science to come in, as it has in the past, with solid facts."

If there are reasonable doubts that a clear-cut superiority of surgery in postponing premature death for large segments of the population with coronary heart disease has been demonstrated, the physician must be concerned as to the possibility of late adverse effects. What happens to the graft over time and what effect does the operation and the established graft have on the native circulation? Unfortunately, the answers to such questions are unknown because the data on which the most favorable claims have been made are for the most part incomplete. The data were not collected in a manner which might prevent the introduction of biases. For example, Lawrie, Morris, Chapman, et al. (1977) have claimed an overall graft patency of 84% with 89% patency rate after five years. Yet these results were based on studying only 11.8% of the patients operated. The patients studied were not stated to be representative of the entire operated population and they probably were not for the graft status of 35 "bodies" examined at autopsy were included. Only 71 patients with 80 grafts were studied more than 60 months after surgery. It would appear that more than 90% of the grafts on which claims for long term graft patency were made were single grafts. Thirty-eight grafts in 27 patients were studied twice and the results were included twice in the calculation of patency. This maneuver appeared to increase overall graft patency by 3.2%.

Data regarding the long term effect of the graft on the native circulation has been equally incomplete and subject to selection biases. For example, Siedes et al. (1978) reported the long term effects in 22 of "30 consecutive patients". But the "30 consecutive patients" were grouped only after excluding 16 patients with occluded grafts that had previously been demonstrated one year after surgery! The careful study of the long term effects of grafts on the native circulation recently reported by Grondin et al. (1979) actually represented data on only 22% of the original cohorts.

It is unfortunate that even after over a decade of experience, not only is the role of bypass surgery in postponing premature death unclear, but the long term graft patency and the effects of the procedure on the native circulation is not well defined. It appears clear that our knowledge regarding the role of bypass surgery is still far from complete. Therefore, my current views are to keep an open mind as to which patients should be selected for surgery.

There is little hesitancy to consider for surgery, if the coronary anatomy and ventricular contractility are appropriate, those patients, who after concerned and conscientious medical management, continue to experience the pain of angina pectoris which interferes with the desired quality of life. The vast majority of such patents who can be operated will enjoy a decline in angina, the need for coronary vasodilators and subsequent hospitalizations. Except in isolated environments, however, it does not appear that the procedure will result in returning large numbers of these patients to gainful employment or insure that those working will remain working. In addition, surgery is recommended for those patients with a markedly limited exercise tolerance that is accompanied by a striking depression of the ST segment and an inappropriate increase in the heart rate and/or blood pressure.

Such patients will include most with significant stenosis of the main left coronary artery and those with three vessel disease and decreased myocardial contractility. Bypass surgery would appear not only to relieve symptoms but to postpone premature death in a significant number of such patients.

With rare exceptions, surgery is not recommended unless we are confident of the skill of the surgeon. Furthermore, surgery is usually not recommended unless the patient has had an adequate trial of comprehensive medical management and unless the patient is normotensive and a nonsmoker with an ideal or near ideal weight and is consuming a prudent diet and is engaged in a regular exercise program. The patient must clearly understand that he will follow such a pattern for the rest of his life. Regardless of how incomplete our data regarding the long term results of bypass surgery might be, it is clear that although the procedure may be a "stay of execution" it is not a "pardon" from the likelihood of progression of coronary atherosclerosis.

References

Brenner H (1979) Estimating the social costs of national economic policy. US Government Printing Office, Washington

DeBakey ME, Lawrie GM (1979) Response to commentary of Hultgren et al on 'Aortocoronary-artery-bypass: assessment after 13 years.' JAMA 2393-2395

Grondin CM, Campeau L, Lesperance J et al.(1979) Atherosclerotic changes in coronary vein grafts six years after operation. Angiographic aspect in 110 patients. Thorac Cardiovasc Surg 77: 24-31

Havlik RJ, Feinleib M (eds) (1979) Proceedings of the conference on the decline in coronary heart disease mortality. October 24-25, 1978 NHLBI, NHI, Bethesda, MD, pp xxiii-xxvi

Hurst JW, King SB III, Logue RB et al.(1978) Value of coronary bypass surgery. Controversies in Cardiology: Part 1. Am J Cardiol 42: 308-329

Lawrie GM, Morris GC Jr, Chapman DW et al.(1977) Patterns of patency of 596 vein grafts up to several years after aortocoronary bypass. J Thorac Surg 73: 443-448

Lawrie GM, Morris GC Jr, Howell JF et al.(1977) Results of coronary bypass more than 5 years after operation in 434 patients. Clinical, treadmill exercise and angiographic conditions. Am J Cardiol 40: 665-672

Lewis T (1974) The medusa and the snail. The Viking Press, New York, New York pp 25-26

McIntosh HD, Buccino RA (1979) Value of coronary bypass surgery; Controversies in Cardiology (continued). Am J Cardiol 44: 387-389

McIntosh HD, Garcia JA (1978) The first decade of aortocoronary bypass grafting, 1967-1977: a review. Circulation 57: 405-431

McMichael AJ (1979) Standardized mortality and the "healthy work effect." Scratching beneath the surface. J Occup Med 18: 165-168

Metropolitan Life Insurance Company (1979) Recent trends in mortality from cardiovascular diseases. Statistical Bulletin 69 (No 2): 2-8

Seides SF, Borer JS, Kent KM et al.(1978) Long term anatomic fate of coronary artery bypass grafts and functional status of patients five years after operation. New Engl J Med 298: 1213-1216

Comparison of Medical and Surgical Mortality in a High Risk Subset of Coronary Patients with Extreme Degrees of Exercise-Induced Ischemia[1]

Richard R. Miller and Craig M. Pratt

Controversy persists concerning indications for coronary artery bypass surgery. Thus, while most workers agree that refractory, disabling angina pectoris, stenosis of the left main coronary artery and severe proximal stenosis of all three major coronary arteries constitute rational reasons to undergo myocardial revascularization (Hurst et al. 1978; Laurie et al. 1979; Takaro et al. 1975), there is disagreement concerning most other anatomic subsets of coronary artery disease (McIntosh and Garcia, 1978; Read et al. 1978). Because properly utilized noninvasive techniques have progressed to a point of relatively high sensitivity and specificity in identifying patients with coronary disease and selective coronary arteriography has achieved a level of expertise and safety to allow wide application, the most pressing clinical question has shifted somewhat from "how to detect the presence of coronary artery disease?" to "how to detect from within a coronary population high risk patients likely to have mortality and morbidity forestalled by surgical intervention?"

In addition to defining certain high-risk subsets of coronary patients according to patho-anatomic criteria, previous studies have correlated specific electrocardiographic and hemodynamic responses to exercise stress with the presence of stenosis of the left main coronary artery or of all three principal coronary arteries (Bruce et al. 1977, 1979; Bruschke et al. 1973; Ellestad and Wan 1975; Lawrie et al. 1977). The presence of prior inferior myocardial infarction also predicts serious disease of the proximal left anterior descending coronary artery in a high percentage of patients (Miller et al. 1977). Despite these studies, with the exception of patients with left ventricular dysfunction or serious ventricular ectopy, non-invasive predictors of mortality within a coronary population have been difficult to define.

The present investigation was undertaken to determine the course of patients with proven coronary artery disease and manifesting extreme degrees of electrocardiographic ischemia during treadmill stress testing.

Study Population

One hundred seventy-five patients were identified with documented coronary artery disease (one or more stenosis > 70%), detailed followup information and manifesting > 2mm horizontal or downsloping ST-segment depression of at least .06 seconds in duration. Of the 175 patients, 124 subsequently underwent coronary bypass surgery while 51 were treated medically. Followup in the surgical group averaged 4.4 years while the mean duration of followup in the medical group was 3.1 years.

---

[1] Supported in part by The National Heart, Lung and Blood Vessel Research and Demonstration Center, Baylor College of Medicine and The Methodist Hospital, NHLBI, HL-17269.

The surgical group was comprised of 116 males and eight females, mean age 55 years. Seventeen (14%) patients had stenosis of the left main coronary artery; forty-five (30%) patients had stenoses of three coronary arteries: 46 (37%) two vessel disease and 33 (27%) stenosis of one coronary artery; 40% had left ventricular dysfunction, defined as resting end-diastolic pressure $\geq$ 20 mm Hg and/or abnormalities of segmental wall motion.

The fifty-one medically treated patients consisted of 43 males and 8 females, mean age 59 years (p=ns vs surgical patients). Twenty-five percent of medically treated patients had three vessel coronary artery disease, 32% two vessel disease and 43% single vessel disease; 34% had left ventricular dysfunction (all p=ns vs surgical group).

RESULTS

The overall mortality among the 124 surgical patients during the 4.4 years of followup was 10.5% (Figure 1). In contrast, the total mortality among the 51 patients in the medically treated group followed for 3.1 years was 21.6% (p<.05 vs surgical therapy) (Figure 1).

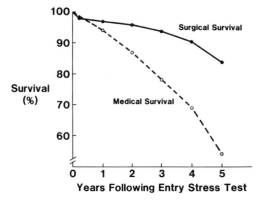

Figure 1.   Comparative surgical vs medical survival in 175 patients with coronary artery disease and severe exertional ischemia.

Perioperative (prior to hospital discharge) mortality was 2.5%. During the followup period 28% of medically treated patients sustained myocardial infarction compared to 11% of the surgical group (p<.05). Further, 59% of the medical group had continuing angina pectoris while 29% of patients undergoing surgery developed angina during the followup of 4.4 years (p<.05). Of the 12 cardiac deaths occurring in the surgical group, four were documented to be sudden(within less than one hour) and eight cardiac deaths were related to repeat myocardial infarction and pump failure. Of the eleven cardiac deaths occurring in the medically treated group, six were documented to have occurred suddenly, while five were related to myocardial infarction and/or congestive heart failure.

The presence of left ventricular dysfunction was predictive of subsequent mortality in both the medical and surgically treated groups. Of 49 patients with impaired left ventricular performance in the surgical group, three died during the perioperative period and seven in the subsequent four years compared to no perioperative and two late deaths in the 75 patients with normal left ventricular function (p<.05). Thus, 83% of all surgical patients who expired during the followup period had abnormal left ventricular function. Among medically treated patients, the mortality during the three years followup was not related (p>.05) to left ventricular dysfunction.

Exercise Predictors of Mortality: Surgical Group

The stated reason for discontinuation of exercise stress was evaluated to determine if this factor was predictive of mortality. Within the surgical group, 65 patients were stopped for either chest pain or marked degree of ST-segment depression and in 47 patients exercise was terminated for other reasons. There was no difference in mortality between these two groups (p= 0.2). Likewise, the duration of treadmill exercise was not predictive of subsequent mortality in the surgical group. Of the 74 patients who exercised less than five minutes on the Bruce protocol, eight(10.8%) subsequently died compared to four of the 47 patients(8.5%) who walked for more than five min- utes (p=0.6). The duration of time for ST-segment normalization after the cessation of exercise was also not predictive of those patients with subse- quent cardiac mortality.

In contrast to the above variables which did not predict subsequent mortal- ity, the presence of ventricular arrhythmias either during or following ex- ercise was predictive of subsequent cardiac mortality during the four year postoperative followup period: five of 26(19%) patients with ventricular ec- topy expired vs seven of 98(7%)patients without ventricular premature beats, (p<.05). Further, by combining both treadmill stress testing data with car- diac catheterization data, seven of the cardiac deaths in the surgical group occurred in the 28 patients who had both evidence of left ventricular dys- function and manifested ventricular arrhythmias during or immediately after exercise (p<.01 vs patients without these findings).

Exercise Predictors of Mortality: Medical Group

Within the medically treated group, cessation of treadmill exercise within five minutes was highly predictive of subsequent cardiac mortality (nine of 22 patients in whom exercise was terminated within five minutes vs two of 29 patients who exercised for longer than five minutes (p<.004). With regard to ventricular arrhythmias, six of 16 patients with ventricular ectopy during or immediately following exercise subsequently expired during the three year followup period vs only five of 35 without ventricular ectopy (p<.05). The total extent of ST-segment depression did not relate to subsequent mortali- ty in this population, all of whom had at least 2 mm ST-segment depression. Additionally, there was no difference (p> .05) in subsequent mortality in patients requiring greater vs those requiring less than four minutes for ST- segment normalization following exercise. Of the 51 patients with coronary artery disease manifesting two mm or more of ST-depression, all of the car- diac deaths occurred in a subgroup who had at least two of the following features during exercise stress testing: 1) chest pain or ST-depression the stated reason for terminating exercise; 2) treadmill exercise duration of less than five minutes; 3) ventricular arrhythmias during or following exer- cise; 4)> 3 mm ST-segment depression at maximal exercise; 5) time for ST- segment normalization after exercise greater than four minutes. The combina- tion that was most highly predictive of subsequent mortality with medical therapy was a duration of treadmill exercise less than five minutes plus time for ST-segment normalization greater than six minutes (mortality in seven of 11 patients with this combination vs four of 40 patients without this combination (p<.001).

Discussion

These data indicate that specific findings indicative of marked degrees of myocardial ischemia provoked by treadmill exercise identify a subset of pa- tients with coronary artery disease who are particularly susceptible to accelerated cardiac mortality. Moreover, in well-matched patients with similar extent of coronary disease, left ventricular function and exercise-induced ischemia who underwent coronary bypass, mortality was markedly lowered compared to medically treated patients.

Previous investigation of exercise predictors of sudden death by Bruce et al. (1977 and 1979) found that while factors relating to left ventricular dysfunction were highly predictive of sudden death, ischemia as defined by 1.0 mm ST-segment depression did not accurately detect patients prone to cardiac events. However, in our population of patients which differed from that reported by Bruce in that all patients had been referred for coronary arteriography and all manifested marked degrees of ischemia during exercise, several factors in addition to ventricular dysfunction were related to subsequent mortality. Further, retrospective data suggests that many patients experiencing sudden cardiac death have no previous symptoms (Roberts and Jones 1979). Therefore, extension of the use of treadmill stress testing from a tool to detect patients with coronary artery disease to a diagnostic modality capable of identifying a subset of patients at high risk of experiencing cardiac mortality, is extremely important and has obvious therapeutic implications.

The predictive value for cardiac mortality of marked degrees of exercise-induced ST-segment depression is enhanced even further by the concomitant findings of chest pain, abbreviated duration of exercise to less than five minutes, ventricular ectopy precipitated by exercise, and prolongation of the ST-segment normalization time beyond four minutes following cessation of exercise. Thus, all cardiac deaths subsequent to the baseline treadmill stress test manifested at least two of these features in addition to > 2 mm segment depression. Conversely, despite the presence of marked ST-segment depression, no patient in the medical group without two or more of the foregoing additional findings experienced a cardiac death.

Thus, patients in whom the number, site or severity of coronary arterial stenoses may be considered equivocal indications for coronary bypass, should be strongly considered as surgical candidates if they demonstrate certain exercise features of severe ischemia as described herein. In this regard, while single vessel coronary artery disease is generally not regarded as an appropriate indication for coronary bypass surgery, we have recently demonstrated great variability in the extent of left ventricular dysfunction following anterior myocardial infarction related to isolated stenosis of the left anterior descending coronary artery (Kumpuris, et al. 1979). Our data documented a close relation between the specific site of stenosis in the left anterior descending coronary and the quantity of left ventricular myocardium disturbed. With stenosis proximal to both the first large septal and diagonal branches, the extent of infarct was markedly greater than with infarctions consequent to stenosis just distal to this site. Accordingly, since post myocardial infarction prognosis relates to the extent of ventricular dysfunction (Bruschke et al. 1973; Reeves et al. 1974), it would appear that the prognosis associated with stenosis isolated to the left anterior descending coronary may differ considerably based on a difference of only a few millimeters in location (Mantle et al. 1979). Consequently if myocardial preservation is a major goal of therapy, strong consideration must be given to coronary bypass surgery in proximally located anterior descending stenosis while it appears that medical therapy is preferable for an isolated lesion slightly more distal. These data strongly suggest that the findings of stenosis of the left anterior descending coronary artery proximal to the first septal branch combined with the exercise predictors of poor prognosis described herein, provide excellent objective rationale for surgical intervention even in the absence of preceding refractory angina pectoris. Utilization of these data with prior data concerning ventricular ectopy (Vismara et al. 1977) may afford means of

accurately detecting high risk subsets of coronary patients likely to benefit from bypass surgery. In conclusion the presence of the specific electrocardiographic and symptomatic findings during exercise described in the
present investigation may greatly facilitate clinical decision making in
patients who, based on coronary anatomy alone, would not meet usual accepted
criteria for coronary bypass surgery.

References

Bruce RA, De Rouen T, Peterson DR, et al. (1977) Noninvasive predictors of
    sudden cardiac death in men with coronary heart disease. Amer J Cardiol
    39:833–840
Bruce RA, De Rouen TA, Hammermeister KE (1979) Noninvasive screening cri-
    teria for enhanced 4-year survival after aortocoronary bypass surgery.
    Circulation 60:638–646
Bruschke AVG, Proudfit WL, Sones FM Jr. (1973) Progress study of 590 con-
    secutive nonsurgical cases of coronary disease followed 5-9 years. Ven-
    triculographic and other correlations. Circulation 47:1154–1157
Ellestad MH, Wan MKC (1975) Predictive implications of stress testing. Fol-
    lowup of 2700 subjects after maximal stress testing. Circulation 51:
    363–369
Hurst JW, King SB, Logue RB, et al. (1978) Value of coronary bypass surgery.
    Amer J Cardiol 42:308–329
Isom WO, Spencer FC, Glassman E, et al. (1978) Does coronary bypass increase
    longevity? J Thoracic Cardiovasc Surg 75:28–37
Kumpuris AA, Miller RR, Kanon DT, et al. (1979) Isolated stenosis of the
    left anterior descending coronary artery: A heterogeneous disease
    with variable surgical implications. Am J Cardiol 43:384
Lawrie GM, Morris GC, Howell JF, et al. (1979) Improved survival beyond 5
    years after coronary bypass surgery in patients with left main coronary
    artery disease. Amer J Cardiol 44:612–615
Lawrie GM,Morris GC, Howell JF, et al. (1977) Results of coronary bypass
    more than five years after operation in 434 patients:Clinical treadmill
    exercise and angiographic correlations. Amer J Cardiol 40:665–671
Mantle JA, Reeves RC, Rogers WJ, et al. (1979) Isolated left anterior de-
    scending occlusion-large infarctions in young men. Clinical Res. 26:749A
McIntosh HD, Garcia JA (1978) The first decade of aortocoronary bypass graft-
    ing 1967-1977: A review. Circulation 57:405–431
Miller RR, De Maria AN, Vismara LA, et al. (1977) Chronic stable inferior
    myocardial infarction: unsuspected harbinger of high-risk proximal left
    coronary arterial obstruction amenable to surgical revascularization.
    Amer J Cardiol 39:959–960
Read RC, Murphy ML, Hultgren HN, et al. (1978) Survival of men treated for
    chronic stable angina pectoris. J Thoracic Cardiovasc Surgery 75:1–16
Reeves JJ, Oberman A, Jones WB, et al. (1974) Natural history of angina pec-
    toris.   Amer J Cardiol 33:423–430
Roberts WC, Jones AA (1979) Quantitation of coronary arterial narrowing at
    necropsy in sudden coronary death. Amer J Cardiol 44:39–45
Takaro T, Hultgren HN, Lipton MJ, et al. (1975) The VA cooperative random-
    ized study of surgery for coronary arterial occlusive disease. II. Sub-
    group with significant left main lesions. Circulation 54:Suppl 3, III-
    107–117
Vismara LA, Miller RR, Price JE, et al. (1977) Improved longevity due to re-
    duction of sudden death by aortocoronary bypass in coronary atheroscle-
    rosis. Amer J Cardiol 39:919–924

Introduction to Epidemiology of Atherosclerotic Lesions[1]

Jack P. Strong and Yuichiro Goto

The participants in this workshop on the Epidemiology of Atherosclerotic
Lesions will be presenting important new information on the relationship
of known and suspected risk factors for coronary heart disease to the
prevalence and extent of atherosclerotic lesions in artery wall.

A workshop session in the IVth International Symposium on Atherosclerosis
held in Tokyo was devoted to the epidemiology of atherosclerotic lesions
with heavy emphasis on the relationship of risk factors to atherosclerosis
per se (Strong and Omae 1977). Strong summarized previous findings concerning the relationship of risk factors and atherosclerotic lesions and provided very preliminary data from a community-wide study of atherosclerosis in
New Orleans (Strong 1977). Interim reports from epidemiological studies
of coronary heart disease which had autopsy follow-ups were included in that
workshop (Garcia-Palmieri et al. 1977; Hatano and Matsuzaki 1977; Solberg
et al. 1977; Stemmermann et al. 1977; Sternby 1977). At that time, autopsy
follow-up with standardized evaluation of atherosclerotic lesions was
available on a relatively small number of subjects in most of the studies.
The consensus of these preliminary studies was confirmation of the positive
association of major coronary heart disease risk factors such as elevated
serum cholesterol levels, elevated blood pressure, and cigarette smoking
with the extent of atherosclerosis as carefully assessed at autopsy. Statistically significant relationship (some highly significant) were demonstrated for some of these risk factors. The three studies with the largest
number of subjects showed statistically significant positive associations
between all three major risk factors and atherosclerosis in at least one
major arterial segment (the aorta or the coronary arteries). It is noteworthy that even in the studies with only a few cases, positive associations
were found for at least two of the three major risk factors. Most of these
studies were continued for variable lengths of time with surveillance and
follow-up. Additional subjects are available at this time to provide further
evidence of the relationship of these risk factors to atherosclerosis. Also,
more subtle significant relationships of atherosclerosis to other suspected
risk factors may become apparent with larger number of cases.

The findings reported in the IVth International Symposium have been summarized in the contex of autopsy evidence for atherosclerosis being preventable
(Strong 1978) and in relationship to risk factors for atherosclerotic
lesions (Strong et al. 1977). The initial findings from the Honolulu Heart
Study have been published (Rhoads et al. 1978). Some of the participants
in the IVth International Symposium (and participants from the Framingham
Study) met in New Orleans in October 1978 to review the status of the epidemiology of atherosclerotic lesions. This Vth International Symposium in
Houston provides an opportunity to expand our knowledge of the epidemiology
of atherosclerotic lesions.

---

[1] See also pp. 719-730: J.P. Strong, W.D. Johnson, M.C. Oalman,
et al., "Community Pathology of Atherosclerosis and Coronary
Heart Disease in New Orleans: Relationship of Risk Factors to
Atherosclerotic Lesions."

References

Garcia-Palmieri MR, Castillo MI, Oalmann MC, Sorlie PD, Costas R Jr (1977) The relation of antemortem factors to atherosclerosis at necropsy. In: Schettler GY, Goto Y, Hata Y, Klose G (eds) Atherosclerosis IV, Springer-Verlag, New York, pp 108-113

Hatano S, Matsuzaki T (1977) Atherosclerosis in relation to personal attributes of a Japanese population in homes for the aged. In: Schettler G, Goto Y, Hata Y, Klose G (eds) Atherosclerosis IV, Springer-Verlag, New York pp 116-123

Rhoads GG, Blackwelder WC, Stemmermann GN, Hayashi T, Kagan A (1978) Coronary risk factors and autopsy findings in Japanese-American men. Lab Invest 38 (3): p 304

Solberg LA, Hjermann I, Helgeland A, Holme I, Leren PA, Strong JP (1977) Association between risk factors and atherosclerotic lesions based on autopsy findings in the Oslo study: A preliminary report. In: Schettler G, Goto Y, Hata Y, Klose G (eds) Atherosclerosis IV, Springer-Verlag, New York, pp 98-102

Sternby NH (1977) Atherosclerosis and risk factors. In: Schettler GY, Goto Y, Hata Y, Klose G (eds) Atherosclerosis IV, New York, Springer-Verlag, pp 102-104

Strong JP (1978) Atherosclerosis, a preventable disease? Autopsy evidence International Symposium: State of Prevention and Therapy in Human Arteriosclerosis and in Animal Models, Westdeutscher Verlag, Munster, Germany

Strong JP (1977) An introduction to the epidemiology of atherosclerosis. In: Schettler G, Goto Y, Hata Y, Klose G (eds) Atherosclerosis IV, Springer-Verlag, New York, pp 92-98

Strong JP, Eggen DA, Tracy RE (1977) The geographic pathology and topography of atherosclerosis and risk factors for atherosclerotic lesions. In: Chandler AB, Eurenius K, McMillan GC, Nelson CB, Schwartz CJ, Wessler S (eds) The Thrombotic Process in Atherogenesis, Plenum Press, New York, 1978, pp 11-31

Strong JP, Omae T (1977) Epidemiology of atherosclerosis and geographic differences in risk factors. In: Schettler G, Goto Y, Hata Y, Klose G (eds) Atherosclerosis IV, Springer-Verlag, New York, pp 92-125

Epidemiology of Coronary Atherosclerosis: Postmortem vs Clinical Risk Factor Correlations. The Framingham Study

W.B. Kannel, Paul Sorlie, Frederick Brand, W.P. Castelli, P.M. McNamara, and G.J. Gherardi

The Framingham Study has followed a cohort of 5209 adults for 26 years examining the relation of cardiovascular risk factors to clinical coronary heart disease (CHD) deaths and to the extent of coronary artery atherosclerosis at autopsy. There were 1519 deaths with acceptable autopsy data on 406 (26%). Of these, 127 were done according to a special protocol which carefully quantified the extent of coronary atherosclerosis (Feinleib et al. in press). From 406 satisfactory routine autopsies, the number of major coronary artery occlusions, associated myocardial infarctions and heart weights were ascertained. Data were also available on 155 clinical CHD deaths over 20 years of follow-up without prior CHD. The coronary artery pathology at autopsy and clinical CHD mortality were each examined in relation to premorbid risk factors measured routinely at biennial intervals.

The bias in making inferences from a population comprised of deaths must be recognized. This is illustrated in Table 1 where age, for example, does not discriminate the CHD deaths from all other deaths, even though it clearly discriminates CHD deaths from survivors. In this case analysis of deaths alone would lead to inaccurate conclusions about the relation of age to the development of CHD. The same applies to many of the other risk factors as indicated in Table 1. Bias can either hide associations or cause spurious results.

The Framingham Study has clearly shown a relationship of serum cholesterol, cigarette smoking, relative weight and blood pressure to the various forms of CHD (Table 2). The associations are no less striking for CHD death than they are for myocardial infarction. The multivariate risk of clinical CHD mortality for the combined effect of blood pressure, serum cholesterol and cigarette smoking is striking, escalating over a 5-fold range in relation to degree of exposure.

Postmortem pathology appeared to correlate better with risk factors the more remote the risk factor measurement from the terminal event. Also the different autopsy methodologies appeared to yield different results on the risk factor relationships.

In the special autopsy series systolic pressure (but not diastolic) correlated strongly with cardiac hypertrophy in both sexes but with the extent of coronary atherosclerosis only in women. Serum cholesterol correlated with the extent of coronary atherosclerosis in both sexes, but this relationship was independent of other risk factors only in men. Body weight correlated with heart size but not atherosclerosis. The degree of coronary atherosclerosis correlated with cardiac hypertrophy in both sexes. Only age was a significant independent correlate of coronary atherosclerosis in women (Table 3).

The general autopsy data showed no relationship between age and the number of coronary artery occlusions found. At any given age men had more severe coronary artery disease than women. Among those with one or more major occlusions, more than 70% had myocardial infarctions. Hearts were found to be heavier in decedents with one or more occlusions. A tendency to higher pressures was noted in women, but not men, in relation to the extent of coronary artery occlusive disease.

The level of serum cholesterol in autopsied subjects who had one or more occlusions appeared to be substantially higher than in those with none. Relative weights in women, but not men were higher in those with one or more occlusions. No clear association between number of occlusions and cigarette smoking or blood glucose was found.

Table 1. Average values of major CHD risk factors at baseline exam. CHD deaths vs. other deaths. Framingham Study 26 year follow-up.

Risk factor at baseline exam	Men			Women		
	CHD deaths	other deaths	survivors	CHD deaths	other deaths	survivors
Age	51	51	43	53	51	45
Systolic pressure	144	139	129	157	147	130
Serum cholesterol	240	226	223	267	238	224
Cigarettes	15	15	14	4.8	5.6	5.0
Blood glucose	88	86	80	91	86	81
No. of subjects	299	506	1443	141	485	2110

Table 2. Impact of risk factors on CHD mortality vs. morbidity. 20 year follow-up. Framingham Study. Men and Women 45-74.

| CHD risk factors | Age-Adjusted Univariate Logistic Coefficients | | | | | |
| | Myocardial Infarction | | Angina Pectoris | | CHD Death | |
	Men	Women	Men	Women	Men	Women
Serum cholesterol	.213[a]	.347[a]	.257[a]	.247[a]	.247[a]	.445[a]
Cigarettes	.224[a]	.127	-.001	-.185	.280[a]	.177
Relative weight	.124	.077	.290[a]	.279[a]	.149	.176
Systolic blood pressure	.279[a]	.530[a]	.310[a]	.462[a]	.408[a]	.538[a]
Diastolic blood pressure	.147[b]	.481[a]	.285[a]	.337[a]	.342[a]	.409[a]

[a] $p = < .01$
[b] $p = < .05$

Table 3. Correlation of cardiac pathology with risk factors. Special Autopsy Study. Framingham Study.

Men	Age at Death	Relative Weight	Systolic Pressure	Serum Cholesterol
Heart weight	-.073	.343[a]	.181	.164
% Intimal involvement	-.026	.180	.036	.321[a]
% Luminal insufficiency	.052	.093	.040	.266[b]

Women				
Heart weight	.249	.423[a]	.418[a]	.084
% Intimal involvement	.609[a]	.222	.322[b]	.260
% Luminal insufficiency	.545[a]	.195	.328[b]	.318[b]

[a] $p = < .01$
[b] $p = < .05$

The inconsistency of the relation of CHD risk factors to coronary artery pathology contrasts with the clear and consistent associations demonstrated for clinical CHD mortality (Feinleib et al. in press; Strong et al. 1968; Scrimshaw and Guzman 1968; Robertson and Strong 1968; Strong and Richards 1976). This may derive from bias in the selection of cases which are autopsied and the influence of the terminal illness on the risk factors, or even possibly on the coronary pathology. It is also possible, that the risk factors may directly contribute to death in subjects with an already compromised coronary circulation.

Table 4. Mean level of risk factors according to number of coronary artery occlusions on standard autopsy. 26 year follow-up.

Coronary risk factors at initial exam	Men Number of Occlusions					
	None			One or More		
	No.	Mean	S.D.	No.	Mean	S.D.
Age	177	48.2	8.1	79	47.1	8.1
Systolic pressure	177	144.7	25.5	79	140.5	19.4
Diastolic pressure	177	89.9	13.3	79	88.4	12.4
Serum cholesterol	151	232.0	55.4	72	247.2	42.7
Blood sugar	145	85.2	20.8	72	85.6	28.9
Relative weight	177	120.8	17.6	78	121.3	16.8
Cigarettes/day	174	15.8	13.5	79	13.7	13.6
	Women					
Age	138	46.4	8.6	33	49.1	8.3
Systolic pressure	138	146.3	33.2	33	157.1	21.9
Diastolic pressure	138	89.2	17.1	33	92.5	10.2
Serum cholesterol	123	236.5	46.5	28	265.8	63.5
Blood sugar	124	90.6	33.2	29	89.6	23.2
Relative weight	138	127.2	26.1	33	134.4	24.2
Cigarettes/day	137	5.8	8.8	33	4.6	7.4

References

Feinleib M et al (in press) The relation of antemortem characteristics to cardiovascular findings at necropsy. The Framingham Study.

Robertson W, Strong JP (1968) Atherosclerosis in persons with hypertension and diabetes mellitus. Lab Invest 18:538–551

Scrimshaw NS, Guzman MA (1968) Diet and atherosclerosis. Lab Invest 18: 623–628

Strong JP et al. (1978) The geographic pathology and topography of atherosclerosis and risk factors for atherosclerotic lesions. In: Chandler AB, Eurenius K, McMillan GC, Nelson CB, Schwartz CJ, Wessler S) The Thrombotic Process in Atherogenesis, Adv Exp Med Biol. Plenum Press, New York, Vol 104

Strong JP, Richards ML (1976) Cigarette smoking and atherosclerosis in autopsied men. Athero 23:451–476.

Risk Factors for Coronary and Cerebral Atherosclerosis in the Oslo Study[1]

Lars A. Solberg, Sven Chr. Enger, Ingvar Hjermann, Anders Helgeland, Ingar Holme, Paul Leren, and Jack P. Strong

The geographic differences in the extent of atherosclerotic lesions suggest that environmental factors are of importance in development of atherosclerosis (McGill 1968). The large variation in the degree of lesions among persons within the same population probably reflects individual susceptibility as well as differences in exposure to risk factors (Tejada et al. 1968). Since coronary atherosclerosis is necessary for the development of coronary heart disease (CHD), the assumption has been made that the risk factors for CHD are identical with those of coronary atherosclerosis. This may be true for some but not necessarily for all factors. Risk factors for CHD may lead to atherosclerotic lesions or to complication of lesions which cause occlusion of vessels. However, risk factors may also act directly on the myocardium and its conductive system, and thus contribute to the development of clinical disease. Since quantitative estimates of atherosclerosis are difficult to obtain in living persons, most information about risk factors have been obtained from retrospective studies on autopsy materials (Strong et al. 1978). More recently a few prospective studies have been initiated with careful documentation of certain risk factors during life, and standardized evaluation of atherosclerotic lesions at autopsy (Solberg et al. 1977; Sternby 1977; Garcia-Palmieri et al. 1977; Stemmermann et al. 1977). These studies show significant relationship between the levels of serum cholesterol, blood pressure and the extent of coronary atherosclerosis. The findings concerning the effect of smoking have so far been more uncertain. In this report we have included more cases from the Oslo Study than in a previous report (Solberg et al. 1977). Additional risk factors have been analyzed. The findings in the cerebral arteries are also included.

Materials and Methods

The Oslo study is an epidemiological investigation of CHD risk factors among men in Oslo. In 1972 all men, aged 40-49 years, were invited to a health examination that included a blood sample for lipid examination, measurement of blood pressure, and questions about smoking habits, physical activities at work and at leisure. The screening procedure and laboratory methods are described elsewhere (Leren et al. 1975; Enger et al. 1979). Among the cases who died in this study, coronary and the main intracranial arteries were collected from 150 men at autopsy. Details about the dissection, preparation, and evaluation of arteries are given elsewhere (Guzman et al. 1968). In brief, the coronary and cerebral arteries were removed, opened longitudinally, fixed in formalin, stained with Sudan IV, and graded for the percentage of intimal surface covered with raised atherosclerotic lesions (RL). The results were then compared with the following previously recorded risk

---
[1]The study is supported by the City of Oslo. Norwegian council on Cardiovascular Diseases. In part by U.S.P.H.S, Grant HL 08974 N.H.L.B.I.

factors: serum cholesterol, HDL-cholesterol, non-fasting triglycerides, systolic and diastolic blood pressure (BP), and physical activity at work and at leisure. A multivariate stepwise linear regression analysis was performed, using the listed risk factors as explanatory variables.

Results

Table 1 shows that the group of cases with CHD at the time of death have more coronary and cerebral RL than a basal group of cases without CHD, other atherosclerotic diseases, diabetes mellitus or hypertension. The CHD cases have higher serum total cholesterol, higher BP and lower HDL-cholesterol than the basal group of cases. The smoking habits seemed to be similar in both subgroups. Figure 1 shows that coronary RL increase with increasing values of total serum cholesterol and systolic and diastolic BP. RL also tend to increase with increasing values of triglycerides. RL decrease with increasing values of HDL-cholesterol and HDL-ratio (HDL-cholesterol divided by total cholesterol minus HDL-cholesterol). The findings are similar for the cerebral arteries (not illustrated). Figure 2 shows that there is large individual variation in coronary RL with increasing total serum cholesterol. Similar individual variation is seen for the other risk factors both in coronary and cerebral RL (data not given). In table 2 RL are compared with the smoking habits in all cases and in the basal group of cases. Smoking habits do not seem to be associated with the extent of coronary RL. Possibly, the degree of cerebral RL is lower in the non-smoking group compared to all daily smokers (p= .06, t-test, total group). Table 3 shows partial and multiple coefficients in the multivariate linear regression analysis using risk factors as explanatory variables. Total serum cholesterol and systolic BP contribute significantly both to coronary and cerebral RL. HDL-cholesterol contributes negatively to coronary RL (p< .01) but not to cerebral RL. The stepwise analysis revealed that 23% of the variation in coronary RL can be explained by serum cholesterol, systolic BP and HDL-cholesterol. When the other risk factors are included, only 3% more of the variation can be explained. Serum cholesterol and systolic BP alone explain 21% of the variation in cerebral RL. When the rest of the listed risk factors are included, an additional 4% of the variation can be explained. Nearly identical figures of partial and multiple correlation coefficients were obtained when diastolic BP or HDL-ratio were used instead of systolic BP and HDL-cholesterol. Analysis of a subgroup of cases without evidence of CHD, diabetes mellitus, and not treated for high blood pressure at the time of screening in 1972, revealed nearly identical results as in the whole material; however, the negative contribution of HDL-cholesterol to coronary RL was weaker in this subgroup compared to the whole material.

Discussion

Even after selecting cases according to race, sex, age, disease and smoking habits, there is much variability in the extent of coronary and cerebral RL (Strong et al. 1978; Solberg et al. 1968). This variability among persons within the most homogeneous subgroups probably reflects the individual differences both in susceptibility to atherosclerosis and in exposure to risk factors. The more we know about the risk factors, the more we can explain the variation in RL. The risk factors recorded in this study explain only 25% of the variation in RL. The study has, however, limitations that may have increased the unexplained part of the variation in RL. Thus, we have used a crude method for estimation of RL. The study is based on <u>one</u> measure-

Table 1. Mean values of risk factors and raised atherosclerotic lesions
(RL) in coronary and cerebral arteries of 150 Oslo men who underwent autopsy,
and in two subgroups of cases: (1) 63 cases with coronary heart disease
(CHD), and (2) 59 cases in a basal group without evidence of CHD or conditions associated with atherosclerosis at the time of death.

Catg.	Coronary RL %	Cerebral RL %	Triglyc. (m mol/1)	Cholest. (mg/dl)	HDL- chol. (mm/dl)	Syst. BP (mm Hg)	Diast. BP (mm Hg)	Ciga- rettes daily (number)
CHD	62	20	2.78	305	28	151	94	13.5
Basal group	28	4	2.67	276	35	132	84	14.0

Table 2. Correlation between mean values of coronary and cerebral raised
atherosclerotic lesions (RL) and smoking in all cases and in a basal group
of cases without evidence of CHD and conditions associated with atherosclerosis. Number of cases are given in parentheses.

Smoking habits	All cases Coronary RL	All cases Cerebral RL	Basal group Coronary RL	Basal group Cerebral RL
Never smoked cigarettes	47 (7)	2 (7)	32 (5)	1 (5)
Previous cigarette smokers	43 (16)	6 (16)	23 (5)	2 (5)
Present cigar/pipe smokers	52 (16)	11 (16)	25 (6)	2 (6)
0 - 9 cigarettes daily	45 (24)	16 (24)	19 (8)	4 (8)
10 - 14 cigarettes daily	44 (35)	11 (35)	30 (13)	5 (13)
15 - 19 cigarettes daily	47 (24)	14 (24)	27 (11)	6 (11)
> 20 cigarettes daily	44 (28)	13 (28)	27 (12)	4 (12)

Table 3. Partial correlation coefficients between risk factors and raised
atherosclerotic lesions (RL) in coronary and cerebral arteries (N=129).

Risk factor	Coronary RL	Cerebral RL
Cholesterol	.30*	.31*
HDL-cholesterol	-.22*	-.11
Systolic BP	.30*	.36*
Triglycerides	-.07	-.16
Cigarettes	-.08	-.08
Physical activity at work	-.14	-.09
Physical activity at leisure	.01	.10
Multiple correlation coeffic.	.51	.50

* $p < .01$

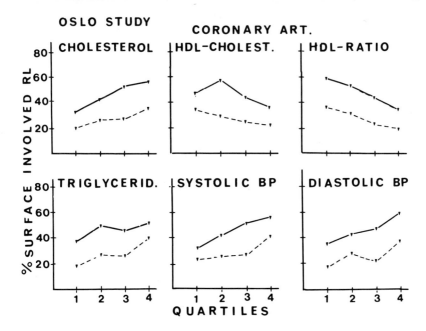

FIG. 1. Mean of raised atherosclerotic lesions in all cases and in
a basal group of cases, by increasing values of risk factors.
------- basal group, _____ all cases. N=150.

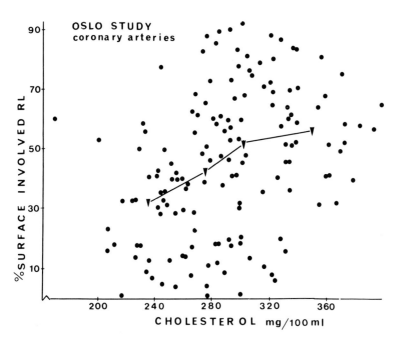

FIG. 2. Raised atherosclerotic lesions in coronary arteries in
individual cases and mean of RL, by increasing values of serum
cholesterol (quartiles). N=150.

ment of risk factors. These risk factors were recorded from a few weeks up to six years before the death. Nothing is known about the risk factors in the decades before the death. Thus, our results indicate only crude estimates of the association between risk factors and RL. This study shows that total serum cholesterol and BP account for most of the explanable variation in coronary and cerebral RL. The negative correlation of HDL-cholesterol to coronary RL is interesting in view of the hypothesis that HDL may remove cholesterol from intima and thus decrease the risk for development of atherosclerotic lesions (Miller and Miller 1975). Clinical studies show negative correlation between HDL and CHD (Forde and Thelle 1979). Why HDL does not have the same effect on cerebral RL cannot be explained from our data. The estimates of HDL were not particularly good, since they were based on analysis of frozen blood samples, stored for more than four years (Enger et al. 1979). Clinical studies indicate that high levels of serum triglycerides increase the risk for CHD (Kannel and Castelli 1972). However, in our study non-fasting triglycerides do not contribute as a significant risk factor either to coronary or cerebral RL. Since LDL (which transport most of the blood cholesterol) is known to be a risk factor by itself and also contains triglycerides, triglycerides may appear as risk factor for CHD because of their interrelation with LDL-cholesterol. There is a tendency in this study for BP to be a stronger risk factor for cerebral RL than for coronary RL, as suggested by higher partial correlation coefficients. Other autopsy studies have indicated that cigarette smoking enhances severity of RL (Strong and Richards 1976; Auerbach et al. 1976). In our prospective study we do not obtain similar results. This may be due to the small number of cases and the large individual variability in RL. However, the possibility exists that the strong clinical association between cigarette smoking and CHD, may be explained by the effect on the myocardium and its conduction system (Bekheit and Fletcher 1976) which may lead to decreased oxygen supply of the myocardium and arrhythmia. Cigarette smoking may also involve the coagulation system and may enhance the formation of the thrombi on the lesions (Hawkins 1972). Smoking may therefore interact with coronary RL in the development of CHD in persons who have extensive coronary RL for reasons other than cigarette smoking.

Conclusion

The study shows that total serum cholesterol, HDL-cholesterol and BP are significantly associated with extent of atherosclerotic lesions. The lack of a significant correlation between RL and the other risk factors may reflect that they are weaker atherogenic factors than total serum cholesterol, HDL and BP. However, a larger study might show significant correlation to these factors also.

Summary

Coronary and cerebral arteries from 150 men in the Oslo Study were collected at autopsy and graded for the extent of intimal raised atherosclertic lesions. The grading results were correlated with risk factors recorded before death. Raised atherosclerotic lesions were significantly correlated to total serum cholesterol, systolic and diastolic blood pressure. HDL-cholesterol was negatively correlated with coronary raised lesions. No significant correlations were found between atherosclerosis and non-fasting serum triglycerides, cigarette smoking, or physical activity at work and at leisure.

References

Auberbach O, Carter HW, Garfinkel L, Hammond EC (1976) Cigarette smoking and coronary artery disease. Chest 70:697-705

Bekheit S, Fletcher E (1976) The effects of smoking on myocardial conduction in the human heart. Am Heart J 91:712-720

Enger SC, Hjermann I, Foss OP, Helgeland A, Holme I, Leren P, Norum KR (1979) High density lipoprotein cholesterol and myocardial infarction or sudden coronary death: A prospective case-control study in middle-aged men of the Oslo Study. Artery 5:170-181

Forde OH, Thelle DS (1979) The Tromso Heart Study. Population studies of coronary risk factors with special emphasis on high density lipoprotein and the family occurrence of myocardial infarction. MD thesis, University of Tromso

Garcia-Palmieri MR, Castillo MI, Oalmann MC, Sorlie PD, Costas R Jr (1977) The relation of antemortem factors to atherosclerosis at necropsy. In: Schettler GY, Goto Y, Hata Y, Klose G (eds) Atherosclerosis IV. Springer-Verlag, New York, pp 108-113

Guzman MA, McMahan CA, McGill HC Jr, Strong JP, Tejada C, Restrepo C, Eggen DA, Robertson WB, Solberg LA (1968) Selected methodologic aspects of the International Atherosclerosis Project. Lab Invest 18:479-497

Hawkins RI (1972) Smoking, platelets and thrombosis. Nature 236:450-452

Kannel WB, Castelli WP (1972) The Framingham Study of coronary disease in women. Med Times (NY) 100:173-175

Leren P, Askeveold EM, Foss OP, Froli A, Grymyr D, Helgeland A, Hjermann I, Holme I, Lund-Larsen PG, Norum KR (1975) The Oslo Study: Cardiovascular disease in middle and young Oslo men. Acta Med Scand (Suppl 588)

McGill HC Jr (ed) (1968) The geographic pathology of atherosclerosis. Lab Invest 18:463-653

Miller NE, Miller GJ (1975) High density lipoprotein and atherosclerosis. Lancet 2:1033

Miller GJ, Miller NE (1975) Plasma high density-lipoprotein concentration and development of ischemic heart disease. Lancet 1:16

Solberg LA, Hjermann I, Helgeland A, Holme I, Leren P, Strong JP (1977) Association between risk factors and atherosclerotic lesions based on autopsy findings in the Oslo Study: A preliminary report. In: Schettler G, Goto Y, Hata Y, Klose G (eds) Atherosclerosis IV. Springer-Verlag, New York, pp 98-102

Solberg LA, McGarry PA, Moossy J, Tejada C, Loken AC, Robertson WB, Donoso S (1968) distribution of cerebral atherosclerosis by geographic location, race and sex. Lab Invest 18:604-612

Stemmermann GN, Rhoads GG, Blackwelder WC (1977) Atherosclerosis and its risk factors in the Hawaiian Japanese. In: Schettler G, Goto Y, Hata Y, Klose G (eds) Atherosclerosis IV. Springer-Verlag, New York, pp 113-116

Sternby NH (1977) Atherosclerosis and risk factors. In: Schettler GY, Goto Y, Hata Y, Klose G (eds) Atherosclerosis IV. Springer-Verlag, New York pp 102-104

Strong JP, Richards ML (1976) Cigarette smoking and atherosclerosis in autopsied men. Atherosclerosis 23:451-476

Strong JP, Eggen DA, Tracy RE (1978) the geographic pathology and topography of atherosclerosis and risk factors for atherosclerotic lesions. In: Chandler AB, Eurenius K, McMillan GC, Nelson CB, Schwartz CJ, Wessler S (eds) The Thrombotic Process in Atherogenesis. Plenum Press, New York, pp 11-31

Tejada C, Strong JP, Montenegro MR, Restrepo C, Solberg LA (1968) Distribution of coronary and aortic atherosclerosis by geographic location, race, and sex. Lab Invest 18:509-526

Atherosclerosis and Its Risk Factors Among Hawaii Japanese[1]

G.N. Stemmermann, G.G. Rhoads, and T. Hayashi

The mortality rate from coronary heart disease (CHD) among Hawaii Japanese
is intermediate between the rates for the indigenous Japanese and the U.S.
Whites (Gordon 1957). Comparative studies of Japanese men in Hiroshima,
Japan and in Honolulu, Hawaii show that the Hawaiian men eat proportionately
more animal fat and animal protein and smaller amounts of carbohydrates than
do indigenous Japanese. A larger proportion of the Hawaii carbohydrate load
is simple (e.g. sugar) rather than complex (e.g. rice, potatoes, etc.) (Kagan
et al. 1974). The Hawaii men are more obese, but only slightly taller than
the Hiroshima men. They also have higher blood cholesterol, uric acid and
glucose levels (Kagan et al. 1974). A comparative autopsy study has shown
that the Hawaii men have substantially more severe degrees of atherosclerosis of the aorta and coronary arteries, as well as a great excess of myocardial infarction (MI) (Stemmermann et al. 1976). In this paper we relate autopsy findings in 45-75 year old Japanese-American men dying in Honolulu to
a series of CHD risk factors and dietary characteristics measured during
life.

Methods

A series of interviews, examinations and laboratory tests were performed on
8006 Hawaii Japanese men with birthdates from 1 January 1900 through 31 De-
cember 1919. The examinations were begun in 1965 and ended in 1968. The
methods employed are described elsewhere (Kagan et al. 1974; Rhoads et al.
1978). Autopsies have been obtained following 302 of the deaths. We are
now able to compare examination data with the findings of protocol dissec-
tions of the heart in 199 cases, of the coronary arteries in 165 cases and
of the aorta in 178 cases. The degree of atherosclerosis of the aorta and
coronary arteries has been assessed by a panel method that matches the vessels with photographs showing increasing degrees of atherosclerosis. The
most appropriate of seven intervals is chosen as the grade of severity
(Rhoads et al. 1978). Myocardial infarction is defined as an area of recent
myocardial necrosis or mural scar larger than 0.5 cm in diameter.

Results

Table 1 indicates that, in univariate analysis, age, serum cholesterol, systolic blood pressure and the 1 hour post prandial glucose are significantly
related to the degree of atherosclerosis of both the aorta and the coronary
arteries. Significant associations were also noted between atherosclerosis
of the aorta and both cigarette consumption and vital capacity; and between
coronary sclerosis and the relative weight. The subscapular skinfold, another measure of obesity, was positively associated with coronary atherosclerosis to the same degree as relative weight.

The dietary questionnaire (Table 2) showed mostly negative associations.
These were statistically significant for total carbohydrate and athero-

---

[1]This study has been funded by Contract NO1-HV-62955.

Table 1. Correlation coefficients between selected examination variables and atherosclerosis score.

		Aorta (N=178)	Coronary arteries (N=165)
Age at death		0.30**	0.16*
Height	(cm)	-0.14	0.00
Relative wt	(%)	-0.03	0.18*
Cigarettes	(mg/dl)	0.15*	0.12
Cholesterol	(mg/dl)	0.21**	0.30**
Triglycerides	(mg/dl)	0.08	0.10
Uric acid	(mg/dl)	0.02	0.08
Glucose	(mg/dl)	0.15*	0.20**
Hematocrit	(%)	0.02	0.14
Vital capacity		-0.20**	0.07
Systolic blood pressure	(mmHg)	0.28**	0.17*

N = Number of specimens.
* = Significant at 0.05 level.
** = Significant at 0.01 level.

Table 2. Correlation coefficients between amounts (and proportions)† of specific nutrients and severity of atherosclerosis.

	Aorta (N=178)		Coronary arteries (N=165)	
Total calories	-0.13		-0.22**	
Protein	-0.08	(0.08)†	-0.15	(0.17*)†
Fat	-0.10	(-0.02)	-0.09	(0.07)
Saturated fatty acids	-0.10	(-0.03)	-0.09	(0.05)
Carbohydrate	-0.14*	(-0.02)	-0.21**	(-0.02)
Sucrose	-0.10	(-0.06)	-0.06	(-0.01)
Starch	-0.08	(0.04)	-0.18*	(0.01)
Cholesterol	-0.04		-0.02	
Alcohol	-0.01		-0.12	

†Figures in parenthesis indicate correlations when dietary variables are computed as a percent of total caloric intake.
*p<0.05
**p<0.01

sclerosis of both the aorta and coronary arteries. Coronary atherosclerosis was also significantly related to total calories per day and starch intake.
Because some clinical variables are inter-correlated, multivariate analyses have been performed. These indicate whether a given clinical variable (e.g. blood pressure) is significantly related to a particular pathologic finding after taking correlated variables (e.g. age and relative weight) into account. In multivariate analysis, the associations of aortic atherosclerosis with glucose and vital capacity became non-significant. The association of coronary atherosclerosis with age and glucose lost significance, while that for cigarette consumption became significant when the other variables were taken into account.

The association of clinical and dietary factors with MI at autopsy is shown in Tables 3 and 4. The significant findings parallel closely those noted for CHD incidence in this population. The absence of a significant association with tobacco use is due to the high mean value for cigarettes/ day in non-MI deaths, a not unexpected finding. Variables associated with MI, but not strongly associated with atherosclerosis, include hematocrit, triglyceride and alcohol intake. Conceivably, they might be related to the precipitation of acute events. In biologic terms, such an interpretation seems to make most sense for hematocrit. However, alcohol consumption in large amounts has been reported to inhibit platelet aggregation (Haut and Cowan 1974), and triglycerides are known to be low in physically active persons who might have larger coronary arteries or better collaterol circulation.

In summary, although these autopsy results suggest that the major known risk factors for myocardial infarction and CHD deaths have their effect primarily on atherosclerosis of both the aorta and coronary arteries, they raise the possibility that other factors may play a role through non-atherogenic mechanisms. These findings require confirmation in other populations.

Table 3.   Relation of exam variables to MI at autopsy.

Variable		MI (N=64)	No MI (N=135)	
		Age-adjusted mean values§		
Cigarette/day		15.1	14.0	
Vital capacity	(L)	2.95	3.04	
Relative wt	(%)	115	109	*
Hematocrit	(%)	45.9	44.0	**
Glucose	(mg/dl)	211	171	**
Cholesterol	(mg/dl)	240	204	**
Triglyceride	(mg/dl)	280	213	*
Systolic BP	(mmHg)	150	141	*
Usual alcohol	(oz/mo)	10.3	21.5	

*p<.05
**p<.01
§Age-adjusted by direct method to age structure of protocol autopsies.

Table 4.   Relation of diet variables to MI at autopsy.

		MI (N=64)	No MI (N=135)
		Age-adjusted mean values§	
Calories		2094	2196
Protein	(g)	90.9	85.7
Fat	(g)	81.8	75.2
Sat fatty acids	(g)	30.3	27.3
Carbohydrate	(g)	233	256
Sugar	(g)	38.3	39.9
Starch	(g)	151	160
Alcohol	(g)	8.3	20.7**
Percent calories as:			
Sat Fatty acids		12.6	11.3*
Protein		17.7	15.7**
Fat		34.1	30.8*
Carbohydrate		45.4	47.1
Sugar		6.8	7.1
Starch		30.1	30.0

*p<.05
**p<.01
§Age-adjusted by direct method to age-structure of protocol autopsies
( )Number of cases

References

Gordon T (1957) Mortality experience among Japanese in the United States, Hawaii and Japan. Pub Health Rep 72: 543

Haut MJ, Cowan DH (1974) The effect of ethanol on hemostatic properties of human blood platelets. Am J Med 56: 22

Kagan A, Harris BR, Winkelstein W et al. (1974) Epidemiologic studies of coronary heart disease and stroke in Japanese men living in Japan, Hawaii and California. Demographic, physical, dietary and biochemical characteristics. J Chron Dis 27: 345

McGill HC Jr, Brown BW, Gore I et al. (1968) Grading human athero-sclerotic lesions using a panel of photographs. Circulation 37: 455

Rhoads GG, Blackwelder WC, Stemmermann GN et al. (1978) Coronary risk factors and autopsy findings in Japanese-American men. Lab Invest 38: 304

Stemmermann G, Steer A, Rhoads GG, et al. (1976) A comparative pathology study of myocardial lesions and atherosclerosis in Japanese men living in Hiroshima, Japan and Honolulu. Lab Invest 34: 592

Atherosclerosis, Smoking and Other Risk Factors

Nils H. Sternby

As previously reported (Isacsson 1972; Lannerstad 1978) 703 men born in even months in 1914 during 1969 participated in a clinical study of cardiovascular and pulmonary diseases in Malmoe, Sweden. They represented 88 % of such males. The aim of the study was to ascertain the role of smoking for the development of various diseases, especially of peripheral arterial disease. Regarding smoking habits the subjects were divided into non- and ex-smokers, light (1-14 cig./day) and heavy (> 14 cig./day) smokers, respectively. During the 9 year follow-up 13.1 % of the clinically studied men died, corresponding figure for non-participating men of the same age was 17.5 %. Of the 92 clinically studied men that died 80 were autopsied. From 60 subjects various arteries were collected. Atherosclerosis was visually estimated on stained specimens preserved in plastic bags according to methods previously reported (McGill 1968; Kagan et al. 1976).

Overall mortality was 13.1 %, but only 4.6 % of the non-smokers died, compared to 12.0 % of the ex-smokers and 15.6 % of the smokers (table 1). Smoking was especially associated with death from diseases related to atherosclerosis but also to death from neoplasia.

Atherosclerosis was studied in the abdominal aorta, the iliac, femoral and lower leg arteries, the left anterior descending coronary artery and the basilar artery, respectively. The extent of raised lesions, i.e., fibrous plaques, complicated and calcified lesions, expressed as the percentage of the intimal area involved, was used for comparison. For coronary, femoral and lower leg arteries stenosis (> 50 %) and/or occlusion was also estimated.

In subjects dying from cardiovascular diseases atherosclerosis was more extensive in all areas, except the abdominal aorta, than in subjects dying from other causes. Stenosis of the coronary, femoral and lower leg arteries was also much more frequent in cardiovascular disease deaths than in other death groups.

The effect of smoking on the development of atherosclerosis was studied in normotensive subjects only since hypertension is well known to increase its extent and severity. Aortic atherosclerosis (table 2) was significantly higher in heavy than in light smokers with ex-smokers in between. The few non-smokers had very little aortic atherosclerosis. The heavy smokers had especially more extensive complicated and calcified lesions than the light smokers, such lesions were practically non existing amongst non-smokers.

In the coronary arteries (table 2) non-smokers had the most extensive raised lesions, even compared to the heavy smokers. However, two of the three studied non-smokers died from myocardial infarction. Coronary stenosis or occlusion was, however, more frequent in smokers, especially in heavy smokers. The previously reported finding in this study (Sternby 1977) of little association between smoking habits and extent of coronary atherosclerosis was thus corroborated. In the basilar artery (table 2) smokers had more extensive raised lesions than non-smokers.

Table 1. Smoking habits and cause of death (1970-78) in 703 clinically studied Malmoe men born in 1914.

Cause of Death Group	Non-smokers N = 108		Ex-smokers N = 159		Smokers N = 436	
	N	%	N	%	N	%
Coronary	2	1.9	4	2.5	25	5.7
Atherosclerosis			2	1.3	5	1.2
Miscellaneous	1	0.9	5	3.2	11	2.5
Neoplasia	1	0.9	7	4.4	23	5.3
Accidental	1	0.9	1	0.6	4	0.9
All	5	4.6	19	12.0	68	15.6

Table 2. Smoking and atherosclerosis in aorta, coronary and basilar arteries.

Smoking Category	N	Abd. aorta Raised lesions	L.A.D. coronary artery Raised lesions	Stenosis (%)	Basilar artery Raised lesions
Non	3	26	65	33	1
Ex	8	63	52	38	6
Light	18	53	45	39	3
Heavy	17	83	54	59	7

In the iliac, femoral and lower leg arteries the smokers had more extensive atherosclerosis than the non-smokers, and especially amongst the heavy smokers atherosclerosis was several times more extensive (table 3). The difference was even more marked regarding the frequency of stenosis: this did not occur in the femoral or the lower leg arteries in the non-smokers but was common amongst the heavy smokers. The ex-smokers had unexpectedly great extent of atherosclerosis and frequency of stenosis in the femoral and lower leg arteries, similar to that of the heavy smokers or even higher. These data may suggest that some of the ex-smokers became smokers again after the clinical examination.

The association between risk of death and original values for systolic blood pressure and serum cholesterol and triglycerides was studied by comparing the death rate in the different quartiles for these variables. No difference was found for the different lipoprotein quartiles, neither in total nor in cardiovascular death rate. Regarding hypertension, however, subjects belonging to the highest quartile died much more frequently than the others, this difference was especially marked amongst the heavy smokers.

Extent of atherosclerosis in relation to these risk factors was studied in smokers only. For aorta (table 4) only hypertensive subjects had an increased extent whereas those with or without hyperlipoproteinemia showed similar values. The hypertensives had especially more complicated and calcified lesions. Regarding coronary atherosclerosis (table 4) subjects with hyperlipoproteinemia had more extensive lesions but the frequency of stenosis was not increased. Hypertensive subjects had much higher frequency of stenosis and more extensive lesions than normotensives. In the basilar artery (table 4) hypertensives had more extensive lesions than the normotensives, but high serum lipid values had no influence. Also in the peripheral arteries (table 5) hypertensives had more extensive lesions than the normotensives, but hyperlipoproteinemia was not associated with either increased

Table 3. Smoking and atherosclerosis in peripheral arteries.

Smoking Category	N	Iliac artery Raised lesions	Femoral artery		Lower leg artery	
			Raised lesions	Stenosis (%)	Raised lesions	Stenosis (%)
Non	3	17	20	0	2	0
Ex	8	18	43	33	18	22
Light	18	29	23	6	3	11
Heavy	17	50	50	35	12	47

Table 4. Aortic, coronary and cerebral atherosclerosis and risk factors.

Smoking Category	Abd. aorta Raised lesions	L.A.D. coronary artery		Basilar artery Raised lesions
		Raised lesions	Stenosis (%)	
Smoking	68	41	50	4
Smoking and hyperlipopro-teinemia	70	47	46	6
Smoking and hypertension	83	52	89	31

Table 5. Peripheral atherosclerosis and risk factors.

Risk Factor	Iliac artery Raised lesions	Femoral artery		Lower leg artery	
		Raised lesions	Stenosis (%)	Raised lesions	Stenosis (%)
Smoking	38	39	23	8	36
Smoking and hyperlipopro-teinemia	43	30	15	5	15
Smoking and hypertension	67	63	33	20	38

extent of atherosclerosis or an increased frequency of stenosis. Adding hypertension to smoking as a risk factor in the femoral and, especially, in the lower leg arteries did not seem to increase the frequency of stenosis, which may indicate that smoking for these arteries is similar to hypertension as a risk factor.

Regarding physical activity and atherosclerosis no consistent differences were observed in the various arterial segments. In aorta low activity was associated with more extensive raised lesions, this was also found in the iliac and cerebral arteries whilst such subjects had less extensive lesions in the coronary and lower leg arteries. For the femoral arteries no diffe- rences were found. Those with low physical activity had, however, more ste- nosis in the coronary and femoral arteries, but not in the lower leg arte- ries. The effect of physical activity on the development of atherosclerosis is thus uncertain, if any.

Summary

Seven hundred and three 55-year old men were followed during 9 years after a health examination to evaluate the role of smoking in relation to cause of death and development of atherosclerosis. Smokers had 3-4 times higher mor- tality than non-smokers and showed more extensive atherosclerosis in the aorta, pelvic, leg and cerebral arteries, but not in the coronary arteries. Coronary stenosis was, however, more frequent among smokers. Heavy smokers had, generally speaking, more extensive atherosclerosis and a higher fre- quency of artery stenosis than light smokers. Of other risk factors hyper- tension increased atherosclerosis in all arterial segments whereas hyper- lipoproteinemia and low physical activity had little influence, if any.

References

Isacsson SO (1972) Venous occlusion plethysmography in 55-year old men. Acta Med Scand Suppl 537

Kagan AR, Sternby NH, Uemura K, Vanecek R, Vihert AM (1976) Atherosclerosis of the aorta and coronary arteries in five towns. Bull World Health Organ 53:483-645

Lannerstad O (1978) Death and disease among middle-aged men in Malmo dissertation, University of Lund, Sweden

McGill HC Jr (ed) (1968) The geographic pathology of atherosclerosis. Williams and Wilkins Company, Baltimore

Sternby NH (1977) Atherosclerosis and risk factors. In: Schettler G, Goto Y, Hata Y, Klose G (eds) Atherosclerosis IV. Springer-Verlag, Heidelberg, pp 102-104

Drug Treatment of Hyperlipidemias[1]

David Kritchevsky

Drug treatment of hyperlipidemia has advanced markedly over the last two decades. Whereas earlier efforts were aimed at reduction of either cholesterol or triglyceride levels (usually the former), today drugs are tested for their effects on specific types of hyperlipidemia and on enrichment or depletion of specific lipoprotein fractions.

Lipoprotein typing (Fredrickson and Lees 1965; Fredrickson et al. 1967), which characterizes hyperlipoproteinemias by elevation in cholesterol level or triglyceride level or both, suggested a more rational means of approaching the problem of diet, drugs and their lipid-lowering effects (Levy et al. 1972). It was clear that drugs could be used specifically to reduce lipoprotein, hence, lipid levels.

In 1951, Barr et al. suggested that the ratio of cholesterol present in the α or β lipoprotein fraction of serum could be a better means of identifying coronary-prone conditions than could the simple measurement of serum or plasma cholesterol levels. This, of course, suggested that a "lipid shifter," a drug that redistributed cholesterol among the plasma lipoprotein classes, could be as effective as a substance which lowered total cholesterol levels without affecting their distribution. Barr's observations were generally ignored until Miller and Miller (1975) reopened speculation in this area. Possible confirmation of alternate roles for the serum lipoproteins was available from the studies of Bailey (1965), Rothblat et al. (1968) and Burns and Rothblat (1969), which showed that HDL could transport cholesterol from cells in culture. Since interest has again been focused on the partition of cholesterol between α and β or HDL and LDL lipoproteins there has been a flood of confirmatory data (Rhoads et al. 1976; Castelli et al. 1977; Gordon et al. 1977).

Elevated HDL cholesterol levels have been found in long-lived populations (Slack et al. 1977; Glueck et al. 1977). A sedentary life style has been associated with decreased levels of HDL (Wood et al. 1976) and with increased risk of coronary disease (Paffenbarger et al. 1977).

Elevations in HDL cholesterol are also seen in persons who drink alcoholic beverages, the level of HDL-cholesterol increasing almost linearly as weekly intake rises from 0 to 20 ounces of alcohol per week (Hulley 1978). A study combining physical work or a sedentary life with alcohol intake has not been carried out at this writing.

Although the approach to increasing HDL-cholesterol levels is appealing, we still must await definitive data concerning the effects of drugs on levels of HDL_2 and HDL_3. At present, it is still not clear whether one or both of these species of HDL is most clearly associated with reduced risk.

[1]Supported, in part, by grants HL-03299, HL-05209 and HL-23625 and a Research Career Award from the National Institutes of Health.

It is not the purpose of this discussion to enumerate the many hypolipidemic drugs which have been developed and are under test. Bencze (1975, 1978) has written excellent reviews on this subject. Some drugs, such as clofibrate, appear to lower LDL cholesterol levels but to have little effect on HDL-cholesterol (Pichardo et al. 1977). Dibenzylcyclooctanone is hypocholesterolemic in the rat but the reduction is in the HDL-cholesterol (Cayen et al. 1976), which brings its use into question. Procetofen, an aryloxyaliphatic acid ester related to clofibrate, has been reported to increase HDL-cholesterol levels while lowering total serum cholesterol (Rossner and Oro 1978). Schurr and Day (1976) have reported that 1-[p-(1-adamantyloxy)-phenyl]piperidine lowers VLDL and LDL levels and raises HDL in rats fed an atherogenic diet.

Another approach to the treatment of hyperlipoproteinemia may lie in the use of drugs which modify apoprotein composition. This is a field which is relatively unexplored. Metformin reduces atherosclerosis in cholesterol-fed rabbits but has no effect on their serum lipids (Marquie and Agid 1968). Sirtori et al. (1977) found that metformin affected the apoprotein composition of the VLDL, with a reduction in levels of the arginine-rich apoprotein and an increase in apo-A I. Metformin also inhibits uptake of VLDL by rabbit aorta (Rodriguez et al. 1976). Another substance which affects arterial uptake of lipoproteins is a sulfated glycosaminoglycans of duodenal origin (Sirtori et al. 1976).

One metabolic manifestation of atherosclerosis is the increase in the esterified/free cholesterol ratio of the aorta. This finding dates back to Windaus (1910) and has stimulated much research on the cholesterol-esterifying and cholesteryl ester-hydrolyzing enzymes of the arterial wall. This field has been the subject of a recent review (Kritchevsky and Kothari 1978). Studies in cholesterol-fed rabbits have shown that drugs such as nicotinic acid, β-sitosterol, clofibrate or D-thyroxine can cause reversion of the increased ratio of cholesterol esterification to cholesteryl ester hydrolysis by arterial tissue towards normal levels (Kritchevsky et al. 1975). Effects on this ratio were not related to changes in serum cholesterol levels.

The foregoing suggests new chemotherapeutic approaches to the control of hyperlipidemias. The studies of HDL/LDL cholesterol ratios are relatively simple and have already been translated to the average laboratory through the medium of several commercially available analytical kits. The analysis of effects of drugs on apoprotein composition is more complicated but will soon probably yield to an electrophoretic or RIA method. Effects of drugs on arterial metabolism are, at the moment, impossible to discern by non-invasive means but, considering the ingenuity displayed by so many investigators in the lipoprotein field, this situation should not persist too much longer.

References

Bailey JM (1965) Exp Cell Res 37:175
Barr DP, Russ EM, Eder HA (1951) Am J Med 11:480
Bencze WL (1975) In: Kritchevksy D (ed) Hypolipidemic Agents. Springer-Verlag, Berlin, p 349
Bencze WL (1978) New hypolipidemic drugs. In: Kritchevsky D, Paoletti R, Holmes WL (eds) Drugs, Lipid Metabolism and Atherosclerosis. Plenum Publishing Corp., New York, p 77
Burns CH, Rothblat GH (1969) Biochim Biophys Acta 176:616
Castelli WP, Doyle JT, Gordon T, Haines C, Hjortland MC, Hulley SB, Kagan A, Zukel WJ (1977) Circulation 55:766
Cayen MN, Dubuc J, Dvornik D (1976) Biochem Pharmacol 25:1537

Fredrickson DS, Lees RS (1965) Circulation 31:321
Fredrickson DS, Levy RI, Lees RS (1967) New Engl J Med 276:32, 94, 148,
    215, 273
Glueck CJ, Gartside PS, Steiner PM, Miller M, Todhunter T, Haaf J, Pucke M,
    Terranna M, Fallat RW, Kashyab LML (1977) Atheroscler 27:387
Gordon T, Castelli WP, Hjortland MJ, Kannel WB (1977) Am J Med 62:707
Hulley SB (1978) In: Kritchevsky D, Paoletti R, Holmes WL (eds) Drugs,
    Lipid Metabolism and Atherosclerosis. Plenum Publishing Corp., New
    York, p 295
Kritchevsky D, Kothari HV (1978) Adv Lipid Res 16:221
Kritchevsky D, Tepper SA, Kothari HV (1975) Artery 1:437
Levy RI, Fredrickson DS, Shulman R, Bilheimer DW, Breslow JL, Stone NJ,
    Lux SE, Sloan HR, Krauss RM, Herbert PN (1972) Ann Int Med 77:267
Marquié G, Agid R, (1968) C R Soc Biol (Paris) 162:563
Miller GJ, Miller NE (1975) Lancet 1:16
Paffenbarger RS, Hale WE, Beard RJ, Hyde RT (1977) Am J Epidemiol 105:200
Pichardo R, Boulet L, Davignon J (1977) Atheroscler 26:573
Rhoads GG, Gulbrandsen CL, Kagan A (1976) New Eng J Med 294:293
Rodriguez J, Catapano A, Ghiselli GC, Sirtori CR (1976) In: Day CE (ed)
    "Atherosclerosis Drug Discovery." Plenum Publishing Corp., New York,
    p 169
Rossner S, Oro L (1978) In: Kritchevsky D, Paoletti R, Holmes WL (eds)
    Drugs, Lipid Metabolism and Atherosclerosis. Plenum Publishing Corp.,
    New York, p 404
Rothblat GH, Buchko MK, Kritchevsky D (1968) Biochim Biophys Acta 164:327
Schurr PE, Day CE (1976) Lipids 12:22
Sirtori CR, Catapano A, Ghiselli GC, Innocenti AL, Rodriguez J (1977)
    Atheroscler 26:79
Sirtori CR, Catapano A, Ghiselli GC, Malinow R (1976) Artery 2:390
Slack J, Noble N, Meade TW, North WRS (1977) Br Med J 2:353
Windaus A (1910) Z Physiol Chem 67:174
Wood PD, Haskell W, Klein H, Lewis S, Stern MP, Farquhar JW (1976)
    Metabolism 25:1249

Drug Treatment of Type II Hyperlipoproteinemia. Effects on Plasma Lipid and Lipoprotein Levels

Donald B. Hunninghake[1]

The primary indication for the use of drugs to alter plasma lipids and lipo-proteins is the expectation that they may decrease the morbidity and/or mor-tality associated with the development of arteriosclerotic vascular disease. Various studies with hypolipidemic agents have suggested that either morbid-ity or mortality associated with coronary heart disease is decreased (Carl-son et al. 1977; Dorr et al. 1978; Newcastle Study 1971; WHO Clofibrate Study 1978), but studies such as the Coronary Drug Project (1975) have not demon-strated a beneficial effect. Since there are no studies, universally ac-cepted by the scientific community, which document a reduction in morbidity and mortality, the results of studies currently in progress, such as the Lipid Research Clinic's Type II Coronary Primary Prevention Trial, are ea-gerly awaited. Increasing attention has been focussed on the importance of the lipoprotein fractions as potential indicators of future risk of develop-ing coronary heart disease. While age and sex differences may exist, there appears to be a positive correlation between low density lipoprotein choles-terol (LDL-C), and an inverse relationship between high density lipoprotein cholesterol (HDL-C) and risk of developing coronary heart disease (Gordon et al. 1977; Rhoads 1976). These observations indicate that the evaluation of hypolipidemic agents should include their effects on both plasma lipids and lipoproteins. Since the efficacy of many hypolipidemic agents is related to the specific lipoprotein disorder being treated (Hunninghake and Probstfield 1977), hypolipidemic agents should specifically be evaluated in patients with either Type IIa or IIb HLP. This paper reports some of our experiences in the treatment of these two lipoprotein disorders.

Methods

All studies were performed in males, age 30-59 years, who had given their consent for participation. All patients were instructed in cholesterol low-ering diets with the minimal dietary restriction being a cholesterol intake of 350 mg per day, a P/S ratio approximating 0.8, and weight reduction, when indicated. Most patients were on more restrictive diets and the results are expressed as changes from steady state diet controls. The criteria for the diagnosis of Type IIa HLP was an LDL-C of $\geq$190 mg/dl and triglycerides (TGG) $\leq$170 mg/dl. No patients with the homozygous defect are included. The re-quirements for Type IIb were an LDL-C of $\geq$190 mg/dl and TGG of $\geq$200 mg/dl. Lipid and lipoprotein analyses were done according to the methods described in the Lipid Research Clinic's Program (1975). Drugs were administered on a twice-daily schedule unless otherwise specified.

Results

Clofibrate produced significant mean reductions in TGG of 33% (p<0.001) and increases in HDL-C of 17% (p<0.01) for the entire group of patients with Type

[1]Work was supported in part by NHLBI contract #N01 HV 2-2195-L and a grant from the Upjohn Co.

Table 1. Type IIb hyperlipoproteinemia. Effect of various drug regimens on plasma lipid and lipoprotein levels.[a]

	Chol	LDL-C	HDL-C	TGG	Wt.(Kg)	% Adherence
Diet control - mean	291.9	199.6	38.3	273.8	83.4	-
$\pm$ S.E.	$\pm$ 2.6	$\pm$ 2.8	$\pm$ 1.0	$\pm$ 9.9	$\pm$1.1	
Per cent change from diet control						
Clofibrate [b]	- 2.4	+ 3.1	$+17.0^c$	-33.3^d	-0.7	94.5
Subgroup A	-10.9	-13.0	+26.1	-34.2		
Subgroup B	+ 9.9	+20.1	+10.0	-27.7		
Colestipol plus	-11.4^d	-14.0^c	$+24.3^d$	-24.6^d	-0.7	90.5
Clofibrate						90.0
Subgroup A	-17.1	-24.9	+32.3	-27.0		
Subgroup B	- 2.2	- 2.2	+18.2	-15.2		
Colestipol	-13.5^d	-24.8^d	+ 3.7	$+16.9^c$	-1.4	90.2
Subgroup A	-13.0	-25.9	+ 3.7	+27.0		
Subgroup B	-15.2	-25.3	+ 5.1	+ 7.5		
Probucol	-14.0	-12.8	-22.6	- 3.3	-0.5	93.8

[a]Twenty-four patients participated in a modified latin-square, crossover study. Each patient received a four month treatment period with each drug regimen. The results are the mean of four determinations during each treatment period. The total daily dose was 20 Gm of colestipol, 2.0 Gm of clofibrate and 1.0 Gm of probucol.

[b]Subgroup A is a group of patients who were noted to have significant reductions in LDL-C with clofibrate administration, while Subgroup B is a group who had significant increases in LDL-C with clofibrate.

[c]$p<0.01$

[d]$p<0.001$

IIb HLP as illustrated in Table 1. There was no significant effect on total plasma cholesterol (TPC) or LDL-C for the entire group. Colestipol therapy alone decreased TPC and LDL-C by 13.5 and 24.8% ($p<0.001$), and increased TGG by 16.9% ($p<0.01$). A significant reduction in TGG of 24.6% and an increase in HDL-C of 24.3% ($p<0.001$) occurred with combination therapy. However, the reduction in LDL-C of 14.0% with combination therapy was significantly less than the 24.8% noted with colestipol ($p<0.01$). Probucol also produced a significant reduction in TPC of 14.0% ($p<0.001$), which was similar to that produced by combination therapy and colestipol. The reduction in LDL-C of 12.8% was significantly less than observed with colestipol ($p<0.01$) and probucol also significantly reduced HDL-C by 22.6% ($p<0.001$). There was no significant difference in weight between treatment groups and adherence to the different drug regimens was comparable. Water was used as the vehicle for administering colestipol.

Two subgroups of responders to clofibrate in terms of its effect on LDL-C were identified. Subgroup A represents a group who had individual mean decreases in LDL-C ranging from 17-62 mg/dl, while Subgroup B had individual mean increases in LDL-C ranging from 21-67 mg/dl. Subgroup A had significant reductions in TPC and LDL-C and a greater increase in HDL-C than Subgroup B. Subgroup B had significant increases in TPC and LDL-C, less increase in HDL-C and no difference in TGG response for the two subgroups was noted. Subgroup B also did not achieve any significant reduction in TPC and LDL-C with combination therapy. The effect of colestipol and probucol on TPC and LDL-C was similar for the two subgroups.

Table 2. Type IIa hyperlipoproteinemia. Effect of various dosing schedules of cholestyramine on plasma lipids and lipoproteins.[a]

	Chol	LDL-C	HDL-C	TGG	Wt.(Kg)	% Adherence
Diet control - mean	280.7	207.6	46.1	133.9	81.8	-
± S.E.	± 4.7	± 4.8	±1.7	± 7.4	±2.3	

Per cent change from diet controls with cholestyramine 24 Gm/day

	Chol	LDL-C	HDL-C	TGG	Wt.(Kg)	% Adherence
Single A.M. dose	-12.2[b]	-21.1[c]	+3.9	+31.7[b]	-1.6	92.9
Single P.M. dose	-18.4[c]	-30.1[c]	+0.8	+40.5[b]	-2.2	91.7
12 Gm B.I.D.	-18.2[c]	-29.2[c]	+2.0	+36.9[b]	-1.8	94.4

[a]Twenty-four males participated in a latin-square, crossover study. Each patient received three treatment periods of nine weeks each with each of the three dosage schedules. The results represent the mean of three observations during each treatment period.
[b]$p<0.01$
[c]$p<0.001$

The importance of appropriate dosage schedules for administering the bile acid sequestering agents is illustrated in Table 2. Approximately 20-25% of patients on chronic resin therapy will elect to take it in a single dose, generally in the A.M. The above results indicate that a single P.M. dose is equally effective to the b.i.d. schedule in terms of lowering TPC and LDL-C. However, the single A.M. dose was not as effective in lowering TPC (difference of 6% or 17 mg/dl, $p<0.01$), and LDL-C (difference of 9% or 17 mg/dl, $p<0.01$) as the other two dosage schedules.

Our cummulative experience in the treatment of Type IIa HLP in recent years with colestipol, cholestyramine and/or clofibrate may be summarized as follows. Controlled studies involving 146 subjects and approximately 600 separate treatment periods with various drugs or dosages have been completed. A representative study is Hunninghake et al. (1978). A dose dependent reduction in TPC and LDL-C occurs with the administration of either colestipol or cholestyramine. Utilizing total daily dosages of 15, 20 and 30 Gm of colestipol (or equivalent doses of cholestyramine) the respective reductions in TPC are 12, 14 and 18% and the reductions in LDL-C are 17, 21 and 28%. The effect of resin therapy on TGG levels is quite variable, but significant increases are generally noted with 4 or 6 packets per day of resin. With 6 packets per day, we generally observe an increase in TGG ranging from 10-25%. The reduction in TPC is generally less than that observed for LDL-C because there is an associated increase in VLDL-C. Resin therapy does not significantly alter HDL-C levels. Clofibrate 2.0 Gm per day decreases TPC, LDL-C and TGG by 11, 14 and 25%, respectively and increases HDL-C by 11%. The addition of clofibrate to a patient receiving more than 4 packets of resin per day does not produce any additional significant decrease in LDL-C, but the TPC may be decreased slightly because of the associated decrease in TGG and VLDL-C.

Discussion and conclusion

Our studies extend the observations of Davignon et al. (1971) that clofibrate was more likely to reduce TPC in Type IIa than IIb HLP and of Fellin et al. (1978) that TPC levels could be increased by clofibrate administration in IIb patients already receiving colestipol. Clofibrate may significantly increase or decrease LDL-C levels or produce no change. In contrast, the response of IIb patients to colestipol and probucol is fairly uniform. In patients who have an increase in LDL-C with clofibrate, combination therapy is also ineffective. The mechanisms for the varied responses to clofibrate were not identified. Future studies will have to assess the significance of the decreased HDL-C levels produced by probucol. The data presented strongly suggests that drug therapy in Type IIb HLP should be monitored with both plasma lipids and lipoproteins. Appropriate dosage schedules of bile acid sequestering agents are essential to maximize their effect. If the population of Type IIa HLP being studied does not include the homozygous patient or a large percentage of the heterozygous patients with tendon xanthomas, the response to clofibrate and the resins is fairly predictable.

Acknowledgements

The author wants to acknowledge the contributions of S.O. Isaacson, M.D., Maureen Kane, M.D., Jeffrey Probstfield, M.D., Florine Peterson, R.N., Marilyn Swenson, R.N., Kanta Kuba, M.S., Lucille Crow, R.N., Linda Olson, R.D., Kay Kurtz, R.D., Catherine Bell, Kay Posthumus and Kathryn LaCroix to these studies.

References

Carlson LA, Danielson M, Ekberg I, Klintemar B, Rosenhamer G (1977) Reduction of myocardial infarction by the combined treatment with clofibrate and nicotinic acid. Atherosclerosis 28: 81-86

Coronary Drug Project Research Group (1975) Clofibrate and niacin in coronary heart disease. JAMA 231: 360-381

Davignon J, Aubry F, Noel C, Lapierre Y, Lafortune M (1971) Heterogeneity of familial hyperlipoproteinemia Type II on the basis of the fasting plasma triglyceride/cholesterol ratio and plasma cholesterol response to chlorophenoxyisobutyrate. Rev Can Biol 30: 307-313

Dorr AE, Gundersen K, Schneider JC, Spencer TW, Martin WB (1978) Colestipol hydrochloride in hypercholesteremic patients - effect on serum cholesterol and mortality. J Chronic Dis 31: 5-14

Fellin R, Baggio G, Briani G, Baiocchi MR, Manzata E, Baldo G, Crepaldi G (1978) Long-term trial with colestipol plus clofibrate in familial hypercholesteremia. Atherosclerosis 29: 241-249

Gordon T, Castelli WP, Hjortland MC, Kannel WB, Dawber JR (1977) High density lipoprotein as a protective factor against coronary heart disease. Am J Med 62: 707-714

Hunninghake DB, Crow L, Isaacson SO, Probstfield J (1978) Effect of clofibrate and colestipol on lipoprotein levels in Type IIa hyperlipoproteinemia. Fed Proc 37: 257

Hunninghake DB, Probstfield JL (1977) Drug treatment of hyperlipoproteinemia. In: Rifkind B, Levy R (eds) Hyperlipidemia, Diagnosis and Therapy. Grune, Stratton

Lipid Research Clinics Program Manual of Laboratory Operations (1975) 1. Lipid and lipoprotein analyses. NHLBI, NIH, Bethesda, Maryland 20014. DHEW publication No(NIH) 75-628

Newcastle Upon Tyne Region Group of Physicians (1971) Trial of clofibrate in the treatment of ischemic heart disease. Br Med J 4: 767-775

Rhoads GG, Gulbransen CL, Kagan A (1976) Serum lipoproteins and coronary heart disease in a population study of Hawaii Japanese men. New Engl J Med 294: 293-298

WHO Report from the Committee of Principal Investigators (1978) A cooperative trial in the primary prevention of ischemic heart disease using clofibrate. Br Heart J 40: 1069-1118

Synergism in Drug Treatment of Familial Hypercholesterolemia[1]

J.P. Kane, P. Tun, M.J. Malloy, and R.J. Havel

The monogenic disorder familial hypercholesterolemia (FH) is associated with a high risk of premature coronary arteriosclerosis, largely attributable to a 2-3 fold increase in levels of low density lipoproteins (LDL) in serum. Heretofore, no regimen of drug therapy or surgical intervention has been reported which is capable of lowering levels of low density lipoproteins consistently to normal in FH heterozygotes. Regimens employing bile acid binding resins, nicotinic acid, neomycin and paraaminosalicylic acid individually have achieved reductions of serum cholesterol of only 25-30%, nearly comparable to the effect of partial ileal bypass, (33%) (Miettinen and Lempinen 1977). Combinations of clofibrate with bile acid resins or neomycin are only slightly more effective than these agents given individually.

Sequestration of bile acids increases conversion of cholesterol to bile acids in liver, with a concomitant increase in hepatic cholesterogenesis, and in some way increases the fractional catabolic rate for LDL in blood (Moutafis et al. 1971; Goodman et al. 1973; Eisenberg and Levy 1975). It is possible that the latter reflects the ability of liver to secure additional cholesterol from circulating LDL. Synergism thus might be expected between bile acid sequestrants and other agents which inhibit production of precursors of LDL, principally very low density lipoproteins (VLDL), or which restrict the availability of cholesterol to the liver either by inhibiting its synthesis or by impeding its absorption via the intestine. To test this hypothesis we studied the effects of three regimens in which the bile acid binding resin, colestipol (30 g/day, in 3 doses) was given to FH heterozygotes with each of three other agents: clofibrate 2 g; β-sitosterol 6 g; or nicotinic acid 4-7 g/day. In order to exclude individuals with other forms of hyperbetalipoproteinemia, patients were admitted to the study only if their serum cholesterol level exceeded 350 mg/dl (mean serum cholesterol 420 mg/dl; triglyceride 122 mg/dl) and if they had tendon xanthomata or an affected first degree relative. Secondary hyperlipidemias were ruled out by appropriate clinical tests.Throughout the study patients were instructed to remain on a diet providing less than 200 mg of cholesterol per day and 10% or less of calories as saturated fat.

In 39 patients (17 men, 21 women, mean age 46) given 20 g/day of colestipol resin alone for one year, the average mean monthly serum cholesterol level was 19.7% below the mean level during 3-12 months of treatment with diet alone. Levels of serum cholesterol fell during the first month to values comparable to the mean for the year and were sustained throughout the year ($p < 0.01$). Increase in dose of the resin to 30 g/day resulted in a significant further decrement in serum cholesterol levels (335 to 319 mg/dl, $p = 0.01$). Though a few individuals had sustained, moderate elevations of serum triglyceride levels, at neither dose were mean levels changed significantly.

---

[1] This research was supported by a Grant from the National Institutes of Health (Arteriosclerosis SCOR HL 14237). Dr. Kane was an Established Investigator of the American Heart Association.

The response to the combination of colestipol (30 g/day) and clofibrate (2 g/day) in 18 patients during 12 months was heterogeneous. In four individuals, levels of serum cholesterol fell 50 to 120 gm/dl whereas the average decrease for the remaining 14 patients was but 10 mg/dl. Serum triglycerides fell, however, in 17 individuals. The mean serum triglyceride level fell from 183 mg/dl to 105 mg/dl for the group (p = 0.001). Changes in levels of cholesterol in low density lipoproteins measured by preparative ultracentrifugation (Myers et al. 1976) were not significantly different from levels during treatment with resin alone (229 mg/dl ± 62 S.D. versus 243 ± 67, p = -.22). Mean HDL cholesterol levels were unchanged at 55 mg/dl (± 11 S.D.).

In nine individuals given colestipol (30 g/day) with β-sitosterol - (6 g/day in two doses) for 1-4 months (gift of Eli Lilly Co.), there was a significant decrease in mean monthly serum cholesterol levels beyond that achieved during a 2-4 month period on resin alone (Table 1).

Table 1. Effect of the combination of colestipol and β-sitosterol on serum lipids and lipoprotein fractions.

	(mg/dl ± S.D.)			
	Colestipol		Colestipol plus β-sitosterol	
	Cholesterol	TG	Cholesterol	TG
Serum total	347 ± 95	162 ± 91	303 ± 51[a]	146 ± 71
VLDL	35 ± 19	102 ± 191	20 ± 18	88 ± 62
LDL	257 ± 78	43 ± 14	228 ± 49[b]	37 ± 8
HDL	53 ± 19	15 ± 7	46 ± 10	15 ± 6

[a] p < 0.02 vs resin alone

[b] p < 0.05 vs resin alone

The effects of colestipol (30 g/day) with nicotinic acid (mean dose 6.5 g/day) on serum lipids and lipoproteins were evaluated in a group of 22 FH heterozygotes for up to one year (mean duration 8 months). Doses of nicotinic acid were started at 300 mg/day and increased at a rate less than 2.5 g/day/month to a maximum of 7.5/g/day. Tachyphylaxis to the cutaneous flushing caused by nicotinic acid occurred in a few days at any dose level. Mild elevations of SGOT and alkaline phosphatase activities were observed only if the rate of increase of dose of nicotinic acid exceeded 2.5 g/day/mo. In order to identify non-compliant individuals, the content of N-methyl-2-pyridone-5-carboxamide, a major metabolite of nicotinic acid, was measured in urine. Data on four patients who excreted less than one third of the mean amount of the metabolite excreted by individuals in the whole group were excluded from analysis.

On the combination of diet, colestipol and nicotinic acid levels of LDL cholesterol were normalized in all compliant patients. Mean serum cholesterol levels fell to 231 mg/dl ± 29.5 S.D. from 314 ± 51 on diet and colestipol and 424 ± 70 on diet alone. The content of cholesterol in LDL fell 55% from the level on diet alone (p < 0.001) (Table 2). Mean serum triglyceride levels fell to 80 mg/dl from 172 mg/dl on diet and resin, and 129 mg/dl on diet alone, reflecting a decrease in triglycerides in all lipoprotein fractions. In addition there was an increase in mean HDL cholesterol from 65 mg/dl and 61 mg/dl on diet, and diet with resin, respectively, to 76 mg/dl (p = 0.05) on the combined drug regimen (Table 2).

For comparison with these data, control values, weighted for age and sex such as to match the patient group, were calculated from data obtained in an epidemiologic survey of a free living industrial population in the San Francisco area. The mean level of LDL cholesterol was substantially lower in the heterozygous FH patients treated with diet, colestipol and nicotinic acid than in the control group (126 vs 150 mg/dl). The mean HDL cholesterol, on the other hand, was substantially higher in the treated FH heterozygotes, than in the matched control population (76 vs 65 mg/dl). That the response of LDL is due to the combination of resin and nicotinic acid rather than to nicotinic acid alone is supported by the appreciable increase observed in LDL cholesterol when the resin was discontinued and treatment with nicotinic acid was maintained. In a group of eight such patients the mean monthly serum cholesterol level increased from 228 mg/dl ± 13 to 289 mg/dl ± 57 during the three month period after discontinuance of the resin.

Table 2. Comparison of the effect of diet, colestipol and nicotinic acid with diet and colestipol and diet alone in heterozygous familial hypercholesterolemia in 11 of the 18 compliant patients in whom complete ultracentrifugal data are available for all three phases of the study.

	Diet	Diet and Colestipol	Diet, Colestipol and Nicotinic Acid
Cholesterol mg/dl			
VLDL	21 ± 12^{a}	36 ± 38	11 ± 12
LDL	278 ± 41	181 ± 45	$126^{b} \pm 27$
HDL	65 ± 16	61 ± 16	$76^{c} \pm 19$
Serum Total	397 ± 61	294 ± 36	220 ± 20
Triglycerides mg/dl			
VLDL	64 ± 46	135 ± 150	55 ± 61
LDL	44 ± 15	39 ± 12	23 ± 10
HDL	19 ± 11	16 ± 7	15 ± 6
Serum Total	141 ± 80	184 ± 140	85 ± 48

[a] denotes S.D.

[b] p < 0.001 vs level on diet and colestipol

[c] p < 0.05 vs levels on diet or diet and colestipol

Discussion

It is clear from the data we have obtained that little synergism occurs between clofibrate and the bile acid binding resin colestipol, whereas moderate synergism is apparent between β-sitosterol and the resin. By contrast the combination of nicotinic acid and colestipol is capable of consistent and complete normalization of levels of low density lipoproteins in compliant patients with heterozygous FH. The lack of apparent synergism between clofibrate and colestipol indicates that clofibrate does not decrease the production of lipoprotein precursors of LDL by liver. This is consistent with data obtained by direct measurement of hepatic triglyceride secretion in humans treated with clofibrate (Wolfe et al. 1973). Further it must be concluded that even though clofibrate may be able to decrease cholesterol biosynthesis under some circumstances (Sodhi et al. 1971) that it is unable to contravene the marked increase in hepatic and intestinal cholesterogenesis induced by the resin (Miettinen and Lempinen 1977).

The decrement in the levels of LDL cholesterol in serum observed when β-sitosterol is added to the treatment regimen with colestipol suggests that dietary cholesterol contributes significantly to the pool of sterol utilized for bile acid synthesis and that interdiction of this source leads to increased catabolism of circulating LDL.

The absence of an effect of nicotinic acid on bile acid production (Miettinen 1968) indicates that the profound effectiveness of the combination of nicotinic acid and colestipol is based upon complementarity of mechanism. Inhibition of synthesis of apolipoproteins in liver (Magide et al. 1975) and reduction of turnover of hepatogenous apolipoproteins (Langer and Levy 1971) by nicotinic acid are consistent with this hypothesis. Data on fatty acid flux in humans during sustained treatment with nicotinic acid are insufficient to determine whether decreased secretion of VLDL may be secondary to suppression of intracellular lipolysis in adipose tissue, with a resulting decrease in fatty acid uptake by liver. Decreased hepatic cholesterogenesis during treatment with nicotinic acid persists even during treatment with bile acid sequestrants and thus may contribute to the synergism of these two agents. The increased HDL cholesterol levels observed on this regimen presumably reflect the ability of nicotinic acid to decrease the fractional catabolic rate of HDL (Blum et al. 1977; Shepherd et al. 1979).

The combination of colestipol and nicotinic acid provides a practical means of achieving completely normal levels of serum LDL in patients with heterozygous familial hypercholesterolemia. We have also observed diminution in the size of tendon xanthomata during treatment in several patients, which indicates that mobilization of cholesterol from tissues attends the decrease in LDL levels. Increases in levels of HDL cholesterol may be important in this regard. Until objective appraisal can be made of the impact of such treatment upon the process of atherogenesis, normalization of lipoproteins with this regimen in FH heterozygotes appears to be the judicious course.

References

Blum CB et al. (1977) High density lipoprotein metabolism in man. J Clin Invest 60: 795-807
Eisenberg S, Levy RI (1975) Lipoprotein metabolism. Adv Lipid Res 13: 1-89
Goodman DS et al. (1973) The effects of colestipol resin and of colestipol plus clofibrate on the turnover of plasma cholesterol in man. J Clin Invest 52: 2646-2658
Langer T, Levy RI (1971) The effect of nicotinic acid on the turnover of low density lipoproteins in type II hyperlipoproteinemia. In: Gey KK, Carlson LA (eds) Metabolic effects of nicotinic acid and its derivatives. Hans Huber, Bern
Magide AA et al. (1975) The effect of nicotinic acid on the metabolism of the plasma lipoproteins of rhesus monkeys. Atherosclerosis 21: 205-215
Miettinen TA (1968) Effect of nicotinic acid on catabolism and synthesis of cholesterol in man. Clin Chim Acta 20:43-51
Miettinen TA, Lempinen M (1977) Cholestyramine and ileal bypass in the treatment of familial hypercholesterolemia. J Clin Invest 7: 509-514
Moutafis CD et al. (1971) Cholestyramine and nicotinic acid in the treatment of familial hyperbetalipoproteinaemia in the homozygous form. Atherosclerosis 14:247-258

Myers LH et al. (1976) Mathematical evaluation of methods of estimation of the concentration of the major lipid components of human serum lipoproteins. J Lab Clin Med 88:491–505

Shepherd J et al. (1979) Effects of nicotinic acid therapy on plasma high density lipoprotein subfraction distribution and composition and on apolipoprotein A metabolism. J Clin Invest 63:858–867

Sodhi HS et al. (1971) Effects of chlorophenoxyisobutyrate on the synthesis and metabolism of cholesterol in man. Metabolism 20:348–359

Wolfe BM et al. (1973) Mechanism of the hypolipemic effect of clofibrate in post absorptive man. J Clin Invest 52:2146–2159

Effect of Plasma Lipoextraction and Infusion of Heterologous HDL on the Development of Experimental Atherosclerosis in Rabbits

A.N. Klimov, L.G. Petrova-Maslakova, G.G. Chetchinachvili, L.M. Tchichatarashvili, V.A. Nagornev, and V.F. Tryufanov

Two new techniques for inhibiting experimental atherosclerosis and for accelerating regression of already developed atherosclerosis in rabbits have been
reported: 1) multiple extraction of plasma lipids (lipoextraction) with subsequent restoration of delipidized plasma and erythrocytes into their own
organism, and 2) multiple intravenous infusion of large doses of heterologous
(horse) HDL.

Methods

The influence of lipoextraction was studied in rabbits with pronounced hypercholesterolemia that was achieved by daily administration for a period of 3
months of 500 mg cholesterol in 5 ml sunflower oil through a tube.

After cholesterol administration was discontinued the animals were divided
into two approximately equal groups according to plasma cholesterol level:
control and experimental. After two months of usual laboratory diet, 20-25
ml blood samples were taken from the experimental group (from the ear vein)
for lipid extraction two to three times per week. After ultracentrifugation,
the erythrocyte suspension in a physiological solution was reinjected into
the original donor; the plasma was delipidated with ethyl ether (Avigan 1957).
The delipidated plasma was dialyzed with a 0.9% NaCl solution, and was restored by means of intravenous infusion to its original donors. Each rabbit
was subjected to 20 procedures of lipoextraction over a period of two and one
half months.

The influence of intravenous infusion of large doses of horse HDL was studied
in rabbits in which hypercholesterolemia has been induced by the daily administration of 350 mg cholesterol in sunflower oil. Horse HDL was isolated
from the plasma by ultracentrifugation at d 1.21 after preliminary removal of
VLDL and LDL. Both native and succinylated HDL were used for intravenous infusions. Succinylation was done with succinic anhydride with the aim of decreasing HDL antigenicity.

Intravenous infusion of HDL was begun from small doses (5 mg HDL protein),
increasing the dose of each successive injection by 5 mg up to the final dose
of 50 mg. Ten rabbits were used in this series; five of them received only
cholesterol, and the other five, cholesterol and intravenous HDL infusions.
In the latter group, two rabbits received native HDL and three rabbits received succinylated HDL. All the animals easily endured the infusion of
both native and succinylated HDL. Both study series, lipoextraction of plasma and intravenous infusion of HDL, were carried out on male Chinchilla rabbits during different seasons of the year. Evaluation of total cholesterol
and triglycerides, and also HDL-cholesterol (after precipitating VLDL and LDL
with heparin in the presence of manganese ions), was carried out on autoana-
lyzers AA-2 "Technicon."

Within two months of discontinuing the feeding of rabbits with cholesterol, there occurred a significant decrease in the plasma cholesterol level, whereas the average level of plasma cholesterol in the experimental group of animals set aside for lipoextraction remained higher than in the control group (376 mg% and 264 mg%, respectively). As a result of multiple lipoextractions, plasma cholesterol content in the experimental group dropped to a lower level in comparison with a spontaneous decrease of cholesterol content over the same period of time in the control group (46 mg% and 105 mg%, respectively, $p < 0.05$). The mean quantity of cholesterol removed by lipoextractions from plasma of one rabbit was 236 ± 58 mg. The degree of aortic lesion in the experimental animals was lower than in the control group (35% and 59%, respectively, $p < 0.05$). Fresh lipid deposition in the superficial plaque layers and the formation of atheromatous foci in the depth of the plaques were observed by microscopic study of atherosclerotic lesions of rabbit aorta in the control group. Lipid resolution and the formation of a dense connective lipid-free covering was observed in the rabbits of the experimental group. Thus, the performance of multiple procedures of plasma lipoextraction not only contributed to a decrease in plasma cholesterol concentration, but also accelerated the regression of experimental atherosclerosis.

During the first hours after the intravenous infusion of horse HDL, a high level of HDL-cholesterol is detected in the rabbits, which gradually drops and in 24 hours reaches approximately the initial level. In our experiments, intravenous infusion of horse HDL was carried out on each of 5 consecutive days for 10 weeks. Analysis of the results showed that both native and succinylated HDL produce a similar influence on the plasma lipid and induced the development of experimental atherosclerosis. This is probably explained by the fact that the bond between the protein amino groups and succinic acid in the organism of the animals undergoes quick hydrolysis. Therefore, in the long run, we study the action of native and succinylated HDL together, but not separately.

As can be seen from the data in Table 1, a higher level of HDL-cholesterol ($p < 0.05$) and a lower level of total cholesterol and triglycerides were observed in the animals which were given horse HDL infusions. It was notable that the plasma of animals that received HDL infusions was always clear in contrast to the lipemic plasma of the animals of the control group. Macroscopic studies of the aortas showed that the degree of lesion in the experi-

Table 1. Effect of repeated intravenous horse HDL administrations to rabbits on the development of experimental atherosclerosis.

Expt. Group	No. of infusions	Total HDL administered (mg HDL protein)	End of trial serum lipid (mg%)			% Aorta Lesions	Horse HDL Antibodies
			TC	HDL-C	TG		
Control (n=5)	–	–	726 ± 235	15 ± 1.7	430 ± 198	4 ± 3	–
HDL recipients (n=5)	58	3145	536 ± 115	26 ± 4.9	156 ± 68	35 ± 15	1:16[a] 1:32[b]

[a]After administration of succinylated HDL.
[b]After administration of native HDL.

mental group was not lower, but considerably higher than in the control group (p<0.05).

It should be added that in the plasma of rabbits infused with horse native succinylated HDL, we detected antibodies against these HDL. Thus, infusion of heterologous HDL enhanced the development of experimental atherosclerosis regardless of the favorable changes in the blood lipids. Apparently, the atherogenic role of the immunologic factors dominated the antiatherogenic HDL action.

Reference

Avigan J (1957) Modification of human serum lipoprotein fractions by lipid extraction. J Biol Chem 226:957–964

New Drug Treatments in Hyperlipidaemia[1]

Anders G. Olsson

The aim of drug treatment of hyperlipidaemia is long-term prevention of
atherosclerosis in most cases. This implies that the drug treatment should
(1) effectively reduce atherogenic i.e. very low (VLDL) and low (LDL) density lipoprotein levels, (2) have few side effects and (3) should be well
tolerated and convenient to use. Available serum lipoprotein-lowering drugs
do not fulfull these criteria. For example clofibrate has a poor LDL cholesterol lowering effect and might cause gall stones. Cholestyramine is in
the long run often inconvenient to take and causes in 25% of cases severe
constipation. Nicotinic acid may cause flushing even during continuous
treatment, etc.

From the lipoprotein point of view an unwanted rise in LDL cholesterol may
occur during treatment of type IV hyperlipidaemia with diet (Strisower et
al.1968; Wilson and Lees 1972), clofibrate (Wilson and Lees 1972) and its
derivatives (Olsson et al 1976, 1977) and nicotinic acid (Carlson et al.
1974). On the other hand treatment of type II hyperlipidaemia with bile acid
sequestrating agents might cause increases in VLDL levels (Miller and Nestel
1975; Olsson and Dairou 1978). We are therefore in urgent need of drug therapies that reduce all atherogenic lipoproteins (VLDL, intermediate density
lipoproteins (IDL) and LDL). They should be more convenient to take. One
way is thereby to find new more efficient compounds, another to try combination therapies with drugs with different modes of action. Examples will be
given of both principles.

Serum lipoprotein cholesterol and triglyceride (TG) analysis was performed
according to the routine at King Gustaf V Research Institute (Carlson 1973).

Bezafibrate (2-{4-|2-(4-chlorobenzamido)-ethyl|-phenoxy}-2-methylpropionic
acid) is a clofibrate analogue which in the dose of 0.6 g daily causes a
20% greater decrease of VLDL TG than does clofibrate (Olsson et al.1977).
In an ongoing long term study bezafibrate was still efficient and without
unwanted effects after 1 year of treatment (Table 1).

A dose response study of **ciprofibrate**, 2{p-(2,2-dichlorocyclopropyl)-phenoxyl}
-2-methylpropionic acid, in 26 hyperlipidaemic patients showed that 100 mg
daily efficiently decreased elevated VLDL TG and LDL cholesterol concentrations (Table 2). Also ciprofibrate increased even those high density lipoprotein (HDL) cholesterol concentrations that initially were not low. No
side effects were noted with the drug. Ciprofibrate is therefore a promising lipid lowering drug and a comparative study with clofibrate is now needed.

We have investigated the possibility of counteracting the unwanted rise in
LDL cholesterol following treatment of type IV hyperlipidaemia with clofibrate by adding a small dose of the bile acid sequestrant cholestyramine
(Questran). Twenty-eight hypertriglyceridaemic subjects (22 type IV, of
whom 8 had a LDL cholesterol below 3.5 mmol/l and 6 type IIB) were given

---

[1] Supported by grants from the Swedish Medical Research Council (19X-204)

dietary advice aiming at decreasing their serum TG levels. Two months later they received clofibrate in the dose of 2 g daily, followed by the addition of cholestyramine in the dose of 4 g twice daily two months later. Fasting serum lipids were analysed monthly and serum lipoprotein analysis was performed after each two month period.

Five subjects did not complete the study, two because of lack of cooperation, one because of sudden death, one because of acute cholecystitis and one because of diabetes starting during the study, illnesses that could not be attributed to the treatment per se. Body weight remained constant through the study.

Clofibrate decreased (Table 3) - as expected - mean total and VLDL TG substantially. A small decrease in total cholesterol could be attributed to a decrease in VLDL cholesterol. Mean LDL cholesterol rose insignificantly. Fig. 1 shows that the effect of clofibrate on LDL cholesterol depended on the initial concentration of the latter. A relation ($p < 0.05$) existed between the LDL cholesterol during diet and the effect, the equation obtained stating a reduction on clofibrate if LDL cholesterol was 5.7 mmol or above and an increase if the concentration was below that level.

The addition of cholestyramine caused a significant decrease of LDL cholesterol and Fig. 2 shows that the decrease even now was highly dependent on the initial LDL cholesterol level. However, the LDL cholesterol level at which no increase could be expected according to the regression equation was considerably lower than for clofibrate.

There was no relation between effect (fall or rise) caused by clofibrate and the effect caused by cholestyramine. Only the LDL cholesterol level itself during clofibrate determined the cholestyramine effect.

The findings are in agreement with a previous study with similar approach using colestipol (Rese et al 1976).

It could thus be concluded that the addition of cholestyramine in the small dose of 8 g daily after treatment of hyper VLDL-aemia has a good LDL cholesterol lowering effect, this being better the higher the LDL cholesterol was. One way of coming round the "LDL cholesterol problem" during treatment of hypertriglyceridaemia with for example clofibrate could therefore be the addition of a small dose of cholestyramine.

Table 1. Serum and lipoprotein cholesterol (chol) and triglyceride (TG) concentrations before and during treatment with 600 mg bezafibrate for one year in 14 patients with type IIA and 20 patients with type IV hyperlipidaemia (mmol, mean±SEM)

	Pretreatment		2 months		12 months	
Type	IIA	IV	IIA	IV	IIA	IV
Serum						
chol	8.4 ±0.2	7.1 ±0.2	6.6 ±0.2^{xx}	5.9 ±0.2^{xx}	6.7 ±0.2^{xx}	6.2 ±0.2^{xx}
TG	1.4 ±0.1	3.3 ±0.4	0.9 ±0.1^{xx}	1.7 ±0.1^{xx}	1.0 ±0.1^{xx}	1.8 ±0.1^{xx}
VLDL TG	0.7 ±0.1	2.7 ±0.3	0.4 ±0.1^{xx}	1.1 ±0.1^{xx}	0.4 ±0.1^{xx}	1.1 ±0.1^{xx}
LDL chol	6.3 ±0.2	4.4 ±0.2	4.7 ±0.2^{xx}	4.0 ±0.2^{x}	4.6 ±0.2^{xx}	4.1 ±0.2
HDL chol	1.51±0.09	1.17±0.05	1.69±0.11^{xx}	1.29±0.06^{x}	1.78±0.11^{xx}	1.35±0.07^{xx}

[1] x, xx, xxx indicate significant differences against pretreatment concentrations on $p < 0.05$, $p < 0.01$ and $p < 0.001$ level respectively (Wilcoxon signed-rank test)

Table 2. Serum and lipoprotein cholesterol (chol) and triglyceride (TG) concentration before and during treatment with 100 and 200 mg ciprofibrate daily in patients with type II and IV hyperlipidaemia (mmol/1 mean±SEM).

	Placebo	100 mg	200 mg
Type IIA+IIB (n=16) Serum			
chol	9.7 ±0.11	7.1 ±0.3 xxx[1]	6.6 ±0.3 xxx
TG	1.4 ±0.1	1.0 ±0.1 xx	0.9 ±0.1 xxx
VLDL TG	0.7 ±0.1	0.4 ±0.04 xx	0.2 ±0.04 xxx
LDL chol	7.3 ±0.5	5.2 ±0.3 xxx	4.5 ±0.2 xxx
HDL chol	1.78±0.1	1.92±0.13 x	1.80±0.1
Type IV (n=10) Serum			
chol	7.3 ±0.2	6.4 ±0.3 x	6.4 ±0.4
TG	4.1 ±0.5	2.2 ±0.2 xxx	2.2 ±0.3 xxx
VLDL TG	3.2 ±0.5	1.5 ±0.2 xx	1.3 ±0.2 xx
LDL chol	4.6 ±0.3	4.7 ±0.3	4.7 ±0.3
HDL chol	0.99±0.11	1.16±0.04	1.05±0.05

[1]See footnote to Table 1.

Table 3. Serum and lipoprotein cholesterol (chol) and triglyceride (TG) concentrations in 23 patients (6 type IIB, 17 type IV) before and during treatment with diet, diet + clofibrate (2 g daily) and diet + clofibrate + cholestyramine (8 g daily) (mean±SEM, mmol/1).

	Diet	+ Clofibrate	+ Cholestyramine
Serum			
chol	7.7 ±0.3	7.2 ±0.3 x[1]	6.6 ±0.3 x
TG	4.3 ±0.3	2.6 ±0.2 xxx	3.1 ±0.3
VLDL TG	3.5 ±0.3	1.8 ±0.2 xxx	2.3 ±0.3
LDL chol	4.6 ±0.3	4.9 ±0.3	4.1 ±0.2 xxx
HDL chol	1.21±0.08	1.30±0.08	1.20±0.09

[1] See footnote to Table 1.

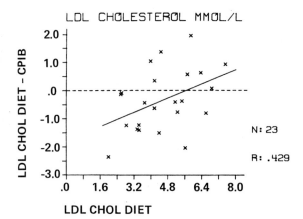

FIG. 1. Change in LDL cholesterol after clofibrate (concentration during diet - concentration during clofibrate) in relation to LDL cholesterol during preceding dietary treatment.

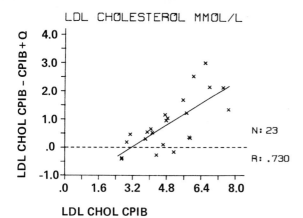

FIG. 2. Change in LDL cholesterol after clofibrate
+ cholestyramine treatment (concentration during
clofibrate - concentration during clofibrate +
cholestyramine) in relation to LDL cholesterol
during preceding clofibrate treatment

References

Carlson K (1973) Lipoprotein fractionation. J Clin Path Suppl 5:32
Carlson LA, Olsson AG, Orö L, Rössner S, Walldius G (1974) Effects of hypo-
        lipidemic regimes on serum lipoproteins. In: Schettler G, Weizel A (eds)
        Atherosclerosis III. Springer-Verlag, Heidelberg, p 768
Miller NE, Nestel PJ (1975) Differences among hyperlipoproteinaemic subjects
        in the response of lipoprotein lipids to resin therapy. Europ J Clin
        Invest 5:241
Olsson AG, Dairou F (1978) Acute effects of cholestyramine on serum lipopro-
        tein concentrations in type II hyperlipoproteinaemia. Atherosclerosis
        29:53
Olsson AG, Rössner S, Walldius G, Carlson LA (1976) Effect of Gemfibrozil
        on lipoprotein concentrations in different types of hyperlipoproteinaemia.
        Proc Roy Soc Med 69, Suppl 2:28
Olsson AG, Rössner S, Walldius G, Carlson LA, Lang D (1977) Effect of BM 15075
        on lipoprotein concentrations in different types of hyperlipoproteinaemia.
        Atherosclerosis 27:279
Rose HG, Haft GK, Juliano J (1976) Clofibrate-induced low density lipoprotein
        elevation therapeutic implications and treatment by colestipol resin.
        Atherosclerosis 23:413
Strisower EH, Adamson G, Strisover B (1968) Treatment of hyperlipidaemias.
        Am J Med 34:488
Wilson DE, Lees RS (1972) Metabolic relationship among the plasma lipopro-
        teins. Reciprocal changes in the concentrations of very low and low
        density lipoproteins in man. J Clin Invest 51:1051

Apoprotein Changes Following Treatments with Hypolipidemic Drugs

C.R. Sirtori, G. Franceschini, M. Sirtori, G. Gianfranceschi, and A. Poli

Changes in plasma lipids and in lipoprotein distribution are well known consequences of the application of hypolipidemic drug regimens. In particular, VLDL lipids decrease with concomitant transient or permanent LDL cholesterol increases (Carlson et al. 1977); according to some reports also HDL cholesterol levels may increase following clofibrate (Wallentin 1978) or nicotinic acid treatments (Blum et al. 1977). Newer clofibrate derivatives appear more likely to increase HDL cholesterol (Olsson and Lang, 1978).

Interest in a separate role for apoproteins in the development of the atherogenic process has been elicited by the observation of a role for specific apoproteins in regulating tissue cholesterol biosynthesis (Goldstein and Brown, 1977) and enzyme activities leading to lipoprotein catabolism (La Rosa et al. 1970). Recent epidemiological findings indicate that the concentrations of specific apoproteins are correlated to the development of peripheral or coronary artery disease (Bradby et al. 1978; Avogaro et al. 1979).

In the past several years, apoprotein patterns have been analyzed in animals and in man following drug treatments in different experimental and clinical conditions. Analyses were carried out by sodium dodecyl sulphate (SDS) gel electrophoresis and by isoelectric focusing (IEF), as well as, when feasible, by appropriate immunological tests. Apoprotein changes are described following treatments with metformin in humans and rabbits and with tiadenol in hypertriglyceridemic patients. A word of caution is also given on rat data pertaining to HDL increases following drug treatments, especially in the case of chlorinated hydrocarbons.

Metformin. This drug, shown by us (Sirtori et al. 1977) to markedly decrease cholesterol atheromatosis in rabbits without significantly reducing plasma cholesterol levels, may significantly reduce the content of apoprotein E both in rabbits and in type III humans (Sirtori et al. 1978). In this latter case, an increased apo A1/A2 ratio may also be observed in HDL(Shore V.G., unpublished results).

An ongoing study on the effects of metformin[1] in patients, both hyper- and normo-lipidemic, with peripheral arterial disease has indicated that changes occur both in VLDL and HDL apoproteins. HDL cholesterol increases following drug treatment both in normo- and hyperlipidemic subjects. Moreover, an increase of A1 is noted in treated patients. Studies on the lymph

---

[1] Glucophage, Spemsa, Florence, Italy.

composition of hypercholesterolemic rabbits also suggest that more apo A1 is present in intestinal lipoproteins of drug treated animals.

Tiadenol. This new hypolipidemic drug is chemically unrelated to clofibrate, but has an apparently similar pharmacological profile (Martin and Feldmann 1974; Crepaldi et al. 1978). In a clinical study on carbohydrate (CHO)$_2$ inducible and non-inducible type IV patients it was noted that Tiadenol significantly lowers VLDL triglycerides, particularly after CHO induction. In this lipoprotein fraction a decrease of apo E, as assessed by SDS electrophoresis and by IEF, is observed in the majority of treated patients, even in the absence of a significant triglyceride reduction (Fig. 1); E isoprotein ratios are not modified. A relative increase of VLDL triglycerides, to the expense of VLDL cholesterol and of VLDL B apoprotein, is also observed. There is thus evidence for a significant enlargement of VLDL particles after treatment. Preliminary data indicate that Tiadenol does not activate lipoprotein lipase, in contrast to clofibrate and similar agents (Nikkila et al. 1977). The apoprotein data suggest a reduced VLDL secretion, rather than an enhanced catabolism, as the most likely mechanism of Tiadenol in hypertriglyceridemia.

Increased HDL levels in rats. In view of the current interest in HDL cholesterol as a protective factor against clinical atherosclerosis, several quantitative studies on these lipoproteins have been carried out in experi-

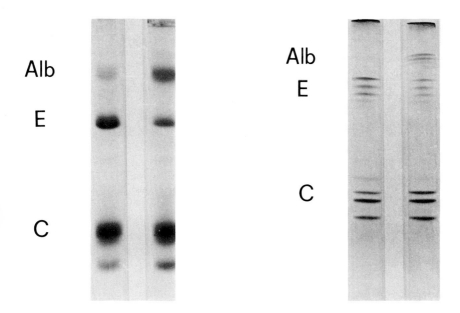

Fig. 1 - SDS (left) and IEF (right) electrophoretic patterns in a type IV patient before and after tiadenol treatment. A reduction of apo E is noted with both techniques, without changes in the E isoprotein ratios.

[2] Tiaterol, Midy, Milan, Italy.

mental animals. A stimulatory effect on HDL cholesterol levels was suggested, among others, for chlorinated hydrocarbons (Ishikawa et al. 1978).
In experimental studies with a highly toxic chlorinated derivative, tetra-
chlorodibenzodioxin (TCDD) (Reggiani 1978) a marked increase of HDL cholesterol levels in normal rats after a single dose of the compound was
noted. However, upon examination of the HDL apoprotein pattern by IEF, a
marked decrease of the CIII-0/CIII-3 ratio was evident (Fig. 2).

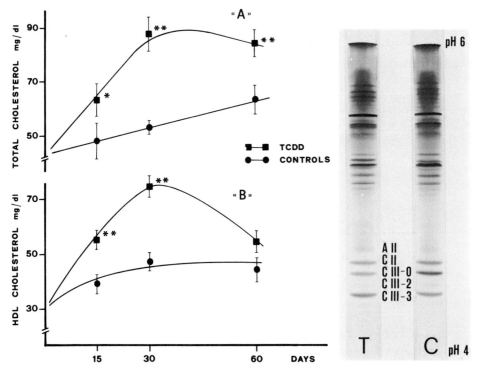

Fig. 2 — Left: plasma total (A) and HDL (B) cholesterol levels after a
single 20 γ/kg dose of TCDD in rats. Right: IEF patterns of HDL
apoproteins from control (C) and TCDD (T) rats 15 days from treatment. A
significant increase of apo CIII-3 with decreased apo CIII-0 is notice-
able, without significant alterations in the other apoprotein components.

This observation is similar to that already reported for streptozotocin
diabetes (Bar-On et al. 1976) and suggests that caution should be applied
to the interpretation of experimental results of a similar type. Rats have,
in fact, a marked expansion of the HDL pool, which may be further increased following treatments which variously affect lipoprotein metabolism.
The detection of HDL apoprotein abnormalities suggests that increased HDL
cholesterol levels may not be simply the result of increased lipoprotein
lipase activity, as generally believed for humans (Nikkila 1978), but the
consequence of as yet unidentified derangements in the lipoprotein synthetic pathway.

In conclusion, clinical and experimental data on plasma apoprotein composition may provide useful information on the mechanism of action of hypolipidemic compounds. They may also indicate whether drug effects may be
considered as beneficial or as indicative of a selective toxicity.

References

Avogaro P, Bittolo Bon G, Cazzolato G and Quinci GB (1979) Are lipoproteins better discriminators than lipids for atherosclerosis? Lancet i: 901-903

Bar-On H, Roheim PS and Eder HA (1976) Serum lipoproteins and apolipoproteins in rats with streptozotocin diabetes. J Clin Invest 57: 714-721

Blum CB, Levy RI, Eisenberg S, Hall M III, Goebel RH and Berman M (1977) High density lipoprotein metabolism in man. J Clin Invest 60: 795-806

Bradby GVH, Valente AJ and Walton KW (1978) Serum high-density lipoproteins in peripheral vascular disease. Lancet ii: 271-1274

Carlson LA, Olsson AG and Ballantyne D (1977) On the rise in low density and high density lipoproteins in response to the treatment of hypertriglyceridemia in type IV and V hyperlipoproteinemias. Atherosclerosis 26: 603-609

Crepaldi G, Briani G, Senin U, Montaguti V, Capurso A and Bondioli A (1978) Multicenter trial with tiadenol in primary hyperlipidemias. In: LA Carlson et al. (eds) International Conference on Atherosclerosis, Raven Press, New York, pp 343-346

Goldstein JL and Brown MS (1977) Atherosclerosis: the low density lipoprotein receptor hypothesis. Metabolism 26: 1257-1275

Ishikawa TT, Mc Neely S, Steiner PM, Glueck CJ, Mellies M, Gartside PS and Mc Millin C (1978) Effects of chlorinated hydrocarbons or plasma α-lipoprotein cholesterol in rats. Metabolism 27: 89-96

La Rosa JC, Levy RI, Herbert P, Lux SE and Fredrickson DS (1970) A specific apoprotein activator for lipoprotein lipase. Biochim Biophys Res Comm 41: 57-62

Martin E and Feldman G (1974) Etude hystologique et ultrastructural du foie chez le rat après administration subaigue d'un nouvel agent hypolipidemiant, le bis (hydroxyethyl-thio) 1-10 decane. Pathol Biol,- 22-II: 179-188

Nikkila EA, Huttunen JK and Ehnholm C (1977) Effect of clofibrate on post-heparin plasma triglyceride lipase activities in patients with hypertriglyceridemia. Metabolism 26:179-186

Nikkila EA (1978) Metabolic endocrine control of plasma high density lipoprotein concentrations. In: AM Gotto Jr et al. (eds) High density lipoproteins and atherosclerosis. Elsevier/North Holland, pp 177-192

Olsson AG and Lang PD (1978) Dose-response study of bezafibrate on serum lipoprotein concentrations in hyperlipoproteinemia. Atherosclerosis 31: 421-428

Reggiani G (1978) Medical problems raised by the TCDD contamination in Seveso, Italy. Arch Toxicol 40: 161-188

Sirtori CR, Catapano A, Ghiselli GC, Innocenti AL and Rodriguez J (1977) Metformin: an antiatherosclerotic agent modifying very low density lipoproteins in rabbits. Atherosclerosis 26: 78-89

Sirtori CR, Catapano A, Ghiselli GC, Shore B and Shore VG (1978) Effects of metformin on lipoprotein composition in rabbits and man. Prot Biol Fluids 25: 379-382

Wallentin L (1978) Lecithin: cholesterol acyl transfer rate and high density lipoprotein in plasma during dietary and clofibrate treatment of hypertriglyceridemic subjects. Atherosclerosis 31: 41-52

Milieu and Function of Arterial Wall—The Clues to Unique Reactivity[1]

M. Daria Haust

Arteries (Burton 1954; McDonald 1960; Abramson 1962) are active organs designed to propel the blood from the heart and distribute it to various tissues and organs. They function unceasingly and are always exposed to a high
blood pressure, deriving the energy necessary for that work from the mural
components themselves.

The large elastic arteries (aorta, innominate, pulmonary, common carotid,
subclavian) maintain the pressure in the diastole and thus effect a relatively constant flow of blood in the arterial system. The mural components concerned with this function are the medial elastic tissue elements. They maintain a tension opposing the expansile force of the blood pressure, and absorb
the impact of the cardiac pump and that of the blood delivered into the circulation.

The medium size or muscular arteries distribute the blood from the elastic
arteries to organs and tissues. The supply of blood is "geared" to the requirement of these various tissues which in turn depends on their functional
status. Pending the demand, the muscular arteries regulate the delivered
blood volume by changing the size of their lumina; this function is governed
by nervous control of the medial smooth muscle cells (Ham 1969).

The structural substratum of the artery is well suited to fulfill the function
of distensibility and "recoiling", to furnish energy for this purpose, and
to provide a smooth surface exposed to the contents of the flowing blood,
aiding even to its fluidity (Todd 1971). Moreover, to prevent a possible
ill-effect that would result if the arterial wall were nourished or "drained"
by conventional means, i.e., by small vascular channels, these necessities
of self-maintenance are all fulfilled by alternative mechanisms. Thus, the
intima of normal arteries is not vascularized and the same applies to the
media of all human arteries with the exception of the external part in the
thoracic aorta. The arterial blood pressure always is high and were the intimal or inner medial capillaries derived from the vasa vasorum they would
collapse since their blood pressure is exceedingly low. To permit an effective diffusion, the wall of the terminal vascular and lymphatic channels of
necessity must be thin. Were the intimal and medial capillaries to originate
from the innermost aspect of the intima, i.e., connecting with the lumen,
the thin walls would rupture upon exposure to the high (luminal) arterial
pressure. The resultant intramural hemorrhage and subsequent repair in such
circumstances would culminate in severe and advancing structural changes and
functional consequences. Similarly absent are the lymphatic capillaries
which usually are concerned with the effective drainage of fluids and substances not returned to the venous circulation (Abramson 1962). It is therefore of interest that the same factor that imposes the constant workload upon
the mural components, i.e., the high blood pressure, is at the same time the
positive force compensating for the structural shortcomings; it effects the

[1] Supported by grants-in-aid of research T.3-11 from The Ontario Heart Foundation, Toronto, Ontario, and MT-1037 from Medical Research Council of
Canada.

94

nourishment and clearing of the arterial wall by "driving" the necessary nutrients from the lumen into the intima, as well as the transmural transport of metabolites by means of pressure and diffusion gradients across the arterial wall (Adams 1970). It is probable that the arterial glycosaminoglycans-rich ground substance aids in the process of take-up, filtration and diffusion of the above substances (Laurent and Persson 1964), facilitating simultaneously the fluctuation of the mural volume with changes of the blood pressure owing to its "spongy" properties. This in turn promotes the movement of substances across the arterial wall.

In addition to the basic nutrients (amino acids, glucose, salt) small amounts of albumin (Haust 1968), alpha-lipoproteins and beta-lipoproteins (Haust 1968; Kao and Wissler 1965; Walton and Williamson 1968), but no fibrinogen enter the intima from the lumen under normal conditions. Apparently, the mechanisms of the transmural transport are operating satisfactorily under normal circumstances, and the influx of blood components is in equilibrium with the forces clearing the wall. This equilibrium may be disturbed easily by a multitude of factors which relate to the blood pressure, constituents of plasma, and the status of mural components, with a resultant focal intimal accumulation of substances that entered from the lumen and of local metabolites.

An important factor in the clearing process of the arterial wall is the thickness of the intima, i.e., the so-called diffuse intimal thickening (DIT). It has been an almost general consensus of opinion that the DIT represents, or is the necessary outcome of normal growth and remodelling of the large and medium size arteries (Jores 1924), and that in fact it is a necessary structural adjustment to postnatally beginning, altered hemodynamics of circulation (Geer and Haust 1972). In the coronary arteries, for example, the DIT acquires even special features not observed in DIT of other arteries, in the form of an intermediary layer (Gross et al. 1934). This layer, interposed between the media and the intima, consists of smooth muscle bundles oriented longitudinally; it replaces segments or a considerable circumference of the internal elastic lamina (IEL). There must be some reason why this phenomenon occurs. Whereas no concrete data exist to explain it, it is reasonable to postulate that such an interposition of contractile elements is an attempt at substituting for a less expendable or more restrictive IEL in muscular arteries that are exposed to an extremely high blood pressure and to patterns of flow imposed by the episodic contractions of the heart. It is tempting to assume that this newly developed layer would allow for an elongation of a given arterial segment without reducing the diameter (Geer and Haust 1972). The DIT, no matter how necessary or useful it may be from the developmental and functional point of view is, on the other hand, an added obstacle to the nutrition of and transport across the arterial wall. Associated with it is the tendency of the connective tissues that constitute the DIT to age prematurely (Movat et al. 1958; Haust 1978). The sclerosed hyalinized collagen and otherwise degenerated elastic tissues are less pliable and less "diffusible", and thus add further to the problems of local nutrition and transmural transport, increasing the already existing tendency to focal accumulation of metabolites and substances which entered from the blood. It is to be expected that such intimal foci will induce in time endothelial changes with consequent disturbed permeability, and such persisting foci themselves will evoke a local tissue reaction, i.e., a process of repair. These features of local difficulties in themselves are injurious to the intima and may be considered as a form of "internal injury", i.e., arising within the arterial wall, largely intima, itself (Haust 1970).

Once the above process sets into a motion tissue reactions of repair at least two features of the arterial wall become detrimental to that intended healing process, i.e., the lack of capillaries which elsewhere in the body aid this process, and the never-ceasing movement of the arterial tissues.

Furthermore, to remain as adapted as possible to the required function, the repair tissue of the inner wall must mimic the structural features of the normal intima. These requirements dictate that the repair tissue also be avascular and composed only of normal intimal elements. Indeed, the organization of blood proteins that gained access to and became arrested within the intima, proceeds by avascular means (Rössle 1944) and smooth muscle cells rather than fibroblasts are the elements concerned with the connective tissue elaboration (Haust et al. 1960). In an ideal situation the outcome of such subtle "maintenance" repair is only a slight focal increase of connective tissues whose composition and structural organization resembles closely those of normal intima. The outcome may be considered to represent a restitutio ad integrum (Haust 1970).

The peculiarities of the arterial wall that determine its unique reactivity not only relate to the features of structure and function discussed above, but in addition reflect, particularly at an age beyond the young adult life, a remarkable premature aging and degeneration of the arterial connective tissues (Yu and Blumenthal 1963; Manley 1965); this applies to both, normal mural components and those acquired in the process of the subtle "maintenance" repair. This premature degeneration has been explained conventionally by the exposure of the wall to continuous tension to which the arteries are subjected, and the difficulties in maintaining an optimal milieu for the mural components by the tissue fluids "bathing" them. Another factor that should be considered is the high oxygen tension to which the intimal connective tissues are constantly exposed. Whereas the high oxygen tension is necessary for the metabolic requirements of the intima and the other mural components, an exposure to it over many years may have an adverse effect upon the connective tissues in analogy to the pathogenesis of retrolental fibroplasia in infants who are therapeutically exposed to a high oxygen tension.

It may be stated in summary that even prior to any influence of injurious elements that set into motion the process of atherosclerosis, the intima of the arterial wall is at a considerable disadvantage. Among other aspects, there is a continuous and "normal" process of sclerogenesis which is promoted by at least two forces, i.e., the growth and remodelling and those of "maintenance". In addition, there is a premature degeneration of these connective tissues with at least three contributing factors: constant tension, mural avascularity and possibly high oxygen tension.

References

Abramson DI (1962) Blood Vessels and Lymphatics. Academic Press, New York
Adams CWM (1970) Local factors in atherogenesis: an introduction. In: Jones RJ (ed) Atherosclerosis. Springer, New York, pp 28-34
Burton AC (1954) Relation of structure to function of the tissues of the wall of blood vessels. Physiol Rev 34: 619-642
Geer JC, Haust MD (1972) Smooth muscle cells in atherosclerosis. In: Pollak OJ, Simms HS, Kirk JE (eds) Monographs on Atherosclerosis, Vol 2. S Karger, Basel
Gross L, Epstein EZ, Kugel MA (1934) Histology of the coronary arteries and their branches in the human heart. Amer J Path 10: 253-274
Ham AW (1969) Histology, 6th edn. JB Lippincott Company, Toronto
Haust MD (1968) Electron microscopic and immunohistochemical studies of fatty streaks in human aorta. In: Miras CJ, Howard AN, Paoletti R (eds) Progr Biochem Pharmacol, Vol 4. S Karger, Basel, pp 429-437
Haust MD (1970) Injury and repair in the pathogenesis of atherosclerotic lesions. In: Jones RJ (ed) Atherosclerosis. Springer, New York, pp 12-20
Haust MD (1978) Atherosclerosis in childhood. In: Rosenberg HS, Bolande RP (eds) Perspectives in Pediatric Pathology, Vol 4. Year Book Medical Publishers, Chicago, pp 155-216

Haust MD, More RH, Movat HZ (1960) The role of smooth muscle cells in the fibrogenesis of arteriosclerosis. Amer J Path 37: 377–389

Jores L (1924) Arterien. In: Henke F, Lubarsch O (eds) Herz und Gefässe. J Springer, Berlin (Handbuch der speziellen pathologischen Anatomie und Histologie, Band II, pp 608–786)

Kao VC, Wissler RW (1965) A study of the immunohistochemical localization of serum lipoproteins and other plasma proteins in human atherosclerotic lesions. Exp Molec Path 4: 465–479

Laurent TC, Persson H (1964) The interaction between polysaccharides and other macromolecules. VII The effect of various polymers on the sediment-ation rates of serum albumin and alpha-crystallin. Biochim Biophys Acta (Amst) 83: 141–147

Manley G (1965) Changes in vascular mucopolysaccharides with age and blood pressure. Brit J Exp Path 46: 125–134

McDonald DA (1960) Blood Flow in Arteries. E Arnold (Publishers), London

Movat HZ, More RH, Haust MD (1958) The diffuse intimal thickening of the human aorta with aging. Amer J Path 34: 1023–1031

Rössle R (1944) Über die serösen Entzündungen der Organe. Virchows Arch path Anat 311: 252–284

Todd AS (1971) Endothelial fibrinolysis and blood flow. Lancet 1: 1179

Walton KW, Williamson N (1968) Histological and immunofluorescent studies on the evolution of the human atheromatous plaque. J Atheroscler Res 8: 599–624

Yu SY, Blumenthal HT (1963) The calcification of elastic fibers. I Biochem-ical studies. J Gerontol 18: 119–126

Atherogenetic Factors Intrinsic to the Artery Wall

Kenneth W. Walton

This Workshop has examined the functional role of various components of
the arterial wall in relation to atherogenesis. My task is now to summarise
the new information which has been presented, to contrast this with existing
knowledge and to consider points which are still the subject of controversy.

Endothelium. This is usually regarded as the primary permeability barrier
although Dr. Smith has stimulated our discussions by dissenting from this
view. It is also widely held that there are regional differences in
permeability in large arteries such as the aorta. This is because Evans
Blue, injected intravenously, gives rise to 'blue' and 'white' areas, each
with a characteristic distribution, even in the normal aorta. The 'blue'
areas have been shown to be localised areas of sub-endothelial oedema, rather
than areas of increased thickness of solid tissue, the colour being accounted
for by the oedema fluid being rich in dye-labelled albumin. In acute
experiments employing agents injurious to endothelial cells this oedema
accounts for the overall increase in thickness of the sub-endothelial space
(intima) as compared with that in 'white' areas.

Dr. Schwartz and his colleagues now draw attention to, and illustrate,
morphological differences in the nature of the intercellular junctions
between endothelial cells and(in confirmation of previous observations)
differences in the thickness of the glycocalyx, between 'blue' and 'white'
areas. One wonders whether such changes might be effect, rather than cause,
in arising because the endothelium is stretched and distended over the
localised regions of sub-endothelial oedema of 'blue' areas.

Passage of Soluble Material Through Intact Endothelium. It is now widely
agreed that macromolecules pass from the blood into the artery wall both by
passing through cells and also between cells. Transcellular passage in
micropinocytotic vesicles from the lumenal to the ablumenal surface (as illustrated by Schwartz et al.) appears to be accomplished without breakdown or
'digestion' of the material being transported through the cell. This can
also be shown, in the case of low-density lipoproteins (LDL), by comparing
photographs of the same field of a frozen section of arterial wall from the
lipid-fed and hyperlipoproteinaemic rabbit where the section has been treated
first by immunofluorescence and then subsequently stained conventionally for
lipid. This allows direct comparison of the tissue, cell for cell and
field for field, by both techniques. Precise correspondence can be shown
for reactivity for apolipoprotein B(apo B) and lipid staining in endothelial
cells and in the immediately subjacent intima (see FIGS. 4A and 4B of
Walton et al. 1976). This allows the inference that LDL is transported in
an intact state through the cell to the underlying intima(see also Walton
1975).

On the other hand, uptake by selective interaction with specific receptors
and the formation of 'coated vesicles' which eventually fuse with lysosomes,
appear to be the stages of a mechanism for the catabolism of macromolecules,

including LDL. It is interesting that Schwartz et al. confirm the virtual
absence or infrequent occurrence of coated vesicles in endothelial cells.
This again suggests that these cells are mainly concerned with the transcellular transfer of macromolecules rather than with their breakdown.

Passage of Cells Through Intact Endothelium. An alternative route for entry,
not only of macromolecules, but also of blood cells, into the intima is via
opened intercellular junctions. It should be recalled that Poole and Florey
(1958) published light microscopic pictures of mononuclear cells apparently
'en passage' between endothelial cells and resembling the SEM appearance
now shown in FIG. 14 of Schwartz et al. The occurrence of 'stomata' between
endothelial cells (possibly representing sites of penetration of the endothelium by blood cells) and resembling the ostia now described, was also
noted by Poole (unpublished observations presented to British Atherosclerosis
Discussion Group Meeting, Oxford 1970) and there are many earlier and similar
observations going back at least a century (see Altschul 1954). The possible
role of mononuclear phagocytic cells entering the wall in this fashion in relation to atherogenesis is discussed below.

Endothelial Injury. Dr. Abel Robertson and Dr. Björkerud have both
discussed the various ways in which endothelial cell damage can arise
naturally or be induced experimentally. Both our contributors have studied
traumatic endothelial damage produced by balloons or mercury-filled
catheters and Dr. Robertson has now illustrated very clearly the stages of
the process leading to endothelial repair following experimentally-induced
osmotic damage. There have been several allusions to the work of Minick
et al.(1977, 1979) which showed that intimal thickening due to new tissue
formation and lipid deposition occur beneath areas of repair rather than in
areas denuded of overlying endothelium. Robertson confirms that lipid
accumulation in medial cells is also most marked beneath areas of re-
endothelialisation in his model.

In this connection it is worth recalling that Hauss et al. (1969) showed that
endothelial damage, however produced, gives rise to a 'non-specific
mesenchymal reaction' involving cell proliferation and glycosaminoglycan
synthesis by arterial wall cells. It seems likely that simple insudation
of plasma into the sub-endothelial tissues in denuded areas is not in itself
of significance but rather it is the firm binding of certain plasma proteins
(especially LDL and fibrinogen) to intimal components which initiates
atherogenesis. Such binding is most likely to occur where the 'mesenchymal
reaction' (i.e. cellular activity) is at its most intense, namely, in
re-endothelialising areas where metabolic activity and glycosaminoglycan
synthesis is high, as Minick et al. (1979) found.

A similar effect is seen in plastic prostheses used for arterial bypass
procedures in humans. Lipid (as lipoprotein) is often demonstrable in
prostheses which have been in position for months or years. But the lipoprotein deposits are strictly confined to areas of the fibrinous pseudo-
intima undergoing transformation to new fibrous tissue and characterised by
glycosaminoglycan-rich interstitial ground substance formation (see Fig. 3
of Walton 1978).

Smooth Muscle Cells and other Cells Involved in Atherogenesis. Dr. Titus
has reviewed for us the evidence relating to the role of the smooth muscle
cell in plaque formation and my co-chairman, together with Dr. Jack Geer,
published an excellent monograph on this topic (Geer and Haust 1972).
However, there is good evidence that mononuclear cells (either blood

monocytes or tissue histiocytes) also play a part by accumulating lipid (lipoprotein) to form fat-filled or foam cells in the intima. Dr. Schwartz has shown us how mononuclear cells can be found in the aortic intima of pigs and baboons in sections examined in the electron microscope and similar observations have been made in other species (e.g. see Joris, Stetz and Majno 1979). Dr. Adams has brought to our attention the way in which histochemical methods (and in particular a technique for detecting the lysosomal enzyme, β-galactosidase, as a marker) for mononuclear phagocytes can be utilised in light microscopy to show these cells in rabbit and human lesions. He has also drawn attention to the particular abundance of mono-nuclear cells in complicated human lesions where they may even fuse to form giant cells.

Walton et al. (1976) drew attention to the apparent functional difference, in capacity to proteolyse lipoprotein, between intimal fat-filled cells and fat-containing cells of the superficial media in experimental atherosclerosis. Rabbit intimal fat-filled cells show variable immuno-reactivity and often a completely negative reaction for apo B (suggesting a capacity completely to degrade the immuno-reactive site which resides in this apoprotein). On the other hand, medial fat-filled cells (which are unmistakeably smooth muscle cells from their morphology, staining reactions, content of organelles and position) often show persistent positive reactivity for apoB (see Figs. 3,4, 5 and 13 of Walton et al. 1976). This suggests that the medial cells, when fully differentiated as myocytes and in position in the artery wall, degrade lipoprotein less readily then intimal mononuclear phagocytic cells. Similar effects can also be seen in human atherosclerotic lesions.

Dr. Sinzinger has presented his findings which suggest that human smooth muscle cell proliferation in the artery wall either induces or enhances prostacyclin generation and that the aortic tissues of species prone to the development of atherosclerosis release less PGI_2 than those of less susceptible species. Diminished prostacyclin production by endothelial cells, he has proposed, may be an important factor in atherosclerosis in influencing platelet adhesion and thrombus formation.

The Internal Elastic Lamina and the Binding of Macromolecules in the Intima.
Dr. Smith's suggestion that the internal elastic lamina, rather than endothelium, is the main permeability barrier to macromolecules, seems at first sight like a revival of the proposal by Gofman and Young (1963) that lipoprotein deposition in arterial intima arises because of arrested filtration of plasma through the artery wall due to blockage of the fenestrations in the internal elastic lamina. However, any barrier offered by the elastic lamina is evidently only a temporary and inefficient one since penetration of LDL into the deeper layers of arteries or of heart valves (Walton et al. 1970) is frequent, especially in the elderly. It seems more likely that Dr. Smith intended to convey the view that the internal elastic lamina appears to act as a boundary for lipoprotein deposition because of the greater binding of LDL that occurs to components of the intima than occurs in the media.

Nevertheless, as Dr. Robert points out, there is evidence for direct binding of LDL to elastin and he has now produced new data which suggest this may be of significance in relation to elastin degradation. While we have been aware of the elastases present in platelets, leucocytes and in pancreatic secretions, Dr. Robert has now characterised the elastase of plasma as being directly associated with the plasma lipoproteins. The binding of LDL to collagen and elastin has been examined ultrastructurally, using the immunoperoxidase technique (Walton and Morris 1977) and other immunohistological methods (Walton and Bradby 1977; Bradby et al. 1979).

It was reported by Larrue et al. (1977) that rabbit fibroblasts, when grown in tissue culture in normal rabbit serum, produce normal collagen whereas the same cells, when grown in hyperlipoproteinaemic serum, produced Fibrous Long Spacing Collagen. Morris et al. (1978) found LDL to be bound directly to Fibrous Long Spacing Collagen in human atherosclerotic plaques and suggested that, since this form of collagen is known to have low tensile strength, the induction by LDL of this abnormality of collagen assembly might explain, at a molecular level, the tendency to weakening, dilation, aneurysm formation etc. known to occur in atheromatous vessels.

In summary, therefore, one may conclude that this Workshop has assembled evidence to show that the insudation of blood components into the artery wall results in a wide range of effects upon the cells and tissues intrinsic to the wall to give rise to what we recognise as atherosclerosis.

References

Altschul R(1954) Endothelium. Macmillan, New York, pp 12-14

Bradby GVH, Walton KW, Watts R (1979) The binding of total low-density lipoproteins in human arterial intima affected and unaffected by atherosclerosis. Atherosclerosis 32: 403-422

Geer JC, Haust MD (1972) Smooth muscle cells in atherosclerosis. Karger, Basel

Gofman JW, Young W (1963) The filtration concept of atherosclerosis and serum lipids in the diagnosis of atherosclerosis. In: Sandler M, Bourne GH(eds) Atherosclerosis and its origin. Academic Press, New York

Hauss WH, Gerlach U, Junge-Hülsing G, Themann H, Wirth W (1969) Studies on the 'non-specific mesenchymal reaction' and the 'transit zone' in myocardial lesions and atherosclerosis. Ann N Y Acad Sci 156: 207-218

Joris I, Stetz E, Majno G (1979) Lymphocytes and monocytes in the aortic intima - an electron microscopic study in the rat. Atherosclerosis 34: 221-231

Larrue J, Daret D, Demond J, Bricaud H (1977) Fibrous long spacing collagen in aortic explants of normal rabbit cultured in hypercholesterolaemic serum. Atherosclerosis 28: 53-59

Minick CR, Stemerman MB, Insull W (1977) Effect of regenerated endothelium on lipid accumulation in the arterial wall. Proc Natl Acad Sci USA 74: 1724-1728

Minick CR, Stemerman MB, Insull W (1979) Role of endothelium and hyper-cholesterolaemia in intimal thickening and lipid accumulation. Am J Pathol 95: 131-158

Morris CJ, Bradby GVH, Walton KW (1978) Fibrous long spacing collagen in human atherosclerosis. Atherosclerosis 31: 345-354

Poole JCF, Florey HW (1958) Changes in the endothelium of the aorta and the behaviour of macrophages in experimental atheroma of rabbits. J Path Bact 75: 245-250

Walton KW (1975) Studies on experimental atherosclerosis by immuno-fluorescence. Adv Exper Med Biol 63: 371-377

Walton KW (1978) Critical re-evaluation of the role of lipids In: Wood C (ed) Cardiovascular Medicine Controversies: Royal Society of Medicine International Congress and Symposium Series No 2. Academic Press and Royal Society of Medicine, London pp 77-81

Walton KW, Bradby GVH (1977) The significance of 'bound' and 'labile' fractions of low-density lipoprotein and fibrinogen in the arterial wall. Adv Exper Med Biol 82: 888-893

Walton KW, Morris CJ (1977) Studies on the passage of plasma proteins across arterial endothelium in relation to atherogenesis. Prog Biochem Pharmacol 13: 138-152

Walton KW, Williamson N, Johnson AG (1970) The pathogenesis of athero-sclerosis of the mitral and aortic valves. J Path 101: 205-220

Walton KW, Dunkerley DJ, Johnson AG, Khan MK, Morris CJ, Watts RB (1976) Investigation by immunofluorescence of arterial lesions in rabbits on two different lipid supplements and treated with pyridinol carbamate. Atherosclerosis 23: 117-139

Arterial Endothelium in the Initial Stages of Atherogenesis

Abel Lazzarini Robertson, Jr.[1]

Atherosclerosis has been regarded as a multifactorial or polyetiologic and polypathogenic family of closely related vascular lesions (McMillan 1973). However, initiating local factors that may explain the anatomical distribution of individual lesions and their great variability on severity and rate of progression are not clearly understood. Recent laboratory data suggest that atherogenesis may be triggered and/or accelerated by the abnormal response of some areas of the vascular wall to the cumulative and often synergistic effects of recurrent injury-repair cycles, producing permanent arterial damage (Robertson 1977).

While Rudolf Virchow (1856) had suggested over a century ago that atherosclerosis may result from the response of the arterial wall to injury,it is only recently that a variety of injurious stimuli have been identified as capable of mimicking experimentally vascular cell responses similar to those found during the initial stages of atherosclerosis. Studies in laboratory models to evaluate hemodynamic stress (Stehbens 1974), immune complexes (Alonso et al. 1977), hypercholesterolemia (Ross and Harker 1976), homocystinemia (Harker et al. 1976), desiccation (Fishman et al. 1975) and mechanical trauma (Baumgartner 1963; Bondjers and Björkerud 1971; Spaet et al. 1975; Schwartz et al. 1975; Moore 1973; Hirsch and Robertson 1977) have demonstrated similarities as well as emphasized species variability on the stages of arterial wall repair following experimental injury. While the final vascular changes to be found include smooth muscle cell proliferation, intra and extracellular deposition of lipids in variable amounts and accelerated synthesis of connective tissue components, particularly glycosoaminoglycans, collagen and elastin, the specific role of different arterial cells during repair has yet to be clearly defined.

If normal endothelium acts as a selective "barrier" to the passage and entrapment of blood components in the arterial wall (French 1966; Bondjers and Björkerud 1973; Hüttner et al. 1973; Robertson and Khairallah 1973; Robertson 1978a) it has been suggested (Ross and Harker 1976) that endothelial desquamation could initiate development of lipid rich lesions in the presence of chronic hyperlipidemia.

The hypothesis that persistent absence of endothelial cells favors intimal thickening, lipid accumulation and accelerated atherosclerosis was recently critically tested in rabbits in a series of well designed experiments by Minick et al. (1977, 1979). Following aortic balloon catheter injury, these authors made the important observation that lipid accumulation and intimal thickening occurred in reendothelialized areas rather than in those where the endothelial lining was still absent, suggesting that under regenerated endothelium, the arterial wall is more prone to hyperplasia and lipid entrapment. These findings cast serious doubts as to the above role of normal endothelium as an effective "barrier" that modulates passage of blood components to the underlying arterial wall while suggesting until now unrecognized characteristics of replicating endothelial cells of considerable potential pathophysiological significance.

---

[1] Supported by Grant HL 20924 from the National Institutes of Health.

It should be noted that the widely used method of deendothelialization by an inflated balloon catheter, as originally described by Baumgartner (1963) requires unphysiological balloon pressures (over 500 mm Hg) to ensure complete endothelial removal, often producing unpredictable injury of underlying arterial layers. The latter may help explain the progressively slower rate of endothelial regeneration followed by asymptotic growth observed by some investigators (Chidi and Insull 1977) after balloon injury with secondary proliferative stimulation of medial smooth cells and protracted vascular repair, lasting from several weeks to months (Spaet et al. 1975).

To summarize current experimental data, direct manipulation of an artery as well as the effects of injurants that distort its size or shape may play important roles in determining the role and characteristics of subsequent vascular repair. Alternative techniques have been suggested that seem to offer considerable advantages for the specific evaluation of the role of the endothelium on vascular repair as well as its interaction with circulating blood cells during regeneration. Hirsch and Robertson (1977) described the use of a thin (1 mm outside diameter) mercury loaded catheter attached to an electric vibrator which induces a predictable and narrow injury tract while it is rapidly withdrawn through a distal arteriotomy. With this method, complete reendothelialization essentially occurred in 72-96 hours after injury with the added advantage of providing uninjured arterial wall for control studies from the same vascular segment. To avoid entirely the use of an intraluminal catheter, while permitting sequential studies in adjacent or distant vascular regions in the same animal, a new method has been recently developed in our laboratory (Robertson et al. 1979) and extensively tested in rabbits and rats. It is based on short-term exposure (1-3 minutes) of temporarily isolated arterial segments of variable length to a hypotonic solution injected at 100 mm Hg pressure, producing predictable and rapid endothelial lysis with ultrastructural preservation of the basal lamina and without morphological evidence of subendothelial, medial or adventitial injury (Figure 1). Deendothelialized arterial segments induced by this method show unusually well defined boundaries by scanning electron microscopy allowing morphometric, cytochemical and biochemical comparisons with the adjacent arterial wall. In contrast to mechanical deendothelialization, the rapid and uniform rate of endothelial regeneration observed by this procedure throughout the entire injured arterial segment, has allowed sequential studies of the interplay of endothelial and blood cells at all stages of vascular repair.

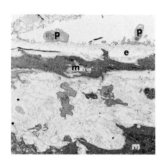

FIG. 1 TEM[2] of carotid artery luminal surface immediately following DEE. Note platelets (p) attached to remanents of basal lamina resting on the underlying internal elastic lamina (e) over unaltered smooth muscle cells (m)

---

[2] In all legends TEM indicates transmission electron micrograph, SEM scanning electron micrograph and DEE deendothelialization or deendothelialized

For the observations to be described herewith, unilateral or bilateral carotid artery osmotic deendothelialization was carried out in normolipemic rabbits or rats followed by periods of observation ranging from 1 minute to 14 days. In vitro perfusion fixation at mean systolic pressure was carried out by modifications of the methods proposed by Schwartz and Benditt (1973) and Clark and Glagov (1976) followed by processing for scanning electron microscopy (Robertson and McKalen 1975), transmission electron microscopy and histochemistry. As shown on Figure 2, single activated and flattened platelets rapidly attached to the deendothelialized surface without significant aggregation or multilayered deposits.

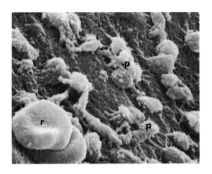

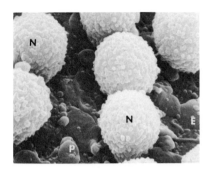

FIG. 2 SEM showing single layer of flattened plate-lets (p) with abundant pseudopods firmly attached to DEE surface 30 minutes after endothelial removal. Some red blood cells (r) are also present.

FIG. 3 SEM demonstrating marginated neutrophils (N) and occasional platelets (p) interdispersed with single endothelial cells (E) 24 hours after DEE

At 24 hours after injury (Figure 3) neutrophils, particularly in the rabbit, appeared in considerable numbers without significant surface ruffling but firmly attached to the deendothelialized surface. Single or multiple plate-lets were usually found in their immediate proximity. These marginated neutrophils remained on the vascular surface for several more hours (Figure 4) even after flat or "plump" single endothelial cells have first appeared by migrating from adjacent uninjured endothelium. Similar findings have recently been described in dog aorta by Ratliff et al. (1979) (Figure 4) weeks after balloon catheter injury, although in their observations the platelet cover was thicker and often multilayered, surrounding polymorphonuclear leukocytes in all sides.

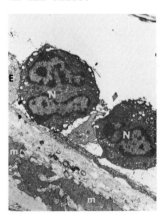

FIG. 4 TEM showing marginated neutro-phils (N) and platelets (p) attached (pavementing) the regenerating arterial surface with portion of a "plump" endo-thelial cell (E) 30 hours after DEE. Note absence of smooth muscle cell changes.

In our own observations, neutrophils were followed by the appearance of esterase positive monocytes showing acid lipase activity and IgG (Fc) receptors (Schaffner et al. 1979). Ultrastructural surface changes were rather characteristic (Figure 5) with long cytoplasmic extensions interspersed with isolated platelets and regenerating ("plump") endothelial cells.

Contrary to previous observations in branched arteries, (Stemerman et al. 1977) carotid artery reendothelialization occurred by migration and proliferation of small "clones" or single endothelial cells that rapidly formed "islets" of plump elements with scattered monocytes and, over 90 hours after injury, with single lymphocytes attached to the regenerating surface (Figure 6). In contrast to mature endothelium, these early stages of endothelial repair often showed cells poorly oriented to the direction of blood flow, a phenomenon already observed with other types of experimental injury (Webster et al. 1974).

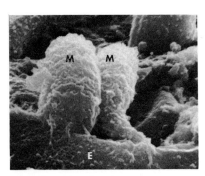

FIG. 5 SEM showing two monocytes (M) attached to regenerated endothelium (E) at 72 hours after DEE

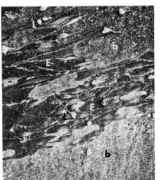

FIG. 6 Low power SEM, 110 hours after DEE showing irregular endothelial "islets" (E) with scattered monocytes and lymphocytes (L) surrounded by still DEE areas of basal lamina (b). Silver staining was used to better demonstrate endothelial cell boundaries.

Over 180 hours after osmotic deendothelialization and seemingly unrelated to the length of the segment under study, endothelial cell confluence was almost completed in most areas of the arterial surface. However, large surface defects containing platelets remained mixed with some "plump" endothelial cells best demonstrated by scanning electron microscopy (Figure 7).

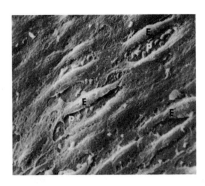

FIG. 7 SEM after 160 hours DEE shows advanced stages of reendothelialization with abundant "plump" endothelial cells (E) separate by surface defects containing isolated platelets (p)

At this stage of arterial repair, transmission electron microscopy demonstrated in normolipemic animals the appearance of cytoplasmic lipid droplets in smooth muscle cells underlying the regenerating endothelium, which could not be found in control arterial segments. These lipid laden cells increased in number and size after 200 hours (Figure 8) and remained in the rabbit intima and the rat media even after endothelial replacement was morphologically completed.

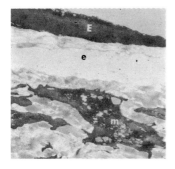

FIG. 8 TEM of repaired arterial lumen 240 hours after DEE. Note electron dense cytoplasm of regenerated endothelial cell (E) overlying unaltered internal elastic lamina (e) and lipid laden smooth muscle cells (m).

The finding of lipid accumulation in the arterial wall following selective endothelial injury in the absence of other recognized atherogenic risk factors in both a highly susceptible (rabbit) as well as a relatively resistant species (rat) is of considerable interest in view of the recent observations by Minick et al. (1979) showing that the intima under regenerating endothelium is significantly thicker and more likely to accumulate lipids in both normo and hyperlipemic rabbits. They also relate to those described by Moore (1979) showing that repetitive endothelial injury, in the absence of hyperlipidemia, leads to the development of lipid containing lesions in the same laboratory model. In the present observations, a single cycle of deendothelialization-repair seems to be sufficient to initiate intracellular lipid deposits in underlying smooth muscle cells. Based on the observations of McMillan and Stary (1968) describing higher rates of ^{3}H-thymidine labelling in endothelial cells overlying experimental rabbit lesions, it is tempting to speculate that once such lipid lesions are induced by injury, they could become rapidly self sustained due to cyclical increased entrapment of lipids under regenerating endothelium with accelerated turnover rates.

STAGES OF ENDOTHELIAL REPAIR FOLLOWING
OSMOTIC DEENDOTHELIALIZATION

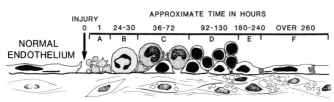

A = Degranulated Platelets
B = Degranulated Platelets plus Neutrophils
C = "Plump" Single Endothelial Cells Plus Activated Monocytes
D = Irregular Endothelial "Islets" Plus Lymphocytes
E = Completed Endothelial Monolayer With Irregular Boundaries
F = Total Repair. Ultrastructural Changes In Underlying Smooth Muscle Cells

FIG. 9 Schematic representation of the stages of rapid endothelial regeneration following osmotic DEE in normolipemic animals. Lipid laden smooth muscle cells are found following endothelial repair (See Figure 8).

Figure 9 schematically describes the sequential appearance of neutrophils, monocytes and lymphocytes attached to the luminal surface in the presence of activated platelets, during the short period required for complete endothelial repair following osmotic deendothelialization (approximately 8-10 days). These findings suggest that circulating leukocytes may play an unsuspected role in the behavior of regenerating endothelium and in the development of accelerated atherosclerosis that deserves further detailed investigation. Leukocytes attached to the luminal surface have been previously described after balloon overdilatation of the rabbit aorta (Haudenschild and Studer 1971), rat carotid following desiccation (Clowes et al. 1978), rabbit aorta after selective mechanical injury (Hirsch and Robertson 1977) and dog aorta after balloon catheter (Ratliff et al. 1979) suggesting that leukotactic stimuli may be elicited by a variety of vascular injurants independent of the method of arterial damage or the laboratory models studied.

Platelets have recently been shown _in vitro_ to specifically enhance human and rabbit monocyte adherence (Musson and Henson 1979) either through release of mediators or by direct platelet-monocyte binding. Platelet factors are, however, unable to affect directly endothelial cell proliferation or migration, in contrast to vascular smooth muscle cells (Thorgeirsson and Robertson 1978 ; Thorgeirsson et al. 1979). Specific chemotactic factors such as complement derived C_3 and C_5 fragments, plasma kallikrein and plasminogen activator as well as several proteases and fibrinopeptides could be locally elicited following vascular injury and induce observed leukotaxis (Ward 1974).

The concept of an endothelial or intimal "barrier" regulating incorporation of plasma components by the arterial wall is not supported by current experimental data. The endothelial vascular lining instead behaves as a selective metabolic boundary easily altered by regeneration and/or replacement and temporarily influenced by marginating leukocytes and platelets.

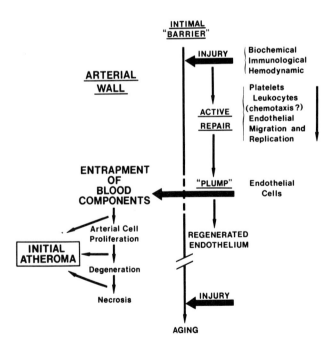

FIG. 10 Summary of suggested role of repetitive endothelial repair during the initial stages of atherogenesis, as described in the text.

To summarize, and as shown diagramatically on Figure 10, a variety of biochemical (hypercholesterolemia, hemocystinemia, cigarette smoking) immunological (antigen-antibody complexes, allograft rejection) or hemodynamic
(hypertension, local flow changes) injurants may induce endothelial injury
and subsequent rapid or protracted vascular repair. Selective osmotic
deendothelialization has shown that during rapid endothelial regeneration by
both cell migration and proliferation, attached platelets and leukocytes are
active participants in the reparative process. Regenerated endothelial
cells remain "plump" and poorly oriented until reendothelialization is completed. During that period, entrapment of blood components occur, with
smooth muscle cell proliferation, degeneration and necrosis initiating a
self-sustained vicious circle resulting in increased endothelial cell turnover and eliciting further entrapment of circulating macromolecules as well
as providing repetitive exposure of underlying smooth muscle cells to mitogenic and/or mutagenic agents.

Summary and conclusions

While current experimental data continue to support Virchow's pioneer and
far-reaching hypothesis on the role of vascular injury in atherosclerosis,
the studies briefly reviewed here suggest that the interplay of regenerated
endothelium with sequentially marginated leukocytes and platelets may be
major contributors to the entrapment of plasma components in the arterial
wall, independent of other atherogenic factors and preceding smooth muscle
cell involvement. Based on these findings, it is further believed that
identification of the cellular events occuring during endothelial repair as
well as the study of specific chemotactic mediators released from plasma,
leukocytes and the vessel wall could provide new vistas to our understanding
of the role of arterial cells in atherogenesis.

References

Alonso DR, Starek P, Minick CR (1977) Studies on the pathogenesis of athero-
    arteriosclerosis induced in rabbit cardiac allografts by the synergy of
    graft rejection and hypercholesterolemia. Am J Pathol 87: 415
Baumgartner HR (1963) Eine neue Methode zur Erzeugung von Thromben durch
    gezielte Uberdehnung der Gefässwant. Z ges exp Med 137:227
Björkerud S, Bondjers G (1971) Arterial repair and atherosclerosis after
    mechanical injury. I. Permeability and light microscopic characteristics
    of endothelium in nonatherosclerotic and atherosclerotic lesions.
    Atherosclerosis 13: 355
Björkerud S, Bondjers G (1973) Arterial repair and atherosclerosis after
    mechanical injury. Atherosclerosis 18:235
Bondjers G, Björkerud S (1973) Arterial repair and atherosclerosis after
    mechanical injury. Part 3. Cholesterol accumulation and removal in
    morphologically defined regions of aortic atherosclerotic lesions in the
    rabbit. Atherosclerosis 17: 85
Chidi CC, Insull W (1977) Rate of regrowth of arterial endothelium in vivo
    after injury. Surg Forum 28: 219
Clark JM, Glagov S (1976) Luminal surface of distended arteries by scanning
    electron microscopy: Eliminating configurational and technical arti-
    facts. Br J Exp Pathol 57: 129
Clowes AW, Breslow JL, Karnovsky MJ (1977) Regression of myointimal thick-
    ening following carotid endothelial injury and development of aortic
    foam cell lesions in long term hypercholesterolemic rats. Lab Invest
    36: 73
Clowes AW, Collazzo RE, Karnovsky MJ (1978) A morphologic and permeability
    study of luminal smooth muscle cells after arterial injury in the rat.
    Lab Invest 39: 141

Clowes AW, Karnovsky MJ (1977) Failure of certain antiplatelet drugs to affect myointimal thickening following arterial endothelial injury in the rat. Lab Invest 36: 452

Fishman JA, Ryan GB, Karnovsky MJ (1975) Endothelial regeneration in the rat carotid artery and the significance of endothelial denudation in the pathogenesis of myointimal thickening. Lab Invest 32: 339

French JE (1966) Atherosclerosis in relation to the structure and function of the arterial intima, with special reference to the endothelium. Int Rev Exp Pathol 5: 253

Harker LA, Ross R, Slichter SJ, Scott C (1976) Homocystine-induced arteriosclerosis. The role of endothelial cell injury and platelet response in its genesis. J Clin Invest 58: 731

Haudenschild C, Studer A (1971) Early interactions between blood cells and severely damaged rabbit aorta. Eur J Clin Invest 2: 1

Hirsch EZ, Robertson AL (1977) Selective acute arterial endothelial injury and repair. I. Methodology and surface characteristics. Atherosclerosis 28: 271

Hüttner I, Boutet M, More RH (1973) Studies on protein passage through arterial endothelium. II. Regional differences in permeability to fine structural protein tracers in arterial endothelium of normotensive rat. Lab Invest 28: 678

McMillan GC (1973) Development of arteriosclerosis. Am J Cardiol 31: 542

McMillan GC, Stary HC (1968) Part II. Preliminary experience with mitotic activity of cellular elements in the atherosclerotic plaques of cholesterol fed rabbits studied by labeling with tritiated thymidine. Ann NY Acad Sci 149: 699

Minick CR, Stemerman MB, Insull W (1977) Effect of regenerated endothelium on lipid accumulation in the arterial wall. Proc Natl Acad Sci USA 74: 1724

Minick CR, Stemerman MB, Insull W (1979) Role of endothelium and hypercholesterolemia in intimal thickening and lipid accumulation. Am J Pathol 95: 131

Moore S (1973) Thromboatherosclerosis in normolipemic rabbits: A result of continued endothelial damage. Lab Invest 29: 478

Moore S (1979) Endothelial injury and atherosclerosis. Exp Mol Pathol 31: 182

Musson RA, Henson PM (1979) Humoral and formed elements of blood modulate the response of peripheral blood monocytes. I. Plasma and serum inhibit and platelets enhance monocyte adherence. J Immunol 122: 2026

Ratliff NB, Gerrard JM, White JG (1979) Platelet-leukocyte interactions following arterial endothelial injury. Am J Pathol 96: 567

Robertson AL (1977) The pathogenesis of human atherosclerosis. In: Gross HL (ed) Atherosclerosis-A Scope publication. TheUpjohn Co Kalamazoo pp 38-54

Robertson AL (1978) The spectrum of arterial disease. In: Paoletti R, Gotto AM (eds) Atherosclerosis Reviews, Raven Press, N.Y., Vol 3 pp 57-68

Robertson AL, Kharillah PA (1973) Arterial endothelial permeability and vascular disease. The "trap door" effect. Exp Mol Pathol 18: 241

Robertson AL, McKalen A (1975) Tissue processing of mammalian vascular endothelium for scanning or scanning-transmission electron microscopy. In: Bailey GW (ed) 33 Ann Proc Electron Micro Soc Amer, Las Vegas pp 632-633

Robertson AL, Ratcliffe MB, Ziats NP (1979) Selective endothelial injury and repair. Fed Proc 38: 1456

Ross R, Harker L (1976) Hyperlipidemia and atherosclerosis: Chronic hyperlipidemia initiates and maintains lesions by endothelial cell desquamation and lipid accumulation. Science 193: 1094

Schaffner T, Vesselinovitch D, Wissler RW (1979) Macrophages in experimental and human atheromatous lesions, immunomorphologic identification. Fed Proc 38: 1076

Schwartz SM, Benditt EP (1973) Cell replication in the aortic endothelium. A new method for study of the problem. Lab Invest 28: 699

Schwartz SM, Stemerman MB, Benditt EP (1975) The aortic intima. II. Repair of the aortic lining after mechanical denudation. Am J Pathol 81: 15

Spaet TH, Stemerman MB, Veith FJ, Lejnieks I (1975) Intimal injury and regrowth in the rabbit aorta. Medial smooth muscle cells as a source of neointima. Circ Res 36: 58

Stehbens WE (1974) Haemodynamic production of lipid deposition, intimal tears, mural dissection and thrombosis in the blood vessel wall. Proc R Soc Lond [Biol] 185: 357

Stemerman MB, Spaet TH, Pitlick F, Cintron J, Lejnieks I, Tiell ML (1977) Intimal healing. The pattern of reendothelialization and intimal thickening. Am J Pathol 87: 125

Thorgeirsson G, Robertson AL (1978) The vascular endothelium: Pathobiological significance – A review. Am J Pathol 93: 803

Thorgeirsson G, Robertson AL, Cowan DH (1979) Migration of human vascular endothelial and smooth muscle cells. Lab Invest 41: 51

Webster WS, Bishop SP, Geer JC (1974) Experimental aortic intimal thickening. II. Endothelialization and permeability. Am J. Pathol 76: 265

Ultrastructure of the Normal Arterial Endothelium and Intima[1]

Colin J. Schwartz, Ross G. Gerrity, Eugene A. Sprague, M. Robin Hagens, Carol T. Reed, and
Daniel L. Guerrero

Notwithstanding numerous intriguing structural and functional aspects of
vascular endothelium, this paper is of necessity limited to selected ultrastructural features of the normal arterial endothelium and intima. For a
recent comprehensive review, the reader is referred to the paper by Majno
and Joris (1978).

Figures 1 and 2 emphasize an important though not well recognized point,
namely that endothelial and intimal ultrastructure may differ significantly
within different segments of the same artery. Such differences are readily
demonstrable utilizing in vivo arterial uptake patterns of the azo dye,
Evans Blue (Gerrity et al. 1977; Schwartz et al. 1978). As an example Fig.
1, derived from the aortic arch of a young pig illustrates elongate endothelial cells with long interdigitating junctions. In contrast, also from
the aortic arch of a young pig, but from a site exhibiting Evans Blue dye
uptake (blue area) Fig. 2 reveals shorter more cuboidal cells with predominantly short end-to-end junctions and little overlap. The latter areas as
observed in the Evans Blue model are sites of increased permeability to
proteins and to ferritin (Bell et al. 1974a, 1974b; Schwartz et al. 1978),
an enhanced endothelial cell turnover (Caplan et al. 1975), together with
various metabolic differences (Schwartz et al. 1978). These blue areas are
also sites of predilection for the development of both spontaneous and
experimental atherosclerosis as shown by Fry (1973). The endothelial surface coat or glycocalyx, visualization of which has been facilitated by
ruthenium red staining (Luft 1966), is seen in Figs. 3 and 4 from white and
blue staining areas respectively. It is apparent that the glycocalyx overlying less permeable or white areas (Fig. 3) is thicker than that over more
permeable or blue areas (Fig. 4). It is tempting to suggest that this
layer may in part account for these permeability differences. Whether the
glycocalyx imparts any antithrombotic characteristics to the endothelium
is unknown. It is interesting to note that the endothelial glycocalyx is
thinned during hypercholesterolemia and early atherogenesis (Weber et al.
1973, 1974; Balint et al. 1974; Gerrity et al. 1979).

Of particular interest is the relatively frequent appearance of blood mono-
cyte-like cells in the aortic subendothelium of both normal young pig and
baboon (P. cynocephalus). Examples of these subendothelial mononuclear
cells are seen in Figs. 5 and 6. These cells, presumably derived from the
circulating blood by passage through or between endothelial cells, have a
large nucleus frequently deeply indented, a prominent Golgi apparatus,
frequent dense granules, and numerous cisternae in the endoplasmic reticulum
(Nichols and Bainton 1975). They are the presumptive macrophages of the
arterial wall and a potential source of foam cells in atherogenesis (Gerrity
et al. 1979). Whether they secrete elastase in the artery has yet to be
determined.

Within the normal aortic subendothelium cell death and lysis with extracellular myelin figures (Fig. 7) and ghost cells (Fig. 8) are not infrequent.

[1]This work was supported in part by Arteriosclerosis SCOR Grant HL-19362

The insert in Fig. 8 shows several so called Weibel-Palade bodies, small membrane bound tubular structures described by Weibel and Palade in 1964. These bodies show considerable species specificity, and are absent in the pig although present in the baboon. Although implicated in a procoagulant role their functional significance is unknown. Nevertheless they are widely used as identity markers in endothelial cell culture.

Pinocytotic vesicles are an important endothelial cellular organelle observed in particularly large numbers en face. They form initially as invaginations of the plasmalemmal membrane with subsequent budding into the cytoplasm. They range in size from 400 to 1500 Å in diameter. Entry of molecules into the caveolae intracellulares may in part be modulated by the presence of a diaphragm across the ostium or stoma. Pinocytotic vesicles are the principal if not exclusive route of transport of large molecules across the endothelium. Figure 9 shows ferritin granules (110 Å) in vesicles and vacuoles 5 minutes after intravenous injection. Granules may also be observed free and within cells in the SES. Another variety of vesicles, namely coated vesicles, deserves brief comment. These are rare in the aortic endothelium of pig and baboon but are prominent in baboon aortic smooth muscle and in human fibroblasts. In the latter they may arise from specialized regions of the plasma membrane containing receptors for low density lipoprotein (Anderson et al. 1977). Coated vesicles from rat aortic endothelium are illustrated in the insert to Fig. 9. As described by Palade and Bruns (1968) these exhibit a coat or corona made up of radiating projections 200 Å in length and some 200 - 250 Å apart. The coated vesicles vary in size and are prominent near the Golgi apparatus. The coating includes clathrin, a major protein of both coated vesicles and the Golgi apparatus. The coating of these specialized vesicles may impart specificity both to packaging and targeting to intracellular organelles.

The surface of normal arterial endothelium as seen by scanning electron microscopy reveals many features of interest. Figure 10 illustrates the polyhedral or ovoid pattern of cells in some areas of the thoracic aorta, together with the prominent cytoplasmic projections which mark the cellular boundaries (Fig. 10 insert). In other regions of the thoracic aorta the cells exhibit a more rugose pattern (Fig. 11) which becomes striking with deep linear folds and prominent cytoplasmic projections in the lower abdominal aorta or at the ostia of branches (Fig. 12 and insert). This latter appearance is not prevented by pressure perfusion fixation. Monocytes, presumably blood derived, are not infrequent in the SES (Figs. 5, 6). Figure 13 illustrates a leukocyte, presumably a monocyte, with prominent ruffles and projections adhering to normal aortic endothelium. In Fig. 14 a similar cell appears to be either entering or leaving the intima. Figures 15 and 16 demonstrate the surface morphology of normal baboon aortic endothelim at much higher magnifications. Spade-like cytoplasmic projections along an intercellular junction are a feature of Fig. 15, together with the presence of a number of pits and ostia having a diameter range of 55 Å to 580 Å on the basis of preliminary measurements. Also visible are relatively large numbers of round or ovoid projections which appear to be overlying indentations or pits on the endothelial surface (Figs. 15, 16). These cap-like structures have a diameter range of 255 Å to 690 Å, not dissimilar to the size of the pits or ostia. Similar pits and ostia and round projections are also seen in normal aortic endothelium grown in tissue culture (insert to Fig. 15). On the basis of size, the pits and ostia could represent caveolae in stages of evolution while the round projections may serve as opercula or caps to some of the vesicles. Further studies are essential to clarify the functional significance of these morphologic observations.

Acknowledgement

The high resolution SEM's were photographed on a JEOL 100CX in Boston, Massachusetts.

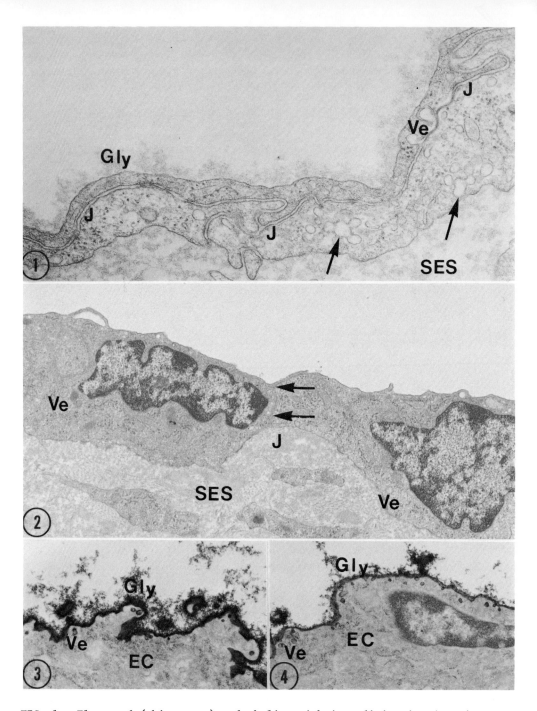

FIG. 1. Elongated (white area) endothelium with interdigitating junctions (J), numerous pinocytotic vesicles (Ve), some showing fusion (arrows), unstained glycocalyx (Gly) and the subendothelial space (SES). (Pig thoracic aorta 48,700X) FIG. 2. Blue area endothelium showing short junctions (J, arrows), vesicles (Ve) and the subendothelial space (SES). (Pig thoracic aorta 12,100X) FIGS. 3, 4. Ruthenium red stained glycocalyx (Gly) overlying endothelial cells (EC) from white (FIG. 3) and blue (FIG. 4) areas. Vesicles (Ve) contain Ruthenium red material. (Pig thoracic aorta 20,600X)

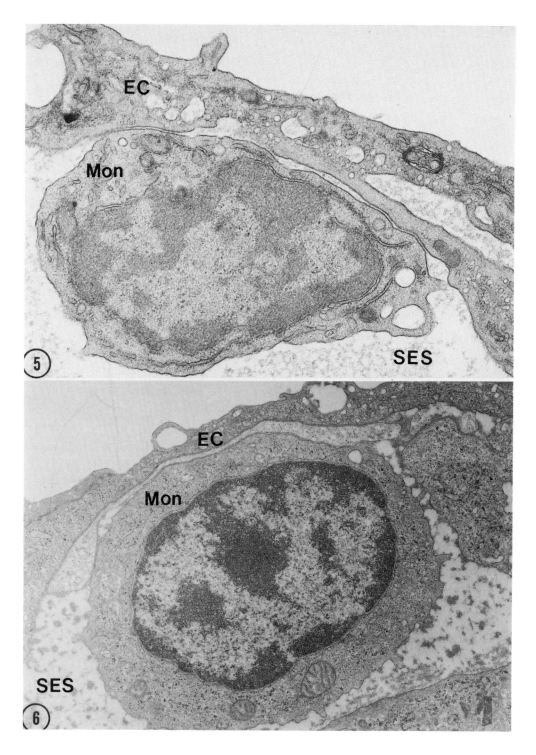

FIG. 5. Mononuclear cell (Mon) in the subendothelial space (SES) of normal baboon aorta. Overlying endothelial cell (EC) is intact. (41,300X) FIG. 6. Mononuclear cell (Mon) in the subendothelial space (SES) of normal pig aorta. Overlying endothelial cell (EC) is intact. (26,300X)

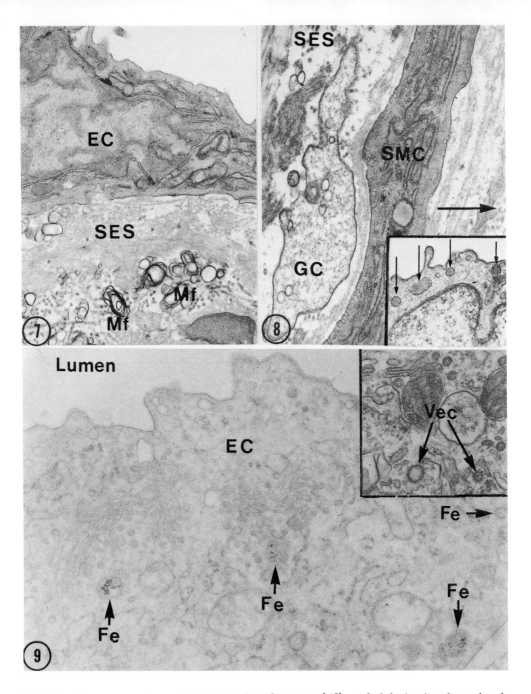

FIG. 7. Numerous extracellular myelin figures (Mf) and debris in the subendothelial space (SES) of normal baboon aorta. Overlying endothelial cell (EC)
appears normal. (50,600X) FIG. 8. Ghost cell (GC) in the endothelial space
(SES) adjoining a smooth muscle cell (SMC). Luminal aspect arrowed. Insert:
Weibel-Palade bodies in transverse and oblique section (arrows) in normal
baboon aortic endothelium. (30,875X, insert 36,100X) FIG. 9. Unstained
normal pig aortic endothelium (EC) showing ferritin-containing vesicles (Fe,
arrows). Insert: 2 coated vesicles (Vec, arrows) from normal rat aortic
endothelium. (47,500X, insert 61,300X)

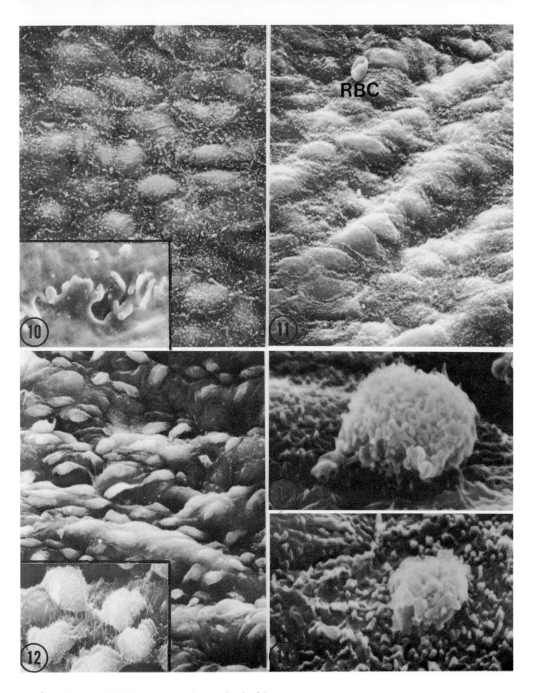

SEM's of normal baboon aortic endothelium.

FIG. 10 shows a polyhedral pattern and prominent cytoplasmic projections at cell boundaries with insert showing a higher magnification of these boundary projections. (1040X, insert 11,300X) FIG. 11 shows an undulating pattern of endothelial cells. (1040X) FIG. 12 shows deep linear folds and prominent cytoplasmic projections with insert showing a higher magnification of these projections. (1040X, insert 1900X) FIG. 13. Mononuclear cell adherant to endothelial surface. (10,000X) FIG. 14. Mononuclear cell either entering or leaving the intima. (5,000X)

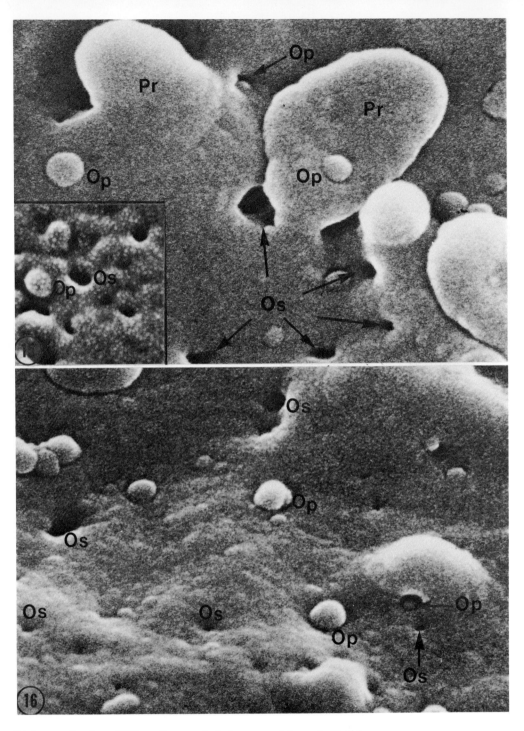

High resolution SEM's of normal baboon aortic endothelium.

FIG. 15 shows projections (Pr) along cell boundary, surface ostia (Os) and opercula (Op). Arrow indicates an operculum within an ostium. Insert: Ostia and opercula in cultured aortic endothelium. (181,250X, insert 337,500X)
FIG. 16 shows ostia (Os) and opercula (Op) of varying size. An operculum within an ostium is arrowed. (181,500X)

References

Anderson RGW, Brown MS, Goldstein JL (1977) Role of the coated endocytic vesicles in the uptake of receptor-bound low density lipoprotein in human fibroblasts. Cell 10, pp 351-364

Balint A, Veress B, Jellinek H (1974) Modifications of surface coat of aortic endothelial cells in hyperlipemic rats. Pathol Eur 9, pp 105-108

Bell FP, Adamson I, Schwartz CJ (1974) Aortic endothelial permeability to albumin: Focal and regional patterns of uptake and transmural distribution of ^{131}I-albumin in the young pig. Exp Mol Pathol 20, pp 57-58

Bell FP, Gallus AS, Schwartz CJ (1974) Focal and regional patterns of uptake and the transmural distribution of ^{131}I-fibrinogen in the pig aorta in vivo. Exp Mol Pathol 20, pp 281-292

Fry DL (1973) Responses of the arterial wall to certain physical factors. In: Atherogenesis initiating factors. Ciba Foundation Symposium 12 (new series) Excerpta Medica, North Holland, Assoc Sci Pub, New York, pp 93-125

Gerrity RG, Naito HK, Richardson M, Schwartz CJ (1979) Dietary induced atherogenesis in swine. Morphology of the intima in prelesion stages. Amer J Pathol 95, pp 775-792

Gerrity RG, Richardson M, Somer JB, Bell FP, Schwartz CJ (1977) Endothelial cell morphology in areas of in vivo Evans Blue uptake in the young pig aorta. II. Ultrastructure of the intima in areas of differing permeability to proteins. Amer J Pathol 89, pp 313-344

Luft JH (1966) Fine structure of capillary and endocapillary layer as revealed by Ruthenium red, Fed Proc 25, pp 1773-1783

Majno G, Joris I (1978) Endothelium 1977: A Review. In: Chandler AB, Eurenius K, McMillan GC, Nelson CB, Schwartz CJ, Wessler S (eds) The thrombotic process in atherogenesis. Plenum Press, New York-London, pp 169-225

Nichols BA, Bainton DF (1975) Ultrastructure and cytochemistry of mononuclear phagocytes. In: Van Furth R (ed) Mononuclear Phagocytes. Blackwell Sci Pub, Oxford, pp 17-54

Palade GE, Bruns RR (1968) Structural modulations of plasmalemmal vesicles. J. Cell Biol 37, pp 633-649

Schwartz CJ, Gerrity RG, Lewis LJ (1978) Arterial endothelial structure and function with particular reference to permeability. In: Gotto AM, Paoletti R (eds) Atherosclerosis reviews. Raven Press, New York, pp 109-124

Schwartz CJ, Somer JB, Gerrity RG (1978) Initial events of atherogenesis. In: McDonald L. Goodwin J, Resnekov L (eds) Very early recognition of coronary heart disease. Excerpta Medica, Amsterdam-Oxford, pp 47-61

Weber G, Fabbrini P, Resi L (1973) On the presence of a concanavalin-A reactive coat over the endothelial aortic surface and its modifications during early experimental cholesterol atherogenesis in rabbits. Virchow's Arch Abt A Path Anat 359, pp 299-307

Weber G, Fabbrini P, Resi L (1974) Scanning and transmission electron-microscopy observations on the surface lining of aortic intimal plaques in rabbits on a hypercholesterolic diet. Virchow's Arch A Path Anat Histol 364, pp 325-331

Weibel ER, Palade GE (1964) New cytoplasmic components in arterial endothelia. J Cell Biol 23, pp 101-112

Biochemical Studies on Permeability and the Interaction Between Blood Constituents and Arterial Components in Atherosclerosis

Elspeth B. Smith[1]

It is now accepted that large amounts of plasma low density lipoprotein (LDL), and cholesterol ester which must be derived from it, accumulate in atherosclerotic lesions, but it is not clear if this is the result of increased endothelial permeability or of increased retention within the intima. In this paper I will try to draw together some of the available biochemical evidence.

Endothelial Permeability

Biochemical studies on endothelial permeability fall into two main groups: those in which the artery has been excised and the uptake of markers measured in response to injury and haemodynamic stresses (for example, Fry 1973; Siflinger et al. 1975) and those in which markers are injected in vivo. Endothelium is easily damaged, and endothelial damage changes the metabolism of the whole wall (Morrison et al. 1976) thus interpretation of results in the first group is uncertain, and here I will discuss only in vivo findings.

Packham et al. (1967) injected Evans blue dye (which binds to plasma albumin) and radio-labelled albumin into pigs and rabbits and found in intimal-medial preparations similar patterns of accumulation. These experiments have been repeated and confirmed in pigs by Bell et al. (1974a,b) using labelled fibrinogen as well as albumin, and sectioning the aortas to obtain the distribution across the wall. They interpret focal increase in uptake as indicating areas of increased endothelial permeability. Stefanovich and Gore (1971) found uptake of labelled albumin into whole rabbit aortas increased by 50% after 3 weeks cholesterol feeding, but thereafter there was no further change in spite of massive increase in lesions. In cholesterol fed cynomolgus monkeys Armstrong et al. (1978) found no consistent increase in "blue" area, but moderate increase in intensity of staining; dye uptake and fatty streak formation were not consistently related. In all experimental studies the amounts of plasma protein entering arterial wall are very low; this is difficult to reconcile with the high concentrations found in normal human aortic intima and, particularly, the concentration of LDL which is approximately the same as the concentration in the patient's plasma (Smith 1974, 1980; Hoff 1978a). In recent studies on the mechanism of accumulation of LDL we found that the internal elastic lamina (IEL) presents an almost total barrier to LDL but allows about 25% of albumin to pass through (Smith 1980). Comparing the results in the layer of media immediately outside the IEL in humans with the results of Bratzler et al. (1977a,b) in rabbit mid-media, the concentration relative to plasma concentration was the same for LDL, but higher than rabbit for albumin suggesting that the IEL in adult humans is "leaky" to smaller proteins. These results suggest that the IEL, and not endothelium, is the main permeability barrier to macromolecules, and this is supported by numerous ultrastructural studies (Thorgeirsson and Robertson 1978).

[1]The author's research is supported by a grant from the Medical Research Council.

Table 1.   Plasma constituents in normal intima, atherosclerotic lesions, thrombi and aortic graft pseudo-intima.

| | Concentration: mg/100mg dry tissue[1] | | | | |
	Free LP	Bound LP	Fibrin-ogen	Fibrin	Residual Choleserol
Normal intima (n = 27)	3.8 $\pm$0.4[2]	0.6 $\pm$0.1	2.5 $\pm$0.4	2.5 $\pm$0.4	3.6 $\pm$0.2
Gelatinous thickenings: low lipid. (n = 25)	13.7 $\pm$ 1.0	1.8 $\pm$0.4	7.7 $\pm$1.0	4.3 $\pm$0.9	5.4 $\pm$0.7
Gelatinous and fibrous plaques: lipid-rich areas.					
Fibrin 0-10mg/100mg. (n = 23)	1.5 $\pm$0.2	3.3 $\pm$0.6	1.9 $\pm$0.2	4.9 $\pm$0.5	72.9 $\pm$ 9.1
Fibrin>10mg/100mg (n = 35)	5.4 $\pm$0.7	7.4 $\pm$0.8	7.7 $\pm$0.9	22.7 $\pm$ 2.0	89.6 $\pm$ 6.8
Translucent mural thrombi					
With endothelium and coll-agen invasion (n = 4)	10.1 $\pm$ 6.9	4.3 $\pm$3.1	21.9 $\pm$ 9.6	47.7 $\pm$ 2.3	5.3 $\pm$1.7
No endothelium (n = 3)	2.0 $\pm$0.6	NIL	2.7 $\pm$1.0	74.3 $\pm$14.1	2.6 $\pm$1.5
Aortic graft pseudo-intima	1.2	0.2	1.4	86.2	2.2

[1] mg/100mg lipid-extracted dry tissue including fibrin.

[2] SEM

In comparative studies of "blue" and "white" areas Bell et al. (1974a,b) measured albumin and fibrinogen uptake into innermost (luminal) sections 100µM thick. In "white" and macroscopically normal areas the thickness of pig intima is 4-8µM (Gerrity et al. 1977; Smith unpublished) thus >90% of the tissue analysed was media outside the IEL, and the distribution of permeability barrier function between IEL and blood/endothelial interface cannot be determined. In "blue" areas the intima is much thicker (Gerrity et al. 1977; in the photograph published by Packham et al. (1967) it is approximately 70µM thick so that 70% of the tissue analysed would lie between the IEL and endothelium.   Thus in "blue" areas labelled protein in the first slice may give a reasonably good measure of endothelial transport whereas in "white" areas it gives no information about endothelial transport, consequently there is no normal baseline from which changes in permeability can be measured. Are "blue" areas blue because of increased permeability to dye/albumin, or because the layer of dye viewed is 10-15 times thicker than in white areas?

Interaction of Macromolecules in Intima

In contrast to the lack of information on endothelial permeability there are now several quantitative studies showing increased retention of free and tightly bound LDL in developing lesions (Hollander 1967, 1976; Smith 1974; Smith et al. 1976, 1978; Hoff et al. 1978b).   Tight binding of lipoprotein (LP) appears to be particularly associated with cholesterol accumulation in developing fibrous plaques (Table 1) but there is no agreement on the arterial

component with which it interacts.   Hoff et al. (1978b) extracted free LP
from intima by homogenization in buffer, and a tightly bound LP fraction from
the residual tissue of lipid-rich lesions with the detergent Triton X-100;
they suggest that LP interacts with cholesterol.   Hollander (1976) obtained
free LP from minces by prolonged extraction with saline, then digested the
residual tissue sequentially with collagenase, elastase and chondroitinase
A,B,C;   28% of the bound LP was released by chondroitinase, and he suggests
that LP is bound to collagen and elastin through glycosaminoglycan-calcium
complexes.   In our studies free LP was extracted and measured by electrophoresis directly from the tissue into antibody-containing gel, the tissue
samples were recovered, incubated with enzyme or buffer and released LP
measured by repeating the immunoelectrophoresis on fresh plates (Smith et al.
1976).   The fibrinolytic enzyme plasmin and a crude collagenase were most
effective in releasing bound LP;   purified collagenase was less effective,
and chrondroitinase A,B,C did not release significantly more LP than incubation with buffer alone.   Brief incubation with plasmin facilitated subsequent
release of LP by purified collagenase but not by chondroitinase.   These results suggest that LP is in some way bound by fibrin;   high concentrations of
fibrin and bound LP are associated in lipid-rich areas of some fibrous and
gelatinous plaques (Table 1) in which, compared with normal intima, there is
a 12-fold increase in bound LP and 10-fold increase in fibrin.   Within these
high-fibrin tissues, however, there is no correlation between bound LP and
fibrin concentrations, suggesting that only part of the fibrin is involved in
LP binding.   To study this relation further we have examined mural thrombi
and aortic graft pseudo-intimas (Smith et al. 1979b).   In partially incorporated mural thrombi the concentration of total LP was about the same as in
gelatinous thickenings, but three times as much was bound (30% compared with
11%;   Table 1).   By contrast, both free and bound LP were very low in mural
thrombi with no endothelium, and in the 2000μM thick, non-endothelialized
pseudo-intima of an aortic graft inserted 6 years before death (Table 1).
The lack of LP accumulation in the absence of endothelium is in striking
agreement with the findings of Minick et al. (1977).

In addition to binding to plaque components, LDL appears to aggregate in lesions (Hollander 1976;   Smith et al. 1979a).   On thin-layer isoelectric focusing 60-70% of LP in normal intima and early gelatinous lesions focused with
plasma LDL, but there was 25% of a larger molecule that failed to enter the
gel and remained at the origin.   In plaques the proportion of normal LDL

Table 2.   Characterization of lipoprotein in different layers of plaques
by isoelectric focusing.

| | | Layer of plaque | | |
	Normal Intima	Surface and edge	Inner Periphery	Lipid-rich centre
Concentration: mg/100mg dry tissue.				
Total free LP	4.6	12.9	13.0	2.0
Bound LP	0.9	2.8	3.0	4.7
Residual cholesterol	3.5	4.2	9.2	84.6
Free LP components: % distribution				
Origin	26.3	36.6	32.5	100
Intermediate peak	5.1	1.6	24.7	Nil
LDL	68.6	61.8	42.8	Nil

decreased in inner layers, and in lipid-rich centres all the free LP, and the bound LP released by incubation with plasmin, were in the aggregated form (Table 2).   Presumably these large LDL aggregates diffuse out of the tissue more slowly than normal LDL thereby adding to the accumulation of LP in lesions.   Thus increased retention of LDL in lesions has been demonstrated by several investigators in several different ways, but there appears to be no unequivocal demonstration of increased endothelial permeability.

References

Armstrong ML, Megan MB, Warner EM (1978) The relation of hypercholesterolemic fatty streaks to intimal permeability changes shown by Evans blue.   Atherosclerosis 31:443

Bell FP, Adamson IL, Schwartz CJ (1974a) Aortic permeability to albumin: focal and regional patterns of uptake and transmural distribution of 131-I-albumin in the young pig. Exp Mol Pathol 20:57

Bell FP, Gallus AS, Schwartz CJ (1974b) Focal and regional patterns of uptake and the transmural distribution of 131-I-fibrinogen in the pig aorta in vivo. Exp Mol Pathol 20:281

Bratzler RL, Chisolm GM, Colton CK, Smith KA, Zilversmit DB, Lees RS (1977a) The distribution of labelled albumin across the rabbit thoracic aorta in vivo. Circulation Res 40:182

Bratzler RL, Chisolm GM, Colton CK, Smith KA, Lees RS (1977b) The distribution of labelled low-density lipoproteins across the rabbit thoracic aorta in vivo.   Atherosclerosis 28:289

Fry DL (1973) Responses of the arterial wall to certain physical factors. In: Atherogenesis: Initiating factors.   Ciba Foundation Symposium (New Series) 12:93

Gerrity RG, Richardson M, Somer JB, Bell FP, Schwartz CJ (1977) Endothelial cell morphology in areas of in vivo Evans blue uptake in the aorta of young pigs. Am J Pathol 89:313

Hoff HF, Gaubatz JW, Gotto AM (1978a) Apo B concentration in the normal human aorta.   Biochem Biophys Res Com 84:1424

Hoff HF, Heideman CL, Gaubatz JW, Titus JL, Gotto AM (1978b) Quantitation of apo B in human aortic fatty streaks.   Atherosclerosis 30:263

Hollander W (1967) Influx, synthesis and transport of arterial lipoproteins in atherosclerosis. Exp Mol Pathol 7:248

Hollander W (1976) Unified concept on the role of acid mucopolysaccharides and connective tissue proteins in the accumulation of lipids, lipoproteins and calcium in the atherosclerotic plaque. Exp Mol Pathol 25:106

Minick CR, Stemerman MB, Insull W (1977) Effect of regenerated endothelium on lipid accumulation in the arterial wall. Proc Natl Acad Sci USA 74:1724

Morrison AD, Berwick L, Orci L, Winegrad AI (1976) Morphology and metabolism of an aortic intima-media preparation in which an intact endothelium is preserved. J Clin Invest 57:650

Packham MA, Rowsell HC, Jorgensen L, Mustard JF (1967) Localized protein accumulation in the wall of the aorta.   Exp Mol Pathol 7:214

Siflinger A, Parker K, Caro CG (1975) Uptake of 125-I-albumin by the endothelial surface of the isolated dog common carotid artery: effect of certain physical factors and metabolic inhibitors.   Cardiovasc Res 9:478

Smith EB (1974)   The relationship between plasma and tissue lipids in human atherosclerosis.   Advan Lipid Res 12:1

Smith EB (1980) Transport of macromolecules across the artery wall.   This volume

Smith EB, Craig IB, Dietz HS (1978)   Factors influencing accumulation and destruction of lipoprotein in atherosclerotic lesions.   In: Carlson LA, Paoletti R, Sirtori CR, Weber G (eds) International Conference on Atherosclerosis, Raven Press, New York, p49

Smith EB, Dietz HS, Craig IB (1979a)   Characterization of free and tightly bound lipoprotein in intima by thin layer isoelectric focusing.   Atherosclerosis 33:329

Smith EB, Massie IB, Alexander KM (1976)   The release of an immobilized lipoprotein fraction from atherosclerotic lesions by incubation with plasmin. Atherosclerosis 25:71

Smith EB, Staples EM, Dietz HS, Smith RH (1979)   Role of endothelium in sequestration of lipoprotein and fibrinogen in aortic lesions, thrombi and graft pseudo-intimas.   Lancet ii:812

Stefanovich V, Gore I (1971) Cholesterol diet and permeability of rabbit aorta.   Exp Mol Pathol 14:20

Thorgeirsson G, Robertson AL (1978) The vascular endothelium - pathobiologic significance.   Am J Pathol 93:803

Smooth Muscle Cells in Atherosclerosis

Jack L. Titus and Donald G. Weilbaecher

This report is an overview of current certain and reasonably certain knowledge of arterial smooth muscle (SM) in the atherosclerotic process. An attempt is made to integrate this information into modern concepts and hypotheses of the pathogenesis of atherosclerosis and to suggest areas of controversy or uncertainty that may merit further study. For brevity only a small number of selected, mainly review-type references are included; a more complete bibliography on the subject is available from the authors.

General Considerations

In examination of the role of the arterial smooth muscle cell in the atherosclerotic (AS) process, at least two normal anatomic features are important. In fetal life the human intima is devoid of smooth muscle cells. As part of the maturation or aging of the vessel, in the first two to three decades of life SM migrates into the intima from the media and may proliferate, creating a musculoelastic intimal layer (diffuse intimal thickening, DIT). This layer (Table 1) is not atherosclerosis but it may be fertile soil for the development of AS. Another normal anatomic fact is that SM is the only cell of the normal media and functions as a multipotential mesenchymal cell.

It is well established that normal arterial SM makes extracellular products including collagen, elastin, and glycosaminoglycans (proteoglycans); can take up and metabolize lipid, principally via the low-density-lipoprotein (LDL) receptor pathway; can release lipid, at least after cell injury or death; and can respond in a proliferative fashion to a wide range of stimuli. The proliferative response includes both increase in numbers of cells and increase of cellular activities in terms of increased production of extracellular products and of intracellular handling (synthesis, degradation) of lipids, cholesterol and cholesteryl esters. These activities may differ either qualitatively or quantitatively for SM in atherosclerosis when compared to SM of the normal vascular wall.

Three morphologic lesions – fatty streak, atheromatous (fibrous, fibrolipid) plaque, and complicated lesion – usually are considered in discussions of atherosclerosis. It appears that there may be more than one type of fatty streak; some may be truly precursors of the atheromatous plaque while many do not appear to have any such pathogenetic relationship. Although the smooth muscle cell in the form of the myogenic foam cell is an integral component of the fatty streak (Table 1), since the bulk of current evidence suggests that fatty streaks do not usually progress to atheromatous plaques, further consideration of SM in this lesion is not warranted in this brief overview. In contrast, SM has a central and crucial role in the development of the atheromatous plaque and of the complicated plaque (Table 1). Morphologically, the relative importance of SM in complicated lesions seems lesser than in atheromatous plaques, perhaps due to the presence of calcification, hemorrhage, ulceration, thrombosis, plasma proteins, and variable amounts of conventional inflammatory-reparative processes. Although the complicated plaque is almost universally regarded as the result of advanced or reactive

Table 1. Morphology of atherosclerotic and related lesions.

Feature	DIT[a]	Streak	Plaque	Complicated
SM[b]	2+	+	3+	2+/3+
Migration	2+	+	+/2+	+/2+
Prolif.	2+	+(?)	3+	2+/3+
Products[c]	+	+	3+	3+
Repair phenomena (non-SM)	0	0	+/2+	3+
Relative role SM	3+	+	3+	+/2+
Clinical Signif.	0	0	2+	3+

[a]Diffuse intimal thickening.
[b]Smooth muscle cell.
[c]Extracellular products of smooth muscle cell.

changes in the atheromatous (fibrous or fibrolipid) plaque, the pathogenesis
of the complicated lesion may involve more than simply progressive and reactive changes of the atheromatous plaque. Some factor(s) may set off an inflammatory-reparative process that differs from, or is additive to, the proliferative SM process that characterizes the fibrous plaque and produce the
complicated lesion.

The importance of smooth muscle cells is recognized in current theories of
the pathogenesis of atherosclerosis. In the response to injury hypothesis,
which in its broadest sense incorporates both the classic lipid and thrombotic theories, SM is assigned a central role. The clonal hypotheses, whether
the monotypic concept or the clonal senescence view, are based upon SM alterations.

Cellular Biology of Arterial Smooth Muscle

The foregoing general considerations of arterial smooth muscle in normal vessels and in the atherosclerotic process established the critical role of SM
in the pathogensis of atherosclerosis. Accordingly, the cellular and subcellular responses of SM that might be important in the development of atherosclerosis have been studied by a wide variety of techniques in invivo and
invitro situations and in both animals and humans. The generally accepted
results of many such studies and some of the areas of uncertainty or controversy are summarized in the following.

Migration of smooth muscle is well recognized; invivo the path is from media
into intima.

Proliferation of smooth muscle can be stimulated in many ways. The proliferative response may be an increase in numbers of cells or an increase in
cellular activities (both intracellular processes and extracellular products)
or both. SM proliferation can be stimulated by lipoproteins (VLDL, LDL, and
to some degree HDL) that may act through the LDL receptor pathway or may
"bypass" it in some circumstances. The proliferative effects of hyperlipidemic blood or serum may occur on the basis of lipoproteins although cholesterol, cholesteryl esters, and some lipids can stimulate SM proliferation.
Platelet-borne growth factors have been well characterized. Hormones, particularly insulin, stimulate SM proliferation.

A variety of agents primarily cause endothelial injury and SM proliferation
occurs secondarily, perhaps as a reparative process. Included in this group
are immunologic reactions, irradiation, chemicals and drugs, endotoxins,

viruses, and probably cigarette smoke. Hemodynamic influences in many instances also belong in this category, but mechanical events may directly stimulate SM proliferation.

Quantitative studies of the stimuli that initiate SM proliferation in a primary fashion are only rudimentary at this time.

Limited information is available concerning factors that might enhance the proliferative responses of SM to various stimuli. Genetic factors of possible significance include controls of cell membrane receptors for LDL and alterations of intracellular, especially lysosomal, enzymes that are involved in lipid synthesis and degradation. Morphologic and biochemical studies have shown that SM in areas of increased glycosaminoglycans content are more susceptible to proliferative responses.

The proliferation of SM can be inhibited by a variety of drugs, chemicals, and conditions, some of which cause cellular injury in non-proliferating as well as proliferating SM cells. Examples include prostaglandins, fatty acids, oxidative derivatives of cholesterol, HDL, heparin, thrombocytopenia in some models, estrogens, and anti-rheumatic drugs. Age itself appears to have a deleterious effect on SM cellular functions, especially on LDL degradation.

No definitive conclusions can be reached at this time regarding continuation of proliferative responses of SM cells after removal of the inciting stimulus, because of different results in different systems and models, particularly when more than one inciting factor is involved. In addition, the initiating events of the proliferative reaction may be removed, but other stimuli become effective as a sort of complication of the proliferated lesion; the major role of platelet and other coagulation factors in the progression of atheromatous plaques is a clear example of this situation.

As suggested previously, knowledge of the quantitative aspects of stimuli for SM proliferation is minimal. For some agents one concentration could stimulate proliferation and another concentration cause cellular injury that may be reversible or irreversible. In the latter-most circumstance, products of the injured or dead cell might provoke the usual inflammatory-reparative processes and thus contribute to the formation of the lesion.

Although considerable information about the pathobiology of arterial SM is available, the effects of multiple factors on the behavior of SM is less well known, particularly in the intact animal and in the environment of a developed or developing plaque. In these exceedingly complex situations, the carefully determined biological reactions now recognized may be significantly altered. Although most likely a minor consideration, it should be recognized that most studies have, appropriately, focused on normal arterial or plaque SM and virtually no studies have insured that SM in complicated lesions behave in the same way.

Summarizing Comments and Tentative Conclusions

Knowledge and study of the smooth muscle cell in the pathogenesis of atherosclerosis can be viewed in four stages. The first and essentially completed phase was the recognition of the central role of SM in atherosclerotic lesions. The second and currently active stage is the study of the cellular biology of the SM cell. The third level of study, which is only beginning, seeks to synthesize the cellular biological information into total concepts that explain the pathogenesis of atheromatous plaques and complicated lesions. The fourth stage, also just beginning, involves identification of ways to modify the cellular response so as to alter the development of the clinically significant lesions.

Current concepts can be diagrammatically summarized as follows:

"Environmental" factors + SM ⟶ SM reactions
                                 (prolif., injury)

SM reactions ⟶ Atheromatous Plaque

Plaque + Cont. SM reaction
             or   ⟶ Complicated Lesion
          Other factors*

*e.g., usual inflammation-repair phenomena

Possible Future Studies

Among the many interesting questions concerning SM in atherosclerosis that may merit further study, the following are singled out to stimulate, titillate, or provoke investigators. For all, some data are available.

1. What is the fate of the SM cell in proliferative reactions, i.e., continued production of products, quiescence, "atrophy" or death? This matter appears important in consideration of regression.
2. Is the biological behavior of the arterial SM cell the same as SM cells in other tissues and organs?
3. Is the fatty streak always or sometimes or never a true precursor of the atheromatous or complicated lesion? SM studies may not provide answers to this problem.
4. Is the complicated lesion definitely just an advanced stage of the atheromatous plaque with secondary changes (that is, a sort of end-stage process) or do factors other than SM responses determine its development?
5. What role, if any, do immunologic reactions play in the SM responses or in the development of atherosclerotic lesions?

Continued study of these and other, perhaps more significant problems will contribute to the resolution of the conundrum of atherosclerosis.

References

Benditt EP (1977) The origin of atherosclerosis. Sci Am 236:74
Geer JC, Haust MD (1972) Smooth muscle cells in atherosclerosis. Monographs in atherosclerosis Vol II. Karger, Basel
Goldstein JL, Brown MS (1977) The low-density lipoprotein pathway and its relation to atherosclerosis. Ann Rev Biochem 46:897
Hauss WH, Mey J, Schulte H (1979) Effect of risk factors and antirheumatic drugs on the proliferation of aortic wall cells. Atherosclerosis 34:119
Haust MD (1978) Light and electron microscopy of human atherosclerotic lesions. Adv Exp Med Biol 104:33
Kottke BA, Subbiah MR (1978) Pathogenesis of atherosclerosis: concepts based on animal models. Mayo Clin Proc 53:35
Ross R, Glomset JA (1976) The pathogenesis of atherosclerosis. New Eng J Med 295:369, 420
Thomas WA, Reiner JM, Florentin RA, Jovakidevi K, Lee KJ (1977) Arterial smooth muscle cells in atherogenesis: births, deaths and clonal phenomena. In:Schettler G et al. (eds) Atherosclerosis IV. Springer-Verlag, Berlin
Wissler RW (1978) Progression and regression of atherosclerotic lesions. Adv Exp Med Biol 104:77

Mononuclear Phagocytes in Atherosclerosis[1]

C.W.M. Adams and O.B. Bayliss-High

The identity of cells in the atherosclerotic plaque has been much discussed in the older histological and ultrastructural literature. More recently histochemical techniques have been used to distinguish cells of the mononuclear phagocyte series from vascular smooth muscle. These techniques depend on the much greater oxidative and lysosomal enzyme activity in mononuclear cells than in vascular smooth muscle, e.g. catalase (Adams et al. 1975), cytochrome oxidase (Adams and Bayliss 1976a,b), acid esterase (Wolman and Gaton 1976; Gaton and Wolman 1977), acid lipase (Schaffner et al. 1977, 1978). In the present presentation it was shown that β-galactosidase gives superior results in identifying mononuclear phagocyte cells than the other methods mentioned above (see Bayliss-High and Adams 1980).

The predominant cell in the early stages of cholesterol-induced rabbit atheroma is known to be a large rounded fat-filled foam cell. This cell reacts strongly with the β-galactosidase technique. Small foci of such activity are occasionally seen in the underlying smooth muscle of tunica media, indicating slight focal induction of lysosomal enzyme activity in these sites.

In the normal human aorta, in the fatty streak lesion and in the uncomplicated human fibro fatty plaque, mononuclear phagocytes stainable by the above techniques either lie in the subendothelial space or enter only relatively superficially into the lesion. Cells at the shoulders of fibro fatty plaques often show a collection of such mononuclear cells. Histiocytes in the tunica adventitia and lining occasionally penetrating vasa vasorum in the outer media also are stained by these methods.

Human atherosclerotic lesions complicated by mural thrombosis, ulceration, subintimal haemorrhage or calcification often show reparative organization accompanied by capillarization. Such capillarization is associated with the entry of monocytes from the blood into the lesion. Thus, mononuclear phagocytes come to pallisade around cholesterol crystals, as shown both with haematoxylin-eosin and with β-galactosidase (Fig. 1). Occasionally, such mononuclear cells form a nearly complete syncytial envelope to the crystal (Fig. 2) and this syncytium goes on to form a typical Langhans giant cell (Fig. 3) (Bayliss-High and Adams 1980). Cholesterol crystals are absent where giant cells are to be found in human atherosclerosis; this constitutes limited evidence of minor lipid regression in man. However, the extent of such regression by giant cells seems to be mainly of theoretical rather than practical importance.

---

[1] Supported in part by a grant from the British Heart Foundation.

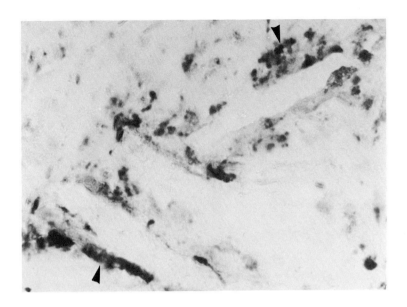

FIG. 1. β-galactosidase activity (arrows) in mononuclear
phagocytes (macrophages) pallisading around cholesterol
clefts. Advanced human aortic atherosclerosis, Lake-Lojda
indigogenic method, X c.250

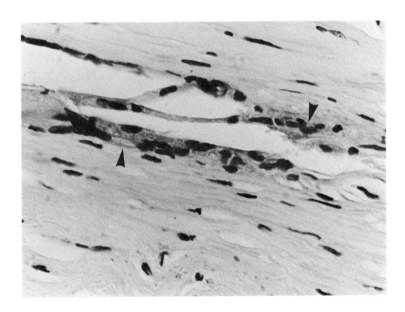

FIG. 2. Mononuclear phagocytes (arrows) forming a syncytium around cholesterol clefts. Advanced human aortic
atherosclerosis. H and E, X c.250

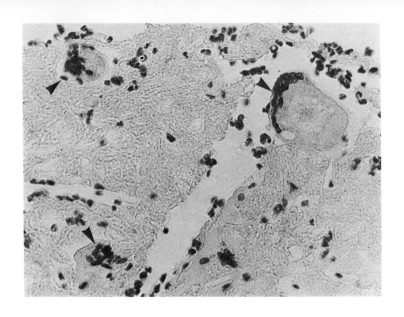

FIG. 3. Giant cells (arrows) in advanced human atherosclerosis. Note: Vascular channel at center. H and E,
X c.200

References

Adams CWM, Bayliss OB (1976a) Detection of macrophages in atherosclerotic le-
    sions with cytochrome oxidase. Br J Exp Pathol 57:30-36
Adams CWM, Bayliss OB, Turner DR (1975) Phagocytes, lipid-removal and regres-
    sion of atherosclerosis. J Pathol 116:225-238
Adams CWM, Bayliss OB (1976b) Succinic dehydrogenase and cytochrome oxidase
    in arterial, venous and other smooth muscle. Atherosclerosis 23:367-370
Bayliss-High, OB and Adams CWM (1980) Macrophages and giant cells in human
    atherosclerotic lesions. Atherosclerosis, in press
Gaton E, Wolman M (1977) The role of smooth muscle cells and haematogenous
    macrophages in atheroma. J Pathol 123:123
Schaffner T, Elner VM, Wissler RW (1977) Histochemical localization of acid
    lipase with naphthyl fatty acid esters. Fed Proc 36:400
Schaffner T, Elner VM, Bauer M, Wissler RW (1978) Acid lipase: A histochemical
    and biochemical study using Triton X-100-naphthyl palmitate micelles. J
    Histochem Cytochem 26:696-712
Wolman M, Gaton E (1976) Macrophages and smooth muscle cells in the pathogene-
    sis of atherosclerosis. J Israel Med Assoc 99:450

Altered Permeability in Atherosclerosis—Morphological Evidence

Sören U. Björkerud

The accumulation in the arterial wall of material from the blood stream is one of the most apparent manifestations of atherosclerosis. Hence, arterial permeability for blood constituents may be of primary importance in atherogenesis.

Several structural entities may function as permeability barriers in the arterial wall. The most apparent - and at present best known - is the endothelium. Other possible candidates as barriers are the intercellular matrix and the elastic constituents (Fig. 1).

Transendothelial passage of material as studied with different tracers occurs via plasmalemmal vesicles and through intercellular junctions as shown by Florey and Sheppard, Stein and Stein, and Hüttner and collaborators. Regional differences were apparent between different segments of the arterial tree.

Fry found that the experimental increase of the hemodynamic flow strain to a level at which histological changes in the endothelium can be detected is followed by increased permeability for certain proteins. The experimental elimination of the endothelium in experiments on rabbits by Bondjers and Björkerud was followed by an increased permeability of ca 30 times for low density lipoprotein (LDL)-cholesteryl ester. Thus, the endothelium is a very prominent permeability barrier for certain proteins and lipoproteins. Injury to the endothelium would consequently impair this barrier (for review see Björkerud 1979).

It is now well established that the integrity of the arterial endothelium varies. Areas with a lowered integrity have larger numbers of injured endothelial cells and are commonly found near branching points, in bends or constrictions, i.e. places where increased hemodynamic strain can be expected to occur (Björkerud and Bondjers 1972; Caplan et al. 1974). Such regions are more permeable for albumin (Packham et al. 1967), LDL-cholesteryl ester (ca 4 times in the normocholesterolemic rabbit; Bondjers and Björkerud 1973) and fibrinogen and accumulate more cholesterol in the cholesterol-fed pig (Bell et al. 1975).

The endothelial permeability barrier is not static. Its efficiency may vary with the magnitude of the load. In hypercholesterolemic rabbits at serum cholesterol levels of about 400 mg% the permeability for LDL-cholesteryl ester in the high-integrity areas is ca 10 times and in the low-integrity areas ca 100 times that in the normocholesterolemic animal (Bondjers et al. 1976). From these data it can be concluded that the importance of the endothelial barrier per se increases with increasing LDL-load. The importance of a high integrity of the endothelium is dramatically augmented when the serum cholesterol level of the animal reaches the human pathophysiological range.

Low integrity areas of arterial endothelium are not devoid of endothelial lining but contain large numbers of injured endothelial cells. The mitotic rate in the endothelium is increased in areas corresponding to low-integrity endothelium (Schwartz and Benditt 1973). It is, therefore, likely that low-integrity areas are characterized by a high turn-over rate and would contain rather immature endothelium. Apart from leakage through injured cells the increased permeability of the low-integrity areas could be due to immaturity of the endothelium, as for young arterial endothelium occurring in other situations (Schwartz and Benditt 1975).

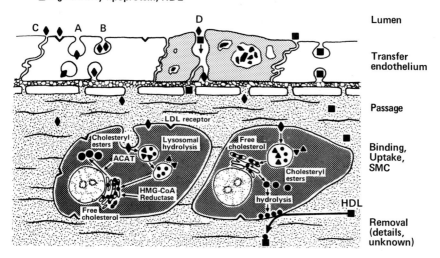

Fig. 1. Scheme depicting different routes for the passage of material from the blood stream into and out from the arterial wall with special emphasis on low density lipoprotein-bound cholesterol. Material is transferred from the lumen through the endothelium via plasmalemmal vesicles bound to receptors (A) or suspended in vesicular fluid (B), through discontinuities in injured endothelial cells (D) or through intercellular clefts (C). The latter route may be more prevalent in immature arterial endothelium where intercellular clefts are broader and have less developed tight junctions (Schwartz et al. 1975). Other structures, such as elastic tissue and intercellular matrix, may act as permeability barriers against passage of material into and out from the wall. Specific mechanisms may be responsible for the mobilization and removal of material, such as high density lipoproteins. HDL has been proposed as carrier for cholesterol out from the arterial tissue. From Björkerud (1979).

Several factors promote the over-all endothelial injury and permeability. Some of these factors are also epidemiological risk factors for atherosclerosis. Hypertension augments the degree of aortic endothelial injury in the rat (Björkerud and Eriksson 1976) and the permeability for certain tracers (Jellinek et al. 1969; Hüttner et al. 1973). Hypoxic endothelial injury, a mechanism that has been suggested as responsible for increased atherogenesis connected to heavy smoking, is accompanied by a marked increase of aortic permeability for certain tracers (Elemér et al. 1975).

A change of the distribution of the low-integrity endothelium is found in cholesterol-induced atherosclerosis with a preponderance to the periphery of the plaques (Bondjers et al. 1977). The periphery of such plaques is also more permeable for albumin (Friedman and Byers 1963). It is possible that this redistribution of high-injury and -permeability endothelium is responsible for the spreading and growth of the plaques.

Other structures than the endothelium such as intercellular matrix and elastic tissue may act as barriers against influx of material from the blood stream. The importance of such factors is, however, poorly known and barrier function and sequestering are difficult to separate. It may be stated that the endothelium can be considered as major permeability barrier towards influx into the non-atherosclerotic arterial wall and maybe also in the early stages of atherosclerosis. This may, however, not be the case in later stages when other constituents such as fibrous capsule may exert a strong barrier function.

"Permeability" in a general sense does not only imply promotion of passage of matter into the arterial wall. Impair of passage of material out from the wall, i.e. elimination, may be just as important or even more important from an atherogenic point of view. Information on this function is, however, virtually non-existent, a fact that seriously limits our understanding of the atherogenic process.

References

Bell FP, Day AJ, Gent M, Schwartz CJ (1975) Differing patterns of cholesterol accumulation and 3H-cholesterol influx in areas of the cholesterol-fed pig aorta identified by Evans blue dye. Exp Mol Pathol 22: 366-375
Björkerud SU (1979) Mechanisms of atherosclerosis. Pathobiology Annual 9:277-301
Björkerud S, Bondjers G (1972) Endothelial integrity and viability in the aorta of the normal rabbit and rat as evaluated with dye exclusion tests and interference contrast microscopy. Atherosclerosis 15:285-300
Björkerud S, Eriksson L-O (1976) Strain, injury, adaption, and repair in hypertensive macroangiopathy. In: Rorive G, Cauwenberge H van (eds) The arterial hypertensive disease. Masson, New York, pp 39-49
Bondjers G, Björkerud S (1973) Cholesterol accumulation and content in regions with defined endothelial integrity in the normal rabbit aorta. Atherosclerosis 17:71-83
Bondjers G, Brattsand R, Hansson GK, Björkerud S (1976) Cholesterol transfer and content in aortic regions with defined endothelial integrity from rabbits with moderate hypercholesterolemia. Nutr Metab 20:452-460
Caplan BA, Gerrity RG, Schwartz CJ (1974) Endothelial cell morphology in focal areas of in vivo Evans blue uptake in the young pig aorta. I. Quantitative light microscopic findings. Exp Mol Pathol 21:102-117
Elemér G, Kerényi T, Jellinek H (1975) Effect of temporary hypoxia on the permeability of the rat aorta. Path Europ 10:123-128
Friedman M, Byers SO (1963) Endothelial permeability in atherosclerosis. Arch Pathol 76:111-117
Hüttner I, Boutet M, Rona G, More RH (1973) Studies on protein passage through arterial endothelium. III Effect of blood pressure levels on the passage of fine structural protein tracers through rat arterial endothelium. Lab Invest 29:536-546
Jellinek H, Nagy Z, Hüttner I, Bálint A, Kócze A, Kerényi T (1969) Investigations of the permeability changes of the vascular wall in experimental malignant hypertension by means of a colloidal iron preparation. Br J exp Path 50:13-16
Packham MA, Rowsell HC, Jørgensen L, Mustard JF (1967) Localized protein accumulation in the wall of the aorta. Exp Mol Pathol 7:214-232.
Schwartz SM, Benditt EP (1973) Cell replication in the aortic endothelium. Lab Invest 28:699-707
Schwartz SM, Stemerman MB, Benditt EP (1975) The aortic intima. II. Repair of the aortic lining after mechanical denudation. Am J Pathol 81:15-42

The Elastic Element in the Arterial Wall: Biosynthesis and Degradation[1]

L. Robert

The elastic fibers are quantitatively and qualitatively important consti-
tuants of the arterial wall. They make up about 40% of the total proteins
in the thoracic aorta, about 20% of the abdominal aorta and about 10% in
most elastic arteries. The degradation of elastic fibers was recognized
by the histopathologists as an early sign of the aging of the arterial
wall and of the development of the arteriosclerotic lesion (Balo 1963).
Elastin is one of the four major macromolecular constituents which make up
the intercellular matrix (the three other families of macromolecules being
the collagens, the proteoglycans and the structural glycoproteins)(Robert
and Robert 1973). It is phylogenetically the "youngest" constituent of
connective tissues because in its present form it can be found only from
the vertebrates on. The other macromolecules appearing much earlier during
phylogenesis, from the first metazoans (collagens, structural glycoproteins) or from the higher invertebrates (proteoglycans).

Elastin is not only the "youngest" of the matrix macromolecules but it
appears also to be the one which is the earliest in being attacked and
lysed during the aging and atherosclerotic process. Histological techniques show an incipient elastolysis (fragmentation of elastic laminae)
starting from the intima and progressing to the adventitia in adolescents
and young adults. This early onset of elastolysis is in an apparent
contradiction with the great chemical and physical stability of the
elastin protein. As a matter of fact it is the most resistent protein of
the organism because it can be obtained in a highly purified form by 45
minutes heating at 100° in 0.1N NaOH (Robert and Hornebeck 1976). Elastin
is however susceptible to hydrolytic attack of H^+ or OH^- ions in the
presence of organic solvents and these findings suggested the hydrophobic
theory of elasticity (Robert and Poullain 1966 ; Kornfeld-Poullain and
Robert 1968). As a matter of fact the lipids can play the same role in
vivo as organic solvents in vitro and play certainly an important role
in the degradation of elastic fibrils (Jacotot et al. 1973 ; Claire et
al. 1976 ; Kramsch 1977).

Elastin is also highly susceptible to some specific proteases, the
elastases, which are capable to degrade it at a relatively high rate.
The results obtained in several laboratories over the last decade enable
us to formulate certain hypotheses concerning the regulation of the
biosynthesis and degradation of elastic tissues as influenced by age and
arteriosclerosis.

Regulation of the Biosynthesis of Elastins

Elastin is synthesised by some specialized mesenchymal cells and in
particular by the smooth muscle cells of the arterial wall. Its probable
precursor is the proelastin molecule of about twice the molecular weight

[1]Supported by C.N.R.S. (GR N° 40), D.G.R.S.T. (Acc Pario Vasculaire),
I.N.S.E.R.M. (ATP Tabac).

of the tropoelastin immediate precursor of crosslinked elastin (Foster
et al. 1976 ; Sandberg et al. 1976). At least too important enzymes
are involved in the processing of the biological precursors of elastin :
tropoelastàse (Foster et al. 1976) and a lysine-oxidase (Harris and
Garcia-de-Quevedo 1978) the first acting on proelastin to yield tropoelastin and the second to catalyze the formation of special covalent
intercatenary bonds, the so-called desmosine and isodesmosine residues
(Partridge 1970). The incorporation of ^{14}C-lysine into desmosine enables
the quantitation of the biosynthesis of crosslinked elastin in aorta
organ cultures or smooth muscle cell cultures. We could show that this
precursor is actively incorporated into crosslinked elastin as well as
in other matrix macromolecules in rabbit aorta organ cultures (Moczar et
al. 1976). This incorporation decreased strongly with the age of the
rabbits. When, however, smooth muscle cells were cultured out of these
aorta explants and their incorporation capacity was studied at the 4th
passage no decrease of the total matrix macromolecule synthesis could be
demonstrated between smooth muscle cells derived from newborn rabbit aorta
and from adult rabbit aorta using radioactive proline and glucosamine as
precursors (Moczar et al. 1976). These findings suggested the hypothesis
that the cell matrix interaction is an important regulatory factor in the
age dependent decrease of the rate of biosynthesis of intercellular matrix
in general and of elastin in particular. The precise nature of the
mechanism by which the matrix can influence the cell function is not yet
known but it is very probable that this informational feedback between
cells synthesising their specific matrix and the matrix influencing on its
turn the cell behaviour is an important part of the regulatory mechanisms
involved in the normal and pathological behaviour of mesenchymal tissues.

Degradation of Elastins

As was mentioned earlier specific proteolytic enzymes called elastases
appear to be responsible for the in vivo degradation of elastic fibrils
(Bieth 1978). Several elastases were isolated, purified and characterized
from a variety of cells and tissues. Several of these elastases were
demonstrated to be present in the circulating blood and elastase activity
could also be extracted and purified from man and pig aorta (Hornebeck
et al. 1975). For the moment, it is difficult to make definitive statements concerning the relative responsibilities of these elastases in the
degradation of arterial or skin elastin. Both the pancreatic elastases
E_1 and E_2, leukocyte elastase, platelet elastase and smooth muscle cell
elastolytic protease may be involved in the degradation of arterial
elastin. Studies actually undertaken in our laboratory tend to determine
the relative roles of these elastases in this process. It is however
probable that several of these enzymes will be found to be involved in
this process. The very recently identified fibroblast metallo-protease
(fibroblast elastase) (Bourdillon et al. unpublished data) and the lipoprotein bound elastase recently isolated from human sera (Bellon et al.
unpublished data) are probably responsible for the early degradation of
skin and aorta elastic fibers confirmed recently by the detailed morphological studies of Bouissou et al. (1976).

We could recently identify a lipoprotein bound elastolytic activity in
human serum and it seems quite possible that this lipoprotein bound
elastase would penetrate with the lipoproteins in the arterial wall and
could contribute actively to the degradation of elastin. It is also
conceivable that the local synthesis of elastase by smooth muscle cells
could be stimulated by some noxious influence and be also strongly
involved in this degradative process.

We could show that there is a simultaneous decrease of crosslinked elastin in the arterial wall as a function of age and arteriosclerosis and an increase of elastolytic activity in these same arterial wall specimens (Hornebeck 1978).

Role of the Lipids

It was shown both by the studies of Kramsch and coworkers (1977) and by our own studies (Szigeti et al. 1972 ; Jacotot et al. 1973 ; Claire et al. 1976) that lipids can strongly interact with elastin and the lipid elastin complexes formed in vivo or in vitro are highly resistent to even strong physicochemical extracting agents. We could thus identify the presence of a whole spectrum of free fatty acids and cholesterol esters in elastin samples isolated from human aorta elastin. As a result of the abovementioned investigations, it can be assumed that this interaction between lipids and elastin is probably involved in the loss of elasticity of elastic fibers and the accelerated degradation by elastases.

Conclusions

Recent studies suggest that the rate of biosynthesis of polymeric elastin decreases with age in the arterial wall and that this decrease is accelerated by arteriosclerosis. The amount of elastolytic enzymes increases in the arterial wall with age and with the gravity of the arteriosclerotic process. The interaction between lipids and elastic tissues is probably an important factor in the acceleration of the elastolytic process and in the loss of the elastic elements of the arterial wall and also in other mesenchymal tissues such as the skin. Several elastases were identified in the circulating blood and in the arterial wall and may be involved in this process.

References

Balo J (1963) Connective tissue changes in atherosclerosis. In : Hall DA (ed) International review of connective tissue research. Academic Press, New York/London, Vol I, pp 241-306

Bellon G, Hornebeck W, Robert L (1978) Méthodes simples pour quantifier l'élastase et ses inhibiteurs dans le sérum humain. Path Biol 26: 515-521

Bieth J (1978) Elastases : structure, function and pathological role. In : Robert L (ed) Frontiers of matrix biology. S. Karger, Basel, Vol 6, pp. 1-82

Bouissou H, Pieraggi MT, Julian M, Douste-Blazy L (1976) Simultaneous degradation of elastin in dermis and in aorta. In : Robert L (ed) Frontiers of matrix biology. S. Karger, Basel, Vol. 3, pp 242-255

Claire M, Jacotot B, Robert L (1976) Characterization of lipids associated with macromolecules of the intercellular matrix of human aorta. Connective Tissue Res 4: 61-71

Foster JA, Mecham R, Imberman M, Faris B, Franzblau C (1977) A high molecular weight species of soluble elastin-proelastin. In : Sandberg LB, Gray WR, Franzblau C (eds) Elastin and elastic tissue. Plenum Press, New York/London (Advances in Experimental Medicine and Biology, Vol. 79, pp 351-369

Jacotot B, Beaumont JL, Monnier G, Szigeti M, Robert B, Robert L
(1973) Role of elastic tissue in cholesterol deposition in the arterial wall. Nutr Metabol 15: 46-58

Harris ED, Garcia-de-Quevedo MC (1978) Reaction of lysyl oxidase with soluble protein substrates : effect of neutral salts. Arch Biochem Biophys 190: 227-233

Hornebeck W, Derouette JC, Robert L (1975) Isolation, purification and properties of aortic elastase. FEBS Lett 58: 66-70

Hornebeck W, Adnet JJ, Robert L (1978) Age dependant variation of elastin and elastase in aorta and human breast cancers. Exp Gerontol 13: 293-298

Kornfeld-Poullain N, Robert L (1968) Effets de différents solvants organiques sur la dégradation alcaline de l'élastine. Bull Soc Chim Biol 50: 759-771

Kramsch DM (1978) The role of connective tissue in atherosclerosis. In : Kritchevsky D, Paoletti R, Holmes WL (eds) Drugs, lipid metabolism and atherosclerosis. Plenum Press, New York/London (Advances in Experimental Medicine and Biology, Vol 109, pp 155-194)

Moczar M, Ouzilou J, Courtois Y, Robert L (1976) Age dependence of the biosynthesis of intercellular matrix macromolecules of rabbit aorta in organ culture and cell culture. Gerontology 22: 461-462

Partridge SM (1970) Isolation and characterization of elastin. In : Balazs EA (ed) Chemistry and molecular biology of the intercellular matrix. Academic Press, London/New York, Vol. 1, pp 593-616

Robert L, Poullain N (1966) Structure de l'élastine. Rôle des forces hydrophobes. Arch Mal du Coeur 59: 121-127

Robert L, Hornebeck W (1976) Preparation of insoluble and soluble elastins. In : Hall DA (ed) The methodology of connective tissue research. Joynson-Bruvvers Ltd, Oxford, pp 81-104

Robert B, Robert L (1973) Aging of connective tissues. General considerations. In : Robert L (ed) Frontiers of Matrix Biology. S. Karger, Basel, Vol. 1, pp 1-45

Sandberg LB, Gray WR, Foster JA, Torres AR, Alvarez VL, Janata J
(1977) Primary structure of porcine tropoelastin. In : Sandberg LB, Gray WR, Franzblau C (eds) Elastin and elastic tissue. Plenum Press, New York/London (Advances in Experimental Medicine and Biology, Vol. 79, pp 277-284)

Szigeti M, Monnier G, Jacotot B, Robert L (1972) Distribution of ingested ^{14}C-cholesterol in the macromolecular fractions of rat connective tissue. Connective Tissue Res 1: 145-152

Prostacyclin Production by Vascular Smooth Muscle and Endothelial Cells

H. Sinzinger, K. Silberbauer, and W. Auerswald[1,2]

It has been shown originally by Moncada et al. (1976) that prostacyclin (PGI_2),
a new metabolite of the arachidonic acid (20:4) metabolism, is formed by vascular tissue. This new prostaglandin has been demonstrated to be the most potent known inhibitor of platelet aggregation (Gryglewski et al. 1976) and a
very strong vasodilator. In their original paper Moncada et al. (1976) pointed out that only vascular endothelium forms prostacyclin which was the base
for their hypothesis that an intact endothelial lining prevents mural platelet
thrombus formation. Later, Moncada et al. (1977), Hornstra et al. (1977) and
Silberbauer et al. (1978) found using different methods that the endothelial
lining is the main source of PGI_2, but subendothelial and medial tissue generate prostacyclin too.

As earlier reports demonstrated (Hornstra et al. 1978), because tissue damage
enhances the PGI_2-synthesis by liberation of enzymes, it is very difficult to
answer the question "How much PGI_2 is formed by various types of vascular
cells?" Moncada et al. (1977) and Herman et al. (1977) showed a continuous decrease of PGI_2-formation from the endothelial layer towards the adventitia.
Until now, no information about cellular prostacyclin formation in tissue cells
has been reported.

The aim of our study was to examine how different preparation and separation
methods influence the total vascular tissue PGI_2-formation. In addition, we
studied the PGI_2-generation of endothelium and resting vascular tissue in
various species. Finally, we looked at the PGI_2-synthesis of human intimal
preparations with different contents of two types of smooth muscle cells.

Methodological Approach

Using Moncada's bioassay (Moncada et al. 1976) in which the inhibitory effect
of prostacyclin formed by the vascular tissue on ADP-induced platelet aggregation in vitro is quantified by means of a synthetic PGI_2-standard (Sinzinger et al. 1978), it can be demonstrated that even after longer incubation
periods, there is still detectable PGI_2-formation (Silberbauer et al. 1978).
At these intervals it can be easily demonstrated by light and scanning electron microscopy that the endothelial layer is almost completely desquamated.
This morphological finding is indicative of the fact that the resting tissue
generates PGI_2 also (Moncada et al. 1977; Herman et al. 1977; Hornstra et al.
1978; Silberbauer et al. 1978).

However, this incubation procedure is not a very useful technique for obtaining reproducible data, though it does not enhance the overall PGI_2-synthesis.

[1]This investigation was supported by the Atherosclerosis and Thrombosis Research Commission of the Austrian Academy of Sciences.
[2]The PGI_2-standard was kindly provided by Dr. John E. Pike.

Table 1. Alteration of PGI$_2$-formation by methodological tissue damage.

	%[a]
Passive desquamation	0
Endothelial removal (Cellulose acetate strip)	10
Micropreparation	20
In vitro ballooning	50
Mincing	>50

[a]% = increase in PGI$_2$-formation.

The most useful method for selective separation of the endothelial sheet seems to be the removal by cellulose acetate strips (Sinzinger et al. 1979b). This procedure enhances PGI$_2$-formation only to about 10% (Table 1). Micropreparation causes an increase in PGI$_2$-formation of at least 20%; this increase is strongly dependent on size, type and lesions of the vessel wall as well as on the technician performing the procedure, and is therefore not sufficiently reproducible. More intensive damaging methods, such as ballooning, lead to very severe tissue damage.

PGI$_2$-formation by Endothelium

From this methodological point of view, the cellulose-acetate-strip method provides a useful methodological approach for the study of endothelial PGI$_2$-synthesis, which we estimated in abdominal aortic tissue of various species. With the exception of rabbits (Figure 1), it appears that the single endothe-

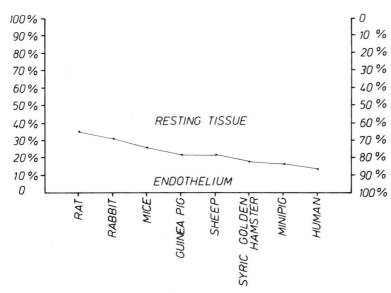

FIG. 1. PGI$_2$-formation by endothelium and resting tissue in various species (pg/mg/min).

lial layer produces the highest amounts of PGI_2 in those species which are resistant to atherosclerosis. The tissues from species which develop very early and severe atherosclerosis, e.g. humans and swine, have a low endothelial PGI_2-synthesizing capacity. These results confirm earlier findings and the hypothesis that the overall PGI_2-generation in vascular tissue from species resistant to the development of atherosclerosis is statistically significantly higher (Sinzinger et al. 1979a). The question of whether various types (morphological and functional stages) of endothelial cells generate different amounts of PGI_2 is still unanswered. However, it seems noteworthy that endothelium of vascular prosthetic grafts implanted in humans and rabbits generate less prostacyclin (Winter et al. unpublished work presented at 7th Congress of Angiology, July 1978) than normal endothelium in neighboring areas.

PGI_2-formation by Vascular Smooth Muscle Cells

To investigate if different PGI_2-generation occurs in different vascular smooth muscles cells (SMC), we used an earlier finding (Feigl et al. 1975) that activated smooth muscle cells (aSMC), characterized by higher chromophilia, increased ^{35}S-incorporation and ^3H-thymidine labeling (Haust and More 1972) and contractiles exhibit a characteristic distribution in human splenic artery specimen. Looking at intimal preparations of human splenic artery with a high and a low aSMC content, a significantly ($p < 0.025$) higher PGI_2-formation could be observed for aSMC (13.77 ± 5.35 pg/mg/min) than for cSMC (8.29 ± 4.36 pg). These studies have not yet been done in other arteries, where the distribution of aSMC is known to be different as well as in different species with and without an experimental lesions.

Recently, Larrue et al. (personal communication) found a significantly depressed PGI_2-formation in cultured cells from atherosclerotic aortas as compared to cultured smooth muscle cells from normal aortas. These findings as well as the data with salicylate in culture (J Mey, personal communication) and Shimamoto's findings (1969) that experimental atheromatosis is c-AMP mediated, suggest that PGI_2 plays an important role in the regulation of SMC-proliferation.

Summary

A high endothelial prostacyclin formation could be a protection mechanism against atherosclerosis in some species. Prostacyclin plays an important role in activation and/or proliferation of SMC. However, it is still unclear, if the enhanced activity of PGI_2 causes the proliferation or is only a side effect or even a secondary phenomenon inhibiting further proliferation.

References

Feigl W, Sinzinger H, Wagner O, Leithner C (1975) Quantitative morphological investigations on smooth muscle cells in vascular surgical specimens and its clinical importance. Experientia 31:1352-1353
Gryglewski R, Bunting S, Moncada S, Flower RJ, Vane RJ (1976) Arterial walls are protected against deposition of platelet thrombi by a substance (prostaglandin X) which they make from prostaglandin endoperoxides. Prosta-

    glandins 12:685-693

Haust MD, More RH (1972) In: Wissler RW, Jones RJ (eds) The pathogenesis of atherosclerosis. Williams and Wilkins, Baltimore

Herman AG, Moncada S, Vane JR (1977) Formation of prostacyclin (PGI$_2$) by different layers of the arterial wall. Arch Int Pharm Int 227:162-163

Hornstra GE, Haddeman E, Don JA (1978) Some investigations into the role of prostacyclin in thrombo-regulation. Thromb Res 12:367-375

Moncada S, Gryglewski R, Bunting S, Vane JR (1976) An enzyme isolated from arteries transforms prostaglandin endoperoxides to an unstable substance that inhibits platelet aggregation. Nature 263:663-665

Moncada S, Herman AG, Higgs EA, Vane JR (1977) Differential formation of prostacyclin (PGx or PGI$_2$) by layers of the arterial wall. An explanation for the anti-thrombotic properties of vascular endothelium. Thromb Res 11: 323-337

Shimamoto T (1969) Experimental study on atherosclerosis. An attempt at its prevention and treatment. Acta Pathol Jap 19:15-21

Silberbauer K, Sinzinger H, Winter M (1978) Prostacyclin production by vascular smooth muscle cells. Lancet 1:1356-1357

Sinzinger H, Silberbauer K, Wagner O, Winter M, Auerswald W (1978) Prostacyclin - Perliminary results with vascular tissue of various species and its importance for atherosclerotic involvement. Atherogenesis 3:123-134

Sinzinger H, Clopath P, Silberbauer K (1979) Is the vascular prostacyclin formation in various species responsible for their susceptibility to atherosclerosis. Experientia, in press

Sinzinger H, Silberbauer K, Auerswald W (1979) Prostacyclin formation by vascular smooth muscle cells. Folia Angiol, in press

Lipid, Apoprotein and Lipoprotein Origin and Synthesis

Barry Lewis and Richard J. Havel

During the last decade, research on the protein moieties of the plasma lipoproteins has provided a major new dimension to research on the origin of
these macromolecules. It is now clear that the triglyceride-rich lipoproteins are synthesized in near final form in the intestinal mucosa and liver,
but the mechanisms of formation of the cholesterol-rich low density lipoproteins (LDL) and high density lipoproteins (HDL) remain uncertain. Several of the approaches to the origin of lipoproteins and the regulation of
lipoprotein biosynthesis were exemplified by the five speakers at this Workshop.

Dr. G. S. Getz reported studies on the biogenesis of apolipoprotein E, a
component of very low density lipoproteins (VLDL), intermediate density
lipoproteins (IDL) and HDL. He described the isolation of a mRNA coding
for apo E and indicated that about 1% of the protein synthesis directed by
rat liver mRNA comprised apo E. The primary translation product, though it
resembled apo E in electrophoretic mobility, resembled other secreted proteins in having an N-terminal extension or "signal peptide." This peptide,
in the case of apo E, appeared to comprise 18 amino acid residues and was
leucine-rich. Partial purification of an mRNA coding for apo E was reported.
The polysomes which react with a monospecific anti-apo E comprised 9-12 ribosomes and represented 0.7% of hepatic polysomes.

Dr. R. L. Hamilton described the isolation of lipoproteins from Golgi apparatus-rich fractions of rat liver. Nascent VLDL have been identified and
characterized from such fractions which differ from plasma VLDL chiefly in
having a smaller complement of C apoproteins, a deficiency which is corrected by transfer of these proteins from HDL after secretion. A small amount
of material was obtained in the HDL density range from Golgi-rich fractions,
some of which appeared as discoidal particles by electron microscopy, but
it is uncertain whether this material represents "nascent" HDL. Well defined discoidal HDL appeared in perfusates of isolated rat livers, which
were rich in apo E and also contained apo A-I and the apo C's. Of importance
is the observation that such discoidal HDL also appeared in undiminished
amounts in perfusates of livers from rats treated with orotic acid, which
almost entirely prevented secretion of nascent VLDL. In this connection,
the observation reported by Dr. Getz that orotic acid did not interfere with
formation of mRNA directed apo E synthesis was of considerable interest.
Dr. Hamilton also found spherical particles that contain apo B in the HDL
density fraction of perfusates of rat livers. Whether these particles, as
well as the discoidal HDL, are directly secreted by the liver, remains uncertain. Discoidal HDL are regularly observed in humans with genetic or
acquired deficiency of lecithin-cholesterol acyltransferase and are converted
to spherical (pseudomicellar) HDL by action of this enzyme.

Dr. D. B. Weinstein dealt with lipoprotein production by isolated hepatocytes maintained in a monolayer. He used an arginine-deficient medium to
inhibit growth of other cell lines. The preparation synthesized VLDL and
HDL, but not LDL. ^{3}H-glycerol was incorporated into triglycerides linearly.
This rate was increased three-fold in cells from sucrose-fed animals. Conversely it was decreased by addition to the medium of macromolecular sub-

stances such as albumin and dextran, an effect not mediated by changes in osmolarity. The isolated hepatocyte preparation has characteristics suggesting that it will provide a valuable model for the study of factors modulating lipoprotein synthesis in a simple system.

The contribution of human intestinal mucosal cells to apolipoprotein production was discussed by Dr. R. M. Glickman. Lymph chylomicrons from both rats and humans contain apolipoproteins B, E, A-I, A-IV and C's. There is evidence from labeled amino acid incorporation of small intestinal synthesis of some (B, A-I and A-IV) but not all of these. By studying the chiefly intestinal lipoproteins excreted in patients with chyluria, the effect of fat-feeding on these particles could be followed: an increase both in triglyceride and protein in the chylomicron fraction was observed. Semi-quantitative estimates suggested that on the order of 50% of circulating apo A-I and A-II might enter plasma on triglyceride-rich lipoproteins of intestinal origin. Apo A-IV also enters plasma from the small intestine, but it is noteworthy that 70% of this peptide in chyluric urine was isolated after ultracentrifugation in the fraction of density >1.21 g/ml. Though it is possible that this is in part an artifact of ultracentrifugation, gel chromatography of plasma also suggested that apo A-IV exists in part in non-lipoprotein form.

It seems clear that LDL normally arise largely, if not entirely, as a product of the degradation of triglyceride-rich lipoproteins. Dr. S. Eisenberg discussed the hypothesis that triglyceride-rich lipoproteins are the only primary secreted particles. Incubation of VLDL with lipoprotein lipase yielded particles resembling, but not identical with LDL; one difference from native LDL was an excess of cholesteryl esters. If HDL_3 were added to this system, the formation of HDL_2-like particles was observed. It was suggested that the conversion of VLDL to LDL requires, not only lipoprotein lipase, but also an interaction with cells and/or the presence of lipid transfer proteins. It was reported that the hepatic lipase rapidly converts VLDL to LDL-like lipoproteins.

The different approaches to the problem of lipoprotein biosynthesis described in the Workshop provide useful methods to evaluate a complex biological problem. To the extent possible, it will be necessary to test in intact animals the conclusions reached from these approaches. The search for inborn human disorders of these events should continue as a means to dissect critical steps in lipoprotein biosynthesis and interconversions.

Origin in Plasma of Low Density and High Density Lipoproteins[1]

Shlomo Eisenberg

A concept that the low density (LDL) and high density (HDL) lipoproteins of the blood plasma are products of triglyceride transport in chylomicrons and very low density lipoproteins (VLDL) and not primary secretory products of cells has been recently developed by us (Eisenberg et al. 1978a, 1978b; Eisenberg 1979a). The concept assumes that chylomicrons and VLDL are the primary lipoproteins synthesized and secreted by cells in normolipidemic states. It is further assumed that both LDL and HDL are by-products of the process of fat transport, the former being a final "core remnant", and the latter a final "surface remnant" of the triglyceride-rich lipoproteins. This concept is presented schematically in Figure 1 and is described and discussed here.

The Origin of Low Density Lipoproteins

Conversion of VLDL constituents to LDL in vivo has been established for the apo B moiety of the lipoprotein (Bilheimer et al. 1972; Eisenberg et al. 1973; Sigurdsson et al. 1975; Berman et al. 1978). Other LDL constituents (cholesterol, phospholipids and the remaining triglycerides) presumably also originate from VLDL. The essential enzymic reaction in LDL formation is triglyceride hydrolysis and removal of hydrolytic products at extrahepatic sites. This reaction is dependent on the presence of and activity of the endothelial bound extrahepatic lipoprotein lipase. Indeed, LDL is practically absent from the plasma of humans with severe defect of lipolysis, Type I hyperlipoproteinemia (Fredrickson et al. 1968) or apo C-II deficiency (Breckenridge et al. 1978).

Studies in vitro, however, have demonstrated that the formation of LDL from VLDL cannot be equated with triglyceride hydrolysis. About 80% of the phospholipids and unesterified cholesterol and almost all of the apo C and apo E molecules are deleted from the surface coat of lipolyzed VLDL during the conversion of the particle to IDL (Eisenberg and Rachmilewitz, 1975) or LDL (Deckelbaum et al. 1979). Most of the triglycerides (>98%) are hydrolyzed and even some cholesterol ester molecules are removed from the VLDL particle. In the in vitro system, the apo C removed from the VLDL is found in HDL. Phospholipids are removed by two pathways, hydrolysis of glycerophosphatides to lysocompounds and distribution of unhydrolyzed phospholipids to HDL (Eisenberg and Schurr 1976). Cholesterol is found mainly with HDL. In this experiment we have attempted to reconstruct the two domains of the intact and post-lipolysis VLDL, i.e., the core and surface coat (Eisenberg 1976). The data show conclusively that the volume of core constituents is in excellent agreement with the calculated core volume of the two lipoproteins, and that the concentration of surface constituents at the outer shell of the two particles remained unchanged. We suggest that the primary event is the decrease of the core volume followed by a coordinated deletion of surface

[1] The author's personal research cited was supported by research grants No. 219 and No. 1189 from the U.S.-Israel Binational Science Foundation and research grant No. HL23864-01 from the U.S. Public Health Service.

constituents. Along this conversion process, a change of the apoprotein profile of the particle takes place, from a predominant apo C to a predominant apo B particle. If the interactions of the particles with lipoprotein lipase are dependent on the concentration of apo C at the lipoprotein surface, and those with tissue cells on that of apo B then it is expected that the biological interactions of the particles will change along the delipidation path. That this is the case, and that the VLDL delipidation path and the LDL receptor path are related has been demonstrated in many experiments, as discussed elsewhere (Eisenberg 1979b).

Can true LDL particles be formed in the test-tube? To answer this question, we have recently attempted to achieve complete lipolysis (triglyceride hydrolysis more than 98%) of human plasma VLDL following incubation in vitro with lipoprotein lipase (Deckelbaum et al. 1979). After the incubation about 80% of the VLDL cholesterol esters were associated with an in vitro produced LDL at density of 1.019-1.063 g/ml. The in vitro LDL was isolated, characterized and compared to circulating LDL isolated from the plasma of the VLDL-donors. The two were very similar in lipid composition, lipid to protein ratio, phospholipid composition and organization of the lipid phase (mainly cholesterol esters). The in vitro LDL differed, however, from the circulating lipoprotein in several respects. The in vitro particle contained twice as many cholesterol ester molecules as the circulating particle, was about 20% larger in average diameter, contained more non-B protein and more phospholipids than the native particle. The data thus demonstrated that LDL can be formed in vitro and is essentially a collapsing product of the core of the lipolyzed VLDL particle. This pathway is shown schematically in Figure 1. However, because of the differences between the two, we suggest that additional interactions of the lipolyzed VLDL with plasma or cell constituents may be involved with the formation of LDL in vivo. These may include lipid exchange proteins, other enzymes (the heparin releasable triglyceride hydrolase of hepatic origin and the lecithin:cholesterol acyltransferase (LCAT), other lipoproteins and cell surfaces.

The Origin of High Density Lipoproteins

The first clue that some or most of the HDL constituents may be derived from the surface coat of lipolyzed triglyceride-rich lipoproteins stemmed from the observation that the apoproteins, phospholipids and unesterified cholesterol content of HDL increase promptly after the injection of heparin to humans or rats (Eisenberg et al. 1973; Eisenberg and Rachmilewitz 1975) and during clearance of alimentary chylomicronemia (Havel et al. 1973). Yet, when we realized that deletion (or exclusion) of surface constituents during lipolysis is an essential feature of the interaction of triglyceride-rich lipoproteins and lipoprotein lipases, that we started to suspect that the relationships between HDL and triglyceride transport may play an important role in HDL formation. To understand these relationships, we started to follow the fate of VLDL surface constituents during lipolysis carried out in the absence of plasma.

In our initial study, we have found that apo C distributed from VLDL to higher density fractions, predominantly that of HDL (d 1.04-1.21 g/ml) and d > 1.21 g/ml, when rat plasma VLDL was lipolyzed in vitro in the absence of plasma (Glangeaud et al. 1977). The appearance of apo C at the buffer density range of HDL in the absence of plasma indicated that a high density lipoprotein particle originated from the lipolyzed VLDL. Subsequent studies carried out during perfusion of the isolated rat heart with labeled VLDL (Chajek and Eisenberg 1978) or during in vitro incubation (Eisenberg and Olivecrona 1979) have substantiated the earlier observations. In these experiments, furthermore, we followed the fate of all lipid constituents of VLDL labeled biosynthetically with [^{14}C]-palmitic acid, [^{3}H]-cholesterol and

[^{32}P]-phospholipids. Both phospholipids (lecithin and sphingomyelin) and unesterified cholesterol were freed from the lipolyzed VLDL and accumulated together with apo C at the HDL density range. We therefore concluded that an HDL precursor ("nascent" HDL) was generated as a by-product of VLDL lipolysis.

The morphology of the HDL precursors generated during VLDL lipolysis was investigated by electron microscopy. As expected, these were discoidal lipoproteins, about 250 x 60 Å in diameter, indistinguishable from other nascent HDL particles isolated from rat liver perfusates (Hamilton et al. 1976) and from intestinal lymph (Green et al. 1978).

A comparison of the hepatic, intestinal and nascent HDL generated during VLDL lipolysis revealed that all three have similar lipid composition but are different in apoprotein profile. The hepatic particles contain predominantly apo E, the intestinal HDL contain apo A-I and apo A-II, whereas the HDL produced during VLDL lipolysis contain predominantly apo C. These differences, however, are reconciled when the nature of the triglyceride-rich lipoprotein present in each of the three systems is considered: the hepatic VLDL contains predominantly apo E, the intestinal chylomicrons apo A-I and the VLDL, apo C. Is it then possible that in each system the nascent HDL is produced from the triglyceride-rich lipoproteins? This question cannot be answered at the present time. Yet, as discussed later, there exists enough circumstantial evidence to assume that "surface remnants" generated during lipolysis of triglyceride-rich lipoproteins are a major source of the circulating HDL lipids and proteins.

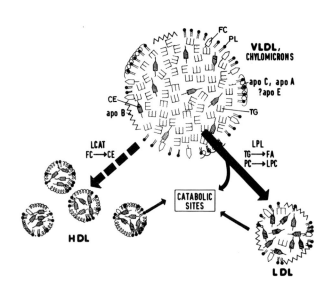

FIG. 1.   Schematic representation of the metabolism of triglyceride-rich lipoproteins, and the formation of LDL ("core remnants") and HDL ("surface remnants") from the lipolyzed lipoprotein.

TG = Triglycerides, CE = Cholesterol esters,   PL = Phospholipids,
FC = Free cholesterol,   FA = Fatty acids,   PC = Phosphatidylcholine,
LPC = Lysophophastidylcholine,   LPL = Lipoprotein lipase,   LCAT =
Lecithin:cholesterol acyltransferase.

How surface fragments are transformed to the spherical circulating HDL is uncertain. The most logical metabolic pathway that could perform this conversion is the cholesterol esterifying pathway, mediated through the LCAT activity, as suggested by Hamilton et al. (1976). It has recently been shown that apo A-I and apo A-II are synthesized and secreted by intestinal absorption cells and are associated with the triglyceride-rich lipoproteins in the intestinal lymph (Imaizumi et al. 1978; Green et al. 1979). Apparently, most of the apo A comes off the chylomicrons only after they circulate in plasma (Schaefer et al. 1978), presumably following their interaction with lipoprotein lipases. Most of the HDL lipids (phospholipids and unesterified cholesterol) however, originate from the continued metabolism of chylomicrons and from lipolyzed VLDL. We suggest that the A proteins and the lipid-rich surface fragments become associated in the HDL density range to form true HDL precursors. These precursors are an ideal substrate for the LCAT reaction and are transformed to spherical HDL particles. We further assume that the amount of apo A and of phospholipids generated from triglyceride transport are such that the initial HDL particles formed are of the HDL_3 subpopulation.

This same pathway, however, provides also an explanation for the existence in plasma of two discernible HDL subpopulations, the HDL_3 and HDL_2. More recently, we have studied in detail the effects of lipolysis on HDL_3, the low molecular weight HDL subpopulation (Patsch et al. 1978). Lipolysis was carried out in vitro as described above, but HDL_3 was included in the incubation mixture. With this system we have consistently observed that phospholipids, unesterified cholesterol and apo C freed from the lipolyzed VLDL distributed to the existing HDL_3 particles. Since the combined density of the VLDL surface constituents transferred to the HDL_3 was lower than that of acceptor lipoprotein, the density of the HDL_3 decreased towards that of HDL_2. Thus, a conversion of HDL_3 to HDL_2-like particles was achieved in the test tube. On the basis of these observations we suggest that indeed HDL_3 is a precursor in plasma for HDL_2, and that this conversion again necessitates the activity of the LCAT system for the final transformation of the HDL_2-like particles to the circulating lipoprotein. We further suggest that the HDL_3 to HDL_2 conversion takes place when the amount of phospholipids and unesterified cholesterol generated exceeds the capacity of the A proteins to form HDL_3.

In summary, the experiments described here support our concept that LDL is a modified "core-remnant" and HDL a modified "surface-remnant" of triglyceride-rich lipoproteins. This concept is presented schematically in Figure 1. There is no doubt that plasma LDL is derived mainly from lipolyzed VLDL although the exact mechanism(s) by which LDL is formed from VLDL, and possibly also from chylomicrons, are still obscure. The views presented with regard to the origin of HDL however are largely speculative and are based on only a few observations. Yet, it is interesting to note that many observations heretofor unexplained, are compatible with the hypothesis. Surface fragments originating from triglyceride-rich lipoproteins have been consistently observed in two genetic diseases when either HDL is absent from the plasma (Tangier disease) or when there is a congenital deficiency of the LCAT system (Herbert et al. 1978; Forte et al. 1979). HDL levels, and in particular HDL_2 levels, are moreover highly correlated with lipoprotein lipase activity and triglyceride transport (Nikkila 1978). Conversely, HDL levels are extremely low, and HDL_2 is absent, from the plasma of patients with lipoprotein lipase deficiency (Fredrickson et al. 1968) or apo C-II deficiency (Breckenridge et al. 1978). In this last situation, HDL levels promptly increase after administration of the apo C-II. Inasmuch as all these and other examples support the concept, they do not prove it. Only by further research will it be possible to prove - or disprove - the concept, and to delineate the pathways involved with the origin of HDL and with the regulation of the circulating levels of the lipoprotein.

References

Berman M, Eisenberg S, Hall MH, Levy RI, Bilheimer DW, Phair RD, Goebel RH
(1978) Metabolism of apoB and apoC lipoproteins in man: kinetic studies
in normals and hyperlipoproteinemics. J Lipid Res 19: 38-56

Bilheimer DW, Eisenberg S, Levy RI (1972) The metabolism of very low density
lipoproteins. I. Preliminary in vitro and in vivo observations. Biochim
Biophys Acta 260: 212-221

Breckenridge WC, Little JA, Steiner G, Chow A, Poapst M (1978) Hypertriglyceridemia associated with deficiency of apolipoprotein C-II. New
Engl J Med 298: 1265-1273

Chajek T, Eisenberg S (1978) Very low density lipoprotein. Metabolism of
phospholipids, cholesterol, and apolipoprotein C in the isolated perfused rat heart. J Clin Invest 61: 1654-1665

Deckelbaum RJ, Eisenberg S, Fainaru M, Barenholz Y, Olivecrona T (1979) In
vitro production of human plasma low density lipoprotein-like particles. A model for very low density lipoprotein catabolism. J Biol Chem
254: 6079-6087

Eisenberg S (1976) Metabolism of very low density lipoprotein. In: Greten H
(ed) Lipoprotein Metabolism. Springer, Heidelberg, pp. 32-43

Eisenberg S (1979a) Plasma lipoproteins interconversion: The origin of
plasma LDL and HDL. Ann N Y Acad Sci In press

Eisenberg S (1979b) Very low density lipoprotein metabolism. Prog in
Biochem Pharmacol, 15: 139-165

Eisenberg S, Olivecrona T (1979) Very low density lipoprotein. Fate of phospholipids, cholesterol, and apolipoprotein C during lipolysis in vitro.
J Lipid Res 20: 614-623

Eisenberg S, Rachmilewitz D (1975) The interaction of rat plasma very low
density lipoprotein with lipoprotein lipase rich (post-heparin) plasma.
J Lipid Res 16: 451-461

Eisenberg S, Schurr D (1976) Phospholipid removal during degradation of rat
plasma very low density lipoprotein in vitro. J Lipid Res 17: 578-587

Eisenberg S, Bilheimer DW, Lindgren FT, Levy RI (1973) On the metabolic conversion of human plasma very low density lipoprotein to low density lipoprotein. Biochim Biophys Acta 326: 361-377

Eisenberg S, Chajek T, Deckelbaum R (1978a) Mode of formation of HDL:
Hypothesis. J Am Oil Chem Soc 55: A256

Eisenberg S, Chajek T, Deckelbaum RJ (1978b) Molecular aspects of lipoproteins
interconversions. Pharmacol Res Commun 10: 729-738

Forte T, Norum KR, Glomset JA, Nichols AV (1971) Plasma lipoproteins in familial lecithin: cholesterol acyltransferase deficiency: Structure of low and
high density lipoproteins as revealed by electron microscopy. J Clin
Invest 50: 1141-1148

Fredrickson DS, Levy RI, Lindgren FT (1968) A comparison of heritable abnormal
lipoprotein patterns as defined by two different techniques. J Clin
Invest 47: 2446-2457

Glangeaud MC, Eisenberg S, Olivecrona T (1977) Very low density lipoprotein.
Dissociation of apolipoprotein C during lipoprotein lipase induced lipolysis. Biochim Biophys Acta 486: 23-35

Green PHR, Glickman RM, Sandek CD, Blum CB, Tall AR (1979) Human intestinal
lipoproteins. Studies in chyluric subjects. J Clin Invest 64: 233-242

Green PHR, Tall AR, Glickman RM (1978) Rat intestine secretes discoid high
density lipoprotein. J Clin Invest 61: 528-534

Hamilton RL, Williams MC, Fielding CJ, Havel RJ (1976) Discoidal bilayer
structure of nascent high density lipoproteins from perfused rat liver.
J Clin Invest 58: 667-680

Havel RJ, Kane JP, Kashyap ML (1973) Interchange of apolipoproteins between
chylomicrons and high density lipoproteins during alimentary lipemia in
man. J Clin Invest 52: 32-38

Herbert PN, Forte T, Heinen RJ (1978) Tangier Disease: one explanation of
lipid storage. New Eng J Med 299: 519-522

Imaizumi K, Havel RJ, Fainaru M, Vigne JL (1978) Origin and transport of
    the A-I and arginine-rich apolipoprotein in mesenteric lymph of rats.
    J Lipid Res 19: 1038-1046
Nikkila EA (1978) Metabolic and endocrine control of plasma high density
    lipoprotein concentration. In: Gotto AM, Miller NE, Oliver MF (eds)
    High Density Lipoproteins and Atherosclerosis. Elsevier, North Holland
    Biomedical Press, Amsterdam, New York, pp 177-192
Patsch JR, Gotto AM, Olivecrona T, Eisenberg S (1978) Formation of high
    density lipoprotein$_2$-like particles during lipolysis of very low den-
    sity lipoprotein in vitro. Proc Natl Acad Sci USA 75: 4519-4523
Schaefer EJ, Jenkins LL, Brewer HB (1978) Human chylomicron apoprotein
    metabolism. Biochem Biophys Res Commun 80: 405-411
Sigurdsson G, Nicoll A, Lewis B (1975) The metabolism of very low density
    lipoproteins in hyperlipidemia: studies of apolipoprotein B kinetics
    in man. Eur J Clin Invest 6: 167-177

Biological and Biochemical Aspects of ML-236B (Compactin) and Monacolin K, Specific Competitive Inhibitors of 3-hydroxy-3-methylglutaryl Coenzyme A Reductase

Akira Endo

Introduction

In anticipation that plasma cholesterol levels may be lowered by inhibiting sterol synthesis in the liver, the major organ that supplies plasma choles- terol, studies aimed at identifying the specific inhibitors of cholesterol synthesis of microbial origin were started in my laboratory in 1971. Since then two novel compounds, ML-236B (compactin) and monacolin K, have been dis- covered and isolated as low-toxic, potent inhibitors of sterol synthesis from ^{14}C acetate in a cell-free enzyme system of rat liver. This paper briefly reviews biological and biochemical data on these two compounds.

Mechanism of Action of ML-236B

ML-236B, which was isolated from cultures of Penicillium citrinum in 1974 and published in 1976 (Endo et al. 1976a), has a chemical structure shown in Fig. 1. The lactone portion of the molecule can be converted to the acid form by saponification which is very similar to HMG (3-hydroxy-3-methylglutarate) in structure (Fig. 1).

The acid form of ML-236B is more active than the lactone form, inhibiting sterol synthesis from ^{14}C-acetate in the cell-free system 50% at a concentra- tion of 10 ng/ml. In cholesterol synthetic pathway, ML-236B inhibits solely the enzymatic step for the conversion of HMG-CoA to mevalonate that is cata- lyzed by HMG-CoA reductase, the rate-limiting enzyme in cholesterol synthetic pathway. As can be expected from its structure, its mode of action in the inhibition of the reductase is competitive with respect to the substrate HMG- CoA (Endo et al. 1976b; Tanzawa and Endo 1979), giving a Ki value of approx- imately 1 nM (Brown et al. 1978; Endo 1979b).

ML-236B is also inhibitory to sterol synthesis in cultured cells (Brown et al. 1978; Doi and Endo 1978; Kaneko et al. 1978). Inhibition of sterol synthesis from ^{14}C-acetate is approximately 50% at a concentration of 20 ng/ml in L cells and at as low as 4 ng/ml in human fibroblasts from normal subjects and patients with homozygous familial hypercholesterolemia when cells are grown in the presence of whole fetal calf serum. Conversion of ^{14}C-mevalonate into

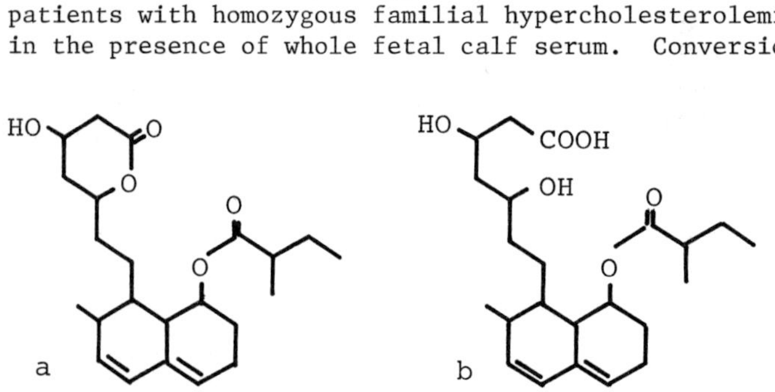

FIG. 1a and b. Structures of lactone form (a) and acid form (b) of Ml-236B.

sterols and syntheses of other lipids and macromolecules like DNA, RNA and protein in cultured cells are, however, not affected even at higher concentrations. The ML-236B-mediated inhibition of sterol synthesis is readily reversible. The complete inhibition of endogenous sterol synthesis at higher concentrations (up to 5μg/ml) of the drug causes a marked inhibition of cell growth even in the presence of exogenous cholesterol contained in whole fetal calf serum as lipoproteins. This inhibition of growth is prevented by the additional presence of mevalonate in the culture medium, thus indicating that ML-236B inhibits cell growth by specifically interferring with mevalonate synthesis, a step that is catalyzed by HMG-CoA reductase. This inhibition of the reductase activity of cultured cells for a longer period results in the production of large amounts of enzyme. The appearance of this HMG-CoA reductase activity cannot be suppressed fully by the addition of LDL (low density lipoprotein) to the culture medium. However, the enzyme can be completely suppressed by the addition of small amounts of mevalonate together with LDL.

ML-236B is readily absorbed into the liver, the major site of cholesterol synthesis, after oral administration to mice; peak concentration of the drug in the liver, which attained within 60 min after administration, is approximately 10% of the dose (Endo et al. 1977). Inhibition of sterol synthesis from ^{14}C-acetate is also observed in tissue slices obtained from rats which previously received ML-236B. Of the sterol synthesis in various tissues tested including the liver, kidney, lung, spleen, ileum, testis, adrenal, prostate, skin, muscle, and aorta, that in the liver and skin is far more strongly inhibited by the drug administration than the other tissues (Endo et al. 1979). Similarly, ML-236B is inhibitory to sterol synthesis in vivo in various tissues of rats in which ^{14}C-acetate was intraperitoneally injected to the animals and labeled digitonin-precipitable sterols formed were isolated and determined (Endo et al. 1977).

Hypocholesterolemic Activity of ML-236B

ML-236B produces no detectable decreases in plasma cholesterol levels in mice, rats (Endo et al. 1979) and hamsters (A Endo et al., unpublished work), when administered for a longer period at a daily dose of as high as 500-2,000 mg/kg either normo- or hypercholesterolemic conditions, except for rats treated with the detergent Triton WR-1339 (Kuroda et al. 1977). Further no changes in plasma lipoprotein composition can be observed in normal rats by the treatment with the drug.

The administration of ML-236B to rats causes a significant decrease in fecal excretion of bile acids and in the hepatic levels of cholesterol 7α-hydroxylase activity, and produces a marked increase in hepatic levels of HMG-CoA reductase activity, resulting in no inhibition of hepatic sterol synthesis, even in the presence of the drug in the active form(s) (Endo et al. 1979). It is likely that the lack of hypocholesterolemic effects of ML-236B in normal rats could, at least partly, be explained by changes in the activity of these two hepatic microsomal enzymes.

On the other hand, ML-236B produces a significant reduction in both plasma cholesterol and phospholipid levels in dogs, when used at a dose higher than 10 mg/kg per day (Tsujita et al. 1979). Triglyceride levels are not consistently changed. Of the lipoprotein classes β-and pre-β-lipoproteins are preferentially lowered. The drug causes no significant changes in the cholesterol content of the liver and aorta and in the activity of serum GOT, GPT, CPK and lecithin: cholesterol acyltransferase under conditions where the drug is administered at a higher dose (100-400 mg/kg) for 5 weeks. Fecal excretion of neutral sterols is unaffected but that of bile acids is markedly elevated in dogs by the drug treatment. Under these conditions, hepatic cholesterol 7α-hydroxylase activity shows no detectable changes. These results are in contrast to those obtained with the rat.

In cynomolgus monkeys, ML-236B is effective in lowering plasma cholesterol levels at a dose of 20-50 mg/kg per day (Kuroda et al. 1979). Concentrations of plasma phospholipids and triglycerides are, however, not significantly reduced by the drug treatment. Of the lipoprotein fractions, a β-lipoprotein corresponding to LDL is preferentially reduced by the drug. ML-236B also causes a slight increase in fecal excretion of bile acids in the monkeys.

Of the other animal species tested, ML-236B is effective in lowering plasma cholesterol levels in hens and rabbits (A Endo, unpublished work). When laying hens are treated with the drug at a 0.06% level in the diet for 4 weeks, a 20% reduction of cholesterol content of egg yolk is also obtained.

Finally, ML-236B has been shown to be highly effective in man (Yamamoto et al. 1979). After 4-8 weeks of the drug treatment at a daily dose of 50-150 mg, plasma cholesterol levels are reduced by 11-37% (27% decrease on average) in patients with heterozygous familial hypercholesterolemia and with combined hyperlipidemia. Cholesterol lowering effects are usually observed within two weeks at a dose of 75-100 mg/day, and this effect is sustained for at least 2-5 months so long as the patients are kept on a maintenance dosage. No significant side effects have so far been observed after using the drug for at least 5 months at doses up to 200 mg/day for adult patients.

Monacolin K

Monacolin K is a new inhibitor of cholesterol synthesis which has recently been isolated in my laboratory from cultures of the fungus Monascus ruber (Endo 1979a, 1979b). The chemical structure of this metabolite is very similar to that of ML-236B (FIG.2). As can be expected from its structure, monacolin K is a specific competitive inhibitor of HMG-CoA reductase, giving a Ki value of 0.49 nM. However, it is far more active than ML-236B in both in vitro and in vivo systems. Thus, monacolin K inhibits sterol synthesis from ^{14}C-acetate in the cell-free system 50% at a concentration of 2 ng/ml. Further, monacolin K produces a significant reduction of both plasma and liver cholesterol levels at a dose of 4 mg/kg in Triton-treated rats, while, under the same conditions, a dose of approximately 20 mg/kg is required for producing a significant effect with ML-236B.

Conclusion

The results of these studies have clearly shown that inhibition of cholesterol synthesis by a specific competitive inhibitor of HMG-CoA reductase is a highly effective means of reducing plasma cholesterol levels in man and also in some animal species except the mice, rat and hamster.

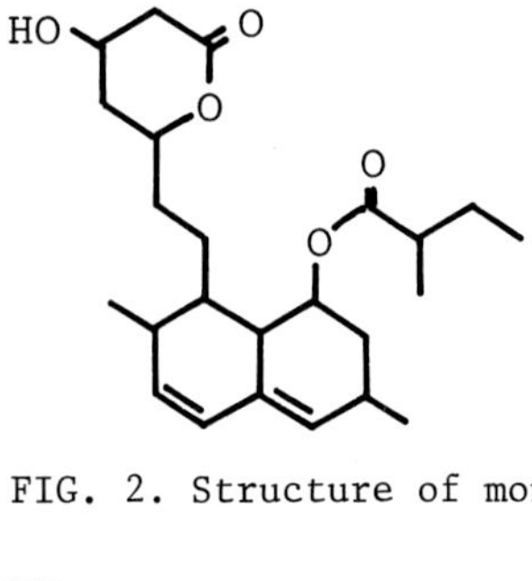

FIG. 2. Structure of monacolin K.

References

Brown MS, Faust JR, Goldstein JL, Kaneko I, Endo A (1978) Induction of 3-hydroxy-3-methylglutaryl coenzyme A reductase activity in human fibroblasts incubated with compactin (ML-236B), a competitive inhibitor of the reductase. J Biol Chem 253: 1121–1128

Doi O, Endo A (1978) Specific inhibition of desmosterol synthesis by ML-236B in mouse LM cells grown in suspension in a lipid-free medium. Japanese J Med Sci Biol 31: 225–233

Endo A (1979a) Monacolin K, a new hypocholesterolemic agent produced by a Monascus species. J Antibiotics 32: 852–854

Endo A (1979b) Monacolin K, a new hypocholesterolemic agent that specifically inhibits 3-hydroxy-3-methylglutaryl coenzyme A reductase. FEBS Letters, in press

Endo A, Kuroda M, Tsujita Y (1976a) ML-236A, ML-236B, and ML-236C, new inhibitors of cholesterogenesis produced by Penicillium citrinum. J Antibiotics 29: 1346–1348

Endo A, Kuroda M, Tanzawa K (1976b) Competitive inhibition of 3-hydroxy-3-methylglutaryl coenzyme A reductase by ML-236A and ML-236B, fungal metabolites having hypocholesterolemic activity. FEBS Letters 72: 323–326

Endo A, Tsujita Y, Kuroda M, Tanzawa K (1977) Inhibition of in vitro and in vivo cholesterol synthesis by ML-236A and ML-236B, competitive inhibitors of 3-hydroxy-3-methylglutaryl coenzyme A reductase. Eur J Biochem 77: 31–36

Endo A, Tsujita Y, Kuroda M, Tanzawa K (1979) Effects of ML-236B on cholesterol metabolism in mice and rats: lack of hypocholesterolemic activity in normal animals. Biochim Biophys Acta, in press

Kaneko I, Hazama-Shimada Y, Endo A (1978) Effects of ML-236B, a competitive inhibitor of 3-hydroxy-3-methylglutaryl coenzyme A reductase, on the lipid metabolism in cultured cells. Eur J Biochem 87: 313–321

Kuroda M, Tanzawa K, Tsujita Y, Endo A (1977) Mechanism for elevation of hepatic cholesterol synthesis and serum cholesterol levels in Triton WR-1339-induced hyperlipidemia. Biochim Biophys Acta 489: 119–125

Kuroda M, Tsujita Y, Tanzawa K, Endo A (1979) Hypolipidemic effects in monkeys of ML-236B, a competitive inhibitor of 3-hydroxy-3-methylglutaryl coenzyme A reductase. Lipids 14: 585–589

Tanzawa K, Endo A (1979) Kinetic analysis of the reaction catalyzed by 3-hydroxy-3-methylglutaryl coenzyme A reductase using two specific inhibitors. Eur J Biochem 98: 195–201

Tsujita Y, Kuroda M, Tanzawa K, Kitano N, Endo A (1979) Hypolipidemic effects in dogs of ML-236B, a competitive inhibitor of 3-hydroxy-3-methylglutaryl coenzyme A reductase. Atherosclerosis 32: 307–313

Yamamoto A, Sudo H, Endo A (1979) Therapeutic effects of ML-236B in primary hypercholesterolemia. Atherosclerosis, in press

Biosynthesis of Rat Apolipoprotein E[1]

Godfrey S. Getz, Rick Hay, and Catherine Reardon

Apolipoprotein E biosynthesis is of particular interest for several reasons. It is a major apolipoprotein of both primary lipoproteins secreted by the liver, namely VLDL and nascent HDL (Marsh 1976; Felker et al. 1977). Unlike the other major apolipoproteins which are made in both the liver and the intestine, significant amounts of apolipoprotein E do not appear to be made in the intestine (Wu and Windmueller 1979). Apolipoprotein E exhibits a genetically influenced polymorphism, which may have a relationship to certain forms of dyslipoproteinemia (Utermann et al. 1977). The plasma concentration of apolipoprotein E and its distribution amongst lipoprotein fractions is significantly modified by the feeding of cholesterol to several species, including rat (Mahley and Holcombe 1977; Weisgraber et al. 1977) and man (Mahley et al. 1978). The most pronounced changes are in the formation of B-VLDL, enriched in apolipoprotein E, and of relatively large quantities of HDL_c, in which apolipoprotein E is the major apoprotein. The latter lipoprotein shows particular affinity for the low density lipoprotein receptor of fibroblasts in culture (Innerarity and Mahley 1978) and readily transports cholesterol into the cell, effecting the same regulation of intracellular cholesterol metabolism first described in association with the incorporation of LDL cholesterol into the cell (Innerarity and Mahley 1978; Goldstein and Brown 1977). Although the detailed function of apolipoprotein E remains obscure, these observations suggest that modulations of its biosynthesis and secretion may be physiologically and pathologically important. Since messenger RNA (mRNA) is the central component in probing the regulation of gene expression and of translational control, our studies have focussed on the characterization of apolipoprotein E-mRNA from rat liver and of its primary translation product.

Both nascent rat liver VLDL and HDL are substantially enriched in apolipoprotein E (Marsh 1976; Hamilton et al. 1976; Sales 1976), suggesting that this may be the most prominent apolipoprotein produced by the liver. Using multiple preparations of total rat liver mRNA to direct protein synthesis in an heterologous wheat germ translation system, 0.9-1.3% of the total protein produced is specifically immunoprecipitable by a purified antibody raised against apolipoprotein E. Antibodies separately obtained from several rabbits and a goat have yielded quantitatively and qualitatively similar results. When the washed immunoprecipitate is dissociated in SDS and analyzed by polyacrylamide gel electrophoresis, the only high molecular weight product comigrates with mature plasma apolipoprotein E (Figure 1) at several gel concentrations, and on gradient slab gels. This was an unexpected finding.

Most secreted proteins are segregated within the lumen of rough endoplasmic reticulum by vectorial translation (Blobel and Dobberstein 1975). In most cases this process involves the synthesis of a hydrophobic N-terminal extension, or "signal peptide," of 15 or more amino acids. Despite the identical electrophoretic mobility of the apoprotein E in vitro translation product and mature apoprotein E, the former does appear to have a leucine-rich N-terminal extension. In demonstrating this we have taken advantage of the known amino-

---

[1] The authors' personal research cited was supported by USPHS research grants SCOR-Atherosclerosis HL 15062, HL 12332, and GM 0093.

terminal sequence of apoprotein E--Glx.Gly.Glx.Leu.Glx.Val.Thr.Asp.X.Leu.Pro. A large-scale in vitro translation was performed with leucine as the isotopic precursor. The translation product having the same electrophoretic mobility as mature apolipoprotein E and immunoprecipitated with specific antibody to apoprotein E was isolated by preparative gel electrophoresis. The electro-eluted radioactive protein was subjected to radiochemical analysis by sequen-tial Edman degradation by Drs. Reddy and Kohler. This experiment has been performed twice with identical results. Radioactivity corresponding to ^{3}H-leucine was found in sequenator cycles 4,7,8,9,12,17,22, and 28 among the first 40 N-terminal residues. Thus, only the leucine residues found at posi-tions 22 and 28 of the in vitro product correspond to the expected interleu-cine spacing (i.e., positions 4 and 10) of the mature molecule (Figure 2). These results suggest that newly translated rat apolipoprotein E includes a leucine-rich (one-third of amino acid residues), and therefore probably hydro-phobic, signal peptide 18 amino acid residues in length. Further chemical confirmation of this inference is in progress. Both the length and leucine content of this signal peptide are consistent with previously analyzed trans-lation products (Strauss et al. 1977; Palmiter et al. 1977). The relatively short sequence is compatible with a similar electrophoretic mobility of pre-cursor and mature protein, especially if differences in glycosylation between translated and secreted proteins are considered.

Initial experiments aimed at isolating apolipoprotein E-mRNA have been per-formed. Affinity-enriched anti-apolipoprotein E labelled with radioactive iodine has been shown to bind to a particular subset of hepatic polysomes (Figure 3). This subset is distinct from that synthesizing serum albumin, and also from that synthesizing apolipoprotein B (latter data not shown). This binding is saturable by a large excess of nonradioactive antibody of the same specificity. These and other findings detailed elsewhere (Hay and Getz 1979) strongly suggest that the antibody binding is to the specific nascent peptides carried on subpopulations of polysomes. The anti-apolipoprotein E binds to polysomes consisting of 9-12 ribosomes, a finding which is consistent with the synthesis of a protein 30,-40,000 daltons in size. When the polysomes complexed with bound antibody are then precipitated with anti-antibody, they are substantially purified from the total polysome population (Hay and Getz

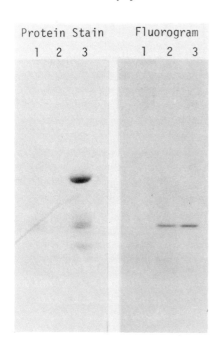

Protein Stain   Fluorogram
  1   2   3   1   2   3

FIG. 1. Electrophoresis of purified in vitro translation products. Protein stain and fluorogram of slab gel containing only mature apolipoprotein E (lanes 1), immuno-precipitated apolipoprotein E translation product (lanes 3), and apoE translation product electroeluted from immunoprecipi-tated material (lanes 2). The two stained but nonradioactive bands in lane 3 repre-sent immunoglobulin in the initial immuno-precipitate; a small amount of unlabelled mature apoE was added as carrier to the material in lane 3 prior to electroelution.

157

1979). Messenger RNA obtained from these precipitated polysomes is 17- to
30-fold enriched, compared to total hepatic mRNA, in its capacity to direct
the in vitro synthesis of the apoprotein E precursor in our heterologous wheat
germ system. The precipitated polysomes represent 0.7% of the total hepatic
polysomes, thus corroborating our other estimates of the proportion of total
in vitro protein synthesis devoted to apoprotein E-like products.

Antibody to apoprotein E also binds specifically to hepatic polysomes and
ribonuclease-generated monoribosomes derived from rats fed 1% orotic acid
for 10 days. Messenger RNA extracted from the livers of these rats contains
molecules directing the synthesis of apoprotein E in the heterologous wheat
germ system, at a level comparable to that obtained with normal rat liver

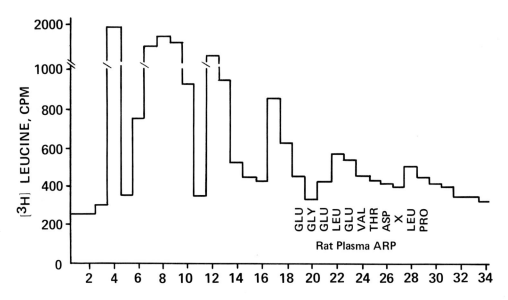

FIG. 2. Amino-terminal radiochemical sequence of apolipoprotein E translation
product. The ^{3}H-leucine-labelled in vitro translation product immunoprecipi-
tated by purified anti-apolipoprotein E and isolated by preparative electrophoresis and electroelution was subjected to sequential Edman degradation.
The abscissa represents the sequenator cycle number. The N-terminal sequence
of mature plasma apolipoprotein E (here designated "ARP" or arginine-rich
peptide) presumably aligns with the radiochemical sequence as shown.

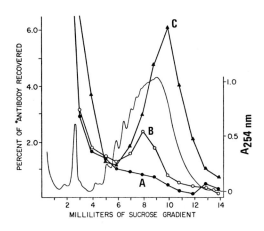

FIG. 3. Reaction of polysomes with
^{125}I-antibody. Radioactive antibody
(*antibody) was incubated with rat
liver polysomes, sedimented on linear sucrose gradients, and the gradients fractionated and counted for
radioactivity. A = preincubation
with excess unlabelled anti-apoE
followed by *anti-apoE; B = *anti-
apoE; C = *anti-serum albumin (shown
to compare the distribution and degree of binding). Sedimentation was
from left to right; the polysomal
ultraviolet absorbance profile is
shown as the thin continuous line.

mRNA. This finding indicates that the deficit in the production of VLDL by orotic acid-fed rats occurs despite an apparently normal level of mRNA coding for apolipoprotein E, and therefore, probably a significant and perhaps normal level of synthesis of this apoprotein in vivo (Pottenger and Getz 1971). Further studies along these lines may elucidate the transcriptional and translational mechanisms operating to regulate the production of apolipoprotein E.

Acknowledgments

We are grateful to Drs. G. Reddy and H. Kohler for their help in the radiochemical sequencing of the precursor of apolipoprotein E, and to Messrs. H. Gershenfeld and J. Ohringer for their help with the orotic acid-fed animals.

References

Blobel G, Dobberstein B (1975) Transfer of proteins across membranes I. Presence of proteolytically processed and unprocessed nascent immunoglobulin light chains on membrane-bound ribosomes of murine myeloma. J Cell Biol 67: 835–851

Felker TE, Fainaru M, Hamilton RL, Havel RJ (1977) Secretion of the arginine-rich and A-I apolipoproteins by the isolated perfused rat liver. J Lipid Res 18: 465–473

Goldstein JL, Brown MS (1977) The low density lipoprotein pathway and its relation to atherosclerosis. Annu Rev Biochem 46: 897–930

Hamilton RL, Williams MC, Fielding CJ, Havel RJ (1976) Discoidal bilayer structure of nascent high density lipoproteins from perfused rat liver. J Clin Invest 58: 667–680

Hay R, Getz GS (1979) Translation in vivo and in vitro of proteins resembling apoproteins of rat plasma very low density lipoprotein. J Lipid Res 20: 334–346

Innerarity TL, Mahley RW (1978) Enhanced binding by cultured human fibroblasts of apo-E-containing lipoproteins as compared with low density lipoproteins. Biochemistry 17: 1440–1447

Mahley RW, Holcombe KS (1977) Alterations of the plasma lipoproteins and apoproteins following cholesterol feeding in the rat. J Lipid Res 18: 314–324

Mahley RW, Innerarity TL, Bersot TP, Lipson A, Margolis S (1978) Alterations in human high-density lipoproteins, with or without increased plasma-cholesterol, induced by diets high in cholesterol. Lancet II: 807–809

Marsh JB (1976) Apoproteins of the lipoproteins in a nonrecirculating perfusate of rat liver. J Lipid Res 17: 85–90

Palmiter RD, Gagnon JG, Ericsson LH, Walsh KA (1977) Precursor of egg white lysozyme. J Biol Chem 252: 6386–6393

Pottenger LA, Getz GS (1971) Serum lipoprotein accumulation in the livers of orotic acid-fed rats. J Lipid Res 12: 450–459

Sales DJ (1976) Lipoprotein abnormalities in streptozotocin-induced diabetic rats. PhD dissertation, The University of Chicago

Strauss AW, Bennet CD, Donohue AM, Rodkey JA, Alberts AW (1977) Rat liver preproalbumin: complete amino acid sequence of the pre-piece. J Biol Chem 252: 6846–6855

Utermann G, Hees M, Steinmetz A (1977) Polymorphism of apolipoprotein E and occurrence of dyslipoproteinemia in man. Nature 269: 604–607

Weisgraber KH, Mahley RW, Assman G (1977) The rat arginine-rich apoprotein and its redistribution following injection of iodinated lipoproteins into normal and hypercholesterolemic rats. Atherosclerosis 28: 121–140

Wu A-L, Windmueller HG (1979) Relative contributions by liver and intestine to individual plasma apolipoproteins in the rat. J Biol Chem 254: 7316–7322

Apoprotein Secretion from the Human Intestine

Robert M. Glickman and Peter H.R. Green

There is mounting evidence that the small intestine is a quantitatively important source of lipoprotein constituents (apoproteins and phospholipids) which eventuate in circulating lipoproteins. This is especially true of apoproteins which are directly synthesized by the intestine and secreted as lipoprotein constituents. Recent work in our laboratory suggests that for certain of these apoproteins the intestine synthesizes and secretes from 30-50% of the total daily synthesis of apoproteins such as apoA-I and apoA-II. We will summarize the evidence for these conclusions.

Composition of Human Mesenteric Triglyceride-Rich Lipoproteins

Prior to the direct analysis of human mesenteric lymph lipoproteins, an incomplete picture of the apoprotein content of chylomicrons was obtained by analysis of "chylomicrons" harvested from post prandial plasma. These particles of d < 1.006 gm/ml, which are now known to be chylomicrons in all stages of catabolism, contain apoB, apoE and the C apoproteins as their major apoproteins (Glickman et al. 1978). When similar analyses are carried out on mesenteric lymph lipoproteins here derived from a patient with chyluria (Figure 1) it is evident that quantitative and qualitative changes in apoprotein content are present when compared to plasma chylomicrons. In Table I are shown representative values for the apoprotein content of these particles.

Evidence for the Active Intestinal Synthesis of Apoproteins

It has been well shown in the rat that the small intestine actively synthesizes apoB, A-I and A-IV during chylomicron formation (Glickman and Kirsch 1978; Imaizumi et al. 1978; Wu and Windmueller 1978). There apparently is little synthesis of apoE or the C peptides and apoA-II is a minor apoprotein in the rat. The evidence for active synthesis of chylomicron apoprotein synthesis in man is less complete. Human duodenal biopsies can incorporate radioactive amino acids into apoB, A-I, A-II (Rachmilewitz et al. 1978). Fluorescent antibody studies from this laboratory have shown a marked increase in fluorescence after fat feeding for apoB (Glickman et al. 1979), apoA-I (Glickman et al. 1978) and apoA-IV (PHR Green, RM Glickman, JW Riley, E Quinet, unpublished data) a newly described human apoprotein. ApoA-IV has a molecular weight of 46,000, is not reduceable, is immunologically distinct and has an amino acid composition analogous to rat apoA-IV. As seen in Table 1, it is a significant apoprotein constituent of intestinal triglyceride-rich lipoproteins.

Table 1. Apoprotein content of d < 1.006 lipoproteins from chylous urine and plasma.[a]

	Chylous Urine n = 7	Plasma n = 5
ApoB	3.4 ± 0.7	17.5 ± 3.3
ApoA-IV	10.0 ± 3.3	4.9 ± 2.1
ApoE	4.4 ± 0.3	17.4 ± 1.4
ApoA-I	15.0 ± 1.8	1.9 ± 0.9
ApoC & A-II	47.3 ±11.3	47.5 ± 4.2

[a]Apoproteins were quantitated by planimetry of densitometric gel scans. Values are mean ± SEM of the percentage area under each apoprotein peak. Plasma chylomicrons were prepared from normal volunteers after lipid feeding (Green et al. unpublished data).

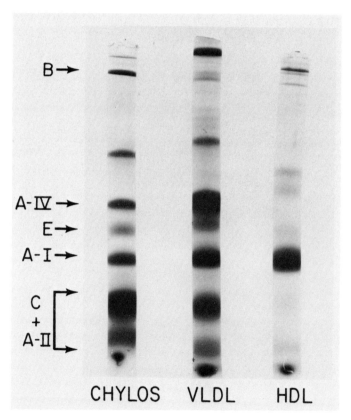

FIG. 1 SDS gels of lipoproteins isolated from chylous urine of one subject after oral corn oil.

Recent studies give some estimate of the quantitative importance of intestinal secretion of these apoproteins. After triglyceride feeding in normal human volunteers there was a rise in plasma apoA-I of 20 mg/dl (161-180 mg/dl) (Glickman et al. 1978), which when calculated for the blood volume amounts to 400-500 mg of apoA-I entering the circulation. More precise estimates of intestinal apoA-I, A-II and A-IV secretion have recently been obtained in two subjects with chyluria (Green et al. 1979). Shown in Table II is the secretion of the indicated apoproteins which were secreted on the d < 1.006 gm/ml lipoproteins after an oral load of corn oil. Although not directly determined in these patients, the figures in parentheses are the estimated daily synthesis rates for these apoproteins in normal individuals of the same weight. It is clear that although we have only considered the apoprotein secretion on the triglyceride-rich lipoproteins, as much as 30-50% of the estimated daily synthesis of apoA-I and A-II were secreted by the intestine. It is probable that these estimates are conservative since the majority of the apoA-I (80%) is found in the d > 1.006 gm/ml fraction of chylous urine or thoracic duct lymph (Green et al. submitted for publication). In view of the known filtration through lymph of plasma HDL it is likely that the greatest portion of this apoA-I is filtered however it remains to be determined whether the human intestine can directly secrete HDL as occurs in the rat (Green et al. 1979).

Also shown in Table II is the quantitative secretion of apoA-IV on triglyceride-rich lipoproteins. Significantly, approximately 50% of apoA-IV in chylous urine was associated with d < 1.006 gm/ml lipoproteins. This is markedly different from the distribution of this apoprotein in plasma where greater than 80% of apoA-IV is found in the d > 1.21 gm/ml fraction. The unusual distribution of this apoprotein and factors which influence its distribution are currently under study. Initial studies suggest that apoA-IV does not parallel other chylomicron apoproteins (apoA-I, A-II) which appear to transfer to and remain with plasma HDL. In several situations of decreased HDL (Tangier disease, alcoholic hepatitis) plasma apoA-IV levels are almost normal despite extremely low levels of apoA-I. These results suggest that different factors determine the metabolic fate of chylomicron apoproteins in the circulation.

Further studies are required to determine which factors are important in modulating the synthesis of apoproteins by the intestine.

Table 2. Apoprotein secretion - chyluria.

Subject	Corn Oil (gm)	Measured Urinary Output			Calculated Intestinal Output (d < 1.006)	
		TG (g)	A-I	A-II	A-I	A-II
			(mg)			
1	40	8.6	199	30	144 (270)[a]	26 (78)
2	100	2.9	44.8	3.2	224 (463)	19 (133)

[a]( ) = Calculated daily synthetic rate from Blum et al. J Clin Invest 60: 795 (1977).

References

Green PHR, Glickman RM, Saudek CD, Blum CB, Tall AR (1979) Human intestinal lipoproteins - Studies in chyluric subjects. J Clin Invest 64:233-242

Glickman RM, Green PHR, Lee RS, Tall A (1978) Apoprotein A-I synthesis in normal intestinal mucosa and in Tangier disease. N Engl J Med 299:1424-1427

Glickman RM, Green PHR, Lees RS, Lux SE, Kilgore A (1979) Immunofluorescence studies of apolipoprotein B in intestinal mucosa: Absence in abetalipoproteinemia. Gastroenterology 76:288-292

Glickman RM, Kirsch K (1973) Lymph chylomicron formation during the inhibition of protein synthesis: Studies of chylomicron apoproteins. J Clin Invest 52:2910-2920

Imaizumi K, Havel RJ, Fainaru M, Vigne JL (1978) Origin and transport of the A-I and arginine-rich apolipoproteins in mesenteric lymph of rats. J Lipid Res 19:1038-1046

Rachmilewitz D, Albers JJ, Saunders DR (1978) Apoprotein synthesis by human duodenojejunol mucosa. Gastroenterology 75:667-682

Wu AL, Windmueller HG (1978) Identification of circulating apolipoproteins synthesized by rat small intestine in vivo. J Biol Chem 253:2525-2528

Nascent VLDL and Nascent HDL from Liver[1]

Robert L. Hamilton

The question explored in this brief discussion is as follows: what are the nascent lipoproteins synthesized and secreted by normal rat liver?

Nascent VLDL

Electron microscopy of rat liver shows that particles of the same size and staining properties as plasma VLDL occur often in cisternae of smooth endoplasmic reticulum (SER) of parenchymal cells and occasionally in the smooth surfaced terminals of rough endoplasmic reticulum (RER), whereas these particles are always concentrated in cisternae and secretory vesicles of the Golgi complex (Hamilton 1972; Hamilton and Kayden 1974). This latter organelle was thus isolated as an intact structure from hepatocytes to test the hypothesis that the contained particles are nascent VLDL (Morré et al. 1970; Mahley et al. 1969). Rupture of the isolated Golgi membranes followed by ultracentrifugation at a density of 1.006 gm/ml yields a pearly-white floating band similar to plasma VLDL. Negatively stained preparations of this fraction contain electron lucent particles with a mean diameter of 460 Å, compared to that of plasma VLDL of 473 Å. VLDL released from Golgi membranes migrate more rapidly than LDL in agarose electropherograms but slightly slower than plasma VLDL. By mass, nascent VLDL contain almost the same amount of triglycerides ($\sim$67%) as plasma VLDL (70%) with only slight differences in cholesteryl-esters; (7-8% for nascent particles and 5-6% for plasma particles). The fatty acid composition of these core lipids is closely similar for nascent and plasma VLDL. Surface constituents differ in the following ways: nascent VLDL contain more phospholipid ($\sim$17%) of mass) and less apoprotein ($\sim$7%) compared to 11% and 10% respectively for plasma VLDL. On SDS electrophoretic gels, nascent VLDL have about equivalent amounts of protein-staining apo B and apo E bands but on urea containing polyacrylamide gels, nascent VLDL are seen to contain substantially less of the 3 apo C bands than plasma VLDL. These differences in surface components are abolished by simply mixing nascent VLDL with plasma HDL at 0°C followed by ultracentrifugal separation (Hamilton 1972; Hamilton et al. unpublished).

Interpretation

The liver synthesizes and assembles nascent VLDL particles that are almost completed within the hepatocyte. The nascent particle possibly begins formation in the SER where triglycerides and cholesteryl-esters are synthesized. The B and possibly E apoproteins may be added to the lipid particle at the smooth surfaced terminals of the RER, the junction between these two compartments (Alexander et al. 1976), whereas most of the C apoproteins are

[1] This work was supported by the U.S. Public Health Service, Arteriosclerosis SCOR grant HL 14237.

transferred to nascent VLDL from plasma HDL in the space of Disse and blood (Hamilton 1972).

Nascent HDL

Although HDL density fractions obtained from disrupted Golgi membranes of liver cells contain lipids and apoproteins, no particles similar in size and chemical composition to plasma HDL are found. Disc-shaped particles are seen by electron microscopy but these have not been successfully separated from membrane fragments of the Golgi fraction. Because discoidal HDL were found in patients with LCAT deficiency (Torsvik et al. 1970; Forte et al. 1971), we perfused rat livers with and without an LCAT inhibitor and compared the HDL particles. Discoidal HDL are the predominant lipoprotein in perfusates in which LCAT is blocked and are present in smaller amounts in perfusates of control livers. These discoidal HDL are the best substrate for highly purified LCAT when compared to other HDL fractions (Hamilton et al. 1976). These findings suggested a model to explain molecular mechanisms by which a lipid bilayer disc, sealed at the edge by apo E and perhaps A-I, could be transformed into a spherical HDL as LCAT generates a core of cholesteryl-esters (Hamilton et al. 1976; Hamilton, 1978).

Others have postulated that discoidal HDL are normally produced by the pinching off of excess surface as chylomicrons and VLDL lose triglycerides from their cores during lipoprotein lipase - induced lipolysis (Tall and Small 1978; Eisenberg, this volume). Nascent VLDL from perfused rat livers might be degraded by hepatic lipase during prolonged recirculation experiments to produce discs by a similar process. Results of single-pass liver perfusions argue against this because discoidal HDL containing newly synthesized apoproteins are synthesized under these experimental conditions (Hamilton, unpublished) that are unfavorable for VLDL degradation (Marsh 1976). Perfused fatty livers of orotic acid fed rats that produce little or no detectable VLDL do produce HDL material (Windmueller and Levy 1976; Marsh 1976). We have recently found that such perfused fatty livers of rats synthesize HDL in quantities equal in mass to that synthesized by normal control livers. The lipid composition of these nascent HDL (from fatty livers) is closely similar to nascent HDL from normal livers whether or not LCAT is inhibited. In addition, nascent HDL produced by fatty livers of orotic acid-fed rats are discoidal when LCAT is inhibited, whereas spherical particles predominate in HDL fractions when LCAT is active. Finally, the apoproteins of these nascent HDL from fatty livers secreting little or no VLDL are similar to those from normal controls, both in the pattern of apoprotein staining on SDS polyacrylamide gels and in distribution of radioactivity in these bands, except for an increased amount and labeling of C apoproteins in nascent HDL from fatty livers (Hamilton et al. unpublished).

Interpretation

The liver is a significant source of discoidal HDL particles that become transformed to spherical HDL by the LCAT reaction. The hepatic mechanism of disc production remains obscure but it apparently occurs independently of VLDL metabolism. The complete formation of mature plasma HDL probably does not occur in isolated liver perfusates in the absence of normal chylomicron and VLDL metabolism in extrahepatic tissues. For example, spherical HDL in perfusates of normal rat livers are smaller than mature plasma HDL (Hamilton, unpublished). Large amounts of apo A I and phospholipid are transferred to HDL from chylomicrons in vivo (Havel 1978). HDL increase in size in vitro after taking up phospholipids from liposomes (Nichols et al.

1978; Jonas 1979) and also after infusion of chylomicrons in vivo (Redgrave and Small 1979; Havel et al. unpublished). Thus, the physiological process of HDL formation may involve the hepatic secretion of nascent discoidal partials enriched in apo E, conversion of these discs to spherical particles by the LCAT reaction (coupled with apo D induced transfers of CE to other particles (Chajek and Fielding 1979), and a subsequent enlargement of pre-existing HDL by uptake of chylomicron surface components (i.e. apo A-I and phospholipid). In the absence or relative deficiency of pre-existing plasma HDL to take up excess chylomicron surface components produced during lipolysis, abnormal particles may be formed, both in vitro and in vivo, that do not reflect physiological processes of lipoprotein metabolism. In the presence of pre-existing HDL_3, controlled lipolysis of human VLDL in vitro forms stable HDL_2-like particles apparently without producing discs (Patsch et al. 1978).

References

Alexander CA, Hamilton RL, Havel RJ (1976) Subcellular localization of B apoprotein of plasma lipoproteins in rat liver. J Cell Biol 69:241-263

Chajek T, Fielding CJ (1979) Isolation and characterization of a human serum cholesteryl ester transfer protein. Proc Natl Acad Sci USA 75:3445-3449

Forte T, Norum KR, Glomset JA, Nichols AV (1971) Plasma lipoproteins in familial lecithin: cholesterol acyltransferase deficiency: structure of low and high density lipoproteins as revealed by electron microscopy. J Clin Invest 50:1141-1148

Hamilton RL (1972) Synthesis and secretion of plasma lipoproteins. In: Holmes WL, Paoletti R, Kritchevsky D(eds) Pharmacological Control of Lipid Metabolism (Adv Exp Med Biol). Plenum, New York, pp 7-24

Hamilton RL (1978) Hepatic secretion and metabolism of high density lipoproteins. In: Dietschy JM, Gotto AM, Ontko JA (eds) Disturbances in Lipid and Lipoprotein Metabolism. American Physiological Society, Bethesda, pp 155-171

Hamilton RL, Kayden HJ (1974) The liver: Normal and abnormal functions. In: Becker FF (ed) The Liver and the Formation of Normal and Abnormal Plasma Lipoproteins. Dekker, New York, Vol 5, Part A, pp 531-572

Hamilton RL, Williams MC, Fielding CJ, Havel RJ (1976) Discoidal bilayer structure of nascent high density lipoproteins from perfused rat liver. J Clin Invest 58:667-680

Havel RJ (1978) Origin of HDL. In: Gotto AM, Miller NE, Oliver MF (eds) High Density Lipoproteins and Atherosclerosis. Elsevier Press, Amsterdam

Jonas A (1979) Interaction of bovine serum high density lipoprotein with mixed vesicles of phosphatidylcholine and cholesterol. J Lipid Res 20: 817-824

Mahley RW, Hamilton RL, LeQuire VS (1969) Characterization of lipoprotein particles isolated from the Golgi apparatus of rat liver. J Lipid Res 10:433-439

Marsh JB (1976) Apoproteins of the lipoproteins in a nonrecirculating perfusate of rat liver. J Lipid Res 17:85-90

Morré DJ, Hamilton RL, Mollenhauer HH, Mahley RW, Cunningham WP, Cheetham RD, LeQuire VS (1970) Isolation of a Golgi apparatus-rich fraction from rat liver. J Cell Biol 44:484-491

Nichols AV, Gong EL, Forte TM, Blanche PJ (1978) Interaction of plasma high density lipoprotein HDL_{2b} (d 1.063-1.100 gm/ml) with single bilayer liposomes of dimyristoylphosphatidylcholine. Lipids 13:943-950

Patsch JR, Gotto AM, Olivecrona T, Eisenberg S (1978) Formation of high density lipoprotein$_2$-like particles during lypolysis of very low density lipoprotein in vitro. Proc Natl Acad Sci USA 75:4519-4523

Redgrave TG, Small DM (1979) Quantitation of the transfer of surface phospholipid of chylomicrons to the high density lipoprotein fraction during the catabolism of chylomicrons in the rat. J Clin Invest 64:162–171

Tall AR, Small DM (1978) Plasma high-density lipoproteins. N Engl J Med 299:1232–1236

Torsvik H, Solaas MH, Gjone E (1970) Serum lipoproteins in plasma lecithin cholesterol acyltransferase deficiency, studied by electron microscopy. Clin Genet 1:139–150

Windmueller HG, Levy RI (1967) Total inhibition of hepatic β-lipoprotein production in the rat by orotic acid. J Biol Chem 242:2246–2254

Synthesis and Secretion of Very Low Density Lipoprotein by Cultured Rat Hepatocytes[1]

David B. Weinstein, Roger A. Davis, Sheldon C. Engelhorn, and Daniel Steinberg

Cells of many animal species and of diverse tissue origins can be grown and maintained under defined and reproducible conditions in cell culture. During the past five years we have gained information and valuable insight from cell culture studies of lipid synthesis, lipoprotein uptake and degradation and factors which regulate the net cholesterol content of cells and tissues. Recent studies on the hepatic contribution to lipoprotein synthesis have utilized either freshly isolated rat hepatocytes (Jeejeebhoy and Phillips 1976) or single-pass and recirculating rat liver perfusions (Marsh 1974, 1976; Hamilton et al. 1976). Primary monolayer cultures of adult rat hepatocytes which maintain hepatic biosynthetic functions for periods of several days, rather than hours, can provide advantages over the short-term isolated cell and organ perfusion systems.

Our laboratory has demonstrated that adult rat hepatocytes which are cultured as primary monolayers secrete very low density lipoprotein (VLDL) for periods of at least seven days. Since triglyceride release into the serum, predominantly in the form of VLDL, is a major hepatic function which is in part controlled by nutritional and hormonal influences, we have examined the effects of nutritional, hormonal and drug-induced perturbations in order to determine whether cultured rat hepatocytes respond to factors which affect VLDL synthesis and secretion in vivo. Cell culture systems have several advantages as in vitro model systems. First, they allow the study of functions which are specific to a single cell type in a complex organ such as the liver. Homogeneous populations of hepatocytes can be used with essentially little or no contamination by non-parenchymal sinusoidal cells. Thus, it should be possible to discrimate between factors which have direct primary effects on hepatocytes and those factors which alter hepatocyte function indirectly as a result of interactions with other cells or tissue systems. Second, up to 80% of the hepatocytes from a single rat liver can be isolated and placed in culture providing multiple samples of cells for both control and test populations from the same donor organ. Third, the environment or cell culture medium can be chemically defined for the metabolic studies and changed as required in order to study effects of different metabolic regulators. Fourth, cells can be maintained for several days under experimental conditions in order to examine both short and long-term responses to the metabolic regulators. Finally, isolated hepatocytes do not metabolize VLDL particles at an appreciable rate, in contrast to the in vivo state, so that accumulation of VLDL in the culture medium represents a good estimate of the rate of secretion of VLDL by the cells.

Preparation of Hepatocyte Cultures

Hepatocytes were prepared as described by Davis et al. (1979). In brief, female Sprague-Dawley rats (100-120 g) were anesthetized with ether and livers

---

[1]This work was supported by NIH research grant HL-14197 awarded by the National Heart, Lung and Blood Institute and by NIH Postdoctoral Fellowship AM-0564 (to RAD).

were perfused by gravity flow at 10 ml/min thru the portal vein with calcium-
free buffer followed by collagenase (50mg/75ml) in buffered saline. The enzyme
solution was recirculated thru the liver for 20 min and the liver was removed,
cut into pieces and treated with 10 ml of fresh collagenase at 37° in a
shaking water bath for 5 min. The isolated hepatocytes were mixed with
arginine-free Dulbecco's modified Eagle's medium (DME medium) containing 20%
fetal calf serum. Hepatocytes were recovered and washed by centrifugation at
150-200 x g for 13-15 sec intervals. Cells were plated in 60 mm dishes at
1×10^6 cells/ml in 3 ml of the arginine-deficient DME medium containing 20%
fetal calf serum, 10µg/ml of insulin and antibiotics. After 24 hours the
medium was changed to the same DME medium without serum.

Experimental Studies

These studies of cultured rat hepatocytes utilized a nutritional selection
technique previously described by Leffert and Paul (1972) which allows the
maintenance of hepatocytes but will not support the maintenance of non-
parenchymal cells. In the presence of ornithine and the absence of arginine,
hepatocytes make sufficient quantities of arginine for survival via the
ornithine transcarbamylase enzyme pathway; whereas other liver cell types
without this synthetic pathway require exogenous arginine for survival and
disappear from the culture within 24-48 hours. Hepatocytes maintained in
arginine-free medium retain their ability to synthesize arginine, urea, albumin and other liver specific proteins for many days under culture conditions
(Leffert and Koch, 1978).

We have studied the secretion of very low density lipoprotein (VLDL) by adult
rat liver hepatocytes either by isolating VLDL from the culture medium for
mass analysis or by measuring the incorporation of (^{3}H)glycerol into newly-
secreted VLDL triglyceride after extraction of the culture medium with lipid
solvents. After a 3 hour pulse of (^{3}H)glycerol in serum-free culture medium
approximately 95% of the radioactivity incorporated into triglyceride was in
the VLDL fraction and about 5% was in the HDL fraction after differential
ultracentrifugation of the culture medium. In contrast, only 29% of the
medium newly-synthesized phospholipids was recovered in the VLDL fraction
and 24% in the HDL density range. Almost half of the newly-synthesized
phospholipid secreted by the cells was not associated with lipoproteins (d>
1.21 g/ml) and may correspond to the biliary phospholipid secretion which
occurs in the intact liver. Subfractionation of the newly-secreted lipoproteins by ultracentrifugation indicated that essentially all of the newly
synthesized apo-B was in the VLDL fraction although ^{3}H-amino acid incorporation studies showed that only 16% of the radioactive apoproteins were in the
VLDL density range and 78% were in the HDL density range. The newly-secreted
VLDL apoproteins were examined by urea-polyacrylamide gel electrophoresis
and it was estimated that apo-E and Apo-B accounted for approximately 60%
and 40%, respectively. The C apoproteins accounted for only a few percent,
at most, of the total VLDL protein after the isolation of the particles from
the medium by ultracentifugation. The VLDL particles were similar in size
and shape to rat serum VLDL (65% of the particles having a diameter of 450-
600A°).

Sufficient quantities of newly-secreted VLDL for analysis of the mass of
the VLDL components could be obtained by pooling culture medium from five
culture dishes containing a total of 7.5 - 10 mg of hepatocyte protein. The
VLDL isolated from the culture medium in the absence of exogenous lipid
sources (no serum or albumin present in the culture medium) contained 6.4
mg of lipid/ mg of protein. The chemical composition of the VLDL secreted
by the cultured hepatocytes is presented in Table 1 along with a comparison

Table 1. Chemical composition of newly secreted VLDL.

Source	Components of VLDL (% by weight)					
	Tri-glyceride	Total cholest-erol	Cholest-erol ester	Free cholest-erol	Phospho-lipid	Prot-ein
Rat serum[a]	70	9	6	3	11	10
Monolayer hepat-ocyte culture[b]	65	11	2	9	11	13
Recirculating liver perfusions #1[a]	67	7	3	4	16	9
#2[c]	71	14	7	7	16	18
Nonrecirculating liver perfusions						
#1[d]	67	10	3	7	23	20
#2[c]	47	20	–	–	10	23

[a]Data from Hamilton et al. (1976).
[b]Data from Davis et al. (1979).
[c]Data from Noel et al. (1979).
[d]Data from Marsh (1974).

Table 2. A comparison of secretion rates of VLDL components by liver systems.

Source[a]	VLDL secretion (µg/g liver/hour)				
	Protein (A)	Triglyc-eride (B)	Total cholest-erol	Phospho-lipid	B/A
Isolated hepatocyte suspensions[b]	35	410	37	–	11.7
Monolayer hepatocyte culture[b]	6	30	5	5	5.0
Recirculating liver perfusion #1	23	160	18	38	7.2
#2	24	75	14	17	3.1
#3	17	97	14	–	5.7
Nonrecirculating liver perfusion #1	39	105	17	36	2.7
#2	29	58	25	12	2.0

[a]The references are the same as in Table 1 with the following additions: the hepatocyte suspension data is taken from Jeejeebhoy et al.(1975) and data for recirculating perfusion #3 is from Witztum and Schonfeld (1978).
[b]Data calculated as µg/g of hepatocyte wet weight/ hour.

of the composition of rat serum VLDL and VLDL isolated from both recirculating and nonrecirculating liver perfusion studies. The lipid and protein distribution of the hepatocyte-secreted VLDL particles is very similar to that of the rat serum VLDL and the VLDL isolated by Hamilton et al. (1976) from liver perfusion studies. The protein content of the VLDL isolated from nonrecirculating perfusions is greater than that of the other liver systems shown.

The average rate of VLDL-triglyceride secretion during a 48 hour incubation of the cultured hepatocytes in lipid-free medium was 0.20 µg/mg cell protein per hour and for VLDL-protein secretion was 0.04 µg/mg cell protein per hour. The rate of secretion of VLDL components by cultured hepatocytes is compared

to VLDL secretion rates of isolated hepatocyte suspensions and liver perfusion
studies in Table 2. Direct comparison of data from these diverse systems is
at best very difficult since the systems and methodology have not been standardized among the various laboratories. For example, some of the studies use
washed red cells or albumin or defatted albumin in the perfusion or incubation
medium and it has been shown that these additions alter the triglyceride output
of perfused livers (Windmueller and Spaeth 1967). Similarly, the rate of VLDL
secretion by hepatocyte suspensions may be an overestimate since synthetic
rates fall with increasing time in vitro (Jeejeebhoy et al. 1975) and hepatocytes maintained in suspension for several hours show significant leakage of
cytoplasmic markers (Bissell et al. 1973). It is evident from inspection of
Table 2 that the secretory rates as measured in the cited references are
scattered over a wide range. The basal VLDL-protein secretory rate for our
hepatocytes cultured in the absence of serum is approximately 25-35% of that
of the 3 circulating perfusion systems; the average triglyceride secretion
rate in our hepatocyte cultures is approximately 20-40% of the rate in these
perfused organ systems. The hepatocyte cultures secrete rat albumin (measured
immunochemically) at a rate of 2.0 µg/mg cell protein per hour which is 60-70
% of the rate measured in perfused organs.

In a series of experiments designed to test the metabolic regulation of VLDL-
triglyceride secretion by cultured rat hepatocytes it was found that the cells
respond to certain metabolic stimuli in the manner which one would predict for
hepatocytes based upon in vivo experiments. For example, feeding rats a sucrose diet for 2 days prior to culturing their hepatocytes resulted in a 2-4
fold stimulation of triglyceride secretion for at least 3 days after the cells
were placed in culture. Orotic acid has been shown to inhibit VLDL secretion
in rat-feeding experiments (Pottenger and Getz 1971) and 5.6mM orotic acid
added dirctly to the culture medium inhibited the secretion but not the synthesis of VLDL-triglyceride. Addition of albumin-bound fatty acids to the
cultures increased VLDL-triglyceride secretion by 4-10 fold compared to the
basal culture conditions without exogenous lipid sources. These experiments
demonstrate that the nutritional and/or hormonal state of the donor animal
or the hepatocyte culture medium has long-lasting effects on the cellular
synthesis of VLDL secretory components. The ability to manipulate the culture
conditions over relatively long time intervals should enable us to use the
hepatocyte culture model to probe the mechanistic questions concerning the
direct effects of nutritional, hormonal and environmental factors on lipoprotein synthesis and its regulation.

References

Bissell DM, Hammaker EL, Meyer UA (1973) Parenchymal cells from adult rat liver
    in nonproliferating monolayer culture. J Cell Biol 59: 722-734
Davis RA, Engelhorn SC, Pangburn SH, Weinstein DB, Steinberg D (1979) Very
    low density lipoprotein synthesis and secretion by cultured rat hepatocytes
    J Biol Chem 254:2010-2016
Hamilton RL, Williams MC, Fielding CJ, Havel RJ (1976) Discoidal bilayer stru-
    ctures of nascent high density lipoproteins from perfused rat liver
    J Clin Invest 58: 667-680
Jeejeebhoy KN, Ho J, Breckenridge C, Bruce-Robertson A, Steiner G, Jeejeebhoy
    J (1975) Synthesis of VLDL by isolated rat hepatocytes in suspension.
    Biochem Biophys Res Commun 66: 1147-1153
Jeejeebhoy KN, Phillips MJ (1976) Isolated mammalian hepatocytes in culture.
    Gastroenterol 71: 1086-1096
Leffert HL, Paul D (1972) Studies on primary cultures of differentiated fetal
    liver cells. J Cell Biol 52: 559-568
Leffert HL, Koch KS (1978) Proliferation of hepatocytes. In: Hepatotrophic
    factors, Ciba Symposium 55. Elsevier, New York, pp 61-94

Marsh, JB (1974) Lipoproteins in a nonrecirculating perfusate of rat liver.
   J Lipid Res 15: 544-550
Marsh JB (1976) Apoproteins of the lipoproteins in a nonrecirculating perfus-
   ate of rat liver. J Lipid Res 17: 85-90
Noel SP, Wong L, Dolphin PJ, Dory L, Fubenstein D (1979) Secretion of chol-
   esterol-rich lipoproteins by perfused livers of hypercholesterolemic rats.
   J Clin Investig 64: 674-683
Pottenger LA, Getz GS (1971) Serum lipoprotein accumulation in the livers of
   orotic acid-fed rats. J Lipid Res 12: 450-459
Windmueller HG, Spaeth AE (1967) De novo synthesis of fatty acid in perfused
   rat liver as a determinant of plasma lipoprotein production. Arch
   Biochem Biophys 122: 362-369
Witztum JL, Schonfeld G (1978) Carbohydrate diet-induced changes in very low
   density lipoprotein composition and structure. Diabetes 27: 1215-1229

Topochemical Studies on Human High Density Lipoprotein[1]

W. Stoffel

Our studies on the supramolecular structure of human serum high density lipoproteins were initiated by the ^{13}C- and ^{31}P-NMR approach (Stoffel et al. 1974, 1977a, 1978a, 1979a, Stoffel and Därr 1976). Using ^{13}C-enriched fatty acids as constituents of phospholipids and cholesterolesters and $25,26-^{13}CH_3-$ cholesterol it was possible by recombination of these lipid classes with the apoproteins AI and AII or by the lipid exchange procedure (Stoffel et al. 1978b, 1979a) to demonstrate that hydrophobic interactions between the acylchains and the apoproteins stabilize the spherical structure of HDL particles whereas the polar head groups of lecithin showed no interaction with apoproteins. Shift reagents furthermore indicated that all polar head groups are accessible at the surface.

In order to get more detailed informations about neighbourhood relationships of lipids and apoproteins the following two chemical approaches were introduced into our structural work on HDL.

Photosensitive Lipids as Tools for
  Studying Nearest Neighbor Relationships

Phospholipids, cholesterol and cholesterolesters of high specific ^{3}H-radioactivity were tagged with the photosensitive azido group in well defined positions and either recombined with single apoproteins (Stoffel et al. 1977b) or exchanged against the genuine HDL-phospholipids and cholesterol. Nitrenes were generated under controlled conditions which crosslinked with their nearest neighbouring lipid or polypeptide sequence.

Lipid-apoAI and -AII crosslinked complexes were separated chromatographically for determining their polypeptide sequences carrying the radioactive crosslinked lipid species. These studies so far not only demonstrate for the first time that our photosensitive chemical azido lipids can be used as an efficient tool to decide about hydrophobic interactions between proteins and lipids, having wide applications in determining intrinsic membrane proteins, but furthermore allow localization of the site of these interactions; e.g. it could be demonstrated in the currently progressing analyses that only the apoAII polypeptide segment between residue 27 to 77 of apoAII was crosslinked to photosensitive lecithin incorporated into the intact HDL particle by our exchange method. This was verified by delipidation of HDL, separation of the lipopolypeptides AI and AII, CNBr-cleavage of the latter and separation and identification of the two fragments 1-26 and 27-77.

---

[1] These studies were supported by Deutsche Forschungsgemeinschaft and Fritz Thyssen Stiftung.

Bifunctional Crosslinkers Allow Insight into the Spatial Arrangement of the Apolipoproteins

This procedure was established by using a model lipoprotein complex. ApoAII-lecithin complexes formed by the recombination procedure (Stoffel et al, 1977a) were reacted with either 1,1'-^{14}C dimethylsuberimidate or 1,1'-[14]C - dithiobisbutyrimidate. The localization of the crosslinked lysines and their surrounding sequences were determined by thermolysin hydrolysis followed by two-dimensional separation of the labelled peptides, their isolation, analysis of stoichiometry and assignment of the crosslinked peptides of apoAII (Stoffel and Preissner 1979c).

The crosslinking pattern indicates a close-neighbour relationship (13-15 Å) of the peptide chains between amino acid residues 3, 23, 46 and 55 of the symmetrical halves of the apoAII molecule. No crosslinking between the halves had occurred.

The surface localization of apoAII in this complex was established by the following approach (Stoffel and Preissner 1979b): A benzimidopolystyrene resin was prepared from the chloromethylated Merrifield resin which had been transformed into the respective nitrile and the above lipoprotein complex passed over this column. It was bound by crosslinks of the apoAII-lysine residues to the resin. Delipidation followed by thermolysin cleavage left only sequences around the lysines covalently bound at the resin. These were finally cleaved of, totally hydrolyzed, their amino acid composition established and assigned to the established primary structure.

The results clearly demonstrated the surface localization of all sequences carrying lysine residues.

Analogous studies are being pursued on genuine HDL.

References

Stoffel W, Därr W (1976) Human high density apolipoprotein AI-lyso-lecithin-lecithin and sphingomyelin complexes. A new method for high yield recombinations to lipoprotein complexes of reproducible stoichiometry. Hoppe-Seyler's Ztschr Physiol Chem 357: 127-137

Stoffel W, Därr W, Salm KP (1977a) Lipid-protein interactions between human apolipoprotein AI and defined sphingomyelin species: A ^{13}C-NMR spectroscopic study. Hoppe-Seyler's Ztschr Physiol Chem 358: 1-11

Stoffel W, Därr W, Salm KP (1977b) Chemical proof of lipid protein interactions by crosslinking photosensitive lipids to apoproteins. Intermolecular cross-linkage between high-density apoprotein AI and lecithins and sphingomyelins. Hoppe-Seyler's Ztschr Physiol Chem 358: 453-462

Stoffel W, Metz P, Tunggal B (1978a) The binding of lysolecithin to human high density apoprotein AI: A ^{13}C-NMR study. Hoppe-Seyler's Ztschr Physiol Chem 359: 465-472

Stoffel W, Preissner K (1979b) Surface localisation of apoprotein AII in lipoprotein-complexes. Hoppe-Seyler's Ztschr Physiol Chem 360: 685-695

Stoffel W, Preissner K (1979c) Conformational analysis of serum apo-
    lipoprotein AII in lipoprotein complexes with bifunctional crosslinking
    reagents. Hoppe-Seyler's Ztschr Physiol Chem 360: 691-707

Stoffel W, Salm KP, Langer M (1978b) A new method for the exchange of
    lipid classes of human serum high density lipoprotein. Hoppe-Seyler's
    Ztschr Physiol Chem 359: 1385-1393

Stoffel W, Salm KP, Tunggal B (1979a) ^{13}C-NMR spectroscopy of human
    serum high density lipoprotein enriched with labelled phospholipids.
    Hoppe-Seyler's Ztschr Physiol Chem 360: 523-528

Stoffel W, Zierenberg O, Tunggal B, Schreiber E (1974) ^{13}C-Nuclear
    magnetic resonance spectroscopic evidence for hydrophobic lipid-protein
    interactions in human high density lipoprotein. Proc Nat Acad Sci USA
    71: 3696-3700

The Associating System of Small Subunits in ApoLDL

Germán Camejo and Lilian Socorro

The Size of ApoLDL

There is controversy about the size and composition of the protein moiety from human low density lipoprotein (LDL, density range 1.019-1.063 g/ml). Bradley et al. (1978) reported results from the partial sequence of CNBr-peptides of apoLDL indicating that the molecular weight was 30,000. Huang and Lee (1979), using a preparation of apoLDL extracted with ether-ethanol, detected polypeptides with molecular weights from 69,000 to 136,000. However, Steele and Reynolds (1979) found that apoLDL delipidated with sodium dodecyl sulfate (SDS) was made of a single component with molecular weight above 200,000 and postulated that proteolysis caused the presence of small components observed upon aging. On the other hand, neither Bradley et al. (1978) nor Huang and Lee (1979) were able to detect the production of new N-terminal amino acids in their preparations. Goldstein and Chapman (1979) examined the competition of peptides, obtained by trypsin digestion of LDL, for the binding sites in antibodies prepared against LDL, indicating that repetition of antigenic sites on the peptides is suggestive of recurrence of similar subunits in apoLDL.

A search on the literature dealing with apoLDL showed that when LDL was delipidated with organic solvents, a high molecular weight was obtained, but when solvent extraction was combined with side-chain modification, intermediate sizes were ascribed to apoLDL (Kane et al. 1970). When studies were conducted without the use of organic solvents, evidence of apoLDL subunits from 8,000 to 30,000 daltons were obtained (Chapman and Kane 1975; Chen and Aladjem 1978; Bradley et al. (1978). The conclusion from these results is that apoLDL can be obtained in different states of aggregation depending on the procedure used for its preparation, requiring strong denaturing agents, as detergents, guanidinium-HCl or urea, to obtain soluble apoLDL. The agents make it difficult to study immunochemical properties, reconstitution and the interaction of apoLDL with cells and tissues.

The Ideal Delipidation Procedure

The ideal depilidation method will be one in which: a. apoLDL is obtained free of lipids; b. apoLDL is quantitatively recovered; c. apoLDL is obtained as a soluble preparation without the use of denaturing agents; d. apoLDL retains conformational properties such as optical characteristics (ORD, CD) and immunological recognition by antisera prepared against plasma or intact LDL. To our knowledge no procedure has been developed that meets these requirements, although progress has been achieved (Huang and Lee 1979; Socorro and Camejo 1979).

Delipidation of LDL Attached to DEAE-Agarose

We have developed a delipidation procedure from which apoLDL is obtained in 50 to 70% yields, lipid-free, soluble in low ionic strength buffers, free of de-

tergent or any other denaturing agent and retaining its immunoreactivity vs.
antisera prepared against human plasma or intact LDL. The drawbacks of the
procedure are that we have failed to obtain total recoveries, that apoLDL is
obtained as dilute solutions, around 0.5 mg/ml, and efforts to concentrate them
in the absence of dissociating agents leads to aggregation. The results in figure 1, present the principle and outcome of the method. Twenty mg of LDL are
loaded in a column packed with 20 ml of DEAE-agarose gel equilibrated with 50
mM Tris-HCl buffer pH 8.6. The lipids from the attached LDL are eluted with a
gradient of the detergent Brij-36 (10-polyoxyethylene lauryl ether). The detergent is washed with 10 column volumes of the initial buffer and the lipid-free
apoLDL is obtained by elution with 1 M NaCl prepared in 50 mM Tris-HCl pH 7.4.
The peak containing the apoLDL was dialyzed vs. 10 mM ammonium carbonate and
concentrated by lyophilization when required.

Electrophoresis of Soluble ApoLDL

Polyacrylamide electrophoresis was performed in 5%, 3 mm thick slabs. The gel
was prepared in 0.25 M Tris-HCl pH 9.0 containing 8 M urea and 0.1% SDS. The e-
lectrodes reservoires were filled with a buffer of 0.2 M glycine and 25 mM
Tris-base pH 8.4, also with 0.1% SDS. Up to 8 mg of apoLDL were dissolved in
a dissociating solution containing 5% SDS, 6 M urea, 0.1% dithiothreitol, 20%
sucrose, buffered to pH 6.8 with 15 mM Tris-HCl and were loaded in the gel. A
segment of the gel was cut and stained for localization of the protein bands,
the corresponding segments were placed in an electrophoretic elutor and the
fractions were separated from the gel. The apoLDL was fractionated into 3 intensively stainable components and 6 minor ones, ranging in apparent molecular
weights (app. mol. wt.) from 8,000 to 200,000 (Figure 2a). The apoLDL fractions were dialyzed vs. 10 mM ammonium carbonate, freeze-dried and labelled
apoLDL-I to apoLDL-IX.

The lyophilized fractions were redissolved in the dissociating solution and
analytical electrophoresis was conducted in a pore-gradient gel from 3 to 20%.

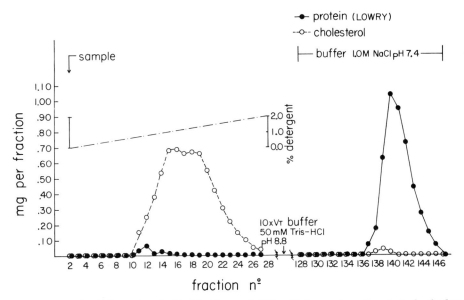

FIG. 1. Method for the delipidation of LDL. Values for the total cholesterol
and protein determinations on each 2 ml fraction. Flow: 20 ml/h.

Table 1. Apparent molecular weights of apoLDL components present in the most prominent fractions isolated with preparative gel electrophoresis.

Band N°	Total apoLDL	Δ app. mol.wt	apoLDL fractions I	II	III	IV	V	VI	VII
1	10200		10200^s	10200					
2	18300	8100	17700^m	17000					
3	20100^m	9900	20100	21000	20800	22000			
4	29700	9000	27000	27000	33000	33800	29700^s		
5	37000^m	7300	38000	38000	38000	37000	37800		
6	46700^s	9700						46000^m	46000
7	60400^m	13700				60400^m			60500
8	73400	13000					80000^s		
9	108000	35000							111000
10	187000	79000							175000^m
11	298000	111000							

^{m} indicates a band of medium intensity in the fraction pattern.
^{s} indicates a band of strong intensity; items without superscript indicate bands of similar weak intensity.

The gel was prepared and run in the SDS–urea buffer system used in the preparative step. In this high resolution gel, each fraction gave multiple bands, indicating that each original band forms an aggregation system clustering around increasing apparent molecular weights. These app. mol. wt. were evaluated with the aid of calibrating proteins and plots of electrophoretic mobility vs. log. mol. wt. $Y=-3.57X+22.3$, $r=0.99$. Table 1 presents the values of individual bands in the more prominent apoLDL fractions, also in this table are given the increments (Δ app. mol. wt.) for consecutive components. Since

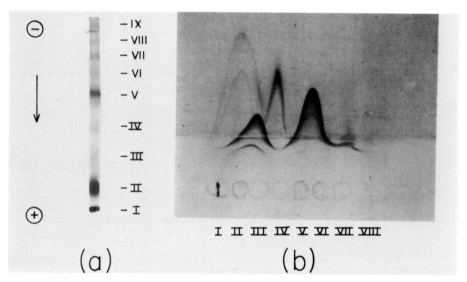

FIG. 2a and 2b. Preparative electrophoresis (a) of soluble apoLDL on a 5% polycrylamide gel containing 8 M urea and 0.1% SDS. (b) Fused rocket immunoelectrophoresis of the fractions from the preparative gel, using antiserum prepared against human plasma. Both gels were stained with Coomassie Brilliant Blue.

in this preparation the formation of new N-terminals could not be detected, and small components of the separated fractions reaggregate into larger ones, the results suggest that apoLDL is mainly made of small subunits with a high tendency to aggregate.

Immunoelectrophoresis of apoLDL fractions

The results presented in figure 2b, indicate that the fractions are heterogenous in their antigenic determinants, there is a major one common to all fractions, but specially centered in II, III, V and VI. However, there are determinants that are exclusive of small mol. wt. fractions. The antiserum used in these experiments detected only one peak in crossed immunoelectrophoresis of the purified LDL, therefore it is the solubilization and fractionation of apoLDL that uncovers at least five antigenic determinants present in different proportions in the fractions of apoLDL.

Conclusions

We have shown that it is possible to obtain soluble apoLDL, free of denaturing agents, that may be useful in studies about its interaction with cells and tissues. The results indicate that apoLDL is made of several polypeptides, the more abundant of approx. 8,000 daltons. We do not know the exact proportion of each component, and methods for their evaluation will have to be developed. A consequence of these findings is that in any structural study of apoLDL, it should be taken into consideration that more than one polypeptide chain can occur in each particle according to the extent of aggregation; this depends upon the delipidation procedure and the conditions used to deaggregate the soluble apoLDL.

References

Bradley WA, Rohde MF, Gotto AM Jr, Jackson RL (1978) The cyanogen bromide peptides of the apoprotein of low density lipoprotein (apoB): Its molecular weight from a chemical view. Biochem Biophys Res Commun 8:928-935
Chapman MJ, Kane JP (1975) Stability of the apoprotein of human serum low density lipoprotein: Absence of endogenous endopeptidase activity. Biochem Biophys Res Commun 66:1030-1036
Chen CH, Aladjem F (1978) Further studies on the subunit structure of human serum low density lipoproteins. Biochem Med 19:178-187
Goldstein S, Chapman MJ (1979) Radioimmunological studies of the surface protein of the human serum low-density lipoprotein: Comparison of the native particle and the products obtained by tryptic treatment. Biochem Biophys Res Commun 87:121-127
Huang SS, Lee DM (1979) A novel method for converting apolipoprotein B, the major protein moiety of human low density lipoproteins, into a water-soluble protein. Biochem Biophys Acta 577:424-441
Socorro L, Camejo G (1979) Preparation and properties of soluble, immunoreactive apoLDL. J Lipid Res 20:631-638
Steele JCH, Reynolds JA (1979) Characterization of the apolipoprotein B, polypeptide of human plasma low density lipoprotein in detergent and denaturant solutions. J Biol Chem 254:1633-1638

Lipoprotein Structure and the Mechanism of Action of Lipoprotein Lipase[1]

Richard L. Jackson, Marja-Riitta Taskinen, Nobuo Matsuoka, Thomas J. Fitzharris, Judith A.K. Harmony, Howard G. Muntz, E.K. Neely, Alan D. Cardin, and J. David Johnson

Introduction

Circulating lipoprotein triglyceride is cleared in extrahepatic tissues by lipoprotein lipase (LpL). The enzyme is normally attached to the capillary endothelium, but is released into the plasma by the injection of heparin. LpL has been purified and characterized from post-heparin plasma, from tissues and from milk (Augustin and Greten 1979). The characteristic feature of LpL is that it is stimulated by apolipoprotein C-II (apoC-II), a protein (Jackson et al. 1977) present in chylomicrons, very low density lipoproteins (VLDL) and high density lipoproteins (HDL). This report describes the role of apoC-II and lipid structure in the mechanism of action of bovine milk lipoprotein lipase.

Effects of LpL on Hydrolysis of Lipoprotein Triglyceride

LpL hydrolyzes triglycerides transported in chylomicrons and VLDL. However, to date there has not been a sensitive method to monitor continuously the rate of hydrolysis. Recently we (JD Johnson, unpublished data) have developed a method utilizing the fluorescent phospholipid dansyl phosphatidyl-ethanolamine (DPE) to monitor lipolysis. Fig. 1a shows the effects of LpL on the fluorescent properties of DPE which had been incorporated into human plasma lipoproteins. The addition of LpL to DPE-labeled chylomicrons or VLDL causes an increase in fluorescence and a 20 nm shift in the wavelenth maxima of the fluorophore (512 to 492 nm). The fluorescence increase and blue shift is due to hydrolysis of DPE to lyso-DPE and the subsequent transfer of lyso-DPE to albumin; the rate of fluorescence increase correlates with the release of free fatty acids. No fluorescence increase or wavelength shift was observed with low density lipoproteins or HDL, indicating that LpL does not catalyze hydrolysis of these lipoproteins. [^{14}C]Triolein was also incorporated into human VLDL using dimethyl sulfoxide (Fielding 1979). As is shown in Fig. 1a (inset), hydrolysis of [^{14}C]triolein catalyzed by LpL correlates directly with the fluorescence changes in DPE. Thus the LpL-induced fluorescence changes provide a facile and accurate means of determining the rate of VLDL catabolism and the effect of apoC-II on this rate.

Role of ApoC-II

The role of apoC-II has primarily been studied using artificial substrates. In these assay systems, it has been relatively easy to demonstrate that apoC-II has an effect on the catalytic rate of hydrolysis. It has, however, been difficult to show that apoC-II plays a similar role in the catabolism

---

[1]This work was supported by NIH grants HL-22619, 23019 and 20882, by Training grant HL-07382 (ADC), by the American Heart Association, by the Lipid Research Clinic Program (NHLBI 72-2914), by GCRC grant RR-00068-15, and by the Muscular Dystrophy Association (JDJ).

of VLDL since lipoproteins normally contain a complement of apoC-II. In a
recent study (Catapano et al. 1979), it was shown that the addition of apo
C-II to VLDL from a patient with apoC-II deficiency resulted in an increased
rate of VLDL-triglyceride hydrolysis in vitro. To show the dependence of
the rate of lipolysis on apoC-II, we have utilized guinea pig VLDL produced
in a perfused liver system (TJ Fitzharris, unpublished data). Guinea pig
VLDL isolated from plasma or by perfusion of liver do not contain the human
equivalent of apoC-II. As is shown in Fig. 1b, the addition of apoC-II to
the reaction mixture increased the rate of VLDL-triglyceride hydrolysis.
The data shown in Fig. 1b together with those of Catapano et al. (1979) suggest that apoC-II affects the catalytic rate of VLDL-triglyceride hydrolysis
by lipoprotein lipase. Whether apoC-II content is also a rate-determining
factor in normal human subjects is still unknown, although the data of
Kashyap et al. (1977) suggest that subjects with plasma triglyceride concentrations >500 mg/dl have decreased apoC-II content per VLDL particle.

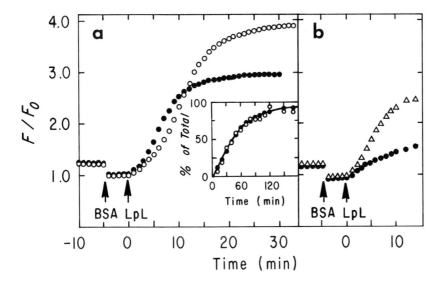

FIG. 1a and b. (a) Effects of LpL on DPE-chylomicrons (—o—o—) and DPE-VLDL
(—•—•—) fluorescence. DPE was incorporated into chylomicrons (1:100, DPE:
triglyceride) and VLDL (1:100, DPE:phospholipid). The reaction mixture contained 0.2 ml of DPE-chylomicrons (3.50 mg/ml triglyceride) or 0.2 ml of
VLDL (3.63 mg/ml phospholipid); 0.65 ml of 50 mM Tris-HCl, pH 7.4, 0.9%
NaCl; 0.15 ml of fatty acid-free bovine serum albumin (BSA) (20%) and 5 μl
of LpL (0.72 mg/ml). Fluorescence excitation was at 340 nm and the emission
as a function of time was monitored at 490 nm. The inset shows the relationship between [^{14}C]triolein released and the fluorescence increase in
DPE-VLDL. DPE-VLDL was labeled with [^{14}C]triolein as described by Fielding
1979. The percent of the total increase in fluorescence (—•—•—) and the
percent of the total [^{14}C]triolein released (—o—o—) is plotted as a function
of time. (b) Effects of apoC-II on the rate of guinea pig VLDL-triglyceride
hydrolysis. Guinea pig VLDL was prepared by perfusion of liver with oleic
acid. The rate of triglyceride hydrolysis was determined by the rate of
fluorescence increase after the addition of LpL (—•—•—) or after the addition of apoC-II (5.0 μg) and LpL (—△—△—). Each reaction contained 0.6 mg
VLDL-triglyceride, 3% BSA and 0.5 μg LpL in 1 ml of 50 mM Tris-HCl, pH 7.4,
0.9% NaCl.

Using monolayer techniques, we (RL Jackson, unpublished data) have demonstrated that LpL and apoC-II are surface active and collect at a lipid interface; apoC-II is not required for penetration of LpL into the lipid interface. To further study the role of lipid structure in LpL action, we have utilized sonicated dimyristoyl phosphatidylcholine (DMPC) vesicles as substrates (Muntz et al. 1979). Fig. 2a shows that the phospholipase activity of LpL is negligible in the absence of apoC-II. The addition of apo C-II to sonicated vesicles in the presence of LpL results in a time-dependent hydrolysis of DMPC; the addition of apoC-III to DMPC vesicles does not activate LpL, nor does apoC-III inhibit the apoC-II-stimulated hydrolysis. To show that apoC-II and apoC-III have similar effects on lipid structure, we (AD Cardin, unpublished data) have studied the effects of the apoproteins upon the fluidity of phospholipid vesicles by measurement of the fluorescence polarization of incorporated fatty acid probes. As Fig. 2b illustrates, both apoC-II and apoC-III increase the rigidity of the phospholipid bilayer to the same extent. Since apoC-III is not an activator of LpL, these data are consistent with the view that apoC-II and apoC-III contain lipid-binding domains but that the interaction of these domains with lipid is not the only factor which accounts for the ability of apoC-II to activate LpL.

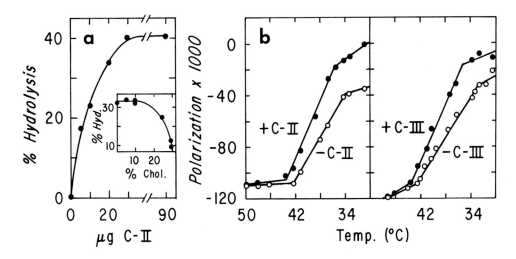

FIG. 2a and b. (a) The effects of apoC-II upon the hydrolysis of dimyristoyl phosphatidylcholine (DMPC). Each reaction mixture contained in the final volume of 0.4 ml of 0.1 M Tris-HCl, 0.15 M NaCl, pH 7.4, the following additions: DMPC vesicles (700 µg), fatty acid-free BSA (5 mg), and apoC-II as indicated. Each reaction mixture was preincubated at 23.4°C for 15 min prior to the addition of LpL (1.4 µg). At the indicated reaction times, the mixtures were extracted and the percent hydrolysis determined after separation of the reaction mixtures by thin layer chromatography. The inset shows the effects of cholesterol on the hydrolysis of DMPC in the presence of apo C-II (20 µg). DMPC vesicles were prepared with varying amounts of cholesterol and the percent hydrolysis was determined. (b) Fluorescence polarization of dipalmitoyl phosphatidylcholine (DPPC) (—o—o—) and DPPC containing apoC-II or apoC-III (—●—●—). The incubation mixtures contained phospholipid (0.1 mg/ml), 12-(9-anthroyloxy) stearic acid (phospholipid/probe molar ratio 100) and apoC-II (10 µg/ml) or apoC-III (23 µg/ml).

In the next experiment the effect of cholesterol on LpL activity was determined. Fielding (1970) showed that the rate of lipolysis of an artificial substrate by LpL was inhibited by cholesterol. In Fig. 2a (inset) is shown the effect of cholesterol on the hydrolysis of DMPC vesicles by LpL. With >10 mol percent cholesterol, there is inhibition of LpL activity even in the presence of excess apoC-II. Whether this decrease in LpL activity is due to altered binding to LpL to the substrate, to altered substrate structure, or to a decreased amount of activator protein per substrate particle remains to be determined. However, since the lipid-binding portion of apoC-II is not required for LpL activation (Kinnunen et al. 1977), inhibition by cholesterol is probably due to less LpL associated with the substrate and not to decreased interaction between apoC-II and LpL.

Summary

We have developed a fluorescence method to monitor continuously the lipolysis of VLDL. Using this technique we find that apoC-II, but not apoC-III, increases the rate of lipolysis of apoC-II-deficient VLDL. ApoC-II, but not apoC-III, also enhances the rate of LpL-catalyzed hydrolysis of DMPC lipid vesicles. ApoC-II and apoC-III have similar effects on lipid structure, suggesting that apoC-II interactions with LpL are responsible for the increased activity of LpL in these systems. Cholesterol inhibits LpL hydrolysis of DMPC lipid vesicles in a manner that is not reversed by apoC-II. Since apo C-II enhances the rate of lipolysis without binding to lipid, inhibition produced by cholesterol may result from decreased binding of LpL to substrate or from altered substrate structure. It will be of considerable interest to determine the role of cholesterol in VLDL catabolism. Experiments along these lines are currently in progress.

Acknowledgements

We acknowledge the assistance of Ms. Gwen Kraft in preparing the figures, and of Ms. Janet Boynton in preparing the manuscript for publication.

References

Augustin J, Greten H (1979) The role of lipoprotein lipase--molecular properties and clinical relevance. In: Paoletti R, Gotto AM (eds) Atherosclerosis Reviews. Raven Press, New York, Vol 5, pp 91-124

Catapano AL, Kinnunen PKJ, Breckenridge WC, Gotto AM, Jackson RL, Little JA, Smith LC, Sparrow JT (1979) Lipolysis of apoC-II deficient very low density lipoproteins: Enhancement of lipoprotein lipase action by synthetic fragments of apoC-II. Biochem Biophys Res Commun 89: 951-957

Fielding CJ (1970) Human lipoprotein lipase inhibition of activity by cholesterol. Biochim Biophys Acta 218: 221-226

Fielding CJ (1979) Validation of a procedure for exogenous isotopic labeling of lipoprotein triglyceride with radioactive triolein. Biochim Biophys Acta 573: 255-265

Kashyap ML, Srivastava LS, Chen CY, Perisutti G, Campbell M, Lutmer RF, Glueck CJ (1977) Radioimmunoassay of human apolipoprotein C-II: A study in normal and hypertriglyceridemic subjects. J Clin Invest 60: 171-180

Jackson RL, Baker HN, Gilliam EB, Gotto AM (1977) Primary structure of very low density apolipoprotein C-II of human plasma. Proc Natl Acad Sci USA 74: 1942-1945

Kinnunen PKJ, Jackson RL, Smith LC, Gotto AM, Sparrow JT (1977) Activation of lipoprotein lipase by native and synthetic fragments of human plasma apolipoprotein C-II. Proc Natl Acad Sci USA 74: 4848-4851

Muntz HG, Matsuoka N, Jackson RL (1979) Phospholipase activity of bovine milk lipoprotein lipase on phospholipid vesicles: Influence of apolipoproteins C-II and C-III. Biochem Biophys Res Commun (In Press).

Structure of High Density Lipoproteins

Gerhard M. Kostner, Peter Laggner, and Helmut Hauser

Composition of High Density Lipoproteins

The high density lipoproteins from human serum comprise some 8-10 individual entities which can be demonstrated by a variety of analytical as well as preparative methods.The basic properties which they have in common is a hydrated density ranging from 1.06-1.20 g/ml and with a few exceptions, the migration in the position of alpha globulins in paper and agarose gel electrophoresis. We have shown as early as 1969(Kostner et al.) that analytical isoelectric focusing separates intact HDL into three major and several minor bands. The protein part of the three major fractions consists primarily of apoAI in addition to various kinds and amounts of other proteins. Experiments published from many laboratories suggest that HDL in fact is a mixture of at least 8 so called lipoprotein families named LpA, LpB.... LpF and Lp(a) (Kostner and Alaupovic 1972; Olofsson et al. 1977; Utermann et al. 1977).In addition some minor antigens can be demonstrated as for example "Thr-poor"-, "Gly-rich"-proteins, $ß_2$glycoprotein-I and others.

Subfractionation of HDL can be achieved by preparative ultracentrifugation most conveniently in a density gradient (Anderson et al. 1977), by affinity chromatography, adsorption and ion exchange chromatography (McConnathy and Alaupovic 1976; Kostner and Holasek 1977) and steric exclusion chromatography (Kostner and Laggner 1979). Applying all these methods it was possible to get some insight into the complexity of HDL structure and composition. It also became evident,that HDL consist of very labile particles which easily alter their composition due to protein and/or lipid loss or exchange with other lipoproteins. During this process a rearrangement of particles may occure giving rise to artificial structures. Thus we have obtained for example from HDL_2 six and from HDL3 seven subfractions using hydroxylapatite column chromatography and stepwise elution with potassium phosphate buffer of increasing molarity. The fractions eluting at low ionic strength contained only apoAI and apoAII; under certain circumstances a small fraction containing apoD only eluted as a first separate peak. Rising amounts of apoC were eluted at higher ionic strength of the elution buffers and finally a fraction containing almost only apoC was demonstrable. A very similar elution profile is obtained by ion exchange column chromatography using DEAE cellulose. The hydrated densities as well as the lipid:protein ratio of the individual subfractions were similar to the parent HDL density class but a characteristic variation within these limits could be observed. Interestingly, total HDL of density 1.063-1.21 gave the same number and kind of subfractions regarding the protein moiety as compared to HDL_2 and HDL_3. Considering the high resolving power of hydroxylapatite one would expect that HDL_2 and HDL_3 resembling subfractions should have been obtained.

In further experiments HDL were subfractionated in a density gradient and divided into 4 fractions (Kostner and Laggner 1979).The parent HDL as well as these 4 subfractions were subjected to steric exclusion chromatography using Sephacryl S-300 superfine, a column medium which optimally separates proteins in the molecular weight range of 10^5-10^6 Daltons. Surprisingly, fresh total HDL gave only one almost completely symmetrical peak. The material eluting first contained apoAI and apoAII at a molar ratio of approx. 10 in addition to all the apoC proteins. At the end of the peak lipoproteins with an AI:AII ratio of ∿ 2 were found which lacked apoC almost completely. The minor constituents of HDL (apoD-apoF) distributed assymetrically over the whole eluate. The individual density subfractions eluted, for the most part, in the form of single symmetrical peaks but their elution volume was shifted to the left(HDL of lower densities) or to the right(HDL of higher densities). In these experiments the protein pattern of individual cuts of the eluate were much more uniform. Although the first part of the eluate of total HDL had a lower and the second part a somewhat higher hydrated density as compared to total HDL, in no case such extreme hydrated densities were found as observed for the ultracentrifugal subfractions. Aging of HDL even in the presence of all kinds of preservatives caused a marked alteration of the elution profile. We conclude form all these observations, that the complexity of the HDL composition is governed by the amount and kind of individual proteins and lipids, rendering the molecules into rather labile particles. Any change of the enviroment gives rise to structural reorganisations. Such enviromental changes comprise the removal of serum proteins, presence or absence of salts, chemical agents used as preservatives as well as aging and enzymatic attacks. These changes however may be of physiological sifnificance for the metabolism of lipids providing a most flexible system.

Physicochemical Structure of HDL

Considering the lability of HDL one is tempted to conclude that structural analyses only in those cases may mirror the in vivo situation where fresh total plasma is used as a sample. Since this in practice is impossible to achieve, we tried to apply only those methods for isolation of HDL fractions which affect the structure to a minimal extent. Thus, only ultracentrifugation and column chromatography using hydroxylapatite were used and special care was taken to use samples as fresh as possible.

Small-angle X-ray studies

Small angle X-ray studies have been performed on the immunochemically defined HDL subfractions LpA from HDL_3 and HDL_2 and LpC from HDL_2 (Laggner and Müller 1978). The results have shown that these subfractions represent fairly homogenous polulations of quasi-spherical particles which are built according to a common structural principle. The diameters of these particles were determined as 9.5 - 10 nm for LpA_3, 11.0 - 11.5 nm for LpA_2, and 13.5 - 14.0 nm for LpC. The structural principle can be inferred from the radial electron density distribution: a low electron density core of diameters ranging from 3.7 nm in LpA_3 to 5.2 nm in LpC is surrounded by a high electron density shell of 1.2 - 1.7 nm thickness. Considering composition and the molecular structure of the individual components, this leads to a model in which the apolar constituents of low electron density form the particle core, most likely in a radial arrangement of the long molecular axes of the cholesteryl esters into which the phospholipid hydrocarbon chains are interdigitated from the external shell. Since the length of a cholesteryl ester molecule in fully extended conformation is about 3.7 nm, full interdigitation has to prevail in LpA_3. This provides an explanation for the fact that LpA_3 is the smallest HDL subfraction of any abundance. The variation in size between the different HDL subfractions is then simply a consequence of the ratio of polar surface apolar core constituents. The upper limit of size is hence given by the minimum of possible interdigitation, which is the case in LpC, where the core radius corresponds almost to the sum of the extended lengths of a cholesteryl ester molecule plus an 18:1 hydrocarbon chain. The external shell thickness is consistent with a model of a two-dimensional, highly α - helical network of the protein into which the polar phospholipid headgroups are intercalated. A schematic representation of these model considerations is shown in Fig. 1.

185

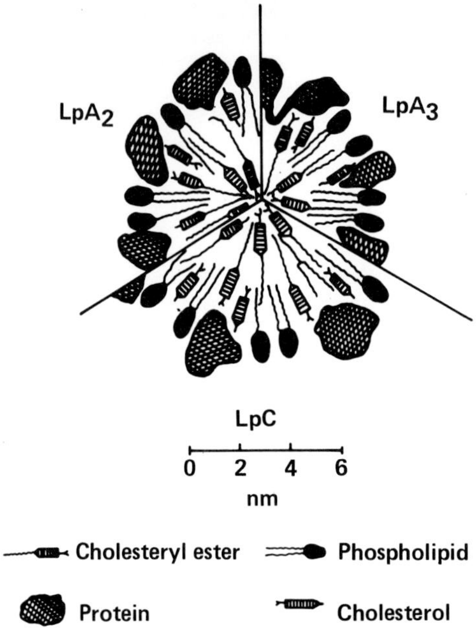

Fig.1. Schematic cross sectional view of the molecular arrangement of proteins and individual lipids within LpA isolated from HDL_2 (LpA_2), LpA isolated from HDL_3 (LpA_3) and of LpC isolated from total HDL. Subfractionations were performed by hydroxylapatite column chromatography.

NMR and ESR studies

In order to obtain further information on the structural organization of individual lipids, ^{13}C nuclear magnetic resonance studies were performed with total HDL as well as with individual density subfractions (Hauser and Kostner, 1979). Experiments were carried out on a Bruker HXS-360 MHz instrument at a magnetic field of 84.5 kG operating in the Fourier transformation mode. We were primarily interested in the distribution of freee (FC) and esterified cholesterol (FC) within the HDL particles. Evaluating the high resolution spectra we were able to distinguish between FC and CE. Table 1 shows the chemical shifts and line widths of C-3, -5 and -6 respectively of the sterol ring. These were the only ones which differed by more than 1 ppm.

Tab.1. Chemical shifts and line widths (in parenthesis) of the C-3, C-5 and C-6 resonances of free and esterified cholesterol present in HDL and other enviroments.

Assignment	HDL	Chemical shift (ppm from $(CH_3)_4Si$)[a]			
		Lipid extract of HDL in $C_6{}^2H_6$	Cholesteryl oleate in $C_6{}^2H_6$	Cholesterol in $C_6{}^2H_6$	Cholesterol in sonicated dispersions of lecithin cholesterol in D2O
C-3 of FC	71.2	71.4		71.7	71.2
C-3 of CE	73.1(23)	73.7	73.7		
C-5 of FC	141.3(27)	141.8		141.3	142.3(56)
C-5 of CE	139.9(16)	139.9	139.8		
C-6 of FC	121.0(30)	121.3		121.6	120.9(60)
C-6 of CE	122.3(15)	122.8	122.6		

[a]Chemical shifts are given in ppm. The number in parentheses are the line width in Hz measured at half high of the signal. The molar ratio of lecithin:cholesterol in the sonicated dispersion was 9:1.

While the C-3 resonance was overlapped by the C-2 glycerol methine signal arising from phospholipids, the C-5 and C-6 resonances were clearly resolved from other signals. These latter signals therefore were used to determine the fraction of FC in intact HDL contributing to the NMR spectrum. The ratio of the peak integral of C-5 and C-6 (CE:FC) was found to be 7 $\pm$ 0.8, whereas the peak integral ratio of protein free HDL lipid extracts was 4 and consistent with the molar ratio CE:FC determined analytically. Thus a certain portion of FC did not contribute to the spectrum. Line width measurements allowed a tentative assignment of the missing fraction. The line width of the C-5 and C-6 FC signals in sonicated dispersions of egg phosphatidycholine:FC at a molar ratio of 8 was significantly larger than the corresponding line widths from HDL. This suggests that the fraction of FC contributing to the spectrum of HDL is mainly in a liquid like environment similar to that of CE. This fraction of FC together with CE forms the hydrophobic core of the HDL particles. The portion of FC not contributing to the NMR spectrum is motionally immobilized similar to the FC present in lecithin bilayers. This fraction is present in the outer layer and in close contact with phospholipids and proteins. Virtually the same results were obtained irrespective of whether measuring total HDL or HDL_2 or HDL_3 subfractions, indicating that this two pool distribution of FC is a general phenomenon in HDL.

In order to substantiate the interpretation of the experiments mentioned above, HDL were investigated by ESR after spin labeling using 4,4'dimethyl-spiro(5 α-cholestane-3,2' oxazolidin)-3'yloxyl as a cholesterol probe. Evaluation of the ESR spectra clearly indicated that the spin label was present in two environments a) interspersed between the external phospholipid monolayer and b) in the liquid hydrophobic core.

In conclusion it can be said that human serum HDL consists of a pool of macromolecules arising from newly formed LpA particles, particles stemming from catabolism of triglyceride rich lipoproteins as well as from catabolic products generated by the action of serum enzymes such as lipases and LCAT. These macromolecules are in a dynamic state exchanging lipids, proteins and lipid:protein adducts. Applying mild separation methods, HDL exhibit a remarkable molecular homogeneity as far as the particle size is concerned. Ultracentrifugation and certain types of chromatography allows the separation of a great variety of subentities. These methods may give some insight into lipoprotein interactions which also are relevant for lipoprotein metabolism. NMR, ESR and small angle X-ray scattering experiments indicate that at least the major subfractions are built according to a common structural principle: The proteins form an outer shell in a quasispherical particle with intercalated polar head groups of phospholipids. The phospholipids form a monolayer and are in close contact of some 60% of free cholesterol. The rest of free cholesterol together with all the cholesteryl ester and the glycerides form the hydrophobic core of HDL.

References

Anderson DW, Nichols AV, Forte TM, Lindgren FT (1977) Particle distribution of human serum high density lipoproteins. Biochim Biophys Acta 493: 55-68

Hauser H, Kostner GM (1979) Structural arrangements of free and esterified cholesterol in human serum high density lipoproteins. A 100.6 MHz ^{13}C NMR study. Biochim Biophys Acta 573: 375-382

Kostner G, Albert A, Holasek A (1969) Analytische Isoelektrische Fokussierung der Humanserum-Lipoproteine. Hoppe Seyler's Z Physiol Chem 350: 1347-1352

Kostner G, Alaupovic P (1972) Studies of the composition and structure of plasma lipoproteins. Separation and quantification of the lipoprotein families occuring in the high density lipoproteins of human plasma. Biochemistry 11: 3419-3428

Kostner GM, Holasek A (1977) The separation of human serum HDL by hydroxyl-apatite column chromatography: evidence for the presence of discrete sub-fractions. Biochim Biophys Acta 488: 417-431

Kostner GM, Laggner P. (1979) Separation of HDL by column chromatography. Proc. of the HDL methodology workshop held in San Francisco, in press

Laggner P, Müller KW (1978) The structure of serum high density lipoproteins as analysed by X-ray small angle scattering. Quarterly Rev Biophys II,3: 371-425

McConnathy WJ, Alaupovic P (1976) Studies on the isolation and partial characterization of apolipoprotein D of human plasma. Biochemistry 15: 515-520

Olofsson SO, McConnathy WJ, Alaupovic P (1978) Isolation and partial characterization of a new acidic apoprotein (apoF) from HDL of human plasma. Biochemistry 17: 1032-1036

Utermann G, Menzel HJ, Langer KH, Dieker P (1975) Lipoproteins in LCAT deficiency II. Further studies on the abnormal HDL. Humangenetik 27: 185-197

Cholesteryl Ester-Rich Very Low Density Lipoproteins: Magnetic Resonance Studies[1]

Joel D. Morrisett,[2] Richard K. Stockton, and Roger D. Knapp

A number of different animals have been used to model human atherosclerosis. Among these are the nonhuman primates, pigs, rabbits, guinea pigs, chickens, and rats. Of these animal models, the rabbit has been the most intensely studied. Although the rabbit has a natural lesion distribution and lipid metabolism which is significantly different from that of man, this animal affords a number of unique advantages including low probability for spontaneous atherosclerosis, fast response to dietary or mechanical intervention, low cost, and facile handling. Furthermore, dietary refinements and careful drug administration have permitted the production of atherosclerotic lesions in the medium and large arteries of the rabbit which closely mimic those found in man. The types and locations of these induced lesions are now well-known. Over the past 50 years, the cholesterol-fed rabbit has been studied extensively as an experimental model for determining the relationship between dietary lipids and atherosclerosis. When the normal chow diet is enriched with 0.5–2.0% cholesterol, rabbits rapidly develop hypercholesterolemia (Duff 1935; Shore et al. 1974; Shumaker 1956) with subsequent appearance of atheromata (Anitschkow 1933; Kritchevsky 1954). While initially the cholesterol diet was utilized only to study induction of atherosclerotic lesions (Duff 1935), during the past 20 years a major focus of interest has been on the characterization of cholesterol-induced changes in the plasma lipoproteins. Gofman et al. (1950) described an initial elevation of lipoproteins with S_f 5–8 followed by the appearance of new particles of S_f 10–30. His data indicated a positive correlation between the extent of atherosclerosis and plasma levels of the S_f 10–30 particles but not with the S_f 5–8 ones. Subsequently, Shumaker (1956) reported that in these animals the S_f 0–400 material was greatly elevated and was enriched in cholesteryl esters while being reciprocally depleted in triglycerides compared to the corresponding lipoprotein fraction of normal rabbit plasma. In a later investigation, Camejo et al. (1973) demonstrated that these chemical changes were restricted to the material of $S_f > 20$. These workers were able to detect two size populations in this flotation fraction designated VLDL-1 ($S_f > 300$) and VLDL-2 (20–300). In our experiments, the larger VLDL-1 are markedly decreased in the plasma of hypercholesterolemic rabbits which have been fasted 24 to 48 hours before bleeding.

Although the metabolism (Camejo et al. 1974) and composition (Shore et al. 1974) of hypercholesterolemic VLDL have been extensively studied, relatively little work has been done on the structure of these particles. A lone exception is the study of Castellino et al. (1977) who used fluorescence polarization to study the temperature dependence of the microviscosity of normal and hypercholesterolemic VLDL. Whereas the microviscosity of the normal triglyceride-rich VLDL at 30° was 0.6 poise, this value was

[1]This research was performed in part under the auspices of the Atherosclerosis and Lipoprotein Section of the National Heart and Blood Vessel Research and Demonstration Center, Baylor College of Medicine, a grant supported research project of the National Heart and Lung Institute, National Institutes of Health, Grant no. 17269.
[2]Established Investigator of the American Heart Association (1974–1979).

increased to 4.6 poise in the hypercholesterolemic cholesteryl ester-rich VLDL. In a subsequent study, these same workers (Ploplis et al. 1979) used pyrene excimer fluorescence to examine further the microviscosity differences in these two lipoproteins.

Studies from these laboratories have indicated the rather marked heterogeneity of cholesteryl ester-rich very low density lipoproteins (CER-VLDL)[3] from hypercholesterolemic rabbit plasma. When these lipoproteins were isolated by ultracentrifugation at d 1.006 g/ml, they consisted of a mixed population found to be heterogeneous with respect to size, density, and chemical composition (Morrisett et al. 1979). DSC thermograms of CER-VLDL revealed reversible endotherms at 41.5° and 47.5° which were tentatively assigned to the smectic → cholesteric and cholesteric → isotropic phase transitions of the cholesteryl esters, the principal species being cholesteryl oleate (40%) which have known transitions at 42° and 47.5° (Small 1970). In this brief report, we describe a further study of the thermotropic properties of intact CER-VLDL. This study focuses sharply on the motion of specific lipid types within these particles as determined by spin label EPR and ^{13}C-NMR. While DSC affords highly instructive information about the macroscopic thermal behavior of CER-VLDL, it became desirable to probe the microscopic structure of this lipoprotein as well. Initially, the overall microscopic fluidity of this particle was studied with the small amphiphilic spin label, TEMPO, which partitions between an aqueous phase and a fluid lipid phase. This partitioning is determined by the measurement of appropriate paramagnetic resonance line amplitudes (Morrisett et al. 1977; Jackson et al. 1977). Increasing distribution of TEMPO into a lipid system implies increasing fluidity for that system. The microscopic fluidity of zonally isolated CER-VLDL increases linearly up to about 40° at which temperature there is an abrupt increase in fluidity which continues to about 48°. At that temperature, the rate of increase falls off significantly (Fig. 1B). This temperature range of 40-48° is the same range over which two thermotropic transitions are observed by DSC (Morrisett et al. 1979). Normal rabbit VLDL does not exhibit this abrupt increase in fluidity (Fig. 1A). The difference in temperature dependence of the microscopic viscosity of these two lipoproteins is easily understood upon examination of their respective lipid compositions (Table 1). Whereas CER-VLDL contains a preponderance of cholesteryl ester which exhibits a well-defined phase behavior, normal VLDL contains almost none of this lipid. Instead, it contains a high proportion of triglyceride which does not possess the thermotropic properties of cholesteryl esters. In fact, triglycerides have the capacity for disrupting the packing of cholesteryl esters which exhibit liquid crystalline behavior (Hamilton et al. 1977; Sears et al. 1976).

While the above described EPR experiment with TEMPO allows probing the total fluid lipid phase of CER-VLDL, NMR has the potential for yielding useful information about the thermal behavior of individual lipid types and even nuclei in different parts of these molecular types. The ^{13}C magnetic resonance spectrum of CER-VLDL at 37° contains relatively few lines; of those present, most are rather broad (Fig. 2). Two single carbon resonance lines which are easily detectable even in this spectrum are attributed to the fatty acyl methyl group (14.1 ppm) and the choline methyl group (54.5 ppm). The fatty acyl olefin envelope in the 128-130 ppm

---

[3]Abbreviations used: DOXYL, 3,3-dimethyloxazolidinyl; TEMPO, 2,2,6,6-tetramethylpiperidine-1-oxyl; CER-VLDL, cholesteryl ester-rich very low density lipoproteins normally isolated from hypercholesterolemic plasma; LDL, low density lipoproteins (human) isolated at d 1.019-1.063; EPR, electron paramagnetic resonance; NMR, nuclear magnetic resonance; DSC, differential scanning calorimetry.

Table 1. Composition of VLDL and CER-VLDL isolated from normal rabbit plasma by zonal ultracentrifugation.

	Normal VLDL	CER-VLDL
Protein	11.4	9.4
Phospholipid	15.9	16.7
Cholesterol	1.6	13.4
Cholesteryl ester	1.4	56.5
Triglyceride	69.7	3.9

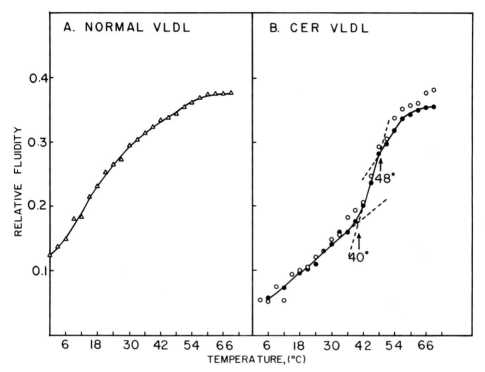

FIG. 1. Plots of microscopic fluidity of (A) normal rabbit VLDL and (B) hypercholesterolemic CER-VLDL as determined by the amphiphilic paramagnetic spin label, TEMPO. Compositional analyses are indicated in Tables 1 and 2. While the fluidity of normal VLDL increases gradually with increasing temperature, the fluidity of CER-VLDL increases abruptly between 40 and 48°, the same temperature range over which the smectic → cholesteric and cholesteric → isotropic phase transitions of the cholesteryl esters are detected by DSC. This transition is not observed in normal VLDL because of the low abundance of cholesteryl ester.

region is detectable but extremely broad. The degree of motion experienced by these nuclei at 37° is not available to the carbon atoms in the steroid ring system (e.g. C3, C5, C6, C9) as evidenced by the absence of their resonance lines from the spectrum. These lines do not appear until the temperature is raised to about 47°, where the cholesteryl esters within the lipoproteins begin to pass into the isotropic phase. A further increase of the temperature is attended by the appearance of additional lines and further narrowing of ones already present. A comparison of the temperature dependence of selected resonance linewidths is presented in Figure 3. It is clear that steroid ring carbons such as C3, C5, C6, and C9 experience an abrupt decrease in linewidth at about 47-48°. This decrease in linewidth

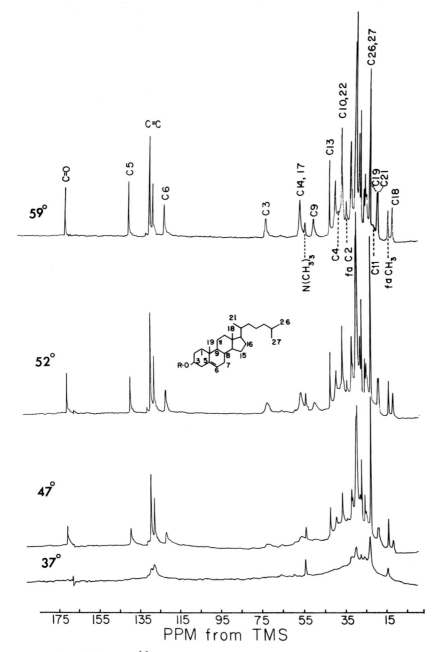

FIG. 2. 25.1 MHz ^{13}C-NMR spectra of CER-VLDL isolated at
d 1.006 g/ml. The same vertical display scale has been used
for all four spectra. These spectra illustrate the temperature
dependence of lines assignable to specific carbon nuclei. The
broad lines observed at 37° indicate slow rotational motion for
the corresponding nuclei. As the temperature is increased above
physiological temperatures, these lines become sharper indicating
increased rotational reorientation of these nuclei within the
particles. The nuclei whose linewidths are most temperature-dependent are those found in the steroid ring system of the cholesteryl esters (e.g. C3, C5, and C6 and C9). A plot of linewidths versus temperature is presented in Figure 3.

Table 2. Fatty acid composition of lipids from CER-VLDL.

Fatty acid	Phospholipid	Cholesteryl ester	Triglyceride	Free fatty acids
14:0	0.30	0.65	4.14	7.82
16:0	23.69	14.50	23.36	26.03
16:1	1.56	7.86	6.35	3.96
18:0	17.27	3.34	3.71	11.75
18:1	13.87	39.64	23.73	14.83
18:2	33.29	22.53	22.21	11.14
18:2-20:4	5.86	10.88	14.74	23.31
20:4	4.14	0.56	1.72	1.13

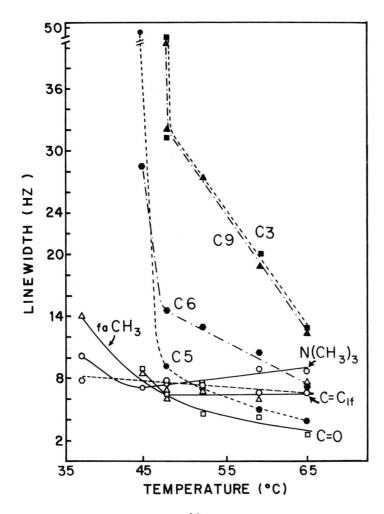

FIG. 3. Plot of 25.1 MHz ^{13}C-NMR linewidths versus temperature for a number of selected nuclei. This plot illustrates that single carbon nuclei within the steroid ring of the cholesteryl esters experience abruptly decreasing motion below 48° C. The motion of nuclei not in these steroid rings is not as strongly affected by temperature.

indicates an increase in rate and/or amplitude of motion for these steroid ring carbons. This effect is not observed for those carbon atoms which already possess a rather high amplitude or rate of motion (fatty acyl CH_3, choline CH_3, fatty acyl olefin, and fatty acyl carbonyl). These results suggest that the higher temperature ($\sim48°$) thermal transition observed previously by DSC, is due to absorbed energy which imparts new degrees of motional freedom to the steroid rings. At present, we do not know how the energy absorbed at the lower DSC endotherm ($\sim41°$) is dissipated among the cholesteryl esters in the smectic phase as it changes to the putative cholesteric phase (e.g. increased fatty acyl chain motion, molecular reorganization within the liquid crystal lattice, etc.).

The observation that the cholesteryl esters in the hydrophobic core of CER-VLDL pass through two well-defined thermotropic changes raises the question of whether this effect is transmitted to the surface of the particle. The answer to this question was sought through the use of 5- and 12-doxylstearate, two paramagnetic fatty acids which localize predominantly in the outer phospholipid monolayer of lipoproteins. The acyl chain order (Hubbell and McConnell 1971; Seelig 1976) of 5-doxylstearate decreases linearly with increasing temperature except at 48-50° where a small inflection is observed (Fig. 4A). The net effect of this inflection is to raise by about 3-4° the remainder of the order parameter curve. This slight, but abrupt elevation in acyl chain order may be the result of newly melted cholesteryl esters interdigitating into the phospholipid monolayer, resulting in a slight rigidifying effect in the latter. This small effect is not observed in the less sensitive 12-doxylstearate (Fig. 4B) whose doxyl ring is more distant from the carboxyl group thought to be anchored near the particle surface. Hence, it appears that the phase change observed in the cholesteryl ester-rich core is only weakly transmitted to the surface phospholipids.

The presence of a rigid, highly-organized neutral lipid core in CER-VLDL at the body temperature of rabbits raises a number of questions regarding how these particles relate to the development of atherosclerosis in these animals. For example, can these particles be degraded by the specific receptor pathway? Will lysosomal enzymes act on such rigid particles? Are these particles deposited in part or in toto in the arterial wall? Answers to these questions are currently being sought in our laboratories.

Acknowledgements

The authors are indebted to Ms. Debbie Mason, Kaye Shewmaker, and Barbara Allen for assistance in the preparation of this manuscript. TTGA.

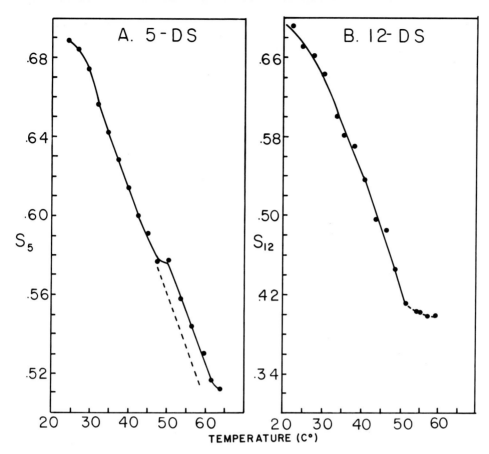

FIG. 4. Plots illustrating the temperature dependence of the acyl chain order parameter of 5-doxylstearate and 12-doxylstearate in CER-VLDL as determined by spin-label paramagnetic resonance. 5- and 12-doxylstearate localize in the outer shell of the lipoprotein and report the motion of fatty acyl chains (primarily of phospholipids) present in this region. The order parameter, S, is a measure of the mean angular deviation of the acyl chain from a line perpendicular to the surface of the particle and is inversely related to acyl chain flexibility. The order of 5-doxylstearate decreases monotonically in the temperature range 25-47°. A small plateau is observed at 48-51°, the temperature at which the cholesteryl esters in CER-VLDL undergo the cholesteric → isotropic transition. Above 53°, the acyl chain order continues to decrease monotonically. In contrast, 12-doxylstearate undergoes a simple decrease in order as the temperature increases from 20° to 50°.

References

Anitschkow A (1933) Experimental arteriosclerosis in animals. In: Cowdry EV (ed) Arteriosclerosis. The Macmillan Company, New York
Camejo G, Bosch V, Arreaza C, Mendez HC (1973) Early changes in plasma lipoprotein structure and biosynthesis in cholesterol-fed rabbits. J Lipid Res 14: 61-68
Camejo G, Bosch V, Lopez A (1974) The very low density lipoproteins of cholesterol-fed rabbits. Atherosclerosis 19: 139-152

Castellino FJ, Thomas JK, Ploplis VA (1977) Microviscosity of the lipid domains of normal and hypercholesterolemic very low density lipoproteins. Biochem Biophys Res Commun 75: 857-862

Duff GL (1935) Experimental cholesterol arteriosclerosis and its relationship to human arteriosclerosis. Arch Pathol 20: 82-123, 259-304

Gofman JW, Lindgren F, Elliott H, Mantz W, Hewitt J, Strisower B, Herring V (1950) The role of lipids and lipoproteins in atherosclerosis. Science 111: 166-171

Hamilton JA, Oppenheimer N, Cordes EH (1977) Carbon-13 nuclear magnetic resonance studies of cholesteryl esters and cholesteryl ester/triglyceride mixtures. J Biol Chem 252: 8071-8080

Hubbell WL, McConnell HM (1971) Molecular motion in spin-labeled phospholipids and membranes. J Amer Chem Soc 93: 314-326

Jackson RL, Morrisett JD, Pownall HJ, Gotto, AM, Kamio A, Imai H, Tracy R, Kummerow FA (1977) Influence of dietary TRANS-fatty acids on swine lipoprotein composition and structure. J Lipid Res 18: 182-190

Kritchevsky D, Moyer AW, Tesar WC, Logan JB, Brown RA, Davies MD, Cox HR (1954) Effect of cholesterol vehicle in experimental atherosclerosis. Am J Physiol 178: 30-32

Morrisett JD, Pownall HJ, Jackson RL, Segura R, Gotto AM, Taunton OD (1977) Effects of polyunsaturated and saturated fat diets on the chemical composition and thermotropic properties of human plasma lipoproteins. In: Holman RT, Kunau W-H (eds) Polyunsaturated fatty acids, American Oil Chemists' Society Monograph #4. AOCA Publishers, Champaign, Illinois, pp 139-161

Morrisett JD, Pownall HJ, Roth RI, Gotto AM, Patsch JR (1979) Structure of rabbit cholesteryl ester-rich very low density lipoproteins (CER-VLDL). Biophys J 25: 286a

Ploplis VA, Thomas JK, Castellino FJ (1979) Comparative studies of the physical state of the lipid phase of normal and hypercholesterolemic very low density lipoprotein. Chem Phys Lipids 23: 49-62

Sears B, Deckelbaum RJ, Janiak M, Shipley GG, Small DM (1976) Temperature-dependent ^{13}C nuclear magnetic resonance studies of human serum low density lipoproteins. Biochemistry 15: 4151-4157

Seelig, J (1976) Anisotropic motion in liquid crystalline structures. In: Berliner LJ (ed) Spin labeling: theory and techniques. Academic Press, Inc., New York, Chapter 10

Shore VG, Shore B, Hart RG (1974) Changes in apolipoproteins and properties of rabbit very low density lipoproteins on induction of cholesterolemia. Biochemistry 13: 1579-1585

Shumaker VN (1956) Cholesterolemic rabbit lipoproteins--serum lipoproteins of cholesterolemic rabbits. Am J Physiol 184: 35-42

Small DM (1970) The physical state of lipids of biological importance: cholesteryl esters, cholesterol, triglyceride. Adv Exp Med Biol 26: 55-83

NOVEMBER 7, 1979

Contributions of Invited Speakers

Plenary Session: Dietary Prevention of Coronary Heart Disease

Co-Chairpersons: Robert I. Levy and Gotthard Schettler
Speakers: Edward H. Ahrens
                        Henry W. Blackburn
                        Michael F. Oliver

Workshop: Hyperlipidemia: Prevalence and Inheritance

Chairperson: Joan Slack
Speakers: Gaetano Crepaldi
                        Jean Davignon
                        William R. Hazzard
                        Basil H. Rifkind
                        Nepomuk Zöllner

Workshop: Risk Factors in Children

Co-Chairpersons: Gerald S. Berenson and Mary Jane Jesse
Speakers: Charles J. Glueck
                        Peter O. Kwiterovitch, Jr.
                        Ronald M. Lauer
                        Richard J. West

Workshop: Diet Treatment of Atherosclerosis

Chairperson: Ivan D. Frantz, Jr.
Speakers: Ralph B. Blacket
                        Tatu A. Miettinen
                        Haruo Nakamura
                        Gunter Schlierf

Workshop: Immunology

Co-Chairpersons: John D. Mathews and C. Richard Minick
Speakers: J.L. Beaumont
                        Carl G. Becker
                        Francis V. Chisari
                        Thomas S. Edgington
                        Anatoli N. Klimov

Workshop: Animal Models

Speakers: David Kritchevsky
                  Robert W. Mahley
                  Sathanur R. Srinivasan
                  Wilbur A. Thomas
                  Draga Vesselinovitch

Workshop: Enzymes of Lipoprotein Metabolism

Speakers: Virgil Brown
                  Christopher J. Fielding
                  Paavo Kinnunen
                  Esko A. Nikkilä
                  Thomas Olivecrona
                  Louis C. Smith

Dietary Prevention of Coronary Artery Disease—A Policy Overview

Robert I. Levy

Coronary artery disease (CAD) represents a medical, social, and economic burden of enormous magnitude to this and other nations around the world (Sixth Director's Report 1979). As the number one killer in the U.S., CAD is responsible for over 650,000 deaths in this country each year, and over 150,000 of these occur before age 65. Nearly 1/3 of deaths from all causes in individuals between 35 and 64 years of age are due to CAD. Over 1 million heart attacks occur each year (of which 750,000 are first events) at a rate of 3,400/day or 2/minute. CAD is also the major cause of Social Security disability. It ranks second in terms of limitation of activity and hospital days spent in bed. Coronary artery disease costs the U.S. an estimated $27 billion per year in lost productivity and medical expenses.

Atherosclerosis is the principal factor responsible for these staggering statistics (Arteriosclerosis Working Group 1977). This insidious process develops silently and secretly in focal areas in blood vessels beginning in the first and second decades of life (Figure 1). It may then proceed for 2-5 decades with no overt clinical signs until after 2/3 of the vessel's lumen is occluded. Symptoms appear suddenly, in a matter of minutes, in the form of heart attack, sudden death, angina, claudication or stroke.

Although advances have been made in the management of CAD (aggressive new concepts of coronary care, the ability to suspend, restore and maintain heart rhythm, sophisticated surgical techniques and equipment to repair or replace damaged hearts, highly effective drugs), sudden death prevents nearly 1/4 of new heart attack victims from receiving definitive medical care. Moreover, our new powerful therapeutic armamentarium is costly and, in many cases, offers help that is either too little or too late. Clearly the ultimate and most cost-effective goal is primary prevention and early detection of CAD (Levy 1978).

In this regard, cardiovascular physiologists are developing non-invasive techniques to diagnose atherosclerosis at an earlier stage, long before any overt manifestations are apparent. Three major non-invasive diagnostic methods (echocardiography, exercise testing, and radionuclear imaging) are still being validated but offer promise for the future.

Parallel to these developments, cardiovascular epidemiologists have made a significant contribution by defining a set of risk factors, traits or habits that help identify those individuals who are at increased risk of premature CAD. Some of these risk factors cannot be reversed at present, namely, age, male sex and family history. We can, however, influence the level of cholesterol or blood pressure, how much an individual smokes and his weight. There is conclusive evidence from prospective studies that the higher the level of cholesterol (more precisely, the level of LDL cholesterol), the higher the level of blood pressure (whether systolic or diastolic), and the more an individual smokes, the more likely he is to sustain a cardiovascular event. In addition, the risk associated

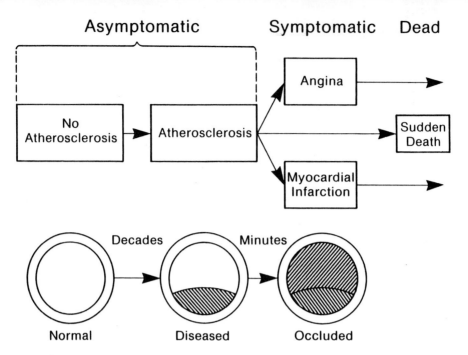

FIG. 1. Natural history of coronary artery disease.

with the presence of more than one risk factor is greater than the
simple combined risk of either factor alone.

Although the predictive power of the risk factors is not open to doubt, a
key question remains unanswered: Will alteration of the risk factors
affect the level of risk? In other words, will aggressive intervention
of these risk factors delay or prevent CAD and its sequelae?

With cigarette smoking, there is no doubt that its relationship to CAD
is dose related − the more one smokes, the greater the risk. Prospective
studies have now shown that with cessation of smoking the risk decreases
rapidly. After one year, it is only some 10% above that of the non-
smoker, and within a 10-year period it falls to normal. Thus we vigor-
ously advocate smoking cessation.

Hypertension is a major risk factor for heart attack; it is the major
risk factor for stroke. Although high blood pressure can now be treated
effectively, we do not yet have all the evidence on the benefits of such
treatment. It is still unclear whether lowering high blood pressure
will prevent heart attack. We do, however, have excellent evidence from
clinical trials of the late 1960's and early 1970's that lowering blood
pressure will prevent stroke, heart failure, and renal failure. For
these reasons, we now also aggressively treat patients with hypertension.

The evidence on the association between serum cholesterol level (and
specifically, LDL cholesterol level) and coronary artery disease is
extensive and unequivocal. (Figures 2a & b)(Arteriosclerosis Working
Group 1977; Stamler 1979). It is equally clear that cholesterol can be
lowered by diet or drugs in most patients. What is still hypothetical
is that LDL-lowering in man will reduce the incidence of heart attack.
A great deal of suggestive epidemiologic data supports this presumption,
but there is no direct clinical trial evidence in man.

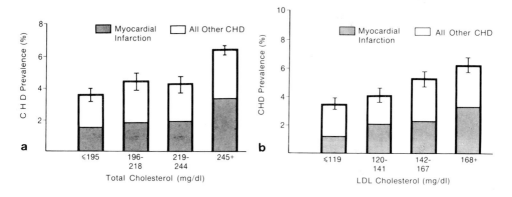

FIG. 2a and b. Estimated prevalence of coronary heart disease (CHD) according to (a) total-serum-cholesterol and (b) LDL-cholesterol quartiles.

The accuracy of predicting the risk of CAD from cholesterol concentrations is higher in the young (below age 65) than in the elderly.   Numerous studies have demonstrated that although subjects with the highest choles- terol levels experience a greater risk for developing CAD, no level encountered seems to be risk-free (Stamler 1978).   The "lipid hypothesis" is further confounded by the need to translate cholesterol level to elevations in the specific lipoproteins. (Figure 3)   In view of the mounting evidence on the inverse relationship of HDL and CAD (Miller et al. 1977; Castelli et al. 1977), it is becoming important to determine whether hypercholesterolemia is caused by increases in the atherogenic LDL or in HDL (Figure 4). Analyses based on data from the Framingham Study suggest that HDL should be integrated into the standard coronary risk profile, together with LDL and VLDL, and that this inclusion would greatly improve our ability to predict coronary heart disease (Gordon et al. 1977).

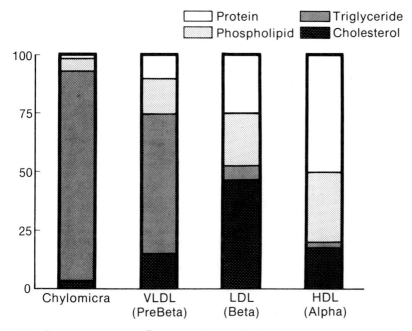

FIG. 3. Approximate % composition of lipoproteins.

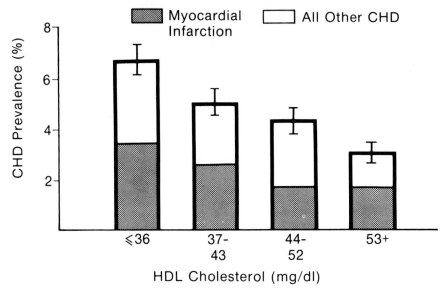

FIG. 4. Estimated prevalence of coronary heart disease (CHD) according
to HDL-cholesterol quartiles.

In the absence of clinical evidence in man, the "lipid hypothesis" is
supported by intriguing animal study data accumulated over the last 10
years. Indeed, data from non-human primates not only show that the
progression of atherosclerosis can be stopped, but they clearly demonstrate that atherosclerosis can be made to regress by lowering the
levels of circulating cholesterol. Such results have been obtained by
at least eight different research groups and there is very little doubt
of the validity of their findings. A limitation of these studies,
however, is that cholesterol levels were raised usually by dietary means
and then lowered again by putting the animals on a second diet very low
in cholesterol and fat, which generally lowered the serum cholesterol in
these non-human primates to below 100 mg/100 ml.

In a recent study by Dr. Tom Clarkson, a group of Rhesus monkeys were
fed a cholesterol-rich diet for 19 months (Clarkson et al. 1977).
Serum cholesterol levels in these animals were close to 800 mg/100 ml.
One-third of the cohort were then sacrificed. One-third were placed on
a modified diet and their cholesterol was maintained at 300 mg/100 ml.
The third group was put on a diet which maintained their cholesterol
levels for a further 24 months at approximately 200 mg/100 ml (a level
that we can hope to achieve in most free-living American subjects).
Those animals whose cholesterol levels were maintained at 300 mg/100 ml
showed advanced coronary stenosis as determined by serial sections.
Although there was less fat in the vessels than in animals sacrificed at
800 mg/100 ml, the amount of medial damage and internal elastic lamina
damage was the same. However, animals which had been maintained at a
level of 200 mg/100 ml showed statistically significant decreases in
stenosis, fat in the vessels, medial and internal elastic lamina damage.
There was no doubt that in these animals when serum cholesterol was
lowered to 200 mg/100 ml regression of lesions occurred (Figure 5).
Although with this diet-induced hypercholesterolemia, the lesions were
not calcified or fibrotic, the results do suggest that regression of
coronary lesions in the species closest to man can be achieved at a
cholesterol level of 200 mg/100 ml (Table 1).

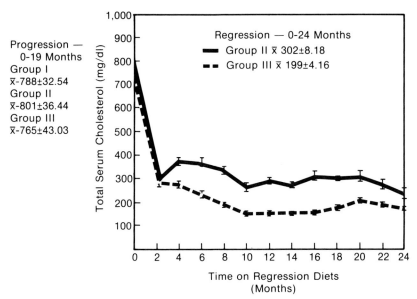

FIG. 5. Primate regression study. Total mean serum cholesterol concentrations.

There is also some presumptive evidence that regression of atherosclerosis can occur in man. Several observations made, often during wartime or in patients with wasting disease or receiving hormonal treatment, have been used to suggest that regression of atherosclerosis can occur. However, all of these studies can be challenged and none of them provide unambiguous proof that the lipid hypothesis is operative. These free-living populations are influenced by a variety of factors which could explain an apparent regression in atherosclerosis.

A number of studies have been performed over the last two decades in an attempt to test the lipid hypothesis (Rifkind and Levy 1978). Between 1955 and 1968 four double blind and eight other studies were reported; since 1970 the results of three large-scale studies have been published. All of the investigations, whether performed on a double blind basis or not, showed that some lowering of serum cholesterol could be achieved. The average cholesterol reduction was approximately 10% in free living populations. But in none of these studies was there a statistically significant difference in terms of the "hard" end-points (heart attack and death). In those studies that were not double blinded there were some changes in "soft" end-points such as angina, but such end-points are difficult to evaluate, especially when a non-blind design is used. Thus there is no firm evidence from diet studies that lowering cholesterol levels will prevent heart disease. However, it is equally important to note that none of these studies show that cholesterol lowering does not prevent heart disease, since none of them had a sample size large enough to prove the null hypothesis (Levy 1977).

The issues involved in attempting to prove the lipid hypothesis were not closely examined until about ten years ago (Table 2). Two factors which are designated as alpha and beta come into the consideration of any clinical trial. Alpha factors are involved in insuring that differences are going to be significant, that an effect will occur only once out of 20, 100 or 1000 times. Beta factors are involved in insuring that a clear difference will be observable between treated and control groups. The major problem with trials attempting to test the lipid hypothesis

Table 1. Primate regression study. Coronary atherosclerosis.

Group	Stenosis %	Fat %	Medial Damage %	IEL Damage %
I	25+5.2	41+3.9	40+8.0	25+5.8
II (Chol 300)	35+4.7	20+2.9	37+5.3	22+3.5
III (Chol 200)	17+4.2	6+1	20+5.4	17+4.1

lies in the end-points that can be measured. These are heart attack and death, since the non-invasive techniques for detecting other events are not yet totally validated or available. Even in a population with existent coronary disease one can only expect a death rate of 5% in one year. Such trials will thus require a large number of patients and a long period of time to generate an adequate number of events.

Other statistical factors relevant to designing such a study include the K value, the fractional lowering of the risk, which varies by the amount that one can lower the cholesterol level. In general, diet studies can only lower the cholesterol level by a maximum of 10%. The best way to consider the F value is to ask the following question: If cholesterol has been lowered from 350 to 250 mg/100 ml, is the risk now equal to that of a subject whose cholesterol has always been at the lower level, or will the risk fall after a period of time? For cigarette smoking we know that the risk decreases very rapidly in the first year and then more slowly thereafter, but the F value for cholesterol lowering is less clear. If it is longer than three years, trials would be particularly difficult to perform. The dropout rate is a problem that occurs in any study and a long-term, large-scale investigation no matter how well-designed, can be destroyed by a dropout rate of 5-15% per year. One can increase the duration of the study and thus take advantage of the greater number of events. In addition, even if the F value is 3-4 years, a study designed to proceed for 7-10 years will still show a difference. But increasing the duration will also increase the number of dropouts, thus threatening the results of the study.

A feasibility study was undertaken in the late 1960's by advocates of a National Diet-Heart Trial. The study was conducted in many centers for a short period of time. Ten percent of adult males volunteered in the areas of the study and a total of 1,211 men aged 45-53 were studied for one year. Specially prepared meats and dairy products were made available to these subjects. The study showed that a double blind design could be maintained, that a cholesterol difference of about 10% could be achieved by diet and that the dropout rate during the year was also about 10%. When the results of the Feasibility Study were looked at in terms of the power and sample size calculations already considered, major problems became obvious. With a dropout rate of 10% and a cholesterol lowering of only 10%, a trial involving patients without existent cardiovascular disease (a primary prevention trial) would require 30,000 - 150,000 subjects to be studied from 1-4 decades. Even before the price of meat increased in the early 1970's, the trial would have required all the resources of the National Heart, Lung, and Blood Institute.

Other practical problems in performing a trial using diet include that of achieving and maintaining dietary change. How can one keep any free living group on a modified dietary regimen for any period of time? Patients generally prefer to have their physician prescribe a drug

Table 2. Factors involved in calculating sample size requirement for clinical trial to prove the "lipid hypothesis".

1. α - (probability of positively interpreting a negative result)

2. β - (probability of not detecting a positive result)

3. - event rate in control subjects

4. $\underline{K}$ - (fractional lowering of risk)

5. $\underline{F}$ - (time taken to achieve maximum treatment effect)

6. $\underline{D}$ - (dropout rate - loss to treatment)

7. - duration of study

rather than to take responsibility for their own welfare.

The lipid hypothesis can also be tested through a variety of drugs (Levy, Rifkind 1977). Many effective hypolipidemic drugs are now available. These can be attractive for use in clinical trials, especially if they can enhance the K factor, the lowering of cholesterol level. On the other hand, all of these drugs have different mechanisms of action and none of them are effective in all types of hyperlipoproteinemia, so that it is necessary to select the patients to be treated (Levy, in press). Moreover, all of the drugs have certain side effects, some more serious than others, but all again posing the problem of adherence to the study regimen within a free-living population for an extended period of time.

The National Heart, Lung, and Blood Institute is at present supporting two major ongoing clinical trials to test the benefits of LDL lowering. The objective of the Lipid Research Clinics Primary Prevention Trial is to determine whether reduction of LDL cholesterol in asymptomatic subjects with Type II hyperlipoproteinemia will prevent or lower the incidence of coronary heart disease. The study is investigating the effects of diet and cholestyramine on 3,800 men aged 35-59 and is expected to be completed in 1983.

For this trial, subjects with hyperbetalipoproteinemia were selected for several reasons. Studies have shown that subjects with familial Type II are at greatly increased risk. Life table analysis of males shows that up to age 20 siblings with hypercholesterolemia do not manifest vascular disease, but after age 30 males with hyperbetalipoproteinemia have a very high incidence of vascular events and by age 60 more than two out of three will have had some incident (Figure 6) (Stone et al. 1974). For this current trial, subjects were selected by age grouping, in part because in primary Type II the incidence of vascular disease increases dramatically in the fourth, fifth, and sixth decade of life.

In the Multiple Risk Factor Intervention Trial (MRFIT), 12,000 subjects are being aggressively treated to achieve cessation of cigarette smoking, to lower high blood pressure with diet and drugs, and to lower cholesterol by 10% with diet.

Because it would be difficult to blind entirely two of these factors (cigarette smoking and the treatment of high blood pressure), 6,000 subjects are being treated by clinic staff, while the remaining 6,000 are under the care of their regular physician. The study is expected to

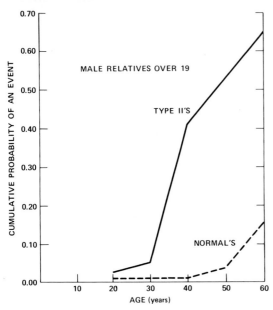

FIG. 6. Cumulative probability by decade of fatal or nonfatal CAD.

be completed in 1982.

Until the results of these trials are available and until the benefits of lipid-lowering can be conclusively demonstrated, what advice can we give the public? How can one achieve and maintain dietary change? The National Heart, Lung, and Blood Institute has launched a Nutrition Education Program aimed at reaching consumers at points of purchase of food. Several projects incorporated under this program include the dissemination of nutrition information at supermarkets, worksetting-based cafeterias, and vending machines. Other projects seek to determine what factors are necessary to achieve and maintain dietary compliance.

The changes that have been occurring in the food consumption patterns are an encouraging sign that the message is getting through. The consumption of milk and cream, butter, eggs, fats and oils of animal origin is decreasing, while the consumption of vegetable fats is increasing (Table 3). Health nutrition surveys (HANES) carried out in 1960-1962 and 1971-1974 suggest a modest lowering of cholesterol in the population over this 10 year period. Comparison with population studies conducted by the Lipid Research Clinics (1972-76) suggests that a 4-8% decrease in plasma cholesterol levels in the U.S. over the past 10 years has occurred, with the most striking changes occurring in the most educated and higher socioecomomic groups (LRC Program 1979).

These dietary changes are associated, at least temporally, with a dramatically decreasing cardiovascular event rate in the U.S. (Proceedings 1979) (Figure 8). During the past 10 years, the rate of heart attack deaths has fallen by over 22% - a rate of over 2% per year. The incidence of stroke has declined more than 33% in this period at a rate since 1972 of over 5% per year. Finally, not only have death rates declined, but the absolute number of cardiovascular deaths in the U.S. has decreased markedly despite an aging and ever increasing population.

In spite of this encouraging evidence, there is still no definitive answer to the question, does cholesterol lowering in man through diet

Table 3. Change in per capita consumption, 1963–75

Product	% Change
Tobacco Products	−22.4
Fluid Milk & Cream	−19.2
Butter	−31.9
Eggs	−12.6
Fats & Oils (Animal)	−56.7
(Vegetable)	+44.1

change the risk of coronary artery disease? Until we do find the answer, it appears wise to recommend a prudent diet change to the American public. The guidelines include avoidance of weight gain and obesity, a moderate reduction in the intake of fat (especially saturated fat) coupled with a prudent decrease in cholesterol intake. If the answer to the question turns out to be negative, there is little likelihood that these dietary changes will have caused any harm. On the other hand, if cholesterol lowering <u>does</u> prove to be beneficial, we will be on our way toward reducing the devastating impact of the mortality, morbidity and suffering associated with premature coronary artery disease.

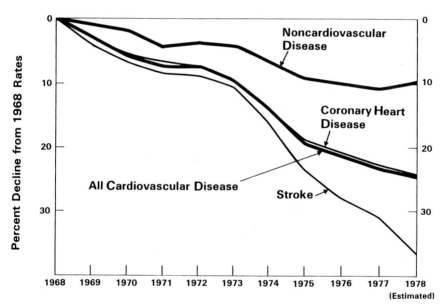

FIG. 7. Trends in cardiovascular disease and noncardiovascular disease decline by age-adjusted death rates, 1968–1978.

References

Arteriosclerosis. Report of the 1977 Working Group to Review the 1971 Report by the National Heart, Lung, and Blood Institute Task Force on Arteriosclerosis. U. S. Department of Health, Education, and Welfare. Public Health Service. DHEW Publication No. NIH 78–1526

Castelli WP, Doyle JT, Gordon T, Haines CG, Hjortland M, Hulley SB,
   Kagan A, Zukel WJ (1977) HDL cholesterol and other lipids in
   coronary heart disease. The Cooperative Lipoprotein Phenotyping
   Study. Circulation 55:767-772

Clarkson TB, Lehner DM, Wagner WD, St. Clair RW, Bond MG, Bullock BC
   (1979) A study of atherosclerosis regression in Macara mulatta.
   I. Design of experiment and lesion induction. Exper and Molec
   Pathol 30:360-385

Gordon T, Castelli WP, Hjortland M, Kannel WB, Dawber T (1977) High
   density lipoprotein as a protective factor against coronary
   heart disease. The Framingham Study. Am J Med 62:707-714

Levy RI (1977) Statement at the Hearings before the Select Committee
   on Nutrition and Human Needs of the United States Senate, 95th
   Congress, First Session. Diet Related to Killer Diseases, II.
   Part I, Cardiovascular Disease. U. S. Government Printing Office,
   Washington, D. C.

Levy RI (1978) Progress in prevention of cardiovascular disease.
   Prev Med 7:464-475

Levy RI (in press) Drugs used in the treatment of hyperlipoproteinemia.
   In: Goodman and Gilman's The Pharmacologic Basis of Therapeutics
   (6th ed.) MacMillan, New York

Levy RI, Rifkind BM (1977) Lipid lowering drugs and hyperlipidaemia.
   In: Avery GS (ed) Cardiovascular Drugs. Vol. 1, Antiarrhythmic,
   Antihypertensive and Lipid Lowering Drugs. ADIS Press Australasia
   Pty Ltd, Sydney

Lipid Research Clinics Program Epidemiology Committee (1979) Plasma
   lipid distributions in selected North American populations: The
   Lipid Research Clinics Program Prevalence Study. Circulation
   60:427-439

Miller NE, Thelle DS, Forde OH, Mjos OD (1977) The Tromso Heart
   Study. High density lipoprotein and coronary heart disease.
   A prospective case-control study. Lancet 1:965-967

Proceedings of the Conference on the Decline in Coronary Heart Disease
   Mortality (1979) U. S. Department of Health, Education, and Welfare.
   Public Health Service. DHEW Publication No. (NIH) 79-1610

Rifkind BM, Levy RI (1978) Testing the lipid hypothesis. Arch Surg
   113:80-83

Sixth Report of the Director of the National Heart, Lung, and Blood
   Institute. U. S. Department of Health, Education and Welfare.
   Public Health Service. DHEW Publication No. (NIH) 79-1605

Stamler J (1978) Lifestyles, major risk factors, proof and public policy.
   Circulation 58:3-19

Stamler J (1979) Diet, serum lipids, and coronary heart disease. The
   epidemiologic evidence. In: Levy RI, Rifkind BM, Dennis BH,
   Ernst N (eds) Nutrition, Lipids and Coronary Heart Disease - A
   Global View. Raven Press, New York

Stone NJ, Levy RI, Fredrickson DS, Verter J (1974) Coronary artery
   disease in 116 kindred with familial type II hyperlipoproteinemia.
   Circulation 49:476-488

Dietary Prevention of Coronary Heart Disease

Gotthard Schettler

Coronary heart disease and other forms of atherosclerosis are still the main cause of death in affluent societies. In the German Federal Republic, a tremendous increase in the number of deaths from coronary heart disease could be observed during the years of 1948 to 1969, and even since then an increase in mortality could be documented (Fig. 1). Though there are no exact statistical data available covering the pre-war and war period, it is very remarkable that in our country myocardial infarction was practically unknown during the years of 1945 and 1948. This applies to morbidity as well as mortality. These times of starvation led furthermore to a decline of fatal thrombo-embolic events and with the normalization of food supply, arterial disease appeared again.

Since the coronary mortality is still very high in our country, we started a screening program for risk factors in two communities of the Heidelberg area. The "Eberbach-Wiesloch" Project is part of the cardiovascular community control program of the WHO-Regional Office in Europe. Survival rates for the 7-year follow-up were extremely low with 68, 58 and 37% (Fig. 2). In spite of intensive care units and early onset of therapy in our country with outstanding medical services through rehabilitation, prognosis for patients suffering from myocardial infarctions is still abysmal. Actually this is even more true for patients above 65 years of age.

In the two communities under study in Germany, 98% of the men and women between 30 and 60 years of age were screened. There was a total of 11,000 men and women. The risk profile consisted of 7 different points (Table 1). Of the subjects studied 17% have hypertension as documented by repeated control. Of the men, 24% had elevated cholesterol values. If one combines hypercholesterolemia and hypertriglyceridemia, more than 30% of the men had hyperlipidemia (Fig. 3). In women of the same age group a similar distribution was found, except for hypertriglyceridemia, which occurred in only 7% and hyperuricemia, which was only found in 1%. Adding up the clinical manifest risk factors which are influenced by nutrition more than half of the men examined aged 30 to 60 showed at least one of these factors.

Obesity occurs rather frequently in the Federal Republic of Germany. Generally speaking, about two-thirds of the male as well as female population are overweight.

In men with ideal weight, hypertension was found in 7% of the cases, in those who were markedly overweight---in 644 persons examined---the rate for hypertension jumped to 29%. To me, the relation between hypercholesterolemia and bodyweight seems of great importance, because even in those persons with an ideal weight 19% were found to be hypercholesterolemic. The strong correlation between hypertriglyceridemia and bodyweight is well known. The differences between men having ideal bodyweight and those who are significantly overweight are extreme. Men having ideal bodyweight had hypertriglyceridemia in 9% of the total cases and their number increased to 41% in those who were overweight. Recapitulating the five clinical manifest risk factors and putting them

Table 1. Seven point check for early detection of risk factors.[a]

	normal	borderline	high
Smoking habits			
Overweight (Broca)	<1.1	between	>1.1
Blood pressure			
systolic	<140	between	>160
diastolic	< 90	between	> 95
Cholesterol	<220	between	>260
Triglycerides	<150	between	>200
Uric acid			
men	<7.0	between	>8.0
women	<6.5	between	>7.5
Sugar (fasting)			
blood	< 90	between	>110
urine	negative		positive
Sugar (postprandial)			
blood	<140	between	>160
urine	negative		positive

[a] Nüssel (1976).

into correlation with bodyweight we find the following (Fig. 4): In 69% of the 443 men examined, those with ideal bodyweight did not have hypertension, hypercholesterolemia, hypertriglyceridemia, hyperuricemia or elevated blood sugar. From those men 20% overweight according to the Broca-index, only 29% were free of the factors mentioned. This shows very clearly that within the scope of the prevention, special emphasis has to be put on hyperalimentation.

Similar findings can be presented from the city of Heidelberg. For the purpose of nutrition and health assessment and as a basis for intervention

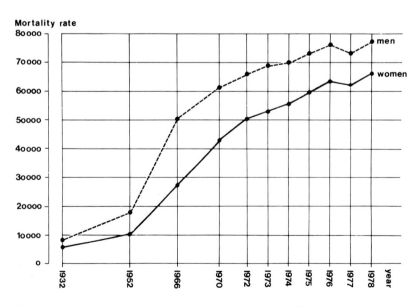

FIG. 1. Mortality rate from coronary heart disease in the Federal Republic of Germany.

Table 2. Nutrition in 20-40 year old Heidelberg men (24-h recall).

	present status	"dietary goals"
Calories	2621	
Fats	44%, P/S 0.3	30%, P/S 1.0
Protein	13%	12%
Carbohydrates	36%	58%
Alcohol	7%	

and prevention a survey was conducted. "Health" was assessed by clinical examination and biochemical measurements as well as nutritional status and nutritional habits (24-hour recall, 7 day diet protocol) in a random sample of 20-40 year old Heidelberg men from 1975 through 1977. In this "healthy" population, the frequency of conventional cardiovascular risk factors was as follows: hypercholesterolemia 11%, hypertension 15% and heavy smoking 32%. In addition a high prevalance of obesity, hyperuricemia and hyperglycemia were found. The main results of dietary assessment are shown in Table 2. Even though total caloric and total protein intake appear to be within an acceptable range, changes as suggested for the United States appear necessary in the area of fat consumption from a high intake of 44% of total calories, from a consumption of mono- and disaccharide of 14% total calories, and from an average alcohol intake of 7% total calories.

We can thus summarize that the so-called risk factors are extemely common. I would like to raise the question: How can we reduce them? What is our evidence that nutrition, especially the fat content of a diet, is an important factor for the development of atherosclerosis and for the mortality from coronary heart disease (Schettler 1978)?

1. In societies suffering from starvation or living on subsistence levels, death from coronary artery disease is very rare.

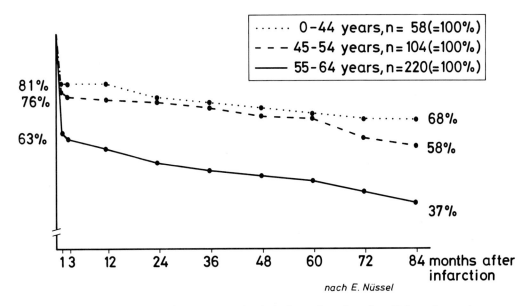

nach E. Nüssel

FIG. 2. Survival-rate after myocardial infarction (men). Taken from the WHO Project (Euro 5010, Heidelberg).

2. During starvation the number of deaths from coronary artery disease in the German Federal Republic and other European Countries was very low. The rate of mortality grew in parallel with better nutrition and increased even more when luxurious food became available. In these first years of starvation after World War II, the food contained only minimal amounts of cholesterol and fat; the plasma cholesterol averaged 130 mg/dl (Fig. 5). Increased intake of fiber and more exercise may have contributed to the lower levels of cholesterol. Autopsies performed on undernourished people and inmates of POW or concentration camps showed predominantly clean arteries. Coronary thrombosis or myocardial infarctions were rare findings. Decreased smoking may have played a role.

3. The number of severe atherosclerosis cases increases with rising luxurious food consumption as shown in studies from Switzerland.

4. Worldwide epidemiological studies show a connection between nutrition, severe forms of atherosclerosis and fatal myocardial infarction.

5. Continuous monitoring of risk factors for the development of atherosclerosis in well-defined cohorts shows that plasma cholesterol, LDL and also VLDL are risk factors of first order. The decline in the death rate of coronary artery disease documented in intervention studies correlates, among others, with the lowering of plasma cholesterol. The reciprocal relationship between LDL-, VLDL-cholesterol versus HDL-cholesterol points in the same direction.

6. Certain hyperlipoproteinemias (HL) cause premature and severe atherosclerosis and coronary artery disease. There is evidence for regression of xanthomas of skin and tendons, xanthomatous valves and coronary atherosclerosis when plasma cholesterol is lowered. The success of lipid-lowering therapy has been shown to improve coronary artery disease as documented by coronary angiography, ECG and treadmill ECG.

7. The studies of Goldstein et al. (1974) on the LDL-receptor are further indications for the relationship between LDL-cholesterol and atherosclerotic lesions. The cholesterol of the arterial intima has its origin predominantly in the plasma. Radioactively labeled LDL-cholesterol accumulates in human coronary arteries as shown in persons undergoing

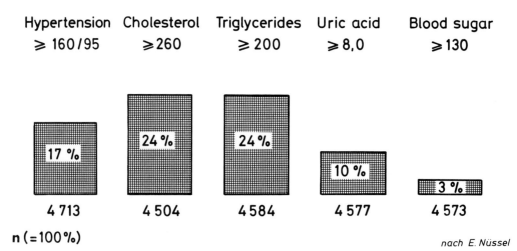

FIG. 3. Risk factors in 30-60 year old men. Taken from the WHO Project (CVD 018, Heidelberg, October 1977).

coronary surgery later on. ApoB has been identified in the human intima by immunochemical methods as well. Below a certain concentration of LDL in plasma, only a very low LDL-flux into the intima can be observed.

8. Experiments, in animals, especially in primates, show that certain modifications of the fat content of diets can influence the development of atheosclerosis. Progression and regression of atherosclerotic lesions have been achieved in these dietary trials.

9. The formation of the initial lesion in atherosclerosis involves closely connected factors and processes such as plasma cholesterol, platelet aggregation, thrombus formation and proliferation of smooth muscle cells. Prostaglandins, their precursors and antagonists, are of crucial importance and can be influenced by linoleic acid.

10. Coagulation processes can cause intramural and intravasal thrombosis leading to incomplete or complete occlusion of the coronary artery. These hemostatic processes frequently determine the course of coronary artery disease.

11. Hyperlipidemias are pacemakers of myocardial infarction in cigarette smokers. The mean age at the time of myocardial infarction in hypercholesterolemic cigarette smokers is 15 years lower than in nonsmoking patients with low blood cholesterol. Hyperlipidemias also represent a cumulative risk factor under risk conditions like hypertension or diabetes and in women taking contraceptives.

Conclusion for Practical Purposes

It is widely accepted that total plasma cholesterol values between 150 and 160 mg/dl and levels of HDL equivalent to the LDL concentration do not promote the process of atherosclerosis. VLDL and chylomicron triglycerides should be as low as possible. It seems therefore reasonable to strive for these concentrations for our preventive trials. Accepting the multifactorial etiology and pathogenesis of atherosclerosis, defects in

Risk Factors:

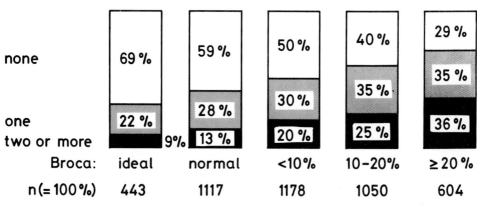

nach E. Nüssel

FIG. 4. Summarized risk factors/body weight in 30-50 year old men (RR 160/ 95, Chol 260, TG 200, UA 8.0, BS 130). Taken from the WHO Project (CVD 018, Heidelber, October 1977).

lipid and lipoprotein metabolism play a key role in nutrition and structural integrity of the arteries. The tight interrelationships between lipids and processes or hemostasis and thrombosis allow us to draw conclusions concerning the pathogenetic mechanisms leading to peripheral and coronary vascular disease. So far we concentrated our attention on plasma lipids; but the plasma lipid pool reflects only a fraction of the total body lipid pool. The input into the plasma pool comes from exogenous sources (food intake) and de novo synthesis. The factors regulating the catabolism and the output of lipids are mostly unknown. There are certainly differences in responses to changes in dietary habits among individuals. We need more information concerning the responses of dietary manipulations in the familial versus environmental forms of HL. We need more data on hormonal regulation of synthesis and removal of lipids and also on the pathogenesis of immune dyslipoproteinemias. Apoprotein concentrations along with the ratios of apoA-I and apoA-II to apoB should be investigated in risk patients. Moreover, we have to consider interactions among different ingredients of our food and not only concentrate on the fat content or cholesterol content of our diet. We know that the cholesterol contents of our diet and the total fat contents in industrialized countries are too high. An average citizen in these industrialized countries gets 40 to 50% of his daily calories from fat. The situation is quite different in countries of the so-called "Third or Fourth World," who make up the majority of the present global population. For this population, atherosclerosis plays no significant factor as a disease or cause of death.

I would like to propose a reduction in calories derived from fat from 40% at the present to 30% in a diet containing 2,600 calories. This measure would reduce the daily fat intake in the average American diet from 159 g/day to 90 g/day. In addition, I would recommend changes in intake of cholesterol, fat composition, protein content, and dietary fiber.

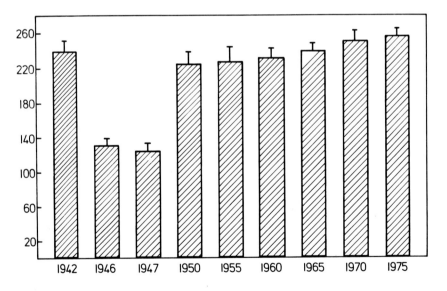

FIG. 5. Blood cholesterol (mg/dl SD) in normal individuals between 1942 and 1975 (n = 19).

Table 3. Dietary influence on plasma cholesterol level.

Reduced and modified fat intake (30%, P/S 1.0)	-20 mg/dl
Reduced cholesterol intake (200 mg)	- 8 mg/dl
Increased fiber intake (6 → 46 g)	-15 mg/dl
Modified protein intake (↑ vegetable)	- 8 mg/dl
Sum Δ cholesterol	51 mg/dl

Cholesterol

Most researchers agree that the daily intake should be lower than 300 mg.

Fatty acid composition

Saturated fatty acids increase plasma cholesterol twice as much as polyunsaturated fatty acids lower cholesterol. For example: If a person gets 30% of his daily calories from fat and the amount of fat calories derived from polyunsaturated, monounsaturated and saturated fats is equal, the plasma cholesterol could be lowered by 18 to 20 mg/dl (calculated for 2,600 calories). We would not recommend an increase in the P/S ratio to 4:1 or 7:1 as performed under certain experimental conditions. P/S ratios of 1:1 have no known side effects.

Dietary fiber

Plant-derived fibers may have a hypocholesterolemic effect. According to Truswell (1978) fibers from vegetable sources can lower the plasma cholesterol by approximately 15 mg/dl.

Protein

The substitution of soy bean proteins for animal proteins can lead to a considerable reduction in plasma cholesterol by 30%. An increase in the protein content derived from vegetable sources from presently 30 to 50% would lead to a reduction of plasma cholesterol of 8 mg/dl. Concomitant alteration of dietary fat, cholesterol, fibers and protein could result in an overall reduction in plasma cholesterol of 50 mg/dl (Table 3).

We could thus lower the average plasma cholesterol from 220 mg/dl to 170 mg/dl and come to close to the antiatherogenic cholesterol level of 150 mg/dl. This goal seems to be attainable, if we start with our effort early on and promote this diet as a guideline, not a strict and inflexible scheme. We have to allow for individual variations, because we think it is not desirable to create a society of diet addicts or fat-manipulated vegetarians. But we think simple appeals for a prudent diet will not work. We should put pressure on the food industry to cooperate along the precepts outlined above. To educate the people in our community and motivate them to follow our dietary guidelines seems to lie within our reach. An important aspect of our work as physicians ofers itself explicitly in preventive medicine.

Table 4. Sterol excretion (mg/24 h stool).[a]

No.	P/S-rich Diet Sterols mg/24 h			18 g of PC Sterols mg/24 h		
	Acid	Net Neutral	Balance	Acid	Net Neutral	Balance
1	112	251	− 363	120	322	− 442
2	225	505	− 730	224	935	−1159
3	485	1352	−1836	258	1596	−1854
4	80	752	− 832	171	941	−1112
5	136	136	− 272	243	1118	−1361
6	−	−	−	−	−	−
7	−	−	−	−	−	−
8	411	343	− 754	892	1078	−1970

[a]Greten et al. (1979).

Yet we must not look only at the plasma lipids. I would like to give you one example from our own experiments (Greten et al. 1979). The study group investigated plasma and lipoprotein composition following oral administration of highly polyunsaturated lecithin in patients with hyperlipidemia and normal subjects under metabolic ward conditions. In addition to these analyses, fecal steroid excretion was measured and bile composition studied. The effect of phosphorylcholine on plasma lipoprotein composition and sterol excretion could be studied. Two dietary periods were applied with similar amounts of calories, cholesterol and polyunsaturated fatty acids in order to evaluate the specific effect of phosphorylcholine. No change in plasma lipid and lipoprotein concentration was observed. However, fecal sterol excretion was substantially increased in all subjects when phosphatidylcholine was added to the diet (Table 4). Bile acids, phospholipids and cholesterol content in bile did not vary.

It has been repeatedly shown that cigarette smoking is a risk factor for coronary heart disease. The question why populations do not have high death rates for myocardial infarctions is of particular interest. Are there certain risk-triggering constellations? We conducted studies to find possible relations between acute smoking and lipoprotein metabolism (Augustin et al. 1979). Compared with the shamsmoker group we found a stimulation of intravascular lipolytic activities directly after inhaling the smoke of two cigarettes. This activation results in the accelerated interconversion of triglyceride-rich VLDL via IDL to atherogenic LDL. In addition, our data demonstrate a fundamental influence of acute smoking on HDL. The amount of phospholipids in this lipoprotein fraction considerably decreases directly after smoking, although the half-life of HDL is supposed to be in the range of three days. The same effect is observed with regard to HDL-cholesterol, which is also reduced directly after smoking (Table 5). Besides a decrease in total plasma HDL our data suggest a considerable change in the structure of this lipoprotein with a loss of surface material after smoking. It has to be evaluated whether this modified HDL is still able to act as a carrier for cholesterol from the periphery to the liver and as a competitor for LDL-binding sites.

Practical prevention

An intervention study has been initiated in Eberbach-Wiesloch which includes community agencies, especially the collaboration with the mayor and the local physicians, as well as the individual cooperation of the citizens. Intensive efforts are made to control the weight of school

Table 5. The effect of acute smoking on lipoprotein metabolism.[a]

Activation of hepatic triglyceride lipase and lipoprotein lipase resulting in increased intravascular lipolysis of VLDL with rise in plasma HDL and LDL.
Decrease in HDL-cholesterol.
Transfer of HDL-phospholipids to LDL.

[a] Augustin et al. (1979)

Table 6. Model of Wiesloch.[a]

Decrease of risk factors	
Uric acid	13.9%
Cholesterol	17.1%
Triglycerides	25.0%

[a] Nüssel et al. (1975).

children and advise them about their dietary habits. We have an exemplary working relationship with bakers, butchers, dairies and restaurant owners. This program, by the way, has been accepted by the World Health Organization as a model for other projects. So far, the results up to 1975 have been very promising (Table 6) and a similar trend has continued to the present.

Certainly the declining death rates for myocardial infarction and stroke are not related to one single cause. The multiple risk concept of atherosclerosis requires the approach of multiple intervention. The success of primary prevention ranks before secondary prevention. I do not agree that atherosclerosis with its clinical complications needs to be accepted as a blow of fate. I do not think that there is any evidence to assume pathogenesis of atherosclerosis is solely the consequence of wear and tear combined with age. I am convinced that lipids play an important key role in the etiology of atherosclerosis, and we have to take this into account in our day-to-day clinical practice.

Conclusions

With our present knowledge we can make recommendations for a prudent diet for our affluent societies (Lewis 1978) while we wait for corroborating results of the ongoing long-term studies dealing with primary or secondary prevention. I believe dietary goals such as the ones defined by the McGovern Committee of the United States Senate can be achieved and should lead to a successful fight against heart attacks and stroke. The achieved decline in death rates may be the result of several processes. Our risk factor hypothesis compels us to work on each risk factor individually. Our research has to be intensified to work on the roles played by our soft data concerning atherogenicity: stress, sedentary life styles, psychological and psychosomatic aspects. We have to pay attention not only to groups posing obvious high risks but also the "no-risk" groups who come down with coronary events and strokes. Medicine was and is practical science. Almost all our success in therapy is derived from the empirical approach. Why should this be different for prophylaxis and rehabilitative measures? The school children in Eberbach-Wiesloch designed an emblem which, I think, could serve as a protective appeal: the sun, in the form of a shield, wards off the rain (risk factors) to ultimately provide for a better life.

Diseases of the heart and blood vessels have assumed the characteristics of an epidemic; therefore, they are also a vital political issue. The eminent pathologist Rudolf Virchow, who published the first comprehensive concept of atherosclerosis, made a proclamation over a century ago: "Epidemics are like important warning signs which a good statesman would interpret as a disturbance in the state of his nation, which even the most carefree policy-maker could not ignore."

References

Augustin J, Pohl J, Schiele A, Geeren U, Greten H (1979) Influence of smoking on lipoprotein metabolism. J Clin Invest 9:2
Goldstein JL, Dana SE, Brown MS (1974) Esterification of low density lipoprotein cholesterol in human fibroblasts and its absence in homozygous familial hypercholesterolemia. Proc Natl Acad Sci USA 71:4288
Greten H, Raetzer H, Stiehl A, Schettler G (1979) The effect of polyunsaturated phosphatidylcholine on plasma lipids and fecal sterol excretion. Atherosclerosis, in press
Lewis B (1978) Hypothesis into theory - The development of aetiological concepts of ischaemic heart disease: A review. J Royal Soc Med 71:809-818
Nüssel E, Buchholz L, Bergdolt H, Ebschner H-J, Kurz E (1979) Übergewicht und risikofaktoren bei 30 bis 60 jährigen Männern und Frauen. Lab Med 3:111 116
Schellenberg B (1979) Erfassung des alkoholkonsums. Ergebnisse der "Heidelberger Männer Studie." In: Auerswald W, Brandstetter B, Gergely S (ed) Probleme um Ernährungserhebungen. Maudrich Verlag, Wien, pp 185-194
Schettler G (1978) Die atiologie der arteriosklerose. Internist 19:611-620
Truswell AS (1978) Effect of different types of dietary fibre on plasma lipids. In: Heaton KW (ed) Dietary Fibre. Newman Publishing Ltd, London, pp 105-112

Evaluation of the Evidence Relating National Dietary Patterns to Disease

E. H. Ahrens, Jr.

In 1978 the American Society for Clinical Nutrition, through the action of its then-president, Dr. Jules Hirsch, and its Council, formed a working group to examine the nature and the strengths of the scientific evidence relating the patterns of our national diet to the genesis of disease. It was mandated that recommendations not be made by this group, but that it confine its attention strictly to the evidence.

The group was chaired by Dr. William E. Connor of the University of Oregon Health Sciences Center and myself. It met on several occasions, and after due consideration of a series of detailed reviews prepared by the committee members, it reached a series of six Consensus Statements that were presented at a Symposium arranged by the Society in Washington, D.C., on May 5, 1979. The six Statements will be published as a supplement to the American Journal of Clinical Nutrition in November 1979, along with an Introduction explaining the aims of the committee and the procedure it followed. In addition, this Introduction presents an evaluation by the committee members of their individual enthusiasms for the consensus statements; this was undertaken as a demonstration of the homogeneity of opinion on each issue (or lack of it) by a group of nine experts who had spent a year reviewing the available evidence.

In addition to Drs. Hirsch, Connor and myself, the working group consisted of Drs. Henry C. McGill, Jr., who prepared the detailed review on cholesterol, Charles J. Glueck (fat), Edwin L. Bierman (carbohydrate), Theodore B. Van Itallie (calories), Norton Spritz (alcohol), and Louis Tobian, Jr. (sodium). These six panelists were advised, in turn, by some 24 outside experts judged to represent the various viewpoints most widely held on the six dietary issues today.

The substance of the Consensus Statements will be presented at this Symposium, along with a discussion of the possible merits of the self-evaluation system referred to above. The six Statements were intentionally not referenced; however, the fully referenced reviews on which the Consensus Statements were based will also be published in full in November 1979 by the American Journal of Clinical Nutrition.

Diet-Lipid-Atherosclerosis Relationship: Epidemiological Evidence and Public Health Implications

Henry Blackburn

The epidemiological evidence about diet, blood lipid levels and atherosclerosis involves population comparisons as well as information on individual risk within populations, and includes their changes over time.

The Seven Countries Study provides contrasts of dietary composition and energy expenditure among men of stable rural, farming, logging and fishing populations having similar socio-economic status (Keys 1970). Data were collected with great attention to adequate sample size, use of standardized measurements, training and quality control, with central and standard chemical analyses of blood lipids and of foods eaten, and central quantitative data analysis. Chemical analysis of the diet was performed on lyophilized specimens shipped from the field, prepared from locally purchased food, in precise quantities as recorded by trained dieticians living in randomly selected households of each geographic area. Diets were measured seasonally in families during one week. Figure 1 shows the large contrast between populations in the fatty acid composition of diet so measured in the late 1950's and the 1960's. The variation is great for the proportion of daily calories as saturated and monounsaturated fat. Dietary cholesterol was not measured. These "natural experiments" include extremely low total fat in Japan, relatively high fat in Greece but of a very different composition than in Northern Europe. In Figure 2a and b the dietary relationships with population levels of total serum cholesterol (TC), and with CHD, are studied across a wide range of saturated fat calories (3 to 22%). Deviations are not great in the linear solution of the relationship of saturated fat calories to average population TC levels of 14 areas depicted in Figure 2a.

In Figure 3 is the correlation between TC median values and the coronary disease rates. Eastern Finland deviates on the high side of the prediction, despite its having the highest average TC level of all the Seven Countries areas. In contrast, West Finland and the Greek Island of Crete are on the low side of the expectation for 16 areas.

Table 1 provides the detailed distributions of TC, ranked by descending order of median TC value, along with 10-year coronary disease and total death rates for Seven Countries populations (Keys 1979). Here a generally unfavorable experience of the northern European countries and the United States is contrasted to the better experience in the Mediterranean Basin and Japan. Again, there is the remarkable absence of clinical atherosclerotic manifestations on the island Crete where the 10-year rate of dying from any cause, among men initially ages 40-59, is only one half to a third that of some areas. All except one of the very low CHD incidence areas, Crete (having CHD deaths from 0.5 to 1.5 per thousand per year) had median TC values under 200 mg/dl. All high incidence areas (having 3-7 cases per 1000 men per year) had TC medians greater than 235 mg/dl. Areas in the intermediate range of average population TC levels show wide variation in CHD rates. All diet analyses are chemical measurements of major nutrients. However, there are differences between Northern Europe, the United States and the other populations in the actual foodstuffs consumed, including simple sugars, complex carbohydrates, dietary fiber, vegetable protein and alcohol.

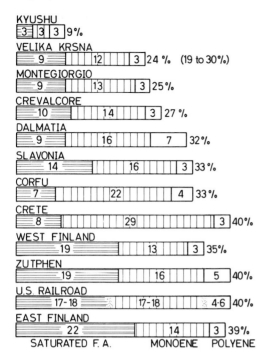

FIG. 1. Average percent calories from fats in men 40-59 years old.

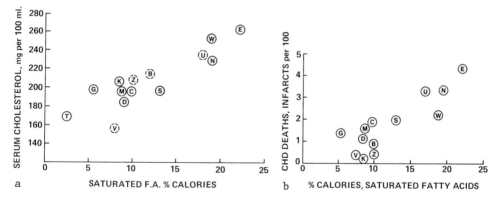

FIG. 2a and b. B = Belgrade Faculty, C = Crevalcore, D = Dalmatia, E = East Finland, G = Corfu, K = Crete, N = Zutphen, M = Montegiorgio, S = Slavonia, U = U.S. Railroad, V = Velika Krsna, W = West Finland, Z = Zrenjanin.

Relevant diet-lipid-atherosclerosis correlations in the Seven Countries data among 14 geographic areas are as follows: TC level is strongly related to CHD deaths and nonfatal infarction, with an r value of 0.76, percent calories from total fats was less strong, r = 0.40, percent calories as saturated fats is the strongest correlate to disease rates, r = 0.84; percent calories as proteins, r = 0.14. Total calories consumed per kg body weight is not correlated to serum cholesterol, r = -0.07, and physical activity calories/kg burned daily is highly negatively correlated with skin-fold obesity, r = -0.75. Thus, with a few interesting departures from prediction, the Seven Countries evidence is consistent. The "dose-effect" relationship of diet and lipids to CHD also supports the diet-lipid-atherosclerosis theory. In sum, to the extent that the study was designed and conducted to characterize diet,

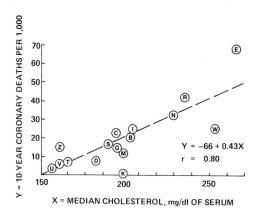

FIG. 3. Median total cholesterol level is related to CHD incidence in men aged 40 to 59 followed 10 years.

Table 1. Seven countries study total serum cholesterol and 10-year CHD incidence - men 40-59

Population	% Sat. fat	TC CENTILE mg/dl			Rates/10,000/10 yrs.		
		5	50	95	CHD deaths	Any CHD	All deaths
E. Finland	22	182	265	356	681	2868	1511
W. Finland	19	184	253	338	251	1582	1270
U.S. Railway	18	173	236	318	416	--	861
Holland	19	169	230	317	317	1066	1134
Crete	8	151	206	279	0	210	627
S. Italy	9	150	198	274	125	966	1007
Corfu	7	141	198	283	149	686	847
W. Yugoslavia	9	128	186	259	74	629	775
T. Japan	3	106	171	304	71	354	1052
Serbia	9	115	156	217	71	452	1136
U. Japan	3	96	141	194	50	458	1349

TC and disease rates across a wide range of each, it confirms the "diet-heart hypothesis."

The baseline TC distributions in the Seven Countries cohorts of Table 1 also provide models for the tentative construction of "existing, feasible and ideal" population TC distribution curves (Figure 4a and b). The curves are thought reasonable and safe because the population data are so congruent with clinical and laboratory evidence and other independent estimates of "ideal" lipid levels. The projected "ideal" TC distributions center around 160 mg/dl as for Velika Krsna, Ushibuka and Tanushimaru and are associated with the lowest CHD rates. "Desirable-feasible" TC curves center around 190 mg/dl as in the Greek Islands and Adriatic coast of Italy and Yugoslavia. These levels are associated with wide variation in CHD rates but which are generally less than half of U.S. and Northern European rates. "Existing" TC curves of adults in the U.S. now center around 215 mg/dl and represent recently measured population samples. It will be recalled that U.S. samples in the 50's and 60's gave TC means around 235 and in Finland and other Northern European countries means were, and still are, around 265 mg/dl for middle-aged adults (Blackburn 1979b).

The U.S.P.H.S. International Study of the relationship of diet, serum lipid levels, and coronary disease rates has made comparisons similar to Seven

Table 2. Japanese emigrant studies

Variable	Japan	Hawaii	California
Relative weight (%)	109	122	126
Calorie intake/wt	40	37	35
Sat. fat % cal.	7	23	26
CHO % cal.	63	46	44
Alcohol % cal.	9	4	3
T. S. cholesterol (mg.dl)	181	218	228
TSC > 260 (%)	3	12	16
S. triglycerides (mg/dl)	134	240	234
CHD deaths/1000	1.3	2.2	3.7

Countries. The Framingham Heart Study, the Honolulu Heart Program and the Puerto Rico Heart Health Project were compared using standardized laboratory and clinical assessments. However, these populations differ widely in socio-economic status and otherwise. Framingham rates of CHD are higher than expectation based on their blood lipids or their combined baseline risk characteristics. Though the comparative data are compatible with a contribution of habitual diet to average population blood lipid levels and to CHD rates, they suggest the absence of a direct effect of serum triglycerides on CHD incidence (Gordon et al. 1974).

The Ni-Hon-San Study provides comparisons based on acculturation of Japanese immigrants from the mainland to Hawaii and California (Marmot et al. 1975). This study is the major present source of epidemiological evidence in which there is a semblance of control for genetic factors. Table 2 summarizes these findings. The acculturation in diet was reported least in elderly mainland Japanese, and most in the California and Hawaiian Japanese. The immigrant populations are seen to take in fewer calories per kg, presumably because they are less active, but to consume substantially more protein, animal protein, fat, saturated fat, dietary cholesterol, and simple carbohydrates while they drink less alcohol than the mainland Japanese. Mean values for TC go up according to the degree of eastward migration and Western acculturation, as

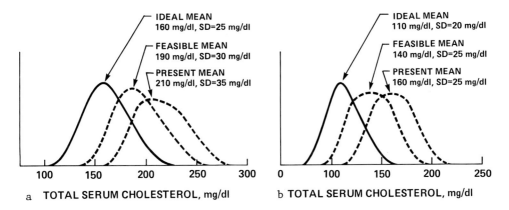

FIG. 4a and b. "Ideal, feasible and existing" total serum cholesterol levels in (a) adults and (b) youth (ages 5-18).

does the frequency of elevated TC and mean levels of triglycerides. There are likely many other aspects of acculturation than diet and activity in these populations, but the data on diet, lipids, and CHD incidence are compatible with a strong dietary and acculturation effect on populations of probable similar genetic composition.

A population's capacity to develop hyperlipidemia as a mass response to habitual differences in diet is thus proposed to be large. Apparently the exhibition of a maximal number of "supermarket" phenotypes among susceptible genotypes is encouraged by mass exposure to high fat diets and caloric abundance.

But there are other types of populations of interest in testing the diet-heart relationship. Truswell has divided humans into four nutritional groups: the hunter-gatherer, the peasant-farming-pastoralist, the urban ghetto dweller, and affluent man. In the Seven Countries, the Minnesota LPH has studied the rural farmer and the affluent man. Primitive populations may provide other important evidence of the relationship between diet and serum lipid levels, but only anecdotal observations exist about their atherosclerosis. For example, the general experience of pathological observations in primitive populations is that they appear to have the same distribution of fatty steaks in younger years, along with moderate amounts of aortic atherosclerosis as adults, but very little coronary atherosclerosis at any age. There is extensive evidence that diets of hunter-gatherers in Africa, Central America and Australia are relatively low in animal foods, extremely low in animal fat because of the composition of wild game, very high in plant protein, complex carbohydrates and fiber, low in simple sugars and salt and, overall, are highly varied. Such diets are consistently associated with remarkably low values for TC, from means of less than 100 to 140 mg/dl and with seasonal differences related to the abundance of calories and weight change. Data on urban construction workers in East Africa also indicate how low TC levels may be in otherwise healthy, active people with average TC levels of 104 mg%. The relevance of anthropological and rural epidemiological studies to the predicament of modern, urban affluent humans may be generally questioned. However, modern man is still a "hunter-gatherer" in respect to major evolutionary metabolic adaptations. The 100,000 or more generations prior to agriculture and civilization were more influential in physical evolution than the mere 500 generations since. The food available and the physical activity patterns required to obtain food during major phases of human development were probably central to physiological adaptations and survival. Thus, while we may be unwilling to return voluntarily to subsistence economies, insights may be gained into the modern maladaptations of hyperlipidemia, hypertension, hyperinsulinemia, obesity, diabetes, and hyperuricemia by study of hunter-gatherers. The evidence suggests they are, compared to affluent man, lean and active, with a more varied diet than agricultural groups, low in blood pressure and blood lipids, with little apparent atherosclerosis and with the capacity for longevity of modern affluent humans (Blackburn 1979b).

How about vegetarians in "high incident" cultures? Studies among Seventh Day Adventists in the United States and New Zealand provide evidence that lipid levels and CHD incidence vary according to classification by diet habits as nonvegetarians, lacto-ovo-vegetarian, and pure vegetarian. Compared to age-matched Californians, non-vegetarian SDA men, aged 35 and over, have CHD mortality rates 44% lower than the general population, the lacto-ovo group 57% lower, and the pure vegetarian group 77% lower. Though these people have pervasive differences in lifestyle other than eating habits, the other factors measured appeared to account for little of the variation in mortality (West and Hayes 1968).

How important are the lipoprotein fractions in population differences? Epidemiological data suggest strongly that average TC values and LDL (or beta-lipoprotein) correlate more strongly with diet and CHD findings in populations

224

Table 3. Population comparisons of serum cholesterol fractions (mg/dl)

	TC	LDL	VLDL	HDL
Norway	250	–	–	51
Maoris	188	122	15	51
New Zealand	176	115	12	49
Koreans	168	–	–	46
Iowa youth	163	103	8	50
Japan	–	120	–	40
Bogaloosa youth	139	–	–	50
U.S. vegetarians	126	73	12	43
Tarahumara adults	134	87	22	25
Tarahumara youth	118	75	20	23
Ethiopian workers	104	48	16	32
Honolulu Japanese	–	183	–	40
Los Angeles Japanese	–	213	–	35

than does HDL or alpha-lipoprotein level (Blackburn 1979b). Table 3 is an attempt to summarize interesting discrepancies between total and HDL cholesterol levels in populations. Generally, HDL values are higher in affluent Western cultures where LDL and TC are also higher, but usually, also, the HDL/TC ratio is lower. One fascinating "natural experiment" departs substantially from this rule. Tarahumara Indians, who have among the lowest TC and LDL values yet measured in adults and youth, also have among the lowest HDL values reported and low HDL/TC ratios (Connor et al. 1978). The Tarahumara are almost entirely vegetarian and are among the more active ethnic groups on earth. Also, they are lean and consume considerable amounts of alcohol as fermented corn beer. They do not smoke heavily. All these characteristics would be associated, in western affluent societies, with higher values of HDL and lower HDL/TC ratios than those found in these Indians. So, the issue of "protective" levels of lipoproteins and their ratios is not yet clear. The data suggest that, generally, LDL and TC follow the population diet and CHD rates more closely than HDL. They may also be more responsive to change than is HDL but data about the effect of dietary composition on HDL cholesterol is still meager. VLDL is assumed to have only an intermediate role. All this evidence of cross-cultural difference is highly important to the public health view and focus on population LDL and TC levels as predictive of the mass diet-hyperlipidemia-atherosclerosis problem. It does not mitigate the clinical predictive value of HDL, for older individuals, living in high CHD incident cultures.

Experimental diets provide other major evidence concerning the relationship between diet and blood cholesterol and lipid fractions. They show mathematically predictable relationships between dietary change and group change in TC levels. They provide classic examples of defining a relationship by a predictive equation, tested for efficiency in populations different from those in which developed. The derivations are nearly identical by independent investigators in four separate laboratories, resulting in equations widely known in "lipid circles" as the Keys, Hegsted, Mattson, and Connor equations relating dietary lipids to blood lipids, as illustrated by the Keys equation:

$$\Delta \text{ CHOL.} = 1.35 \ (2\Delta S - \Delta P) + 1.52 \ \Delta Z$$

Where Δ CHOL. = estimated change in serum cholesterol in mg/dl; ΔS = change in percent daily calories from saturated fat; ΔP = change in percent daily calories from polyunsaturated fat; ΔZ = change in the square root of daily dietary cholesterol in mg/1000 kcal.

Work is needed to establish prediction equations involving not only other components of diet than fatty acids and cholesterol, but their effects on lipoprotein fraction cholesterol levels. Whether the equations will be greatly improved upon depends on the incompletely known HDL response to diet, the proportion of LDL and TC changes obtainable by dietary manipulation, and the likelihood of significant effects of other diet factors, in the range of usual affluent diets. It is possible that the contribution to TC change of vegetable protein, fiber and complex carbohydrates may give relatively small coefficients of partial correlation in the presence of the major contributions of dietary fatty acids and cholesterol. The individual and population importance of other dietary components is not denied. Dietary fat composition fails to explain all of the variation in population levels of TC or CHD. It is not clear whether the unexplained TC differences have to do with the early age of onset of a given diet pattern and the duration of that pattern, or of the usually encountered association of low saturated fat diets with high vegetable protein, complex carbohydrate and fiber diets and absence of excess calories. Alternatively, the relatively greater energy expenditure of most rural populations studied may be involved. These are important areas for detailed research not now being adequately studied (or approved, or funded!).

Why are zero correlations found between individually measured diet intake and serum lipid level in U.S. studies? Does this negate the importance of the diet-lipid-atherosclerosis relationship? Powerful links in the chain of epidemiological evidence are correlations between a personal characteristic and subsequent disease, and between personal behavior and level of the characteristic. In all reported North American studies, the relationship between measured individual diet and TC levels is near zero. This has been interpreted by a few to negate the "diet-heart theory". Such an interpretation is probably in error and surely misleading because a) dietary intake varies, along with its measurement and that of blood lipid levels. Intra-individual variation in diet is about equal to the variation between individuals in the U.S. Under these circumstances, even several measurements of diet and blood lipids would be unlikely to demonstrate a true relationship if it existed. The solution to this problem includes the development of diet methods which reduce technical sources of variability to a minimum and which more accurately characterize current individual eating patterns. This might be obtained by experimentally controlling that pattern, by chemical diet analysis, and by other more reliable, precise and representative measures of individual diet. The usual 24-hour dietary recall meets none of these criteria, nor do 3-day or 7-day diaries. It is likely that a dozen such measurements is required to improve individual diet characterization (Liu et al. 1978); b) there is an insufficient range of the variables correlated. The range of dietary fat intake or fatty acid composition of the diet in U.S. population studies of the 1950's and 60's, in which these zero correlations with TC were derived, is small. Diets in these affluent, volunteer participants were characterized by homogeneity in an excess of calories and fat. The solution for this problem might be 1) to seek cultures and populations in which there is a much wider range, or 2) to specifically select subgroups in the U.S. population to represent a physiologic range in intake from, say, total vegetarianism and fat intake of less than 10% of total calories, up to 40 and 50% levels. Under the first condition, significant correlations of individual diet intake and serum cholesterol levels have been demonstrated in Italy, among the Tarahumara Indians and among Seventh Day Adventists in New Zealand and the United States, where differences in TC levels are related to pure vegetarian, lacto-ovo-vegetarian, and nonvegetarian eating practices. The following factors, then, "guarantee" the near zero correlation found between individual blood lipid levels and diet in the U.S.: high individual variability due to technical and biological sources; poor reliability and validity of the instrument

Table 4. Serum cholesterol. Standardized incidence ratio, risk ratio V/(I+II) number of men, person years of experience, and number of first events by quintile of level: pool 5 and individual studies.

Quintile and level (mg/dl)		Study group								
		Pool 5	ALB	CH-GAS	CH-WE	FRAM	TECUM	LA	MI-EX	MI-RR
All	All	100	100	100	100	100	100	100	100	100
		Standardized incidence ratio:								
I + II	<218	66	70	79	60	62	49	(42)	70	49
I	<194	72	72	100	62	74	(10)	(37)	(64)	(47)
II	194–218	61	67	61	57	50	(83)	(46)	(78)	50
III	218–240	78	72	89	70	88	(56)	116	(117)	77
IV	240–268	129	129	124	99	160	145	73	(117)	96
V	>268	150	177	118	159	167	242	143	(189)	194
Risk ratio: V/(I+II)		2.4	2.5	1.5	2.7	2.7	4.9	( )	( )	4.0
95% confidence interval:	low	1.9	1.7	0.9	1.7	1.7	2.0	( )	( )	3.4
	high	2.9	3.8	2.4	4.6	4.0	13.1	( )	( )	7.6
Number of men at risk		8,274	1,765	1,264	1,980	2,130	1,135	1,104	283	2,551
Person years of experience		70,781	16,878	11,064	16,505	19,480	6,854	10,137	4,008	12,484
Number of first events		647	156	123	142	177	49	72	28	112

( ) Based on fewer than 10 first events.

to characterize a person's diet; the homogeneity of the U.S. diet in respect to lipid-raising characteristics.

Blood cholesterol levels are strongly correlated with individual CHD risk. Pooling Project data are among the more relevant and representative sources of epidemiological evidence from the United States, or from any high CHD incidence population, about personal levels of TC in relation to subsequent risk of a coronary event (Pooling Res. Grp. 1978). In all eight U.S. studies shown in Table 4 there is greater CHD risk for higher levels of TC. Risk ratios between the top quintile and lower two quintiles vary from 1.5 to 4.9, averaging 2.4. When quintiles 1 and 2 are combined, the risk increases uniformly and smoothly with TC level, and the findings are consistent with a <u>continuous</u> relationship between TC level and CHD risk. But it is also noted that there is no statistically significant difference in the rates of CHD events between the first three quintiles of TC values and a slight but insignificantly greater number of events occur in the lowest quintile in 4 of 5 studies.

In Figure 5, across all areas and TC levels in the Seven Countries Study, the individual risk of CHD death rises from TC levels of 160 mg/dl upward, over a wide range of age-adjusted values and different populations. These data are also consistent with an assumption of a continuous increase in risk with TC level. Israeli and Honolulu studies show low rates overall for CHD deaths. Their mean TC value and CHD rate correspond rather closely to those of Mediterranean cohorts of the Seven Countries Study. Together, they illustrate TC distributions approaching those considered here as "desirable" in respect to CHD risk and "feasible" in regard to palatable, nutritious eating patterns.

HDL cholesterol is also strongly associated with individual CHD risk, based on evidence from clinical, experimental and population studies. Epidemiological studies show that the future individual risk of coronary disease in middle-aged and older men and women in high risk societies is significantly lower the greater the level of HDL cholesterol (HDL-C) (Gordon et al. 1977). They all find little correlation between individual HDL-C values and those

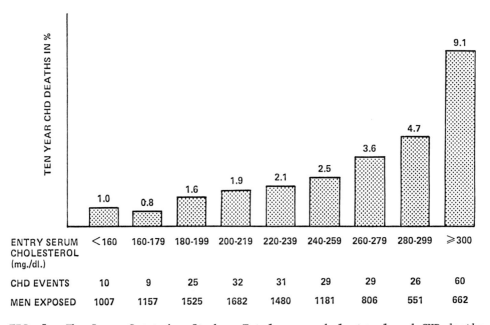

FIG. 5. The Seven Countries Study. Total serum cholesterol and CHD deaths.

for LDL-C or TC. Individual CHD risk prediction is improved by use of the ratio of HDL-C to either TC or LDL-C. These data are compatible with experimental evidence but not with population comparisons, as shown in Table 3.

Change in CHD incidence, diet and blood lipid levels is another indirect but important epidemiological source of evidence bearing on optimal lipid levels for populations and on the diet-lipid-atherosclerosis relationship. Cultural differences and results of changes in these measures may provide a rational basis for diet and lipid recommendations in preventive action and public policy when they are confirmatory of other findings, and when they converge with evidence from clinical and experimental disciplines. When all is congruent, the whole is a powerful confirmation of the hypothesis. It thus establishes a working theory without the largely unobtainable "definitive answer", "experimental proof" or "ultimate truth."

Epidemiological data on change come from government data on diet and on Vital Statistics on Causes of Death, from sample surveys showing "spontaneous" time trends in diet, lipid levels and disease rates, from "natural experiments" such as wars and immigration, and from man-made experiments such as large preventive trials.

These countries appear to have experienced an increase in CHD deaths reported in their Vital Statistics between 1968 and 1976:

Sweden	Poland	Bulgaria	Republic of Ireland
Denmark	Yugoslavia	Hungary	Northern Ireland
France	Romania		

These have experienced no apparent change:

Czechoslovakia	Netherlands	Switzerland
New Zealand	F. R. Germany	Austria
Italy		

These countries have apparently experienced a significant decrease in annual reported CHD mortality rates for the period:

United States	Finland	Israel (males)
Canada	United Kingdom	Japan
Australia	Belgium	Norway

The decreasing U.S. cardiovascular mortality trend graphed in Figure 6 is established for every age group, sex, race, and type of cardiovascular event (Havlik and Feinleib 1979). Thus, there appears to be no group impermeable to preventive influences, whatever they may be. Some of these trends are uncertain, and in no case are representative data available on national CHD incidence or on case-fatality rate. Nevertheless, some evidence exists that risk factor and risk behavior changes may precede or accompany the changes in CHD mortality.

The epidemiological evidence about change in population TC distributions derives from several sources: different populations examined at intervals, from true national samples taken at intervals, and from population cohorts followed over time. HES and HANES studies in the U.S. are national probability samples while Lipid Research Center data are from representative local samples (Blackburn 1979b). Age-adjustment of their data results in the suggestion that a 2 to 6 mg/dl or 1 to 3 percent difference exists in representative U.S. groups measured at two different times. But methodologic questions render it uncertain whether the difference is real. TC trends in cohorts followed in the Tecumseh Community Study, in Framingham and Minnesota, and in Framingham children, suggest a 10 to 20 mg/dl (5-10%) lowering over

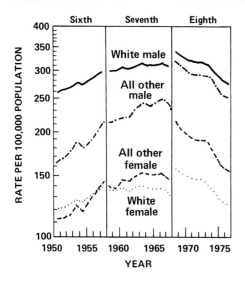

FIG. 6. Age-adjusted death rates for ischemic heart disease by color and sex: United States, 1950-76.

the last 10-15 years, perhaps preceding the same inflection in national CHD mortality data. In contrast, a significant 10 year increase from, roughly, 1960 to 1970, occured in average TC in the Seven Countries Study. The mean increase from 1,939 Northern European men was 6.9 mg/dl and among 3,928 Southern European was 28.4 mg/dl (Keys 1979). The Northern European findings are compatible with the known age TC trend between 50 and 60 years in the West and with no major environmental change. In contrast, the highly significant change in Southern Europeans is compatible with a documented rapid change in their lifestyle and economy. Thus, population surveys, having little or no intervention on health practice, indicate that mean values and distributions of TC can, and do change among entire populations and that the change has been in the same direction as CHD death rates, downward.

Change in TC as a result of experimental changes in diet is "mathematically" established for small groups under metabolic ward conditions and for large numbers in the mass preventive trials of Diet-Heart, LRC and MRFIT and is well documented elsewhere.

The observed population TC lowering corresponds well to predicted experience, based on the Keys equation applied to reported national food consumption data (Stamler 1979). Stamler applies a multivariate model of the change predicted in CHD mortality from observed risk factor changes. A substantial part of the predicted CHD mortality change is "accounted for" by the decrease in mean TC.

The interaction of genetic and environmental factors in lipid regulation is among the more difficult and controversial issues in the diet-heart matter (Blackburn 1979a). A simplistic model is given here for pedagogical purposes of the relative importance to the individual of genetic factors in Table 5 and in Table 6 for the relative importance to population differences of environmental factors. These models can help clarify the matter and reduce controversy even if they are imprecise. In Table 5 it is suggested that a hypothetical individual having "ideal" heredity in respect to cholesterol level in childhood, who is exposed to maximally cholesterol-elevating diets during life and who responds in the predicted way, might end up with an adult average TC of 175 mg%, thus below average for the U.S. population. Similarly, individuals who inherit the major gene defect of hypercholesteremia may eat the world's best (non-cholesterol raising) diet for a lifetime and yet have

Table 5. A model of individual diet-serum cholesterol relations, with individual examples

Minimum genetic value (mg/dl)	Mean diet effect (mg/dl)				
	0	+25	+50	+75	+100
75	75	100	125	150	175
150	150	175	200	225	250
300	300	325	350	375	400

Table 6. A model of population diet-serum cholesterol relationships with population examples

	Mean diet-cholesterol effect (mg/dl)				
	Japan	Greece	Italy	U.S.	Finland
	0	+25	+50	+75	+100
Population mean	150	175	200	225	250
Lower limit (2.5%)	75	100	125	150	175
Upper limit (97.5%)	225	250	275	300	325

an adult blood cholesterol level in the upper 1% of the population. This slide demonstrates why individuals on the same diet may have different cholesterol levels or why individuals with the same cholesterol level may have different diets, due to their instrinsic cholesterol regulation and response. It emphasizes the important effect of inherent lipid regulatory factors in determining the individual mean TC level. In contrast, Table 6 makes the assumption that there are no "magnitude" differences between large heterogeneous populations (such as North America, Europe and Asia) in the distribution of the many genes which affect regulation of blood lipids. This assumption may well be challenged. However, under these conditions, the habitual diet of the whole population influences the number of hyperlipidemias exhibited, and in addition determines, in effect, the population TC mean and distribution. This model emphasizes therefore the overriding importance to population differences of environmental, cultural, behavioral and dietary factors. These latter are the factors which are the major concern of the public health, i.e., the determinants of mass phenomena, mass disease, and of the potential for primary prevention.

In respect to the nature of this epidemiological evidence, medical science tends to accept as "proof" only the combinations of observation and experiment which fulfill Koch's postulates or other experimental models of causation. They partially ignore the history of causal inference, the development of sound and durable theories, for example, in the sciences of evolution, mathematics, astronomy and gravity, geology and archeology, and other disciplines which rely almost entirely on observation, induction and inference rather than on experiment. True, epidemiological associations in themselves provide only clues and suggestions. However, when congruent with clinical and experimental evidence, they provide powerful tests of causal hypotheses. The popular derogation of evidence as "only epidemiological and statistical" is naive. It misses the profound significance of a discipline which seeks causes and provides useful bases of decision-making in preventive practice and in the public health. It may, therefore, be worthwhile to summarize the guidelines that distinguished scientists have come to use to arrive at causal inference from statistical associations found in epidemiological studies. The logic is sound, and causal inference reasonable, when such findings and associations have the following characteristics:

Strength. The 20-fold excess in risk of lung cancer in 40 year old individuals who smoke 2 packages of cigarettes a day, compared to age-matched non-smokers, suggests a direct causal effect. The significant but only 2 to 3 fold difference in death rates between divorced and married persons, for example, is both less strong and less specific; thus inference of cause is not made without other evidence.

Graded Relationships. If the data show a significant graded increase in risk according to the duration, frequency or intensity of the exposure, the inference of cause is abetted, without eliminating the possibility of curvilinear or more complex relationships.

Temporal Sequence. The measure of a characteristic in health and its association with the subsequent development of a manifestation or disease carries greater strength in causal inference than cross-sectional associations, or measurements made after the event.

Prediction. Causal inference is strengthened when the prediction derived from one body of data, applied to an independent population, successfully discriminates individual cases.

Independence. Causal inference is strengthened when the contribution of a given risk factor to the prediction of events is found, by analytical groupings and statistical adjustments, to be independent of any significant association it has with other characteristics of risk.

Consistency. Causal inference is strengthened by the similarity of observations from different populations and cultures, by different investigators, using systems having different techniques and measurement errors. Inconsistencies in relationships may lead to very important new clues of causation without negating a theory which is based on the preponderance of evidence.

Congruence. If what is found in clinical observations and at the pathological table is consistent with what can be produced under laboratory experimental conditions, and these findings, in turn, are congruent with results of hypothesis testing in epidemiological studies, the whole adds up to a strong inference of causation. A part of causal inference is thus based on the existence of phenomena and mechanisms, which may or may not be completely elucidated, but which are logical and rational and congruent.

These guidelines, useful in evaluating the statistical associations found in population studies, are encouraged to be used to examine the epidemiological evidence linking diet, blood lipids, other risk factors and mass atherosclerosis. The inference of cause here is strong because of congruent evidence from all disciplines. The implications are clear for desirable, safe and feasible preventive measures and public policy on the atherosclerotic diseases.

Finally, the excellent strategy proposed and being carried out at the Rockefeller and elsewhere is highly appropriate to the clinical treatment of the monogenic hyperlipidemias and of the small proportion of the population having the severest polygenic types. These are extremely important clinical issues, but major areas of evidence about the diet-lipid-atherosclerosis relationship, and the public health action implied, require attention. "Defini-

232

tive proof of benefit and safety" of therapy in clinical hyperlipidemic patients is not directly relevant to the remarkable <u>population</u> differences in
distributions of blood lipid levels, or in the habitual diets which are the
principal influence on these population differences. Diet is uninvolved in the
rare expression of monogenic types. It may be more involved in the frequency
and the degree of exhibition of the polygenic types. But habitual diet of a
population largely determines the wide variation in population means and distributions of lipid levels which are, in turn, accompanied by widely varying
rates of atherosclerotic disease. This evidence, widely recognized and accepted in the scientific community, is congruent with clinical and experimental findings on the causes of atherosclerosis. These "natural experiments"
are important criteria confirming the "acceptability, adherance and safety"
of wide differences in natural diets.

Actually, substantial changes are now occuring in the eating pattern of many
cultures; these changes appear to have an effect on the population means and
distributions of blood lipid levels. Another change of similar magnitude
(about 5%) in the means and resulting distributions of total or LDL cholesterol levels would put the U.S. adult population values in the range of those
cultures now having half the disease rates of ours.

References

Blackburn H (1979a) Diet and mass hyperlipidemia: a public health view. In:
    Levy R, Rifkind B, Dennis B, Ernst N (eds) Nutrition, lipids, and coro-
    nary heart disease. Raven Press, New York
Blackburn H (1979b) Workshop report: epidemiological section. Conference on
    the health effects of blood lipids: optimal distributions for popula-
    tions. Prev Med 8 no. 6
Connor WE, Cerqueira MT, Connor RW, Wallace RB, Malinow MR, Casdorph HR (1978)
    The plasma lipids, lipoproteins and diet of the Tarahumara Indians of
    Mexico. Am J Clin Nutr 31:1131-1142
Gordon T, Castelli WP, Hjortland MD, Kannel WB, Dawber TR (1977) High density
    lipoprotein as a protective factor against coronary heart disease. Am
    J Med 63:707-714
Gordon T, Garcia-Palmeri MR, Kagan A, Kannel WB, Schiffman J (1974) Differen-
    ces in coronary heart disease in Framingham, Honolulu and Puerto Rico.
    J Chronic Dis 27:329-344
Havlik RJ, Feinleib M (eds) (1979) Proceedings of the conference on the de-
    cline in coronary heart disease mortality. U.S. Dept H.E.W., NIH pub-
    lication 79-1610
Keys A (ed) (1970) Coronary heart disease in seven countries. Circulation
    41:Suppl 1
Keys A (1979) Seven countries: death and coronary heart disease in ten years.
    Harvard University Press
Liu K, Stamler J, Dyer A, McKeever J, McKeever P (1978) Statistical methods
    to assess and minimize the role of intra-individual variabiiity in ob-
    scuring the relationship between dietary lipids and serum cholesterol.
    J Chronic Dis 31:399-418
Marmot MG, Syme SL, Kagan A, Kato H, Cohen JB, Belsky J (1975) Epidemiologic
    studies of coronary heart disease and stroke in Japanese men living in
    Japan, Hawaii and California: prevalence of coronary and hypertensive
    heart disease and associated risk factors. Am J Epidemiol 102:514-525
The Pooling Project Research Group (1978) Relationship of blood pressure,
    serum cholesterol, smoking habits, relative weight and ECG abnormalities
    to incidence of major coronary events: final report of the pooling pro-
    ject. J Chronic Dis 31:201-306

Stamler J (1979) Public health aspects of optimal serum lipid-lipoprotein levels. Prev Med 8 no. 6

West RO, Hayes OB (1968) Diet and serum cholesterol levels. A comparison between vegetarians and non-vegetarians in a Seventh Day Adventist group. Am J Clin Nutr 21:853-862

Dietary Prevention of Coronary Heart Disease: The Role of Essential Fatty Acids

M.F. Oliver

To Act or Not to Act?

Anyone who writes on this subject of diet and coronary heart disease (CHD) is instantly classified as a believer or non-believer. So polarized are the views (Mann 1977; Hegsted 1978) that credit is seldom given to one who wishes to try and dissect the facts and not embrace any extreme view. It is particularly the responsibility of professional investigators to try to derive a balanced view. It is equally our responsibility to guide the media. We should not complain if the press and television distort, when we ourselves are unclear.

It is not always our fault that appraisal of the role of diet in the causation and prevention of CHD has been confused and confusing. Other forces are operating, often for entirely non-scientific reasons, to make objective appraisal even less easy. Those who lobby for and against butter and milk fats, or for and against polyunsaturated margarines, are regretably frequently less interested in determining perspective than in prosletysing their own case for financial gain.

Another factor which is influencing accurate appraisal of the situation is a classic non sequitur. This is that, because 16 out of 18 national committees have advised a reduction of saturated fat and an increase in polyunsaturated fats (F.A.O. Report), it follows that the case in favour of such advice is clear cut; but, of course, the 18 national advisory committees have all had to evaluate more or less the same evidence, and it is not surprising that they have reached rather similar conclusions. Most of the evidence is not of the quality which we are accustomed to expect from laboratory investigations or clinical studies of precision and much derives from extrapolations from epidemiological studies, many of which are soundly based and valid in their conclusions but which are, nevertheless, epidemiological pointers and no more.

An argument in favour of making major dietary changes which is heard more and more is that ideal testing of the effect of dietary change on the primary prevention of CHD is logistically so complicated and so costly that it will never be done. Therefore, the argument runs, let us take action now. This is another non-sequitur because it presumes that we know what to do and that what we decide to do has been proved to be safe. The argument derives from the wish of doctors to do good or to be seen to be doing good rather than from a dispassionate scientific assessment of how much and how little we know.

It is redundant to review the evidence of a graded positive relationship between increasing serum concentrations of cholesterol and low density lipoproteins with CHD morbidity and mortality. It is redundant also to reconsider the lipid hypothesis in any detail except to re-emphasize Ahrens' conclusions in his paper (Ahrens 1976) "The management of hyperlipidaemia: whether, rather than how" that that part of the lipid hypothesis which claims that redution of hyperlipidaemia should reduce CHD is only inferential and not based on direct evidence.

It is, however, necessary to emphasize that the three major primary prevention trials of the effectiveness of lowering raised serum cholesterol concentrations, which have been reported so far, have three findings in common: (1) no significant reduction in CHD mortality, (2) a significant reduction in non-fatal myocardial infarction morbidity, (3) a slight and not always significant increase in non-cardiovascular mortality. None of these trials---two using polyunsaturated fat diets (Dayton et al. 1969; Miettinen et al. 1972), and one using clofibrate (Report from the Commitee of Principal Investigators 1978)---achieved a striking reduction in serum cholesterol concentrations; this was, on the average, less than 10% during the duration of the trials compared with starting values. In the WHO clofibrate (Report from the Committee of Principal Investigators 1978), the reduction in non-fatal myocardial infarction was of the order expected in relation to the degree of reduction of serum cholesterol. The increased non-cardiovascular mortality in these trials needs to be taken more seriously than at present and is not yet explicable.

How to Act - Dietary Goals

The Senate Select Committee on Nutrition and Human Needs has proposed dietary goals for the United States (Dietary Goals for the United States 1977). So far as fat consumption is concerned, they amount to a reduction of 30% of energy intake from fats and modification of the composition of dietary fat to provide equal proportions of saturated, monounsaturated and polyunsaturated fatty acids. They include recommendations to reduce cholesterol consumption to 300 mg/day. These goals have been endorsed by the Council for Responsible Nutrition (1977), a trade association of food supplement manufacturers which has stated "We live in the present and cannot afford to await the ultimate proof before correcting trends we believe to be detrimental."

But the onus of proof is as much on the shoulders of the innovators as on those who take no action. Both courses could lead to detrimental results. While there is little disagreement that reduction of the total saturated fat content is desirable in most affluent countries, the extent to which an unselective increase in polyunsaturated fat content should be recommended requires much more examination. Although these U.S. goals have been broadly endorsed by 16 out of 18 national committees (reviewing the same evidence), the U.K. Committee (COMA Report, 1974) disagreed and expressly stated that they could not recommend an increase in the intake of polyunsaturated fats.

Essential Fatty Acids or Polyunsaturated Fatty Acids?

One valid proposition with regard to the decreasing CHD mortality in the U.S.A. and Australia is that it is due to the increased consumption of polyunsaturated fatty acids. It is not necessary to increase the total P/S ratio to high levels to follow the specific recommendation of the FAO Committee (FAO Report 1977) to provide one-third of fat calories from linoleic acid, particularly since polyunsaturated fatty acids might be harmful under certain circumstances. Thus, co-carcinogenecity of polyunsaturated fatty acids has been related to hydroperoxide formation and can be reduced by synthetic anti-oxidants. Trans-isomers occur with hydrogenation in some margarines and can increase EFA requirements. Some polyunsaturated fatty acids appear to be slowly metabolized. Until recently, comparatively little attention has been given to the advantages and disadvantages of some polyunsaturated fatty acids over others. Current interest in EFA and atherosclerosis derives partly because of the key role played by linoleic (Vergroesen 1977) and arachidonic acids (Moncada and Vane 1978) in prostaglandin synthesis and the consequent relationship of these essential fatty acids to prostacyclin and thromboxane A2 interaction as determinants of intravascular coagulability, and partly because of population studies of dietary EFA in relation to CHD mortality.

Many years ago, Sinclair (1956), suggested that atherosclerosis might be due to a chronic deficiency of arachidonic acid, when diets are high in saturated fat or unnatural fats and low in EFA. He asked: Are such diets encountered? If his question is extended to linoleic acid ($18:2\omega6$) which is the precursor EFA of arachidonic acid ($20:4\omega6$), then the answer would appear to be "yes." With the exception of the Eskimos, an approximate inverse relationship can be identified between the percent composition of these EFA in serum cholesteryl esters with mortality rates from CHD (Table 1). A significantly lower proportion of linoleic acid has previously been reported in the adipose tissue of two populations dying suddenly (Insull et al. 1969); it was 6% lower in Japanese dying in Tokyo than in Americans dying in Cleveland and the latter showed a much higher incidence of myocardial infarction or coronary occlusion as the cause of death. In Table 2, the ratio of $\omega6/\omega3$ fatty acids in serum cholesterol esters is shown for various populations in relation to international CHD mortality rates. The $\omega3$ acids are competitive inhibitors of the $\omega6$ acids and the ratio of triene ($20:3\omega3$) to tetraens ($20:4\omega6$) is used as a measure of EFA status. It is important to stress that the results presented in these tables have been accrued from unconnected studies made over a considerable span of years and from laboratories in which the methods of chromotagraphic analysis to fatty acids are not made to a common standard, and, therefore, the observations should only be regarded as a pointer to a putative relationship. It is interesting also to note from Table 2 that there is comparatively little variation in the total polyunsaturated fatty acid content of serum cholesterol esters in these populations and the overall P/S ratios present in various tissues may not be a sensitive method of assessing the biological importance of polyunsaturated fatty acids.

Dietary essential fatty acids

While the effects of deficiency of dietary EFA have been studied for many years in animals, their role in human atherosclerosis has been under-evaluated probably because of the considerable methodological difficulties in obtaining any accurate account of dietary fatty acid composition. Most dietary surveys involve a 24 hour recall or prospective 24 hour assessment and, while adequate for evaluation of some dietary components, these are almost valueless for appraisal of dietary fatty acids for which a 7-10 day weighed record is recommended (Marr 1973). If this can be backed up by homogenation of all food taken during this period with chromatographic analysis of fatty acid composition, an even more accurate assessment is possible. An example of the importance of such an approach is shown in Table 3, where the Scots diet (assessed from a 7 day weighed record) is different from that in England (obtained from a 24 hour recall through the National Food Survey). Thus, national returns can confuse. Even allowing for major differences in survey methods, it appears that the area of the U.K. with the highest CHD mortality has a low EFA intake. Is this also true elsewhere? The dietary analysis recently reported in the NHLBI survey (1979) of the declining CHD mortality in the U.S.A. gives no

Table 1. Distribution of polyunsaturated fatty acids (%) in serum cholesterol esters in relation to CHD mortality.

Populations	18:2	ω6 18:2+20:4	ω3 18:3+20:5+22:6	CHD Mortality
Eskimos (Greenland)[a]	20	21	17	0
Danes (Copenhagen)[a]	53	54	7	+
Swedes (Stockholm)[b]	59	65	3	++
Americans (Berkeley)[c]	55	61	3	+++
Scots (Edinburgh)	50	56	3	++++
Finns (Tampere)[d]	43	48	2	++++
Males with atherosclerosis[e]	39	41	3	+++++
Males with hyperlipidemia[e]	33	36	4	++++

[a](Dyerberg and Bang 1975).
[b](Logan et al. 1977; G Walldius, personal communication).
[c](Lindgren et al. 1961).
[d](T Nikkari, personal communication).
[e](Schrade et al. 1961).

Table 2. Polyunsaturated fatty acids in serum cholesteryl esters and CHD.

	Eskimos[a]	Danes[a]	Swedes[b]	Scots[b]	Finns[c]	M.I. patients[d]
CHD rates	0	+	++	++++	++++	
$\dfrac{\omega3^{e}}{\omega6^{f}}$	0.9	0.1	0.06	0.05	0.04	0.03
Sums of polyunsaturated fatty acids	44%	59%	68%	60%	60%	62%

[a](Dyerberg and Bang 1975).
[b](Logan et al. 1977; G Walldius, personal communication).
[c](T Nikkari, personal communication).
[d](Kirkeby et al. 1972).
[e](18:3, 20:5, 22:5, 22:6).
[f](18:2 + 20:4).

lead to permit evaluation of any relationship between dietary EFA and regional CHD mortality, although the consumption of linoleic acid has risen as a proportion of total fat (Page and Marston 1979).

Our own interest in a possible relationship between a "deficiency" of certain dietary EFA and high CHD mortality derives from two studies: the Edinburgh-Scotland Study (Logan et al. 1978), and one of regional differences in CHD mortality in the U.K. (Fulton et al. 1978).

Essential fatty acids and CHD risk

A study (Logan et al. 1978) was made in 1976 of men aged 40 selected at random from the Edinburgh and Stockholm populations in order to determine

Table 3. Analysis of dietary fat in the United Kindgom.

	England[a]	Scotland (Edinburgh)[b]
CHD Mortality/100,000 (35-44)[c]	66	95
Total fat: g/day	135	120
Saturated: g/day	61	49
Monounsat: g/day	51	43
Polyunsat: g/day	23	<12
Linoleic	20	9
Linolenic	3	1.5
Arachidonic	?	0.8
Eicosapentanoic	0.1	?

[a]National Food Survey, 1977 (24 hour recall)
[b](M Thomson, RL Logan, RA Riemersma, MF Oliver, unpublished data), 7 days weighed record.
[c]Males.

whether risk factors other than the expected ones (raised serum cholesterol, raised blood pressure and greater cigarette smoking) could explain a difference in CHD mortality, which is three times in excess in Edinburgh compared with Stockholm in men of this age. This study was conducted at the same time in each city with standardized clinical methods and with analysis of any given biochemical measurement conducted blind in one laboratory (for details, see publication). The principal findings were that the Edinburgh population had higher serum triglyceride and VLDL triglyceride concentrations, a lower precentage of serum cholesteryl linoleic acid, a lower P/S ratio in adipose tissue and a very strikingly lower percent of linoleic acid in adipose tissue (Figure 1). Other findings included similar serum cholesterol and LDL concentrations and relatively low total levels (median less than 220 mg/ml), and minor differences in HDL cholesterol. In Edinburgh, there were more men with raisd blood pressure, more cigarette smokers, higher serum uric acid level, less physical fitness as measured by bicycle ergometry and a significant shortness of stature.

Adipose tissue fatty acid composition is not influenced by recent food habits and is a good reflection, in view of the very slow turnover, of sustained dietary habits. While the recommendations of the Swedish government in 1972 that there should be an increase in polyunsaturatd fat intake may have exaggerated the difference between the two populations, the low percent of linoleic acid recorded in Edinburgh men should be considered as an absolute finding on its own.

Mortality from CHD in Scotland is more than twice that for England for both sexes and all ages (Fulton et al. 1978). The difference for men aged 45-54 can reach as much as three times between south-west Scotland and south-east Engand. While similar differences have been reported between East Finland (Karelia) and West Finland, there are more obvious differences in life-style in these two areas of Finland then between the Scots and the English in the areas under consideration. This observation, taken in conjunction with a report (Crawford and Crawford 1967) suggesting that there is no excess of coronary atheroma in Glasgow compared with London (these are the main cornubations associated with the greatest gradients of difference in CHD mortality), other pathogenic explanations need to be invoked. Assuming that the mortality data is sound---and there is every reason to believe it is---and that the conclusion from the pathological study (Crawford and Crawford 1967) is true, then two possible explanations arise. One is that Scots, particularly those living in the south-west (where the incidence is the highest in the world), there is a greater thrombogenic tendency and another is that there is a higher incidence of fatal arrhythmias.

Preliminary observations (S Renaud, personal communication) do indeed suggest that a greater thrombogenic tendency may exist, since platelet aggregation occurs more readily in Scots farmers in areas where CHD mortality is particularly high. Possibly, this may be elated to a low dietary P/S ratio but inadequate information exists, however, concerning the dietary EFA intake in the different populations under study. These observations support findings (Renaud 1979) from farmers in the Var and Moselle, where a low dietary P/S ratio was associated with increased platelet aggregation. The relation of individual EFA to CHD rates has come into focus recently with Dyerberg and Bang (1979) recommending that an increase in dietary ω-3-eicosapentaenoic acid (EPA), which might be partially substituted for ω-6-arachidonic acid in order to reduce thrombogensis. This would be easy to achieve since 10 g (two teaspoons daily) of cod liver oil contribute 1 g of EPA to the diet. Based on the remarkable record of the Eskimos (Greenland Report 1963) who rarely get CHD and have a high EPA content in their diet, this makes sense. EPA competitively inhibits the production of thromboxane A2 from platelets but what effect it has either on endothelial cell production of prostacyclin or on the platelet stimulatory effect on prostacyclin production in not clear.

The possibility of an increased CHD case fatality rate should not be dismissed too quickly and is certainly a viable alternative hypothesis, although there is not evidence yet available of differential rates for sudden cardiac death and non-sudden cardiac deaths in communities other than Japan, where sudden death is not necessarily atherosclerotic in

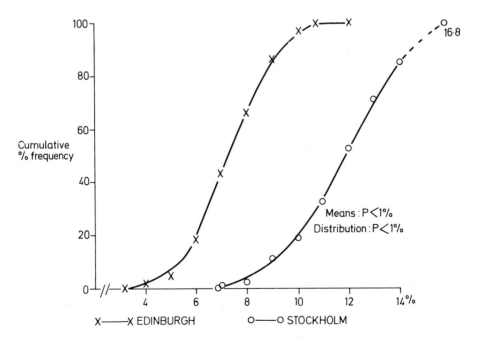

FIG. 1. Edinburgh-Stockholm Study II. Adipose tissue - C 18:2 (%).

240

origin. There is abundant evidence that a heart attack is associated with rapid elevation of plasma free fatty acids (FFA) as a result of mobilization of stored adipose triglyceride due to catecholamine stimulation and to indicate a relationship between raised serum FFA and the occurrence of lethal ventricular arrhythmias (Kurien and Oliver 1970).

Catecholamine-induced myocardial lipolysis contributes significantly, and there is much experimental data that accumulation on long-chain acyl CoA is "bad" for ischaemic myocardial metabolism, while an increase in available glucose is "good" for maintained viability of the ischaemic myocardium (Oliver 1978; Opie 1975).

However, there is practically no information to suggest that one or the other fatty acid - essential or otherwise - is more or less associated with the development of lethal ventricular arrhythmias. This is because appropriate studies have not been made. When the effects of individual fatty acids on electrophysiological parameters have been studied, it is their addition which has been investigated. In terms of the argument being developed here, it would be a deficiency of linoleic or arachidonic acid relative to other fatty acids that might be of greater interest. In respect of arrhythmogenesis analysis of phospholipid fatty acid is more relevant than analysis of adipose or cholesterol ester fatty acids, since membrane integrity and maintenance of normal gradients of ions across membranes is crucial. Less dodocosahexanoic ($22:6\omega3$) is present in serum phospholipids of patients with atherosclerosis compared with controls (Gudbjarnason et al. 1978) although Gudbjarnason found an excess of $22:6\omega3$ in the heart muscle of patients who have died from a heart attack compared with controls and argues that in some way this may not be metabolized. Significantly higher values for serum phospholipid $22:6\omega3$ have previously been reported in patients with myocardial infarction compared with controls (Kirkeby et al. 1972). Clearly, this area requires intensive investigation.

Conclusion

While the basis for recommending a reduction in total saturated fat intake is reasonably sound, that for recommending an increase in polyunsaturated fats is much less so.

Compared with the volume of research given to polyunsaturated fats as a whole, little attention has been given to the relative importance of the two main essential fatty acids families - the 6 and 3 series - in relation to CHD mortality. Arguments are advanced, mostly on epidemiological data, to suggest that deficiency of both these EFA relative to the saturated fat intake may exist in populations with a high CHD mortality: in particular, attention again is drawn to the potential importance of a low dietary linoleic acid level. A relative EFA eficiency could contribute to CHD mortality by leading to a greater thrombogenic tendency and by increasing the vulnerability of the ischaemic myocardium to lethal ventricular arrhythmias.

It is suggested that much more attention should be given to the relationship of individual EFA to the total problem of CHD mortality and that specific supplementation of the diet with linoleic and perhaps eicosapentaenoic acids might be more acceptable than a general increase in polyunsaturated fats.

References

Ahrens EH (1976) The management of hyperlipidemias: Whether rather than how. Ann Intern Med 85:87

Annual Report from the Chief Medical Officer in Greenland (1963-1967)

COMA Report, Department of Health and Social Security (1974) Diet and coronary heart disease. HMSO, London

Council for Responsible Nutrition (1977) Comm Nutr Inst 21:4

Crawford T, Crawford MD (1967) Prevalence and pathological changes in ischaemic heart disease in hard water and soft water areas. Lancet 1:229

Dayton S, Pearce ML, Hashimoto S, Dixon WJ, Tomiyasu U (1969) A controlled clinical trial of a diet high in unsaturated fat in preventing complications of atherosclerosis. Circulation 40, Suppl II, 1

Dietary Goals for the United States (1977) US Government Printing Office

Dyerberg J, Bang HO (1975) Fatty acid composition of the plasma lipids in Greenland Eskimos. Am J Clin Nutr 28:958

Dyerberg J, Bang HO (1979) Haemostatic function and platelet polyunsaturated fatty acids in Eskimos. Lancet II:433

FAO Report (1977) Dietary fats and oils

Fulton M, Adams W, Lutz W, Oliver MF (1978) Regional variations in mortality from ischaemic heart and cerebrovascular disease in Britain. Br Heart J 40:563

Gudbjarnason S, Oskarsdottir G, Doell B, Hallgrimsson J (1978) Myocardial membrane lipids in relation to cardiovascular disease. In: Proceedings of the 6th World Congress on Cardiology. Tokyo, in press

Hegsted DM (1978) Dietary goals – A progressive view. Am J Clin Nutr 31:1504

Insull W Jr, Dieter Lang P, Hsi BP, Yoshimura S (1969) Studies of atherosclerosis in Japanese and American men. I. Comparison of fatty acid composition of adipose tissue. J Clin Invest 48:1313

Kirkeby K, Ingvaldsen P, Bjerkedal I (1972) Fatty acid composition of serum lipids in men with myocardial infarction. Acata Med Scand 192:513-519

Kurien VA, Oliver MF (1970) A metabolic cause of arrhythmias during acute myocardial hypoxia. Lancet 1:813

Lindgren FT, Nichols AV, Wills RD (1961) Fatty acid distribution in serum lipids and serum lipoproteins. Am J Clin Nutr 9:13

Logan RL, Riemersma RA, Thomson M, Oliver MF, Olsson AG, Rossner S, Callmer E, Walldius G, Kaijser L, Carlson LA (1978) Risk factors in ischaemic heart disease in normal men aged 40. Lancet 1:949

Mann GV (1977) Diet-heart: End of an era. N Engl J Med 297:644

Marr JW (1973) Surveys: Aims and methods. Nutrition 27:239

Miettinen M, Karvonen MJ, Turpeinen O, Elosuo R, Paavilainen R (1972) Effect of cholesterol-lowering diet on mortality from coronary heart disease and other causes. A twelve year clinical trial in men and women. Lancet 2:835

Moncada S, Vane R (1978) Unstable metabolites of arachidonic acid and their role in haemostasis and thrombosis. Br Med Bull 34:129

Oliver MF (1978) Metabolism of the normal and ischaemic myocardium. In: Dickinson CJ, Marks J (eds) Developments in Cardiovascular Medicine. MTP, London

Opie LH (1975) Metabolism of FFA, glucose and catecholamines in acute myocardial infarction. Am J Cardiol 36:938

Page L, Marston RM, (1979) Food consumption patterns – US Diet. In: Proceedings of Conference on Decline in CHD Mortality. US Dept HEW, 236

Proceedings of the Conference on Decline in Coronary Heart Disease Mortality (1979) US Dept of HEW

Renaud S, Dumont E, Godsey F, Suplisson A, Thevenon C (1979) Platelet functions in relation to dietary fats in farmers from two regions of France. In: Biggs R (ed) Thrombosis and Haemostasis. Verlag, Stuttgart

Report from the Committee of Principal Investigators (1978) A co-operative trial in the primary prevention of ischaemic heart disease using clofibrate. Br Heart J 40:1069

Schrade W, Biegler R, Bohle E (1961) Fatty acid distribution in the lipid fractions of healthy persons of different age, patients with atherosclerosis and patients with idiopathic hyperlipidaemia. J Atheroscl Res 1:47

Sinclair HM (1956) Deficiency of essential fatty acids and atherosclerosis. Lancet 1:381

Vergroesen AJ (1977) Physiological effects of dietary linoleic acid. Nutr Rev 35:1

Identification of Children Who Are Heterozygotes for Familial Hypercholesterolaemia

Joan Slack, Michael Preece, and Peter Giles

The risks of death from coronary heart disease among heterozygotes for familial hypercholesterolaemia are well known and
are so high that attempts at prevention are usually undisputed.
The earlier diagnosis can be established the sooner treatment
can be started and the ideal must be to diagnose the heterozygous state during childhood. However, where the diagnosis
carries such a serious prognosis and treatment will be inst-
igated for life it is important that the diagnosis should be
correct. The best chance of making a correct diagnosis is
among the children of known heterozygotes in whom there is a
1 in 2 chance that they will be affected; but among these
children measurement of total serum cholesterol as well as
low density lipoprotein cholesterol segregates into two overlapping Gaussian distributions of normal and heterogous
individuals.

In the Lipid Clinic at Great Ormond Street Children's Hospital
London the intercept of the two overlapping distributions
among children of heterozygotes entering the clinic was at a
serum cholesterol level of 261 mg/100ml, and at that level
4.25 percent of the children would be misdiagnosed (Leonard
et al. 1977). The number of misdiagnoses increases rapidly as
the prior probability, or the 1 in 2 chance falls; and if
screening of the general population were contemplated, a
situation in which the prior probability is likely to be about
1 in 500, the likelihood of making a correct diagnosis even
using higher cut-off points would be very small indeed.

The extent of the overlap and hence the accuracy of the diagnosis depends upon the variance of the two distributions as
well as the distance between the two means and the variance
will be increased by differences between the sexes and by
changes with age. We have examined these two factors in a longitudinal series of serum cholesterol levels measured in 120
schoolchildren, 63 girls and 57 boys between 11 and 15 years
of age who volunteered to take part in a wider investigation
of biochemical changes taking place during puberty. A total
of 380 observations have been made. Measurements were at six
monthly intervals and have so far been continued over a period
of 2 years. The data have been used to compare the changes in
mean serum cholesterol level with age and with puberty staging
in each sex.

Serum cholesterol concentration appears to be unaffected by
age in girls. There appears to be a decrease with age in boys
between 11 and 14 years of age, but the trend fails to reach
conventional levels of significance probably because numbers
are so small in the 14 year age group. When the girls and boys
are divided into groups according to their puberty stage the
girls show a significant reduction in serum cholesterol as

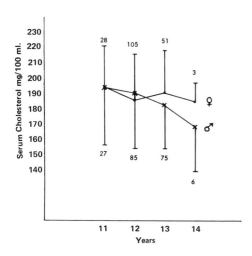

SERUM CHOLESTEROL
IN BOYS AND GIRLS BY AGE

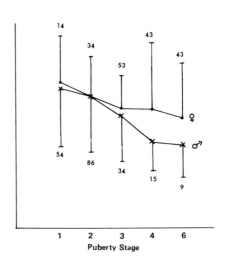

SERUM CHOLESTEROL
IN BOYS AND GIRLS BY PUBERTY STAGE

Fig. 1 shows a comparison of the changes in serum cholesterol concentration with age and with puberty stage. The levels in boys are indicated by crosses and in girls by dots. The vertical axis shows the serum cholesterol concentration and the horizontal axis the age in years and the puberty stage. The vertical lines indicate the standard deviations around the means and the number of observations is shown above and below each of these lines.

puberty progresses and in the boys the same trend is more marked reaching a significance of less than 1 in 500. The variance around the mean levels in each group remains unchanged whether the data are analysed by age or by puberty stage. It would seem therefore that when serum cholesterol levels are examined in boys or girls during puberty, allowance should be made for the puberty stage of the child but that it is unlikely that the allowance will help to distinguish those affected with familial hypercholesterolaemia since the variance of the control group is not reduced by allowing for either age or puberty stage. The need for a test to distinguish children who are heterozygous for familial hypercholesterolaemia from those who are not remains, particularly in families of patients who are known to be affected.

Goldstein and Brown (1974) have shown that when cultured skin fibroblasts are incubated in lipoprotein deficient serum there is an increase in the incorporation of 14C labelled acetate into sterols but that whereas in normal cells the addition of low density lipoproteins results in repression of sterol synthesis, no repression occurs in fibroblasts from patients with familial hypercholesterolaemia. Furthermore they later showed (Goldstein et al 1975) that fibroblasts from heterozygotes in the presence of low density lipoprotein incorporate 14C labelled oleate into cholesteryl ester at a rate mid-way between homozygotes and normals. Fogelman et al.(1975), using leucocytes have shown that incubation with delipidated serum results in induction of sterol synthesis from 14C labelled acetate at a rate which was greater in cells from heterozygotes than normals and suggested that this resulted from increased release of endogenously synthesised sterol into lipid free incubation medium.

We have used cultured skin fibroblasts from 4 normals, 3 homozygotes, 3 obligate heterozygotes, all parents of homozygotes and 5 other heterozygotes to examine the possibility of distinguishing heterozygotes from homozygotes and normals using 14C labelled acetate incorporation into sterols in cultured skin fibroblasts after incubation with delipidated serum. Delipidated serum was used in preferance to lipoprotein deficient serum because we found it to be more active in inducing sterol synthesis, that its preparation was simpler and that it gave more reproducible results.

Cultured skin fibroblasts were incubated in delipidated serum. After 24 hours the medium was changed and low density lipoprotein added to half the dishes for a total of 26 hours to produce maximum repression of sterol synthesis. 14C labelled acetate was added to all dishes for the final 20 hours incubation. The medium was then removed and saved, and the cells washed and harvested. The radio active label incorporated into digitonin precipitated sterols was assayed in both cells and medium and the results were calculated as nanomoles of precipitated sterols/mg of cell protein. A normal cell line was used as a quality control in each set of experiments.

Fig. 2 shows the findings in the cells alone.
Fig. 3 shows the findings in the cells and the medium.
The percentage repression of sterol synthesis after the addition of the LDL is shown on the vertical axes. Percentage repression has been calculated as the difference between induced and repressed sterol synthesis over synthesis in the induced state. The three groups are shown, from left to right, homozygotes, heterozygotes and normals. Obligate heterozygotes are shown by open circles and the quality control is shown by the crosses.

Cells from the normal cell lines consistently showed more than 90 percent repression of sterol synthesis and the experiments repeated on one normal cell line showed good reproducibility. All the homozygotes showed less repression of sterol synthesis than the normals, one showed 30 percent, but the results were variable and others showed substantially more. These results are in broad agreement with Fung et al. (1977). The repression of sterol synthesis found in the cells of heterozygotes overlapped the other two groups. They could not therefore be distinguished from either homozygotes or normals by this method. In this finding we are in agreement with Kayden et al. (1976) who used 14C labelled oleate incorporation into cholesteryl esters in his attempt to distinguish heterozygotes from normals.

Using both cells and medium to measure percentage repression of sterol synthesis the separation of normals and homozygotes shown in Fig. 3 was complete but the repression in the heterozygotes overlapped both normals and homozygotes.

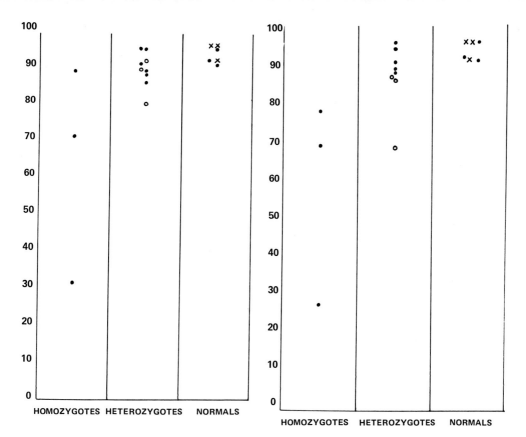

FIG. 2. Percent repression of sterol synthesis in familal hyhypercholesterolaemia in cells alone. x, repeats; o, obligates.

FIG. 3. Percent repression of sterol synthesis in familal hypercholesterolaemia in cells plus medium. x, repeats; o, obligates.

We conclude therefore that in the conditions we have measured repression of sterol synthesis neither the cells alone nor cells and medium together can be used to distinguish heterozygotes for familial hypercholesterolaemia from normals.

Using leucocytes from a single heterozygote and normal Fogelman et al. (1975) found that when these cells were transferred from a full serum to a lipid free medium there was an increased efflux of sterol from the cells into the medium in the heterozygote compared to the normal.

We have therefore examined this index of efflux, calculated in the same way as Fogelman, that is the sterol in the medium over the total sterol in both cells and medium, and found that while heterozygotes showed greater mean efflux than normals there was still no clear distinction between the groups. These findings are shown in Fig. 4.

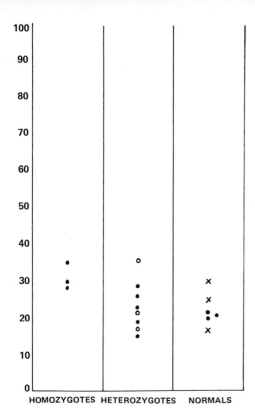

FIG. 4. Percent efflux of sterol into medium in familial hypercholesterolaemia, calculated as the sterol in the medium alone divided by the total sterol in cells plus medium. x, repeats; o, obligates.

We therefore conclude that while measurement of total serum cholesterol, even allowing for the reduction of serum cholesterol in boys and girls with advancing puberty stages fails to allow a clear diagnosis of familial hypercholesterolaemia, there is no better separation between normals and heterozygotes when repression of sterol synthesis or efflux is measured in cultured skin fibroblasts after induction with delipidated serum.

References

Fogelman AM, Edmond J, Seager J and Popjak G (1975) Abnormal induction of 3 Hydroxy-3 methyl glutaryl Coenzyme A Reductase in Leukocytes from subjects with heterozygous Familial Hypercholesterolaemia . Journ. Biol. Chem 250: 2045-2055

Fung CH, Kachadurian AK, Wang C-H and DurrBF. (1977)Regulation of lipid synthesis by low density lipoproteins in cultured skin fibroblasts in homozygous familial hypercholesterolaemia Biochim et Biophys Acta. 487 445-457

Goldstein JL, Dana SE and Brown M (1974) Esterification of low density lipoprotein cholesterol in human fibroblasts and its absence in homozygous Familial Hypercholesterolaemia Proc. Nat. Acad. Sci. USA 71. 4288-4292

Goldstein JL, Dana SE, Brunschede GY and Brown MS (1975)
Genetic heterogeeity in Familial Hypercholesterolaemia: Evidence for two different mutations affecting functions of low density lipoprotein receptor. Proc. Nat. Acad. Sci. U.S.A. 72. 1092-1096

Kayden HJ, Hatam L and Beratis NG. (1976) Regulation of 3-Hydroxy-3-methylglutaryl Coenzyme A Reductase Activity and the esterification of cholesterol in human long term lymphoid cell lines. Biochemistry 15 521-528

Leonard JV, Whitelaw AGL, Wolff OH, lloyd JK and Slack J. (1977) Diagnosing Familial Hypercholesterolaemia in childhood by measuring serum cholesterol. Brit. Med. Journ. 1 1566-1568

Lipoprotein and Apoprotein, Adipose Tissue and Hepatic Lipoprotein Lipase Levels in Patients with Familial Hyperchylomicronemia and their Immediate Family Members[1]

G. Crepaldi, R. Fellin, G. Baggio, J. Augustin, and H. Greten

The object of this study was to evaluate:

a) Levels of adipose tissue lipoprotein lipase (T-LL) and hepatic triglyceride lipase (H-LL) in 6 patients with familial hyperchylomicronemia from three different families, as well as in their immediate family members.

b) Concentration and composition of different lipoprotein fractions in the patients with specific attention to HDL_2, HDL_3, and apoproteins AI and B.

c) Distribution of CII and CIII peptides in the chylomicrons and VLDL of the 6 patients.

Materials and Methods

Six patients with familial hyperchylomicronemia from three different families (1 brother and 1 sister from each family) were studied following a two months period of free diet. Blood samples were taken after an overnight fast, and 10 minutes after intravenous injection of 60 U/Kg heparin (Liquemin, LaRoche). Cholesterol, triglyceride and phospholipids were determined on fasting plasma and in VLDL (including both chylomicrons and VLDL), LDL, HDL_2 and HDL_3, obtained by sequential preparative ultracentrifugation. AI and B apoproteins were measured in serum with rocket electrophoresis. Post-heparin triglyceride lipase (T-LL and H-LL) were both partially purified, and characterized by selective precipitation of hepatic triglyceride lipase with specific antibody. CII and CIII peptides were evaluated by polyacrylamid gel electrophoresis (PAGE) according to the method of Kane.

Results

Normal or slightly increased cholesterol levels (Table 1) were confirmed in the plasma of the patients, as well as the marked hypertriglyceridemia. LDL cholesterol was rather low, but the percentage of triglycerides in that fraction was relatively elevated, compared to normal LDL composition. HDL_2 and HDL_3 subfractions were rather low. Apoprotein B was decreased in plasma and LDL (Table 2), but was increased in the fraction with d < 1.006 g/ml in all patients. Apo AI was also decreased in plasma, and was very low in HDL_2 and HDL_3.
Table 3 reports the distribution of CII and CIII peptides in chylomicrons and VLDL. While patients 1,2,3, and 4 have CII peptides, patients 5 and 6 (belonging to the same family) have

---

[1] Programma Finalizzato CNR, Medicina Preventiva, Subprogetto Aterosclerosi, Rome (Italy) Unità operative RF_1, Padova.

Table 1. Distribution of cholesterol (CH), triglyceride (TG) and phospholipids (PL (mg/dl)) in plasma and different lipoprotein classes of six patients with familial hyperchylomicronemia.

Patients	Sex	Age yrs	Plasma			"VLDL"[a]			LDL			HDL2		HDL3	
			CH	TG	PL	CH	TG	PL	CH	TG	PL	CH	PL	CH	PL
1 - C.D.	M	36	353	3000	325	260	2510	191	19	29	23	3.5	bs[b]	6	26.5
2 - C.R.	F	49	289	2226	257	215	1665	158	16	29	16	2	bs[b]	6	25
3 - D.P.G.	M	32	258	2070	252	182	1785	95	13	21	3	3	bs[b]	5	15
4 - D.P.V.	F	48	248	1472	272	125	1106	114	19	17	19	4	bs[b]	9	31
5 - S.A.	M	37	235	2020	304	180	1503	228	21	21	23	2.3	bs[b]	9.1	28
6 - S.F.	F	35	183	1985	296	136	1539	148	10	28	12	2.4	bs[b]	5.4	17
M[c]		39.5	261	2128.8	284.3	183	1684.6	155.6	16.3	24.1	16.1	2.9	-	6.7	23.7
SEM[d]		±2.9	±23.2	±202.9	±11.7	±20.4	±189.8	±19.9	±1.7	±2.1	±3.1	±0.3	-	±0.7	±2.6

[a] "VLDL" = including both VLDL and chylomicrons.
[b] bs = below sensibility of the method.
[c] M = mean.
[d] SEM = standard error of mean

Table 2. Concentration of apolipoprotein B and AI (mg/dl) in plasma and different lipoprotein fractions of six patients with familial hyperchylomicronemia.

Patients	Apo B			Apo AI		
	Plasma	"VLDL"[a]	LDL	Plasma	HDL_2	HDL_3
1 - C.D.	74	24	20	77	1.7	28
2 - C.R.	74	24	16	88	3	20
3 - D.P.G.	44	19	16	65	2.5	13
4 - D.P.V.	72.5	21.5	13	83	4	15
5 - S.A.	88	43.5	19.5	115	1	17
6 - S.F.	66	30.5	11.5	90	2.5	7
M[b]	69.75	27.08	16	86.33	2.45	16.67
SEM[c]	±5.93	±3.64	±1.38	±6.81	±0.42	±2.88

[a]"VLDL" = including both VLDL and chylomicrons.

[b]M = mean.

[c]SEM = standard error of mean.

no immunological or electrophoretical evidence of CII peptide. In the first four patients, moreover, CIII-0 and CIII-3 were absent in chylomicrons, but present in VLDL. Triglyceride and cholesterol plasma values, T-LL and H-LL levels in the patients and their immediate family members are reported in Table 4.

Family C.: One sister (C.An.) has mild hypertriglyceridemia and hypercholesterolemia in addition to a maturity onset diabetes. A brother has slight hypertriglyceridemia. All the immediate members of this family had T-LL values near the limit of the lower normal range (4-8 μmol/ml). H-LL was normal (normal range = 10-25 μmol/ml).

Family D.P.: All the immediately family members of the two patients have normal blood lipid levels. T-LL was normal in two brothers and one sister of this family, but it is below normal in the mother, as well as in the three children of one patient.

Family S.: All immediate family members are normolipaemic. The two patients, in contrast to the others, have normal T-LL, however, they do not show CII peptide in any lipoprotein fraction.

Table 3. Distribution of CII and CIII peptides in chylomicrons and VLDL of 6 patients with familial hyperchylomicronemia.

Patients	Chylomicrons					VLDL				
	CII	$CIII_0$	$CIII_1$	$CIII_2$	$CIII_3$	CII	$CIII_0$	$CIII_1$	$CIII_2$	$CIII_3$
1 - C.D.	+	−	+	+	−	+	+	+	+	+
2 - C.R.	+	−	+	+	−	+	+	+	+	+
3 - D.P.G.	+	−	+	+	−	+	+	+	+	+
4 - D.P.V.	+	−	+	+	−	+[a]	+	+	+	+
5 - S.A.	−	−	+	+	−	n.e.	n.e.	n.e.	n.e.	n.e.
6 - S.V.	−	−	+	+	−	n.e.	n.e.	n.e.	n.e.	n.e.

[a]n.e. = not evaluated

Table 4. Plasma triglyceride and cholesterol (mg/dl), adipose tissue lipoprotein lipase (T-LL) and hepatic lipoprotein lipase (H-LL) in the 6 patients with familial hyperchylomicronemia and their immediate family members.

	Relation to patients	Age	Sex	Plasma		T-LL	H-LL
				TG	CH	µmol/ml	µmol/ml
Family C							
C.D.	Propositus	36	M	3000	353	0	25
C.R.	Propositus	49	F	2226	289	0	8.5
C.M.	Mother	75	F	143	167	3.8	13.8
C.An.	Sister	51	F	269	255	4.8	13.7
C.L.	Sister	50	F	77	164	4.5	11.2
C.Al.	Brother	45	M	219	186	4.3	16.4
G.A.	Son	24	M	115	166	3.8	13.1
G.L.	Daughter	21	F	72	138	4.7	11
G.D.	Daughter	18	F	71	122	3.0	9.4
C.Ad.	Son	7	M	73	157	4.5	25
Family DP							
DP.G.	Propositus	32	M	2070	258	0	13.8
DP.V.	Propositus	48	F	1472	248	0	15.1
DP.F.G.	Mother	78	F	154	175	2.6	7.3
DP.G.	Brother	53	M	56	195	8.1	11.9
DP.G.	Brother	51	M	113	224	7.1	19.3
DP.M.	Sister	47	F	75	200	6.5	11.8
DP.S.	Sister	39	F	59	152	4.3	19.9
DP.M.	Daughter	8	F	105	158	4.2	13.2
DP.M.	Daughter	6	F	136	160	1.9	18.7
DP.C.	Son	2	M	95	169	2.4	14.6
Family S							
S.A.	Propositus	37	M	2020	235	6.4	32.3
S.F.	Propositus	35	F	1985	183	4.5	17.4
S.F.	Father	64	M	91	260	6.2	26.6
C.M.	Mother	60	F	101	210	6.5	25.9
F.W.	Son	17	M	120	122	7.6	35.7
F.A.	Daughter	9	F	54	199	11.4	32.2

Conclusion

The above data indicate that familial hyperchylomicronemia is characterized by a lack of lipoprotein lipase activity that is not necessarily due to the absence of T-LL. In the first two families, the patients showed a complete absence of T-LL, while in the third family, the patients had no detectable CII apoprotein (the physiological T-LL activator) and a normal T-LL level. Lack of T-LL activity (due either to its absence or CII absence) in the patients may explain the very low levels of VLDL, LDL, HDL$_2$, and HDL$_3$. The low levels of these lipoprotein fractions in turn explain the low concentrations of Apo B and AI. In all three families H-LL was normal.

In Family C, the tendency of all immediate family members to have a T-LL within lower normal values or slightly decreased

is relevant. This is still more evident in some members of the
D.P.family where in three children and the mother of the patient
a decreased T-LL was found. In the S.family, instead, T-LL was
normal in both patients and all immediate family members. The
absence of the CII apoprotein is most likely the cause of the
lack of adipose tissue lipoprotein lipase activity. From these
results it may be concluded that the phenotypes of familial hyperchylomicronemia correspond to different genotypes.

References

Breckenridge WC, Little JA, Steiner G, Chow A, Poapst M (1978)
    Hypertriglyceridemia associated with deficiency of apolipo-
    protein C-II. New Engl J Med 298: 1265-1273
Fredrickson DS, Goldstein JL, Brown MS (1978) The familial hyper-
    lipoproteinemias. In: Stanbury JB, Wyngaarden JB, Fredrick-
    son DS (eds) The metabolic basis of inherited disease.
    McGraw-Hill, New York, pp 604-617
Greten H, DeGrella R, Klose G, Rascher W, de Gennes JL, E Gjone
    (1976) Measurement of two plasma triglyceride lipases by an
    immunochemical method: studies in patients with hypertrigly-
    ceridemia. J Lipid Res 17: 203-209
Krauss RM, Levy RI, Fredrickson DS (1974) Selective measurement
    of two lipase activities in post-heparin plasma from normal
    subjects and patients with hyperlipoproteinemia. J Clin
    Invest 54: 1107-1124
Yamamura T, Sudo H, Ishikawa K, Yamamoto A (1979) Familial type
    I hyperlipoproteinemia caused by apolipoprotein C-II defi-
    ciency. Atherosclerosis 34:53-65

Studies of a Large French-Canadian Kindred with Two Forms of Hyperlipoproteinemia[1]

J. Davignon, S. Lussier-Cacan, A. Gattereau, P.P. Moll, and C.F. Sing

Familial hypercholesterolemia (FH) is characterized by a very high plasma low density lipoprotein (LDL) cholesterol level, the presence of tendon xanthomas in some of the affected subjects, premature atherosclerosis and a decreased number of cell surface LDL-receptors (Fredrickson et al. 1978). Although plasma cholesterol is always strikingly elevated, plasma triglycerides and their major carrier, very low density lipoproteins (VLDL), may be either normal (phenotype IIa) or elevated (phenotype IIb).

We initiated a study to examine the genetic basis for plasma lipid levels and lipoprotein patterns in a large French-Canadian kindred identified by a proband with the IIb phenotype, as well as with tendon xanthomas and premature coronary heart disease (CHD). Specifically, this kindred was studied to determine whether hypercholesterolemia and hypertriglyceridemia are inherited independently, what is the contribution of the various concomitant variables associated with plasma lipid levels to hyperlipidemia and what are the contributions of the factors responsible for the proband's phenotype to the hyperlipidemia and morbidity among his siblings and their descendants.

We have identified 508 individuals of whom 379 span 4 generations and have been extensively studied for over 175 variables. A systematic evaluation was carried out to record clinical manifestations of hyperlipidemia and atherosclerosis, to assess the major influences on plasma lipid levels, to detect secondary causes of hyperlipidemia and to document risk factor phenotypes of healthy and diseased individuals. Plasma cholesterol (CH), triglycerides (TG), glucose, uric acid, LDL-cholesterol, VLDL-cholesterol and high density lipoprotein (HDL) cholesterol were measured according to standard techniques used in our laboratory (Pichardo et al. 1977). The proband was a 36 year old French-Canadian police officer whose father had died of a myocardial infarction at 57. He had FH with a IIb phenotype, CHD, arcus corneae and Achilles' tendon xanthomas. He had 370 mg/dl of CH, 283 mg/dl of TG, 80 mg/dl of VLDL-CH, 261 mg/dl of LDL-CH and 29 mg/dl of HDL-CH when first seen at our lipid clinic.

The 379 individuals examined included 142 (71 females) maternal relatives (M subset) of the proband, 135 (72 F) paternal relatives (P subset), 27 (13 F) codescendants (C subset) including the proband, his siblings and their children, and 75 (37 F) unrelated non-members (NM) who married into the kindred (35, 34 and 6 into the M, P and C subsets, respectively). The 379 individuals were distributed among 103 households. Fifty-four percent lived in the proximity of Grand Falls, New Brunswick. We report here preliminary findings on the distribution of hyperlipoproteinemia and disease among the four subsets of the kindred, the heterogeneity in the relationship between age and lipid levels in the four subsets and, finally, the differences among lipid levels of children from different mating types. These pre-

---

[1] Supported by grants from Health and Welfare Canada (# 604-7-759), the Medical Research Council of Canada (MA-5427), the Quebec Heart Foundation, and grant US-DoE 2828

liminary findings provide valuable directions to the formal genetic analysis
of this kindred which is underway.

Combined effects of two forms of hyperlipidemia

Using standard cut off points to identify the hyperlipidemic individuals we
found FH in the P subset (27 IIa, 6 IIb, 1 IV) and familial hyperprebetalipo-
proteinemia (FHPB) in the M subset (14 IV, 3 IIb). Both parents of the
proband were affected (phenotypes II + IV) and there was high prevalence of
plasma lipid abnormalities in the codescendants (Fig. 1). Indeed hyperlipidemia was present in 13.8% of the M subset, in 27.6% of the P subset, and
in 63.0% (12 IIa, 5 IIb) of the C subset. The clinical manifestations of
hyperlipidemia and atherosclerosis were also most frequent in the C subset.
Combined angina pectoris, myocardial infarction and intermittent claudication
frequencies were, respectively, 2.1%, 8.1% and 18.5% in the M, P and C subsets. Xanthelasma and/or arcus corneae were present respectively in 2.1,
5.9 and 33.3% of the same subsets. Tendon xanthomas occurred in the P subset
(9.6%) and in the C subset (25.9%). Obesity was more frequent in the M
(11.2%) than in the P subset (6.6%). Overt diabetes occurred in 4.2% of the
M subset. In the generation of the proband in the C subset (Fig. 1, III)
7 of 8 siblings were hyperlipidemic (87.5%; 4 IIb, 3 IIa) and had tendon
xanthomas. Unexpectedly the NM subset had a high prevalence of hyperlipidemia (26.4%; 12 IV, 2 IIa, 2 IIb, 3 V), atherosclerosis (13.8%), obesity
(23.6%), arcus corneae and/or xanthelasma (13.3%). There was also one case
of diabetes among them. The IIb phenotype found in 18.5% of the codescendants will probably increase in frequency as the 19 individuals under 20
years of age mature. The high frequency of hyperlipidemia and cardiovascular
morbidity among codescendants is consistent with the cosegregation of alleles
determining two distinct lipid abnormalities with a possible contribution
from factors influencing glucose metabolism.

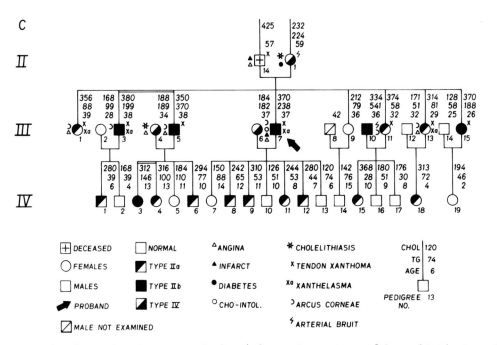

FIG. 1 Plasma lipids, age and clinical manifestations of hyperlipidemia and
atherosclerosis in the codescendants and their spouses (CHO: carbohydrate)

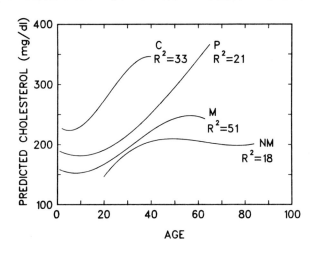

FIG. 2. Regression curves for cholesterol and age in the various subsets of the kindred (see text).

Heterogeneity in the age-lipid relationship

The large number of subjects in the kindred distributed equally between the paternal and the maternal sides as well as the large number of variables explored allowed us to study the heterogeneity in the expression of lipid phenotypes among the major subsets of the pedigree. In most methods used to test for the presence of bimodality in plasma lipid and lipoprotein distributions an age-correction is required which assumes that the relationship with age is the same for all individuals. Significant differences in the age-lipid relationship were detected among the various subsets. This is illustrated in figure 2 where plasma cholesterol values predicted from a third order polynomial regression were plotted against age. The presence of FH in the P subset, of FHPB in the M subset and their combination in the codescendants results in uniquely different cholesterol-age relationships. The shape and displacement of the regression curves are not significantly different among the four subsets when only normocholesterolemic individuals are considered. The displacement, but not the shape, of the regressions estimated using hyperlipidemics only varied significantly among the subsets. The amount of variability attributable to age (R^2) given in Figure 2 also varies for each part of the kindred. Regression differences are attributable to different types of abnormal subjects in the various subsets. The curve drawn for the NM subset was not significantly different from one derived from a normative Canadian population above age 20 (Hewitt et al. 1977). Similar findings were obtained when LDL-CH, TG, and VLDL-CH were related to age. These results indicate that caution should be exercised in the interpretation of data derived from standard age-correction procedures for the study of frequency distribution of plasma lipids in a given kindred.

Influence of parents' triglycerides on plasma lipids of the offspring

The differences between kindred parts in the age-lipid relationship in childhood and at relatively low levels of plasma cholesterol or triglyceride concentrations suggested that the lipid mating types could markedly influence the plasma lipids of children, even in situations where detection of "affected" individuals is delayed as in hypertriglyceridemia. This kindred enabled us to evaluate the ability to predict the lipid profiles of children from the triglyceride concentrations of their parents. Data were compiled from 49 matings with 146 children. The variables in Table 1 all have significantly different means for children from the different mating types. Significantly higher TG and VLDL-CH and significantly lower uric acid levels were found for children of a normal father and a hypertriglyceridemic mother (N x H) compared to offspring of the reciprocal mating (H x N). The difference in plasma TG in the children of these reciprocal mating types is not

Table 1. TG mating types (Father x Mother) and plasma lipids of children.

	H x H	H x N	N x H	N x N	Total
Number of matings	5	10	7	27	49
Number of children	20 (10M)	24 (14M)	28 (9M)	74 (40M)	146
Total chol	241 ±72*	183 ±55	171 ±42	159 ±45	p <0.001
LDL-chol	191 ±66	138 ±54	120 ±45	110 ±41	p <0.001
Triglycerides	66 ±29	47 ±18	67 ±48	49 ±23	p =0.013
VLDL-chol	§21 ±8	12 ±7	18 ±8	§16 ±9	p =0.007
HDL-chol	35 ±4	39 ±7	37 ±8	34 ±6	p =0.031
Uric acid	4.4 ±0.8	4.6 ±1.7	3.6 ±1.0	4.4 ±1.0	p =0.008

* mean ± S.D., the values underlined with a full line differ from those underlined with a dotted line, those marked with § also differ from one another. The p value is given for the test of the hypothesis that the offspring from the 4 mating types are equal. H = high TG, N = normal TG

associated with differences in sex distribution, age, body mass index (weight/height^2), part of the pedigree or dietary habits of the children. In addition, parents in these reciprocal matings did not differ in terms of age, prevalence of obesity, hypertension, cigarette smoking habits, distribution among pedigree parts or electrophoretic types. Analysis of variance among groups of "high TG" parents (H x H group, high fathers alone and high mothers alone) and among groups of "normal TG" parents (N x N group, normal fathers and normal mothers) failed to show a difference in the means for CH, TG, VLDL-CH, LDL-CH, HDL-CH, uric acid, glucose, blood pressure, age or body mass index. Adjustments for differences in height and weight in the children failed to alter the maternal effect on triglycerides. On the other hand exclusion of the subjects with a glucose abnormality and their offspring completely abolished the differences between children from H x N and N x H matings. Except for uric acid, the means of the other variables in Table 1 were still significantly different. The 24 children excluded had higher mean TG and glucose and were heavier than the other children. Their 8 excluded parents had higher glucose levels and were older than the other parents. Thus, in this large pedigree, what appeared at first to be evidence for a significant maternal effect could be accounted for by the presence of a glucose abnormality which was associated with a higher mean plasma TG in the children when the mother rather than the father was hypertriglyceridemic.

The preliminary results suggest that several assumptions about large kindreds need to be investigated before commencing formal genetic analyses. Heterogeneity in the relationship between lipids and concomitant variables, the effects of associated diseases such as diabetes on lipid levels and the increased information in quantitative lipid levels rather than normal or affected status when multiple generations are considered will be incorporated into the analyses of etiology of hyperlipidemia and morbidity in this large kindred.

References

Fredrickson DS, Goldstein JL, Brown MS (1978) The familial hyperlipoproteinemias. In: Stanbury JB, Wyngaarden JB, Fredrickson DS (eds) Metabolic basis of inherited disease. McGraw-Hill, New York pp 604-655

Hewitt D, Jones GJL, Godin GJ et al (1977) Normative standards of plasma
cholesterol and triglyceride concentrations in Canadians of working age
Canad Med Assoc J 117: 1020-1024

Pichardo R, Boulet L, Davignon J (1977) Pharmacokinetics of clofibrate in
familial hypercholesterolemia Atherosclerosis 26: 573-582

The Complex Genetics of Type III Hyperlipoproteinemia: Influence of Co-inherited Monogenic Hyperlipidemia upon the Phenotypic Expression of Apolipoprotein E3 Deficiency

William R. Hazzard, G. Russell Warnick, Gerd Utermann, John J. Albers, and Barry Lewis

The genetic basis of Type III hyperlipoproteinemia remained unclear until the demonstration by Utermann et al. (1975) of the uniform lack of isoapolipoprotein E3 in very low density lipoproteins (VLDL) from patients with this disorder. Subsequent studies have disclosed that the content of this peptide in VLDL (relative to E2) is determined by autosomal codominant inheritance (Utermann et al. 1979).

This was confirmed in Seattle in the O'D kindred (Warnick et al. 1977), the largest pedigree of a propositus with Type III hyperlipoproteinemia described to date (Figure 1). While previous studies of this family, using β-VLDL to denote the presence of Type III, had suggested that the disorder was transmitted by an autosomal dominant mechanism (Hazzard et al. 1975), re-study of the kindred in 1977 using a modification of the isoelectric focusing technique of Utermann (Warnick et al. 1979) disclosed the following: (1) the E3/E2 ratio was trimodally distributed in the O'D family, ratios of $\leq$ 0.2, 0.3 - 1.1, and $\geq$ 1.2 corresponding to the E3 deficient (apo E3-DD), partially deficient (apo E3-ND), and normal (apo E3-NN) patterns described by Utermann; (2) when family members were classified according to these patterns, the pedigree clearly demonstrated non-sex-linked codominant transmission of the E3/E2 ratio; i.e., that the ratio in a given member reflected that in both parents in a classical, Mendelian fashion (apo E3-DD x apo E3-NN → apo E3 ND); apo E3-DD x apo E3-ND →apo E3-ND or apo E3-DD ("pseudodominant transmission"); apo E3-ND x apo E3 NN → apo E3-ND or apo E3-NN; apo E3-NN x apo E3-NN → apo E3-NN).

Additional inspection of the pedigree suggested that the E3/E2 ratio and the hyperlipidemia segregated independently. When hyperlipidemia and the apo E3-DD pattern coincided, Type III hyperlipoproteinemia resulted; when lipid levels were normal but VLDL apo E3 was absent, the lipoprotein pattern (by standard Lipid Research Clinic Techniques) was normal; when hyperlipidemia coexisted with an intermediate or high E3/E2 ratio, it was expressed in a pattern other than Type III (IIa, IIb, or IV). The occurrence of these multiple lipoprotein patterns in the O'D pedigree in a distribution consistent with autosomal dominant transmission of the hyperlipidemia suggested the presence of familial combined hyperlipidemia (Goldstein et al. 1973). Inspection of the distribution of lipoprotein patterns in families of other Seattle patients with Type III hyperlipoproteinemia has also almost invariably disclosed the likely presence of familial combined hyperlipidemia.

An important exception was noted during the senior author's sabbatical stay in London, where S.D., a white prepubertal girl was referred from her family physician at age 12 for bilateral planar popliteal xanthomas, later appearing in the right antecubital fossa and left thumb interdigital web. The Achilles tendons were also suspiciously hard and thickened. Lipid analysis demonstrated both hypercholesterolemia (409 mg/dl) and hypertriglyceridemia (266 mg/dl), and lipoprotein electrophoresis showed increases in both β and pre-β lipoproteins. Family history (Figure 2) disclosed that her mother was healthy at age 48, while both her father and paternal uncle had persistent, severe hypercholesterolemia and had died prematurely of coronary heart disease (at 43 and 35, respectively). Her paternal grandfather was alive but disabled by angina pectoris at age 74 and had extensive nodular thickening of the Achilles tendons and tuberous xanthomas over the elbows. Of note, the latter had recently regressed significantly during treatment with clofibrate, which reduced cholesterol levels from as high as 520 mg/dl to as low as 163 mg/dl.

Assessment of the family by measurement of VLDL apo E3/E2 ratios demonstrated that both S.D. and her paternal grandfather had apo E3-DD patterns, while her grandmother was apo E3-NN and her mother was apo E3-ND. Hence, according to Mendelian genetics and the mode of inheritance of the E3/E2 ratio demonstrated by Utermann et al. and in the O'D kindred, both her father and uncle had been obligate heterozygotes (apo E3-ND). Of note, both had been resistant to clofibrate. The patient, by contrast, rapidly normalized on clofibrate (cholesterol 136 mg/dl, triglyceride 97 mg/dl), and her xanthomas disappeared. Furthermore, when clofibrate was withdrawn 31 months later (the patient meanwhile having passed menarche), lipid levels re-stabilized at an intermediate level (cholesterol 241 mg/dl, triglyceride 154 mg/dl) with moderate elevations in both VLDL and low density lipoproteins (LDL).

While this pedigree is small and definitive studies (of LDL receptors) remain to be performed, it does appear to represent the clearest demonstration to date of the phenotypic expression of the combination of apo E3 deficiency and (heterozygous) familial hypercholesterolemia (FH) (LDL receptor deficiency). Presumptive evidence for the letter includes expression of hyperlipidemia during childhood (rare in Type III, invariable in FH), the predominant hypercholesterolemia (hypertriglyceridemia is usually predominant in Type III), and the tendinous xanthomas in the paternal grandfather (and possibly in the propositus), plus the severe, intractable hypercholesterolemia in her father and uncle, who were heterozygous for E3 deficiency.

The pathophysiological implications of these two pedigree studies (and the far more extensive studies of Utermann et al.) include the following: (1) In the absence of a co-inherited (or acquired) abnormality in lipoprotein metabolism, apo E3 deficient VLDL (remnants) are cleared by an alternative, non-E3-dependent pathway which does not generate LDL; hence in this circumstance LDL (and cholesterol) levels are low; (2) Familial combined hyperlipidemia, which is not frequently expressed in childhood, is commonly the co-inherited abnormality which converts hypocholesterolemic apo E3 deficiency ("dysbetalipoproteinemia") to Type III hyperlipoproteinemia, most likely via increased VLDL apo-B production and saturation of this non-E3-dependent pathway; (3) the LDL (apo-B) receptor is normally involved in this non-E3-dependent pathway, since apo E3-deficient lipoproteins (both VLDL and LDL) accumulate when it is reduced (in heterozygous FH); (4) Clofibrate, which is only modestly effective in heterozygous FH, is markedly effective in this rare form of Type III hyperlipoproteinemia resulting from the coincidence of familial hypercholesterolemia with apo E3 deficiency. However, since it does not affect the E3/E2 ratio, this drug may exert its hypolipidemic effect on a catabolic subpathway dependent on neither apolipoprotein E3 nor apolipoprotein B.

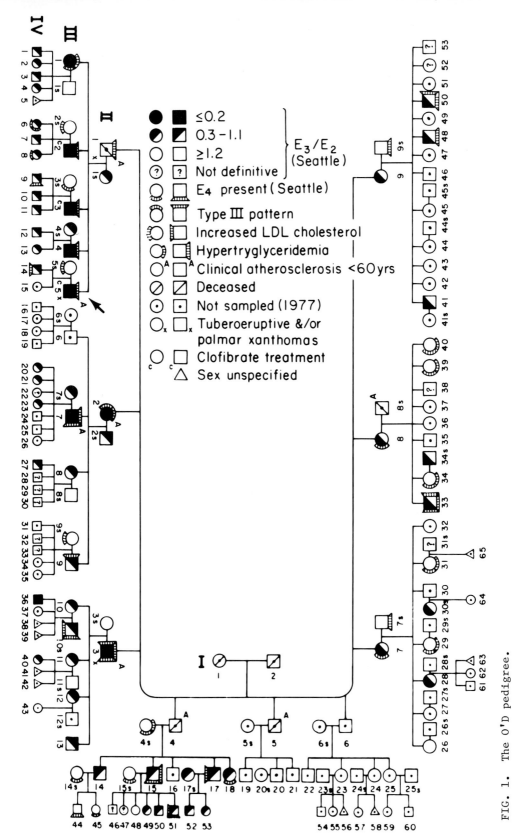

FIG. 1. The O'D pedigree.

262

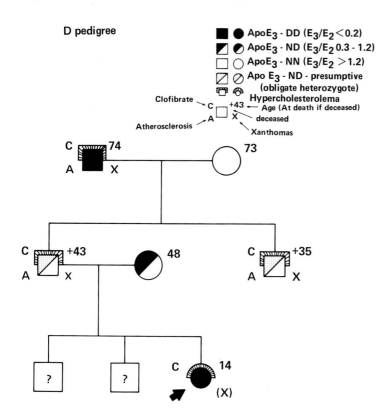

FIG. 2. The FD pedigree.

References

Goldstein JL, Hazzard WR, Schrott HG, et al. (1973) Hyperlipidemia in coronary
heart disease. II. Genetic analysis of lipid levels in 176 families
and delineation of a new inherited disorder: combined hyperlipidemia.
J Clin Invest 52:1544–1568

Hazzard WR, O'Donnell TF, Lee YL (1975) Broad-β disease (type III hyperlipoproteinemia) in a large kindred: evidence for a monogenic mechanism. Ann
Int Med 82:141–149

Utermann G, Jaeschke M, Menzel J (1975) Familial hyperlipoproteinemia type
III: deficiency of a specific apolipoprotein (apo-E-III) in the very
low density lipoproteins. FEBS letters 56:352–355

Utermann G, Vogelberg KH, Steinmetz A, et al. (1979) Polymorphism of apolipoprotein E II. Genetics of hyperlipoproteinemia type III. Clinical Genetics
15:37–62

Warnick GR, Albers JJ, Hazzard WR (1977) Genetics of type III hyperlipoproteinemia: "pseudodominant" transmission in a large kindred. Circulation 56:
(Suppl. III): 56

Warnick GR, Mayfield C, Albers JJ, et al. (1979) Gel isoelectric focusing method
for specific diagnosis of familial hyperlipoproteinemia type 3. Clin
Chem 25: 279–284

Prevalence of Hyperlipoproteinemia in Selected North American Populations

B.M. Rifkind, J. LaRosa, and G. Heiss for The Lipid Research Clinics Program

Lipoprotein typing is a widely used method for the broad classification of plasma lipoprotein disorders encountered in clinical practice, though the caveat put forth by its originators, that typing is not equivalent to genotyping (Fredrickson et al. 1967), has been amply demonstrated. Genotypes are, as yet, incompletely described and the techniques required to assign genotype are not easily applicable in large-scale population surveys. Lipoprotein typing depends on relatively simple procedures and thus is also a useful tool for the description of the distribution of lipoprotein abnormalities in large populations.

The prevalence of the lipoprotein types has been described for several populations in the United States and Western Europe (Gustafson et al. 1972; Wood et al. 1972; Gibson and Whorton 1973; Nikkila and Aro 1973). These studies report that Types II and IV, especially the latter, are most common (Table I). However, substantial differences in their prevalence are apparent. For example, almost a five-fold difference is reported for Type II in males. Some of this difference may reasonably be attributed to intrinsic variability between populations. A considerable amount, however, is undoubtedly due to differences in arbitrarily chosen limits (or cut points) for plasma lipid and lipoprotein levels as well as differing laboratory methods.

The Lipid Research Clinic Program (LRC) Prevalence Study provides an opportunity to examine the prevalence of different types of hyperlipoproteinemia in a large series of epidemiologically defined North American populations.

Methods

The populations surveyed and the epidemiologic methods used in the LRC Prevalence Study are detailed elsewhere (The Lipid Research Clinics Program Epidemiology Committee, 1979). The data presented here derived from the 15% random sample (13,852) of white individuals recalled for a second visit (Visit 2) after an initial screening visit (Visit 1) of the target population (60,502). Lipid and lipoprotein methodology was performed according to the standardized procedures of the LRC Program (Lipid Research Clinics Program, 1974). Lipoprotein types were assigned according to algorithms which depended on the following: upper and lower cut points were specified for LDL- and HDL-cholesterol, and for triglyceride. Other parameters included the presence of "floating beta" lipoprotein and the VLDL-cholesterol:plasma triglyceride ratio to assign the type III phenotype, and a qualitative estimation of post-heparin lipolytic activity by lipoprotein electrophoresis to separate Types I and V. For this study individuals were either classified as "normal", as having Types I-V hyperlipoproteinemia, or as having "hypobeta-", "hypoalpha-" or hyperalphalipoproteinemia. These categories were mutually exclusive.

This report deals with the prevalence of Types I-V hyperlipoproteinemia. It utilizes two separate sets of "cut-points". One set consisted of the age-,

---

[1] For References and Appendix, see p. 829.

Table 1. Reported prevalence (%) of major hyperlipoproteinemia types.

		NORMAL	II	IV
GUSTAFSON et al. 1972	76 males	77.0	13.0	8.0
NIKKILÄ and ARO 1973	263 males+ females	82.7	10.0	7.3
WOOD et al. 1972	494 males	82.2	2.8	13.0
	503 females	88.8	4.6	4.8
GIBSON et al. 1973	142 males	76.0	3.0	21.0
	148 females	83.0	6.0	10.0

Table 2. NHLBI and LRC 95th percentile points of plasma triglyceride and LDL cholesterol.

	Triglyceride			LDL-cholesterol		
	NHLBI[1]	LRC		NHLBI[1]	LRC	
Age		Male	Female[2]		Male	Female[2]
6-7		69	142		129	124
8-9		99	116		123	142
10-11		96	113		131	140
12-13	140[3]	107	122	170[3]	129	133
14-15		128	122		130	129
16-17		144	121		129	138
18-19		144	123		142	143
20-24	140[4]	165	---	170[4]	148	---
25-29		204	128		165	151
30-34	150	253	138	190	185	150
35-39		316	174		190	172
40-44	160	318	179	190	186	174
45-49		279	192		202	187
50-54	190	313	214	210	197	215
55-59		262	280		203	213

[1]Males + females.
[2]Females not taking sex hormone preparations.
[3]Age band: 6-19 yrs.
[4]Percentiles are shown for 10 yr age bands.

sex-, and race-specific 95th percentile points for LDL-cholesterol, HDL-cholesterol and triglyceride derived from the LRC Prevalence Study (Table II) (Heiss et al. 1979). The other set employed the 95th percentile points previously published by Fredrickson et al. (1967) and widely applied since then as the "normal" levels for the North American and other populations. The latter cut-points, often labelled "NHLBI" criteria (Table II), were in-cluded both because of their wide previous usage in clinical and investigative work and to draw attention to the profound effect that differing cut-points can have on the estimation of distribution of hyperlipoproteinemia types, even when the same scheme for typing is used.

Table 3. Prevalence (%) of types by NHLBI and LRC cutpoints (preliminary estimates).

	Males, 20-59 yrs. (n = 2456)		Females, 20-59 yrs. (n = 1661) No sex hormones		Females,20-59yrs. (n = 647) On sex hormones	
	NHLBI	LRC	NHLBI	LRC	NHLBI	LRC
Normal*	75.48	91.04	90.01	93.50	79.29	87.01
I	0	0	0	0	0	0
IIA	2.81	4.60	2.17	3.91	1.55	4.17
IIB	1.26	0.08	0.90	0.30	0.93	0.93
III	0.41	0.41	0.24	0.24	0	0
IV	19.95	3.79	6.68	2.05	18.24	7.88
V	0.08	0.08	0	0	0	0

*Includes hypobeta-, hyperalpha- and hypoalphalipoproteinemia, and "other" categories.

Discussion

It is apparent that estimates of prevalence of Types II and IV hyperlipoproteinemia are markedly influenced by the cut-points used to define them. The use of the 95th percentile for LDL-cholesterol or triglyceride to define Types II and IV hyperlipoproteinemia, respectively, should automatically lead to each of these types having an approximate prevalence of 5% in each age- sex- and race-specific group for which cut-points are generated. In general, the NHLBI cut-points yield high prevalence rates, up to 20%, for Type IV in the present and in other studies. Such rates suggest that the NHLBI estimate of the 95th percentile for triglyceride were set unduly low.

Another consequence of using population based age- and sex-specific cut-points is their impact on prevalence rates by age. In contrast to previous reports and to the rates observed with the NHLBI cut-points, the prevalence of normal and Type II and IV patterns does not significantly alter with age in any of the sex categories.

The LRC cut-points yield prevalence rates for Type IIA + IIB and Type IV each close to 5% in the males, and in the females when they are not distinguished by hormone use. It should be noted that subgroups of these populations defined by attributes which are associated with changes in lipoprotein distribution can lead to departures from the expected overall prevalence of 5%. This is exemplified by the rates reported for women according to hormonal usage (Table III).

The present findings indicate the desirability of deriving accurate cut-points from representative and well-defined populations. They also, however, emphasize the inherent difficulty in separating "normal" from "abnormal" on the basis of measurements which are continuously distributed in populations.

Table 4. Influence of age on prevalence (%) of types using NHLBI and LRC cutpoints (preliminary estimates).

	MALES (n = 3227)		FEMALES (n = 2998)	
	NHLBI	LRC	NHLBI	LRC
NORMALS				
0-19	74.58	73.67	81.30	73.77
20-39	63.55	75.96	71.85	73.41
40-59	60.75	75.23	63.70	72.86
IIA + IIB				
0-19	0.52	4.54	0.29	4.49
20-39	3.94	4.81	1.29	4.52
40-59	4.20	4.57	3.89	4.41
IV				
0-19	3.24	3.50	2.75	3.91
20-39	19.32	3.76	8.08	3.30
40-59	20.50	3.81	11.75	4.06

Results

Table III presents the prevalence of hyperlipoproteinemia according to either NHLBI or LRC cut-points, for three groups: males aged 20-60 years, females aged 20-60 years not taking sex hormones and females aged 20-60 years taking such medication either as oral contraceptives or post-menopausal estrogens. Both NHLBI and LRC cut-points result in a distribution in which Types II and IV predominate. The LRC criteria, however, classify considerably more males, and females on sex hormones, as normal and slightly more females not on hormones. This is mainly due to the considerable reduction in males and females on hormones classified as Type IV. On the other hand, somewhat more subjects are classified as Type IIA + IIB, according to the LRC criteria.

Use of either set of criteria results in classification of about three times as many females taking hormones as Type IV, as compared with females not taking hormones, which reflects previously reported effects of these medications on triglyceride and VLDL levels (Wallace et al. 1979). The LRC criteria also have the effect of substantially reducing the number of subjects classified as Type IIB, resulting in a prevalence of only 0.08% in males, 0.30% in females not on hormones, and 0.93% in females on hormones.

Types III and V hyperlipoproteinemia also were uncommon and no one in any of the three groups met the criteria for Type I.

Table IV summarizes the effect of age on the classification according to the two sets of cut-points. When NHLBI criteria are used, the fraction of both males and females classified as "normal" declines progressively with increasing age. This reflects a marked age-related increase in the prevalence of Type IV together with a moderate increase in that of Type IIA + IIB. When the age- and sex-specific LRC Program cut-points are employed, little or no change in prevalence is seen.

(continued on p. 829)

Hypercholesterolemia Type IIa: Incidence of Secondary, of Familial and of Non-Familial Forms in Central Europe[1]

N. Zöllner, F. Spengel, and G. Wolfram

Research into the pathogenesis of hyperlipidemias and their clinical consequences as well as into their therapy depends to a large extent on the establishment of their etiology, genetic and/or environmental. Among the hyperlipidemias those with elevated levels of cholesterol and LDL in the plasma, i.e. the diseases with the lipoprotein pattern type II carry a particularly unfavourable coronary prognosis. We have therefore studied the incidence of one of these hyperlipidemias, namely type IIa, further on called hypercholesterolemia type IIa, in a population in München, Bavaria.

Primary and Secondary Hypercholesterolemia

In the year of 1978, 11,246 consecutive admissions to the Medizinische Poliklinik of the University of München were studied. The patients were of all age groups and both sexes; in most cases complaints or diseases were minor, not necessitating hospitalization.

Upon admission, cholesterol and triglyceride levels were determined and compared with our own normal values, determined earlier in a healthy local population (table 1). From patients whose serum cholesterol was above the age specific average plus two standard deviations and whose serum triglycerides ranged below the age specific upper ninetieth percentile repeat blood samples were obtained. If the earlier findings were confirmed and LDL (Burstein et al. 1970) were elevated, the diagnosis of hypercholesterolemia type IIa was considered to be established. Table 2 exhibits the results.

Among the 480 patients with hypercholesterolemia type IIa, 344 had objective evidence of diabetes, hepatic, biliary, renal or thyroid disease. Since it could not be decided whether in these cases the hypercholesterolemia was secondary or whether there was solely a coincidence, all of them were classified to be secondary and only the rest of the cases was considered to be primary, i.e. not due to another disease. From this for primary hypercholesterolemia an incidence of 1.21 per cent may be calculated. If the data are reorganized and the above named disease groups commonly leading to hypercholesterolemia are excluded much the same incidence, 1.25 per cent, results (table 3). Thus we may safely assume that about 40 per cent of all cases of hypercholesterolemia type IIa are primary. About the other 60 per cent occuring in diseases which may produce lipid abnormalities we are on less safe grounds. Of course we must not consider that primary hypercholesterolemia causes diabetes or

[1] Supported by Deutsche Forschungsgemeinschaft.

Table 1. Upper limits of normal serum cholesterol (age specific average plus two standard deviations) and of normal serum triglycerides (upper ninetieth percentile) as derived for this study from 681 healthy industrial employees.[a]

Sex	Age group	Cholesterol[b] (mg/dl)	Triglycerides[c] (mg/dl)
m	20 - 29	228	218
	30 - 39	254	252
	40 - 49	266	264
	50 - 59	269	254
	above 60	283	303
f	20 - 29	221	166
	30 - 39	245	151
	40 - 49	246	151
	50 - 59	285	205
	above 60	295	238

[a] Henze et al, unpublished work from our laboratory.
[b] Method of Röschlau et al (1974).
[c] Method of Eggstein and Kreutz (1966).

Table 2. Hypercholesterolemia combined with normal serum triglycerides in 11 246 consecutive admissions to the Medizinische Poliklinik München

Description	Number of cases	Percentage
Cases examined	11,246	
Cholesterol elevated, triglycerides normal	480	4.27
Among these:		
Patients with diabetes, hepatic, biliary, renal or thyroid disease	344	3.06
Primary hypercholesterolemia	136	1.21

Table 3. Incidence of primary hypercholesterolemia type IIa in 10,902 consecutive admissions (excluding patients with diabetes, hepatic, biliary, renal or thyroid disease) to the Medizinische Poliklinik München

Description	Number of cases	Percentage
Cases examined	10,902	
Primary hypercholesterolemia	136	1.25

hepatic, biliary, renal or thyroid disease, but the manifestation of a primary metabolic disorder may be aided by one of the mentioned disorders. Studies using cell cultures are necessary and only with that reservation may we set the incidence of secondary hypercholesterolemia at about 1.8 per cent.

Familial and Non-Familial Hypercholesterolemia

A group of our patients with primary hypercholesterolemia were subjected to family and to tissue culture studies. The selection was based on availability and a sufficient size of the family. Familial hypercholesterolemia was considered to be established when two or more first degree relatives of the propositus had the same lipid disorder. On this basis, six out of nine propositi had familial hypercholesterolemia.

The propositi with familial hypercholesterolemia and 23 family members were studied by fibroblast cultures. An elevated activity of HMGCoA-reductase and a low cholesterol ester content of the cells grown in fetal calf serum were considered as proof of the genetic disease. The results from all persons from the families studied fitted into the clouds of data obtained from our total material of families with hypercholesterolemia type IIa (figure 1). In the cases of this study, heterozygosity by family study and by cell biochemistry coincided completely. However, in our total material there are 7 per cent discrepancies between phenotyping by clinical and genetic evaluation on the one hand, cell biochemistry on the other (Spengel et al. unpublished work from our laboratory).

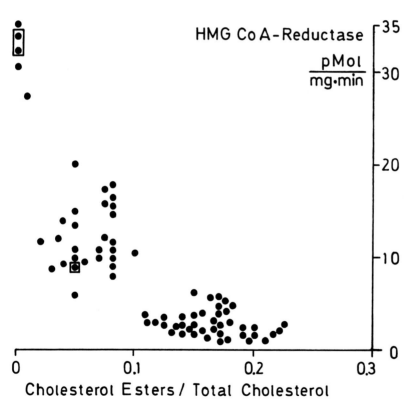

FIG. 1. HMGCoA-reductase activity and cholesterol esters of fibroblasts from members of families with hypercholesterolemia type IIa. Each point denotes one of our cases, the rectangles describe findings in fibroblasts (two homozygous, one heterozygous) from a reference laboratory.

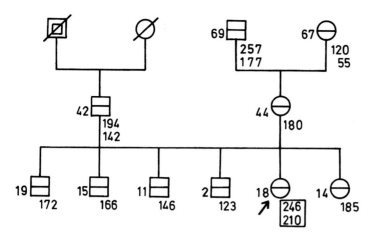

FIG. 2.   Family tree of a eighteen year   old
healthy girl with primary hypercholesterolemia
type IIa. Her paternal grandfather died early
from a coronary infarction, her grandmother at
a high age from a stroke. The rest of the family
is alive and well. To the left of the symbols age
at study, right below the symbols serum cholesterol and, in the propositus and her father LDL
cholesterol.

In three patients, family studies indicate a sporadic disease.
In one of these, ten members were studied. All of them but the
propositus had normal serum lipids, and on tissue culture all
their fibroblasts including those of the propositus showed
HMGCo-reductase activity and cholesterol esters in the normal
range (figure 2). The propositus, an eighteen years old girl,
was repeatedly studied; her serum cholesterol and her LDL
cholesterol were always above the upper limit. In all other
respects she was completely healthy. This case reminds of the
cases described by Morganroth et al. (1974); it certainly is
further evidence that not all cases of primary hypercholesterolemia are familial and that not all may be explained by
the hypothesis of Goldstein and Brown. Preliminary results
favour the hypothesis that these seemingly sporadic cases are
caused by some other hereditary metabolic lesion.

References

Burstein M, Scholnick HR, Morfin R (1970) Rapid method for the
    isolation of lipoproteins from human serum by precipitation
    with polyanions. J Lipid Res 11: 583
Eggstein M, Kreutz FH (1966) Eine neue Bestimmung der Neutral-
    fette im Blutserum und Gewebe. Klin Wschr 44: 262
Morganroth J, Levy RI, McMahon AE, Gotto AM Jr (1974) Pseudo-
    homozygous type II hyperlipoproteinemia. Pediatrics 85: 639
Röschlau P, Bernt E, Gruber W (1974) Enzymatische Bestimmung
    des Gesamt-Cholesterins im Serum. Z klin Chem klin Biochem
    12: 403

Clues to Mechanisms of Cardiovascular Disease from an Epidemiologic Study of Children—The Bogalusa Heart Study

G. S. Berenson, S. R. Srinivasan, A. W. Voors, and L. S. Webber

Since atherosclerosis and essential hypertension are believed to begin asymptomatically in early life, much interest has recently been shown in the study of risk factor variables in children. Extensive information is now available on cardiovascular (CV) disease risk factor variables of children in a general population, somewhat comparable to information from similar studies of adults (Monograph 1978). Additional research is now providing longitudinal observations following time-course changes of CV risk factor variables (Voors et al. 1979b, Frerichs et al. 1979) and determining how levels during the pediatric years may relate to adulthood, when the risk of coronary heart disease or essential hypertension can be judged by morbid events. Although there is a lack of understanding of the clinical significance and aftermath of disease in children, such as it occurs in adults, there are certain advantages to studying children. Heretofore, most of the epidemiologic studies described adult disease during a time when biologic changes of risk factors are less obvious. For example, in adults, stature, body weight, and serum total cholesterol change relatively little when compared to the dramatic changes that occur in the developing infant or child (Berenson et al. in press). These temporal changes in children occur during life periods when clues to mechanisms responsible for different levels of risk factor variables are available. The observation of race and sex contrasts enhances the potential usefulness of a pediatric study.

It is well known that there are race and sex differences in the occurrence of CV disease (Gordon and Devine 1966). For example, hypertension is more prevalent and is a much more severe disease in blacks than in whites living under comparable environmental conditions. Although CV disease at an anatomic level is greater in young black than white men (Oalmann et al. 1971), it is generally recognized that coronary heart disease events are more common in middle-aged white men. Such events occur at a later age in white women (Grove and Hetzel 1965). This raises the question, "can information be obtained about children to help understand these selective differences?" Observations from the Bogalusa Heart Study on growing black and white children bear on CV disease in adults. Interesting and dynamic changes occur during developmental phases that provide insight into biologic mechanisms contributing to the development of CV disease. From such observations, it becomes possible to generate hypotheses for future investigations.

Methods

The total population of 5,000 children in Bogalusa, Louisiana, ages birth to seventeen years, is being examined in a mixed epidemiological design of cross sectional and longitudinal studies. Participation in the various studies has included over 90% of the population of a well-defined geographic area of approximately 22,000 people. The racial mixture is 1/3 black and 2/3 white.

A series of examinations are conducted that include anthropometric measurements of height, weight, and skinfold, sexual maturation of secondary characteristics, a general physical examination, blood pressure measurements, and a venipuncture for serum lipids and lipoproteins.

Based on observations from a study of 3,524 children, ages 5-14, a subsample (N=272) was stratified according to diastolic blood pressure levels and was examined in a Special Blood Pressure Study, 1 to 1½ years later (Berenson et al. 1979, Voors et al. 1979a). This study included collection and analysis of 24-hr urine samples and blood samples for multiple laboratory analyses, plasma renin, dopamine β-hydroxylase, fasting glucose and insulin, serum and urine creatinine and electrolytes. A repeat blood sample was obtained 1 hr after a glucose load and a series of CV response tests were conducted measuring heart rate and blood pressure during orthostatic changes, submaximal voluntary hand contractions and a cold pressor test.

Observations

Population characteristics of risk factor variables

Observations on height and weight of the children for comparable ages were essentially similar to those of the National Health Examination Survey. The black and white boys were of similar height and weight and black girls were slightly heavier than white girls of older ages (Foster et al. 1977). Although heights and weights were very similar in both race groups, white children demonstrated considerably more body fat based on skinfold measurements and densitometric studies of body fat compositions. A greater body density and a larger muscle mass were noted in black children (Harsha et al. 1978).

Judged from a sample of children, dietary consumption of black and white children was similar, with two-thirds of the calories being supplied by school lunches and snack foods (Frank et al. 1978). In general, the diet was high fat, with a low P/S ratio, high cholesterol, high sucrose, and high salt content.

Careful measurements of blood pressure revealed levels 2 to 6 mm greater for systolic and diastolic pressures in black children than white beginning at 5 years of age, detectable with a Physiometric automatic blood pressure recorder. In the older children, 10 years and up, this difference could be shown with a mercury Sphygmomanometer (Voors et al. 1976). Higher levels are particularly evident at the 95th percentile for the population. Black boys, particularly in the high blood pressure group, demonstrated higher supine systolic blood pressures in a resting state.

Significant lipid and lipoprotein differences were apparent in the race and sex groups. Black children had higher serum total cholesterol due to higher α-lipoprotein levels. β-lipoproteins were quite similar in both racial groups, while pre-β-lipoproteins were somewhat higher in white children, especially white girls. Although there were slight differences of serum lipids and lipoproteins in early infancy, the significant racial differences of the α-lipoprotein and pre-β-lipoprotein levels only became apparent in the school age (Srinivasan et al. 1976).

An interrelationship of the risk factor variables similar to that known for adults was noted; for example, body weight correlates closely with blood pressure levels (Voors et al. 1977). The clustering of multi-risk factor variables suggests that greater selective associations occur, particularly in white boys and black girls. A greater relationship of serum total cholesterol and triglycerides with increased body weight was observed in the white children.

Observations of risk factor variables with implications for biologic mechanisms related to CV disease

<u>Essential hypertension</u>. The study of selected children, stratified by levels of blood pressure, indicated interesting racial differences. These are summarized in Table 1. Ambulatory peripheral renin activity tended to be

Table 1. Racial differences related to blood pressure of children. Higher values for characteristics noted in:

All blood pressure strata

Whites	Blacks
Percent body fat	
Plasma renin activity	
Serum dopamine β-hydroxylase (DβH)	
24-hr urine K^+	
Fasting serum glucose	

High blood pressure strata

Resting heart rate	Sitting blood pressure levels
Renin activity and DβH combined	Pos. association 24-hr urine Na^+ versus sitting blood pressure
One-hr serum glucose	Systolic blood pressures in boys
	Neg. association of plasma renin versus systolic blood pressures (black boys only)

---

lower in the black children, especially at the high blood pressure strata, with lower values for dopamine-β-hydroxylase in all blood pressure groups. Plasma insulin and glucose after a 1 hr glucose load tended to be higher in the white children.

Creatinine clearance tended to be less in the black boys in the higher blood pressure strata. Although 24 hr urine sodium excretion was comparable in the race/sex groups, black children excreted one-third less potassium than white children at all blood pressure levels.

Observations of resting levels and responses to various CV stress tests showed faster heart rates in white children, especially those at the high blood pressure level. A slightly greater response to cold pressor tests was observed in the black children.

Certain implications from these observations are possible. Subtle racial differences are likely in the renal handling of sodium and potassium. Blacks have a greater intolerance to the sodium chloride in our diet; i.e., a greater sensitivity to salt exposure. The observations on electrolytes and the greater muscle mass in blacks suggest blood volume may be an important early determinant of essential hypertension, especially in blacks. On the other hand,

the more rapid heart rates and higher 1 hr insulin and blood sugar levels
suggest subtle neuro-hormonal and adrenergic influences in the pathogenesis
of hypertension in whites. Such differences were proposed earlier by studies
in adults by Brunner et al. (1973) and conceptually by Guyton et al (1974).

Coronary artery disease. Beginning with puberty, a decrease in serum total
cholesterol levels occurs (Lee 1967). We examined the decrease of a serum
total cholesterol in 1600 children by age and maturation and noted a somewhat greater decrease in levels of boys; perhaps, beginning at slightly
earlier ages in girls and in black children (Fig. 1). A more detailed examination demonstrated significant lipoprotein changes, indicating that α-
and β-lipoproteins accounted for the decrease. The ratio β/α lipoprotein

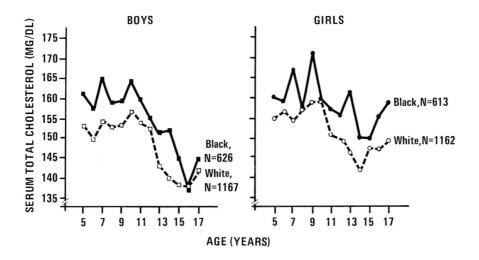

Fig. 1. Serum total cholesterol levels in children: Bogalusa Heart Study,
1976–1977.

cholesterol (Fig. 2) indicated that the ratio was essentially constant with
age in girls and in black males. However, an inordinate drop in the α-lipoprotein fraction occurred in white boys, with an earlier rise in the β-lipoproteins. The relationship of α- to β-lipoproteins results in a rather
dramatic ratio increase in white boys. If such changes can be extrapolated
to the significance of high density lipoprotein (HDL) and low density lipoprotein (LDL) levels in adults, it is as if the white boys are programmed
early for coronary heart disease.

It is interesting to speculate on mechanisms producing the serum lipoprotein
changes, especially in white children. A comparison to hormonal data obtained on a cross-section of Caucasian children (Bidlingmaier and Knorr 1978)
suggests sex hormonal changes during puberty modify the dynamic metabolic
changes observed for serum lipoproteins with potential implications for
coronary heart disease.

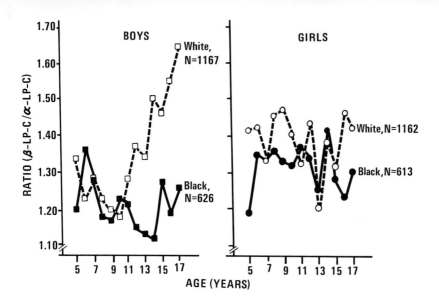

Fig. 2. Ratios of mean β-LP-cholesterol/mean α-LP-cholesterol in children:
Bogalusa Heart Study, 1976-1977.

Summary

Observations on a large biracial population of children from birth to 17
years reveal dramatic changes in risk factor variables. Studies of determinants of the risk factors in children provide an opportunity to explore
mechanisms contributing to levels of risk factors. These mechanisms, in all
likelihood beginning early in life, are operative in the development of
CV disease in adulthood.

References

Berenson GS, Blonde CV, Farris RP, Foster TA, Frank GC, Srinivasan SR, Voors
AW, Webber LS (In press) Cardiovascular disease risk factor variables during
the first year of life. Am J Dis Child

Berenson GS, Voors AW, Dalferes ER Jr, Webber LS, Shuler SE (1979) Creatinine clearance, electrolytes, and plasma renin activity related to the blood
pressure of white and black children--The Bogalusa Heart Study. J Lab Clin
Med 93:535-548

Bidlingmaier F, Knorr D (1978) Oestrogens Physiological and Clinical Aspects,
Pediatric and Adolescent Endocrinology. V 4, S. Karger, Basel

Brunner HR, Sealey JE, Laragh JH (1973) Renin subgroups in essential hypertension. Circ Res 33, Suppl: 99-109

Foster TA, Voors AW, Webber LS, Frerichs RR, Berenson GS (1977) Anthropometric and maturation measurements of children, ages 5-14 years, in a
biracial community--The Bogalusa Heart Study. Am J Clin Nutr 30:582-591

Frank GC, Berenson GS, Webber LS (1978) Dietary studies and the relationship of diet to cardiovascular disease risk factor variables in ten-year-old children--The Bogalusa Heart Study. Am J Clin Nutr 31:328-340

Frerichs RR, Webber LS, Voors AW, Srinivasan SR, Berenson GS (1979) Cardiovascular disease risk factor variables in children at two successive years-- The Bogalusa Heart Study. J Chron Dis 32:251-262

Gordon T, Devine B (1966) Hypertension and hypertensive heart disease in adults. Vital Health Stat PHS Pub No 1000, series 11 no 13. Public Health Services, Washington: US Government Printing Office

Grove LD, Hetzel AM (1965) Vital Statistics Rates in the United States, 1940-1960. PHS Pub No 1677 Washington: US Government Printing Office

Guyton AC, Cowley AW Jr, Coleman TG, DeClue JW, Norman RA, Manning DA (1974) Hypertension: a disease of abnormal circulatory control. Chest 65: 328-338

Harsha DW, Frerichs RR, Berenson GS (1978) Densitometry and anthropometry of black and white children. Hum Biol 50: 261-280

Lee VA (1967) Individual trends in the total serum cholesterol of children and adolescents over a ten-year period. Am J Clin Nutr 20: 5-12

Monograph (1978) Cardiovascular Profile of 15,000 Children of School Age in Three Communities, 1971-1975. National Heart, Lung and Blood Institute DHEW Pub No (NIH) 78-1472

Oalmann MC, McGill HC, Strong JP (1971) Cardiovascular mortality in a community: Results of a survey in New Orleans. Am J Epidemiol 94: 546-555

Srinivasan SR, Frerichs RR, Webber LS, Berenson GS (1976) Serum lipoprotein profile in children from a biracial community--The Bogalusa Heart Study. Circulation 54: 309-318

Voors AW, Berenson GS, Dalferes ER Jr, Webber LS, Shuler SE (1979a) Racial differences in blood pressure control. Science 204: 1091-1094

Voors AW, Foster TA, Frerichs RR, Webber LS, Berenson GS (1976) Studies of blood pressure in children, ages 5-14 years in a total biracial community-- The Bogalusa Heart Study. Circulation 54: 319-327

Voors AW, Webber LS, Berenson GS (1979b) Time course studies of blood pressure in children--The Bogalusa Heart Study. Am J Epidemiol 109: 320-334

Voors AW, Webber LS, Frerichs RR, Berenson GS (1977) Body height and body mass as determinants of basal blood pressure in children--The Bogalusa Heart Study. Am J Epidemiol 106:101-108

Cigarette Smoking: A Risk Factor for Atherosclerosis in Childhood?

Mary Jane Jesse

Three issues are pertinent in the discussion of cigarette smoking as a risk factor for atherosclerosis. First, the evidence which links the smoking of cigarettes to the development of atherosclerosis. Second, the relationship between cigarette smoking and the occurrence of coronary artery, cerebral vascular, and peripheral vascular disease. Third, in the face of positive relationship for the first two issues, what can be done to remove this risk factor from the population before it begins.

The evidence correlating the development of atherosclerosis with smoking of cigarettes is not great in quantity, but in quality is rather substantial.

Autopsy studies relating cigarette smoking and atherosclerosis are not common. In six studies reviewed for this paper, including studies from the United States, from Russia and from Chile, all of which were retrospective, the trend is uniformly that cigarette smoking history is associated in a dose related manner with the severity or extent of aortic and coronary artery atherosclerosis. Unfortunately, these studies have not generally permitted analysis for other risk factors nor have they permitted multi-variate analysis common in prospective studies. Despite that caveat, the report of Jack Strong and his colleagues in 1969 of the study of 747 males 25 through 64 years of age who were autopsied between 1963 and 1966 at Charity Hospital in New Orleans provided the conclusion that atherosclerotic involvement of aorta and coronary arteries is greatest in heavy smokers and least in non-smokers. Five of the six studies reviewed reached the same conclusion.

In 1978, Dr. Kagan and his colleagues in Honolulu reported in Laboratory Investigation a prospective study relating cigarette smoking to atherosclerosis. This group is engaged in a prospective study of cardiovascular risk factors among 8,000 Japanese-Americans living on the Island of Oahu. The variables were measured during life and the extent of atherosclerosis in the coronary arteries and the aorta were studied at necropsy. In this published report, systematic, pathological findings on the vessels in 137 autopsies from the cohort were reported. Cigarettes smoked per day were positively and independently associated with the extent of atherosclerosis affecting both the aorta and the coronary arteries. The aortic regression co-efficient was statistically significant at the 0.05 level and the coronary co-efficient at the 0.01 level.

At the present time, animal experiments on atherogenesis and carbon monoxide as well as nicotine have provided conflicting data and must be regarded as unsatisfactory. Experiments have variously employed continuous and intermittent exposure, have estimated the lesions biochemically and morphologically, and have used diverse short or long term dietary loads so that the comparisons of the results are difficult. Animal experiments remain to be done in which carbon monoxide or nicotine are varied in a setting of whole smoke administered by inhalation, without stress and in a suitable atherogenic context.

In man, additional findings in autopsy studies of individuals who have been heavy smokers indicate that the small arteries and arterioles in the myocardium have undergone fibrotic and hyaline changes more predominately than in non-smokers.

In summary then, cigarette smoking has been shown to enhance the prevalence and extent of atherosclerosis of the aorta and coronary arteries in men. The experimental results in animals have produced conflicting results and are inconclusive. Chronic inhalation of cigarette smoke appears to enhance fibrotic and hyaline changes in small myocardial vessels.

As regards the second issue, that of cigarette smoking and its relation to coronary artery disease and myocardial infarction, numbers of epidemiologic studies both prospective and retrospective indicate that the three major risk factors, the level of cholesterol, the level of blood pressure, and the smoking of cigarettes, are independent and strong predictors of coronary heart disease. In all of these studies which were done in adults, it has been assumed that reducing the level of the risk factor, and in the case of smoking cigarettes eliminating it, will reduce the risk of coronary artery disease.

In studies which involved populations (1) which never smoked, (2) which currently were smoking cigarettes, and (3) individuals who had stopped smoking, the risk is less than in those who continue to smoke. The risk among non-smokers remains lower than those who have stopped smoking, and based on this evidence it would appear that the cessation of smoking will indeed reduce the risk in those persons under the age of 65.

Of particular interest to those of us who care for the younger population are the three reports, two from England and one from the United States, which indicate that population studies have determined that the risk of non-fatal myocardial infarction among women during child-bearing ages is increased by a factor of about two times by the use of estrogen containing oral contraceptives, and that it is increased to about ten times the expected value when the users also smoke. In Lancet July 1978, Wingerd and his colleagues report that oral contraceptives also increases the risk of subarachnoid hemorrhage about six times and that the additional use of cigarettes increased the risk to about twenty times.

The data regarding the correlations between cigarette smoking and cerebral vascular disease as well as peripheral vascular disease are equally impelling.

In view of all the evidence presented regarding the first and second issues relating atherosclerosis development to cigarette smoking and overt coronary artery disease to cigarette smoking, the third issue, that of how to accomplish elimination of the risk factor becomes one of high importance. Clearly the evidence indicates that the non-smoker has a much less risk than that of the smoker. It would, therefore, appear that our efforts should be directed toward the avoidance of smoking, that is preventing it from becoming a habit at the outset.

In spite of a decrease in adult smoking since the dissemination of the 1964 Surgeon General's report on smoking and health, there is discouraging evidence that smoking among teenage boys is remaining virtually constant and among teenage girls is actually increasing. It is apparent that more knowledge is needed concerning the way in which psychosocial factors contribute to the initiation of smoking and how such knowledge can be applied to the development of effective strategies to deter the onset of smoking.

Prevention programs directed at children in adolescence have generally placed a great confidence in communicating knowledge about the dangers of smoking.

Indeed there is evidence to indicate that by the time children reach junior high school almost all of them believe smoking is dangerous. This paradox is illustrated by the fact that even teenage smokers seldom consider the decision to smoke a wise decision. Data from the National Clearing House for Smoking and Health indicate that, for example, 77% of smokers believe that it is better not to start smoking than to have to quit. Over half of the teenage smokers believe that cigarette smoking becomes harmful after just one year of smoking. 84% reported that smoking is habit forming, while 68% agreed that it is a bad habit. Of all teenagers, 78% believed that cigarette smoking can cause lung cancer and heart disease. 87% of all teenagers and 77% of teenage smokers believe that smoking can harm their health. The vast majority of teenagers consider smoking as habit forming, but almost two-thirds do not feel that becoming addicted to smoking is an imminent threat to their health. Experimental smoking is considered safe.

These findings, among many others, would indicate that knowledge or beliefs about the dangers of smoking are often confused with attitudes towards smoking. Attitudes are clearly much more complex than simple beliefs about the harmful effects of smoking. Factors which appear to influence the complexity of attitudes towards smoking include such things as the adverse effects of smoking on an individual's health and on the environment, that is pollution, the psychological and sociological benefits of smoking (it makes you feel good), rationalizations that allow smoking, perceptions of reasons for smoking and for smoking initiation, attitudes toward authority, and even control over one's destiny.

It would appear that our efforts toward prevention of the onset of smoking have not been terribly successful. Obviously the psychosocial factors that influence the initiation of smoking are varied and complex. Except for a few promising prevention programs, most of such programs fail to encompass psychosocial conceptual frameworks. It may be that health education, and smoking education in particular, must take into consideration the multiplicity of factors which are related, not only physical, but mental and social. It may be that the "one size fits all" approach is contraindicated in terms of this kind of health education. It may be essential that several distinct approaches to smoking education be explored for social sub groups which have demonstrably different backgrounds of exposure, involvement and maturation.

It would appear that the best efforts at present possess at least some conceptual basis, are long term, are multiphasic studies attempting to establish good baseline data. Once this is done the development of specific hypotheses which can be tested arise. Obviously such testing must employ carefully controlled methods of investigation. Of high priority is the development of objective measurements of smoking, that is, a dosimetry measure, which could validate self-reporting. Clearly in such studies, evaluations of the program should be done regularly through several years of implementation. Failure to incorporate rigorous evaluation procedures emerges as a significant limitation of nearly all of the intervention programs reviewed.

It would, therefore, appear that in our efforts to eliminate smoking as a risk factor, the most effective way would be to eliminate it at the outset. The methodology to achieve this goal has currently escaped us. However, the range of possibilities appears vast. At this point it would appear that large efforts should be expended in research into the developing life style of children and adolescents. The development of such programs using the initiation of smoking as its keystone may indeed provide critical new knowledge about those life styles and their development.

From the evidence presented, the most effective way to eliminate smoking as a risk factor will be to prevent its initiation. It is hoped that the health leaders of this Country will provide the impetus for such research. There is little doubt that the smoking of cigarettes is a true risk factor. It is one of the risk factors which we impose completely on ourselves. Understanding why we elect at any age to impose upon ourselves, from the outside, a risk factor of this proportion, may be extraordinarily difficult. It would appear that the thrust of research in this area must be directed toward that question. The question will most likely be answered when we direct it in the proper framework to the children themselves.

Nutrient Intake, Lipids, and Lipoproteins in 6−19-Year-Old Schoolchildren[1]

John A. Morrison, Rhea Larsen, Lenora Glatfelter, Donna Boggs, Kathryn Burton, Charlene Smith, Kathe A. Kelly, Margot J. Mellies, Phil Khoury, and Charles J. Glueck

Nutrient Intake and Coronary Heart Disease Risk

Dietary intake of cholesterol, saturated and polyunsaturated fats, and (perhaps) carbohydrates and total calories may relate to lipid and lipoprotein levels and to the ultimate development of coronary heart disease (CHD) (InterSociety Commision, 1970; National Diet Heart Study 1968; Connor and Connor 1972). However, the strength, consistency, and predictability of nutrient-CHD risk associations remains controversial (Mann 1977; Glueck et al. 1978).

Two recent studies in children have assessed relationships of pediatric nutrient intake and plasma lipids, and lipoproteins, (Frank et al. 1978, 1977; Weidman et al. 1978). In the Bogalusa study, in a rural bi-ethnic population, nutrient information was obtained by use of a 24-hour diet recall in 185 ten-year old children (Frank et al. 1978). There were few significant correlations between dietary components, lipids, and lipoproteins. However, when children were grouped into quartiles for serum cholesterol, children in the top quartile ingested more total fat, more saturated fat, and less polyunsaturated fat than children in the lowest quartile. In the Rochester study, nutrient information was obtained from 103 healthy white schoolchildren (ages 6-16) using a seven-day diet record (Weidman et al. 1978). No significant correlations were observed between the level of serum cholesterol and the mean daily intake of total calories, cholesterol, fats, saturated fats, or sugar.

Nutrients, Lipids, and Lipoproteins in 949 Children Ages 6-19 in the Cincinnati Lipid Research Clinic's Princeton School Survey

This report focuses upon the relationships between nutrient intakes and plasma lipids and lipoproteins in 949 children ages 6-19 in the Cincinnati Lipid Research Clinic's Princeton School Survey (Morrison et al. 1977, 1978). The data displayed are abstracted from and contained in a recent description of nutrient intake, lipids, and lipoproteins in the Princeton School Study (Morrison et al. 1979). The final data set for this report comprises 949 children; 372 white males, 120 black males, 331 white females, and 126 black females. From the initial study group of 7430 schoolchildren (seen at a first visit, Visit 1), ages 6-19 years, the targeted random recall group (for resampling) comprised 1,114 students. The overall proportion of eligible children participating at a second visit, Visit 2, was 86%. The nutrient data was collected on all subjects by means of the standardized Lipid Research Clinic's collaborative 24-hour diet recall (Lipid Research Clinics, unpublished data). The data collection took place six days a week, twelve

---

[1]From the Lipid Research Clinic and General Clinical Research Center, University of Cincinnati, College of Medicine. Supported in part by NHLBI Contract N01 HV-2-2914 L and the General Clinical Research Center Grant RR 00068-17.

months a year, from October, 1973, to October, 1975. The recall was done on the day of the Visit 2 sampling and covered the 24 hours prior to the 14-hour fasting period, which was a requisite for blood sampling. Each recall was conducted by a Lipid Research Clinic's program certified nutritionist to ensure uniformity of data collection (Lipid Research Clinics program 1974). Dietary recalls were obtained on all days of the week except Sunday; 26% of the children were seen on Mondays to reflect weekend food patterns in accordance with the collaborative LRC protocol.

Relationships Between Lipids, Lipoproteins, and Nutrients in the Cincinnati LRC Study in Schoolchildren

Table 1 (Morrison et al. 1979) provides partial correlation coefficients summarizing the relationships between lipids, lipoproteins, and nutrients after covariance adjustment for age, sex, race, weight, height, in 949 children. Plasma cholesterol and C-LDL were inversely correlated with the dietary P/S ratio (p$\leq$.05). Plasma cholesterol and C-LDL were also inversely correlated with dietary carbohydrate intake. The only significant correlation between nutrient intake and plasma triglyceride was a positive one with sugar intake (p<.01). Plasma C-HDL levels were positively correlated to dietary cholesterol (p<.05) and inversely correlated with dietary sugar (p<.01).

Relationships Between Daily Nutrient Intake and Plasma Lipids and Lipoproteins in Children at the Extremes and in the Middle of Lipid and Lipoprotein Distributions

Covariance adjusted mean daily nutrient intake was assessed for children (Morrison et al. 1979) having low (<5th percentile), intermediate (48 to 52 percentile), and high (>95th percentile) plasma cholesterol, triglyceride, C-HDL, and C-LDL respectively. Covariance adjustment was carried out for age, sex, race, and Quetelet index. Children having the highest percentile C-HDL ingested less calories, less polyunsaturated fat and less carbohydrate than children having intermediate, or lower rank C-HDL values, (p<.05). Although there was a progressive increase in dietary cholesterol from the lowest to the intermediate to the highest percentile groups for both plasma cholesterol and C-LDL, these differences were not significant.

Covariance adjusted mean daily nutrient intake for children from low, intermediate, and high lipoprotein groups was further studied after adjustment for age, sex, race, Quetelet index, and calories. There was a progressive increase in dietary cholesterol from the lowest to the intermediate to the highest groupings of plasma cholesterol (p<.025), and a relatively similar pattern of change in protein intake.

Nutrient Intake Patterns, Age, Sex, and Race (Morrison et al. 1979)

Overall for males, nutrient intake increased with age; however, age associated increases in nutrient ingestion were much less consistent, or were not significant for female schoolchildren.

In the 6-9 and 10-12 year old age groups, white children ingested more total calories, saturated fats, a lower ratio of polyunsaturated to saturated fat, more total carbohydrate, sucrose, starch, and other carbohydrates and more protein than black children, (p<.05)(Morrison et al. 1979). As had been the case in the Bogalusa study, there were no black-white differences in dietary cholesterol intake (Frank et al. 1978).

Table 1. Partial correlation coefficients of lipids and lipoproteins with nutrients, adjusting for anthropometric[a] and demographic variables in 949 children from the random recall group.

	Cholesterol	Triglyceride	C-HDL	C-LDL
Calories	-.021	-.001	-.015	-.027
Fat	.015	-.037	.011	.015
Saturated Fat	.021	-.036	.007	.026
Polyunsaturated Fat	-.04	-.037	-.015	.038
P/S	-.065[b]	-.012	-.024	-.066[b]
Dietary Cholesterol	.038	-.018	.074[c]	.015
Protein	.017	-.047	.002	.034
Total Carbohydrate	-.066[b]	.037	-.037	-.079[c]
Starch	-.037	.022	-.038	-.044
Sucrose Sugar	-.045	.078[d]	-.074[c]	-.038

[a]Partial correlation coefficients obtained after adjustment for age, sex, race, weight, and height.
[b]$p \leq .05$.
[c]$p \leq .025$.
[d]$p \leq .01$.

In the Bogalusa studies (Frank et al. 1978) also observed an inverse dietary carbohydrate-plasma cholesterol relationship. The Bogalusa group also observed that sucrose and plasma triglyceride levels were positively correlated and that dietary sucrose was inversely related to HDL cholesterol. In both the Bogalusa study (Frank et al. 1978) and the current study (Morrison et al. 1979) there were no significant positive relationships between dietary cholesterol and C-LDL.

In a generally similar fashion to the studies of Rochester (Weidman et al. 1978) and Bogalusa schoolchildren (Frank et al. 1978), correlations between nutrient intake and plasma lipids and lipoproteins were few, and generally of low magnitude. This may reflect not so much a lack of biologic association (Glueck et al. 1978a,b) but may reflect limitations of the tools utilized for dietary recall (Garn et al. 1978; Liu et al. 1978, Diamond et al. 1972). Since diet represents a major "environmental" factor subject to modification, the findings of this report (Morrison et al. 1979) particularly in regard to total cholesterol, C-LDL, and C-HDL, reinforce the need for a serious evaluation and consideration of modifications of food patterns in children.

References

Connor WE, Connor SL (1972) The key role of nutritional factors in the prevention of coronary heart disease. Prev Med 1:49-83
Diamond EL, Lilienfeld AM (1962) Effects of errors in classifications diagnosis in various types of epidemiological studies. Am J Public Health 52:1137-1144
Frank GC, Berenson GS, Schilling, PE, Moore MC (1977) Adapting the 24 hour recall for epidemiologic studies of schoolchildren. J Am Diet Assoc 71:26-31
Frank GC, Berenson GS, Webber LS (1978) Dietary studies and the relationship of diet to cardiovascular disease risk factor variables in ten-year old children - The Bogalusa Heart Study. Am J Clin Nutr 31:328-340
Garn SM, Larkin FA, Cole PE (1978) The real problem with one day records. Am J Clin Nutr 31:1114-1116
Glueck CJ, Mattson FH, Bierman EL (1978a) Diet and coronary heart disease: another view. N Engl J Med 298:1471-1474

Glueck CJ, McGill H, Shank R, Lauer R (1978b) The value and safety of diet modification to control hyperlipidemia in childhood and adolescence. American Heart Association, Position Statement. Circulation 58:A381-385

Lipid Research Clinics Program (1974) Reference Manual for Lipid Research Clinics Program Prevalence Study. University of North Carolina, Chapel Hill, Central Patient Registry and Coordinating Center for Lipid Research Clinics, Department of Biostatistics

Lipid Research Clinics Program (1979) Nutrition data collection in the LRC and MRFIT programs. Collaborative manuscript of the Lipid Research Clinics, in preparation.

Liu K, Stamler J, Dyer A, McKeever J, McKeever P (1978) Statistical methods to assess and minimize role of intra-individual variability in obscuring relationships between dietary lipids and serum cholesterol. J Chron Dis 31:399-418

Mann G (1977) Diet-heart: end of an era. N Engl J Med 297:644-650.

Morrison JA, deGroot I, Edwards BK, Kelly KA, Mellies MJ, Khoury P, Glueck CJ (1978) Lipids and lipoproteins in 927 schoolchildren, ages 6-17 years. Pediatrics 62:990-995

Morrison JA, deGroot I, Edwards BK, Kelly KA, Rauh JL, Mellies MJ, Glueck CJ (1977) Plasma cholesterol and triglyceride levels in 6,775 school-children, ages 6-17. Metabolism 26:1199-1211

Morrison JA, Larsen R, Glatfelter L, Boggs D, Burton K, Smith C, Kelly KA, Mellies MJ, Khoury P, Glueck CJ (1979) Interrelationships between nutrient intake and plasma lipids and lipoproteins in schoolchildren, ages 6-19: The Princeton School District Study. Pediatrics, in press

Primary Prevention of the Arteriosclerotic Disease (1970) Report of the InterSociety Commission for Heart Disease Resources. Circulation 42: A55-A95

The American Heart Association. (1968) The National Diet-Heart Study, Final Report. Circulation 37-38 (Suppl 1): 1-125

Weidman WH, Elveback LR, Nelson RA, Hodgson PA, Ellefson RD (1978) Nutrient intake and serum cholesterol level in normal children 6-16 years of age. Pediatrics 61:354-359

Pediatric Lipoprotein Metabolism and Atherosclerosis: A Prospectus[1]

Peter O. Kwiterovich, Jr.

The purpose here will be to summarize briefly the recent advances in the area of lipid and lipoprotein metabolism in pediatrics and, in view of the newer data, to discuss a number of questions that remain unanswered. A recurrent theme will be the relation of atherosclerosis to lipoprotein metabolism in early life, with an emphasis on identification of susceptible children, modification of risk and, ultimately, prevention of atherosclerosis. The discussion will be confined to humans. Other "risk factors" such as hypertension will not be considered since they are covered elsewhere in this workshop.

There appear to be four basic questions:
1. What are the "risk factors" for atherosclerosis in childhood?
2. What are the "determinants" of these "risk factors"?
3. How can these factors be detected and then modified?
4. Will treatment in childhood prevent the development of atherosclerosis?

Risk Factors for Atherosclerosis in Childhood and Lipid and Lipoprotein Metabolism

Plasma lipid and lipoprotein cholesterol levels

Since children only very rarely develop ischemic heart disease (IHD), most of the studies relating risk for IHD to lipid and lipoprotein levels have been performed in adults. The importance of plasma levels of certain lipids and lipoproteins in the pathogenesis of atherosclerosis has been supported by a number of epidemiologic and genetic studies that have been recently summarized by Chase and co-workers (1979). Briefly, increased levels of total plasma cholesterol and the major cholesterol-carrying lipoproteins, low density (beta) lipoproteins (LDL), are associated with an increased risk of developing IHD. Whether an elevated level of plasma triglyceride is a separate risk factor for IHD is controversial; conflicting evidence has been presented in both epidemiological surveys and in studies in kindreds with familial hypertriglyceridemia (Chase et al. 1979). Low concentrations of another lipoprotein, high-density (alpha) lipoproteins (HDL), appear to be a separate risk factor for IHD, while high levels of HDL may have a protective effect (Chase et al. 1979). A relation between adult coronary mortality and the levels of total plasma cholesterol in school children has recently been reported by Schrott and co-workers (1979). Still, a demonstration of direct, longitudinal relation between IHD and certain lipid and lipoprotein levels in childhood will require well-defined prospective studies that: first, assess tracking of lipid and lipoprotein levels at various times of early life; second, determine the relation between levels of lipids and lipoproteins and the kind and extent of atherosclerotic lesions by pathological examination in young subjects whose risk factors have previously been defined.

[1] Supported in part by a Contract NHLBI, HV-1-2158L.

Because prospective studies are very difficult, the initial approach has been to describe lipid and lipoprotein cholesterol levels in cord blood, infancy, childhood and adolescence, using cross-sectional surveys in groups with different racial and socioeconomic characteristics. For example, the Specialized Centers of Research for Arteriosclerosis (1978) have studied 15,000 school-aged children in Bogalusa, Louisiana, Iowa, and Rochester, Minnesota. The Lipid Research Clinics (LRC) have accumulated data from five different populations of children (LRC Data Book 1979). From the results of these surveys and several others, certain trends are emerging. Levels of lipids and lipoproteins are low in cord blood where HDL transports as much of the plasma cholesterol as LDL (Glueck et al. 1977a; Frerichs et al. 1978). The concentrations of total plasma and LDL cholesterol increase considerably in the first four weeks of life and then more slowly throughout the first two years of life; after the age of two years, the levels of lipids and lipoproteins in both sexes remain relatively constant until the second decade (Kwiterovich 1977). In the second decade, mean total plasma and LDL cholesterol levels fall while VLDL and triglyceride levels increase. These changes are most marked in the male. In addition, males have a mean fall in HDL cholesterol of about 10 mg% after the age of 15 years, while females have little change in the mean HDL cholesterol levels (LRC Data Book 1979). Finally, there are significant differences between black and white children, perhaps starting as early as the preschool years (Berenson et al. 1978). White school-aged children have higher LDL and VLDL cholesterol levels but lower HDL cholesterol levels than black children (Srinivasan et al. 1976; Morrison et al. 1978a). Whether racial differences in lipid and lipoprotein levels are present at birth is controversial (Glueck et al. 1977a; Frerichs et al. 1978). Several of these well-studied populations are already being utilized as a base from which to do prospective, longitudinal studies of tracking of lipid and lipoprotein levels. For example, in the Bogalusa population, the correlation coefficients (r) for the plasma lipid and lipoprotein levels obtained during two successive years ranged from 0.34 to 0.82; the variability (r^2) in the second measurement that could be explained by the first measurement ranged from 11% to 67% (Frerichs et al. 1979).

Plasma apoprotein levels

At least eight polypeptides have been found to be associated with the plasma lipoproteins. The initial research effort has been to characterize the structure and function of these molecules (Smith et al. 1978). ApoA-I and apoA-II are major apoproteins of HDL. ApoB constitute most of the protein of LDL. ApoB is also found in VLDL, the metabolic precursor of LDL. Four apoproteins, apoC-I, apoC-II, apoC-III and apoE are found in VLDL, LDL and HDL. ApoD is confined to HDL. ApoA-I is a cofactor for lecithin cholesterol ester transferase (LCAT) and may play a role in transporting cholesterol from peripheral cells to the liver for re-utilization or excretion. ApoB is the binding protein for the LDL receptor. ApoE, the arginine-rich apoprotein also binds to the LDL receptor and also inhibits lipoprotein lipase. ApoC-II is cofactor for lipoprotein lipase, the major enzyme that hydrolyzes triglycerides. ApoD is involved with exchange of cholesterol ester between lipoproteins.

The association between risk for IHD and lipoprotein concentration has classically been studied by using lipoprotein levels measured in terms of their cholesterol content. This approach assumes that, in general, the composition of the major lipoprotein classes are constant and that the determination of the cholesterol accurately reflects the number of lipoprotein particles in the circulation. It has recently been suggested that apoproteins may be better discriminators than lipids for IHD. We have described, in collaboration with Dr. Allan Sniderman (1980), a group of patients with coronary atherosclerosis who have normal levels of LDL cholesterol but elevated levels of

LDL B protein. The elevated LDL B protein concentrations are as high as those found in patients with type IIa hyperlipoproteinemia and we have chosen to term this group "hyperapobetalipoproteinemia" to distinguish them from the patients who have elevations in both LDL cholesterol and LDL protein levels (Sniderman et al. 1980). Avogaro and co-workers (1979) recently reported that normocholesterolemic survivors of myocardial infarction had significantly higher apoB but lower apoA-I levels than the control group. Further, Rossner et al. (1978) have also found in young patients with ischemic cerebrovascular disease the presence of normal serum cholesterol but low HDL cholesterol levels. It therefore seems most important to determine the apoprotein levels in children, their natural history, their relationship to plasma lipids and lipoprotein levels and what determinants may affect their concentration in plasma.

Determinants of Plasma Lipid, Lipoprotein and Apoprotein Levels

Determinants of the lipid, lipoprotein and apoprotein levels may be exogenous (e.g., diet, hormone use), endogenous (genetic or hormonal regulation of the synthesis and catabolism of lipoproteins and their constituents) or a combination of these two factors (e.g., genetically determined response to dietary factors).

Exogenous factors

Human or cow's milk contain a larger amount of cholesterol than commercially available formulas. Infants fed human or cow's milk have higher plasma cholesterol levels than those fed commercial formulas. However, whether the amount of cholesterol in the milk fed in infancy has any effect on later total plasma cholesterol, apoprotein or lipoprotein levels has not been resolved. mean cholesterol levels (173 mg/100 ml) at ages 7 to 12 years than those fed commerical formulas (157 mg/100 ml). In another study (Friedman and Goldberg 1976), infants fed a modified cholesterol and saturated fat diet from 2-3 months of age had statistically significant lower mean cholesterol levels at two years of age than those fed a "regular" diet; there was no difference between the groups in their growth and development. In a cross-sectional survey of school-aged children, Frank and co-workers (1978) found no significant correlation between intake of dietary cholesterol and saturated fat and plasma cholesterol levels; however, when the children were grouped by qunitiles for plasma cholesterol, those in the upper and middle qunitiles had significantly higher intakes of cholesterol, saturated and polyunsaturated fat than those children in the lower quintile. The significant inverse correlation (r=-0.189) between dietary sucrose and HDL cholesterol levels in this study is of interest. More information is certainly needed on the relation between various dietary constituents and plasma lipoprotein and apoprotein levels from infancy throughout young adulthood. These data would best be obtained in prospective studies. Indeed, Jacobs and co-workers (1979) have recently shown that if certain variances are sufficiently great, even when there may be a cause and effect relation between diet and plasma cholesterol, correlation coefficients close to zero would be expected from the actual data of cross-sectional study.

Other exogenous factors that may affect lipid and lipoprotein levels include the use of birth control pills that can produce hyperlipidemia and affect blood lipoprotein levels (Wallace et al. 1979). Smoking may be associated with significantly lower HDL cholesterol levels in adolescent school children (Morrison et al. 1979b).

Endogenous factors

We have recently presented strong evidence for familial aggregations of plasma cholesterol and triglyceride levels in 242 families selected through a pediatric proband from a free living population (Chase et al. 1979). While it is clear that there are mixed genetic and environmental (also termed multifactorial) influences on plasma lipid and lipoprotein cholesterol levels, little is known about the factors that regulate the synthesis and catabolism of LDL and HDL in normal children or those with mild forms of primary hypercholesterolemia. For ethical reasons, these metabolic studies cannot be performed in the healthy pediatric age group. Certain clues can be taken from metabolic studies in children with homozygous familial hypercholesterolemia, precocious atherosclerosis before the age of 20 years and a deficiency of functional cell surface receptors for LDL (Bilheimer et al. 1979). Bilheimer and co-workers (1979) recently reported that the fractional catabolic rate for apoB of LDL was only one-third of normal in 7 FH homozygotes and appeared fixed at about 17%/day. Despite the similarity in the catabolic rate, the plasma LDL levels varied and the level was highly correlated (r = 0.94) with the synthetic rates of apoB of LDL. The endogenous synthesis of cholesterol in these homozygous FH children was not increased and the choleserol must therefore be re-utilized to maintain the increased synthesis of apoLDL. If these studies may be extrapolated to normal children, the synthetic rate of apoB of LDL may play an important role in determining the level of total plasma and LDL cholesterol, provided that the catabolic rates of LDL are approximately equal.

Less is known about the endogenous metabolism of HDL in children. Male hormones probably affect either the synthesis or catabolism of HDL since HDL levels fall significantly in post-adolescent males. Thus, adolescence may provide an important clue to determinants of plasma HDL levels and there is now a need for good prospective, longitudinal studies throughout this period of life that might profitably include the careful measurement of both sex and trophic hormones, as well as plasma lipoprotein and apoprotein levels. Other clues may be derived from newborns and children heterozygous for FH who have lower HDL cholesterol levels than normal children; the persistence of these low HDL levels in adults with FH has been found to be associated with IHD, an effect separate but not necessarily independent of the elevated LDL levels (Streja et al. 1978). Familial aggregation of high HDL cholesterol levels has been described and this "hyperalphalipoproteinemia" can be expressed in infancy and childhood (Glueck et al. 1977b).

Undoubtedly, a number of genes are involved in the regulation of these complex processes. The development of biological assays to assess the synthesis and catabolism of lipoproteins in children will be paramount for future studies on endogenous factors that affect lipoprotein metabolism in children.

Interaction of exogenous and endogenous factors

The extent of heterogenous response to dietary factors, such as cholesterol, in the general population of children is, for the most part, undocumented. For example, it is not known if there is a human equivalent to some non-human primates who have a genetic predisposition to handle increased dietary cholesterol differently; some animals have a marked rise in the plasma cholesterol levels (hyper-responders) while others have little change at all (hypo-responders).

It is important to understand further changes in the composition of the lipoproteins with dietary modification. For example, in animals fed high cholesterol diets, an altered HDL, termed HDL_c, is induced. HDL_c has an increased content of the arginine rich apoprotein, apoE, and competes with LDL for the

LDL receptor site in cultured fibroblasts (Mahley et al. 1978). Mahley and co-workers (1978) recently showed that the daily consumption of large (4 to 6) numbers of eggs by young adults, whether or not it lead to an increase in plasma cholesterol, altered the properties of human HDL. The dietary induced HDL contained a subfraction enriched in apoE. The competitive binding of this HDL to the LDL receptor site was enhanced 2.6 to 4 fold compared to HDL obtained from the subjects before diet. Further studies are required to learn about the possible significance of HDL_c in human lipoprotein metabolism and atherosclerosis.

Detection and Modification of Risk Factors

Detection of risk factors and screening

Some of the questions concerning the detection of children "at risk" for atherosclerosis are still investigational and need to be pursued in longitudinal studies of free-living populations, or on the metabolic ward or on the cellular level. In view of the currently available knowledge, there is some urgency, however, to "identify" certain "risk factors" such as hyperlipidemia in children. Several different approaches have been taken at detecting these hyperlipidemic children. From 16 to 33% of children who have one parent with premature IHD have been found to have hyperlipidemia (Kwiterovich 1977). Screening the pediatric offspring of "hyperlipidemic" parents from a general population is less efficient. For example, in Columbia, Maryland, we found that the enrichment in screening children of hyperlipidemic parents was confined to a two-fold increase in hypercholesterolemia in offspring of hypercholesterolemic fathers (Chase et al. 1979). Further, Morrison and co-workers (1978b) found that children from a "high cholesterol level household" were only 2.7 times more likely than children from the total pediatric population to have cholesterol levels above 205 mg/100 ml, the pediatric 95th percentile in the Cincinnati population. Screening entire pediatric populations for hyperlipidemia is a third approach. General screening is fraught with multiple difficulties including methodological problems, interpretation of results, followup and treatment. For example, several methods that are currently used to determine cholesterol levels provide significantly different results (Albers et al. 1978). Further, Morrison et al. (1979a) found that 16% of hypercholesterolemic school children (above 95th percentile) had elevated HDL cholesterol but normal LDL cholesterol levels. These children would not warrant treatment. When the immunochemical measurement of apoprotein levels using microtechniques becomes feasible for large scale application, screening may become more cost-efficient. When combined with cholesterol measurements, the use of immunochemical techniques may identify subsets of children with normal lipid levels but with elevated or depressed apoproteins or lipoproteins of abnormal composition. Apoprotein measurements may yet provide some usefulness for cord blood screening.

Treatment of disorders of lipoprotein metabolism

There is a reasonable consensus that children with primary hyperlipidemia should be treated with diet modification (American Heart Association, 1978). Children with hypercholesterolemia have been usually treated with a diet low in cholesterol and saturated fats but enriched in polyunsaturated fats. Possible side effects of the diets require long-term monitoring; these include the effects of phytosterols and polyunsaturated fats on gallstone production, carcinoma of the gastrointestinal tract and maturation and growth and development. Sheperd and co-workers (1978) found that a diet containing a ratio of polyunsaturated to saturated fats of 4:1 significantly depressed

HDL cholesterol and apoA-I levels, presumably through decreased apoA-I synthesis. Some espouse a dietary change for all American children regardless of their plasma lipid and lipoprotein levels, as an across-the-board public health measure. At the other extreme are those who believe that no intervention is indicated because the diet-heart hypothesis has not been proven. Some theoretical and practical concerns about these approaches have been previously discussed in more detail and will not be repeated here (Kwiterovich and Salz 1979).

When indicated, drug of choice for FH in childhood has been cholestyramine and a dosage schedule modified for children has been worked out (Farah et al. 1977). Although quite effective, especially over the short term, there are problems with long-term compliance to an agent that is both expensive and difficult to take. Further research on the problem of motivation and its solution is necessary. Finally, newer and more practical lipid-lowering drugs need to be developed.

Effect of Treatment in Childhood on the Development of Atherosclerosis

An answer to this question in the near furture will most likely be confined to observing the effects of surgical intervention (portacaval shunt) or plasmapheresis on lowering total plasma and LDL cholesterol levels and regression of coronary atherosclerosis in children homozygous for FH (National Heart and Lung Institute 1974, Thompson et al. 1975). The development of non-invasive techniques to detect atherosclerosis may allow a more general approach to answering this question in future years.

References

Albers JJ, Warnick GR, Chenng MC (1978) Quantitation of high density lipoproteins. Lipids 13: 926-932
American Heart Assocation (1978) The value and safety of diet modification to control hyperlipidemia in childhood and adolescence. A statement for physicians. Circulation 58: 381A-387A.
Avogaro P, Bon GB, Cazzolato G, Quinci GB (1979) Are apolipoproteins better discriminators than lipids for atherosclerosis? Lancet 1: 901-903
Berenson GS, Foster TA, Frank GC, Frerichs RR, Srinivasan SR, Voors AW, Webber LS (1978) Cardiovascular disease risk factor variables at the preschool age -- the Bogalusa Heart Study. Circulation 57: 603-612
Bilheimer DW, Stone NJ, Grundy SC (1979) Metabolic studies in familial hypercholesterolemia (evidence for a gene-dosage effect in vivo). J Clin Invest 64: 524-533
Chase G, Kwiterovich PO, Bachorik P (1979) Columbia Population Study. II. Familial aggregation of plasma cholesterol and triglycerides. Johns Hopk Med J 145: 150-156
Farah R, Kwiterovich PO, Neill CA (1977) A study of the dose-effect of cholestyramine in children and young adults with familial hypercholesterolemia. Lancet 1: 59-63
Frank GC, Berenson GS, Webber LS (1978) Dietary studies and the relationship of diet to cardiovascular disease risk factor variables in 10-year-old children -- the Bogalusa Heart Study. Am J Clin Nutr 31: 328-340
Frerichs RR, Srinivasan SR, Webber LS, Rieth MC, Berenson GS (1978) Serum lipids and lipoproteins at birth in a biracial population: The Bogalusa Heart Study. Pediat Res 12: 858-863

Frerichs RR, Webber LS, Voors AW, Srinivasan SR, Berenson GS (1979) Cardiovascular disease risk factor variables in children at two successive
years -- the Bogalusa Heart Study. J Chron Dis 32: 251-262
Friedman G, Goldberg SJ (1976) An evaluation of the safety of a low saturated
fat, low cholesterol diet beginning in infancy. Pediatrics 58: 655-657
Glueck CJ, Gartside PS, Tsang RC, Miller M, Steiner PM (1977a) Black-white
similarities in cord blood lipids and lipoproteins. A preliminary report.
Metabolism 26: 347-350
Glueck CJ, Tsang RC, Mellies MJ, Steiner PM (1977b) Neonatal familial hyper-
alphalipoproteinemia. Metabolism 26: 469-472
Hodgson PA, Ellefson RD, Elveback LR, Harris LE, Nelson RA, Weidman WH (1976)
Comparison of serum cholesterol in children fed high, moderate, or low
cholesterol milk diets during neonatal period. Metabolism 25: 739-746
Jacobs Jr PR, Anderson JT, Blackburn H (1979) Diet and serum cholesterol.
Do zero correlations negate the relationship? Am J Epid 110: 77-87
Kwiterovich PO (1977) Pediatric aspects of hyperlipoproteinemia. In: Rifkind
BM, Levy RI (eds) Hyperlipidemia, Diagnosis and Therapy. Grune and
Stratton, New Jersey, pp 249-280
Kwiterovich PO, Salz K (1979) Pediatric aspects of the diet-heart hypothesis.
In: Bond J (ed) Proceedings of an International Symposium on Infant
and Child Feeding. In press
Lipid Research Clinic Data Book (1979) Selected variables in eleven North
American populations. Vol I. Physiologic and socio-demographic charac-
teristics. DHEW, in press
Mahley RW, Innerarity TL, Bersot TP, Lipson A, Margolis S (1978) Alterations
in human high-density lipoproteins, with or without increased plasma-
cholesterol, induced by diets high in cholesterol. Lancet: 807-809
Morrison JA, deGroot I, Edwards BK, Kelly KA, Mellies MJ, Khoury P, Glueck
CJ (1978a) Lipids and lipoproteins in 927 schoolchildren ages 6 to 17
years. Pediatrics 62: 990-995
Morrison JA, Kelly KA, Mellies M, deGroot I, Glueck CJ (1978b) Parent-child
associations at upper and lower ranges of plasma cholesterol and triglyc-
eride levels. Pediatrics 62: 468-477
Morrison JA, deGroot I, Kelly KA, Edwards BK, Mellies MJ, Tillett S, Khoury
P, Glueck CJ (1979a) High and low density lipoprotein cholesterol levels
in hypercholesterolemic school children. Lipids 14: 99-104
Morrison JA, Kelly K, Mellies M, deGroot I, Khoury P, Gartside P, Glueck CJ
(1979b) Cigarette smoking, alcohol intake, and oral contraceptives:
Relationships to lipids and lipoproteins in adolescent school-children.
Metabolism, in press
National Heart and Lung Institute. Workshop on Portacaval Shunt in the
Management of Homozygous Familial Hypercholesterolemia, August 1974
Rössner S, Kjellin KG, Mettinger KL, Sidén A, Söderström CE (1978) Normal
serum cholesterol but low HDL cholesterol concentration in young patients
with cerebrovascular disease. Lancet 1: 577-579
Schrott HG, Clarke WR, Wiebe DA, Connor WE, Lauer RM (1979) Increased coronary
mortality in relatives of hypercholesterolemic school children: the
Musatine study. Circulation 59: 320-326.
Shepherd J, Packard CJ, Patsch JR, Gotto AM, Taunton OB (1978) Effects of
dietary polyunsaturated and saturated fat on the properties of high
density lipoproteins and the metabolism of apoA-I. J Clin Invest 61:
1582-1592
Smith LC, Pownall HJ, Gotto Jr AM (1978) The plasma lipoproteins: structure
and metabolism. Ann Rev Biochem 47: 751
Sniderman A, Shapiro S, Marpole D, Malcolm I, Skinner B, Teng B, Kwiterovich
PO (1980) The association of coronary atherosclerosis and hyperapobetalipoproteinemia (increased protein but normal cholesterol content in
human plasma low density lipoprotein). Proc Natl Acad Sci, in press.
Specialized Centers of Research in Arteriosclerosis (1978) Cardiovascular
profile of 15,000 children of school age in three communities. 1971-1975.
DHEW Publicat-on No. (NIH) 78-1472

Srinivasan SR, Frerichs RR, Weber LS, Berenson GS (1976) Serum lipoprotein profile in children from a biracial community -- the Bogalusa Heart Study. Circulation 54: 309-318

Streja D, Steiner G, Kwiterovich Jr PO (1978) Plasma high density lipoproteins and other lipids and lipoproteins and ischemic heart disease in a large Newfoundland pedigree with familial hypercholesterolemia. Ann Int Med 89: 871-880

Thompson GR, Lowenthal R, Myant NB (1975) plasma exchange in the management of homozygous familial hypercholesterolaemia. Lancet 1: 1208-1211

Wallace R, Hoover J, Barrett-Connor E, Rifkind BM, Hunninghake DB, Mackenthun A, Heiss G (1979) Altered plasma lipid and lipoprotein levels associated with oral contraceptive and estrogen use. Lancet 2: 111-114

Tracking of Coronary Risk Factors in Children: The Muscatine Study[1]

Ronald M. Lauer and William R. Clarke

Physicians routinely plot the heights and weights of children on charts. In using these charts it has been noted that children tend to maintain their percentile rank with increasing age. Children who have high percentiles tend to stay high as they mature, and children who begin low tend to stay low. A child who deviates from his or her percentile rank for height or weight over time may be suspected of having some chronic growth perturbing disease. The phenomenon of children maintaining their rank within their age-sex group is herein referred to as "tracking". Height and weight are said to "track with age". This study describes and compares the degree of tracking that occurs for measures of height, weight, triceps skinfold thickness, blood pressures, cholesterol and triglyceride over the school age in order to examine their consistency in childhood.

Subjects and Methods

The school children of Muscatine, Iowa have participated in a screening program for coronary risk factors since 1970. The great majority of children in the schools of Muscatine are white (96.4%). The children sampled were in kindergarten through twelfth grade and ranged in age from 5-18 years. Other data relating to this population and their measurements have been published previously by Lauer et al. (1975), and Clarke et al. (1978).

To date, four cross sectional screenings at two-year intervals have examined 8,909 children. Of these, 3,848 have been seen only once, 2,409 twice, 1,368 three times and 1,284 have been examined in all four school screens. Since the initial school screen took two school years, there are observations six years apart on only 820 children. Of the 1,284 children sampled in all four school screens, 662 have been followed six years and 622 for five years.

Height and Weight

Pearson correlations between measurements made on the same individuals two, four, and six years apart are displayed in Table 1. Correlations between repeated observations of height and weight were high (approximately 0.88 for two years, 0.80 for four years, and 0.74 for six years). A high proportion of children in the extreme percentiles were still there on follow-up.

---

[1]The author's research cited was supported by an Atherosclerosis Specialized Center of Research grant from the National Heart, Lung and Blood Institute, National Institutes of Health, HL 14230 and a research grant HL 20124.

Table 1. Pearson correlations between repeated measurements.*

Initial age	Number		Height		Weight		Skinfold		Cholesterol	
	Male	Female	Male	Female	Male	Female	Male	Female	Male	Female
Observations 2 Years Apart										
5	48	52	0.78	0.88	0.88	0.92	0.50	0.62	0.63	0.64
6	217	204	0.89	0.87	0.90	0.89	0.60	0.65	0.66	0.73
7	288	297	0.87	0.88	0.89	0.92	0.70	0.72	0.71	0.65
8	381	387	0.92	0.89	0.90	0.90	0.74	0.77	0.73	0.66
9	446	478	0.88	0.86	0.93	0.91	0.80	0.76	0.62	0.68
10	458	492	0.88	0.87	0.91	0.91	0.74	0.82	0.70	0.69
11	422	462	0.87	0.84	0.92	0.90	0.76	0.74	0.70	0.66
12	403	443	0.86	0.80	0.92	0.89	0.74	0.75	0.65	0.68
13	315	368	0.87	0.88	0.89	0.88	0.67	0.68	0.66	0.69
14	261	336	0.81	0.93	0.90	0.89	0.71	0.70	0.72	0.67
15	204	251	0.84	0.96	0.88	0.93	0.57	0.69	0.73	0.71
16	78	80	0.89	0.99	0.89	0.83	0.68	0.74	0.71	0.67
Overall	7371		0.87		0.90		0.73		0.68	
Observations 4 Years Apart										
6	57	63	0.89	0.89	0.80	0.90	0.46	0.57	0.63	0.65
7	127	156	0.78	0.80	0.84	0.88	0.70	0.66	0.67	0.69
8	204	213	0.80	0.82	0.81	0.81	0.63	0.69	0.70	0.71
9	260	264	0.79	0.81	0.85	0.85	0.68	0.71	0.65	0.64
10	255	274	0.84	0.75	0.87	0.84	0.60	0.71	0.64	0.60
11	223	255	0.74	0.68	0.85	0.77	0.70	0.65	0.63	0.62
12	192	222	0.74	0.64	0.83	0.76	0.63	0.65	0.61	0.60
13	151	170	0.67	0.80	0.79	0.83	0.47	0.71	0.54	0.58
14	89	93	0.68	0.88	0.82	0.80	0.71	0.64	0.64	0.60
Overall	3268		0.77		0.83		0.65		0.63	
Observations 6 Years Apart										
8	67	76	0.76	0.78	0.64	0.76	0.50	0.70	0.69	0.48
9	109	117	0.83	0.68	0.79	0.72	0.72	0.68	0.63	0.63
10	103	100	0.84	0.65	0.83	0.73	0.62	0.75	0.65	0.61
11	96	83	0.77	0.52	0.70	0.74	0.64	0.59	0.66	0.67
12	33	32	0.81	0.78	0.69	0.72	0.63	0.65	0.66	0.48†
Overall	816		0.74		0.74		0.65		0.61	

Table 1. (continued)

Initial age	Fasting triglyceride		Systolic blood pressure		Diastolic blood pressure	
	Male	Female	Male	Female	Male	Female
	Observations 2 Years Apart					
5	0.38*	0.34*	0.27(NS)	0.35†	0.38†	0.22(NS)
6	0.42	0.47	0.34	0.37	0.18†	0.27
7	0.39	0.51	0.42	0.36	0.28	0.17†
8	0.39	0.46	0.34	0.40	0.13†	0.27
9	0.34	0.50	0.44	0.41	0.22	0.27
10	0.42	0.47	0.32	0.42	0.22	0.24
11	0.48	0.43	0.46	0.44	0.28	0.24
12	0.46	0.46	0.40	0.42	0.26	0.35
13	0.34	0.40	0.45	0.42	0.42	0.21
14	0.42	0.42	0.53	0.42	0.41	0.28
15	0.57	0.40	0.42	0.42	0.39	0.36
16	0.54	0.48	0.57	0.59	0.28†	0.39
Overall	0.44		0.41		0.27	
	Observations 4 Years Apart					
6	0.39†	0.44	0.39	0.32†	0.04(NS)	0.11(NS)
7	0.30†	0.52	0.47	0.27	0.28†	0.04(NS)
8	0.27†	0.26†	0.35	0.35	0.14*	0.24
9	0.31	0.41	0.44	0.41	0.25	0.19†
10	0.43	0.40	0.35	0.28	0.27	0.21
11	0.35	0.41	0.35	0.33	0.18†	0.22
12	0.59	0.53	0.28	0.27	0.20†	0.21
13	0.50	0.24*	0.42	0.38	0.33	0.23†
14	0.40*	0.55	0.28†	0.36	0.32†	0.14(NS)
Overall	0.40		0.35		0.21	
	Observations 6 Years Apart					
8	—	—	0.11(NS)	0.40	0.28*	0.21(NS)
9	—	—	0.41	0.22	0.25†	0.22*
10	—	—	0.50	0.08(NS)	0.09(NS)	0.07(NS)
11	—	—	0.34	0.29†	0.06(NS)	0.31†
12	—	—	0.02(NS)	0.53†	0.33(NS)	0.15(NS)
Overall			0.30		0.18	

*0.01<p<0.05   †0.001<p<0.01   p<0.05 (NS); otherwise p<0.001

Even though the correlations for height and weight were high, some variation in percentile ranks with time was observed. About 60% of those children were again in the lowest quintile of height six years later, while 26% had risen to the second quintile and nearly 14% were above the third quintile. Similarly, of those children who were initially in the highest quintile for height, 60% were again there six years later, 26% had dropped to the fourth quintile and 14% had dropped below the fourth quintile. Of those children initially in the middle quintile for height, 33% were again there six years later, while 10% were found in the lowest quintile and 12% were found in the highest quintile. This symmetry of the highs becoming lower and the lows becoming higher is an example of the phenomenon called "regression toward the mean" (Ederer 1972).

Triceps Skinfold Thickness

Triceps skinfold is presented as an example of a measure of obesity. Results for other measures of obesity, including ponderal index ($Ht/\sqrt[3]{Wt}$) and relative weight (weight corrected for age, sex and height), were similar. Most two-year correlations were between 0.7 and 0.8 for both males and females (Table 1). Four-year and six-year correlations ranged between 0.46-0.71 with most values being greater than 0.6.

Cholesterol

Overall, two, four, and six-year correlations for cholesterol were 0.68, 0.63, and 0.61, respectively, and age-sex specific correlations ranged between 0.48 and 0.73. The differences between two-year and six-year correlations were generally small. Greater variability in percentile ranks with time was observed for cholesterol than for height or weight. After a six year interval, 57% of children initially in the lowest quintile were again in the first quintile, 17% were in the second quintile, 14% were in the third quintile, and 12% were above the third quintile. Similarly, of those subjects initially in the highest quintile, 50% were there again, 26% were in the fourth quintile, 15% in the third quintile and 9% below the third quintile. Two-year and four-year quintile distributions were very similar. The effect of time on the magnitudes of correlations between repeated observations and changes in percentile ranks was less pronounced than for height or weight. (Clarke et al. 1978)

Triglyceride

Large changes in percentile ranks with time were observed. One-third of those children initially in the lowest quintile were found there four years later while 21% were above the 60th percentile. Of those children initially in the highest quintile, 40% were again there after four years and 19% had dropped below the 40th percentile. After a four year interval, the distribution of quintiles of those children initially in the middle quintile was very nearly a random 20% in each of the five quintiles.

Blood Pressure

Overall correlations for systolic blood pressure were 0.41 for observations separated by two years, 0.35 for observations separated by four years and 0.30 for observations six years apart. Overall correlations for diastolic blood pressure were 0.27, 0.21 and 0.18 for observations two, four and six years apart, respectively. Four-year and six-year correlations were usually smaller than two-year correlations. Although correlations for both systolic and diastolic blood pressure were generally significant (P<0.001), all were relatively small and several of the age- and sex-specific correlations for diastolic blood pressure were not statistically significant (P>0.05). Although weaker than observed for height and weight, there was still a tendency for children in the extreme percentiles of systolic blood pressure to maintain their rank orderings. The middle quintile distribution closely resembled a random 20% in each quintile. The distributions of follow-up diastolic blood pressure quintiles after six years was nearly a random scatter for all five quintiles.

Persistence of High Values

In clinical practice one is usually interested in patients who have consistently high levels of obesity, serum lipids or blood pressure. Figure 1 displays the estimated probability of a child who was initially found in the upper quintile of being there consistently on repeated measurement.

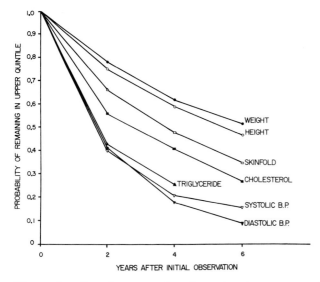

Figure 1. Persistence of values in the upper quintile. Entries in this figure are estimates of the probabilities that a child in the upper quintile for a variable will continue to be there on repeated examinations spaced at two year intervals. If a child fell below the 80th percentile at any stage then he was not considered in subsequent steps. Approximately 900 children were in the upper quintile of a variable, initially. Since the rate at which children dropped below the 80th percentile was different for each variable, the numbers of children eligible to continue at each stage was also differed. (Courtesy of Clarke et al 1978)

When those with values in the upper quintile of blood pressure were examined over a period of six years at two-year intervals, it was noted that with each succeeding examination subjects emerged who were tracking well. This is indicated by the nearly horizontal slope of systolic and diastolic blood pressure in Figure 1 between the fourth and sixth years. Thus, repeated blood pressure measurement can identify subjects who are tracking with persistently high blood pressures.

In order to characterize the subjects whose cholesterols and blood pressures remained in the upper quintile of the distribution on four occasions over six years, corrected scores (standard deviation units for age, sex and survey year) were calculated for their descriptive variables measured on the initial examination. Table 2 shows these scores. In those with persistently high cholesterols, triglycerides were elevated (P<0.01) and they tended to have higher blood pressures. In those with persistently high systolic blood pressures, the subjects were taller, heavier, and more obese as indicated by higher relative weights and triceps skinfold thickness. They also had higher diastolic pressure (P<0.01) for age. The subjects with persistently high diastolic pressure showed similar features. Of those with persistently high relative weights, triglyceride levels, as well as systolic and diastolic blood pressure were elevated (P<0.01). In addition they tended to have higher cholesterols (p<0.06).

Discussion

Measurement of children's heights, weights and skinfold thicknesses is clearly a useful assessment tool for physicians. There is a high correlation of early measurements to future levels, and only a small percentage of children in the extremes of the distributions show large changes in percentile ranks. The practice of plotting a child's height and weight against percentile grids is useful in distinguishing a child who is growing well from one who has growth difficulties. Measures that are used as indices of obesity (skinfold thickness, relative weight and ponderal index) show similar tendencies because they also exhibit high correlations between measurements repeated over time.

Cholesterol measurements also track reasonably well. Nearly 60% of subjects initially in the highest quintile were found there again six years later. The probability of remaining in the upper quintile for four consecutive screens was estimated to be 0.27.

Triglyceride and casual blood pressure showed a lower correlation between early and future levels. Triglyceride levels yielded correlations over two years approximately 0.4; 65% of upper quintile subjects stayed in the upper two quintiles, and 35% dropped to the lower three. Systolic blood pressure had an overall six-year correlation of 0.30 with 60% of upper quintile subjects staying in the upper two quintiles. Diastolic blood pressure showed six-year correlations of 0.18 and, except for the upper quintile, distributions of percentile ranks were nearly random.

The children who tracked persistently in the upper quintile of cholesterol did not appear to have features of height, weight or ponderosity which distinguish them from the general population. However, those with blood pressures which tracked in the upper quintile were significantly taller and heavier and more obese than other children. Those whose relative weight tracked in the upper quintile had significantly higher triglycerides and blood pressures initially.

The observation in adults that risk for coronary heart disease is related to a single elevated cholesterol or blood pressure, despite the fact that these measurements have considerable variability with time, raises the question of whether the same may also be true in children. In both children and adults, casual blood pressures are highly variable in their measurement and require repetitive observation to identify those who have persistent pressure elevations (Rames et al. 1978; Report of the Task Force 1977). In adults, pressures are more variable in persons with higher levels, and there is no correlations between the degree of variability at one point in time to another time. Despite this variability which does not allow a precise characterization for an individual, single blood pressure measurements are predictive of future cardiovascular disease (Gordon and Shurtleff 1973). There is no

Table 2. Initial character of those with levels in the upper quintiles over six years.

	Height	Weight	Relative Weight	Triceps Skinfold	Cholesterol	Triglycerides	Systolic BP	Diastolic BP
High Cholesterol n=78								
Mean Z*	-0.03	0.05	0.06	0.12	1.65	0.29	0.19	0.21
SE	0.11	0.12	0.13	0.12	0.07	0.11	0.11	0.11
p	0.80	0.66	0.65	0.33	0.001	0.01	0.09	0.06
High Systolic BP n=41								
Mean Z	0.67	1.22	1.01	0.85	0.09	0.34	1.76	0.73
SE	0.13	0.24	0.25	0.19	0.14	0.20	0.14	0.18
p	0.001	0.001	0.001	0.001	0.55	0.11	0.001	0.001
High Diastolic BP n=32								
Mean Z	0.53	1.01	0.87	0.91	-0.04	-0.01	1.08	1.49
SE	0.16	0.32	0.34	0.19	0.22	0.23	0.22	0.13
p	0.002	0.003	0.02	0.001	0.88	0.97	0.001	0.001
High Relative Weight n=104								
Mean Z	0.34	1.75	2.04	1.60	0.21	0.50	0.66	0.51
SE	0.10	0.14	0.11	0.08	0.11	0.12	0.10	0.09
p	0.001	0.001	0.001	0.001	0.06	0.001	0.001	0.001

* Z=age, sex, initial survey year standard deviation unit.

longitudinal study of children relating casual blood pressure measurements at an early age to the risk of future cardiovascular disease. Until such information is obtained, the significance of casual elevation of blood pressure in childhood will remain in doubt.

References

Clarke WR, Schrott HG, Leaverton PE, Connor WE and Lauer RM (1978): Tracking of Blood Lipids and Blood Pressure in School Age Children: The Muscatine Study. Circulation 58:626-634

Ederer F (1972): Serum cholesterol changes: effects of diet and regression toward the mean. J Chronic Dis 25:277

Gordon T, Shurtleff D (1973): Means at each examination and interexamination variation of specified characteristics: Framingham Study, Exam 1 to Exam 10. Washington, D.C., Section 29 DHEW Publication No (NIH) 74-478

Lauer RM, Connor WE, Leaverton PE, Reiter MA, Clarke WR (1975): Coronary heart disease factors in school children: The Muscatine Study. J Pediatr 86:697

Rames L, Clarke W, Reiter MA, Lauer RM (1978): The prevalence of hypertension in school age children: The Muscatine Study. Pediatrics 60:493

Report of the Task Force on Blood Pressure Control in Children (1977). Pediatrics 59 (suppl): 797

Risk Factors in Children: Role of Hereditary Hyperlipoproteinemia

Richard J. West and June K. Lloyd

In some inherited disorders characterized by hyperlipoproteinemia, the risk of development of ischemic heart disease (IHD) in early or middle adult life is high, and attempts during childhood aimed at the prevention of IHD should concentrate on these individuals.

The major inherited diseases predisposing to IHD are

a. Familial hypercholesterolemia (Type IIa, familial hyperbetalipoproteinemia)
b. Familial combined hyperlipidemia (Type IIb)
c. Familial (endogenous) hypertriglyceridemia (Type IV).

Familial hypercholesterolemia (FH) is a common, dominantly inherited condition with biochemical features expressed from early childhood; familial combined hyperlipidemia is probably also dominantly inherited. In childhood it is usually expressed as hypercholesterolemia rather than as hypertriglyceridemia or combined hyperlipidemia (Glueck et al. 1973). Familial hypertriglyceridemia is only infrequently manifest in childhood.

Biochemical study of individuals with premature IHD and their families will identify those with inherited hyperlipoproteinemias. FH can be detected in childhood but if the primary disease is thought to be hypertriglyceridemia or combined hyperlipidemia children apparently unaffected should be retested after puberty. With such family studies case detection will inevitably be incomplete but the diagnostic problems and practical and ethical difficulties associated with treatment rule out population screening for hyperlipidemia in children at the present time.

As FH is the major hyperlipidemia to occur in children further discussion will be limited to this condition. The population incidence of FH, based on screening and family studies on large numbers in the U.S. (Tsang et al. 1974; Goldstein et al. 1974) and in Germany (Greten et al. 1974), suggest an incidence of 0.2-0.5%, and smaller studies from other countries are in general agreement with these estimates.

The risks of developing IHD for individuals with FH are high (Slack 1969; Stone et al. 1974). In the British study 51% of affected males had had symptoms of IHD, and 24% had died by the age of 50 (Slack 1969). This should be compared with a risk for men of dying from IHD by the age of 50 of 1.7% for the general British population. Women with FH are at less risk of IHD than are affected males, but for them the risks are still considerable. Individuals with FH are at much greater risk of IHD than individuals who are hypercholesterolemic for other reasons.

Children with FH are at considerable risk of developing IHD in adult life. Early diagnosis and intervention therapy to lower serum cholesterol would seem to offer the best chance of delaying the development of atherosclerosis. It is equally important to avoid other adverse risk factors in these children by encouraging an active lifestyle, avoidance of smoking, and the maintenance of a normal body weight and blood pressure.

Table 1. Results of cholestyramine treatment in 35 children with FH.

| | Start | Completed years of Cholestyramine treatment | | | | | |
		1	2	3	4	5	6
No. on treatment	35	26	25	22	21	16	15
Mean cholesterol mg/dl	357	251	250	255	269	263	258
% reduction	–	30	31	30	26	28	30
No. off drug treatment	–	6	7	10	10	13	13
No. transferred	–	3	3	3	4	6	7
Compliance %	–	81	78	69	68	55	54
Mean dose g/kg/day	–	0.42					0.38

Initially, lowering of plasma cholesterol should be attempted by dietary means by altering the amount and type of dietary fat. Utilizing diets it is possible in the short term to lower plasma cholesterol in FH by about 20%, although there is wide variation between individuals (Segall et al. 1970; Kwiterovich et al. 1970; Schlierf et al. 1977; Glueck et al. 1977a). Even with a significant reduction, plasma cholesterol concentrations remain above the normal range in many patients.

In the longer term, dietary treatment of FH is less successful (West et al. 1975; Schlierf et al. 1977). Compliance with the diet is difficult, especially if the individual eats away from home. In our own series only about 20% of children with FH maintained satisfactory cholesterol lowering with diet as the only form of treatment. Nevertheless, we feel dietary fat modification should be the first treatment tried in all patients with FH.

When dietary treatment alone is inadequate, or if compliance with the diet is poor, drug treatment may be needed. The anion exchange resin cholestyramine is probably the drug of choice, and there is now prolonged experience on the use of cholestyramine in children with FH. In the short term cholesterol is lowered by 18-39% (West and Lloyd 1973; Farah et al. 1977; Glueck et al. 1977b). Cholestyramine is somewhat unpalatable, being a bulky powder which must be mixed with water or fruit juice. Our practice is to start with a small dose of 2 or 4 g twice daily before meals, and gradually increase the dose until the plasma cholesterol is within the normal range, or until the maximum tolerated dose is being taken. Having previously shown that cholestyramine without diet is as effective in lowering plasma cholesterol concentrations as is cholestyramine with diet (West and Lloyd 1973), when the drug is started the diet is liberalized, and most of our patients are on a full normal diet.

Up until July 1973, we had recommended cholestyramine to 35 children aged 1 to 17 years with the heterozygous form of FH, and follow-up of this group permits long term evaluation of the drug. Most of the patients were referred because of a family history of IHD, but 9 were detected while being investigated for intercurrent problems, or by screening, and had no close family history of IHD.

The results are summarized in Table 1. Of the 35 children being recommended cholestyramine, 6 abandoned treatment and 3 others transferred to the care of other physicians during the first year. The remaining 26 children had a reduction in mean plasma cholesterol from a pre-treatment value of 360 mg/dl to 251 mg/dl on treatment, a reduction of 30%, on a mean cholestyramine does of 12.2 g/day, or 0.42 g/kg/day.

By the end of 6 years, 15 patients were known to remain on cholestyramine while 13 had stopped the treatment or defaulted from our clinic, a compliance of 54%. For 7 patients who had transferred to the care of other physicians, data was not available. In the 15 known to remain on cholestyramine, the mean dose was 17.7 g/day (0.38 g/kg/day) and the mean reduction in plasma cholesterol was 30%.

Compliance with therapy was better in those with family history of IHD than in those without, but compliance is not apparently influenced by age or sex of the child. Although both efficacy and compliance using cholestyramine is better than with dietary fat modification, as therapy in FH must inevitably be prolonged, new approaches to treatment are needed.

References

Farah JR, Kwiterovich PO, Neill CA (1977) Dose effect relation of cholestyramine in children and young adults with familial hypercholesterolemia. Lancet 1:54
Glueck CJ, Fallat R, Buncher CR, Tsang R, Steiner P (1973) Familial combined hyperlipoproteinemia: Studies in 91 adults and 95 children from 33 kindreds. Metabolism 22:1403
Glueck CJ, Tsang RC, Fallat RW, Mellies MJ (1977a) Diet in children heterozygous for familial hyercholesterolemia. Am J Dis Child 131:162
Glueck CJ, Tsang RC, Fallat RW, Mellies M (1977b) Therapy of familial hypercholesterolemia in childhood: Diet and cholestyramine resin for 24 to 36 months. Pediatrics 59:433
Goldstein JL, Albers JJ, Schrott HG, Hazzard WR, Bierman EL, Motulsky AG (1974) Plasma lipid levels and coronary heart disease in adult relatives of newborns with normal and elevated cord blood lipids. Am J Hum Genet 26:727
Greten H, Wagner M, Schettler G (1974) Frühdiagnose und Häufigkeit der familiaren hyperlipoproteinamie typ II. Dtsch Med Wochenschr 99:2553
Schlierf G, Hueck CC, Oster P, Raetzer H, Shellenberg B, Vogel G (1977) Dietary management of familial type II hyperlipoproteinemia in children and adults – a feasibility study. In: Manning GW, Haust MD (eds) Atherosclerosis. Plenum Press, New York
Segall MM, Fosbrooke AS, Lloyd JK, Wolff OH (1970) Treatment of familial hypercholesterolemia in children. Lancet 1:641
Slack J (1969) Risks of ischaemic heart disease in familial hyperlipoproteinaemic states. Lancet 2:1380
Stone NJ, Levy RI, Fredrickson DS, Verter J (1974) Coronary artery disease in 116 kindred with familial type II hyperlipoproteinemia. Circulation 49:476
Tsang R, Fallat R, Glueck CJ (1974) Plasma cholesterol at birth and age 1. Pediatrics 53:458
West RJ, Lloyd JK (1973) Use of cholestyramine in treatment of children with familial hypercholesterolemia. Arch Dis Childh 48:370
West RJ, Fosbrooke AS, Lloyd JK (1975) Treatment of children with familial hypercholesterolemia. Postgrad Med J 51 (Suppl 8):82

Diet Treatment of Atherosclerosis

Ivan D. Frantz, Jr.

When this workshop was held, the diet treatment of atherosclerosis was in an unsettled state. Although effective diets were available for lowering blood lipid concentrations, proof of their efficacy in reducing the rate of progression of atherosclerosis or preventing its complications was not fully convincing. A further complicating factor was the general acceptance of high density lipoproteins as a negative risk factor. All recommended diets now required reevaluation for their effect on the individual lipoproteins. Even at this meeting, some of the data presented had been collected before the methodology for such evaluation had been adopted by the laboratories involved. The presentations emphasized the effect of dietary modification on the blood lipids, with little mention of their effect on atherogenesis. The pendulum had swung back towards the low fat, low cholesterol diet, and away from the addition of large quantities of polyunsaturated fat. Fear of doing harm by feeding a diet never consumed by large populations over a long span of time seemed to have pervaded all workers in the field. The importance of dietary cholesterol was no longer questioned.

Dr. Connor presented evidence that a high carbohydrate diet providing 20% of calories from fat (5% saturated) and not more than 100 mg of cholesterol daily is very effective for the treatment of almost all cases of hyperlipoproteinemia, regardless of type. An occasional case, complicated by the accumulation of chylomicrons, must be treated with even less dietary fat. Elevations of triglycerides sometimes produced by such a diet subside after a short time.

Dr. Blackett demonstrated the importance of body weight as a determinant of serum cholesterol. Persons placed on cholesterol lowering regimens who lose weight generally show an additional fall in serum cholesterol not accounted for by the changes in dietary fat and cholesterol. An implication of his results seemed to be the likelihood that much of the rise in serum cholesterol with age seen in American men may be accounted for by weight gain.

Dr. Miettinen presented extensive studies of the effect of various types of fiber on serum cholesterol and lipoprotein concentrations, and on cholesterol and bile acid metabolism. Gel-forming, purified fiber increases bile acid excretion and lowers serum cholesterol. The fiber generally found in human food, however, has little effect on serum cholesterol. Dr. Miettinen did not recommend fiber as a useful tool for cholesterol lowering at this time.

Dr. Nakamura described a technique making use of heparin followed by protamine, for the study of the VLDL production rate. This rate was not affected by an isocaloric diet high in polyunsaturated fat, but it was decreased by caloric restriction. Diets with P:S ratio lowered LDL+VLDL, but had little or no effect on HDL. Severe caloric restriction reduced HDL, while mild caloric restriction raised it.

Dr. Schlierf presented data of practical importance in connection with the relationship of obesity, weight reduction, and cholesterol lowering dietary regimens to gallstone formation. He collected bile from his subjects and calculated a "lithogenic index" based on the bile composition. No increase in lithogenicity occurred with cholesterol lowering diets high in either polyunsaturated or monounsaturated fat. Six hundred calorie diets also caused no change in the lithogenic index, but complete fasting in obese subjects caused a fall calculated to be sufficient to promote the dissolution of gallstones.

Body Weight, Dietary Fat, Hyperlipidemia, and Coronary Heart Disease

R.B. Blacket, P.J. Brennan, B. Leelarthaepin, C.A. McGilchrist, A.J. Palmer, J.M. Simpson, and J.M. Woodhill

Western nations with a high incidence of premature CHD consume a high fat, high calorie diet and gain weight from adolescence and maturity to the middle of the sixth decade. The main preoccupation in dietary prevention of CHD over the last 25 years has been with reduction of saturated fats in the diet and the use of polyunsaturated oils (Intersociety Commission, 1970). The role of overweight in generating hypercholesterolemia, hypertriglyceridemia, glucose intolerance, hyperuricemia and hypertension, all putative risk factors for CHD, seems to have been underestimated. In this paper we present data which support the idea that energy balance as reflected in body weight, may be more important than dietary fat in the pathogenesis of hyperlipidemia and premature CHD.

Effects of weight reduction

Our first evidence came from a study of the effect of weight reduction on hypercholesterolemia and hypertriglyceridemia in middle aged moderately overweight men (Leelarthaepin et al. 1974). More recently (Blacket et al. 1979) we compared the response of the serum lipids to a low fat high polyunsaturate, low cholesterol diet and to a slightly modified normal diet in 41 men who lost weight with 20 similarly overweight hypercholesterolemic men who did not lose significant weight over a 3 year period. At steady state after weight loss the diet of the weight losers was not significantly different from that of the non-weight losers. The diet of the men on the low P/S diet contained 15.0% saturated fat and 7.3% polyunsaturates; for the high P/S men corresponding figures were 9.7% and 15.8%

Table 1 shows the overall effect on serum lipids, regardless of diet, when the 61 subjects were subdivided by lipoprotein phenotype. In Group 1 a mean weight loss of 10.3 kg was accompanied by a mean fall of 65 mg/dl in serum cholesterol. The response in type 2A and 2B was identical; the triglyceride response was greater in type 2B. In Group 2, whose weight loss was insignificant, but whose steady state diet was the same, the mean fall in serum cholesterol was 31 mg/dl and there was no significant change in triglycerides.

Could the greater response in the weight losers be accounted for by greater changes in the fat and cholesterol content of their diet? As all the necessary information was available in 55 of the 61 subjects we compared the observed falls in serum cholesterol with those predicted by the equations of Keys et al. (1965) and Hegsted et al. (1965). The results are shown in Table 2.

There are some discrepancies which are discussed elsewhere (Blacket et al. 1979). In the weight losers the observed falls of serum cholesterol exceeded the predictions, particularly in the low P/S group. The addition of polyunsaturates generated high predicted falls but in the event had no significant effect. The combined fall for low P/S and high P/S patients of 61.6 mg/dl was 1.57 times greater than predicted by the Keys equation. In those who did not lose weight the mean fall of 29.9 mg/dl agreed well with the predictions of 32.3 mg/dl and 31.8 mg/dl. The mean steady state diets conformed well with

Table 1. Response of body weight and serum lipids to dietary change. Mean±SD

	Group 1		Group 2	
Phenotype	2A	2B	2A	2B
Number	19	22	9	11
Body weight (kg)				
Entry	84.3 ± 8.5	83.2 ± 10.7	83.0 ± 6.6	85.9 ± 9.7
Steady State	73.6 ± 8.1	73.2 ± 7.2	82.4 ± 6.8	84.9 ± 8.6
Difference	10.7 ± 3.7[b]	10.1 ± 4.7[b]	0.6 ± 1.1	1.0 ± 1.0[a]
% Change	12.8	12.0	0.7	1.2
Serum Cholesterol (mg/dl)				
Entry	303 ± 28	316 ± 44	282 ± 21	323 ± 61
Steady State	240 ± 26	249 ± 21	251 ± 26	292 ± 61
Difference	63 ± 38[b]	67 ± 40[b]	31 ± 17[b]	31 ± 15[b]
% Change	20.8	21.2	11.0	9.6
Serum Triglyceride (mg/dl)				
Entry	139 ± 24	277 ± 138	116 ± 13	253 ± 60
Steady State	100 ± 42	135 ± 44	121 ± 36	223 ± 74
Difference	36 ± 45[a]	142 ± 132[b]	−5 ± 39	30 ± 67
% Change	25.9	51.3	−4.3	11.9

[a] $P < 0.01$; [b] $P < 0.001$.

the prescribed diets thus giving confidence in the method. Reduction of serum cholesterol by the amount observed in the weight losers through change in dietary saturated fat alone would require that approximately 5% of calories came from that source. This is unlikely.

To examine the effect of change in body weight the regression of ΔC (change in serum cholesterol) on ΔW (change in body weight) was calculated for the low P/S and the high P/S subsets of Group 1 and for the two subsets together. The three regression equations were not significantly different; all showed a significant linear regression of ΔC on ΔW. When the non-weight losers of Group 2 were included similar results were obtained. The regression equation describing the data in the 55 men with reliable dietary data is $\Delta C = 3.67 \Delta W + 25.69$ (F ratio 27.08, $P < 0.01$). There was considerable variability in individual response. Change in body weight appeared to cause a proportional change in serum cholesterol over the whole range of weight examined. The regression equation should give an independent estimate of the change in serum cholesterol in the non-weight losers of Group 2. The predicted value from the regression equation is 27.4 mg/dl. The observed value was 29.9 mg/dl. Thus the observed changes in serum cholesterol, the estimates based on the prediction equations of Keys and of Hegsted, and the regression of ΔC on ΔW all indicate that weight loss accounted for about 40 to 50% of the observed fall in serum cholesterol in this group of men. The relative contribution of weight loss and change in dietary lipids will vary with the amount of change in each. After weight reduction the mean weight of our men still lay at the 35th per-

Table 2. Observed and predicted changes in serum cholesterol.

Group	1			2		
P/S	<1.0	>1.0	All	<1.0	>1.0	All
Number	18	18	36	10	9	19
ΔW kg	9.7	10.3	10.0	1.0	0.7	0.8
ΔSC mg/dl	65.8	57.6	61.6	25.8	34.4	29.9
ΔSC (Keys)[a]	30.7	49.0	39.3	18.4	47.3	32.3
ΔSC (Hegsted)[b]	33.3	52.0	42.0	16.1	50.5	31.8

[a] predicted change according to Keys et al. (1965).

[b] predicted change according to Hegsted et al. (1965).

centile of American men in the U.S. National Diet-Heart Study (1968). If they had reached truly ideal weight, their serum cholesterol, according to the regression equation, would have been 210 mg/dl.

Cross-sectional study of body weight and coronary risk factors

If reduction in body weight leads to a fall in serum cholesterol and serum triglycerides and in blood pressure (Reisin et al. 1978), then the prevalence of high values for these variables should be higher in the overweight than in the lean. Brennan et al. (1979) have re-examined this in 600 men and 400 women age 20 to 49 who were healthy blood donors in Sydney. The results differed for men and women and only the former will be discussed here. In each of the three decades 20-29, 30-39 and 40-49, there were highly significant correlations of serum cholesterol, triglyceride, urate and blood pressure with body mass index, ranging from 0.18 to 0.30. The separate effects of age and weight on the prevalence of high levels were determined by logit analysis. High levels of all four variables were associated with high values for body mass index. After adjusting for the latter, age had no effect on the prevalence of hypertriglyceridemia or hypertension. Age and body mass index had interacting effects on serum cholesterol. The rise in serum cholesterol with age and body mass index can be modelled best by an inverse polynomial incorporating these two variables.

If one adopts the 40th percentile of body mass index as an arbitrary division between acceptable weight and overweight, 9% of the men below this division had hypercholesterolemia (>250 mg/dl) compared with 17% above it. For hypertriglyceridemia (>160 mg/dl) the figures were 4% and 14%. 75% of men aged 20 to 49 with hypercholesterolemia and 85% of men with hypertriglyceridemia lay above the 40th percentile of weight.

Overweight was also associated with "clustering" of high values. Only 2.5% of men below the 40th percentile of body mass index had two or more risk factors compared with 13.0% of men above that level. Of the 120 men who lay below the 20th percentile and thus came closest to ideal weight, 99 were free of high values, 18 had one and only 2 had two.

Discussion

These studies provide good evidence that weight gain in adult life promotes hypercholesterolemia and hypertriglyceridemia and that weight reduction reverses this. Weight gain also promotes hypertension, hyperuricemia and glucose intolerance all of which have been linked to premature coronary disease. While none of these facts are new the very considerable contribution that weight gain makes to the coronary profile appears to have been underplayed. Maintenance of truly ideal weight, that is below the 20th percentile, does not guarantee freedom from risk; however, it makes multiple risk improbable. Risk, both single and multiple, becomes much more common above the 40th percentile of weight. This represents a gain of less than 7 kg above "ideal" weight by the sixth decade. Coronary men are only slightly if at all, fatter than their peers. However, the high prevalence of risk factors which coronary men show and their reversability in part or in whole by weight reduction suggests that response to weight gain has played an important part in their illness. Bodyweight is the resultant of input and output. Evidence from British civil servants indicates that when weight is kept constant increased physical activity in leisure is protective against future CHD. (Morris et al. 1973). Thus turnover and other effects of physical activity may be important also. In our Diet-Heart Study (Woodhill et al. 1978) physical activity in leisure was the most significant determinant of survival, when all other factors were controlled. An intervention which reduces one risk factor only is less likely to be successful than one which controls many. Weight gain after maturity is clearly contributory to a significant degree to high serum cholesterol, to high blood pressure and to diabetes which are generally accepted as prime risk factors. Although the contribution of high serum triglycerides and high serum urate levels to risk is controversial, the almost complete dependence of the former on excess body weight and the partial dependence of the latter is notable. Thus control of body weight is likely to be more rewarding than change of dietary lipids. The two measures should be seen as complementary.

Acknowledgments

This work was supported by grants-in-aid from the Life Insurance Medical Research Fund of Australia and New Zealand and the National Heart Foundation of Australia. Table 1 is reproduced by courtesy of the Australian and New Zealand Journal of Medicine. We thank Mrs. L. Bernstein for dietary counselling and Miss. J. Aitken, Miss L. Abbott and Mrs. D. Moham for lipid estimations.

References

Blacket RB, Leelarthaepin B, McGilchrist CA, Palmer AJ, Woodhill JM (1979) The synergistic effect of weight loss and changes in dietary lipids on the serum cholesterol of obese men with hypercholesterolemia. Aust N Z J Med 9: in press
Brennan PJ, Simpson JM, Blacket RB, McGilchrist CA (1979) The effects of body weight on serum cholesterol, serum triglycerides, serum urate and systolic blood pressure. Aust N Z J Med 9: in press
Hegsted DM, McGandy RB, Myers ML, Stare FJ (1965) Quantitative effects of dietary fat on serum cholesterol in man. Am J Clin Nutr 17: 281-295
Intersociety Commission for heart disease resources. Primary prevention of the atherosclerotic disease (1970) Circulation 42: A55
Keys A, Anderson JT Grande F (1965) Serum cholesterol response to changes in the diet. Metabolism 14: 747-758
Leelarthaepin B, Woodhill JM, Palmer AJ, Blacket RB (1974) Obesity, diet and type II hyperlipidemia. Lancet ii: 1217-1221
Morris JN, Chave SPW, Adam C, Sivey C, Epstein L, Sheehan DJ (1973) Vigorous exercise in leisure-time and the incidence of coronary heart-disease. Lancet i: 333-339
National diet-heart study. Final report (1968) Circulation 37: suppl 1.
Reisin E, Abel R, Modan M, Silverberg DS, Elihou HE, Modan B (1978) Effect of weight loss without salt restriction on the reduction of blood pressure in overweight hypertensive patients. N Engl J Med 298: 1-6
Woodhill JM, Palmer AJ, Leelarthaepin B, McGilchrist C, Blacket RB (1978) Low fat low cholesterol diet in secondary prevention of coronary heart disease. In: Kritchevsky D, Paoletti R, Holmes WL (eds) Drugs, Lipid Metabolism and Atherosclerosis. Plenum Press, New York, pp 317-330

Effects of Dietary Fiber on Serum Lipids and Cholesterol Metabolism in Man

Tatu A. Miettinen[1]

Dietary fiber consists of plant cell wall materials which are not digested by enzymes of the human upper gastrointestinal tract. Chemically they are mostly noncarbohydrate lignin or polysaccharides, i.e. cellulose, hemicellulose, pectic substances, gums, mucilages or algal polysaccharides. Fibers hold water and when purified they can form gel (or mucilages) in water as, e.g., pectin, guar gum and plantago ovata preparations. Natural fiber products, such as vegetables, salads, fruits and bran, also hold water but do not usually form gel. Accordingly, dietary fibers can be divided into gel-forming and nongel-forming ones. Since fibers also have adsorptive capacity and cation exchange nature they can interfere with many absorptive function in the small intestine. In fact, cholesterol and bile acid absorption has been assumed to be disturbed by a high fiber diet, resulting via enhanced fecal elimination of cholesterol in a decrease in serum cholesterol. On the basis of epidemiological studies dietary fiber deficiency has been claimed to promote development of coronary heart disease by modifying cholesterol metabolism. The present paper deals with the effects of dietary fibers on serum cholesterol, serum lipoproteins and some measures of cholesterol metabolism.

Vegetarians

A vegetarian diet increases markedly the intake of dietary fiber and plant sterols (Connor et al. 1978; Miettinen and Tarpila 1978). The daily intake of the vegetable sterols (400-600 mg) is hardly high enough to interfere with cholesterol absorption in vegetarians. In fact, the few studies on fecal steroids have indicated that the neutral sterol output is within normal limits (Miettinen 1978). A low serum cholesterol level, a characteristic finding in vegetarians (Burslem et al. 1978) and in studies on populations consuming a high fiber diet (Connor et al. 1977; Walker and Walker 1978), is then hardly caused by plant sterols. The low serum cholesterol is due to decreased low density lipoprotein (LDL). The high density lipoprotein (HDL) concentration is also usually low (Burslem et al. 1978; Connor et al. 1978) but exceptions are found (Walker and Walker 1978), very low density lipoprotein (VLDL) being normal or even increased. The percentage of total serum cholesterol transported by HDL is usually increased. Fecal analysis showed that vegetarians eliminate cholesterol as bile acids at a low normal rate (Miettinen 1978). Kinetic bile acid analysis gives similar results (Hepner 1975), low fractional turnover of cholate suggesting that a fiber-rich diet conserves bile acids. Some evidence is available that Indians and Ugandans consuming a vegetarian type of diet actually have a low fecal bile acid output (Hill and Aries 1971). Since the vegetarian diet and the diet of primitive populations are low in fat, saturated fat in particular, in simple sugars and to some extent also in calories, the differences in cholesterol metabolism may not be solely caused by the high dietary fiber. The effects of addition of supplementary fiber will therefore be dealt with.

---

[1] Supported by the National Council for Medical Sciences, Finland.

Bran is the most defined and most widely used mixed fiber preparation tested
in human experiments. Short term studies have not shown any consistent hypocholesterolemic effect, however (Table 1). In a 1-year trial the serum cholesterol of the bran group was significantly decreased but the final values
were not different from those of the controls (Angelico et al. 1978), while
in another 1-year study no consistent bran effect was detectable, even though
the change in serum cholesterol showed a significant negative correlation
with the initial serum cholesterol levels in the bran group but not in the
controls (Tarpila et al. 1978). Other recent studies on addition of mixed
natural fiber to a regular diet or low fiber diet, low or rich in cholesterol,
have failed to demonstrate any consistent change in serum cholesterol (Table
1). The serum lipoprotein concentrations have changed inconsistently by bran
or mixed fiber although the initially low HDL values have increased slightly,
and may thus prevent development of arterial atheromatosis.

On the other hand, many purified plant polysaccharides or their mixtures,
e.g. pectin, guar gum, hydrophilic seed preparations and less consistently
cellulose, decrease serum cholesterol when fed in large quantities to human
subjects (Tables 1 and 2). The mean decrease, mainly caused by lowered LDL
cholesterol with unchanged or increased HDL and VLDL, is usually, however,
about 15% or less, and accordingly these gel-forming or mucilaginous polysaccharides are clearly inferior to actual hypocholesterolemic anion exchangers in the treatment of hypercholesterolemia. The changes in serum cholesterol indicate that the fibers alter cholesterol metabolism to some extent
at least.

Effects of Fibers on Cholesterol Metabolism

Despite the inconsistent hypocholesterolemic effect of bran and mixed dietary
fiber they can modify cholesterol metabolism. Short term bran experiments have
revealed variable changes in fecal steroid elimination. A long term consumption
of bran decreased fecal bile acids in patients with the diverticular disease
of the colon proportionately to the initial bile acid production, decreased
biliary deoxycholate, decreased equally cholic acid and chenodeoxycholate
synthesis, and lowered cholesterol synthesis proportionately to the baseline
values and to the changes in serum cholesterol (Tarpila et al. 1978). A decrease in biliary deoxycholate, in pool size of deoxycholate and in biliary
cholesterol saturation has been found in short term studies (Pomare et al.
1976). Administration of a mixed natural fiber on a zero or high cholesterol
formula diet revealed that the fecal bile acid and neutral sterol excretions
were not affected but the sum of the two was slightly increased during the
zero cholesterol formula (Raymond et al. 1977). The plot of the changes in
steroid eliminations against the initial values indicated that the fiber
reduced the fecal output of bile acid and total endogenous steroids in the
cases with high initial values. Cholesterol absorption was not altered. On
a solid food diet normal or low in baseline fiber content the mixed natural
fiber also conserved bile acids and may have interfered with cholesterol absorption with no consistent increase in fecal neutral sterols (Table 2).
Thus, in agreement with the results in vegetarians, nongel-forming dietary
fiber appears to conserve bile acids (See Table 1) and to decrease formation
of secondary bile acids.

Strikingly different results have been obtained with the gel-forming or
mucilaginous polysaccharides (Tables 1 and 2). The decrease in serum cholesterol by these substances is associated with a usually proportionate increase

Table 1. Changes caused by dietary fiber additions in serum cholesterol and fecal steroids. Percent change from control.

Fiber material	Serum cholesterol				Fecal steroids		References
	Total	Free	LDL	HDL	Acidic	Total	
Vegetarian[1]	-30[x]	-	-32[x]	-18[x]	-	-	Burslem et al. 1978
Vegetarian[2]	+31[x]	-	-	+33[x]	-32[x]	-18	Miettinen 1978
Bagasse	0	-	-	-	+49[x]	-6	Walters et al. 1975
Bran	0	-	-	-	-2	+3	Walters et al. 1975
Bran	0	-	-	-	-23	-	Eastwood et al. 1973
Bran	-3	-	-	+36	-44[x]	-45[x]	Tarpila et al. 1978
Wheat fiber	+4	-	-	-	-25[x]	-19	Kay and Truswell 1977
Mixed fiber[3]	-2	-	-10	+2	+37	+29[x]	Raymond et al. 1977
Mixed fiber[3]	-4	-	0	+2	-5	-4	Raymond et al. 1977
Apples + mixed	+7	+2	-	-3	-45[x]	-22[x]	Miettinen 1978
Mixed fiber[4]	0	-2	-1	+11[x]	-20[x]	-1	Table 2
Guar gum[4]	-7[x]	-5	-11[x]	+7	+77[x]	+32[x]	Table 2
Guar gum	-16[x]	-	-	-	+84[x]	-	Jenkings 1978
Pectin	-15[x]	-	-	-	+36[x]	-	Jenkings 1978
Pectin	-9[x]	-12[x]	-	-11	+57[x]	+27[x]	Miettinen 1978
Pectin	-13[x]	-	-	-	+33[x]	+24[x]	Kay and Truswell 1977
Psyllium colloid	-17[x]	-	-	-	+195[x]	+65	Forman et al. 1968
Psyllium colloid	-6	-7[x]	-	+16[x]	+35[x]	+9	Miettinen 1978
Cellulose	-25[x]	-30[x]	-	-	+45[x]	-	Shurpalekar et al. 1971

[1] Mean percent difference from matched control groups.
[2] Difference from a younger control group on a normal home diet.
[3] The first study on a zero cholesterol, the second one on an 1 g/day cholesterol formula.
[4] Changes calculated from the low fiber period of Table 2.
[x] Statistically significant (p<0.05 at least) difference or change.

Table 2. Effects of guar gum and high mixed fiber on serum and fecal steroids in patients with diverticular disease of the colon. Mean±SE.

Period	Serum cholesterol, mmol/l				MS, µmol/l	Fecal steroids, mg/day			Cholesterol absorption,%
	Total	VLDL	LDL	HDL		Acidic	Neutral	Total	
Guar	4.73[x]	0.52	3.34[x]	0.87	2.66[x]	669[x]	796	1465[x]	26
Low	5.09	0.54	3.74	0.81	2.00	377	737	1112	26
High	5.11[*]	0.49	3.72[*]	0.90[x]	2.27	320[**]	786	1105[*]	21[x]

[x] p<0.05 from the low fiber period and [*] from the guar gum period. MS = serum free total methyl sterols; serum levels of these cholesterol precursors reflect cholesterol synthesis in many clinical conditions. Eight patients were put on a standard solid food diet low in fiber (low = crude fiber 3 g/day) and cholesterol (120 mg/day/2400 kcal); to this diet guar gum (guar; 40 g/day) or mixed natural fiber (high; crude fiber 15 g/day from bran, beans, vegetables, salad) were added in random order; the lipid values were obtained at the end of each 10 to 13-day period; ultracentrifugation was performed in 7 cases only. The decrease in fecal bile acids by the high fiber diet showed a negative correlation (r = -0.748; P<0.05) and the increase by the guar gum addition a positive correlation (r = 0.829; P<0.05) with the fecal bile acid values of the low fiber period (Tarpila and Miettinen, unpublished observations).

in cholesterol elimination as fecal bile acids. Neutral sterol excretion and cholesterol absorption may not be disturbed, but cholesterol synthesis appears to increase as a consequence of enhanced bile acid loss and synthesis. No consistent change is seen in biliary bile acid or lipid composition, indicating that the elimination of all the major bile acids is enhanced at a similar rate.

Summary

Administration of nongel-forming mixed dietary fiber, including bran, to human subject has an inconsistent effect on serum cholesterol but it may increase initially low HDL. This type of fiber conserves bile acids, particularly in cases with high initial fecal bile acid output, and may in this way normalize biliary lipid composition and decrease cholesterol synthesis. Large amounts of gel-forming or mucilaginous polysaccharide fibers fed to human subjects cause quite consistently a modest decrease in serum cholesterol by increasing cholesterol elimination as fecal bile acids. This is balanced by enhanced cholesterol synthesis. It is the LDL cholesterol level which is lowered, while the HDL cholesterol may even increase slightly.

References

Angelico F, Clemente P, Menotti A, Ricci G, Urbinati G (1978) Bran and changes in serum lipids: Observations during a project of primary prevention of coronary heart disease. In: International Conferences on Atherosclerosis. Carlson LA et al. (eds) Raven Press, p 205

Burslem J, Schonfeld G, Howald MA, Weidman SW, Miller JP (1978) Plasma apoprotein and lipoprotein lipid levels in vegetarians. Metabolism 27: 711

Connor WE, Cerqueira MT, Connor RW, Wallace RB, Malinow MR, Casdorph HR (1978) The plasma lipids, lipoproteins and diet of the Tarahumara Indians of Mexico. Am J Clin Nutr 31: 1131

Eastwood MA, Kirkpatrick JR, Mitchell WD, Bone A, Hamilton T (1973) Effects of dietary supplements of wheat bran and cellulose on faeces and bowel function. Brit Med J 4: 392

Forman DT, Garvin JE, Forestner JF, Taylor CB (1968) Increased excretion of fecal bile acids by an oral hydrophilic colloid. Proc Soc Exp Biol Med 127: 1060

Hepner GW (1975) Altered bile acid metabolism in vegetarians. Am J Dig Dis 20: 935

Hill MJ, Aries VC (1971) Faecal steroid composition and its relationship to cancer of the large bowel. J Pathol 104: 129

Jenkings DAJ (1978) Action of dietary fiber in lowering fasting serum cholesterol and reducing post-prandial glycemia: Gastrointestinal mechanisms. In: Carlson LA et al. (eds) International Conference on Atherosclerosis. Raven Press, p 173

Kay RM, Truswell AS (1977) The effect of wheat fibre on plasma lipids and faecal steroid excretion in man. Br J Nutr 37: 227

Kay RM, Truswell AS (1977) Effect of citrus pectin on blood lipids and fecal steroid excretion in man. Am J Clin Nutr 30: 171

Miettinen TA (1978) Effects of dietary fibers on ion-exchange resins on cholesterol metabolism in man. In: Carlson LA et al. (eds) International Conference on Atherosclerosis. Raven Press   p 193

Miettinen TA, Tarpila S (1978) Fecal β-sitosterol in patients with diverticular disease of the colon and in vegetarians. Scand J Gastroent 13: 573

Pomare EW, Heaton KW, Low-Beer TS, Espiner HJ (1976) The effect of wheat bran upon bile salt metabolism and upon the lipid composition of bile in gallstone patients. Am J Dig Dis 21: 521

Raymond TL, Connor WE, Lin DS, Warner S, Fry MM, Connor SL (1977) The interaction of dietary fibers and cholesterol upon the plasma lipids and lipo-

proteins, sterol balance, and bowel function in human subjects. J Clin
    Invest 60: 1429
Shurpalekar KS, Doraiswamy TR, Sundaravalli OE, Narayana Rao M (1971) Effect
    of infusion of cellulose in "atherogenic" diet on the blood lipids of
    children. Nature 232: 554
Tarpila S, Miettinen TA, Metsäranta L (1978) Effects of bran on serum choles-
    terol, faecal mass, fat, bile acids and neutral sterols, and biliary
    lipids in patients with diverticular disease of the colon. Gut 19: 137
Walker ARP, Walker BF (1978) High high-density-lipoprotein cholesterol in
    African children and adults in a population free of coronary heart
    disease. Brit Med J 2: 1336
Walters RL, McLean Baird I, Davies PS, Hill MJ, Drasar BS, Southgate DAT,
    Green J, Morgan B (1975) Effects of two types of dietary fibre on faecal
    steroid and lipid excretion. Brit Med J 2: 536

Effects of Dietary Changes on Plasma Lipoprotein Lipids

Haruo Nakamura, Toshitsugu Ishikawa, and Naoki Suzuki

Abnormal lipoprotein profile has been known to be closely related to atherosclerosis based on epidemiological and experimental data. Increased VLDL and
LDL, and decreased HDL are the most characteristic features leading to coronary atherosclerosis.

The present study was performed to investigate the effect of polyunsaturated
fat diet on the production of VLDL triglycerides (TG) and the composition of
VLDL, and to examine the changes of VLDL and LDL-cholesterol and HDL-cholesterol on the different dietary alterations.

Material and Methods

VLDL analysis

Six normal controls and 6 hypertriglyceridemic subjects (Type IV) were used
in this experiment. Alteration of diets was made isocalorically and 80% of
fat (40% of total energy) was composed of coconut oil and safflower oil respectively. TG secretion rate was measured by the method of Kaye and Galton
(1975) and newly secreted VLDL was separated by ultracentrifugation.

Lipoprotein cholesterol analysis

Three to five control (normal plasma lipids) subjects and five obese subjects
were used in this part of the experiment. HDL-cholesterol was measured with
the precipitation procedure using 2 M manganese solution with heparin.

Results

VLDL analysis

Table 1 shows the plasma lipids of the control and hypertriglyceridemic subjects with secretion rate of VLDL-TG. Mild hypertriglyceridemia revealed
significantly increased VLDL-TG secretion rate. Caloric restriction (1000
Kcal/day) decreased plasma TG level with concomitant decrease of TG secretion rate. However, TG level also decreased on the safflower diet without
changing TG secretion rate (Table 2). TG and cholesterol-ester (CE) which
are rich in the core part of VLDL, phospholipid (PL) and free cholesterol (FC)
primarily distributed in the surface part of VLDL-lipid are shown in the control and calorie-restricted diet in Table 3 and in the coconut and safflower
diet in Table 4. Composition of VLDL remained unchanged on the control and
calorie-restricted diet. However, PL and FC, which are mainly located in the
surface of VLDL-lipids, significantly diminished on the safflower diet. This
change showed that on the safflower diet, core lipids increased compared with
surface lipids, indicating compositional change of VLDL.

Table 1. Plasma lipids and triglyceride production rate in control and hypertriglyceridemic subjects.

	Body Weight (Kg)	Triglyceride (mg/dl)	Cholesterol (mg/dl)	Triglyceride Production(mg/dl)
Control (N=6)	58.5 + 5	104 + 9	202 + 18	32 + 13 ⎤ **
Hypertriglyce-ridemia(N=6)	67.2 + 7	238 + 38	254 + 26	78 + 21 ⎦

** P < 0.01   Mean + S.D.

Table 2. Plasma lipids and triglyceride production rate in hyper-triglyceridemia on different diets.

	Triglyceride (mg/dl)	Cholesterol (mg/dl)	Triglyceride Production(mg/dl)
Control Diet	237 + 38 ⎤ ⎤	254 + 26 ⎤ ⎤	78 + 21 ⎤
Safflower Diet Isocaloric	162 + 21 ⎦ ** ⎥ **	220 + 19 ⎦ ** ⎥ **	62 + 19 ⎥ **
Restricted Calorie(1000Kcal)	159 + 22 ⎦	215 + 23 ⎦	41 + 11 ⎦

** p < 0.01   Mean + S.D.

Table 3. Composition of secreted VLDL and triglyceride production rate in the control diet and the restricted calorie diet.

	Composition of Secreted VLDL				Triglyceride Production Rate (mg/h)
	Core		Surface		
	Trigly-ceride	Cholesterol - ester	Free Chol-esterol	Phospho-lipid	
Control Diet Coconut : Safflower (1 : 1)	100	17.9 + 2.5	3.1 + 1.3	10.2 + 2.1	78 + 21 ⎤ **
Restricted Calorie Coconut : Safflower (1 : 1)	100	18.1 + 2.7	3.0 + 1.1	10.6 + 1.9	41 + 11 ⎦

** P < 0.01   Mean + S.D.

Postheparin lipolytic activity (PHLA) was measured using these separated VLDL as the substrates. PHLA increased significantly when VLDL obtained from the subjects on the safflower diet was used as the substrate (Table 5).

Lipoprotein cholesterol analysis

HDL-cholesterol and (LDL-VLDL)-cholesterol were measured on the basis of different energy without changing the dietary composition. HDL-cholesterol de-

Table 4. Composition of secreted VLDL.

| | Core | | Surface | |
	Triglyceride	Cholesterol – ester	Free Chol- esterol	Phospho- lipid
Coconut Oil	100	18.4 $\pm$ 2.8	3.2 $\pm$ 1.5*	15.1 $\pm$ 2.2**
Safflower Oil	100	16.7 $\pm$ 3.5	2.6 $\pm$ 1.8*	8.8 $\pm$ 2.7**

$* P < 0.05$ $** P < 0.01$ Mean $\pm$ S.D.

Table 5. Postheparin lipolytic activity.

Substrate	PHLA(μEqFFA/ml/h)
VLDL (Saturated Fat)	5.9
VLDL (Polyunsaturated Fat)	9.2*

$* P < 0.05$

Table 6. Effect of overnutrition (N = 5).

Lipoprotein (mg/dl)	0 (1)	1 (2)	(W)
(LDL+VLDL)-Cholesterol(a)	161 $\pm$ 21	194 $\pm$ 32	
HDL-Cholesterol (b)	64 $\pm$ 7	61 $\pm$ 7	
(b) / (a)	0.40	0.31	

(1) 1800Kcal (Protein 15%, Fat 35%, Carbo. 50%)
(2) 2600Kcal (Protein 15%, Fat 35%, Carbo. 50%)

creased on the 2600 Kcal diet with the elevation of (LDL+VLDL)-cholesterol (Table 6). On the contrary to this dietary alteration, reduction of energy showed the opposite change on HDL depending upon the magnitude of energy restriction. Marked energy restriction revealed the reduction of HDL-cholesterol while mild restriction increased HDL-cholesterol level, with concomitant decrease of (LDL+VLDL)-cholesterol (Table 7).

Effect of cholesterol ingestion (1.0 g/day) on the lipoprotein cholesterol is shown in Table 8. Cholesterol of (LDL+VLDL) increased initially and HDL-cholesterol increased subsequently. Alteration of the P/S ratio in the diet also changed HDL-cholesterol. Both marked decrease and increase of the P/S ratio reduced the HDL-cholesterol level. There seemed to exist optimum P/S ratio to maintain the elevated HDL-cholesterol (Table 9).

Discussion and Summary

Polyunsaturated fat diet has been widely known to decrease plasma lipids. In the present study, TG decrement is considered to occur with latered composition of VLDL, leading to the increase of susceptibility to hydrolysis. How-

Table 7. Effect of undernutrition (N = 5).

Energy	Lipoprotein(mg/dl)	0 [†]	1-2 (W)
20-25 Kcal/Kg	(LDL+VLDL)-Cholesterol(a)	185 + 23	176 + 21
	HDL-cholesterol (b)	48 + 6	54 + 5
	(b) / (a)	0.26	0.31
10-15 Kcal/Kg	(LDL+VLDL)-Cholesterol(a)	179 + 20	172 + 19
	HDL-Cholesterol (b)	49 + 5*	42 + 3*
	(b) / (a)	0.27	0.24

[†] 30-35 Kcal/Kg   * P< 0.05

Table 8. Effect of cholesterol ingestion (N = 4).

Lipoprotein (mg/dl)	0	1-2(W)	3-4(W)
(LDL+VLDL)-Cholesterol (a)	164 + 13	179 + 9	179 + 8
HDL-Cholesterol (b)	52 + 5	49 + 4	55 + 4
(b) / (a)	0.32	0.36	0.31

Table 9. Effect of fatty acid polyunsaturation (N = 5).

Lipoprotein (mg/dl)	P / S		
	0.3-0.4	1.0-1.5	3.0-
(LDL+VLDL)-Cholesterol(a)	192 + 14*	181 + 11	173 + 10*
HDL-Cholesterol (b)	50 + 9	54 + 6	51 + 5
HDL-Free Cholesterol / (b)	0.21	0.24	0.22
(b) / (a)	0.26	0.30	0.29

* P< 0.05

ever, extremely increased polyunsaturated fat feeding reduced the HDL-cholesterol level in the plasma which has been known to be antiatherogenic.

HDL-cholesterol seemed to depend on either energy or P/S ratio. Therefore,
in order to prevent against atherosclerosis, various dietary compositions
should be carefully considered to reduce (LDL+VLDL)-cholesterol and to ele-
vate the diminished HDL-cholesterol level.

Reference

Kaye JP, Galton DJ (1975) Triglyceride-production rates in patients with
    type-IV hypertriglyceridemia. Lancet 1:1005

Hypolipidemic Diets and Biliary Lipid Composition[1]

G. Schlierf, A. Stiehl, C.C. Heuck, M. Kohlmeier, P. Oster, and B. Schellenberg

Introduction

Prevalence and incidence of cholelithiasis has been increasing in industrialized countries. Of the nutritional factors, high cholesterol intake (DenBesten et al. 1973) and factors causing overweight may play an important role in gallstone formation. In obese subjects, studies by Bennion and Grundy (1975) and by Shaffer and Small (1977) have shown increased biliary cholesterol secretion and saturation which result in an elevated "lithogenic index". Conversely, following weight reduction, biliary cholesterol secretion was diminished and the lithogenic index lowered. The greatest rate of weight loss in obesity can be achieved by complete fasting. Since, however, bile after an overnight fast was found to be more lithogenic than during feeding (Metzger et al. 1973), and lithogenicity increased when fasting was extended from 9 - 16 hours (Williams et al. 1977) it was of interest to study bile lipid composition with prolonged fasting and to compare the results to those obtained during weight reduction with low calorie diets.

A second question concerned possible lithogenic effects of a fat-modified diet, as suspected by Grundy in 1974. This question was studied in 10 normal volunteers comparing the conventional diet of these young males with a low cholesterol, highly unsaturated (corn oil) diet and with a similarly low cholesterol "olive oil" diet.

Material and methods

The first study was performed on in-patients of the metabolic ward who had given their informed consent. 11 obese patients (weight index 1.3 - 1.79) were fasted 20 days. Bile lipid composition was determined before and at 10 and 20 days of fasting. Samples were obtained by duodenal intubation and cholecystokinin administration. Biliary cholesterol was measured enzymatically using a test kit of Boehringer Mannheim, total bile acids were also measured enzymatically (Sterognost Nyegaard), and lipid phosphorus was measured following extraction with chloroform/methanol. Calculation of the lithogenic index (Admirand and Small) was performed as proposed by Thomas and Hofmann (1973). Statistical evaluation was done using the Wilcoxon test. Bile lipids were studied in a similar manner with 600 calorie diet in 9 pa-

---

[1] Supported by Deutsche Forschungsgemeinschaft.

tients (weight index 1.01 - 1.46) for the same period of 20 days.

The second study was performed in 10 healthy young males of normal body weight, who were given, in randomized order, low cholesterol diets containing corn oil and olive oil, respectively (30 - 35 calorie %). Gallbladder bile was obtained after an overnight fast at the end of the control period and the end of the two oil periods as described above. In addition, in these subjects, plasma lipids and lipoproteins were analyzed using standardized methodology; apo-lipoproteins A-I and A-II were determined using a radioimmuno assay (Riesen et al. 1978).

Results

The effects of fasting and 600 calorie diet on bile lipid composition is shown in table 1.

Table 1. Effects of fasting and 600 calorie diet on "lithogenic index" of human gallbladder bile (medians and ranges).

Fasting:	before	after 10	after 20 days
	1.0	0.8	0.7 *
	(0.7-1.8)	(0.4-1.4)	(0.3-1.3)
600 calorie diet:	before	after 10	after 20 days
	0.9	0.8	0.9
	(0.6-1.1)	(0.3-1.1)	(0.5-1.3)

* Significantly ($p < 0.01$) different from 0-value

After 10 days fasting, biliary cholesterol saturation fell from 10.1 to 8.4 mol %, after 20 days to 6.9 mol %. The lithogenic index according to Admirand and Small fell from 1.0 to 0.8 and 0.7 ($p < 0.01$). The individual values, at ten days, showed a fall in 8 of 11 and at 20 days in all patients. With 600 calorie diet, there were no significant changes of individual bile lipids or of the lithogenic index. For both fasting and 600 calorie diets, the amount of weight loss in 20 days was correlated with change of biliary cholesterol concentration and with a change of the lithogenic index ($p < 0.01$).

The oil diets in normal subjects markedly affected plasma lipids and lipoproteins. Plasma total cholesterol fell by 16 % with the olive oil and by 23 % with the corn oil diet due to significant decreases of LDL cholesterol by 17 % and 27 % respectively. There also was a significant and comparable fall of HDL cholesterol by 25 % and 26 % respectively, while apo-lipoproteins A-I and A-II remained unaffected. Both diets, therefore, resulted in a significant increase of the apo A-HDL/cholesterol ratio pointing to a decreased cholesterol content of individual HDL particles. Biliary lipid composition, as shown in table 2 in spite of this marked alteration of plasma lipids and lipoproteins were not affected significantly.

Table 2. Effects of plasma lipid lowering diet on "lithogenic index" in normal volunteers (n = 10, medians and ranges).

normal diet	corn oil diet	olive oil diet
0.43	0.38	0.42
(0.29 – 0.60)	(0.31 – 0.65)	(0.32 – 0.79)

Discussion

In agreement with findings by Bennion and Grundy (1975) and by Schreibmann et al. (1974), there was no change of the lithogenic index in 9 obese patients during weight loss on a 600 calorie reducing diet. Complete fasting, in contrast, appears to give a different response of biliary lipid composition. The significant fall of the lithogenic index by 30 % is comparable in magnitude with changes obtained during chenodesoxycholic acid treatment for dissolution of gallstones and in fact, dissolution of gallstones has, in the meantime, been described following significant weight reduction (Thornton. 1979).

Contrary to the suspicion raised by Sturdevant et al. (1973) from the Los Angeles Veterans administration study and by Grundy from the study of biliary lipid secretion and bile lipid composition in patients with hyperlipidemias, isocaloric "prudent diets" either highly polyunsaturated or of the olive oil type, according to our data do not result in significant changes of the lithogenic index. Since this is true for subjects in whom plasma lipid and lipoprotein concentration fell by almost 30 %, gallstone formation does not appear to be among the possible side effects of such lipid lowering diets. We do realize, however, that patients may behave differently from normal subjects and that studies of longer duration could modify our conclusions. Thus, if there is any doubt as to the risk for cholelithiasis with measures aimed at lowering plasma cholesterol concentration, biliary lipid composition should be monitored by appropriate methods.

Acknowledgements: The skilled assistance of Miss M. Lenz and Miss G. Rudolf and Miss G. Vogel is appreciated.

References

Admirand WH, Small DM (1968) The physico-chemical basis of cholesterol gallstone formation in man. J clin Invest 47:1043-1052

Bennion LJ, Grundy SM (1975) Effects of obesity and caloric intake on biliary lipid metabolism in man. J clin Invest 56:996-1011

DenBesten L, Connor WE, Bell S (1973) The effect of dietary cholesterol on the composition of human bile. Surgery 73: 266-273

Grundy SM (1974) Dietary management of hyperlipoproteinemias. in: Atherosclerosis III, Ed G Schettler and A Weizel, Springer Verlag, Heidelberg, p 761 - 792

Metzger AL, Adler R, Heymsfield S, Grundy SM (1973) Diurnal variation in biliary lipid composition. New Engl J Med 288:333-336

Riesen WF, Mordasini RC, Middelhoff GW (1978) Quantitation of the two major apoproteins of human high density lipoproteins by solid phase radioimmunoassay. FEBS Letters 91:35-39

Schreibman PH, Pertsemlidis D, Liu GCK, Ahrens jr. EH (1974) Lithogenic bile: a consequence of weight reduction. 66th annual meeting of the American Society for Clinical Investigation, Atlantic City, May 6, 1974, p 72a

Shaffer EA, Small DM (1977) Biliary lipid secretion in cholesterol gallstone disease. J Clin Invest 59:828-840

Sturdevant R, Pearce ML, Dayton S (1973) Increased prevalence of cholelithiasis in men ingesting a serum cholesterol lowering diet. New Engl J Med 288:24

Thomas PJ, Hofmann AF (1973) A simple calculation of the lithogenic index of bile: expressing biliary lipid composition on rectangular coordinate. Gastroenterology 65:698-700

Thornton JR (1979) Gallstone disappearance associated with weight loss. Lancet II:478

Williams CN, Morse JWI, MacDonald IA, Kotoor R, Riding MD (1977) Increased lithogenicity of bile on fasting in normal subjects. American J of Digestive Disease 22:189-194

Interaction of Genetic and Environmental Factors Causing Atherosclerosis by Immunologic Mechanisms

John D. Mathews[1]

Summary

Animal experiments support epidemiologic evidence for the view that the immune response to autoantigens or to environmental antigens can cause human atherosclerosis. Some environmental factors (including infections, vasectomy) could cause atherosclerosis by contributing to autoimmunity in genetically susceptible individuals; infections and dietary factors could also cause atherosclerosis by providing "extrinsic" antigens. Human antibody responses to influenza and polio virus antigens are higher in individuals with high levels of plasma cholesterol, and plasma cholesterol levels increase during the course of the immune response. Immunogenetic loci (including Gm, HLA and possibly ABO blood groups) affect the immune response to particular environmental antigens and auto-antigens, and have been shown to be correlated with the risk of atherosclerotic disease in individuals. A model is proposed for genetic-environmental interactions causing coronary heart disease (CHD); geographical gradients in the frequencies of immunogenetic alleles are attributed to past natural selection by infectious agents; the pattern of correlation of CHD death rates with genetic gradients leads to the conclusion that (similar) infectious agents are still active as causes of CHD. A prediction of the hypothesis that environmental agents interact with immunogenetic alleles to cause cardiovascular disease has been successfully tested by showing that among patients presenting with acute myocardial infarction, individuals with similar HLA phenotypes tend to be affected at similar times.

Introduction

Immunological abnormalities such as autoantibodies to thyroid and other tissue autoantigens, autoantibodies to lipids and lipid cofactors, increased levels of immunoglobulins, rheumatoid factors, food antibodies and immune complexes have been found to be associated with atherosclerosis and/or with its risk factors including hypertension, obesity, hypercholesterolaemia and smoking (Mathews et al. 1974; Poston and Davies 1974; Mathews et al. 1976a; Lancet 1977, 1978a; Fust et al. 1978). The human data and animal data reviewed elsewhere in these proceedings support the view that immunological mechanisms can contribute to spontaneous atherosclerosis in man. However it is important to consider whether the immunological changes are merely epiphenomena or secondary to human atherosclerosis. To help answer this question, it is useful to find out whether the genetic loci controlling the human immune response are also correlated with susceptibility to vascular disease. There is also a need to identify those environmental factors which can interact with genetic factors to cause immunological changes in susceptible individuals, and to search for pathogenic mechanisms. Thirdly, there

---

1 Supported by N.H.M.R.C., U.S. Public Health Service (grant HL 19984) and the Victor Hurley Medical Research Fund.

324

is a need to relate these factors (and immunologic mechanisms) to the recognised risk factors and to the ecology and evolutionary biology of human
populations.

Immunogenetic Studies

The human immune response may be controlled by at least three main groups of
genes linked to the major histocompatibility complex (HLA), to immunoglobulin
allotypes and to the X chromosome (Lancet 1978a). In essential hypertension,
the frequencies of HLA-A locus antigens differ from those in control subjects.
The most constant finding is an increase of HLA-A28 in hypertensive subjects
(Mathews et al. 1976b; Kristensen et al. 1977). In family studies, HLA-
haplotype frequencies in hypertensive subjects differ significantly from
those in non-hypertensive subjects. In both case-control and family data,
blood pressure levels are related to interactions between Ig allotypes at
the Gm locus and HLA-A locus alleles. In survivors of myocardial infarction,
the pattern of HLA-B locus alleles differs significantly from that in controls,
and there is also a significant increase in the frequency of the Gm a+x+b+
phenotype (Mathews et al. 1978, unpublished observation). A polymorphism
at the C3 locus (C3F) has also been associated with atherosclerosis and its
complications (Kristensen and Petersen 1978). Hypercholesterolaemia has been
found to be more frequent in subjects with particular HLA-B locus alleles,
notably HLA-B5 and HLA-B35, and in subjects with Gm a+x+b+ (Mathews et al.
1978; Raffoux et al. 1978; Mathews unpublished observations). HDL-cholesterol
levels have also been found to be correlated with the HLA-B and Gm loci;
levels were lowest in subjects with Gm a+x+b+ (Table 1). Earlier studies
found that atherosclerotic disease, hypercholesterolaemia and hypertension
were related to ABO blood groups; in general, risks were higher for blood
group A than for O.

Geographic gradients in coronary heart disease (CHD) mortality in European
populations are strongly correlated with gradients in HLA, Gm and blood
group allele frequencies (Mathews 1975a, unpublished observations; Mitchell
1977); these effects are highly significant and can explain most of the
variation in CHD mortality between European countries. A critical finding
however, is that the particular alleles which are positively associated
with CHD mortality rates in comparisons between populations, tend to be
negatively associated with CHD in individuals (Table 2). Thus for example,
there is a high death rate from CHD in countries such as Scotland where
blood group O is at high frequency; however, as the risk of CHD in an individual with blood group O is less than average, the high risk of CHD in
Scotland cannot be explained as a direct effect of the blood group or other
genetic constitution of the population. This paradox can be explained in
terms of an evolutionary model. The model assumes firstly that natural
selection by (infective) environmental agents (EA) has contributed to the
geographic gradients of immunogenetic alleles and blood groups through
Europe. Thus, the high frequency of blood group O in Scotland is interpreted to mean that individuals with blood group O had a survival advantage
after exposure to EA which were more dangerous in Scotland than elsewhere.
This assumption is not novel. However, the key to the evolutonary model is
provided by the novel conjecture that the environmental agents (EA) causing
natural selection in evolutionary time may be closely related to environmental agents (EA') causing CHD in contemporary time. Thus for example,
the high frequency of blood group O in Scotland indicates intense natural
selection by environmental agents (EA) against which blood group O was protective; this implies that these EA were particularly dangerous in Scotland.
By conjecture, the frequency of CHD is high in Scotland because similar environmental agents (EA') are still active as causes of CHD in Scotland. By
analogy, it is conjectured that an individual with blood group O is also protected against CHD caused by environmental agents EA'. The positive assoc-

Table 1. Immunogenetic markers and mean HDL-cholesterol levels (mM/1)

HLA – B7	1.14	Gm b+	1.04
B8	1.06	a+x–	1.14
B12	1.02	a+x+	1.19
B7/B8	1.15	a+x–b+	1.07
B7/B12	1.24	a+x+b+	0.93
B8/B12	1.02		
Other	0.98	$F_{10,350}$ = 3.69	p<0.001

Table 2. Associations of CHD with immunogenetic markers

Marker	Frequency in populations at high risk of CHD*	Frequency in individuals with CHD
Gm a+x–	Increased	Decreased
a+x+	Decreased	Increased
Blood group O	Increased	Decreased
A	Decreased	Increased
HLA–B8	Increased	Unchanged

* Adjusted for other markers

Table 3. Regression of systolic blood pressure on age, time since vasectomy and acrosomal autoantibody (Mathews, Law, Bodmer, Skegg and Vessey – unpublished observations).

SBP = 121 + 0.313 x (age in years)
      + 1.332 x (years since vasectomy)
      + 1.816 x (grade of acrosomal antibody (0-4))

Overall significance: $F_{3,261}$ = 6.36 (P < 0.001)

Increment due to vasectomy and autoantibody: $F_{2,261}$ = 4.48, p < 0.02

Increment due to autoantibody alone: $F_{1,161}$ = 3.68, p < 0.06

iation of blood group O frequencies with CHD death rates observed in comparisons between populations is explained as an effect of natural selection by EA in increasing the frequency of a protective gene. The negative association of blood group O with CHD in individuals is explained as a direct consequence of the protective effect of O against EA'. Detailed analyses show that similar arguments apply to other blood groups and immunogenetic alleles.

Environmental Agents Causing Natural Selection and CHD

It is almost axiomatic that past natural selection has not been caused by death from CHD, as most such deaths occur in post-reproductive life. Pre-reproductive deaths have largely been caused by infectious diseases. In developed countries, with declining mortality from infectious diseases following improvements in nutrition and hygeine, there has been a complementary increase in CHD; these two trends could be causally related. For example, changes in herd immunity or nutrition have shifted the host-parasite balance so that the number of pre-reproductive deaths from infection is markedly reduced; one of the costs of this may be that genetic susceptibles die from CHD in adult life. If, as seems indicated, higher levels of plasma cholesterol are associated with the ability to produce higher antibody titres (Mathews and Feery 1978), the observed substitution of adult CHD deaths for earlier infective deaths may be partly due to nutritional changes affecting those later born cohorts. This "trade-off" of infective deaths for CHD deaths may also occur in reverse, as evidenced by dietary intervention trials in CHD which show a tendency for infective and other deaths to be increased when CHD deaths are decreased.

Temporal fluctuations in the incidence of acute myocardial infarction can correlate with cold weather and/or with influenza epidemics (McFarlane 1978). To provide a specific test of the genetic-environmental interaction model, we have examined the HLA-phenotypes of 516 consecutive patients admitted to hospital over a 16 month period with a diagnosis of acute myocardial infarction (AMI). It was possible to show that there were clusters (or micro-epidemics) of patients with similar HLA phenotypes who were admitted at similar times. The overall effect was highly significant ($P < 0.0001$), and independent of the temporal clustering of the whole series of cases. It is suggested that persons with particular HLA phenotypes show susceptibility to particular (infectious) environmental agents which cause or precipitate AMI; each cluster of patients with similar HLA types would reflect the effect of a micro-epidemic of a particular infectious agent in selecting out a sub-group of individuals with the most susceptible HLA types for that infectious agent.

Detailed geographical studies suggest that two (or more) environmental components are correlated with immunogenetic allele frequencies and with CHD mortality rates: the first increases with (northern) latitude and may reflect the influence of latitude and temperature on susceptibility to infection with respiratory pathogens such as influenza virus. The second component decreases with latitude and may reflect the effect of temperature and hygeine on the transmissibility of enteric pathogens. These tentative conclusions are in accord (respectively) with the observation that influenza epidemics are correlated with AMI admissions rates (McFarlane 1978) and with a report of coxsackie virus infection in association with AMI (Nichols and Thomas 1977). Animal studies have already shown that coxsackie and herpes viruses can cause atherosclerotic lesions in the coronary arteries and elsewhere (Lancet 1978b; these proceedings); the challenge is to identify the precise role of viral and other pathogens in man. A critical problem is to discover whether the persistence of foreign genetic material or foreign antigens is of importance for the progression of vascular lesions; the alternative view is that pathogens may play an important initiating role in triggering autoimmune responses or in causing cell transformation.

Other Human Evidence

Toxaemia of pregnancy is characterised by hypertension and vascular lesions associated with circulating immune complexes (Stirrat et al. 1978). A normal or toxaemic first pregnancy protects against toxaemia in later pregnancies, possibly because of the production of blocking or enhancing antibodies (Mathews 1975b; Feeney et al. 1978). Although women are more resistant to CHD than men, antibody responses are generally higher in women (Mathews et al. 1974). These two situations raise the possibility that augmented antibody responses may sometimes protect against vascular damage, possibly by helping to clear pathogenic immune complexes formed in antigen excess.

Autoantibodies to sperm antigens are induced by vasectomy. Although this immune response has usually been thought to be harmless, some data suggest that blood pressures may be elevated after vasectomy, particularly in men with autoantibodies to sperm acrosome (Table 3). Experiments in monkeys indicate that diet-induced atherosclerosis is enhanced by prior vasectomy (Alexander and Clarkson 1978).

Immunologic sensitisation to food antigens is well recognised. The claimed association of milk and egg antibodies with AMI has not been confirmed (Scott et al. 1976). A controversial report that circulating immune complexes are more prevalent in bottle-fed than in breast fed infants (Delire et al. 1978) is of interest in view of the claimed importance of bottle feeding as a risk factor for AMI in later life. Monoclonal antibodies to ethinyl oestradiol have been identified in women using oral contraceptives, and may prove to be important in causing the vascular complications associated with pill use (Beaumont and Lemort 1976).

Relation to Other Risk Factors

Cigarette smoking modifies the immune response during influenza infection, and it may predispose to autoantibody formation (Mathews et al. 1974). Obesity is associated with thyrogastric autoimmunity in young men, but not in older men, possibly because of excess mortality in obese men who have auto-antibodies (Mathews et al. 1976a). Plasma cholesterol fractions can change during the immune response to influenza and poliovirus antigen in man, and the magnitude of the antibody response is higher in individuals with higher total cholesterol levels prior to immunisation (Mathews and Feery 1978; Mathews unpublished observations). There is an extensive literature on the effects of lipids as antigens and immunologic adjuvants in experimental systems and new data, summarised in this workshop, on the immunoregulatory role of specific lipoprotein fractions from human plasma. The precise connections of plasma lipids with membrane lipids and with membrane functions related to immunologic responses need further study.

Acknowledgment

I thank Professor R.R.H. Lovell, University of Melbourne and the Royal Melbourne Hospital for facilities and accommodation; Mr. I.D.Mathieson, and Drs. D.Campbell, D.Cowling, D.Hunt, D.Propert, J.Shaw, G.Sloman, B.Tait, B.Ungar helped with various aspects of this work.

References

Alexander NJ, Clarkson TB (1978) Vasectomy increases the severity of diet-induced atherosclerosis in Macaca Fascicularis. Science 201: 538-541

Beaumont JL, Lemort N (1976) Oral contraceptive, pulmonary artery thrombosis and anti-ethinyl-oestradiol monoclonal IgG. Clin Exp Immunol 24: 455-463

Delire M, Cambiaso CL, Masson PL (1978) Circulating immune complexes in infants fed on cow's milk. Nature 272: 632

Feeney JG, Tovey LAD, Scott JS (1977) Influence of previous blood transfusions on the incidence of pre-eclampsia. Lancet 1: 874-875

Fust G, Szondy E, Szekely J, Nanai I, Gero S (1978) Circulating immune complexes in vascular diseases. Atherosclerosis 29: 181-190

Kristensen BO, Andersen PL, Lamm LU, Kissmeyer-Nielsen F (1977) HLA antigens in essential hypertension. Tissue Antigens 10: 70-74

Kristensen BO, Petersen GB (1978) Association between coronary heart disease
    and the C3F-gene. Circulation 58: 622-625
Lancet (1977) Thyroiditis, autoimmunity and coronary risk factors. Lancet
    2: 173-175
Lancet (1978a) Immunogenetics and essential hypertension. Lancet 2: 409-410
Lancet (1978b) Virus infections and atherosclerosis. Lancet 2: 821-822
McFarlane A (1977) Daily mortality and environment. Brit J Prev Soc Med 31: 54
Mathews JD, Whittingham S, Mackay IR (1974) Hypothesis: Autoimmunity and
    vascular disease. Lancet 2: 1423-1426
Mathews JD (1975a) Ischaemic heart disease: possible genetic markers. Lancet
    2: 681-682
Mathews JD (1975b) Immune mechanisms in vascular disease. Lancet 1: 1298
Mathews JD, Rodger BM, Stenhouse NS (1976a) The association of rheumatoid
    factor and tissue autoantibodies with angina. J Chronic Dis 29: 345-353
Mathews JD et al. (1976b) Antigen and haplotype frequencies in essential
    hypertension and ischaemic heart disease. Abstracts, HLA and Disease,
    Paris, Inserm. p.257
Mathews JD, Tait BD, Mathieson ID (1978) Immunological and immunogenetic
    factors in atherosclerosis. In: Proceedings 1st International Symposium
    on Immunological Factors in Atherosclerosis (in press)
Mathews JD, Feery BJ (1978) Cholesterol and the immune response to influenza
    antigens. Lancet 2: 1212-1213
Mitchell JRA (1977) ABO blood group distribution and geographical differences
    in death rates. Lancet 1: 295-297
Nichols AC, Thomas M (1977) Coxsackie virus infection in acute myocardial
    infarction. Lancet 1: 883-884
Poston RN, Davies DF (1974) Immunity and inflammation in the pathogenesis of
    atherosclerosis. Atherosclerosis 19: 353-367
Raffoux C, Pointel JP, Drouin P, Streiff F, Debny G, Sauvanet JP (1978) Type
    IIa hyperlipoproteinaemia and the HLA system. Tissue Antigens 11: 55-58
Scott BB, McGuffin P, Swinburne ML, Losowsky MS (1976) Dietary antibodies
    and myocardial infarction. Lancet 2: 125-126
Stirrat GM, Redman CWG, Levinsky RJ (1978) Circulating immune complexes in
    pre-eclampsia. Brit Med J 1: 1450-1451

Immunologic Arterial Injury and Atherogenesis

C. Richard Minick[1]

Arterial injury has been shown to be a primary causative factor in arterio-sclerosis (Minick et al. 1976; Ross and Glomset 1976). Arterial injury, and the resulting necrosis, inflammation, intimal thickening and other reparative features may favor the deposition of blood-borne lipid at sites of injury and lead to atherosclerosis. It is important to our understanding of the etiology and pathogenesis of human atheorsclerosis to identify those causes of arterial injury and the nature of the reactive change that may be important in etiology and pathogenesis of atherosclerosis in man and other animals. There is considerable evidence to suggest that inflammation of the arterial wall and in particular that resulting from immunologic injury may be important in the development of arteriosclerosis in man. The following observations support this suggestion:

1. Inflammation and atherogenesis share major pathogenic features. Inflammation is a reaction to injury in which there is increased permeability of endothelium of the microcirculation, accumulation of protein-rich fluid in the intersitium, migration of leukocytes, and repair characterized by proliferation of mesenchymal cells and increased connective tissue synthesis. Similarly, necrosis of arterial smooth muscle cells, increased permeability of endothelium, migration of leukocytes, proliferation of mesenchymal cells and increased connective tissue synthesis are all features of atherosclerosis (Joris and Majno 1978).

2. Immunological vascular injury and atherosclerosis also share pathogenic features. Increased endothelial permeability resulting from IgE mediated release of vasoactive amines from basophils and platelets is believed to be essential for localization of immune complexes in the arterial wall. Such IgE mediated increases in endothelial permeability may enhance transport of other macromolecules, e.g., lipoproteins, into the arterial wall (Henson and Cochrane 1971). Alterations in endothelium are also important in other types of immunological injury such as graft rejection (Alonso et al. 1977).

3. Premature atherosclerosis or atherosclerosis of increased severity has been found in human in association with arterial diseases that have a major inflammatory or immunological components. Saphir et al. (1950) noted evidence of healed arteritis in hearts of humans with premature atherosclerosis and ischemic heart disease. Syphilis, rheumatic heart disease, lupus erythematosus and organ transplantation may be associated with vascular injury, arteritis and premature or unusually severe atherosclerosis (Zeek et al. 1932; Bulkley and Roberts 1975; Rider et al. 1975). There is evidence to indicate that arterial injury in syphilis, rheumatic heart disease, lupus erythematosus and organ transplantation are immunologically mediated.

---

[1] The authors' personal research cited was supported by Grant HL-19109 from the National Heart, Lung and Blood Institute of the National Institutes of Health and by The Cross Foundation.

For several years, we have investigated the role of immunologic arterial injury and subsequent reparative changes in atherogenesis (Minick et al. 1966; Minick and Murphy 1973; Hardin et al. 1973; Minick, 1976, Alonso et al. (1977). In these experiments immunologic arterial injury was induced in rabbits by repeated intravenous injections of foreign serum protein or by graft rejection in heterotopically placed cardiac allografts. Hypercholesterolemia was induced by feeding cholesterol-supplemented or semisynthetic, lipid rich, cholesterol-poor diets. Results of our experiments indicate the following:

1. The synergy of immunological arterial injury and simultaneous dietary hypercholesterolemia led to atherosclerosis that was not seen in comparably hypercholesterolemic controls fed lipid-supplemented diets alone.

2. Although immunological arterial injury alone led to a few lipid-containing arterial lesions, most arterial lesions were characterized by fibromuscular intimal thickening with little lipid. Severity of arterial change was considerably enhanced in rabbits with immunological arterial injury fed lipid-supplemented diets as compared to those fed lipid-poor diets.

3. Sites of healed immunological arterial injury induced many weeks previously in the presence of normal serum cholesterol were predisposed to atherosclerosis as compared to the normal artery in rabbits subsequently fed cholesterol-supplemented diets.

4. Arterial lesions induced by the synergy of immunological arterial injury and hypercholesterolemia bore striking resemblance to chronic human atherosclerosis with regard to the amount of hypercholesterolemia necessary to induce them, distribution of lesions in the arterial system, and morphological features of the arterial change. In contrast, lesions in hypercholesterolemic controls bore little resemblance to human atherosclerosis.

5. Chronic atherosclerosis, induced in rabbits by the synergy of immunologic arterial injury and hypercholesterolemia did not regress following dietary modifications similar to those recommended for man (Minick, 1979, unpublished observations).

6. Endothelial injury and denudation are early features of arterial injury induced by both immune complex disease and graft rejection (Minick, 1976; Alonso et al. 1977; Minick 1979 unpublished observations).

Results of experiments of Van Winkle and Levy, (1968) and Lamberson et al. (1974) also indicate that the synergy of immunological arterial injury due to immune complex disease and hypercholesterolemia leads to atherosclerosis not found in rabbits receiving dietary lipid supplement alone. Similar observations have recently been made in swine (Clopath, 1978). Recently, reported experiments of Alexander and Clarkson, (1978) suggest that immune complex disease induced by vasectomy will lead to atherosclerosis in Macaca fasicularis fed a lipid supplemented diet. Results of further experiments indicate that vasectomy was also associated with increased atherosclerosis in normocholesterolemic nonhuman primates fed lipid-poor monkey chow over a period of many years (Clarkson and Alexander, 1979).

In searching for causes of arterial injury that may lead to atherosclerosis in man, it has been proposed that reaction to antigens in infecting microorganisms and vaccines, foreign serum, antibiotics and drugs, tobacco, foodstuffs and the individuals own tissue maybe causative of arterial disease that can evolve as atherosclerosis (Minick et al. 1966). Persistent hepatitis B antigenemia is associated with an increased incidence of vasculitis and intimal hyperplasia which may evolve as atherosclerosis. Infection with virus may lead to arterial disease in many animals and in some instances these arterial changes may lead to atherosclerosis (Minick et al. 1979). Results of recent experiments in our laboratories, indicate that infection with Marek's disease herpesvirus will lead to atherosclerosis in both normocholesterolemic and hypercholesterolemic chickens (Fabricant et al. 1978; Minick et al. 1979). Such arterial lesions could result from a direct effect of the virus of Marek's disease or an immunologic reaction to the virus. Harkavy and Perlman (1964) have shown that patients with coronary disease who smoked have an increased incidence of positive skin tests to tobacco leaf protein, as compared to smokers without coronary disease. Becker et al. (1976) have recently isolated a small glycoprotein from cured tobacco leaves and from cigarette smoke condensate to which approximately one third of smokers and nonsmokers exhibited immediate cutaneous hypersensitivity.

In conclusion, results of experiments summarized here indicate that immunologic arterial injury will lead to atherosclerosis in man and experimental animals. Results suggest that immunologic reaction to many antigens in man's environment may lead to repeated or protracted immunologic arterial injury and local reactive changes that may favor deposition of lipid in the arterial wall and thus lead to an even greater amount of atherosclerosis.

References

Alexander NJ, Clarkson TB (1978) Vasectomy increases the severity of diet-induced atherosclerosis in Macaca fasicularis. Science 201:538-541

Alonso DR, Starek PK, Minick CR (1977) Studies on the pathogenesis of atheroarteriosclerosis induced in rabbit cardiac allografts by the synergy of graft rejection and hypercholesterolemia. Am J Pathol 87:415-442

Becker CG, Dubin T, Wiedeman HP (1976) Hypersensitivity to tobacco antigen. Proc Natl Acad Sci (USA) 73:1712-1716

Bulkley BH, Roberts WC (1975) The heart in systemic lupus erythematosus and the changes induced in it by corticosteroid therapy. Am J Med 58:243-264

Clarkson TB, Alexander NJ (1979) Effect of long-term vasectomy on the occurrence and extent of arteriosclerosis in Rhesus monkeys fed monkey chow. Fed Proc 38:1346

Clopath P (1978) Immunologic arterial injury in swine. In: Peptides of the Biological Fluids. H. Peters (Ed) Proceedings of the 26th Colloquium Pergamon Press, New York, pp 437-440

Fabricant CG, Fabricant J, Litrenta MM, Minick CR (1978) Virus-induced atherosclerosis. J Exp Med 148:335-340

Hardin NJ, Minick CR, Murphy GE (1973) Experimental induction of athero-arteriosclerosis by the synergy of allergic injury to arteries and lipid-rich diet. III. The role of earlier acquired fibromuscular intimal thickening in the pathogenesis of later developing atherosclerosis. Am J Pathol 73:301-326

Harkavy J, Perlman E (1964) Tobacco allergy in coronary artery disease. N.Y. State J Med 64:1287-1296

Henson PM, Cochrane CG (1971) Acute immune complex disease in rabbits: the role of complement and of a leukocyte-dependent release of vasoactive amines from platelets. J Exp Med 133:554-571

Joris I, Majno G (1978) Atherosclerosis and inflammation. Adv Exp Med Biol 104:227-233

Lamberson HV, Fritz KE (1974) Immunological enhancement of atherogenesis in rabbits. Persistent susceptibility to atherogenic diet following experimentally induced serum sickness. Arch Pathol 98:9-16

Minick CR, Murphy GE, Campbell WG, Jr (1966) Experimental induction of athero-arteriosclerosis by the synergy of allergic injury to arteries and lipid-rich diet. I. Effect of repeated injections of horse serum in rabbits fed a dietary cholesterol supplement. J Exp Med 124:635-652

Minick CR, Murphy GE (1973) Experimental induction of atheroarteriosclerosis by the synergy of allergic injury to arteries and lipid-rich diet. II. Effect of repeatedly injected foreign protein in rabbits fed a lipid-rich, cholesterol-poor diet. Am J Pathol 73:265-300

Minick CR (1976) Immunologic arterial injury in atherogenesis. Ann N Y Acad Sci 275:210-227

Minick CR, Fabricant CG, Fabricant J, Litrenta MM (1979) Atheroarteriosclerosis induced by infection with a herpesvirus. Am J Pathol (In Press)

Rider AK, Copeland JC, Hunt SA, Mason J, Specter MJ, Winkle RA, Bieber CP, Billingham ME, Dong E, Greipp RB, Schroeder JS, Stinson EB, Harrison DC, Shumway NE (1975) The status of cardiac transplantation. Circulation 52: 531-539

Ross R, Glomset JA (1976) The pathogenesis of atherosclerosis. N Engl J Med 295:369-377, 420-425

Saphir O, Gore I (1950) Evidence for an inflammatory basis for coronary atherosclerosis in the young. Arch Pathol 49:418-426

Sharma HM, Geen JC (1977) Experimental aortic lesions of serum sickness in rabbits. Am J Pathol 88:255-266

Van Winkle M, Levy L (1968) Effect of removal of cholesterol diet upon serum sickness cholesterol-induced atherosclerosis. J Exp Med 128:497-516

Zeek P (1932a) Studies in atherosclerosis. I. Conditions in childhood which predispose to the early development of atherosclerosis. Am J Med Sci 184:350-356

Zeek P (1932b) Studies in atherosclerosis II. Atheroma and its sequelae in rheumatic heart disease. Am J Med Sci 184:356-364

Autoimmune Hyperlipidemia and Autoimmune Xanthomatosis

J. L. Beaumont, M. F. Baudet, C. Dachet, and V. Beaumont

Autoimmune hyperlipidemia (AIH) is a metabolic disease of immune origin, in which the lipoprotein clearance is inhibited by circulating autoantibodies (Beaumont 1965).

In AIH different types of antibodies may react with different types of antigens to induce different types of hyperlipidemia and hyperlipoproteinemia. The hyperlipidemia is usually of the mixed type, and all patterns of hyperlipoproteinemia were already seen except type IIa. According to the antigen implicated in the reaction, three main varieties of AIH may be indentified: AIH with antibody to lipoproteins, to enzymes, and to acceptors of lipids.

Atherosclerosis, thrombosis and ischemic diseases are frequently associated with AIH. In some cases, tuberous and tendonous xanthomas may appear.

In the IgA antilipoprotein type of AIH, the variety first reported (Beaumont and Lorenzelli 1967), the monoclonal IgA kappa reacts with a site present on LDL and HDL, and forms with these lipoproteins cholesterol- and triglyceride-rich complexes, which may be visualized in the microscope and are easily precipitated. Atherosclerosis and tuberous xanthomas are often associated.

Hyperlipidemia in this type is secondary to the blood accumulation of lipoprotein/IgA complexes, which clearance seems to be reduced, as indicated by the vitamin A tolerance test, in which the clearance of the ingested liposoluble vitamin is decreased and delayed (Beaumont and Beaumont 1977). However an increase of cholesterol synthesis by extrahepatic tissue was demonstrated in one case (Ho et al. 1976).

Atherosclerosis and xanthomas might be due either to an infiltration of complexes in the tissues, either to an overproduction of lipids by fibroblasts and smooth muscle cells. The infiltration of the arterial wall by IgA/lipoprotein complexes was observed (Lewis and Lazzarini-Robertson 1974). On the other hand, we have found that antilipoprotein IgA interfered in vitro with the LDL degradation and with the endogenous cholesterol synthesis regulation by fibroblasts in culture (Baudet et al. 1978).

In the latter work, we have studied the in vitro activity of 3 myeloma IgA kappa associated with a mixed hyperlipidemia and a delayed clearance of circulating IgA/lipoprotein complexes (Table 1). Atherosclerosis was present in all 3 cases. Numerous xanthoma tuberosa could be seen in case SOR and GER, but none in case BAR.

The IgA kappa SOR and GER were shown to reduce in vitro the degradation of LDL by cultured human skin fibroblasts, and to interfere with the LDL regulation of cholesterol synthesis in the cells (Table 2). In case BAR, the antilipoprotein IgA had no effect on LDL degradation nor on the inhibitory effect of fibroblasts on cell cholesterol synthesis.

Table 1. Antilipoprotein myelomas.

Cases	Antibody	Antigen		Lipidemia mg/100 ml		Athero-sclerosis	Xanthomatosis	
				Chol.	Triglyc.		Tuberous	Tendinous
GER	IgA	LDL HDL	} Pg	400 to 900	180 to 1 440	+	+	+
SOR	IgA	LDL HDL	} Pg	770 to 1 120	430 to 1 350	+	+	-
BAR	IgA	LDL HDL	Not identi- fied	560	345 to 445	+	-	-

Table 2. In vitro interference of different human immunoglobulins with the interaction of cultured human skin fibroblasts and human LDL.

Human proteins added to the cell culture		LDL degradation by the cells after 22 hours	Regulation of intra-cellular free cholesterol synthesis by LDL
LDL	Immunoglobulins		
+	None	Control	Control
+	Standard Igs	Unchanged	Unchanged
+	IgA SOR	Decreased	Decreased
+	IgA GER	Decreased	Decreased
+	IgA BAR	Unchanged	Unchanged

According to these results, it may be infered : 1) that xanthomas may form when the circulating LDL, complexed with the IgA kappa, have lost their power to regulate cholesterol synthesis in extrahepatic tissues (Brown and Goldstein 1975). This mechanism, which may be called autoimmune xanthomatosis (AIX), could explain cases of AIH with xanthomas, like cases SOR and GER ; 2) that the hyperlipidemia of AIH may be partly independent of the above mechanism, as may be seen in case BAR, with hyperlipidemia, antilipoprotein antibodies, but no xanthomas, and normal fibroblast regulation; 3) reversely, that AIX without AIH may be expected, as demonstrated by cases of xanthomatosis without hyperlipidemia (Kodama et al. 1972).

Further research will be needed to assess the relative atherogenic potency of AIH and AIX in antilipoprotein IgA kappa myelomas with atherosclerosis.

References

Baudet MF, Dachet C, Beaumont JL (1978) In vitro interaction of LDL, antilipoprotein IgA, and human fibroblasts. Biomedicine 29: 217-220

Beaumont JL (1965) L'hyperlipidémie par auto-anticorps anti-beta-lipoprotéines. Une nouvelle entité pathologique. Comptes-Rendus Acad Sci Paris Série D 261: 4563-4566

Beaumont JL, Lorenzelli L (1967) L'auto-anticorps anti-lipoprotéines (anti-Pg) du gamma-A myélome avec hyperlipidémie. Méthode d'isolement et de purification à partir des complexes circulants. Ann Biol Clin 25: 655-675

Beaumont JL, Beaumont V (1977) Autoimmune hyperlipidemia. Atherosclerosis 26: 404-418

Brown MS, Goldstein JL (1975) Regulation of the activity of the low density lipoprotein receptor in human fibroblasts. Cell 6: 307-316

Ho KJ, de Wolfe VG, Siler W, Lewis LA (1976) Cholesterol dynamics in autoimmune hyperlipidemia. J Lab Clin Med 88: 769-779

Kodama H, Nakagawa S, Tanioku K (1972) Plane xanthomatosis with antilipoprotein autoantibody. Arch Derm 105: 722-727

Lewis LA, Robertson AL Jr (1974) Hyperimmuno-globulinemia-lipoprotein-emia and atherogenesis. In: Schettler G, Weizel A (eds) Atherosclerosis III. Springer-Verlag, Heidelberg, pp 595-603

Tobacco, Immunologic Injury, and Cardiovascular Disease[1]

Carl G. Becker and Theodore Dubin

Cigarette smokers are at greater risk of developing peripheral vascular disease and of suffering heart attacks than are nonsmokers. The pathogenetic mechanisms underlying these epidemiologic associations are unknown. A clue to these mechanisms may be provided from the observation that younger smokers are at relatively greater risk of suffering heart attacks than are older smokers (The Framingham Study, 1970, 1971).

This observation could be interpreted as indicating that among the population of younger smokers are a certain number who are allergic to constituents of tobacco smoke and that repetitive immunologic challenge when these individuals smoke results in acceleration of cardiovascular disease and increased mortality, resulting in decreased representation of hypersensitive subjects in the older population.

This hypothesis receives support from experimental observations indicating that:

1. IgE mediated release of vasoactive amines from basophils and platelets enhances permeability of blood vessels to macromolecules such as immune complexes (Henson and Cochrane, 1971).
2. Immune complex mediated injury to blood vessels acts synergistically with modest hyperlipidemia to induce atherosclerosis in coronary and other arteries (Minick and Murphy, 1973).
3. The heart can be a target organ for anaphylactic reactions, responding to antigenic challenge with a variety of changes including sinus tachycardia, atrioventricular conduction block, increased ventricular automaticity, including ventricular fibrillation, decreased contractility, and decreased coronary perfusion (Capurro and Levi 1975), and
4. Hypersensitivity to extracts of tobacco leaves had been described by Harkavy, et al. (1932) who suggested that allergy to constituents of tobacco may underlie the relationship between tobacco smoking and coronary artery disease and peripheral vascular disease.

We set out to purify and characterize an antigen from cured tobacco leaves from cigarette smoke condensate (tar) and to study its allergenicity in humans and in animals. The results of these experiments are summarized below:

1. A glycoprotein of molecular weight 18,000 - 26,000 can be purified from saline extracts of tobacco leaves (TGP-L) by ammonium sulfate fractionation, molecular sieve chromatography, and continuous flow, preparative electrophoresis on polyacrylamide gel to which approximately one-third (16/50) of human volunteers, smokers and nonsmokers, exhibit immediate cutaneous hypersensitivity (Becker et al. 1976). Further fractionation of this material yields preparations capable of eliciting an immediate

---

[1] The authors' personal research cited was supported by Grant HL -01803 and Thrombosis SCOR Grant HL-18828 from the National Institutes of Health, and The Cross Foundation.

cutaneous hypersensitivity (wheal and flare) reaction in doses of as little as 10 pcg (Becker, unpublished observations, 1979). Electrophoretically, tinctorially, and immunochemically identical material can be isolated from cigarette smoke condensate (TGP-CSC)(Becker et al. 1976). Antigenically similar material can be identified in commonly ingested Solanaceae such as eggplants, green peppers, potatoes and tomatoes (Becker et al. 1976).

2. Both TGP-L and TGP-CSC contain a polyphenol hapten identical to or closely resembling rutin which enables them to activate the factor XII dependent pathways of coagulation, fibrinolysis, and kinin generation (Becker and Dubin 1977). Activation of factor XII can be demonstrated in vivo and in vitro. Antigens cross reactive with TGP, also containing polyphenol haptens and capable of activating factor XII can be isolated from ragweed pollen and cocoa, common respiratory and food allergens, but not members of the plant family Solanaceae (Becker and Dubin, unpublished work, 1979).

3. Neonatal sensitization of rabbits with TGP-L induces preferential synthesis of IgE antibodies to TGP. These antibodies can mediate cutaneous anaphylactic reactions on challenge with either TGP-L or TGP-CSC or with cross reactive antigens from ragweed and cocoa. No blocking antibodies are formed by these animals, even after continued immunization (Becker et al. 1979).

4. Cardiac anaphylaxis can be induced in hearts of rabbits neonatally sensitized with TGP-L or hearts of adult guinea pigs sensitized with TGP-L on challenge with either TGP-L or TGP-CSC (Levi et al. 1978 and Levi et al. unpublished work).

These results, taken together, indicate that exposure to TGP in inhaled tobacco smoke may be related to cardiovascular disease through the mechanisms or events diagramed below.

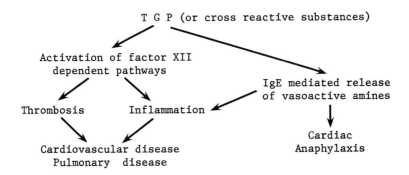

It is implicit in this diagram that activation of factor XII dependent pathways in the hypersensitive smoker would act synergistically with IgE-mediated mechanisms to induce tissue injury. These data also point to the possibility that smoking mothers sensitize their children early in life to TGP and a wide variety of antigens cross reactive with TGP, perhaps rendering them more susceptible to cardiovascular and pulmonary disease mediated by allergic mechanisms. Neonatal or earlier sensitization of children to tobacco antigen through maternal smoking may also account in part for the high incidence of immediate cutaneous hypersensitivity to tobacco. The high incidence of hypersensitivity to tobacco may also be related to the ubiquity of antigens similar to TGP in commonly ingested plants.

References

Becker CG, Dubin T, Wiedemann HP (1976)   Hypersensitivity to tobacco antigen.   Proc Natl Acad Sci USA 73:1712

Becker CG, Dubin T (1977)   Activation of factor XII by tobacco glycoprotein.   J Exp Med 146:457

Becker CG, Levi R, Zavecz J (1979)   Induction of IgE antibodies to antigen isolated from tobacco leaves and from cigarette smoke condensate. Am J Path 96:249

Capurro N, Levi R (1975)   The heart as a target organ in systemic allergic reactions.   Circ Res 36:520

The Framingham Study: An epidemiologic investigation of cardiovascular disease. Monograph. Sections 26 and 27. DHEW, Natl Heart Institute, 1970 and 1971

Harkavy J, Hebald S, Silbert S (1932)   Tobacco sensitiveness in thromboangiitis obliterans.   Proc Soc Exp Biol Med 30:104

Henson PM, Cochrane CG (1971)   Acute immune complex disease in rabbits: the role of complement and of a leukocyte-dependent release of vasoactive amines from platelets.   J Exp Med 133:554

Levi R, Zavecz, Holland B, Becker CG (1978)   Cardiac and pulmonary anaphylaxis induced by tobacco glycoprotein.   Fed Proc 37, no. 3:590

Minick CR, Murphy GE (1973)   Experimental induction of atheroarteriosclerosis by the synergy of allergic injury to arteries and lipid rich diet. Am J Path 73:265

Immunoregulatory Lipoproteins, Viral Hepatitis, and Cancer[1]

Francis V. Chisari

A large number of metabolically important proteins involved in multisystem transport, storage and nutritional functions throughout the body are known to originate in the liver. We (Chisari 1977) and others (Morse et al. 1977) have shown that one of these, namely very low density lipoproteins (VLDL), can modulate an assortment of inductive, recognitive, proliferative and differentiative cellular processes in vitro. The in vivo correlates of these cellular functions are thought to contribute directly to the pathogenesis and control of several liver diseases including viral hepatitis B (Chisari et al. 1978), primary and metastatic liver disease (Hellstrom et al. 1968), and primary malignant transformation of hepatitis B virus (HBV) - infected hepatocytes (Goudeau et al. 1978). Recognition of the anatomic coexistence of these pathogenetically important cellular mechanisms and the bioregulatory lipoproteins potentially capable of modulating them spawned the hypothesis that the local release of bioregulatory molecules within the hepatic extracellular microenvironment may abrogate immune surveillance mechanisms responsible for the control of intrahepatic neoplastic proliferation and suppress immunopathogenetic hepatocytotoxic effector pathways in viral hepatitis. The studies reported herein represent the seminal observations responsible for the generation of this hypothesis.

VLDL are synthesized in the liver (Eisenberg and Levy 1975) and are normally secreted into the plasma where they are catabolized. We have isolated VLDL from fresh human plasma by preparative ultracentrifugation and molecular exclusion chromatography according to standard techniques (Chisari 1977). The resulting preparation has been demonstrated to be free of serum contaminants and, in particular, free of other immunoregulatory molecules (Chisari 1977). This material routinely has pre-beta electrophoretic mobility, a density of less than 1.006 gm/cm^3, a triglyceride:protein ratio of 4.7 ± 1.6 and a triglyceride:cholesterol ratio of 3.8 ± 1.0.

We have found that VLDL are potent inhibitors of phytohemagglutinin (PHA) stimulated peripheral blood lymphocyte (PBL) DNA synthesis. Fifty percent inhibition of this response is produced by as little as 1.03 ug of VLDL protein per culture (this represents $1.2-3.6 \times 10^{-12}$M in culture). Inhibition is not due to cytotoxicity.

Suppression does not require the continuous presence of VLDL throughout the culture period (Figure 1). In this experiment PBL were preincubated with VLDL or buffer for varying intervals, then they were washed extensively resuspended in complete culture medium and PHA was added. The cultures were harvested 72 hr later after 18 hr ^{3}H-thymidine pulse. Significant suppression (relative to buffer control) is detectable after a brief 1 hr VLDL pulse; 50% inhibition occurs within a 2 hr pulse period whereas between 6 and 24 hr preincubation is necessary for complete inhibition.

In separate studies VLDL were found to preferentially inhibit early inductive events. In these experiments, VLDL were added to cultures at varying intervals before, coincident with, or after the addition of PHA and remained

[1]Supported by NIH grant AI-13393, RCDA 5 KO4 AI-00174. Publication #1897.

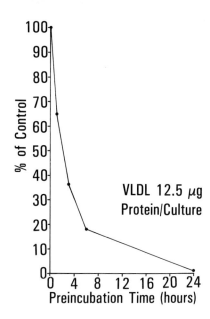

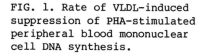

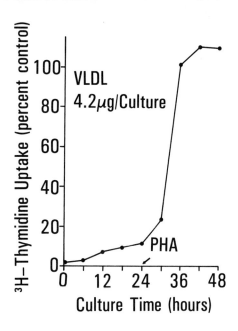

FIG. 1. Rate of VLDL-induced
suppression of PHA-stimulated
peripheral blood mononuclear
cell DNA synthesis.

FIG. 2. Temporal aspects of
VLDL-induced inhibition of
PHA-stimulated lymphocytes.

present in the culture system for the duration of the experiment. Maximal
inhibition is observed when VLDL are added to PBL coincident with or prior to
the addition of PHA (Figure 2). Inhibition decreases rapidly with time when
VLDL are added after PHA and is absent by 12-18 hr after PHA demonstrating
the resistance of ongoing DNA synthesis to suppression by VLDL.

The suppressive effect of VLDL on mitogen-induced lymphocyte DNA synthesis
is not due to fluid phase binding of PHA by VLDL since VLDL suppress the DNA
synthetic response of PBL to an equivalent degree over a wide PHA dose range.
The fact that VLDL are also equally potent inhibitors of lymphocyte activation by pokeweed mitogen (PWM) and by allogeneic cells and that they also
inhibit PHA-induced protein synthesis further suggests that a common central
metabolic event in the activation process is the target of VLDL induced
suppression.

This attests to the potential general bioregulatory properties of VLDL and
suggests that they may profoundly affect a variety of immune effector functions which are dependent on de novo protein synthesis for expression.

VLDL inhibit the in vivo immune response of mice to immunization with sheep
red blood cells (Figure 3). A single injection of VLDL administered on day
-1 suppressed the primary and secondary immune response to SRBC injected on
days 0 and +21 to an equivalent degree. The temporal characteristics of each
response were unaffected.

Assuming a mean molecular weight of 10×10^6 daltons and 10% (w/w) protein
composition (Eisenberg and Levy 1975), 50% inhibition of the day 5 hemagglu-
tinin response was accomplished with as little as 2.6 picomoles of VLDL per
mouse. This compares favorably with other immunoregulatory molecules such
as LDL-In (10 picomoles)(Curtiss et al. 1977) but is substantially more
potent than other described immunosuppressive molecules such as fibrinogen
peptides (Girmann et al. 1975) which display equivalent immunosuppressive

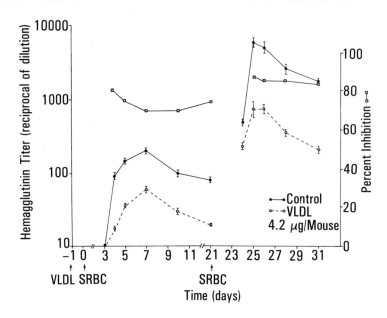

FIG. 3. Temporal characteristics of the inhibitory effect of human VLDL on the in vivo murine immune response to sheep red blood cells.

activity only after administration of 10,000 and 200,000 picomoles respectively.

We have also examined the ability of VLDL to influence Epstein-Barr virus (EBV) induced transformation and immortalization of human B lymphocytes in vitro. EBV has been shown to stimulate irreversible DNA synthesis and blast transformation in human adult and fetal B lymphocytes (Thorley-Lawson et al. 1977).

Preliminary experiments in our laboratory indicate that VLDL suppress EBV-induced transformation of human B lymphocytes in a dose-dependent fashion (Table 1). EBV was grown in B95-8 lymhocytes derived from an EBV-induced marmoset lymphoma (Miller and Lipman 1973). B lymphocytes were isolated from human umbilical cord blood. The B cells were preincubated with varying dilutions of VLDL and buffer for 24 hr prior to the addition of an optimally mitogenic concentration of EBV. The cultures were maintained for 14 days (with refeeding on day 7) whereupon they were harvested after an 8 hr pulse with ^{3}H-thymidine. Others (Thorley-Lawson et al. 1977) have clearly demonstrated that the DNA synthesis measured at 14 days represents a marker for the irreversible transformation and immortalization of the B lymphocytes by

Table 1. Effect of VLDL on Epstein-Barr virus-induced ^{3}H-thymidine uptake by cultured fetal B lymphocytes

VLDL (ug protein/culture)	^{3}H-thymidine uptake (cpm)
26.0	72
13.0	861
5.2	5,931
2.6	10,740
0	13,554

342

EBV. These observations are provocative because they imply the existence of natural non-immune molecular mechanisms potentially capable of preventing DNA virus-induced neoplasia in vivo. They are of further interest because considerable evidence (Goudeau 1978) suggests that the hepatitis B virus (another human DNA virus) may be responsible for the induction of primary hepatocellular carcinoma in long-term HBV carriers in Africa. Thus, the EBV-human B lymphocyte model is analogous to the putative transforming relationship between HBV and human hepatocytes and the in vitro effects of VLDL on the former process may presage their in situ in vivo effects on the latter.

Since VLDL are synthesized and released by the liver it is likely that its intracellular and extracellular intrahepatic concentration far exceeds that normally found in plasma. Since all the aforementioned inhibitory effects are achieved by concentrations of VLDL far below those in plasma, it is very likely that sufficient amounts of VLDL exist in the hepatic microenvironment to suppress the biological processes under consideration. We therefore predict that VLDL may represent an important candidate mechanism whereby: 1) generally intact immune surveillance mechanisms are bypassed in the liver, the commonest site of tumor growth and metastasis; 2) autoaggressive hepatocytolytic effector mechanisms are suppressed in situ thereby limiting HBV-induced hepatocellular necrosis to areas of focal distribution, and 3) potential neoplastic transforming signals by intrahepatocellular HBV may be suppressed.

Critical examination of these hypotheses is currently underway.

References

Baird S, Raschke W, Weissman IL (1977) Evidence that MuLV-induced thymid lymphoma cells possess specific cell membrane binding sites for MuLV. Int J Cancer 19: 403

Chisari FV (1977) Immunoregulatory properties of human plasma in very low density lipoproteins. J Immunol 119: 2129

Chisari FV, Edgington TS, Routenberg JA, Anderson DS (1978) Cellular immune reactivity in HBV induced liver disease. In: Vyas GN, Cohen HN, Schmid R (eds) Viral Hepatitis. Franklin Institute Press, Philadelphia, pp 245–266

Curtiss LK, DeHeer DH, Edgington TS (1977) In vivo suppression of the primary immune response by a species of low density serum lipoprotein. J Immunol 118: 648

Eisenberg S, Levy RI (1975) Lipoprotein metabolism. Adv Lipid Research 13: 1

Girmann G, Pees H, Schwarze G, Scheurlen PG (1975) Immunosuppression by micromolecular fibrinogen degradation products in cancer. Nature 259: 399

Goudeau A, Maupas PH, Coursaget P, Drucker J (1978) Detection of HBV antigens and DNA in hepatoma tissue. In: Vyas GN, Cohen HN, Schmid R (eds) Viral Hepatitis. Franklin Institute Press, Philadelphia

Hellstrom I, Hellstrom KE, Pierce GE, Yang JPS (1968) Cellular and humoral immunity to different types of human neoplasms. Nature 220: 1352

Miller G, Lipman M (1973) Release of infectious Epstein-Barr virus by transformed marmoset leukocytes. Proc Natl Acad Sci 70: 190

Morse JH, Witte LD, Goodman DS (1977) Inhibition of lymphocyte proliferation stimulated by lectins and allogeneic cells by normal plasma lipoproteins. J Exp Med 146: 1791

Occhino JC, Glasgow AH, Cooperband SR, Mannick JA, Schmid K (1973) Isolation of an immunosuppressive peptide fraction from human plasma. J Immunol 110: 685

Thorley-Lawson DA, Chess L, Strominger JL (1977) Suppression of in vitro Epstein-Barr virus infection. J Exp Med 146: 495

Regulation of Pathways of Lymphocyte Differentiation by the Serum Lipoprotein: LDL-In

Thomas S. Edgington, Dennis K. Fujii, and Linda K. Curtiss

Introduction

Serum lipoproteins serve physiologically critical transport functions. As a consequence of the non-covalent nature of these particles and the resultant capacity to exchange constituent lipids and peptides, the existence of specific cell surface receptors, and the central role of lipids in membrane synthesis and function these particles possess an important potential to influence cell metabolism. Although LDL has been relatively well-characterized with respect to regulation of cholesterol metabolism, a number of other bioregulatory functions of various lipoproteins have only recently been recognized. Among some newer bioregulatory functions have been the effects of subsets of normal and acquired serum lipoproteins on the lymphoid system (Chisari and Edgington, 1975; Waddel et al., 1976; Curtiss and Edgington, 1976). Perhaps the most extensively characterized, though still incompletely understood regulatory lipoprotein, is a subset of intermediate density lipoprotein (IDL) designated LDL-In. The physical and biochemical characteristics, biological effects and mechanistic features of LDL-In will be considered in order to identify the potential significance of this immunoregulatory serum lipoprotein and broader perspectives regarding the functions of serum lipoproteins.

Physical and biochemical characteristics of LDL-In

Following observations that LDL fractions of normal plasma could suppress mixed lymphocyte reactions (Chisari and Edgington, 1975), a fraction from the light edge of LDL, referred to by Morse et al. (1977) as IDL, was isolated by three methods and found to be enriched in immunosuppressive activity. Whereas LDL-In activity was originally recovered on the low density edge of LDL (1.006–1.063 gm/cm^3), systematic isolation of density 1.006–1.019 gm/cm^3 fractions (IDL) has provided the same lipoprotein subset. It is a spherical particle of 246 Å compared with 210 Å for LDL. This fraction contains apolipoprotein B as well as smaller chains consistent by SDS polyacrylamide gel electrophoresis with E, AI, AII and one or more C chains; however the chain composition requisite for biological activity has not been established. The biologically active lipoprotein is bound by Con A and precipitated by dextran sulfate (Curtiss and Edgington, 1976) consistent with apolipoprotein B content; however, the biologically active particle is not bound by selected antibodies to apolipoprotein B indicating that it may differ in the surface presentation of Apo B antigenic determinants. LDL-In particles are devoid of detectable peroxidation byproducts by thiobarbituric acid assays and of oxygenated sterols (<1%) by thin-layer chromatography.

---

[1] This is publication number 1929 from the Immunology Departments. These studies were supported by NIH research grants CA-14346 and AI-14921.

The bioregulatory properties of LDL-In have been characterized in respect to suppression of lymphocyte function. LDL-In enriched fractions require approximately 20-24 hr to exert a maximal effect on the lymphocyte in culture (Curtiss and Edgington 1976), but the lipoprotein can be removed before stimulation without loss of suppression. LDL-In is not toxic to lymphoid cells, nor is more activity generated upon culture with lymphoid cells. This is a serious consideration since the oxidation of sterols, or the hydrolysis of triglycerides to yield free fatty acids could occur during culture, and both are capable of suppressing lymphocyte function. LDL-In appears to have a direct effect on the responding lymphocyte rather than functioning via an intermediate regulatory cell (Fujii and Edgington in press). LDL-In appears to affect only the inductive phase of the lymphocyte response, block-ing re-entry of the resting lymphocyte into the cell cycle by a variety of stimuli including lectins and allogeneic stimuli. However, it appears to have no effect on subsequent proliferative or metabolic events once trigger-ing of the lymphocyte has been accomplished. Its effect is not mediated via the macrophage, a requisite for many immune functions and in vitro lymphocyte responses (Curtiss and Edgington 1977). Its effect is selective on lympho-cyte subpopulations and is most striking in attenuation of T suppressor cell function in vitro. Attenuation of T suppressor cell function probably re-sults from inhibition of proliferation which appears to be required for expression of T suppressor cell function (Curtiss and Edgington 1979). At somewhat higher doses, B cells are suppressed with respect to immunoglobulin synthesis; but T helper cells which do not require re-entry into the prolif-erative cell cycle to express biological activity are relatively insensi-tive. LDL-In has also been demonstrated to suppress the primary cellular and humoral immune response in vivo (Curtiss et al. 1977), where its major effect appears to be suppression of the proliferative expansion of both B and T antigen-binding lymphocytes rather than suppression of differentiation (Curtiss et al. in press). Although it has no effect on the effector function of cytolytic T cells (Edgington et al. 1977) (a function that is sensitive to LDL and oxygenated sterols) it will suppress the primary but not the secondary generation of these cytolytic T cells. In vivo studies have also shown modification of the induction of protective immunity to murine fibrosarcoma, SaD2. Low doses of LDL-In given i.v. before immune sensitiza-tion augment tumor rejection, whereas higher concentrations suppress tumor rejection. The dose profiles correspond with the low dose suppression of T suppressor cells which would permit a greater protective immune respone to this syngeneic tumor.

Mechanism

Elucidation of the mechanistic basis for the biological effects await con-clusive characterization of the protein and lipid composition of LDL-In. The demonstration of a lymphocyte surface membrane receptor specific for LDL-In (Curtiss and Edgington 1978) has led to speculations that the biological effects may require interaction with this receptor. This saturable recep-tor, present at maximum density of approximately 4,800 per lymphocyte is reduced in number to about 2,400 on cells directly recovered from peripheral blood (Robin et al. unpublished). The receptor is clearly modulated by available concentrations of this lipoprotein, but is not suppressed by oxy-genated sterols in contrast to the LDL receptor. The LDL-In receptor is independent of the LDL receptor since neither lipoprotein is capable of significant blocking of binding of the other in competitive inhibition studies. Recent studies have suggested that lysosomal catabolism of LDL-In is not required for the expression of biological activity. Chloroquine, at concentrations sufficient to suppress the catabolism of LDL, did not dimin-ish suppression of the lymphocyte response to lectins in vitro. This clearly distinguishes it from LDL. Most recent studies have indicated that receptor specificity and biological activity remain quantitatively intact following removal of triglycerides and cholesterol from the LDL-In particle by partial delipidization with heptane in the presence of starch. This reduces the potentially biologically active moieties within the LDL-In particle to: a) protein, b) free fatty acids, c) phospholipids, and d) glycolipids.

Issues

The major molecular issues rest first with the precise and unequivocal identification and characterization of the biologically active LDL-In particle. Second, the structure and characteristics of the biologically active moiety within the LDL-In particle must be resolved. The requirement for receptor binding and clarification as to whether LDL-In can act directly via surface membrane effects or requires internalization must be examined. Systematic delineation of the mechanism of biological activity of LDL-In should provide not only an exposition of the molecular and cell biology of this system, but may also serve to elucidate more general principles of the regulation of cell function by lipoproteins. The questions as to molecular origin and ultimate immunobiological significance await resolution of the basic issues and a precise assay for LDL-In

Significance

The significance of LDL-In lies not only in the possibility that it may be a participant in regulation of immunologic hemostasis of the host, but also that yet unrecognized quantitative or qualitative aberrations in LDL-In may be associated with specific diseases. Principles of cell regulation also may be better understood as this model is characterized in further detail.

References

Chisari FV, Edgington TS (1975) Lymphocyte E rosette inhibitory factor: a regulatory serum lipoprotein. J Exp Med 142: 1092

Curtiss LK, Edgington TS (1976) Regulatory serum lipoproteins: regulation of lymphocyte stimulation by a species of low density lipoprotein. J Immunol 116: 145

Curtiss LK, DeHeer DH, Edgington TS (1977) In vivo suppression of the primary immune response by a species of low density serum lipoprotein. J Immunol 118: 648

Curtiss LK, Edgington TS (1977) Effect of LDL-In, a normal immunoregulatory human serum low density lipoprotein, on the interaction of macrophages with lymphocytes proliferating in response to mitogen and allogeneic stimulation. J Immunol 118: 1966

Curtiss LK, Edgington TS (1978) Identification of a lymphocyte surface receptor for low density lipoprotein inhibitor, an immunoregulatory species of normal human serum low density lipoprotein. J Clin Invest 61: 1298

Curtiss LK, Edgington TS (1979) Differential sensitivity of lymphocyte sub-populations to suppressionn by low density lipoprotein inhibitor, an immunoregulatory human serum low density lipoprotein. J Clin Invest 63: 193

Curtiss LK, DeHeer DH, Edgington TS (1979) Influence of the immunoregulatory serum lipoprotein LDL-In on the in vivo proliferation and differentiation of antigen-binding and antibody-secreting lymphocytes during a primary immune response. Cell Immunol, in press

Edgington TS, Henney CS, Curtiss LK (1977) The bioregulatory properties of low density lipoprotein inhibitor (LDL-In) on the generation of killer T cells. In: Lucas DO (ed) Regulatory Mechanisms in Lymphocyte Activation: Proceedings of the Eleventh Leukocyte Culture Conference. Academic Press, New York, p 736

Fujii DK, Edgington TS (1979) Direct suppression of lymphocyte induction by the immunoregulatory human serum low density lipoprotein, LDL-In. J Immunol, in press

Autoimmune Mechanisms in the Development of Atherosclerosis

A.N. Klimov, V.A. Nagornev, Yu N. Zubzhitsky, and A.D. Denisenko

The development of atherosclerosis is closely associated with an increase in plasma LDL and VLDL concentrations. These lipoproteins probably acquire auto-antigenic properties. Some authors (Beaumont 1970; Lewis and Robertson 1974; Noseda et al. 1972) have identified autoimmune complexes containing LDL as antigens and IgA or IgM as antibodies in plasma of atherosclerotic patients. It is also known that a specific immunologic lesion of the arterial wall in-duces or aggravates the development of atherosclerosis as has been shown by Minick and Murphy (1973). On the other hand, sensitization to structural antigens of the vessel wall, desequestered in the course of degenerative changes on the sites of atherosclerotic lesions, probably enhances the patho-logic process. This trend is being successfully studied by Gerö et al. (1975).

Over a period of 10 years we have intensively studied the role of immunologic factors in the formation and development of experimental atherosclerosis in rabbits. The results of these studies permitted the formulation of the auto-immune theory of the pathogenesis of atherosclerosis, which has been reported in detail in the review by Klimov et al. (1979). For the past several years, our studies of atherosclerosis in man have been directed toward the validation of this theory. An attempt was made to isolate a specific autoimmune complex from the blood serum and arterial wall of humans. This complex was detected in the blood plasma of 12 of 15 men, 45-55 years of age, without any clinical manifestations of atherosclerosis. In all cases the antibodies isolated from the complex were related to class IgG according to the data of immunodiffusion in agar. In all cases the antigen was VLDL, and in 1 case it was lipoprotein d >1.006. Moreover, no connection between cholesterol and triglyceride con-centrations in the blood and the presence of an autoimmune complex was detec-ted. In addition, in all of 7 cases studied, autoimmune complex IgG–lipopro-tein was detected in the tissue fluid of the aorta wall with atherosclerotic lesions, but was not detected in the unaffected aorta.

Thus in the majority of studied cases, VLDL was the antigen in the isolated autoimmune complexes. It is not excluded that VLDL was the antigen in those cases with a complex density of more than 1.006.

Another aspect of the work was to perform autolymphocytic tests on patients with different manifestations of atherosclerosis and ischemic heart disease (IHD). The results of this reaction were evaluated in conjunction with other immunologic studies. A direct correlation between the number of patients who survived myocardial infarctions and the number of positive skin reactions to autolymphocytes has been noted in this work. Thus, out of 212 patients di-vided into groups according to the number of myocardial infarctions experi-enced, it was found that in the presence of angina pectoris without infarc-tion in the anamnesis, the number of positive tests did not exceed 23%; in cases of one or more survived infarctions the number of positive tests approx-imated 40%. In the control groups of healthy subjects of the same age, not suffering from any other diseases, the number of positive tests did not ex-ceed 6%.

From this study it follows that atherosclerosis, both with and without mani-festations of IHD, is accompanied by an active reaction to administered auto-

lymphocytes. This result is more reliable and more frequently obtained in
patients who have had myocardial infarction. Also, at the present time it
is not possible to say which factor in the manifestation of the reaction is
the primary one: the presence of atherosclerosis or the development of sensitization, which precedes the atherosclerosis or develops at certain stages
of the disease. At the same time we carried out an immunomorphologic study
of coronary artery segments (bioptates) taken during operation on coronary
vessels of patients with IHD. This investigation enabled us to detect deposits of lipoproteins containing apoB, γ-globulin fixation and CI_3-complement
fractions in the superficial sections of the dissected plaques in 16 of 22
cases. Detection of lipoproteins, γ-globulin and complement on parallel sections of the same site, permits the presumption that in these cases a fresh
deposition of immune complex occurred and the course of atherosclerosis and
IHD on the whole was exacerbated (Fig. 1).

Finally, the third component of the work was an immunomorphologic study of
γ-globulin fixation in the aortic wall of man with diverse manifestations of
atherosclerosis. Quantitative immunoluminescent analyses (70 cases) showed
that fixation of γ-globulin and fibrin in the subendothelial layer at the
site of lipoprotein accumulation can already be observed in the initial stages
of atherosclerotic lesion formation.

In cases of progression of atherosclerotic lesions the content of fixed
γ-globulin and fibrin in the aortic wall exceed the quantity of the same proteins in normal tissue by 5 or 6 times, and by 3 times those in the fatty
streaks. Significant deposition of fibrin and albumin in the superficial
and deep sections of the atherosclerotic plaques attest to a sharp permiabi-
lity disturbance of the vascular wall.

In highly marked stages of atherosclerosis γ-globulin fixation was also revealed in sections of elastic and collgenic fiber destruction and was accompanied by an expansion of connective tissue and marked macrophage and lympho-
histocyte infiltration. This does not exclude the simultaneous occurence of
an antibody fixation with the formation of an autoimmune complex in situ contributing to a further development of destructive changes in the arterial
wall. This observation is supported by: 1) the data obtained by Gëro et al.
(1975) that in approximately 50% of cases a sensitization to structural antigens of the vascular wall is observed in patients with atherosclerosis,
2) our results of a blood serum serologic study of IHD patients utilizing
vascular wall structural components of man (elastin, collagen, and structural glycoproteins) as antigens.

Thus, the data discussed above indicate the significance of the role of immunologic factors in the genesis of atherosclerosis in man. It appears to

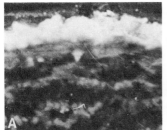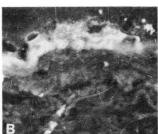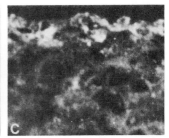

FIG. 1. Fresh deposits of apoB containing lipoproteins (A), γ-globulin (B)
and CI_3-fraction of complement (C). Parallel sections of the plaque of the
left coronary artery. X640

us that this pertains primarily to cases with a quickly progressing or undulatory course of atherosclerosis already diagnosed in people of a young age.

References

Beaumont JL (1970) Autoimmune hyperlipidemia. An atherogenic metabolic disease of immune origin. Rev Eur Etud Clin Biol 15:1037–1041
Gëro S, Szekely J, Szondy E, Seregelyi E (1975) Immunological studies with aortic and venous tissue antigens. Arterial Wall 3:89–92
Klimov AN, Zubzhitsky YuN, Nagornev VA (1979) Immunochemical aspects of atherosclerosis. Atherosclerosis Rev 4:119–156
Lewis LA, Robertson AL (1974) Hyperimmuno-globulinemia-lipoprotein and atherogenesis. In: Schettler G, Weizel A (eds) Atherosclerosis III. Springer-Verlag, Heidelberg, pp 595–603
Minick CR, Murphy GE (1973) Experimental induction of athero-arteriosclerosis by synergy of allergic injury to arteries and lipid-rich diet. Am J Pathol 73:265–300
Noseda G, Riesen W, Schlumpf E, Morell A (1972) Hypolipoproteinemia associated with autoantibodies against β-lipoproteins. Europ J Clin Invest 2: 342–347

Nutritional Factors in Atherosclerosis[1]

David Kritchevsky

Most approaches to the study of the effects of diet on experimental atherosclerosis have involved manipulation of a single dietary component, usually
fat. Studies have shown that saturated fat is more cholesteremic than unsaturated fat for man (Ahrens 1957) and more atherogenic for rabbits
(Kritchevsky et al. 1954, 1956). However, the influence of dietary fat is
not solely dependent on its fatty acid composition. Cocoa butter, iodine
value 35, is considerably less atherogenic than either coconut oil, iodine
value 10, or palm oil, iodine value 53 (Kritchevsky and Tepper 1965a).
Peanut oil, iodine value 93, is surprisingly atherogenic for rats (Gresham
and Howard 1960), rabbits (Kritchevsky et al. 1971) and rhesus monkeys
(Vesselinovitch et al. 1974). Peanut oil contains 4-6% of long-chain saturated fatty acids (arachidic, behenic and lignoceric) which have been
suggested as the possible source of the atherogenicity of peanut oil. PGF,
fat made by mixing olive, safflower and cottonseed oils (55:35:10), resembled
peanut oil in composition, minus the long-chain fatty acids, and was significantly less atherogenic than peanut oil (Kritchevsky et al. 1971).
Interesterification of PGF with triarchidin and tribehenin yielded a fat
whose iodine value and fatty acid composition were virtually identical with
those of peanut oil but PGF was considerably less atherogenic. It was then
shown that autointeresterification (randomization) of peanut oil significantly reduced its atherogenicity (Kritchevsky et al. 1973b).

Saturated fat was impugned as the principal atherogenic factor in a semipurified, cholesterol-free diet (Lambert et al. 1958; Malmros and Wigand
1959) but collation of the literature suggested that the fiber in the diet
may have played the deciding role (Kritchevsky 1964). The importance of
the fiber in the diet was shown in subsequent experiments (Kritchevsky and
Tepper 1965b, 1968; Moore 1967).

These experiments led to the formulation of a cholesterol-free, semipurified
diet which was hyperlipoproteinemic for rabbits and resulted in development
of atherosclerosis. The diet contained 40% carbohydrate (41.5% of calories),
75% protein (25.9% of calories), 14% fat (32.6% of calories), 15% fiber,
5% salt mix and 1% vitamin mix. In the basic diet the carbohydrate, protein,
fat and fiber were sucrose, casein, coconut oil and cellulose, respectively.

Experiments in which fat was varied showed that coconut oil was more atherogenic than butter oil (Kritchevsky et al. 1976). When carbohydrate was
manipulated it was shown that sucrose and fructose were more atherogenic
for rabbits than glucose or lactose (Kritchevsky et al. 1968, 1973a). In
baboons or vervet monkeys fructose was considerably more sudanophilic than
sucrose, glucose or lactose (Kritchevsky et al. 1974, 1977a). However,
addition of 0.1% cholesterol to this diet rendered the lactose severely
atherogenic for baboons, even though lipid levels were comparable to those
of animals fed the other carbohydrates (Kritchevsky et al. 1979a).

─────────
[1]Supported, in part, by grants HL-03299, HL-05209, HL-23625 and a Research
Career Award from the National Institutes of Health.

Ignatowski (1909) first suggested that animal protein might be a major factor in atherosclerosis. Newburgh and his collaborators (1920, 1923) found that rabbits fed powdered beef developed atherosclerosis. To answer the criticism that their results were due to the cholesterol content of the beef, the investigators fed rabbits the same amount of cholesterol in a diet containing no beef and found much less atherosclerotic involvement. Meeker and Kesten (1940) showed that casein was more atherogenic than soy protein in rabbits fed small amounts of cholesterol. Carroll and Hamilton (1975) showed that vegetable protein was less cholesteremic than animal protein but there was a wide range of activity within each protein class. Kritchevsky et al. (1977b) have reported that soy protein is much less cholesteremic and atherogenic than casein in diets containing cellulose as the fiber, but when the cellulose is replaced by alfalfa the two proteins are virtually identical in their effects. Rabbits fed casein and dextrose exhibit much higher cholesterol levels than those fed soy protein and dextrose. However, diets containing either protein result in normal cholesterol levels when the carbohydrate is raw potato starch (Carroll and Hamilton 1975).

The level of dietary protein is also important; high protein diets are more atherogenic than low protein diets for pigeons (Lofland et al. 1966) and baboons (Strong and McGill 1967).

Animal protein, such as beef or casein, is more atherogenic for rabbits than vegetable protein, such as soy. However, a 1:1 mixture of beef and soy proteins gives serum lipid levels and levels of atherosclerosis similar to those seen in rabbits fed soy protein (Kritchevsky 1979). The cause of this phenomenon may lie in a change in the amino acid content of the diet. One of the major differences between animal and vegetable protein is in the ratio of lysine to arginine which is considerably higher in animal protein. We have shown (Kritchevsky 1979) that addition of lysine to soy protein will increase its atherogenic potential. The serum lipoprotein spectra of rabbits fed casein or soy protein are markedly different. Lipoprotein spectra of rabbits fed soy protein plus lysine resemble those of casein-fed rabbits (Czarnecki and Kritchevsky 1979).

In summary, saturated fat is more atherogenic than unsaturated fat and the atherogenicity of some fats can be affected by altering their structure. High protein diets are generally more atherogenic than low protein diets. Animal protein is generally more atherogenic than vegetable protein but the effect can be vitiated by the type of carbohydrate or protein present in the diet. The effect of carbohydrate can be changed dramatically by addition of 0.1% cholesterol to the diet. Finally, the type of fiber present will affect atherogenicity.

Still, the combination of these ingredients within a particular food (as distinct from being mixed into a diet) may not give the expected results. A good example is milk which contains casein, lactose, cholesterol, saturated fat and still is hypocholesteremic in man (Mann 1977; Howard and Marks 1977) and in rats (Malinow and McLaughlin 1975; Nair and Mann 1977; Kritchevsky et al. 1979b). The probable mechanisms are discussed in a recent review (Richardson 1978).

References

Ahrens EH (1957) Nutritional factors and serum lipid levels. Am J Med 23: 928
Carroll KK, Hamilton RMG (1975) Effects of dietary protein and carbohydrate on plasma cholesterol levels in relation to atherosclerosis. J Food Sci 40: 18

Czarnecki SK, Kritchevsky D (1979) The effect of dietary proteins on lipoprotein metabolism and atherosclerosis in rabbits. J Am Oil Chem Soc
56: 388A

Gresham GA, Howard AN (1960) The independent production of atherosclerosis
and thrombosis in the rat. Br J Exp Pathol 41: 395

Howard AN, Marks J (1977) Hypocholesterolaemic effect of milk. Lancet 2: 255

Ignatowski A (1909) Über die Wirkung des tierischen Eiweisses auf die Aorta
und die parenchymatösen Organe der Kaninchen. Virchows Arch Pathol Anat
Physiol Klin Med 198: 248

Kritchevsky D (1964) Experimental atherosclerosis in rabbits fed cholesterol-
free diets. J Atheroscler Res 4: 103

Kritchevsky D (1979) Vegetable protein and atherosclerosis. J Am Oil Chem
Soc 56: 135

Kritchevsky D, Davidson LM, Kim HK, Krendel DA, Malhotra S, Vander Watt JJ,
duPlesses JP, Winter PAD, Ipp T, Mendelsohn D, Bersohn I (1977a) Influence of semipurified diets on atherosclerosis in African green
monkeys. Exp Mol Pathol 26: 28

Kritchevsky D, Davidson LM, Malhotra S, Mendelsohn D, Krendel DA, Vander
Watt JJ, Winter PAD (1979a) Atherosclerosis in baboons fed semipurified
diets plus 0.1% cholesterol: Effect of carbohydrate. Fed Proc 38: 445

Kritchevsky D, Davidson LM, Shapiro IL, Kim HK, Kitagawa M, Malhotra S,
Nair PP, Clarkson TB, Bersohn I, Winter PAD (1974) Lipid metabolism and
experimental atherosclerosis in baboons: Influence of cholesterol-free,
semi-synthetic diets. Am J Clin Nutr 27: 29

Kritchevsky D, Moyer AW, Tesar WC, Logan JB, Brown RA, Davies MC, Cox HR
(1954) Effect of cholesterol vehicle in experimental atherosclerosis.
Am J Physiol 178: 30

Kritchevsky D, Moyer AW, Tesar WC, McCandless RFJ, Logan JB, Brown RA,
Englert M (1956) Cholesterol vehicle in experimental atherosclerosis.
II. Effect of unsaturation. Am J Physiol 185: 279

Kritchevsky D, Sallata P, Tepper SA (1968) Experimental atherosclerosis in
rabbits fed cholesterol-free diets. 2. Influence of various carbohydrates. J Atheroscler Res 8: 697

Kritchevsky D, Tepper SA (1965a) Cholesterol vehicle in experimental atherosclerosis. VII. Influence of naturally occuring saturated fats. Med
Pharmacol Exp 12: 315

Kritchevsky D, Tepper SA (1965b) Factors affecting atherosclerosis in
rabbits fed cholesterol-free diets. Life Sci 4: 1467

Kritchevsky D, Tepper SA (1968) Experimental atherosclerosis in rabbits fed
cholesterol-free diets: Influence of chow components. J Atheroscler
Res 8: 357

Kritchevsky D, Tepper SA, Kim HK, Story JA, Vesselinovitch D, Wissler RW
(1976) Experimental atherosclerosis in rabbits fed cholesterol-free
diets. 5. Comparison of peanut, corn, butter and coconut oils. Exp
Mol Pathol 24: 375

Kritchevsky D, Tepper SA, Kitagawa M (1973a) Experimental atherosclerosis in
rabbits fed cholesterol-free diets. 3. Comparison of fructose and lactose
with other carbohydrates. Nutr Rep Int 7: 193

Kritchevsky D, Tepper SA, Morrissey RB, Czarnecki SK, Klurfeld DM (1979b)
Influence of whole or skim milk on cholesterol metabolism in rats. Am J
Clin Nutr 32: 597

Kritchevsky D, Tepper SA, Vesselinovitch D, Wissler RW (1971) Cholesterol
vehicle in experimental atherosclerosis. 11.Peanut oil. Atherosclerosis
14: 53

Kritchevksy D, Tepper SA, Vesselinovitch D, Wissler RW (1973b) Cholesterol
vehicle in experimental atherosclerosis. 13. Randomized peanut oil.
Atherosclerosis 17: 225

Kritchevsky D. Tepper SA, Williams DE, Story JA (1977b) Experimental atherosclerosis in rabbits fed cholesterol-free diets. 7. Interaction of animal or vegetable protein with fiber. Atherosclerosis 26: 397

Lambert GF, Miller JP, Olsen RT, Frost DV (1958) Hypercholesteremia and atherosclerosis induced in rabbits by purified high fat rations devoid of cholesterol. Proc Soc Exp Biol Med 97: 544

Lofland HB, Clarkson TB, Rhyne L, Goodman HO (1966) Interrelated effects of dietary fats and proteins on atherosclerosis in the pigeon. J Atheroscler Res 6: 395

Malinow MR, McLaughlin P (1975) The effect of skim milk on plasma cholesterol in rats. Experientia 31: 1012

Malmros H, Wigand G (1959) Atherosclerosis and deficiency of essential fatty acids. Lancet 2: 749

Mann GV (1977) A factor in yogurt which lowers cholesteremia in man. Atherosclerosis 26: 335

Meeker DR, Kesten HD (1940) Experimental atherosclerosis and high protein diets. Proc Soc Exp Biol Med 45: 543

Moore JH (1967) The effect of the type of roughage in the diet on plasma cholesterol levels and aortic atherosis in rabbits. Br J Nutr 21: 207

Nair CR, Mann GV (1977) A factor in milk which influences cholesteremia in rats. Atherosclerosis 26: 363

Newburgh LH, Clarkson S (1923) The production of atherosclerosis in rabbits by feeding diets rich in meat. Arch Intern Med 31: 653

Newburgh LH, Squier TL (1920) High protein diets and arteriosclerosis in rabbits: A preliminary report. Arch Intern Med 26: 38

Richardson T (1978) The hypocholesteremic effect of milk: A review. J Food Protect 41: 226

Strong JP, McGill HC (1967) Diet and experimental atherosclerosis in baboons. Am J Pathol 83: 145

Vesselinovitch D, Getz GS, Hughes RH, Wissler RW (1974) Atherosclerosis in the rhesus monkey fed three food fats. Atherosclerosis 20: 303

Cholesterol-Induced Hyperlipoproteinemia and Atherosclerosis in Dogs, Swine and Monkeys: Models for Human Atherosclerosis

Robert W. Mahley

Hypercholesterolemia has been clearly implicated in the development of accelerated atherosclerosis. Clinical and population studies have directly correlated
the level of dietary lipids and plasma cholesterol with the mortality and
morbidity associated with human atherosclerosis (for review see Mahley 1979).
Experimental animal studies not only support and extend inferences from the
clinical and epidemiologic data but also provide opportunities to explore the
mechanisms by which dietary fat and cholesterol lead to alterations in arterial
tissue (broadly termed atherosclerosis). There is no one ideal animal model.
Each of the different species highlights specific components of the atherosclerosis process and allows us to study certain aspects of the disease process as
it relates to human atherosclerosis. The description of a few selected animal
models will be presented to illustrate the effects of dietary lipids on the
development of atherosclerosis and on the types of hyperlipoproteinemia associated with the accelerated atherosclerosis.

Dietary-Induced Atherosclerosis

The dog has proven to be an interesting and important model (for review see
Mahley 1979). Dogs are resistant to the development of hypercholesterolemia
and do not have naturally occurring atherosclerosis. However, the dog may
well provide considerable insight into the mechanisms of lipid deposition in
arterial tissue. Two different protocols have been utilized to produce a
hypercholesterolemia in excess of 750 mg/dl, the level required to produce
canine atherosclerosis (Mahley et al. 1974). One protocol requires that the
dog be made hypothyroid by thyroidectomy and then be fed a diet composed of
fat, cholesterol, and bile salts. Hypercholesterolemia can also be produced
in dogs without thyroid suppression by feeding a semisynthetic diet containing
hydrogenated coconut oil as the only fat and high levels of cholesterol.

It is our experience that, regardless of which protocol is used, the responses
of the arterial tissue to the hypercholesterolemia are generally similar (Mahley 1979). Canine atherosclerosis involves the aorta and the coronary and
intracranial arteries. In addition, peripheral small artery involvement is
sometimes very extensive and may, in fact, be far more severe than the disease
seen in the aorta (Mahley et al. 1976, 1977). Intimal proliferative atheromatous lesions closely resembling human atherosclerosis do occur commonly in
the abdominal aorta and in the entrance to the internal carotid artery. However, in other locations, the medial component of the disease may be most
prominent (Mahley et al. 1977). Histologically, many of the lipid-laden cells
have characteristics resembling those of macrophages.

A potentially important observation in the dog is that the severity and the
associated complications of the arterial lipid deposition vary in the hypothyroid dog model depending on the type of fat (saturated vs. unsaturated) fed
in association with the cholesterol (Mahley et al. 1976). The results
obtained with hypothyroid dogs fed saturated fat and cholesterol are similar
to those obtained with the highly saturated coconut oil-cholesterol diet

(Mahley et al. 1977). Diets containing the saturated fats produce much more widespread and severe atherosclerotic lesions than occurs with the unsaturated fats, even when the cholesterol levels are similar. Furthermore, thrombosis is associated with the atheromatous lesions induced by the saturated fat-cholesterol diet in both the hypothyroid and the coconut oil-cholesterol-fed dogs. The sequelae of thrombosis have been noted, i.e., visceral organ infarction, gangrene of the lower extremities, and myocardial infarction. Thrombosis has never been noted in hypothyroid dogs fed unsaturated fat (cottonseed oil or corn oil) plus cholesterol. The dog may thus provide a model for the study of the primary or secondary role of thrombosis in the development of atherosclerosis.

Swine, particularly the miniature breeds, are excellent models for the study of dietary-induced experimental atherosclerosis (for review see Mahley 1979). Swine develop atherosclerosis spontaneously with age, and the distribution of the lesions in the aorta and coronary and intracranial arteries is similar to that seen in man. Accelerated atherosclerosis can be produced simply by the addition of cholesterol to the diet. Characteristically, the high cholesterol diet increases the plasma cholesterol from a control level of approximately 100 mg/dl to 250–400 mg/dl. Complicated atheromatous lesions develop within 6 to 8 months of the induction of the cholesterol-induced hyperlipoproteinemia.

The dietary-induced atherosclerosis involves the aorta, with the most severe and complicated lesions occurring in the abdominal region. Coronary artery atherosclerosis is often severe and involves primarily the major epicardial arteries or major branches as they penetrate the myocardium. Myocardial infarctions have been observed. Other investigators have induced severe coronary artery atherosclerosis and infarction by cholesterol feeding in combination with irradiation of the coronaries or damaging the endothelial surface of the coronaries with balloon catheters (Lee et al. 1971; Lee and Lee 1975). These same results can be obtained by diet alone in miniature swine (Mahley 1979).

The Erythrocebus patas monkey appears to be an excellent model for the study of dietary-induced atherosclerosis (Mahley et al. 1979). When a semisynthetic diet containing 0.5% cholesterol is fed to the patas monkeys for 1–2 years, the plasma cholesterol levels are elevated from ∿120 mg/dl to 300–600 mg/dl. After 2 years of cholesterol feeding, the animals develop extensive atherosclerosis with many advanced lesions. The abdominal aorta is most severely involved. These lesions are often advanced and are characterized by intimal proliferation, a well-developed fibrous cap, lipid accumulation with crystal formation, necrosis, calcification, and hemorrhage. Severe coronary artery atherosclerosis occurs in some animals with the highest cholesterol levels. These atherosclerotic lesions closely resemble human atherosclerosis (Mahley et al. 1979).

Dietary-Induced Changes in the Plasma Lipoproteins

Associated with the development of atherosclerosis in the various species, there is a remarkable consistency in the types of lipoprotein changes induced by the high cholesterol diets (for review see Mahley 1978). Although there are differences among different species with respect to the amount of cholesterol transported by a specific type of lipoprotein in response to a high cholesterol diet, it appears that the qualitative changes in the lipoproteins are similar from species to species. These changes include: (a) the occurrence of B-VLDL in the d < 1.006 fraction; (b) an increase in LDL; (c) a decrease in the typical HDL; and (d) the appearance of a lipoprotein referred to as HDL_c. The association of B-VLDL with lipid accumulation in smooth muscle cells and macrophages and the potential role of B-VLDL in the development of the athero-sclerotic lesion are discussed elsewhere in these Proceedings (Mahley 1980). The discussion to follow focuses on changes in the HDL. The appearance of a specific cholesterol-induced HDL (HDL_c) has provided insight into the effects of cholesterol feeding on HDL metabolism (Mahley 1978). Furthermore, HDL_c have served as useful probes in the determination of the properties of lipopro-teins responsible for specific interaction with cell surface receptors of cultured fibroblasts and smooth muscle cells (Mahley and Innerarity 1978).

The HDL_c occur at various ultracentrifugal densities overlapping both LDL and HDL and are cholesterol-rich lipoproteins with a chemical composition and particle size similar to those of LDL. HDL_c and LDL are distinctly different, however, with respect to their apoprotein contents. Whereas LDL contain primarily the B apoprotein, HDL_c lack apo-B and contain the A-I apoprotein and the arginine-rich (apo-E) apoprotein as major constituents or, in some cases, contain exclusively apo-E. Comparisons between LDL and HDL_c from cholesterol-fed dogs and swine have proven to be valuable in ascertaining the properties of lipoproteins responsible for specific high affinity binding to the cell surface receptors of fibroblasts and smooth muscle cells. We have demonstrated that the protein moiety is the determinant responsible for receptor binding and that either the apo-B of LDL or the apo-E of HDL_c can mediate the high affinity binding to the same cell surface receptors (Mahley and Innerarity 1978). Furthermore, it has been shown that the apo-E has a greatly enhanced binding activity as compared to apo-B (Innerarity and Mahley 1978; Pitas et al. 1979). The apo-E HDL_c are 100-fold more active in displacing iodinated LDL from the receptors than are LDL at the same concentration. Therefore, a lipoprotein which contains apo-E, even as a minor apoprotein constituent, can be as potent as LDL with respect to receptor binding activity and the regulation of intra-cellular cholesterol metabolism. Typical HDL, which lack apo-E, do not bind to the high affinity cell surface receptors.

Based on an understanding of the properties of apo-E HDL_c, it has been possible to demonstrate that there are two metabolically distinct subclasses of HDL, not only in lower species, but also in man. One subclass contains primarily the A-I (A-II) and C apoproteins (lacks apo-E) and represents the most common type of HDL (typical HDL). This HDL subclass (e.g., human HDL_3) does not bind to the cell surface receptors of fibroblasts. The other subclass of HDL, which also occurs in man and lower animals, contains the E apoprotein in addition to the A-I (A-II) and C apoproteins. The two subclasses can be isolated by Geon-Pevikon block electrophoresis or heparin affinity chromato-graphy (Weisgraber and Mahley 1978 and unpublished data). The apo-E-contain-ing HDL bind with high affinity to the cell surface receptors of fibroblasts (Innerarity et al. 1978). Furthermore, earlier data had indicated that these apo-E-containing HDL are increased following cholesterol feeding in man (Mah-ley et al. 1978). Thus, it appears that HDL_c production can be induced by high cholesterol diets in man, as previously described in lower animals.

Summary: Accelerated atherosclerosis can be produced in a variety of animals by feeding diets which cause hypercholesterolemia. The hypercholesterolemia is associated with various changes in the plasma lipoproteins. A major change includes the production of B-VLDL (β-migrating, cholesterol-rich lipoproteins in the d < 1.006 fraction) and an increase in LDL. Changes also occur in the HDL and include an increase in the apo-E-containing subclass (HDL_c) and a decrease in typical (non-apo-E-containing) HDL.

Acknowledgments

Experimental atherosclerosis studies were performed in collaboration with Drs. D. L. Fry, J. E. Pierce and D. K. Johnson at the National Institutes of Health.

References

Innerarity TL, Mahley RW (1978) Enhanced binding by cultured human fibroblasts
    of apo-E-containing lipoproteins as compared to low density lipoproteins.
    Biochemistry 17: 1440-1447
Innerarity TL, Mahley RW, Weisgraber KH, Bersot TP (1978) Apoprotein (E-A-II)
    complex of human plasma lipoproteins. II. Receptor binding activity of a
    high-density lipoprotein subfraction modulated by the apo(E-A-II) complex.
    J Biol Chem 253: 6289-6295
Lee WM, Lee KT (1975) Advanced coronary atherosclerosis in swine produced by
    combination of balloon-catheter injury and cholesterol feeding. Exp Molec
    Path 23: 491-499
Lee KT, Jarmolych J, Kim DN, Grant C, Krasney JA, Thomas WA, Bruno AM (1971)
    Production of advanced coronary atherosclerosis, myocardial infarction and
    "sudden death" in swine. Exp Molec Path 15: 170-190
Mahley RW (1978) Alterations in plasma lipoproteins induced by cholesterol
    feeding in animals including man. In: Dietschy JM, Gotto AM, Jr, Ontko JA,
    (eds) Disturbances in lipid and lipoprotein metabolism. American Physio-
    logical Society, Bethesda, MD pp 181-197
Mahley RW (1979) Dietary fat, cholesterol, and accelerated atherosclerosis.
    In: Paoletti R, Gotto AM, Jr (eds) Atherosclerosis Reviews. Raven Press,
    New York Vol 5, pp 1-35
Mahley RW (1980) Cholesterol feeding: Effects on lipoprotein structure and
    metabolism. In: Proc 5th international symposium on atherosclerosis
Mahley RW, Innerarity TL (1978) Properties of lipoproteins responsible for
    high affinity binding to cell surface receptors. In: Kritchevsky D, Pao-
    letti R, Holmes WL (eds) Advances in experimental medicine and biology,
    Sixth international symposium on drugs affecting lipid metabolism. Plenum
    Press, New York Vol 109, pp 99-127
Mahley RW, Weisgraber KH, Innerarity TL (1974) Canine lipoproteins and athero-
    sclerosis. II. Characterization of the plasma lipoproteins associated with
    atherogenic and nonatherogenic hyperlipidemia. Circ Res 35: 722-733
Mahley RW, Nelson AW, Ferrans VJ, Fry DL (1976) Thrombosis in association with
    atherosclerosis induced by dietary perturbations in dogs. Science 192:
    1139-1141
Mahley RW, Innerarity TL, Weisgraber KH, Fry DL (1977) Canine hyperlipopro-
    teinemia and atherosclerosis. Accumulation of lipid by aortic medial cells
    in vivo and in vitro. Am J Pathol 87: 205-225
Mahley RW, Innerarity TL, Bersot TP, Lipson A, Margolis S (1978) Alterations
    in human high-density lipoproteins, with or without increased plasma-
    cholesterol, induced by diets high in cholesterol. Lancet II: 807-809
Mahley RW, Johnson DK, Pucak GJ, Fry DL (1979) Atherosclerosis in the Erythro-
    cebus patas, an old world monkey. Am J Pathol, in press
Pitas RE, Innerarity TL, Arnold KS, Mahley RW (1979) Rate and equilibrium
    constants for binding of apo-E HDL_C (a cholesterol-induced lipoprotein)
    and low-density lipoproteins to human fibroblasts: Evidence for multiple
    receptor binding of apo-E HDL_C. Proc Natl Acad Sci USA 76: 2311-2315
Weisgraber KH, Mahley RW (1978) Apoprotein (E-A-II) complex of human plasma
    lipoproteins. I. Characterization of this mixed disulfide and its identi-
    fication in a high-density lipoprotein subfraction. J Biol Chem 253:
    6281-6288

Dietary Animal Models for Studying Cardiovascular Disease Risk Factors

S.R. Srinivasan, B. Radhakrishnamurthy, E. R. Dalferes, Jr., and G. S. Berenson

Although the significance of Yudkin's (1972) observation relating morbidity
from coronary heart disease (CHD) to excessive intake of dietary sucrose
remains controversial, the metabolic effects of sucrose on CHD risk factor
variables such as serum lipids, glucose and insulin are well recognized.
We observed that the average intake of sucrose in Bogalusa children consti-
tuted 50% of the total carbohydrate (Frank et al. 1978). It is also generally accepted that excessive salt intake is an etiologic factor in the
development of hypertension, another major CHD risk factor. In rats dietary
sucrose has been shown to potentiate salt induced hypertension (Hall and
Hall 1966). While manipulation of dietary fat and cholesterol continues to
be extensively applied in experimental atherosclerosis, only a few studies
have been concerned with the effect of dietary sucrose on the accepted CHD
risk factors, viz., hyperlipidemia and hypertension, under experimental
conditions, especially in nonhuman primates. In these studies we investigated the response of different nonhuman primates to the potentiating effects
of sucrose on hyperlipoproteinemia and salt induced hypertension (Srinivasan
et al. 1978, 1979a, 1979b).

Methods

Serum lipid and lipoprotein responses to diets with a high level of sucrose
and a low level of saturated fat (butter-coconut oil mixture, 1:1) with and
without cholesterol (1 mg/kcal) were studied in squirrel (Saimiri sciurea),
spider (Ateles sp.) and rhesus (Macaca mulatta) monkeys. Semi-synthetic
diets were prepared with the carbohydrate representing 76.5% of the calories,
the protein (casein) 11%, and the fat 12.5%. Variations in the response
produced by altering the nature of dietary carbohydrate (sucrose vs. dextrin)
in the above diet was also observed in spider monkeys. In addition, varied
effects of dietary sucrose and cholesterol on serum apolipoproteins, glucose
and insulin were studied in rhesus monkeys. Effects of sucrose on salt induced hypertension were also studied in three groups of spider monkeys.
They were fed chow-based diets containing no added NaCl, 3% NaCl (9.9 mg/
kcal) or 3% NaCl and sucrose at 38% of calories. Serum lipoprotein levels
and apolipoprotein ratios were determined as described previously (Srinivasan
et al., 1979b). Blood pressure measurements were taken with a Physiometrics[R]
automatic blood pressure recorder (Sphygmetric Inc., Woodland Hills, Ca.).

Results

Sucrose and hyperlipoproteinemia

Dietary sucrose with or without cholesterol had varied effects on serum
lipids and lipoproteins in the different nonhuman primate species (Table 1).
In the absence of exogenous cholesterol, feeding a sucrose-saturated fat
diet for six weeks produced a consistent increase in serum total cholesterol
in all three species, whereas serum triglycerides showed significant increases
only in squirrel and rhesus monkeys. On the other hand, we observed that

Table 1. Effects of dietary sucrose and cholesterol on serum lipids (means±S.E.) in nonhuman primates.

Species (No. animals)	Diet	Lipoprotein cholesterol, mg/100 ml				Triglyceride, mg/100 ml
		Total	Beta	Pre-Beta	Alpha	
Spider (5)	Basal	152.2 ± 6.9^a	102.9 ± 4.2^a	2.0 ± 0.2^a	48.1 ± 4.7^a	73.8 ± 8.2^a
	Sucrose w/o chol.	208.8 ± 4.2^b	141.8 ± 2.3^b	$3.3\pm0.5^{b,c}$	$64.2\pm 4.2^{b,c}$	68.2 ± 9.4^a
	with chol.	327.6 ± 34.8^c	242.2 ± 24.5^c	$2.4\pm0.4^{a,c}$	$80.4\pm12.5^{a,c}$	34.4 ± 8.4^b
Squirrel (4)	Basal	191.5 ± 17.0^a	82.3 ± 9.7^a	1.0 ± 0.3^a	108.8 ± 10.8^a	62.2 ± 13.2^a
	Sucrose w/o chol.	332.0 ± 9.6^b	167.8 ± 24.4^b	2.0 ± 1.1^a	165.0 ± 20.4^b	135.5 ± 37.0^a
	with chol.	589.4 ± 61.0^c	260.2 ± 18.2^c	1.9 ± 0.4^a	328.9 ± 55.6^c	49.9 ± 4.0^a
Rhesus (9)	Basal	131.1 ± 9.0^a	55.5 ± 9.7^a	7.6 ± 3.4^a	68.2 ± 3.6^a	26.9 ± 4.1^a
	Sucrose w/o chol.	163.9 ± 15.5^b	62.0 ± 13.8^b	8.7 ± 2.8^a	93.5 ± 11.2^b	$74.8\pm26.4^{b,c}$
	with chol.	311.1 ± 50.3^c	172.2 ± 36.3^c	10.9 ± 2.8^a	128.4 ± 15.9^c	$44.7\pm15.8^{a,c}$

Chol.: Cholesterol

a-c Means within a column without a common superscript differ significantly at the p<0.05 level.

substitution of complex carbohydrate (dextrin) in the semi-synthetic diet did not induce a serum cholesterol response in spider monkeys. Exogenous cholesterol had a remarkable synergistic effect on the high sucrose diet in increasing the serum total cholesterol and had an unexpected suppressing effect on serum triglycerides in all three species. These observations are consistent with the concept that endogenous cholesterol synthesis related to carbohydrate metabolism plays an equally important role in modulating serum total cholesterol levels (Schreibman and Ahrens 1976). When rhesus monkeys were fed sucrose diets with cholesterol, there was a strong relationship between the basal or initial serum total cholesterol levels and the magnitude of response ($r=0.73$). Dietary sucrose with or without exogenous cholesterol consistently increased the serum β- as well as α-lipoprotein cholesterol in all species. However, none of the nutrition models elicited a carbohydrate induced mixed hyperlipoproteinemia (Type IIb) or pre-beta-lipoproteinemia (Type IV) similar to man, although significant inter-species differences in individual responses to sucrose diets were noted. Overall, the lipoprotein response (especially α-lipoprotein) of squirrel monkeys was far greater than spider and rhesus monkeys.

Dietary sucrose with exogenous cholesterol also had a profound effect on the composition of lipoproteins. Sucrose feeding seemed to increase ApoB more than non-ApoB proteins (Table 2). The ratio of ApoC-II/ApoC-III increased

Table 2. Effect of dietary sucrose and cholesterol on serum apolipoproteins and glucose (G), insulin (I) and I/G ratios in rhesus monkeys.

Variable	Diet		
	Basal	Sucrose	Sucrose + Cholesterol
Apolipoprotein ratio			
B/AI+AII	0.42±0.11 (4)[*]	0.67± 0.26 (4)	0.64± 0.20 (4)
AI/AII	1.85±0.13 (4)[a]	1.35± 0.41 (4)[b]	1.66± 0.09 (4)[c]
CII/CIII	0.08±0.03 (4)[d]	0.80± 0.22 (4)[e]	2.84± 0.95 (4)[f]
Glucose, mg/100 ml	52.8 ±1.4 (9)	60.2 ± 1.8 (9)	56.8 ± 2.1 (9)
Insulin, μU/ml	27.8 ±5.3 (9)	60.2 ±22.4 (9)	52.9 ±10.2 (9)
I/G Ratio	0.52±0.10 (9)	1.03± 0.41 (9)	0.94± 0.19 (9)

[*] Means±S.E. (number of animals)

Mean levels of variables differed significantly among dietary groups (F-test): b and c<a ($p<0.05$); e and f>d ($p<0.0001$); f>e ($p<0.01$).

in each animal and exogenous cholesterol further increased this trend. The above alterations in C peptides may facilitate efficient lipid clearing through activation of the enzyme lipoprotein lipase. That dietary sucrose and cholesterol may have opposite effects on high density lipoprotein subfractions is suggested from the changes in ApoA-I/ApoA-II ratios. Dietary sucrose increased the plasma glucose (G), insulin (I) and I/G ratios of most rhesus monkeys, whereas the addition of cholesterol tended to decrease plasma glucose and insulin levels. It is noteworthy that the above changes paralleled serum triglyceride levels. We observed in a separate set of experiments in rabbits that hepatic triglyceride secretion rate and VLDL total protein synthesis, including ApoB, was suppressed by dietary cholesterol

when added to the sucrose diets but not to the basal chow diet. These observations suggest that exogenous cholesterol results in secretion of apoprotein and triglyceride poor and cholesterol rich VLDL in sucrose fed animals
and thus could be a possible mechanism of the effect of exogenous cholesterol
on serum triglycerides.

Sucrose and Salt Hypertension

Unlike observations on a basal diet, both systolic and diastolic blood pressures of spider monkeys increased following 8 weeks of experimental diets
(Table 3). The increase was more pronounced for salt and salt-sucrose diets.

Table 3. Effect of salt and sucrose on blood pressures in spider monkeys
(mean±S.E.).

Experimental dietary groups (no. animals)	Blood Pressure, mm Hg			
	Systolic*	Δ Systolic	Diastolic*	Δ Diastolic
I Control (6)	141.9±1.2	8.9±1.2	96.0±1.1	5.6±0.8
II Salt (6)	163.0±2.6	19.4±1.3[a]	108.2±0.9	6.7±1.1[b]
III Salt-Sucrose (6)	165.8±2.6	24.0±1.5[a,x]	108.4±1.5	10.4±0.7[b,x]

* Differences among dietary groups were significant at $p<0.0001$ level (F-test).
Δ Experimental values minus mean basal value.
II and III >I; a : $p <0.001$; b : $p <0.01$ (F-test)
III >II; x : $p <0.01$

For example, systolic/diastolic blood pressures for salt and salt-sucrose
diets reached an average maximum level of 174/116 and 178/111 mm/Hg, respectively, compared to 155/100 mm/Hg noted on the control diet. The mean rise
in blood pressures (blood pressure response Δ, calculated by subtracting
mean basal diet values from the corresponding individual experimental diet
values) for salt-sucrose diet was significantly greater than for the salt
diet. Monkeys with high or low initial mean blood pressure levels remained
more or less on the same order throughout the experimental period, although
their absolute blood pressure levels varied with time and diet (Fig. 1).

Feeding salt and salt-sucrose diets resulted in significantly higher serum
Na^+ levels and lower serum K^+ in animals given salt-sucrose than in animals
receiving salt alone. Body weight correlated positively with serum Na^+,
and negatively with K^+. Both systolic and diastolic blood pressures correlated positively with body weight and negatively with K^+. The significant
differences observed in blood pressure but not in body weight gain between
animals in experimental and control diets suggest that effects of dietary
salt and sucrose on blood pressure may be independent of the effect of body
weight on blood pressure.

Discussion

The observations of the potentiating effects of dietary sucrose on serum
lipids and blood pressure in nonhuman primate models and the different responses of species are rather interesting to the relationship of human diets
and cardiovascular diseases. Sucrose in relatively high content in human

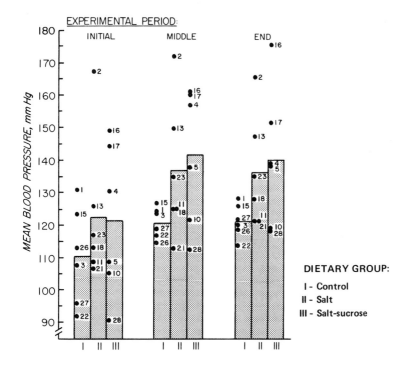

FIG. 1. Mean blood pressure levels in spider monkeys at different stages of feeding of experimental diets.

diets in the United States differs markedly from other carbohydrates by decreasing the glucose tolerance and increasing the fasting insulin levels in humans as well as in experimental animals (Yudkin 1972). Such conditions are known to augment hepatic lipogenesis and lipoprotein synthesis. An increased insulin level has been also shown to facilitate sodium retention by renal tubular reabsorption (Defronzo et al. 1975), which apparently is occurring in the study of monkeys as seen from the relatively high serum Na^+ levels during the salt-sucrose diet compared to the diet of salt alone. Salt retention not only results in expanded extracellular fluid volume and plasma volume but contributes to an increased peripheral resistance leading to elevated blood pressure levels. Sucrose-rich diets must exert a profound effect not only on lipid, but on salt and water metabolism as well.

References

Defronzo RA, Cooke CR, Andres R, Faloona GR, Davis PJ (1975) The effect of insulin on renal handling of sodium, potassium, calcium and phosphate in man. J Clin Invest 55: 845–855

Frank GC, Berenson GS, Webber LS (1978) Dietary studies and the relationship of diet to cardiovascular disease risk factor variables in 10-year-old children – the Bogalusa Heart Study. Am J Clin Nutr 31: 328–340

Hall CE, Hall O (1966) Comparative effectiveness of glucose and sucrose in enhancement of hypersalimentation and salt hypertension. Proc Soc Exp Biol Med 123: 370–374

Schreibman PH, Ahrens EH (1976) Sterol balance in hyperlipidemic patients after dietary exchange of carbohydrate for fat. J Lipid Res 17: 97–106

Srinivasan SR, Berenson GS, Radhakrishnamurthy B, Dalferes ER, Jr, Underwood D, Foster TA (1979) Effects of dietary sodium and sucrose in the induction of hypertension in spider monkeys. Am J Clin Nutr (in press)

Srinivasan SR, Clevidence BA, Pargaonkar PS, Radhakrishnamurthy B, Berenson GS (1979b) Varied effects of dietary sucrose and cholesterol on serum lipids, lipoproteins and apolipoproteins in rhesus monkeys. Atherosclerosis 33: 301-314.

Srinivasan SR, Radhakrishnamurthy B, Webber LS, Dalferes ER, Jr, Kokatnur MG, Berenson GS (1978) Synergistic effects of dietary carbohydrates and cholesterol on serum lipids and lipoproteins in squirrel and spider monkeys. Am J Clin Nutr 31: 603-613

Yudkin J (1972) Sucrose and cardiovascular disease. Proc Nutr Soc 31: 331-337

Transformation of Naturally Occurring Quiescent Intimal Smooth Muscle Cell Masses into Atherosclerotic Lesions in Swine Fed a Hyperlipidemic Diet[1]

W.A. Thomas, J.M. Reiner, R.A. Florentin, R.F. Scott, and K.T. Lee

We have become increasingly aware that cholesterol diet-induced atherosclerosis
in the abdominal aorta of young swine begins frequently (and perhaps exclusively) in pre-existing collections of intimal cells. The rather quiescent
collections in the intima prior to feeding the atherogenic diet metamorphose
into rapidly proliferating cell masses. It is too early to generalize that
atherosclerosis will begin in this way in all arteries of all species including man; but it is a reasonable possibility. Pathologists have noted
that atherosclerotic lesions often seem to arise in intimal smooth muscle
cell (SMC) "cushions", which begin to develop in fetal life near the orifices
of branch vessels. They have also noted the presence of diffuse intimal
thickening at points far removed from orifices, but have usually considered
this a result of aging and probably not related to atherosclerosis. In recent
studies of abdominal aortas of pre-adolescent swine, we found, in sites far
removed from orifices, collections of intimal SMC indistinguishable from
those near orifices. We also found continuous sheets of SMC similar to those
observed in adult man ("diffuse intimal thickening").

We usually start experiments with male Yorkshire swine about 2 months old,
weighing 8-12 kg. The entire abdominal aorta is divided into 15-25 segments
for microscopy. We count all intimal SMC in sections; and from the counts,
we calculate total intimal SMC in the aorta from celiac axis to trifurcation
(Thomas 1979; Scott 1979). Mathematical treatments of data from tritiated
thymidine studies (Thomas 1971, 1976a, 1976b, 1979; Scott 1979) gives loss
of cells (probably by death) and multiplication rates of survivors over a
selected period, usually 60 days. We currently arbitrarily divide the collections of intimal SMC in normal animals into 2 classes: (1) continuous
layers less than 20 microns thick, which we have called intimal cell sheets
(ICS), and (2) layers 20 or more microns thick, called intimal cell masses
(ICM). Most of this report is concerned with the latter which may be as
much as several hundred microns thick.

The ICM and ICS are usually not visible grossly in the unstained aorta.
However, if the swine is injected with Evans Blue prior to sacrifice, most
of the blue areas are over ICS or ICM, although less than 50% of their total
surface is stained. The ICM tend to run longitudinally with respect to vessel
axis and may be as much as several cm long. Some are at or near branching
vessel orifices, but many others are not. The extent of ICM varies from
swine to swine, but they usually occupy 20-30% of total surface area. In
the 8-12 kg swine, the total number of cells in ICM of the abdominal aorta
averages approximately 1.6 million (total number of medial SMC in same abdominal aortas about 70 million). We have on occasion divided the abdominal
aorta into proximal and distal halves and then divided each half into ventral,
dorsal, and right and left quadrants. In proximal half, about 50% of the
ICM cells were in the dorsal quadrant; in distal half, about 50% are in the

---

[1]Supported by PHS Grant No. HL-20993

ventral quadrant. The cells in ICM are usually arranged randomly and are not oriented parallel to one another as the SMC in the media generally are. The ICS occupy an additional 20-30% of the surface and contribute about 0.2 million cells. We have not attempted to determine their preferred location; but they appear to be more randomly distributed than ICM. The overwhelming majority of cells in ICM and ICS are SMC. We previously reported (Lee 1970) on other types of cells occasionally found in the intima of swine aortas; but the current presentation focuses on SMC and particularly those in ICM.

We have studied cell kinetics (births and deaths) of SMC in ICM, and of their overlying endothelial cells (EC), during a 60-day period starting from about 8 weeks of age in normal mash-fed swine using tritiated thymidine techniques (Thomas 1979; Scott 1979). Values were compared with values for underlying medial SMC and for EC not over ICM. In a recent study (Thomas 1979; Scott 1979), about 50% of SMC originally present in ICM and a similar percentage in the overlying EC were lost over the subsequent 60 days without surviving progeny. This compares with significantly lower losses from the media and among SMC not over ICM. Many survivors did not divide in 60 days while others divided 1 to 4 times. The net result was a population of cells in ICM on day 60 not significantly greater than that present on day 0. Meanwhile, in these growing swine, medial SMC increased in number about 2-fold. Total EC also increased over ICM and elsewhere so that the entire surface remained covered. The remains of the lost SMC (presumed dead) were apparently largely removed, since necrotic cellular debris was not seen by light microscopy. However, in studies by transmission electron microscopy we have observed in aortas tiny foci of cellular debris even in normal animals (Imai 1970).

In early studies in swine fed atherogenic diets, we thought that atherosclerosis originated at focal points within ICM. This hypothesis implies that in atherogenic diet-fed swine we would find some ICM that were sites of early lesions and others that were quiescent as in normal animals. However, our accumulated studies of ICM cell kinetics with tritiated thymidine do not support this view, and instead suggest another. The hypothesis we favour at present is that all ICM become activated by the diet; hence, ICM metamorphose into atherosclerotic lesions in toto, although activity may be greater in some sites than in others. The activated ICM in diet-fed swine are in the same locations as quiescent ICM in controls, i.e., largely in dorsal quadrant in proximal half and in ventral in distal half. Even in swine subjected to balloon-catheter-denudation of virtually 100% of EC of the abdominal aorta prior to feeding an atherogenic diet, the same predominance of certain quadrants is seen in early stages. In later stages, lesions grow to cover most of the aorta and localization is blurred.

Studies of population changes in SMC of ICM of the abdominal aorta of swine over a 60-day period from beginning of the atherogenic diet are presented in Tables I & II along with values for mash-fed controls. The terminal cholesterol levels for the hyperlipidemic (HL) groups averaged 582 mg/dl, for the controls (NL) 75 mg/dl. It is apparent from the data in the tables that more SMC are in the dividing population in HL group during the 60-day period than in NL group. Also, there is a small but significant shift in cycle times in HL swine. Somewhat to our surprise, loss rates of cells were not significantly greater in HL group than in controls. Net result was a 3-fold increase in cells of ICM-cum-lesions over the 60-day period in the HL group while there was no statistically significant increase among controls. At this stage of atherogenesis, then, our evidence suggests that some mitogenic effect of the cholesterol diet is the decisive factor, although injury or loss of cells may be important for manifestation of the mitogenic effect. As for cell loss rates from the ICM-cum-lesions, we predict that these will become greater than in ICM of NL swine as the lesions increase in size till

Table 1. Population dynamics of smooth muscle cells in and of endothelial cells over intimal cell masses of swine abdominal aortas during 60 days on a hyperlipidemic (HL) diet compared with values for controls.

Items[a]	Smooth muscle cells in intimal cell masses avg (n=5)		Endothelial cells over intimal cell masses avg (n=5)	
	Control	HL	Control	HL
A. No. of cells present on day 0	15.9		3.1	
B. No. of day 0 cells lost in 60 days without surviving progeny	6.1 ←ns→	6.4	1.8 ←ns→	1.4
C. No. of day 0 cells surviving for 60 days without dividing	5.0 ←$p<0.04$→	0.0	0.8 ←ns→	0.5
D. No. of day 0 cells dividing at least once in 60 days	4.8 ←$p<0.03$→	9.5	0.5 ←$p<0.01$→	1.1
E. Avg. no. of progeny per dividing day 0 cell in item D	3.7 ←$p<0.05$→	5.3	5.6 ←$p<0.05$→	3.8
F. Total no. of progeny present on day 60 (items D times E)[b]	15.6 ←$p<0.001$→	47.3	2.1 ←$p<0.04$→	3.7
G. Total no. cells present on day 60 (items C + F)	20.6 ←$p<0.001$→	47.3	2.9 ←$p<0.05$→	4.3

[a]All except item E are times 10^{-5}. Statistics were obtained with the Mann-Whitney-U test.
[b]Items involving combinations of other items (esp. multiplication, as in F) were calculated for individual animals and then averaged; combining averages does not necessarily give the same result.

frank necrosis becomes apparent.

Data on EC from the same study are presented in Table 1. We found a significant loss of EC over ICM in both HL and NL swine. Unexpectedly, the losses did not differ significantly, although we had anticipated greater losses of EC in HL than in NL swine. We found no significant losses over non-ICM areas in either dietary group. The EC over the ICM in the HL group divided somewhat less frequently than those in the NL group, but this was more than offset by a larger division fraction. The result was a significantly greater terminal number of EC over ICM in the HL group, as would be expected since the ICM are larger. These data provide limited support for the idea that alterations in EC are among the earliest factors in atherogenesis. The fact that lesions develop selectively at sites where EC are turning over fairly rapidly suggests a possible role for EC in atherogenesis; e.g., there may be transient changes in permeability during the time of turnover. On the other hand, the fact that we found similar losses over ICM in the mash-fed controls suggests that such changes alone are not sufficient for initiation

Table 2. Approximate cycle times of smooth muscle cells present at day 0 that divided during the 60-day period.

Cycle times	Number of cells[a] with specified cycle times X 10^{-5}			
	In intimal cell masses		In media	
	Control	Hyperlipidemic	Control	Hyperlipidemic
12–19 days	0.3	2.1	55	41
20–37 days	0.9	1.9	48	14
38–75 days	1.7	1.1	75	123
76+days	1.9	4.4	151	151
Totals	4.8 $\xrightarrow{p<0.03}$	9.5	329 $\xleftrightarrow{ns}$	329

[a]Total cells on day 0 15.9 X 10^{-5} as shown in Table 1.

of atherogenesis although they may be necessary for manifestation of the mitogenic effect. Observations on more advanced lesions suggest a role for EC in later stages (Thomas 1968, 1976). Also, we have data using other methods suggesting a more important role of EC even in early atherogenesis than was indicated in the current study. This aspect needs further investigation.

References

Thomas WA, Reiner JM, Florentin RA, Scott RF (1979) Cell kinetics of arterial cells during atherogenesis. VIII. Separation of the roles of injury and growth stimulation in early aortic atherogenesis in swine originating in pre-existing intimal smooth muscle cell masses. Exp & Molec Path 31: 124–144

Scott RF, Thomas WA, Reiner JM, Florentin RA (1979) Cell kinetics of arterial cells during atherogenesis. IX. Similarity of endothelial cell loss over intimal smooth muscle cell masses (cushions) in aortas of swine fed normolipidemic and hyperlipidemic diets for 60 days. Exp & Molec Path 31:145–153

Thomas WA, Florentin RA, Nam SC, Reiner JM, Lee KT (1971) Cell kinetics of arterial smooth muscle cells during atherogenesis. I. Activation of interphase cells in cholesterol-fed swine prior to gross atherosclerosis demonstrated by "postpulse salvage labeling". Exp & Molec Path 15: 245–267

Thomas WA, Florentin RA, Reiner JM, Lee WM, Lee KT (1976a) Cell kinetics of arterial smooth muscle cells during atherogenesis. IV. Evidence for a polyclonal origin of hypercholesterolemic diet-induced atherosclerotic lesions in young swine. Exp & Molec Path 24: 244–260

Thomas WA, Reiner JM, Florentin RA, Lee KT, Lee WM (1976b) Cell kinetics of arterial smooth muscle cells. V. Cell proliferation and cell death during initial 3 months in atherosclerotic lesions induced in swine by hypercholesterolemic diet and intimal trauma. Exp & Molec Path 24: 360–374

Lee KT, Lee KJ, Lee SK, Imai H, O'Neal RM (1970) Poorly differentiated subendothelial cells in swine aortas. Exp & Molec Path 13: 118–129

Imai H, Lee SK, Pastori SJ, Thomas WA (1970) Degeneration of arterial smooth muscle cells: Ultrastructural study of smooth muscle cell death in control and cholesterol-fed animals. Virchows Arch Path Abt A Path Anat 350: 183–204

Thomas WA, Florentin RA, Nam SC, Kim DN, Jones RM, Lee KT (1968) Preproliferative phase of atherosclerosis in swine fed cholesterol. Arch Path 86: 621–643

Reversal of Atherosclerosis: Comparison of Non-Human Primate Models[1]

D. Vesselinovitch and R. W. Wissler

Numerous reports attest to the usefulness of non-human primates for the study of experimental atherogenesis. During the past decade monkeys have also been utilized for investigations of lesion reversal (Wissler and Vesselinovitch 1977). Dietary regimens designed to reduce serum lipids as well as pharmacological and surgical interventions have been tested in six species. These include one new world species, the squirrel monkey (Saimuri sciureus), and five old world species, i.e., rhesus (Macaca mulatta), cynomolgus (Macaca fascicularis), stumptail (Macaca arctoides), African green monkeys (Cercopithecus aethiops), and baboon (Genus Papio). The approaches used thus far to influence the fate of experimentally induced atherosclerotic lesions are summarized in Table 1 (Armstrong and Megan 1974; Clarkson et al. 1979; De Palma et al. 1977; Hollander et al. 1979; Howard and Patelski 1974; Malinow et al. 1978; Maruffo and Portman 1968; Pick et al. 1978; Stary et al. 1977; Strong et al. 1977; Tucker et al. 1971; Vesselinovitch et al. 1979; Wissler 1979). Each of the primate models has shown special features of lesion configuration and composition during both induction and regression. The rhesus monkey has been the most widely studied (Armstrong and Megan 1974; Clarkson et al. 1979; Stary et al. 1977; Strong et al. 1977; Vesselinovitch et al. 1976; Wissler and Vesselinovitch 1977). Regression of "diet-induced" atherosclerosis in this species is characterized by a decrease in lipids and collagen within lesions as well as resolution of both necrosis and calcification. These regressive or healing changes are associated with a substantial reduction in degree of lumen obstruction. Although the lesions may be reduced readily by any one of several regimens, induction of severe coronary artery atherosclerosis appears to require specially severe atherogenic regimens for extended periods and/or special ancillary models of vessel injury. Lesions induced in the cynomolgus differ from those noted in the rhesus or in humans. In the cynomolgus large numbers of foam cells accumulate in the media and adventitia in association with marked fibroplasia and calcification. Intimal lesions are similar in composition and appear to heal after therapy, but there is little associated reduction of luminal narrowing of affected coronary or peripheral arteries (Hollander et al. 1979; Vesselinovitch and Wissler 1979). In contrast to the rhesus, however, induction of severe coronary artery lesions in the cynomolgus can be achieved in a relatively short time and may result in cardiovascular complications similar to those seen in man. These include coronary stenosis (M Kramsh 1979, personal communication) and development of severe cerebral artery atherosclerosis (Malinow et al. 1978). Lesion regression in the cynomolgus includes decrease of cholesterol content and disappearance of foam cells from the vessel wall. It may be speculated that great preponderance of "foam cells" represents a different cellular pathogenesis which results in a lesion type that is much less responsive to regression by means of serum cholesterol reduction. Despite the dissimilarities from human disease, the cynomolgus model would appear to be useful for the study of matrix protein in lesion regression and for the study of

---

[1] The authors' personal research cited was supported by Atherosclerosis SCOR Grant HL-15062-08.

the role of calcium in lesion histogenesis (Armstrong and Megan 1974; Hollander et al. 1979).

Table 1. Regimens utilized for treatment of athersclerosis in primates.

Specific Regimen	Investigators
Nutritional:	
Primate chow[a,b,c]	Maruffo et al. 1968; Kramsh 1979
Low-fat, basal diet[b]	Tucker et al. 1971; Stary et al. 1977; Strong et al. 1977
Low-fat, low cholesterol diet[b]	Vesselinovitch et al. 1974, 1976
Low-fat, cholesterol-free[b,c]	Armstrong et al. 1972, 1974
Corn oil enriched diet (18%)	Vesselinovitch et al. 1977
Corn oil enriched diet (40%)	Armstrong et al. 1972
Semi-synthetic diets with definite cholesterol levels	Clarkson et al. 1979
Alfalfa enriched diet	Malinow et al. 1978
Cholesterol conc. as in American diet	Malinow et al. 1978
Chemical:	
a. Hypocholesterolemic drugs	
N-y-phenylpropyl-N-benzyloxy acetamide[b]	Vesselinovitch et al. 1976
Cholestyramine[b,c,d,f]	Wissler et al. 1975, 1979 Malinow et al. 1978
Dextrathyroxine	De Palma 1972; Malinow 1978
b. Platelet activity inhibitory drugs	
Dipyridamole,[c] aspirin[c]	Hollander et al. 1979
c. Antihypertensive drugs[d]	
Hydrochlorothiazide; alpha-methyldopa; minoxidil; guanethidine; hydralazine[d]	Pick et al. 1978
d. Polyunsaturated phosphatidyl choline (EPL)[e]	Howard, Paletski 1974
Surgical:	
Biliary diversion	De Palma 1972

[a]S. siurcus (Squirrel m.)
[b]M. Mulatta (Rhesus m.)
[c]M. Fascicularis (Cynomolgus)

[d]M. Arctoides (Stumptail m.)
[e]Papio P. (Baboon)
[f]Cereopithecus Aethiops (African green m.)

Although the stumptail has been tested in only one study, it promises to be a satisfactory model for the study of lesion reversal, for therapeutic dietary regimens have resulted in lesion changes suggestive of repair (Pick et al. 1978). Furthermore, the distribution of coronary artery lesions appear to resemble those seen in patients with atherosclerotic heart disease (Bullock et al. 1969). Data is as yet insufficient to evaluate the suitability of the two remaining species (African green and baboon) for regression studies. Additional studies under different experimental conditions are needed to evaluate properly the potential of the stumptail for study of this aspect of atherosclerosis.

It is evident that the relative merits of each of these models of the human disease and/or for the illumination of various aspects of lesion morphogenesis and resolution requires further detailed exploration. Comparative studies conducted under identical conditions are particularly indicated in order to delineate these features which are attributable to species differences. Such studies are in progress in our laboratory (Vesselinovitch et al. 1979). We report here results obtained recently in our laboratory from studies designed to compare the responses of rhesus, cynomolgus and African green monkeys with identical induction and regression regimens. Specifically, we evaluated susceptibility to a peanut oil-cholesterol diet during induction and the effects of subsequent substitution of a prudent diet with cholestyramine on regression. The plan of this study is shown in Figure 1. At the end of a 12-month induction period, 4 of 8 animals of each species were autopsied to assess the severity of the disease; the remaining 4 were treated with a prudent diet and 2.5% cholestyramine and autopsied 12 months later. Fasting cholesterol (Abell et al. 1952) and lipoprotein profiles (Noble 1968) were determined initially and at monthly intervals thereafter. At the end of the 12-month induction period, average serum cholesterol levels for the African green was 300 mg/dl while the values for cynomolgus and rhesus were about twice as high, i.e., 600 mg/dl. By the second month of the treatment period, serum cholesterol levels had returned to nearly normal levels in all three species. Plasma lipoproteins showed a consistent increase in the β-lipoprotein fraction and a decrease in α-lipoprotein during induction in both macaque species. But this was not the case in African green monkeys. The incidence and severity of cutaneous xanthomas observed during the experimental period were closely correlated with serum lipoprotein levels in the two macaque species; no xanthomas were evident in African green monkeys (Vesselinovitch et al. 1979). At autopsy, striking species differences were observed in both aortic and coronary artery atherosclerosis (Table 2). The extent of intimal disease as judged grossly by percent of surface involved was quite high in both cynomolgus (91%) and rhesus (70%) at the end of the induction period. After 12 months of a prudent diet and cholestyramine, surface involvement was only mildly reduced in the cynomolgus (80%), but was moderately reduced in the rhesus monkeys (46%).

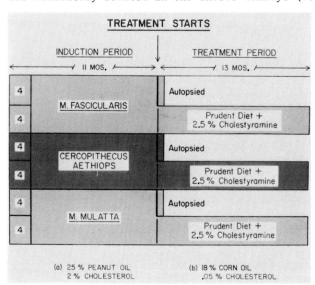

FIG. 1. Plan of the experiment of comparative study in three primate species.

Table 2. Major microscopic findings in artery lesions.

Regimen	Species	Aorta Gross surface area involved (%)	Severity ratings	Coronary Arteries	Luminal narrowing
Group I: Induction					
Peanut Oil (25%)	M. fascicularis	91	2.0±0.2	1.6±0.1	37±3.3
	C. aethiops	13	0.2±0.0	0.1±0.1	2±0.7
Cholesterol (2%)	M. mulatta	70	1.0±0.1	0.7±0.2	11±1.9
Group II: Therapy					
Prudent diet	M. fascicularis	80	1.2±0.2	1.5±0.1	37±3.2
	C. aethiops	4	0.1±0.0	0	1±0.8
Cholestyramine (2.5%)	M. mulatta	46	0.5±0.1	0.3±0.1	7±1.4

Mean ± standard error; measured by Hewlett-Packard digitizer and basic computer.

In contrast, gross aortic lesions of the African green monkey involved only 13% of the intimal surface after induction and were reduced to 4% after therapy. Microscopic evaluation of the aortic lesions showed evidence of lesion resolution in the cynomolgus, but this effect was more pronounced in lesions of the rhesus and African green monkeys. Coronary disease was distinctly more occlusive after induction than after treatment in rhesus monkeys, but there was little or no difference in degree of coronary artery stenosis before and after treatment in the cynomolgus (Table 2). Representative cynomolgus coronary artery lesions after the 12-month induction period and after treatment are shown in Figures 2 and 3. Marked intimal proliferation, abundant accumulation of foam cells throughout the vessel wall, intra- and extra-cellular lipid in both intima and media and foci of necrosis and calcification were evident after induction (Fig. 2). In contrast, coronary artery lesions of the treated cynomolgus showed a substantial decrease of stainable lipid, in the foam cells, in the necrotic areas and generalized transmural fibrosis (Fig. 3). Thus, although lesion composition changed considerably in the cynomolgus after 12 months of treatment, the size of the lesions were unchanged. Coronary lesions of rhesus monkeys, both before and after therapy, were confined mainly to the intima. Before therapy, lesions were rich in both intra-cellular and extra-cellular lipid, but foam cells were few. After therapy, lesions were fibrocellular and reduced in size (Vesselino-vitch et al. 1979). Aortic and coronary artery lesions of African green monkeys never advanced beyond fatty streaks during the induction period and only small foci of intimal thickening remained after therapy.

Thus lesions of different composition but equal severity were found in the aortas of the cynomolgus and rhesus after the 11-month induction period, but coronary lesions were somewhat more severe in the cynomolgus. Treat-

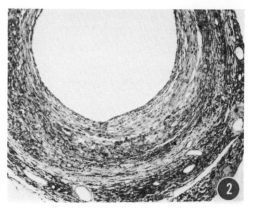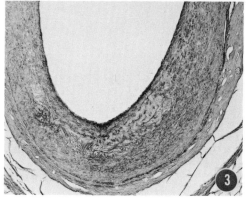

FIGS. 2 and 3. Photomicrograph of the coronary artery lesions in the
cynomolgus monkey fed atherogenic diet for 12 months (1) and in animal
after treatment with cholestyramine and prudent diet for the same period
of time. Oil red O. x16

ment with a "prudent" diet and cholestyramine resulted in the reduction of
lesion size and widening of the lumen in the rhesus. In the cynomolgus,
morphologic changes suggestive of repair were observed, but the lesions
did not diminish in size and lumenal narrowing persisted. The disappearance of lipid from the lesions of the African green indicated that the
fatty streaks present at the end of induction had regressed.

In summary, different species showed different response patterns to identical atherogenic and therapeutic regimens. The significance of these differences is not yet clear. Although primate models are proving useful for
studies of lesion regression for the investigation of functional complications of atherosclerosis and for the evaluation of various therapeutic
approaches, some of the species offer much more adequate reflection of the
human disease. On the other hand, the various models may well provide
complimentary data which could help to illuminate some of the aspects of
the induction and regression process in humans. The influence of genetic
factors in the different types of experimental diets and the anatomic
features related to animal size and arterial distribution all merit detailed
consideration.

References

Abell IL, Levy BB, Bradie BB, Kendall FB (1952) A simplified method for the
estimation of total cholesterol in serum and demonstration of its specificity.
J Biol Chem 195: 375.

Armstrong ML, Megan MB (1974) Responses of two macaque species to atherogenic diet and its withdrawal. In: Schettler G., Weizel A (eds) Atherosclerosis III. Springer-Verlag, Berlin, p 336.

Bullock, BC, Clarkson TB, Lehner NDM, Lofland HB, St. Clair RW (1969)
Atherosclerosis in Cebus albifrons monkeys III. Clinical and pathological
studies. Exp Mol Pathol 10: 39.

Clarkson TB, Lehner NDM, Wagner WD, St. Clair RW, Bond MG, Bullock, BC
(1979) A study of atherosclerosis regression in Macaca mulatta. I. Design
of experiment and lesion induction. Exp Mol Pathol 30: 360.

DePalma RG, Bellon EM, Klein L, Koletsky S, Insull W Jr (1977) Approaches to evaluating regression of experimental atherosclerosis. Adv Exp Med Biol 82: 459.

Hollander W, Kirkpatric B, Paddock J, Colombo M, Nagraj S, Prusty S (1979) Studies on the progression and regression of coronary and peripheral atherosclerosis in the cynomolgus monkey. Exp Mol Pathol 30: 55.

Howard AN, Patelski J (1974) Hydrolysis and synthesis of aortic cholesterol esters in atherosclerotic baboons. Effect of polyunsaturated phosphatidyl choline on enzyme activities. Atherosclerosis 20: 225.

Malinow RM, McLaughlin P, Naito WH, Lewis LA, McNulty WP (1978) Effect of alfalfa meal on shrinkage (regression) of atherosclerotic plaques during cholesterol feeding in monkeys. Atherosclerosis 30: 27.

Maruffo CA, Portman OW (1968) Nutritional control of coronary artery atherosclerosis in the squirrel monkey. J Atheros Res 8: 237.

Noble RP (1968) The electrophoretic separation of plasma lipoproteins in agarose gel. J Lipid Res 9: 963.

Pick R, Prabhu R, Glick G (1978) Diet-induced atherosclerosis and experimental hypertension in stumptail macaques (Macaca arctoides). Effects of antihypertensive drugs and a non-atherogenic diet in the evaluation of lesions. Atherosclerosis 29: 405.

Stary HC, Eggen DA, Strong JP (1977) The mechanism of atherosclerosis regression. In: Schettler G, Goto Y, Hata Y, Cose GK (eds) Atherosclerosis IV. Springer-Verlag, Berlin, pp 394–404

Strong JP, Stary HC, Eggen DA (1977) Evolution and regression of aortic fatty streaks in Rhesus monkeys. In: Atherosclerosis: Metabolic morphological and clinical aspects. Adv Exp Mol Med 82: 915.

Tucker CF, Catsulis C, Strong JP, Eggen DA (1971) Regression of early cholesterol-induced aortic lesions in Rhesus monkeys. Am J Pathol 65: 493.

Vesselinovitch D, Wissler RW, Hughes R, Borensztajn J (1976) Reversal of advanced atherosclerosis in Rhesus monkeys. I. Gross and light microscopic studies. Atherosclerosis 23: 155.

Vesselinovitch D, Wissler RW, Harris L (1979) The relationship between lipoprotein profiles and xanthomata in three species of non-human primates during development and regression of atherosclerosis. Fed Proc 38: 1347.

Vesselinovitch D, Wissler RW, Schaffner TJ (1979) Quantitation of lesions during progression and regression of atherosclerosis in Rhesus monkeys. In: Cardiovascular disease in nutrition, Symposium of American College of Nutrition. Spectrum Publications, New York. In press.

Wissler RW (1979) Evidence for regression of advanced atherosclerotic plaques. Artery 5(5): 398.

Wissler RW, Vesselinovitch D (1977) Atherosclerosis in nonhuman primates. In: Advances in Veterinary Science and Comparative Medicine Vol 21. Academic Press, New York, p 351.

Triglyceride Hydrolysis by Lipoprotein Lipase Bound to Endothelial Cells in Culture

Patsy Wang-Iverson, Eric A. Jaffe, and W. Virgil Brown

The location of lipoprotein lipase (LPL) on the lumenal surface of the vascular endothelium is supported by much experimental data. In this site it is responsible for the hydrolysis of the triglyceride of circulating plasma lipoproteins (Scow et al. 1976). Studies of the endothelial cells in culture however, have failed to demonstrate the presence of endogenous lipoprotein lipase activity (Howard 1977). The adipocyte has been shown to synthesize and to secrete the enzyme (Stewart and Schotz 1971). It is thus postulated that LPL originates in the parenchymal cells such as adipocytes or muscle cells and migrates to the endothelium. The functional activity in tissues is almost certainly controlled through synthesis and secretion (Garfinkel et al. 1976) but may also be dependent on regulation of specific binding to the external aspect of the endothelial cell.

Methods

Endothelial cells were isolated from human umbilical cords and cultured by previously reported methods (Jaffe et al. 1973). The study was initiated two days after the third passage by plating 9×10^4 cells into 12 mm diameter wells in Costar trays. Each well is maintained with 0.5 ml of overlying medium (Medium 199 containing 20% human serum). LPL was partially purified from bovine milk via binding to heparin/Sepharose 4B (Egelrud and Olivecrona 1972; Kinnunen 1977), and its activity assayed as previously described (Baginsky and Brown 1977). The specific activity of the enzyme preparation used in these studies was 4.2 mmoles FFA released/mg/protein/hr. To each well were added 17.2 U enzyme activity (1 U = 1 umole FFA released/hr) into 0.5 ml medium and incubated at 27° for 30 min. Control cells were simultaneously incubated in medium without added enzyme. After incubation, the wells were washed 6 times with medium, following which the bound enzyme activity was measured by adding 1 mg triolein substrate (labelled with [^{3}H] in the 9,10 position of the fatty acid) in 0.5 ml of medium. The substrate was prepared by sonicating the triolein (Nu-Chek Prep) with 15% egg yolk phosphatidylcholine (Sigma Chem. Co.) and activated with human serum as previously described (Baginsky and Brown 1979). After incubation for varying time periods (up to four hours), the medium was removed and the free fatty acids were quantitated by liquid scintillation counting (Pittman et al. 1975). The cells were then washed three times with medium, and total cell associated radioactivity was quantitated directly by adding an aliquot of suspended cells in buffer to liquid scintillation fluid. The remainder of the cells was extracted to determine the content of radioactive free fatty acid (Pittman et al. 1975).

Results

As shown in Fig. 1, the human endothelial cells do not exhibit intrinsic surface bound lipase activity under the conditions of these experiments.

When the triolein substrate was incubated with cells which had previously been exposed to lipoprotein lipase, free fatty acids were released into the medium for at least four hours at 27ºC (Fig. 1). Cell bound activity was approximately four fold greater than activity bound to empty dishes. The medium overlying the cells contained no measurable activity before addition of substrate.

Addition of heparin at 1 u/ml in the medium caused release of lipoprotein lipase activity into the medium which was 3 to 4 fold greater than that measured in the cell bound state. Addition of heparin at this concentration did not activate the purified soluble enzyme (Table 1).

The possibility that the enzyme might be released from the cell surface by the substrate prior to hydrolysis was examined by removing the medium containing the triolein emulsion after 5 min. of incubation with the cells containing bound enzyme. No further hydrolysis was observed with this mixture during a four hour incubation separate from the cells. Fresh substrate was added to the same cells and was hydrolyzed during parallel incubations indicating that the enzyme remained bound to cells.

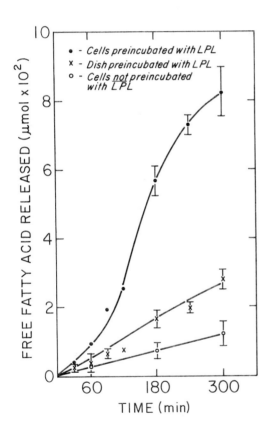

FIG. 1. Hydrolysis of Triglyceride Emulsion.
Endothelial cell monolayers and empty dishes
were preincubated with lipoprotein lipase
for 30 min. prior to addition of substrate.
Control monolayers were preincubated under
identical conditions in the absence of enzyme.

Table 1. Release of Cell Associated Lipoprotein Lipase
          Activity by Heparin.[a]

Condition	Activity (μmol x 10^2)
Cell associated LPL	7.3
Heparin-solubilized LPL	21.0
Cell associated LPL after heparin wash	1.6

[a]Endothelial cell monolayers were preincubated with partially purified bovine milk LPL for 30 min followed by
extensive washing (see Methods). Heparin (1 unit/ml)
was added to some monolayers and incubated for 15 min.
After quantitative removal of the heparin medium, the
monolayers were washed twice with medium containing no
heparin and substrate added and assayed for cell bound
LPL activity. Monolayers not exposed to heparin were
assayed under identical conditions. The heparin wash
was assayed for released LPL activity.

Examination of the endothelial cells after incubation with substrate revealed no significant association of radioactivity with the cell pellet,
suggesting no sequestration of the lipid within the cells.

Discussion

These studies establish that lipoprotein lipase can bind tightly to endothelial cells and remain active for periods of several hours. Although repeated washing with the medium and incubation with serum activated trigly-
ceride-phospholipid emulsions failed to remove the lipase activity, it cannot be concluded that the binding occurred at specific sites. Similar to
the in vivo situation, heparin added to the medium resulted in release of
the enzyme and the hydrolytic rates were clearly greater following heparin
release. Increased activity is compatible with the marked accentuation of
intravascular hydrolysis observed after intravenous heparin (LaRosa et al.
1971).

The addition of VLDL to endothelial cell monolayers has resulted in accumulation of triglyceride within cells (Howard 1977). In these experiments
no lipoprotein lipase was added and no endogenous lipase activity was
found. Radioisotopic double labelling experiments indicated that the uptake of triglyceride was not associated with hydrolysis. In the present
experiments, the failure of the endothelial cells to accumulate significant
quantities of labelled lipid during the active hydrolysis of triglyceride
by bound enzyme may be due to the ongoing rapid transcellular movement of
fatty acids and partial glycerides. However, documentation of the relevance of this approach to the study of lipoprotein degradation requires
demonstration of this transport process in the cultured cells.

References

Baginsky ML and Brown WV (1977) Differential characteristics of purified
hepatic triglyceride lipase and lipoprotein lipase from human postheparin
plasma. J Lipid Res 18: 423-437

Baginsky ML and Brown WV (1979) A new method for the measurement of lipo-protein lipase in postheparin plasma using sodium dodecyl sulfate for the inactivation of hepatic triglyceride lipase. J Lipid Res 20: 548-556

Egelrud T and Olivecrona T (1972) The purification of a lipoprotein lipase from bovine skim milk. J Biol Chem 247: 6212-6217

Garfinkel AS, Nilsson-Ehle P and Schotz MC (1976) Regulation of lipoprotein lipase: Induction by insulin. Biochim Biophys Acta 424: 264-273

Howard BV (1977) Uptake of very low density lipoprotein triglyceride by bovine aortic endothelial cells in culture. J Lipid Res 18: 561-571

Jaffe EA, Nachman RL, Becker CG and Minick CR (1973) Culture of human endo-thelial cells derived from umbilical cords. J Clin Inves 52: 2745-2756

Kinnunen PKJ (1977) Purification of bovine milk lipoprotein lipase with the aid of detergent. Med Biol 55: 187

La Rosa JC, Levy RI, Brown WV and Fredrickson, DS (1971) Changes in high density lipoprotein composition after heparin induced lipolysis. Am J Physiol 220: 785-791

Pittman RC, Khoo JC and Steinberg D (1975) Cholesteryl esterase in rat adipose tissue and its activation by cyclic adenosine 3':5'-monophosphate dependent protein kinase. J Biol Chem 250: 4505-4511

Scow RO, Blanchette-Mackie EJ and Smith LC (1976) Role of capillary endo-thelium in the clearance of chylomicrons. Circ Res 39: 149-162

Stewart JE and Schotz MC (1971) Studies in release of lipoprotein lipase activity from fat cells. J Biol Chem 246: 5749-5753

LDL-mediated Endocytosis and Cholesteryl Ester Transfer—Alternative Metabolic Pathways for the Regulation of Cellular Cholesterol Synthesis[1]

C.J. Fielding and P.E. Fielding

Cholesteryl esters in human plasma are derived in large part by the action of lecithin:cholesterol acyltransferase (LCAT). This is well shown by the very low levels of such esters in the plasma of human subjects with congenital LCAT deficiency (Glomset et al. 1970; Frohlich et al. 1978). However, analysis of the reactivity of LCAT with the major plasma lipoprotein classes indicated that neither low density lipoprotein (LDL) nor very low density lipoprotein (VLDL) were significant substrates for the enzyme, although containing the major part of plasma cholesteryl esters (Akanuma and Glomset 1968; Fielding and Fielding 1971). This paradox has recently been elucidated by the identification and isolation of a cholesteryl ester transfer protein in human plasma (apo D) which catalyses the net transport of LCAT-derived cholesteryl ester to VLDL and LDL (Chajek and Fielding 1978). The apparent Michaelis constant for reaction with VLDL is significantly lower, and hence the extent of transfer of sterol ester to LDL via the two available pathways, directly and via VLDL, will depend on the concentrations of each in the plasma and the turnover rate of VLDL. In normolipidemic man by far the greater part of LDL is derived by catabolism of VLDL (Sigurdsson et al. 1975).

The rate of cholesteryl ester transfer to VLDL and LDL under these conditions is approximately 2.2 nmoles min^{-1} ml^{-1} plasma (Chajek and Fielding 1978; Fielding and Fielding, unpublished). According to the hypothesis by which plasma lipoproteins, particularly LDL, are catabolized by endocytosis of the intact lipoprotein particle (Goldstein and Brown 1977) this rate should therefore equal the rate of irreversible catabolism of LDL protein, which is degraded in the lysosomes following receptor-mediated uptake. The rate of turnover of LDL protein has been measured in a number of studies (Langer et al. 1972; Simons et al. 1975). For a cholesteryl ester/protein weight ratio of 2.1 for LDL (Skipski 1972) this is equivalent to 1.0 nmoles min^{-1} ml^{-1} catabolized via the irreversible degradation of LDL and this estimate ignores endocytosis at any except the hepatic receptor systems since in the peripheral cells, LDL cholesteryl ester is recycled not degraded, while the protein after endocytosis is catabolized to peptide fragments (Goldstein and Brown 1977). The irreversible degradation of cholesterol in the adrenals and reproductive organs (probably < 100 mg day^{-1}) is negligible in terms of total body cholesteryl ester transfer. On the other hand the reported rates for the irreversible catabolism of cholesterol in man are in good agreement with those for the catabolism of lipoprotein protein (Grundy and Ahrens 1969).

Accordingly, the available data suggests that a large proportion of cholesteryl ester transferred to VLDL and LDL from the reaction of LCAT and through the activity of the cholesteryl ester transfer protein is not metabolized by endocytosis, either in the peripheral or hepatic cells, but is taken up without degradation or interiorization of lipoprotein apoprotein, is hydrolysed, and then recycles through the plasma compartment. In the case of VLDL,

---

[1] This research was supported by grants from the National Institutes of Health (HL 23738 and Arteriosclerosis SCOR 14237).

this loss of cholesteryl ester without endocytosis, is also indicated from the chemical composition of circulating VLDL and product LDL (Havel 1975).

A mechanism for such a pathway has recently been described (Fielding 1978). The coronary bed takes up cholesteryl ester from triglyceride-rich lipoproteins by a mechanism involving interiorization of steryl ester without detectable uptake or degradation of lipoprotein apoprotein. In these studies the cholesteryl ester was shown to be hydrolysed to the free sterol within the tissue after a rapid interiorization process ($t_{1/2}$ approximately 3 min). More recently an apparently identical mechanism has been identified in cultured endothelial cells (Fielding et al. 1979). In these studies it was shown that endothelial cells contain a chylomicron binding site at which chylomicron cholesteryl ester was interiorized without uptake or degradation of chylomicron protein. Furthermore, this cholesteryl ester was hydrolyzed in the lysosomes and as free cholesterol, was highly reactive in suppressing endothelial cell cholesterol synthesis; indeed, the system was almost completely coupled for suppression: uptake of each cholesterol molecule was accompanied by the suppression of synthesis of 0.6 cholesterol molecules within the cells. This slow process (about 150 ng cholesterol per 10^6 cells per 24 h) was fully expressed in whole plasma i.e. did not require preincubation with lipoprotein-depleted serum for significant effect. Moreover regulation was not accompanied by significant accumulation of cholesterol within the cells, indicating an ongoing regulatory process whose entry component must be balanced by an equivalent exodus of cholesterol into the plasma. This receptor, and its regulatory activity, therefore had all the properties required for the recycling pathway for LCAT-derived cholesteryl ester predicated by the excess of cholesteryl ester synthesis over lipoprotein apoprotein degradation. It is distinct from the LDL receptor of endothelial cells, (Fielding et al. 1979) which is in any case not expressed in contact-inhibited endothelium owing to the specific block in interiorization previously

ACTIVE PATHWAYS OF NORMAL PLASMA CHOLESTEROL METABOLISM

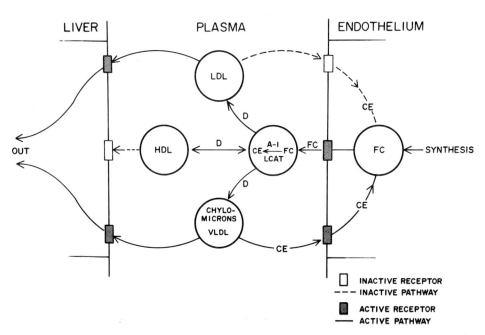

FIG. 1. Metabolic pathways related to LCAT and cholesteryl ester transfer protein.

reported (Vlodavsky et al. 1978). Thus not only can the endothelium regulate its cholesterol content via interiorization from triglyceride-rich lipoproteins, but it effectively lacks the LDL pathway by which other cells may limit their sterol content.

For a whole body endothelial content of 0.015 body weight (derived from Altman and Dittmer 1971) and an endothelial cell protein content of 0.36 mg per 10^6 cells (Vlodavsky et al. 1978) the uptake of cholesteryl ester from triglyceride-rich lipoproteins would equal 468 mg day^{-1} for a 75 kg human, equivalent to about 0.30 nmoles cholesterol min^{-1} ml^{-1} plasma. This would therefore represent about one third of the excess esterified cholesterol produced by the LCAT and transfer reactions. For the reasons given above, this may represent a minimal value. It therefore seems probable that major and previously undetected flux of cholesterol recycles through the vascular bed, which regulates endothelial cholesterol synthesis. Evidently quite modest imbalance in entry and output of cholesterol would result in the rapid accumulation of sterol in the vascular bed. The coincidence of rates of irreversible degradation of cholesterol and irreversible degradation of apoprotein in man probably indicates that the major site of endocytosis is via receptors in the liver (Figure 1).

References

Akanuma Y and Glomset JA (1968) In vitro incorporation of cholesterol-^{14}C into very low density lipoprotein cholesteryl esters. J Lipid Res 9:620-626

Altman PL and Dittmer DS (1971) Respiration and Circulation. In: Handbook of Physiology. Bethesda, Md. (Federation of American Societies for Experimental Biology, pp 357-359)

Chajek T and Fielding CJ (1978) Isolation and characterization of a human serum cholesteryl ester transfer protein. Proc Natl Acad Sci 75:3445-3449

Fielding CJ (1978) Metabolism of cholesterol-rich chylomicrons. Mechanism of binding and uptake of cholesteryl esters by the vascular bed of the perfused rat heart. J Clin Invest 62:141-151

Fielding CJ et al. (1979) Characteristics of chylomicron binding and lipid uptake by endothelial cells in culture. J Biol Chem 254:8861-8868

Fielding CJ and Fielding PE (1971) Purification and substrate specificity of lecithin:cholesterol acyltransferase from human plasma. Fed Eur Biochem Soc (FEBS) Letters 15:355-359

Fielding PE et al. (1979) Effect of contact inhibition on the regulation of cholesterol metabolism in cultured vascular endothelial cells. J Biol Chem 254:749-755

Frohlich J et al. (1978) Familial LCAT deficiency. Report of two patients from a Canadian family of Italian and Swedish descent. Scand J Clin Lab Invest Suppl 150:156-161

Glomset JA et al. (1970) Plasma lipoproteins in familial lecithin cholesterol acyltransferase deficiency: lipid composition and reactivity in vitro. J Clin Invest 49:1827-1837

Goldstein JL and Brown MS (1977) The low density lipoprotein pathway and its relation to atherosclerosis. Ann Rev Biochem 46:897-930

Grundy SM and Ahrens EH (1969) Measurement of cholesterol turnover, synthesis, and absorption in man, carried out by isotope kinetic and sterol balance methods. J Lipid Res 10:91-107

Havel RJ (1975) Lipoproteins and lipid transport. In:Kritchevsky D, Paoletti R, Holmes WL (eds) Lipids, lipoproteins and drugs. Plenum Press, New York

Langer T et al. (1972) The metabolism of low density lipoprotein in familial Type II hyperbetalipoproteinemia. J Clin Invest 51:1528-1536

Sigurdsson G et al. (1975) Conversion of very low density lipoprotein to low density lipoprotein. A metabolic study of apolipoprotein B kinetics in human subjects. J Clin Invest 56:1481-1490

Simons LA et al. (1975) The metabolism of the apoprotein of plasma low density lipoprotein in familial hyperbetalipoproteinemia in the homozygous form. Atherosclerosis 21:283-298

Skipski VP (1972) Lipid composition of lipoproteins in normal and diseased states. In: Nelson GJ (ed) Blood lipids and lipoproteins; quantitation, composition and metabolism. Wiley-Interscience, New York

Vlodavsky I et al. (1978) Role of contact inhibition in the regulation of receptor-mediated uptake of low density lipoprotein in cultured vascular endothelial cells. Proc Natl Acad Sci (USA) 75:356-360

Mode of Action of the Hepatic Endothelial Lipase: Recycling Endocytosis via Coated Pits

Paavo K.J. Kinnunen and Ismo Virtanen

Within the last few years our understanding on the role of lipoprotein lipase (LPL) acting on the capillary endothelium of the extrahepatic tissues
in the plasma lipoprotein metabolism has been markedly improved. The overall reaction of LPL with VLDL and HDL_3 can be presented as follows (Kinnunen 1979):

$$VLDL + HDL_3 \xrightarrow{\text{LPL}} 'LDL' + 'HDL_2'.$$

The particles generated in the LPL reaction in _in vitro_ experiments appear
very similar to the particles isolated from plasma. However, the lipid content (per protein) of the in vitro lipolytic products is slightly higher
(Catapano et al. 1978; Patsch et al. 1978).

Far less is known about the function of the other lipolytic enzyme of plasma lipoprotein metabolism, the hepatic heparin-releasable lipase. We recently localized this enzyme in rat exclusively on the liver endothelial
cells (Kuusi et al. 1979). Inhibition of the hepatic endothelial lipase
in vivo after intravenous injection of a specific antibody causes no change
in VDL composition or lipoprotein triacylglycerols, but results in an enrichment in the LDL and HDL phospholipids and cholesterol (Kuusi et al.
1979), the content of protein remaining virtually unaffected. The increase
in HDL phospholipids and cholesterol has been specified to occur in the
HDL_2-subfraction with a slight decrease in the concentration of HDL_3 (Jansen et al., unpublished data). Hepatic catabolism of both LDL and HDL
lipids has been shown to occur mainly in the non-parenchymal cells of
liver (Van Berkel and Van Tol 1979). Partial hepatectomy decreases the half
life of HDL but does not affect the decay of HDL-protein (Jansen et al.
submitted for publication). The minor hepatic uptake of both LDL and HDL
protein has been shown earlier (Sigurdsson et al. 1978, Van Berkel and Van
Tol 1978).

The above listed findings suggest that part of the HDL_2 and LDL lipids (phospholipids and cholesterol) are removed by the hepatic endothelial cells in
a process involving the action of the hepatic endothelial lipase. The removal of lipids from HDL_2 and LDL by this enzyme occurs independently from
the catabolism of the protein moiety of these lipoproteins.

Ultrastructural examination of the livers of rats perfused with rabbit antibodies against rat hepatic lipase, followed by perfusion with ferritin-
coupled anti-rabbit IgG antibodies as described earlier (Kuusi et al. 1979)
revealed that ferritin particles were localized only in hepatic endothelial
cells (Figure 1a) in regions with the characteristic appearance of coated
pits (Figures 1a,b)(Goldstein et al. 1979). The pits invaginate and form
typical coated vesicles (Figure 1c).

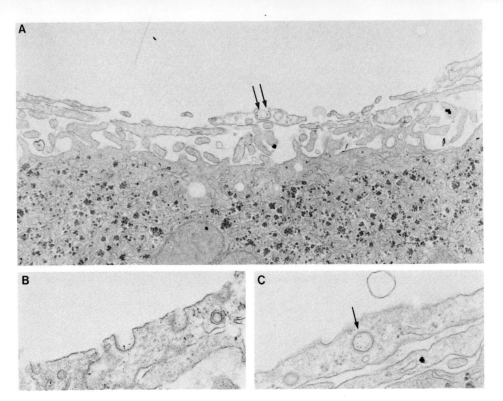

FIG. la-c. Electron micrographs of rat liver perfused with rabbit anti-rat hepatic lipase antibodies followed by ferritin-coupled anti-rabbit IgG antibodies. Thereafter the specimens were perfusion fixed with glutaraldehyde and Epon-embedded thin sections were post-stained with uranyl acetate and lead citrate. (a) Ferritin particles are seen only on an invagination of the sinusoidal surface of an endothelial cell (arrows). The surface of the liver parenchymal cell lacks the label. (b) At higher magnification the cytoplasmic surface of the invagination of the endothelial cell surface is seen to be covered with a knob-like fuzzy coat. (c) Also the cytoplasmic surface of vesicles containing the ferritin particles (arrow) is seen to be covered by a knobbed fuzzy coat.

Based on the concept of receptor-mediated endocytosis via coated pits (Brown et al. 1979; Goldstein et al. 1979) we propose a cellular model on the action of the hepatic endothelial lipase on 'LDL' (or intermediate density lipoprotein, IDL; Deckelbaum et al. 1979) and 'HDL'$_2$ (Patsch et al. 1978) derived from the LPL reaction with VDL and HDL$_3$. The schema presented in Figure 2 shows the pathway of 'LDL'-particles in the liver endothelial cells, depleting part of the surface phospholipids (and cholesterol) and resulting in the formation of LDL. By analogy, we propose a similar conversion of 'HDL$_2$' to HDL$_2$ by the same mechanism, involving the action of the hepatic endothelial lipase. The model involves recycling of the enzyme. Once the enzyme has acted on the lipoprotein particle, the coated vesicle opens at the surface and releases the modified particle, containing all of the protein originally in the lipoprotein, back to the circulation.

The recycling endocytotic action of the hepatic endothelial lipase via coated pits is in agreement with all the experimental results summarized above. Several aspects still need to be investigated in more detail. One possibility is that this process converts HDL$_2$ to HDL$_3$ as suggested by Jansen et al. (submitted) and Kuusi et al. (1979). This would, however,

SINUSOID

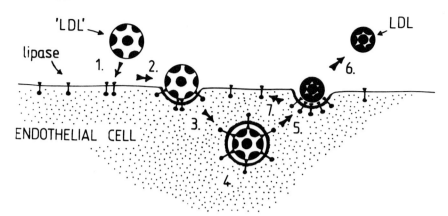

FIG. 2.   Mode of action of hepatic endothelial lipase on 'LDL'. Recycling
receptor-mediated endocytosis via coated pits. 1. Binding of the lipoprotein to the cell surface-bound lipase. 2. Aggregation of the lipases with
the bound lipoprotein with a subsequent invagination of the cell membrane
to coated pits. 3. Internalization to form coated vesicles with (4) action of the lipase. 5. Association of the coated vesicle with the cell
surface membrane and opening of the vesicle. 6. Release of the modified
lipoprotein and dissociation of the membrane-bound lipases of the coated
pits.

require the dissociation of apoC from HDL_2. Hydrolysis of phospholipids by
phospholipase A_2 is not sufficient to dissociate apoC from VLDL (Eisenberg
1977). The half-time of HDL-protein was not affected by partial hepatectomy
(Jansen et al. unpublished data).   Another possibility may thus be
considered, taking into account the heterogeneity of HDL_2 (Patsch et al.
1979). The hepatic lipase would merely modify HDL_2 within its density
range, probably removing the excess lipids remaining in the HDL_2-like particles generated in the $LPL-VLDL-HDL_3$-reaction (Patsch et al. 1978).

We do not know if any of the apoproteins is involved in the recognition/in-
teraction between the hepatic endothelial lipase and the lipoprotein particle. Binding of the antibody and anti-IgG-ferritin to the lipase seems
to be enough to induce the concentration of hepatic endothelial lipase to
coated pits with subsequent internalization.

Uptake of apoE (arginine-rich protein, ARP) containing lipoproteins (HDL
and HDL_c) by rat liver has been shown (Mahley et al. 1979). In contrast to
HDL_3 and LDL, chemical modification causes retardation of this uptake. One
obvious possibility would thus be the conversion of HDL (=HDL_c) to HDL_2,
and B-VLDL to LDL, by the action of the hepatic endothelial lipase via recycling receptor-mediated endocytosis. In this process the coated vesicles
should fuse with lysosomes and result in the degradation of part of the
apoE and hydrolysis of cholesterol esters by lysosomal enzymes. The phospholipase A_1 activity of the hepatic lipase may therefore be needed to expose
the cholesterylesters. High concentrations of HDL_c (and B-VLDL) could be
expected to cause the observed decrease in the activity of heparin-releasable hepatic-lipase, possibly due to an enhanced lysosomal degradation
(Mahley 1978). However, also this process would require the recycling of
the vesicles, opening back to the cell surface and release of the modified
lipoproteins.

References

Brown MS, Goldstein JL (1979) Receptor-mediated endocytosis: Insights from the lipoprotein receptor system. Proc Nat Acad Sci USA 76: 3330-3337

Catapano AL, Kinnunen PKJ, Packard CL, Gotto AM, Smith LC (1978) Action of lipoprotein lipase on very low density lipoprotein subclasses in vitro. In: Carlson LA et al. (eds) International Conference on atherosclerosis. Raven Press, New York, 315-318

Deckelbaum RJ, Eisenberg S, Fainaru M, Barenholz Y, Olivecrona T (1979) In vitro production of human plasma low density lipoprotein-like particles. J Biol Chem 254: 6079-6087

Eisenberg S (1977) Hydrolysis of phosphatidylcholine by phospholipase A_2 does not cause dissociation of apolipoprotein C from rat plasma very low density lipoprotein. Biochim Biophys Acta 489: 337-362

Goldstein JL, Anderson RGW, Brown MS (1979) Coated pits, coated vesicles, and receptor-mediated endocytosis. Nature 279: 679-685

Kinnunen PKJ (1979) High-density lipoprotein may not be anti-atherogenic after all. Lancet II: 34-35

Kuusi T, Kinnunen PKJ, Nikkilä EA (1979) Hepatic endothelial lipase antiserum influences rat plasma low and high density lipoproteins in vivo. FEBS Lett 104: 384-388

Kuusi T, Nikkilä EA, Virtanen I, Kinnunen PKJ (1979) Localization of the heparin-releasable lipase in situ in the rat liver. Biochem J 181: 245-246

Mahley RW (1978) Alterations in plasma lipoproteins induced by cholesterol feeding in animals including man. In: Dietschy JM, Gotto AM, Ontko JA (eds) Disturbances in lipid and lipoprotein metabolism. American Physiological Society, Bethesda, 181-197

Mahley RW, Weisgraber KH, Innerarity T, Windmueller HG (1979) Accelerated clearance of low-density and high-density lipoproteins and retarded clearance of E apoprotein-containing lipoproteins from the plasma of rats after modification of lysine residues. Proc Nat Acad Sci USA 76: 1746-1750

Patsch JR, Gotto AM, Olivercrona T, Eisenberg S (1978) Formation of high density lipoprotein$_2$-like particles during lipolysis of very low density lipoproteins in vitro. Proc Nat Acad Sci USA 75: 4519-4523

Patsch W, Schonfeld G, Gotto AM, Patsch JR (1979) Characterization of human high density lipoprotein subfractions obtained by zonal ultracentrifugation. Abstracts of V International symposium on atherosclerosis, Houston, n. 91

Sigurdsson G, Noel S-P, Havel RJ (1978) Catabolism of the apoprotein of low density lipoproteins by the isolated perfused rat liver. J Lipid Res 19: 628-634

Van Berkel TJC, Van Tol A (1978) In vivo uptake of human and rat low density and high density lipoprotein by parenchymal and nonparenchymal cells from rat liver. Biochim Biophys Acta 530: 299-304

Van Verkel TJC, Van Tol A (1979) Role of parenchymal and nonparenchymal rat liver cells in the uptake of cholesterol-labeled serum lipoproteins. Biochim Biophys Res Commun 89: 1097-1101

Lipoprotein Lipase and Hepatic Endothelial Lipase are Key Enzymes in the Metabolism of Plasma High Density Lipoproteins, Particularly of HDL$_2$[1]

Esko A. Nikkilä, Timo Kuusi, Kari Harno, Matti Tikkanen, and Marja Riitta Taskinen

In spite of the close association of plasma high density lipoproteins (HDL) with atherosclerotic vascular disease there is still relatively little knowledge on the pathways of HDL synthesis and degradation and on the factors which regulate the concentration of HDL and of its subfractions HDL$_2$ and HDL$_3$. It is becoming increasingly evident that circulating HDL particles are formed by a stepwise assimilation of constituents derived from different sources (Nikkilä 1978a,b). The primary HDL particle ("nascent" HDL) is elaborated by intestine and liver but immediately after its delivery to the circulation it becomes associated with apoprotein A-I and is transformed to HDL$_3$. Another step in HDL synthesis takes place during degradation of the triglyceride-rich lipoproteins (VLDL and chylomicrons) at peripheral capillary beds by the action of lipoprotein lipase (LPL). Recently, preliminary evidence has been obtained for a role of yet another endothelial lipolytic enzyme, hepatic lipase (HEL), in the metabolism of HDL. The present paper summarizes some of the data indicating that the two heparin-releasable endothelial enzymes are important in the regulation of plasma HDL (HDL$_2$) levels.

Lipoprotein Lipase Activity and Plasma HDL Concentration

Early observations indicated that during heparin-induced intravascular lipolysis of triglycerides, cholesterol was transferred from beta (VLDL) to alpha lipoprotein (HDL) (Nikkilä 1952, 1953) and that an increase of HDL phospholipids occurred during clearance of alimentary lipemia (Havel 1957). These findings lacked physiological interpretation and until recently it was believed that HDL acts as a donor of apoproteins and perhaps also of cholesterol esters and phospholipids to triglyceride-rich lipoproteins during their degradation. Newest evidence indicates, however, that HDL rather than being a donor acts as an acceptor of lipid and protein material released during hydrolysis of chylomicron and VLDL triglycerides, a concept which fits to the findings mentioned above.

During the hydrolysis of chylomicrons _in vivo_ their surface phospholipids and apoproteins are transferred to HDL (Havel et al. 1973; Redgrave and Small 1979). A similar transfer process occurs when VLDL is incubated with purified LPL in the presence of HDL$_3$ (Patsch et al. 1978). Upon assimilation of phospholipids, cholesterol and apoproteins from degraded VLDL the HDL$_3$ is transformed to particles resembling HDL$_2$.

The possibility that part of HDL could be a product of VLDL and chylomicron hydrolysis and that the rate of this reaction might be an important determinant of plasma HDL level was first raised by finding of a close positive association between plasma HDL cholesterol concentration and LPL activity in postheparin plasma (Nikkilä et al. 1977) or in adipose tissue (Nikkilä

---
[1]Supported by grants from the National Research Council for Medical Sciences, Finland, the Finnish Foundation for Cardiovascular Research and the Lions Organization of Finland.

Table 1. Lipoprotein lipase activity of tissues and serum HDL cholesterol in short-distance and long-distance runners.

| | LPL activity µmol FFA.h^{-1} per gram | | HDL-C |
	Adipose tissue	Skeletal muscle	mg/dl
Males			
Sedentary	2.2	0.85	47
Short-distance runners	2.4	0.82	50
Long-distance runners	6.1	1.46	66
Females			
Sedentary	7.9	0.90	61
Long-distance runners	11.4	1.39	74

et al. 1978) of man. In normal healthy subjects a correlation coefficient of the order of r = + 0.60 was found between HDL cholesterol and adipose tissue LPL activity.

The above hypothesis has been further supported by data accumulated from several studies. Since it is known that physically highly active people have higher total HDL and HDL$_2$ levels than sedentary subjects (Wood and Haskell 1979) we determined the LPL activity in biopsies taken from adipose tissue and skeletal muscle of active runners. It was revealed that long-distance runners undergoing continuous endurance training showed remarkably high LPL activities not only in their thigh muscle but also in subcutaneous adipose tissue whereas the activity in the same tissues of short-distance runners was similar to that of sedentary controls (Table 1). The HDL cholesterol levels were also much higher in the distance runners than in sprinters and in sedentary subjects. These findings suggest that endurance training causes an adaptive increase in the tissue LPL activity, which in turn leads to an accelerated turnover of circulating endogenous and exogenous triglycerides and this results in an increased formation and plasma concentration of HDL$_2$.

An opposite situation, viz. a low turnover of endogenous and exogenous triglycerides is present in people undergoing weight reduction. After reduction of caloric intake to about one-third of the actual need the LPL activity in adipose decreases to about 20 % and that in skeletal muscle to 50 % of the corresponding values present in caloric steady-state. At the same time the HDL levels start to decrease and end at a level which is, on an average, 20 to 30% lower than the starting value. This might be accounted for by a diminished formation of HDL$_2$ from triglyceride-rich lipoproteins.

Another condition where LPL activity and plasma HDL concentration are both decreased is insulin deficient diabetes. Recently we determined the LPL activity in adipose tissue and skeletal muscle of patients with untreated ketotic diabetes and of matched non-diabetic controls. The diabetic patients had markedly reduced activity of LPL in both tissues and also a low HDL cholesterol concentration (Table 2). In diabetic patients individual HDL cholesterol values did not show a significant correlation with corresponding tissue LPL activities but in the combined group of diabetics and controls a highly significant positive correlation emerged between the HDL cholesterol and adipose tissue LPL activity (r = + 0.58, p < 0.001). After initiation of insulin treatment the LPL activity rose in both tissues but still after two weeks of treatment the values were below those of controls but also the HDL cholesterol concentrations remained subnormal.

The LPL activity in adipose tissue rises also after initiation of regular use of alcohol about at the time when plasma HDL concentration starts to increase (Belfrage et al. 1977). Yet, it is uncertain whether the alcohol-

Table 2. Lipoprotein lipase activity of tissues and plasma HDL cholesterol concentration in insulin dependent diabetes.

Group	LPL activity μmol FFA h^{-1} per gram		HDL-C
	Adipose tissue	Skeletal muscle	mg/dl
Diabetics			
Untreated	1.09	0.42	43.0
On insulin (2 weeks)	1.79	0.72	44.1
Controls	3.21	0.92	53.1

induced hyper-HDL-emia is accounted for by increased LPL activity or rather by hepatic microsomal induction and concomitant stimulation of HDL production.

There are, however, a number of conditions in which plasma HDL levels are abnormally low or high without corresponding changes in LPL activity. One of these is obesity, where HDL concentration is often low in spite of the fact that the flux of exogenous and endogenous triglycerides (i.e. chylomicrons and VLDL) through plasma compartment is increased and the activity of LPL in adipose tissue (and in postheparin plasma) is not subnormal. A similar "discordance" is also present in many patients who have type IV or IIb hyperlipoproteinemia associated with overproduction of VLDL. In spite of presumably high production rate of HDL_2 in these patients they usually have low HDL levels. Furthermore, many hormonal steroids have profound influences on plasma HDL levels without affecting postheparin LPL activity. These include estrogens which increase HDL and norethisterone (Table 4) and oxandrolone (Tamai et al. 1979) which decrease HDL concentration. All these compounds share the feature, however, that in addition to changing the plasma HDL levels they have remarkable influences on the heparin-released hepatic lipase activity (Ehnholm et al. 1975; Tikkanen et al. 1979).

Heparin-Releasable Hepatic Lipase and the Metabolism of HDL

Localization of hepatic lipase in rat liver. Using antiserum prepared against highly purified heparin-releasable rat liver lipase and anti-IgG-ferritin complex we have shown that the lipase is located on luminal surface of hepatic endothelial cells (Kuusi et al. 1979). In electron micrographs (Fig. 1) the ferritin granules are clustered to certain areas of external surface of the endothelial cells and they are seen to enter the cell in the form of coated vesicles, a process much resembling the endocytosis of LDL-ferritin complexes in fibroblasts (Goldstein et al. 1979). It is tempting to speculate that the hepatic endothelial lipase (HEL) could act as receptor for some lipoproteins, which are then internalized with the enzyme and herewith removed from circulation and transferred further to hepatocytes for excretion and catabolism. It seems likely that the hepatic lipase located on endothelial cells represents the functional enzyme but the actual synthesis of the enzyme protein occurs in hepatocytes (or in the endothelial cell itself) from which it is transported to cell surface, a situation equivalent to the events of LPL synthesis in peripheral tissues and transport to endothelial cells. This view is supported by the release of lipase from perfused liver in two separate phases, rapid and slow, and by the inhibition of the slow release phase by colchicine (Kuusi 1979).

Table 3. Cholesterol and phospholipid concentrations (mg/dl) in rat serum lipoproteins after two injections of anti-hepatic lipase serum (AHS) or normal rabbit serum (NRS).

	VLDL		LDL		HDL	
	NRS	AHS	NRS	AHS	NRS	AHS
Cholesterol	traces		25	42^{xxx}	46	65^{x}
Phospholipids	10	13	22	35^{x}	110	157^{xx}

$^{x}p < 0.05$, $^{xx}p < 0.01$, $^{xxx}p < 0.001$

Changes of rat plasma lipoproteins produced by hepatic endothelial lipase antiserum.   Availability of a specific rat anti-HEL serum offered an opportunity to study the influence of selective HEL inactivation on serum lipoproteins. After injection of anti-HEL serum to intact rats the postheparin plasma HEL activity was completely inhibited while the LPL activity remained uninfluenced. Five hours after selective inactivation of HEL by antiserum in vivo the rats showed a significant increase of plasma LDL and HDL cholesterol and phospholipid concentrations above the corresponding values of control serum treated rats (Table 3). This observation suggests that HEL could function in removal of LDL and HDL. In other experiments we have found that depletion of HEL by heparin does not influence the removal of chylomicron remnants in the rat.

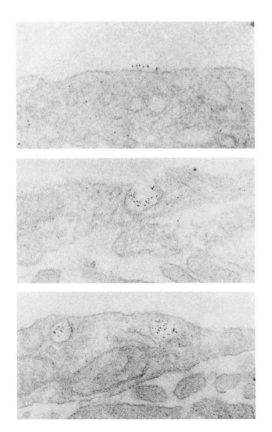

FIG. 1. Electron micrographs of rat liver endothelial cells demonstrating ferritin granules as indicators of location of hepatic lipase. The rats were injected with anti-hepatic lipase serum and the isolated liver was perfused with sheep antirabbit IgG-ferritin conjugate and fixed 5 min later with glutaraldehyde. Note the cluster of granules in upper figure and the formation of endocytotic vesicles in the middle and lower figures.

Table 4. Postheparin plasma lipase activities and serum HDL cholesterol during administration of estradiol valerate (2 mg/day) or d-norgestrel (250 μg/day) to normal women.

| | Lipase activity μmol FFA.h^{-1} per ml | | | | HDL-C mg/dl | |
| | LPL | | HEL | | | |
	Before	After	Before	After	Before	After
Estradiol	34.6	30.6	21.4	15.4[xxx]	61	73[xxx]
D-norgestrel	24.5	23.9	19.7	26.8[xxx]	58	46[xxx]

[xxx] $p < 0.001$

Is plasma HDL concentration related to hepatic lipase activity? The HEL activity is influenced by several hormones. The postheparin HEL activity is lower in women than in men (Huttunen et al. 1976) and it is further decreased upon administration of estrogens to fertile-age or postmenopausal women (Applebaum et al. 1977; Tikkanen et al. 1979). On the contrary, the progestin d-norgestrel significantly increases the HEL activity (Table 4) and an anabolic steroid oxandrolone has a similar effect (Ehnholm et al. 1975). All these hormones influence also the HDL levels but to an opposite direction than that of HEL activity. Thus, a decrease of HEL is associated with an increase of HDL (estrogens) and a fall of HDL accompanies rise of HEL activity (progestins, anabolic steroids, androgens?). Yet, we have not been able to demonstrate a significant correlation between the individual absolute or percentile changes of HEL and total HDL cholesterol during sex steroid administration. Our recent data indicate, however, that there is a significant inverse correlation between the increase of postheparin HEL activity and decrease of HDL$_2$ during progestin administration.

Postheparin plasma HEL activity is often increased in patients with type IV or IIb hyperlipoproteinemia (Huttunen et al. 1976). Obesity is also associated with a trend to higher HEL activities although the difference from the values of normal weight people is not significant. We have found that HDL cholesterol in obese population shows a significant negative correlation with postheparin plasma HEL activity ($r = -0.40$, $p < 0.01$). On the other hand, the postheparin HEL activity is positively correlated with fasting and two-hour plasma insulin values in obese subjects ($r = +0.47$, $p < 0.001$ for both). Thus, insulin may be one of the hormones regulating HEL activity.

Conclusions

The concentration of plasma HDL (HDL$_2$) is determined by the activity of two endothelial lipolytic enzymes, viz. lipoprotein lipase and hepatic lipase. In a variety of circumstances the HDL level is associated with lipoprotein lipase activity (normal men and women, high physical activity, caloric restriction, insulin-deficient diabetes). However, there is also preliminary evidence for a role of hepatic lipase in the removal of HDL from the circulation. The enzyme is located on luminal surface of hepatic endothelial cells and is thus well adapted to function as a removal enzyme for circulating lipoproteins.

References

Applebaum DM, Goldberg AP, Pykälistö OJ, Brunzell JD, Hazzard WR (1977) Effect of estrogen on post-heparin lipolytic activity. Selective decline in hepatic triglyceride lipase. J Clin Invest 59: 601-608

Belfrage P, Berg B, Hägerstrand I, Nilsson-Ehle P, Törnqvist H, Wiebe T (1977) Alterations of lipid metabolism in healthy volunteers during long-term ethanol intake. Eur J Clin Invest 7: 127-131

Ehnholm C, Huttunen JK, Kinnunen PJ, Miettinen TA, Nikkilä EA (1975) Effect of oxandrolone treatment on the activity of lipoprotein lipase, hepatic lipase and phospholipase A_1 of human postheparin plasma. N Engl J Med 292: 1314-1317

Goldstein JL, Anderson RGW, Brown MS (1979) Coated pits, coated vesicles, and receptor-mediated endocytosis. Nature 279: 679-685

Havel RJ (1957) Early effects of fat ingestion on lipids and lipoproteins of serum in man. J Clin Invest 36: 848-854

Havel RJ, Kane JP, Kashyap ML (1973) Interchange of apolipoproteins between chylomicrons and high density lipoproteins during alimentary lipemia in man. J Clin Invest 52: 32-38

Huttunen JK, Ehnholm C, Kekki M, Nikkilä EA (1976) Post-heparin plasma lipoprotein lipase and hepatic lipase in normal subjects and in patients with hypertriglyceridemia: correlations to sex, age and various parameters of triglyceride metabolism. Clin Sci Mol Med 50: 249-260

Kuusi T (1979) Heparin-releasable lipase of rat liver. Purification of the enzyme and studies on its function in lipoprotein metabolism. Dissertation, University of Helsinki

Kuusi T, Kinnunen PKJ, Nikkilä EA (1979) Hepatic endothelial lipase antiserum influences rat plasma low and high density lipoproteins in vivo. FEBS Lett 104: 384-388

Nikkilä EA (1952) The effect of heparin on serum lipoproteins. Scand J Clin Lab Invest 4: 369-370

Nikkilä EA (1953) Studies on the lipid-protein relationships in normal and pathological sera and the effect of heparin on serum lipoproteins. Scand J Clin Lab Invest 5: Suppl 8: 1-101

Nikkilä EA (1978a) Metabolic and endocrine control of plasma high density lipoprotein concentrations. Relation to catabolism of triglyceride-rich lipoproteins. In: Gotto AM Jr, Miller NE, Oliver MF (eds) High density lipoproteins and atherosclerosis. Elsevier, Amsterdam, pp. 177-192

Nikkilä EA (1978b) Metabolic regulation of plasma high density lipoprotein concentration. Eur J Clin Invest 8: 111-113

Nikkilä EA, Hormila P, Huttunen JK (1977) Increase of high density lipoprotein levels and of postheparin plasma lipoprotein lipase activity in insulin-treated diabetics. Circulation 56: suppl 3: 23

Nikkilä EA, Taskinen M-R, Kekki M (1978) Relation of plasma high-density lipoprotein cholesterol to lipoprotein-lipase activity in adipose tissue and skeletal muscle of man. Atherosclerosis 29: 497-501

Patsch JR, Gotto AM Jr, Olivecrona T, Eisenberg S (1978) Formation of high density lipoprotein$_2$-like particles during lipolysis of very low density lipoproteins in vitro. Proc Natl Acad Sci USA 75: 4519-4523

Redgrave TG, Small DM (1979) Quantitation of the transfer of surface phospholipid of chylomicrons to the high density lipoprotein fraction during the catabolism of chylomicrons in the rat. J Clin Invest 64: 162-171

Tamai T, Nakai T, Yamada S, Kobayashi T, Hayashi T, Kutsumi Y, Takeda R (1979) Effects of oxandrolone on plasma lipoproteins in patients with type IIa, IIb and IV hyperlipoproteinemia: occurrence of hypo-high density lipoproteinemia. Artery 5: 125-143

Tikkanen MJ, Kuusi T, Vartiainen E, Nikkilä EA (1979) Treatment of postmenopausal hypercholesterolaemia with estradiol. Acta Obstet Gynecol Scand Suppl 88: 83-88

Wood PD, Haskell WL (1979) The effect of exercise on plasma high density lipoproteins. Lipids 14: 417-427

How Does Lipoprotein Lipase Bind to Substrate Lipoproteins and How Is Its Activity Regulated?[1]

Thomas Olivecrona and Gunilla Bengtsson

A major step in the metabolism of triglyceride-rich lipoproteins is hydrolysis of their triglycerides and some of their phospholipids by lipoprotein lipase at the capillary endothelium. However, little is known about how the binding between the enzyme and the lipoprotein takes place. Binding of pancreatic lipase to lipid droplets in the intestine is dependent on colipase (Chapus et al. 1978; Borgström 1978). By analogy, binding of lipoprotein lipase to the lipoproteins might be mediated by its activator apolipoprotein. To explore this we carried out model experiments using a phosphatidylcholine stabilized triglyceride emulsion (Table 1). These experiments demonstrated that the enzyme adsorbs well to this emulsion even in the absence of the activator protein. Under other experimental conditions binding of the enzyme was less efficient but even in those situations the activator had little or no effect on the binding (Table 1). This suggests that a main interaction is between the enzyme itself and the lipoproteins. This conclusion is in accord with the recent demonstration that fragments of apolipoprotein CII which do not bind to dimyristoylphosphatidylcholine liposomes (Sparrow and Gotto 1978) retain the ability to activate the enzyme (Kinnunen et al. 1977).

A corollary is that the activator protein enhances hydrolysis by making the enzyme at the interface more effective in hydrolysis. How this is accomplished is presently not known. An interesting possibility is that the activator protein binds with highest affinity to the catalytically most effective form of the enzyme, thus changing the equilibrium between more or less effective forms in favour of the most effective one. According to this hypothesis the effect of the activator is analogous to that of a positive ligand operating on an allosteric enzyme. However, it can not be ruled out that the action of the activator also involves interaction with the substrate and/or product molecules.

The fatty acids and monoglycerides produced by the action of lipoprotein lipase are rapidly transferred into the tissue cells and metabolized there. Scow, Blanchette-Mackie and Smith (1976) have proposed an elegant model for how this transfer may take place by lateral diffusion in the membranes of endothelial cells, pericytes and tissue cells. The overall process of transport and reesterification must be highly efficient, but the capacity is presumably limited. It has long been known that lipoprotein lipase is subject to product inhibition. This provides a feed-back regulation of its action so that lipolytic products are not generated more rapidly at the endothelium than they can be taken up and utilized by the tissue. However, the mechanism of this inhibition is not well understood. We have studied the product inhibition in model systems and have found that at least three factors contribute:

1. Since the fatty acids and monoglycerides are more surface active than the triglycerides they locate at the lipid-water interface. With rat chylomicra this extends the surface into bilayer protrusions (Scow et al. 1976).

[1] Supported by the Swedish Medical Research Council (B13X-00727).

Table 1. Binding of ^{125}I-labeled lipoprotein lipase to triglyceride emulsions.[a]

Emulsion	Albumin	Ca^{2+}	CII	[125]I in top phase[b]	Initial rate of hydrolysis[c]
Triglyceride-egg yolk PC	+	−	−	92	74
"	+	−	+	96	470
"	−	+	−	53	62
"	−	+	+	58	270
"	−	−	−	36	n.d.
"	−	−	+	35	n.d.
Triolein-gum arabic	+	−	−	55	200
"	+	−	+	59	730
No emulsion	+	−	−	8	−

[a] Conditions: Triglyceride emulsion corresponding to 4 mg/ml triglyceride in 0.13 M Tris-Cl, 0.1 M NaCl, 1 mg/ml heparin at pH 8.5. Where indicated the medium also contained 60 mg/ml albumin, 20 mM Ca^{2+}, 5 µg/ml apolipoprotein CII. To measure binding 20 ng/ml ^{125}I-labeled lipoprotein lipase was added and after about 10 min at 25° 5 ml of the medium was separated by centrifugation in a SW 50:1 rotor at 30,000 rpm for 20 min in a Spinco L2 centrifuge at 15^oC. The tubes were sliced to give a top layer of about 0.5 ml and ^{125}I-radioactivity was determined in top and bottom layers. The total recovery of radioactivity was in all cases better than 95%. To measure the initial rate of hydrolysis a suitable amount of enzyme was selected for the anticipated rate and incubated in 1.5 ml of medium at 25°. Serial samples were taken so that a time curve was obtained for each experiment. Methods for purification and iodination of the lipase, preparation of apolipoprotein CII from human plasma, and preparation of the triglyceride emulsions will be detailed elsewhere (G Bengtsson and T Olivecrona, unpublished data).
[b] percent of total
[c] µmol fatty acid/min x mg

The fatty acids and the monoglycerides are substrates for the enzyme which compete with the triglycerides for its active site. Thus, the inhibition can be seen as due to a change in composition of the substrates available for the enzyme from predominantly triglycerides to a mixture containing predominantly fatty acids and monoglycerides. Presumably this factor is operative in product inhibition of other lipases also. However, the two following factors are more specific for lipoprotein lipase.

2. Small amounts of lipolytic products interfere with binding of the enzyme to the emulsion droplets. In a model experiment with a phosphatidylcholine-stabilized triglyceride emulsion more than 90% of the lipase adsorbed to the emulsion when the medium also contained albumin (Table 1). In contrast, when albumin was omitted, the amount of lipase which adsorbed to the droplets decreased to less than 40%. There is indirect evidence that lipoprotein lipase forms complexes with fatty acids (Fielding 1968; Baginsky and Brown 1977). Direct evidence for binding of another anionic detergent, deoxycholate, has been obtained in our laboratory by equilibrium dialysis and by charge shift electrophoresis. It is therefore likely that the enzyme was displaced from the emulsion droplets as enzyme-fatty acid complexes. Some of the enzyme which remained on the droplets may have been associated

with the extensions of the surface layer, which according to Scow, Blanchet-te-Mackie and Smith (1976) are composed primarily of fatty acids. If a major mechanism of the product inhibition is sequestration of the enzyme into complexes with fatty acids, than a major mechanism through which albumin relieves the inhibition is by preventing the formation of such complexes.

3. The activator protein does not enhance triglyceride hydrolysis unless a fatty acid acceptor is present. For instance, the activator enhanced the rate of triglyceride hydrolysis about 5-fold in the experiment in Fig 1 when albumin was present but it had no effect when albumin was omitted. Clearly this must be a major factor in the product inhibition. A consequence is that an efficient fatty acid acceptor, e.g. albumin, increases the apparent initial rate of hydrolysis in incubations with activator or with native lipoproteins but not in incubations without activator (Fig 1). To further study the influence of fatty acids on the effects of the activator we turned to a monoolein-Triton X-100 dispersion (Bengtsson and Olive-

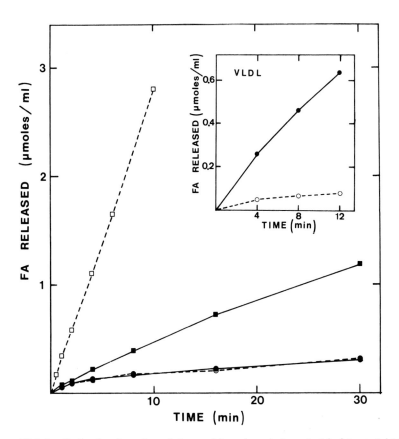

FIG 1. Hydrolysis of triglycerides in a phospholipid stabilized emulsion. Effect of activator in the presence and absence of albumin. Conditions as in Table 1. 0.7 µg/ml lipoprotein lipase was added. (□) 5 µg/ml CII, 60 mg/ml albumin. (■) albumin but no CII, (O) CII but no albumin, (●) no CII or albumin. The inset shows an experiment under the same conditions, but with human very low density lipoproteins (VLDL) as substrate (1 mg/ml triglyceride), 0.16 µg/ml lipoprotein lipase was added. (●) 60 mg/ml albumin, (O) no albumin. In the experiment with VLDL the fatty acids were determined by titration.

crona 1979). In this system the activator increased the initial rate of hydrolysis, but the rate decreased as hydrolysis progressed until the rate with activator was the same as that without. The decrease in the effect of the activator by fatty acids formed on hydrolysis could be reproduced by addition of oleate to the medium before the enzyme. The mechanism by which the fatty acids interfere with the effect of the activator can presently not be resolved. One possibility is that the activator effect involves interaction with the substrate and/or product molecules, e.g. that it facilitates separation of the product fatty acids from the enzyme and their transfer to a fatty acid acceptor. Another possibility is that the binding of fatty acids to the enzyme interferes with binding of the activator to the enzyme. However, the relationship between the site on the enzyme which binds fatty acids and the site which binds the activator is not known.

The effect of products on the activity of the enzyme and on its binding to the emulsion droplets has interesting and important implications for lipoprotein metabolism. When the lipoprotein attaches to the endothelium, hydrolysis is initially rapid and the products are efficiently utilized by the tissue cells. However, as soon as the capacity for rapid utilization of the lipolytic products is exceeded, hydrolysis slows down primarily because the lipolysis-promoting effects of the activator apolipoprotein are abolished. Furthermore, enzyme-particle binding is weakened by the fatty acids which facilitates for the lipoprotein to go back into the circulation and search for a new site. The length of each such cycle may be limited by the capacity of the tissue to utilize the lipolytic products. There is evidence in the literature that each lipoprotein goes through several such attachment/hydrolysis/detachment cycles until it is finally depleted of triglycerides or is removed from the circulation as a remnant lipoprotein (reviewed by Schaefer, Eisenberg and Levy 1978).

References

Baginsky ML, Brown MW (1977) Differential characteristics of purified hepatic triglyceride lipase and lipoprotein lipase from human post-heparin plasma. J Lipid Res 18:423-437
Bengtsson G, Olivecrona T (1979) Apolipoprotein CII enhances hydrolysis of monoglycerides by lipoprotein lipase, but the effect is abolished by fatty acids. FEBS Lett In press
Borgström B (1978) Mode of action of pancreatic colipase. Adv Exp Med Biol 101 (Enzymes Lipid Metab) 69-78
Chapus C, Sémériva M, Charles M, Desnuelle PP (1978) Adsorption and activation of pancreatic lipase at interfaces. Adv Exp Med Biol 101 (Enzymes Lipid Metab) 57-68
Fielding CJ (1968) Inactivation of lipoprotein lipase in buffered saline solutions. Biochim Biophys Acta 159:94-102
Kinnunen PKJ, Jackson RL, Smith LC, Gotto AM, Sparrow JT (1977) Activation of lipoprotein lipase by native and synthetic fragments of human plasma apolipoprotein CII. Proc Natl Acad Sci USA 74:4848-4851
Schaefer EJ, Eisenberg S, Levy RI (1978) Lipoprotein apoprotein metabolism. J Lipid Res 19:667-687
Scow RO, Blanchette-Mackie EJ, Smith LC (1976) Role of capillary endothelium in the clearance of chylomicrons. A model for lipid transport from blood by lateral diffusion in cell membranes. Clin Res 39:149-162
Sparrow JT, Gotto AM (1978) Synthetic fragments of apolipoprotein CII: Phospholipid binding studies. Abstract 294, Am Heart Ass Monograph no 61, suppl to Circulation vol 58

Activation of Lipoprotein Lipase by Synthetic Fragments of ApoC-II[1]

Louis C. Smith, John C. Voyta, Alberico L. Catapano, Paavo K.J. Kinnunen, Antonio M. Gotto, Jr., and James T. Sparrow[2]

Lipoprotein lipase hydrolysis of triglyceride at capillary endothelium is the key event in removal of circulating triglyceride from the plasma. In humans, there appears to be little, if any, uptake of intact triglyceride-rich lipoproteins (Robinson 1970, Jackson et al. 1975, Scow 1977, Fielding and Havel 1977). In man under normal circumstances, greater than 95% of the circulating LDL originates from the triglyceride-rich lipoproteins by the action of lipoprotein lipase (Sigurdsson et al. 1975). The mechanism by which apolipoprotein C-II (apoC-II), a protein component of the surface film of chylomicrons, VLDL and HDL, activates lipoprotein lipase (LaRosa et al. 1970, Havel et al. 1973) has not yet been established. The hydrolysis of triglyceride by lipoprotein lipase in the absence of apoC-II (Egelrud and Olivecrona 1973, Kinnunen et al. 1976, Catapano et al. 1979) excludes a true coenzyme function of the apoprotein.

Studies with both native and synthetic fragments of apoC-II have identified the minimum sequence required for activation of lipoprotein lipase and some of the structure:function relationships in the apoprotein (Kinnunen et al. 1977, Smith et al. 1978). The carboxyl terminal CNBr fragment containing residues 60-78 of apoC-II increases hydrolysis 4-fold, about 40% of the activation by apoC-II. The corresponding synthetic peptide prepared by solid phase techniques enhances the lipolysis 3-fold. Addition of five residues produces a synthetic fragment apoC-II (55-78), containing residues 55 through 78, that gives complete activation. By contrast, removal of the three carboxyl terminal residues from CNBr fragment 60-78 decreases the ability to activate lipoprotein lipase by greater than 95%. Therefore, activation of lipoprotein lipase by apoC-II requires a minimal sequence contained with residues 55-78.

A discrete α-helical lipid binding region in apoC-II has been identified with VLDL from an individual deficient in apoC-II (Catapano et al. 1979). Normal rates of lipoprotein lipase dependent fatty acid release could be achieved in vitro with native apoC-II and by three shorter synthetic peptides, apoC-II(55-78), apoC-II(50-78) and apoC-II(43-78); each peptide produces a 7-fold activation. ApoC-II(43-78), but not apoC-II(55-78), associates with VLDL as shown by separation of unbound ^{125}I peptides and the lipoproteins. Thus, residues 43-50 of apoC-II are part of a lipid binding region. The difference in the abilities to bind to the apoC-II deficient VLDL indicates that high affinity binding of the apoprotein to the lipoprotein surface is not required for lipoprotein lipase action on

[1]Support was provided by the Robert A. Welch Foundation Grant Q-343; the National Heart and Blood Vessel Research and Demonstration Center, Baylor College of Medicine, a grant supported research project of the National Heart, Lung and Blood Institute, HL-17269; U.S. Public Health Service Grant HL-15648; The American Heart Association, Texas Affiliate; and a grant from the Finnish Cultural Foundation to PKJK.
[2]JTS is an Established Investigator of the American Heart Association.

triglyceride and makes no apparent contribution to the enhancement of lipoprotein lipase activity. The lipid binding region has also been identified by isolation and characterization of a complex of apoC-II(43-78) and dimyristoylphosphatidylcholine (Sparrow and Gotto 1978). Shorter peptides do not form isolatable complexes.

The empirical rules developed by Chou and Fasman (1978a, 1978b) for prediction of the secondary structure of proteins from the amino acid sequence have been used to identify possible structural domains in the carboxyl terminal region of apoC-II. The following secondary structure for apoC-II(35-78) serves as a working hypothesis and provides the rationale for synthesis of the individual synthetic fragments.

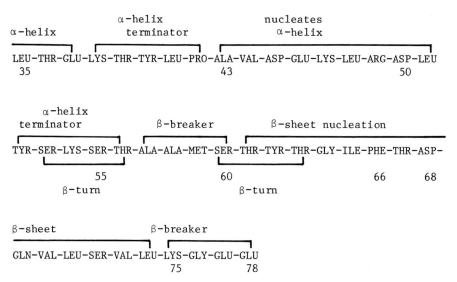

In the present studies, a series of related peptides that differ by a single amino acid or in the number of amino acid residues has been prepared as an experimental approach to study the structure:function relationships in apoC-II and to determine a requirement for the phenolic hydroxyl group of TYR_{62}. Modified peptides, apoC-II(50-78 PHE_{62}), apoC-II(50-78 TRP_{62}) and apoC-II(50-78 GLY_{62}) with phenylalanine, tryptophan and glycine, respectively, substituted for tyrosine at position 62 have been synthesized. The substitution of these amino acids for TYR in apoC-II(55-78) reduces the activation of lipoprotein lipase mediated triglyceride hydrolysis about 60-78%. The lower activity of apoC-II(55-78 PHE_{62}) may have reflected the functional importance of the phenolic hydroxyl group, which may be a hydrogen-bond donor or acceptor. Alternatively, insertion of PHE in lieu of TYR may have disrupted an essential β-turn involving residues 60-63 in apoC-II(55-78), thereby reducing the activation of lipoprotein lipase. This latter possibility is not likely, since ApoC-II(55-78 GLY_{62}) activation is comparable to the enhancement by apoC-II(55-78 PHE_{62}) and apoC(55-78 TRP_{62}), about 1/3 as much as the native sequence. There is an extremely high conformational potential of GLY for stabilizing a β-turn (Chou and Fasman, 1978a). The presence of an aromatic nucleus at position 62 is not sufficient for activation of lipoprotein lipase. The similar but lower level of activation by the substituted peptides apparently can be accomplished through hydrogen-bonding by residues adjacent to TYR_{62} in apoC-II(55-78).

Since the apoC-II(60-75) derived from CNBr apoC-II(60-78) by tryptic removal of the terminal tripeptide is not active, apoC-II(50-75) has been synthesized and tested. This fragment is fully active (AL Catapano, PKJ

Kinnunen, AM Gotto, LC Smith, and JT Sparrow 1979 unpublished experiments). Furthermore, the activation by apoC-II and the synthetic peptides apoC-II(43-78), apoC-II(50-78) and apoC-II(50-75) is abolished by 1M NaCl in the reaction mixture. These results exclude competition of the salt anion with the carboxyl terminal GLU residues as a simple explanation for the inhibition of lipoprotein lipase by salt high concentrations.

Differences in the activity of apoC-II(60-78) and apoC-II(60-75), the inhibition by high salt and the inactivity of apoC-II(66-78) suggest that a minimum critical length of the activator sequence between residues 60-78 is required for activation. This possibility is supported by the pattern of activation obtained with a series of synthetic peptides with ASP$_{68}$ as the carboxyl terminus: apoC-II(60-68), apoC-II(55-68), apoC-II(50-68), apoC-II(43-68) and apoC-II(35-68).

At low concentrations of peptides, where there is a linear increase in triglyceride hydrolysis with increasing amounts of activator, apoC-II(60-68) and apoC-II(55-68) give virtually no enhancement of lipoprotein lipase activity. By contrast, apoC-II(55-78) gives complete activation, identical to that produced by the entire apoC-II. Extension of the peptide chain, as in apoC-II(50-68), apoC-II(43-68) and apoC-II(35-68), increases the ability to activate. The stimulation by these peptides at concentrations up to 4 μM is 50, 100 and 100 percent of that of the native peptide. The presence of residues 50-55 in apoC-II(50-78) has no detectable effect on lipoprotein lipase catalysis, since apoC-II(55-78) gives complete activation. Whether the increased activity of apoC-II(50-68), as compared to apoC-II(55-68), results from stabilization of β-turn comprised of SER$_{60}$ THR$_{61}$ TYR$_{62}$ THR$_{63}$ or from direct interaction of ASP$_{50}$ LEU$_{51}$ TYR$_{52}$ SER$_{53}$ LYS$_{54}$ with the enzyme remains for future study. The inclusion of a lipid binding region in the activator peptide allows complete activation, even when the sequence region 69-78 is absent.

Full activation of lipoprotein lipase by apoC-II can be achieved if two different sequence regions are present. We postulate that the putative β-sheet of residues 63-74 of apoC-II forms hydrogen bonds with a corresponding β-sheet of the enzyme. If this β-sheet forms, it is reasonable to envision orientation of the peptide backbone parallel to the plane of the interface. Juxtaposition of space filling molecular models of apoC-II and a β-sheet region of a protein suggests that hydrophobic interactions between the carboxyl terminal region of the apoprotein and the enzyme seem to be sterically prohibited. The association of apoC-II with lipoprotein lipase may occur only through electrostatic and hydrogen bond interactions. Alternately, if the carboxyl terminal of the putative β-sheet of apoC-II is too short for high affinity interaction with the enzyme, the presence of a lipid binding region consisting of residues 43-52 could increase the concentration of the activator at the surface of the macromolecular substrate, where the lipoprotein lipase could interact laterally with the activator sequence region including TYR$_{62}$, thereby enhancing catalysis. We conclude that enhancement of lipoprotein lipase catalysis depends on specific structural features in apoC-II that concentrate the apoprotein at the interface with the enzyme and the substrate. Both protein:protein and lipid:protein interactions appear to contribute to this process.

Acknowledgements

We are indebted to Drs. William A. Bradley and William W. Mantulin for valuable discussions and to Mrs. Karen Pogue for preparation of the manuscript.

References

Catapano AL, Kinnunen PKJ, Breckenridge WC, Gotto AM Jr, Jackson RL, Little JA, Smith LC, Sparrow JT (1979) Lipolysis of apoC-II deficient very low density lipoproteins: enhancement of lipoprotein lipase action by synthetic fragments of apoC-II. Biochem Biophys Res Comm 89: 951-957

Chou PY, Fasman GD (1978a) Empirical predictions of protein conformation. Ann Rev Biochem 47: 251-276

Chou PY, Fasman GD (1978b) Prediction of the secondary structure of proteins from their amino acid sequence. In: Meister A (ed) Advances in Enzymology. John Wiley & Sons New York, NY pp 45-148.

Egelrud T, Olivecrona T (1973) Purified bovine milk (lipoprotein) lipase: activity against lipid substrates in the absence of exogenous serum factors. Biochim Biophys Acta 306: 115-127

Fielding CJ, Havel RJ (1977) Lipoprotein lipase. Arch Pathol Lab Med 101: 225-229

Havel RJ, Fielding CJ, Olivecrona T, Shore VG, Fielding PE, Egelrud T (1973) Cofactor activity of protein components of human very low density lipoproteins in the hydrolysis of triglycerides by lipoprotein lipase from different sources. Biochemistry 12: 1828-1833

Jackson RL, Morrisett JD, Gotto AM Jr (1976) Lipoprotein structure and metabolism. Physiol Rev 56: 259-316

Kinnunen PKJ, Huttunen JK, Ehnholm C (1976) Properties of purified bovine milk lipoprotein lipase. Biochim Biophys Acta 450: 342-351

Kinnunen PKJ, Jackson RL, Smith LC, Gotto AM Jr, Sparrow JT (1977) Activation of lipoprotein lipase by native and synthetic fragments of human plasma. Proc Natl Acad Sci USA 74: 4848-4851

LaRosa JC, Levy RI, Herbert PN, Lux SE, Fredrickson DS (1970) A specific apoprotein activator for lipoprotein lipase. Biochem Biophys Res Commun 41: 57-62

Robinson DS (1970) The function of the plasma triglycerides in fatty acid transport. In: Florkin M, Stotz E (eds) Comprehensive Biochemistry. Elsevier, Amsterdam, Vol 18, pp 51:116.

Scow RO (1977) Metabolism of chylomicrons in perfused adipose and mammary tissue of the rat. Fed Proc 36: 182-185

Sigurdsson GA, Nicoll A, Lewis B (1975) Conversion of very low density lipoprotein to low density lipoprotein. J Clin Invest 56: 1481-1490

Smith LC, Kinnunen PKJ, Jackson RL, Gotto AM Jr, Sparrow JT (1978) In: LA Carlson, R Paoletti, G Weber (eds) International Conference on Atherosclerosis. Raven Press, New York, pp 269-273.

Sparrow JT, Gotto AM Jr (1978) Synthetic fragments of apolipoprotein C-II: phospholipid binding studies. Circulation 58: II-77

Contributions of Invited Speakers

Plenary Session: The Vessel Wall in Atherosclerosis
Co-Chairpersons: James F. Mustard and Robert W. Wissler
Speakers: Michael A. Gimbrone, Jr.
                       Salvador Moncada
                       Russell Ross

Workshop: Non-Dietary, Non-Pharmacological Treatment of Hyperlipidemia
Co-Chairpersons: Thomas E. Starzl and Gilbert R. Thompson
Speakers: G.M.B. Berger
                       Henry Buchwald
                       Paul-J. Lupien
                       Tatu Miettinen
                       Evan A. Stein

Workshop: HDL: Negative Risk Factor for Coronary Heart Disease
Co-Chairpersons: William P. Castelli and Frederick H. Epstein
Speakers: Charles J. Glueck
                       Tavia Gordon
                       N.E. Miller

Workshop: Clinical Trials
Speakers: William L. Holmes
                       Robert H. Knopp
                       James A. Schoenberger

Workshop: The Arterial Wall—II
Co-Chairpersons: Donald M. Small and Elspeth B. Smith
Speakers: Yoshiya Hata
                       Henry F. Hoff
                       Fujio Numano
                       Richard W. St. Clair

Workshop: Vessel Wall—Platelet Interaction
Co-Chairpersons: Hans R. Baumgartner and G.V.R. Born
Speakers: Laurence A. Harker
                       C. Richard Minick
                       Michael B. Stemerman

Workshop: Catabolism of Lipids, Apolipoproteins and Lipoproteins

Co-Chairpersons:	DeWitt S. Goodman and Paul J. Nestel
Speakers:	David W. Bilheimer
	Scott M. Grundy
	James Shepherd
	Allan Sniderman
	Donald B. Zilversmit

The Vessel Wall and Atherosclerosis

James Fraser Mustard

In this session, consideration will be given to some aspects of the mechanisms in thrombosis, particularly as they relate to the arachidonic acid pathway in platelets and the cells of the vessel wall. The first two presentations provide an overview of the arachidonic acid, thromboxane A_2, PGI_2 pathways and their effects on thrombosis and the vessel wall. The final two presentations are concerned with the endothelium, its normal physiology, the effects of endothelial injury, and the response of the smooth muscle cells to vessel wall injury in relation to the development of proliferative intimal lesions.

Platelets do not adhere to the normal endothelium but if it is removed, the subendothelium rapidly becomes covered with platelets which adhere to microfibrils, basement membrane and collagen (Mustard et al. 1977). When the platelets adhere to collagen they are stimulated to release their granule contents, including the mitogenic factor for smooth muscle cells. In addition, the arachidonic acid pathway is activated and thromboxane A_2 forms. If blood flow is not disturbed and there is a high shear, only a thin layer of platelets will form on the subendothelial surface; few thrombi will be present.

In regions of disturbed flow, platelets and activated clotting factors that promote thrombus formation can accumulate (Goldsmith and Karino 1978). It should be emphasized that thrombosis in arteries is only a significant problem at sites of disturbed flow such as vessel bifurcations or stenoses.

In conditions of disturbed flow in arteries, all the pathways that are involved in thrombus formation come into play, leading to the formation of a platelet-rich mass with fibrin and red cells associated with it. The pathways involved include release of ADP from platelets which causes circulating platelets to change shape and adhere to each other, and the formation of thromboxane A_2 from arachidonic acid freed from platelet membrane phospholipids which also causes platelet aggregation and induces the platelet release reaction (Mustard et al. 1980). Perhaps most important for the growth and stability of a thrombus is the acceleration of coagulation that occurs on the surface of the aggregated platelets. The thrombin which forms can cause further platelet aggregation independently of released ADP and the thromboxane A_2 pathway (Kinlough-Rathbone et al. 1977), as well as causing the release reaction and stimulating further formation of thromboxane A_2. In addition, thrombin causes fibrin to form which binds tightly to adherent platelets (Niewiarowski et al. 1972) and is probably responsible for keeping the platelet mass together since platelets rapidly deaggregate if fibrin does not form. The fibrin can be lysed if plasminogen, particularly the plasminogen associated with the fibrin, is activated by plasminogen activator. Plasminogen activator can be released from an injured vessel wall and plasminogen can be converted to plasmin through activation of the intrinsic pathway of coagulation (Mustard and Packham 1979). It should be realized that the thromboxane A_2 pathway is not essential for thrombus formation and in circumstances where thrombin formation is extensive, thromboxane A_2 is probably not important.

The vessel wall contributes to thrombus growth not only through platelet contact with the wall but also through activation of coagulation. The original evidence that when platelets interact with collagen, Factor XI is activated (Walsh 1972a) has recently been questioned (Østerud et al. 1979), as has the report that the aggregation of platelets by ADP activates Factor XII (Walsh 1972b; Vicic et al. 1979). It has been demonstrated recently that stimulated platelets release Factor Va which binds Factor Xa at the surface of the platelets (Miletich et al. 1978). Platelet membrane phospholipids are undoubtedly involved in coagulation reactions (Zwaal 1978) and it is well accepted that damaged cells release tissue thromboplastin that activates the extrinsic coagulation pathway (Nemerson and Pitlick 1972). The relative importance of vessel wall stimulation of thrombin formation in the initiation and growth of thrombi in arteries has not been defined but it may be important in some circumstances. Since a variety of mechanisms are involved in thrombosis, the thromboxane A_2 pathway may not be important in all thrombotic episodes.

The endothelium is responsible for maintaining the integrity of the vessel wall. An interesting aspect of endothelial injury is the resultant increase in vessel permeability. One way of locating sites of increased endothelial permeability is to examine blood vessels for sites where Evans blue bound to albumin accumulates (Packham et al. 1967; Mustard et al. 1978). Examination of sites of increased permeability where Evans blue accumulates shows endothelial cell alterations that are often associated with small thrombi and white cells. How these 'spontaneous' lesions occur in normal animals is not known. However, many studies have now shown that they occur around vessel orifices and bifurcations. Blood flow changes are probably important in contributing to the endothelial injury at these sites.

One of the key findings concerning the vessel wall and injury is the demonstration that the endothelium and smooth muscle cells can form PGI_2 from arachidonic acid. PGI_2 inhibits platelet aggregation and the platelet release reaction and causes relaxation of arterial smooth muscle cells. This is in direct contrast to the thromboxane A_2 formed by the platelets which causes platelet aggregation and contraction of arterial smooth muscle cells (Mustard et al. 1980; Moncada and Vane 1979; Gerrard and White 1978).

The role of PGI_2 in preventing thrombus formation is important, particularly in circumstances in which PGI_2 formation is extensive. The work of Kelton and his associates (Kelton et al. 1978) has shown the effect of aspirin, in doses that block PGI_2 formation, on thrombus formation in injured rabbit jugular veins. In these experiments a low dose of aspirin had no effect on the PGI_2-like activity produced by the vein segments or on the amount of thrombus formed as measured by ^{125}I-fibrinogen accretion. However, when high doses of aspirin were given, PGI_2 formation was blocked and thrombus formation was dramatically enhanced. These data suggest that under the conditions of these experiments in a damaged jugular vein the formation of PGI_2 by the injured vessel wall is an important factor in limiting thrombus formation and if PGI_2 formation is blocked, thrombus formation is enhanced.

In contrast, in circumstances where blood flow is rapid and thrombin formation is minimal, such as in the aorta of the rabbit, inhibition of PGI_2 formation by the vessel wall does not lead to increased platelet accumulation on the subendothelium (Dejana et al. 1979). Thus the effect of PGI_2 on thrombus formation may be dependent upon the site of injury, the patterns of flow and the extent to which PGI_2 formation is stimulated.

An important aspect of platelet accumulation on the subendothelial surface
of a vessel is that the ability of the surface to attract fresh platelets
rapidly decreases (Groves et al. 1979). One of the unresolved questions
about the mechanisms involved in this is whether PGI_2 formation by the vessel wall is one of the factors that reverses the thrombogenicity of the
initial injury site.

Finally, the story of vessel injury, platelets and atherosclerosis (Mustard
et al. 1978) was greatly stimulated by the observations of Ross and his
colleagues that platelets can release a mitogen that stimulates smooth
muscle cell proliferation (Ross and Vogel 1978). There is considerable
experimental evidence supporting the role of platelets as one source of a
factor causing smooth muscle cell proliferation following endothelial injury (Moore et al. 1976; Friedman et al. 1977).

Summary

The role of endothelial injury in thrombosis and the development of atherosclerosis involves platelet interaction with the vessel wall and the platelet release reaction. The mitogen released by platelets is one of the
factors involved in the proliferation of arterial smooth muscle cells in
the intima. Thromboxane A_2 formed from arachidonic acid by platelets promotes platelet aggregation and thrombosis while PGI_2 formed from arachidonic acid by cells in the vessel wall inhibits thrombosis.

References

Dejana E, Cazenave J-P, Groves HM, Kinlough-Rathbone RL, Mustard JF (1979)
The effect of inhibition of PGI_2 production on platelet adherence to damaged and undamaged rabbit aortae in vitro and in vivo. Fed Proc 38: 1271

Friedman RJ, Stemerman MB, Wenz B, Moore S, Gauldie J, Gent M, Tiell ML,
Spaet TH (1977) The effect of thrombocytopenia on experimental arteriosclerotic lesion formation in rabbits: I. Smooth muscle cell proliferation
and re-endothelialization. J Clin Invest 60: 1191

Gerrard JM, White JG (1978) Prostaglandins and thromboxanes: "Middlemen"
modulating platelet function in hemostasis and thrombosis. In:Spaet TH
(ed) Progress in Hemostasis and Thrombosis, Grune and Stratton, New York,
Vol 4, p.87

Goldsmith HL, Karino T (1978) Mechanically induced thromboemboli. In:
Quantitative Cardiovascular Studies, Clinical Research Applications of
Engineering Principles, University Park Press, Baltimore, Md, p.1

Groves HM, Kinlough-Rathbone RL, Richardson M, Moore S, Mustard JF (1979)
Platelet interaction with damaged rabbit aorta. Lab Invest 40: 194

Kelton JG, Hirsh J, Carter CJ, Buchanan MR (1978) Thrombogenic effect of
high-dose aspirin in rabbits. Relationship to inhibition of vessel wall
synthesis of prostaglandin I_2-like activity. J Clin Invest 62: 892

Kinlough-Rathbone RL, Packham MA, Reimers H-J, Cazenave J-P, Mustard JF
(1977) Mechanisms of platelet shape change, aggregation and release induced
by collagen, thrombin or A23,187. J Lab Clin Med 90: 707

Miletich JP, Majerus DW, Majerus PW (1978) Patients with congenital factor V deficiency have decreased factor Xa binding sites on their platelets. J Clin Invest 62: 824

Moncada S, Vane JR (1979) The role of prostacyclin in vascular tissue. Fed Proc 38: 66

Moore S, Friedman RJ, Singal DP, Gauldie J, Blajchman MA, Roberts RS (1976) Inhibition of injury-induced thromboatherosclerotic lesions by anti-platelet serum in rabbits. Thromb Haemost 35: 70

Mustard JF, Kinlough-Rathbone RL, Packham MA (1980) Prostaglandins and platelets. Annu Rev Med: In Press

Mustard JF, Packham MA (1979) The reaction of the blood to injury. In:Movat HZ (ed) Inflammation, Immunity and Hypersensitivity, 2nd Edition, Harper & Row, New York, p.557

Mustard JF, Packham MA, Kinlough-Rathbone RL (1977) Platelets and thrombosis in the development of atherosclerosis and its complications. Adv Exp Med Biol 102: 7

Mustard JF, Packham MA, Kinlough-Rathbone RL (1978) Platelets, thrombosis and atherosclerosis. Adv Exp Med Biol 104: 127

Nemerson Y, Pitlick FA (1972) The tissue factor pathway of blood coagulation. In:Spaet TH (ed) Progress in Hemostasis and Thrombosis, Vol 1, p.1

Niewiarowski S, Regoeczi E, Stewart GJ, Senyi A, Mustard JF (1972) Platelet interaction with polymerizing fibrin. J Clin Invest 51: 685

Østerud B, Harper E, Rapaport SI, Levine KK (1979) Evidence against collagen activation of platelet-associated factor XI as a mechanism for initiating intrinsic clotting. Scand J Haematol 22: 205

Ross R, Vogel A (1978) The platelet-derived growth factor. Cell 14: 203

Packham MA, Rowsell HC, Jørgensen L, Mustard JF (1967) Localized protein accumulation in the wall of the aorta. Exp Mol Pathol 7: 214

Vicic WJ, Ratnoff OD, Saito H, Goldsmith GH (1979) Platelets and surface-mediated clotting activity. Br J Haematol 43: 91

Walsh PN (1972a) The effects of collagen and kaolin on the intrinsic coagulant activity of platelets. Evidence for an alternative pathway in intrinsic coagulation not requiring factor XII. Br J Haematol 22: 393

Walsh PN (1972b) The role of platelets in the contact phase of blood coagulation. Br J Haematol 22: 237

Zwaal RF (1978) Membrane and lipid involvement in blood coagulation. Biochim Biophys Acta 515: 163

The Artery Wall and the Pathogenesis of Progressive Atherosclerosis[1]

Robert W. Wissler

Introduction

A decade has passed since I served as organizing secretary for the Second
International Symposium on Atherosclerosis in Chicago, the first one held
in the United States. I chaired the session on pathogenesis at that meeting
and opened it by focusing on the artery wall and its reaction to multiple
pathophysiologic stimuli. By means of a diagram (Wissler 1970) I reviewed
evidence suggesting that one of the most characteristic features of atherogenesis in both human and animal disease was the accumulation of low density
(LDL) and very low density lipoproteins (VLDL) in the intima and inner media.
The evidence was strong then, and I submit that it is stronger now, that this
is a phenomenon which precedes any evidence of endothelial damage or sticking
of platelets in most human and experimental lesions.

I included in the diagram the formulation that "platelet sticking" and release of platelet factors exerted effects on lesion development. We were
cognizant at the time that substantial endothelial damage, with evidence of
platelet sticking was present in some progressive plaques, and that platelets
carried vasoactive amines. If they adhered to, spread and released these factors in areas of arterial intimal injury these amines would be expected to
lead to profound effects on endothelial permeability.

The other factors affecting arterial endothelial permeability which were reasonably well formulated at that time and which were reflected in the diagram
were hypertension and anoxia and "toxins". These factors are still considered to be important in the acceleration of atherosclerosis, but in most instances in human or experimental animals none of them appear to be atherogenic in the absence of some degree of hyperlipidemia involving LDL or VLDL.
In that diagram we also called attention to metabolic changes in the plaque
cells and these received the most emphasis in that program I chaired in 1969.
They were the subject of three outstanding presentations (Bowyer and Gresham
1970; Geer 1970; and Haust 1970).

Perhaps the three most important facets of this diagram and my brief presentation on pathogenesis are contained in the next three lines: cell proliferation, poorly metabolized lipoproteins accumulating in medial cells, and necrosis of medial smooth muscle cells (SMC) due to accumulating lipids. In
1968 Drs. Kao and I had reported results which indicated that LDL from hyperlipemic serum stimulated arterial smooth muscle cell proliferation in stationary cultures of outgrowths from primary explants of aortic media (Kao
et al. 1968). We and others had published immunohistochemical evidence that
Apo B localizes and accumulates in the artery wall both intra- and extracellularly (Watts 1963; Kao and Wissler 1965). The pathogenesis of necrosis
was, and is, largely inferred although Chen et al. have since demonstrated

[1]Supported by USPHS Grants HL 15062-08 and HL 17648-05, by the Block Fund at
the University of Chicago and by the Heart Research Foundation, Inc.

that cell death is increased when arterial SMC cultures are exposed to ingress and accumulation of LDL from hypercholesterolemic serum (Chen et al.
1977b). Accelerated cell death has been demonstrated in experimental plaques
(Thomas et al. 1976, 1977) and probably is correlated with accumulated cholesteryl ester in those cells. It has also become more evident that feeding
some kinds of food fats in a high cholesterol, high fat ration is likely to
produce evidence of endothelial injury after rather brief intervals (Jones et
al. 1972). Furthermore, at least some lesions resulting from sustained high
levels of LDL and VLDL are accompanied by rather striking evidence of endothelial cell necrosis and loss (Weber et al. 1974; Ross and Harker 1976; Weber
et al. 1977).

Some Highlights of Knowledge in 1979-80

The artery wall is a much better understood histologic and metabolic unit in
1979 that it was 10 years ago (Figure 1). Studies at this institution (Clark
and Glagov 1979) have furnished evidence that the fundamental structural units
of the media are groups of integrated arterial SMC. This organization may
form the basis for the large colonies of monospecific cells of the plaque
which seem to become evident relatively late in the development of the atherosclerotic process in human aortas (Benditt 1977; Pearson et al. 1977; Thomas
et al. 1978).

Furthermore, results both of ultrastructural studies and functional studies
(Simionescu et al. 1976; Stein and Stein 1979) suggest that the normal arterial endothelium can be expected to admit molecules of the size and shape of
low density lipoproteins (LDL) at a regulated rate so that the concentration
of these macromolecules reaching the artery wall is comparable to their concentration in lymph. Nevertheless, we now appreciate more completely the
"trapping" mechansims that operate to support the accumulation of molecules
such as LDL and fibrinogen in the artery wall, often at levels rivaling plasma concentrations (Smith et al. 1978; Camejo 1978; Srinivasan et al. 1978).

We are approaching the time when it will become clearer how these "trapping"
mechanisms operate. In some controlled circumstances we should be able to
determine how much of the accumulated cholesteryl ester involves smooth muscle cellular LDL ingress and egress by means of cell death or defective or
inadequate cell metabolism. On the other hand, it may be that most of the
measureable LDL cholesteryl ester building is due to interstitial accumulation with little or no intracellular passage (Wissler et al. 1976).

We do have abundant evidence at present which indicates that the preliminary
observations reported by us in 1968 (Kao et al. 1968) are reproducible (Fischer-Dzoga et al. 1976a, 1976b, 1977). We also know that the cell prolifera-
tion-stimulation that occurs so regularly when arterial SMC in stationary outgrowths of primary aortic explants are exposed to LDL from hyperlipemic serum
can be largely traced to the action of one special family of LDL particles.
This type of LDL is usually present in small quantities in normal serum of the
male rhesus monkey and it is found in much larger quantities when these animals are fed an atherogenic ration (Fless et al. 1978).

These observations along with the time course studies underway in our laboratory suggest that a relatively brief interval is required for this LDL fraction to become predominant and active in the male rhesus moneky after an atherogenic ration is initiated (Fless et al. unpublished work, 1979). They
also suggest that one should carefully investigate the origin of this fraction.

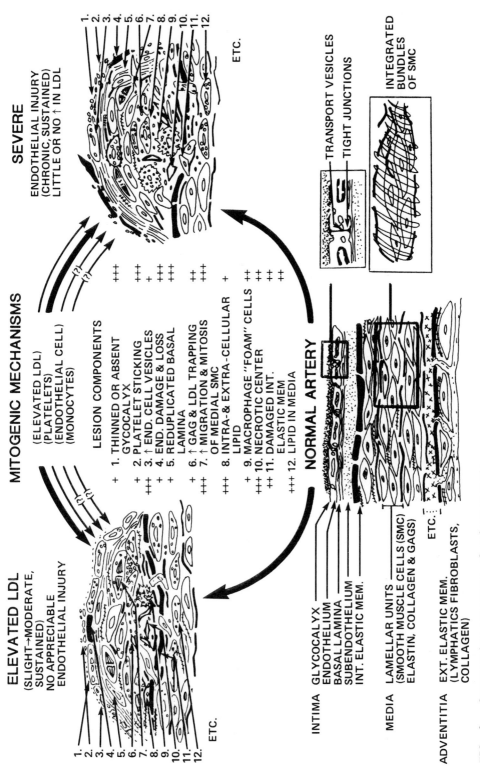

FIG. 1. Contrasting patterns of atherogenesis.

This type of LDL may be coming from intestinal synthesis - a source that seems more likely in view of recent studies in this Atherosclerosis Center by Getz and co-workers using rats fed an atherogenic ration (Krishnaiah et al. unpublished work, 1979).

The characteristics of the LDL moiety that support the greater accumulation of cholesteryl ester in arterial SMC are not nearly so clear. The development of the animal's serum factor which will produce excess "cell proliferation" response requires about 4 weeks after an atherogenic ration is started. In contrast, the excess accumulation and storage of cholesteryl ester in arterial SMC subcultures, being studies in detail in our laboratory (Bates and Wissler 1976; Chen et al. 1977; Bates and Wissler 1979), as well as at Bowman-Gray (St. Clair et al. 1977, 1978), has a gradual development following initiation of an atherogenic ration. It is evident that additional work is necessary in order to understand the mechanisms by which excess cholesteryl ester accumulates both intracellularly and extracellularly. Furthermore, the mechanisms besides cell death by which cholesteryl ester is excreted by the cell must have further attention.

The decade following the Chicago Symposium in November of 1969, and in particular the 3 intervening years since the Tokyo Symposium in 1976, have witnessed increasing attention to the study of arterial intimal-endothelial injury and its contribution to atherogenesis, especially by means of the platelet growth factor (Ross and Glomset 1976; Ross et al. 1977).

Few would doubt, I think, the contribution of endothelial injury, either acute or chronic, as an accelerator of atherogenesis when it is added to the insult provided by sustained hypercholesterolemia. On the other hand there are legitimate doubts as to whether endothelial injury alone is likely to lead to the development of progressive atherosclerosis or only to a "cushion" type lesion of intimal thickening. The attempts, thusfar, to produce progressive atherogenesis in hypercholesterolemic von Willebrand swine in which the platelet-derived cell proliferation stimulating factor is presumably not active seems to be leading to conflicting results. Similarly the thrombocytopenic rabbit with elevated cholesterol levels appears to develop rather striking raised lesions in spite of the virtual absence of circulating platelets (Brinkhous and Bowie 1978).

Equally intriguing is the experimental model developed by Minick et al. (1977a). Their studies indicate that the lesions which most resemble progressive atherosclerosis in the balloon catheter endothelial injury rabbit are in the areas where the endothelium has regenerated, not where the adherent platelets are most likely to be found. This paradoxical finding is receiving the additional study that seems indicated with the result that the accumulated GAG seems to be correlated with the more progressive character of the raised lesion under the regenerated endothelium (Minick et al. 1977b).

Recent studies in our Center have suggested that in primate models of dietarily induced, progressive atherosclerosis (Taylor et al. 1979; Jones et al. 1979) the evidence (at the center of the most prominent lesions) of endothelial injury or platelet adherence based on scanning electron microscopy is very slight during the period when the lesions are developing rapidly. These observations suggest that the platelet-derived growth factor may be most important after the lesions have progressed and when considerable lipid deposition and cell proliferation have taken place.

The recent in vitro studies in this laboratory on the effects of the platelet factor and the SMC proliferation produced by LDL from hyperlipidemic serum (HLDL) indicate that these phenomena are independent. The HLDL stimulates SMC proliferation in the presence of abundant platelet factor. Furthermore, the HLDL seems to be quite effective in stimulating SMC proliferation in the absence of platelet factor when one confines one's studies to the stationary outgrowth preparations from primary explants (Fischer-Dzoga et al. 1976).

All of these findings suggest that artery wall interactions with a number of plasma constituents deserve additional attention. At present with the relatively crude tools that we have available, the results indicate that hyperlipemic serum in the absence of appreciable endothelial injury probably is sufficient to support progressive atherogenesis in most instances. They also indicate that slight and intermittent endothelial injury will not lead to progressive atherosclerosis unless the blood lipids are elevated. On the other hand, both the experimental and epidemiological data would seem to indicate that atherogenesis can be prevented or reversed if the blood lipids are reduced to basal levels even though some degree of endothelial damage is present. It appears likely, nevertheless, that certain paradoxical phenomena which are characterized by severe, sustained arterial endothelial damage such as lupus erythematosis (Tsakraklides et al. 1974) in humans, or antigen-antibody complexes (Minick and Murphy 1973) in animals, or homocystinemia (Harker et al. 1976) in humans or animals are able to support the development of atheromatous lesions, even when the blood lipids are very low. These unusual situations are of great value, it seems, because they may help explain the occasional exceptional cases in which advanced human atherosclerosis develops in the absence of the usual classical risk factors of hypercholesterolemia, hypertension or cigarette smoking.

Questions That Need Answering

The curent understanding of the interaction of low density lipoproteins, as well as platelet derived growth factor with the artery wall offers great opportunities for further study of human atherogenesis, animal models of atherosclerosis and the cellular pathobiology of atherosclerosis.

It is evident that we need to know more about:
1. The precise function of the endothelial glycocalyx in atherogenesis?
2. The relative potential of cell proliferation stimulating factors from HLDL, platelets, endothelial cells and macrophages in atherogenesis and the mechanisms by which each factor acts?
3. The LDL fractions that are most likely to lead to artery wall proliferation, the conditions under which they are produced and the mechanisms by which they induce an excess of cell division?
4. The interaction of factors leading to increased cell death in the progressive plaque?
5. The mechanisms by which hypercholesterolemic LDLs damage endothelium?
6. The mechanisms by which regenerating endothelium sustains LDL "trapping" and cholesteryl ester accumulation?
7. Improved ways to quantitate arterial endothelial damage in the intact human subject (or animal model) by non-invasive means?
8. The relative proportion of the total lipid accumulating in advanced plaques that has been intracellular?
9. The major ways in which cholesteryl ester egresses from the SMC cytoplasm?
10. The source of cholesteryl ester in those unusual plaques that develop without elevated LDL levels?

Acknowledgements

The author is grateful for the excellent help he has had from Barbara Ann Baxter and Lauren Brown in preparing this manuscript and for the conscientious help with the art work he received from Manjula Haksar.

References

Bates SR (1979) Accumulation and loss of cholesterol esters in monkey arterial smooth muscle cells exposed to normal and hyperlipemic serum lipoproteins. Atherosclerosis 32:165-176

Bates SR, Wissler RW (1976) Effect of hyperlipemic serum on cholesterol accumulation in monkey aortic medial cells. Biochim Biophys Acta 450:78-88

Benditt EP (1977) Implications of the monoclonal character of human atherosclerotic plaques. Am J Pathol 86:693-702

Bowyer DE, Gresham GA (1970) Arterial lipid accumulation. In: Jones RJ (ed) Atherosclerosis II. Springer-Verlag, New York, pp 3-5

Brinkhous KM, Bowie EJW (1978) Summary of workshops 4a and 4b: Animal models of atherosclerosis involving the thrombotic process. In: Chandler AB, Eurenius K, McMillan GC, Nelson CB, Schwartz CJ, Wessler S (eds) The Thrombotic Process in Atherogenesis (Adv Exp Med Biol, Vol 104). Plenum Press, New York, pp 385-407

Camejo G (1976) Interaction of low density lipoproteins with arterial constituents: Its relationship with atherogenesis. In: Day CE, Levy RS (eds) Low Density Lipoproteins. Plenum Press, New York, pp 351-370

Chen RM, Fischer-Dzoga K (1977a) Effect of hyperlipemic serum lipoproteins on the lipid accumulation and cholesterol flux of rabbit aortic medial cells. Atherosclerosis 28:339-353

Chen RM, Getz GS, Fischer-Dzoga K, Wissler RW (1977b) The role of hyperlipemic serum on the proliferation and necrosis of aortic medial cells in vitro. Exp Mol Pathol 26:359-374

Clark JM, Glagov S (1979) Structural integration of the arterial wall. I. Relationships and attachments of medial smooth muscle cells in normally distended and hyperdistended aortas. Lab Invest 40:587-602

Fischer-Dzoga K, Kuo YF (1976) Investigation of the role of platelets in the proliferation response to hyperlipemia of arterial smooth muscle cells in vitro. Circulation (Suppl II) 54:54

Fischer-Dzoga K, Wissler RW (1976a) Stimulation of proliferation in stationary primary cultures of monkey aortic smooth muscle cells. II. Effect of varying concentrations of hyperlipemic serum and low density lipoproteins of varying dietary fat origins. Atherosclerosis 24:515-525

Fischer-Dzoga K, Fraser R, Wissler RW (1976b) Stimulation of proliferation in stationary primary cultures of monkey and rabbit aortic smooth muscle cells. I. Effects of lipoprotein fractions of hyperlipemic serum and lymph. Exp Mol Pathol 24:346-359

Fischer-Dzoga K, Wissler RW, Scanu AM (1977) The lipoproteins and arterial smooth muscle cells: Cellular proliferation and morphology. In: Manning GW, Haust MD (eds) Atherosclerosis: Metabolic, Morphologic, and Clinical Aspects (Adv Exp Med Biol, Vol 82). Plenum Press, New York, pp 86-93

Fless GM, Kirchhausen T, Fischer-Dzoga K, Wissler RW, Scanu AM (1979) Relationship between the properties of the apo B containing low-density lipoproteins (LDL) of normolipidemic rhesus monkeys and their mitogenic action on arterial smooth muscle cells grown in vitro. This volume

Geer JC, Panganamala RV, Newman HAF, Cornwell DG (1970) Mural metabolism. In: Jones RJ (ed) Atherosclerosis II. Springer-Verlag, New York, pp 5-12

Harker LA, Ross R, Schlichter SJ, Scott CR (1976) homocystine-induced arteriosclerosis. The role of endothelial cell injury and platelet response in its genesis. J Clin Invest 58:731-741

Haust MD (1970) Injury and repair in the pathogenesis of atherosclerotic lesions. In: Jones RJ (ed) Atherosclerosis II. Springer-Verlag, New York, pp 12-23

Jones RM, Hughes R, Vesselinovitch D, Wissler WR (1972) Ultrastructural changes in the aortas of rhesus monkeys fed large quantities of food fats for short periods. Fed Proc 31:273

Jones RM, Schaffner TJ, Chassagne G, Glagov S, Wissler RW (1979) Comparison of coronary with aortic fatty streaks in rhesus monkeys. Scanning Electron Microscopy 1979/III SEM Inc, AMF O'Hare, pp 829-834

Kao VCY, Wissler RW (1965) A study of the immunohistochemical localization of serum lipoproteins and other plasma proteins in human atherosclerotic lesions. Exp Mol Pathol 4:465-479

Kao VCY, Wissler RW, Dzoga K (1968) Influence of hyperlipemic serum on the growth of medial smooth muscle cells of rhesus monkey aorta in vitro. Circulation 38:6-12

Minick CR, Murphy GE (1973) Experimental induction of atherosclerosis by the synergy of allergic injury to arteries and lipid-rich diet. II. Effect of cholesterol-poor diet. Am J Pathol 73:265-300

Minick CR, Stemerman MB, Insull W Jr (1977a) Effect of regenerated endothelium lipid accumulation in the arterial wall. Proc Natl Acad Sci USA 74:1724-1728

Minick CR, Litrenta MM, Alonso DR, Silane MF, Stemerman MB (1977b) Further studies on the effect of regenerated endothlium on intimal lipid accumulation. Prog Biochem Pharmacol 13:115-122

Pearson TA, Kramer EC, Solez K, Hepinstall RH (1977) The human atherosclerotic plaque. Am J Pathol 86:657-664

Ross R, Glomset J (1976) The pathogenesis of atherosclerosis. N Engl J Med 295:369-377, 420-425

Ross R, Harker L (1976) Hyperlipidemia and atherosclerosis. Science 193:1094-1100

Ross R, Glomset J, Harker L (1977) Response to injury and atherogenesis. Am J Pathol 86:675-684

Simionescu N, Simionescu M, Palade GE (1976) Recent studies on vascular endothelium. Ann NY Acad Sci 275:64-75

Smith EB, Craig IB, Dietz HS (1978) Factors influencing accumulation and destruction of lipoprotein in atherosclerotic lesions. In: Carlson LA, Paoletti R, Sirtori CR, Weber G (eds) International Conference on Atherosclerosis. Raven Press, New York, pp 49-56

Srinivasan SR, Radhakrishnamurthy B, Dalferes ER Jr, Berenson GS (1978) Interactions of lipoproteins and connective tissue components in human atherosclerotic plaques. In: Carlson LA, Paoletti R, Sirtori CR, Weber G (eds) International Conference on Atherosclerosis. Raven Press, New York, pp 585-588

St Clair RW, Leight MA (1978) Differential effects of isolated lipoproteins from normal and hypercholesterolemic rhesus monkeys on cholesterol esterification and accumulation in arterial smooth muscle cells in culture. Biochim Biophys Acta 530:279-291

St Clair RW, Smith BP, Wood L (1977) Stimulation of cholesterol esterification in rhesus monkey arterial smooth muscle cells. Circ Res 40:166-173

Stein Y, Stein O (1979) Interaction between serum lipoproteins and cellular components of the arterial wall. In: Scanu AM, Wissler RW, Getz GS (eds) Biochemistry of Atherosclerosis. Dekker, New York, pp 313-344

Taylor K, Schaffner T, Wissler RW, Glagov S (1979) Immuno-morphologic identification and characterization of cells derived from experimental atherosclerotic lesions. Scanning Electron Microscopy 1979/III SEM Inc, AMF O'Hare, pp 815-822

Thomas WA, Reiner JM, Florentin RA, Lee KT, Lee WM (1976) Population dynamics of arterial smooth muscle cells. V. Cell proliferation and cell death during initial 3 months in atherosclerotic lesions induced in swine by hypercholesterolemic diet and intimal trauma. Exp Mol Pathol 24:360-374

Thomas WA, Reiner JM, Florentin RA, Janakidevi K, Lee KJ (1977) Arterial smooth muscle cells in atherogenesis: Births, deaths and clonal phenomena. In: Schettler G, Goto Y, Hata Y, Klose G (eds) Atherosclerosis IV. Springer-Verlag, New York, pp 16-23

Thomas WA, Janakidevi K, Florentin RA, Reiner JM (1978) The reversibility of the human atherosclerotic plaque. In: Hauss WH, Wissler RW, Lehmann R (eds) International Symposium: State of Prevention and Therapy in Human Arteriosclerosis and in Animal Models. Westdeutscher Verlag, Opladen, Germany, pp 73-80

Tsakraklides VG, Glieden LC, Edwards JE (1974) Coronary atherosclerosis and myocardial infarction associated with systemic lupus erythematosus. Am Heart J 87:637

Watts HF (1963) Role of lipoproteins in the formulation of atherosclerotic lesions. In: Jones RJ (ed) Evolution of the Atherosclerotic Plaque. University of Chicago Press, Chicago, pp 117-138

Weber G, Fabbrini P, Resi L (1974) Scanning and transmission electron microscopy observations on the surface lining of aortic intimal plaques in rabbits on a hypercholesterolic diet. Virchows Arch Path Anat Histol 364:325-331

Weber G, Fabbrini P, Resi L, Jones R, Vesselinovitch D, Wissler RW (1977) Regression of arteriosclerotic lesions in rhesus monkey aortas after regression diet: Scanning and transmission electron microscope observations of the endothelium. Atherosclerosis 26:535-547

Wissler WR (1970) Introduction to the pathogenesis of atherosclerosis. In: Jones RJ (ed) Atherosclerosis II. Springer-Verlag, New York, pp 2-3

Wissler RW, Vesselinovitch D, Getz GS (1976) Abnormalities of the arterial wall and its metabolism in atherogenesis. Prog Cadiovasc Dis 18: 341-369

Endothelial Dysfunction and the Pathogenesis of Atherosclerosis

Michael A. Gimbrone, Jr.[1]

Vascular endothelium is a structurally simple but functionally complex tissue, the integrity of which is essential to the health of the arterial wall. Since the classical theories of Rokitansky and Virchow, various roles have been ascribed to endothelium in the atherosclerotic process, but only recently have many relevant aspects of its biology been appreciated. In part this is due to the development of new experimental tools, but more importantly it reflects a renewed interest in the functional capabilities of vascular cells, their mutual interactions, and the potential consequences of their dysfunction.

In general, early studies of endothelium tended to be limited to the structural features of this simple squamous membrane (Majno 1965), while more recent approaches have explored its biochemical capabilities (Majno and Joris 1978; Gimbrone 1977, 1980). Thus, our concept of endothelium has progressively evolved from that of a passive anatomical barrier to a functionally active component of the blood vessel wall. At the present time, knowledge of endothelial cell biology is increasing rapidly. A major factor has been the development, and widespread application of reliable methods for cultivating pure populations of vascular endothelial cells in vitro. Such cultures permit direct study of metabolic, synthetic and physiological properties under controlled conditions, which often are unattainable in vivo (Gimbrone 1976). Data obtained in several laboratories on the biology of vascular smooth muscle, blood platelets and leukocytes, and the response of the arterial wall to experimental injury, have provided fresh insights into the pathogenesis of atherosclerosis.

This report will briefly update selected aspects of endothelial biology, especially certain functional capabilities, which are relevant to atherosclerosis and its complications. As will become apparent, our working concept of "endothelial injury", which is the keystone of the modern "Response-to-Injury Hypothesis" of atherogenesis (Ross and Glomset 1976), needs to be broadened to encompass various types of endothelial dysfunction.

Endothelial Functions

Structurally, endothelium is a very simple tissue: a broad, flat, ultra-thin cellular membrane. Even when viewed by transmission electron microscopy there is little to indicate all that is going on along this dynamic interface between circulating blood and the vessel wall. However, from various physiological and biochemical approaches, it is clear that endothelium performs important functions in at least three basic areas; it acts as

[1] The author's research is supported in part by grants from the National Heart, Lung and Blood Institute (HL 20054, HL 22602) and an Established Investigatorship Award from the American Heart Association.

a: 1) Selective permeability barrier; 2) Synthetic-metabolic-secretory tissue; and 3) Blood-compatible "container".

Selective permeability barrier

Data from several lines of investigation indicate that the role of the endothelium in regulating the influx of plasma macromolecules into the arterial wall is complex (Gimbrone 1980). Clearly, the endothelial membrane functions as more than a passive molecular sieve. Structurally, it provides multiple, parallel routes to the subendothelial space: transcellular (pinocytotic vesicles, transendothelial channels), pericellular (intercellular junctional complexes and spaces), and intramembranous (diffusion in the lipid phase of the cell membrane). Each of these pathways presumably has its own capacity, selectivity and regulatory mechanisms. Enzymatically, endothelium also can directly alter certain molecules during their passage from blood to subendothelial space, as well as secrete extracellular matrix materials, which can influence the retention of plasma components within the intima.

The latter two aspects of endothelial metabolism may be especially relevant to lipid accumulation in the arterial wall. For example, lipoprotein lipase, an enzyme which hydrolyzes the triglyceride component of plasma chylomicrons, appears to be bound to the glycoprotein coat of the luminal endothelial surface (Olivecrona et al. 1976; Dicorleta and Zilversmit 1975). According to a novel model of transendothelial lipid transport proposed by Scow and co-workers (1976), the relatively water-insoluble products of lipolysis (diglycerides, monoglycerides and free fatty acids) would preferentially dissolve in the outer leaflet of the endothelial cell membrane. Having entered this lipid phase, they could rapidly diffuse along the cell surface to reach the abluminal side, where binding to extracellular matrix or transfer to other cells might occur. Further experimental verification of the details of this hypothetical scheme is needed; however, it serves to emphasize the potential for active involvement of endothelium in the transport of complex lipids into the arterial wall.

The fate of plasma lipids and other macromolecules which have reached the subendothelial space may also be influenced by endothelial-associated connective tissue elements. For example, certain glycosaminoglycans (GAGs) can selectively bind low-density lipoproteins (Iverius 1972), and lipoprotein-GAG complexes have been isolated from samples of human aortic intima (Srinivasan et al. 1975). The increased intimal GAG content observed in human fatty streaks and early fibromuscular lesions (Stevens et al. 1976), as well as in various experimental models of atherosclerosis (Wight and Ross 1975; Curwen and Smith 1977) thus may be an important factor contributing to intimal lipid accumulation. Cultured aortic endothelial cells appear to exhibit a unique pattern of GAG synthesis, compared to aortic smooth muscle (Gamse et al. 1978). More needs to be learned about the factors which regulate extracellular matrix synthesis by endothelium, in both normal and pathologic settings.

In a unique fashion, endothelium also may influence its own permeability characteristics through the local secretion or degradation of vasoactive mediators. The endothelial lining of large blood vessels can release prostaglandins (Gimbrone and Alexander 1977), degrade bradykinin and generate angiotensin II (Johnson and Erdős 1977; Hial et al. 1979), and synthesize histamine (Hollis and Rosen 1972). Each of these hormones has been implicated in the control of vascular permeability. Aortic endothelium, in particular, has an active "histamine-forming capacity" (histidine decarboxylase system), which appears to be responsive to hemodynamic (wall shear) stresses. This mechanically coupled enzymatic mechanism for histamine generation may explain the focal increases in aortic permeability often observed in areas of increased hemodynamic stress (DeForrest and Hollis 1978).

Thus, as the above observations indicate, the abnormal permeation, and subsequent retention, of plasma constituents in the arterial wall may result from metabolic dysfunction, as well as frank anatomical discontinuity, of the endothelial lining.

Synthetic-metabolic-secretory activities

The vascular endothelium is the most expansive simple endothelium in the body. In the aggregate, this tissue measures several hundred square meters in surface area, and has a total mass comparable to other vital organs of the body. This organization of endothelium as a broad monolayer serves to amplify its impact as a metabolically active, secretory tissue. Various blood-borne substrates are efficiently delivered to ectoenzymes present on the luminal endothelial surface and the resulting metabolites can diffuse into surrounding tissues or be carried by the circulation to distant sites. Substances synthesized and secreted by endothelial cells similarly can have local or systemic effects. In addition, all materials entering or leaving the blood vessel wall are potentially susceptible, in transit, to biochemical alteration by the endothelium.

Several laboratories using cell cultures, have now established that the endothelial cell is capable of synthesizing most of the extracellular matrix components of the arterial wall, including basement membrane collagen, other types of collagen, elastin, glycosaminoglycans and fibronectin (Jaffe et al. 1976; Howard et al. 1976; Jaffe and Mosher 1978; Macarak et al. 1978; Birdwell et al. 1978). Such connective tissue elements are essential for the normal mechanical properties of the vessel wall, and the anchorage of the endothelial monolayer in the face of constant hemodynamic stress. As noted above, endothelial-derived matrix also may be involved in the extracellular trapping of lipid in the diseased intima. In addition, cytochemical and biochemical studies have documented the presence of multiple enzymes important in the intermediary metabolism of carbohydrates, lipids and proteins (Thorgeirsson and Robertson 1978). The demonstration of specific receptors for neurotransmitters, as well as polypeptide and steroid hormones also suggests that endothelium is a hormonally responsive tissue. Many of these metabolic activities of endothelium undoubtedly are relevant to total body homeostasis, as well as local vessel wall function.

Blood-compatible container

Endothelium is Nature's prototype for blood-compatible surfaces. Under normal circumstances, the vascular lining does not promote blood clotting or the adherence of circulating platelets, leukocytes or red blood cells. Several properties of endothelium appear to be essential to this vital function. Conceptually, they comprise two broad categories: first, physicochemical characteristics of the endothelial cell surface that allow it to act as "insulation" between circulating blood elements and highly thrombogenic subendothelial connective tissues; and, second, more active, metabolic influences on platelet function and blood clotting. As will become apparent, the endothelial cell can promote, as well as inhibit, hemostasis and thrombosis; thus, the net outcome in a given situation will reflect the dynamic interplay of these antagonistic functions.

The most basic, and least well understood, aspect of endothelial thromboresistance is the failure of platelets, and the products of blood coagulation to deposit on the intima. Studies of the distribution of anionic sites on the endothelial cell surface (Skutelsky et al. 1975; Pelikan et al. 1979) indicate that non-specific electrostatic repulsion is not the explanation. However, heparin-like proteoglycans (Buonassisi and Root 1975; Gamse et al. 1978), which can interact with plasma antithrombin, and alpha-2 macroglobulin (Becker and Harpel 1976) are associated with the endothelial surface; these anti-protease activities can inhibit several enzymes in the coagulation, fibrinolytic and kinin-generating systems, and therefore may be involved in the control of hemostatic and inflammatory reactions at the vessel wall-blood interface. Endothelial cells also contain plasminogen activator(s) and inhibitor(s) (Loskutoff and Edgington 1977) and thus may be an important source of fibrinolytic activity for the resolution of intravascular thrombi and the clearing of fibrin deposits from the intimal surface.

In contrast to these anti-thrombotic activities, endothelial cells can promote hemostasis and thrombosis through the synthesis and release of procoagulant substances. Thromboplastin, or tissue factor, the particle-bound lipoprotein which activates the extrinsic clotting system, appears to be present in a latent form in endothelium, and can be released by certain pharmacologic stimuli and sublethal forms of cell injury (Maynard et al. 1975). Endothelial cells also produce vonWillebrand factor (Factor VIII-VWF) (Jaffe et al. 1974), a cofactor involved in the adherence of platelets to subendothelial connective tissues (Sakariassen et al. 1979). Experiments with cultured porcine aortic endothelium (Booyse et al. 1977) suggest that secreted Factor VIII-VWF becomes associated with extracellular microfibrils to which platelet attachment can occur. Animals deficient in vonWillebrand factor have a markedly reduced incidence of spontaneous and dietary-induced atherosclerosis (Fuster et al. 1978).

The collagenous components of the subendothelium, synthesized and secreted by endothelium, provide a highly thrombogenic substrate for platelet adhesion at sites of intimal injury. Immunofluorescent studies with endothelial cultures (Birdwell et al. 1978) show a definite organizational pattern in the extracellular matrix, with localization beneath, but never on top of, the confluent monolayer. Failure to maintain this structural polarity in vivo, conceivably could result in loss of endothelial attachment or the promotion of thrombosis.

The rapid aggregation of platelets at a site of vascular injury is mediated by the local generation or release of proaggregatory substances. There is increasing evidence that endothelium can influence this process indirectly, through degradation of platelet agonists, and directly, through secretion of platelet antagonists. Endothelial cells can actively interiorize and/or degrade catecholamines, serotonin, bradykinin and other mediators of platelet aggregation (Thorgeirsson and Robertson 1978). In addition, they exhibit an ecto-ADPase activity, which can convert pro-aggregating adenosine diphosphate, released from platelets, to adenosine, a potent platelet inhibitor (Habliston et al. 1978; Pearson and Gordon 1979).

While each of the above mechanisms can influence platelet aggregation, the most profound effect of endothelium on platelet function appears to be exerted via a unique product of arachidonic acid metabolism: prostacyclin or PGI$_2$. Originally described by Moncada and coworkers (1976) as an unstable derivative of prostaglandin endoperoxides generated by aortic microsomes, prostacyclin is the most potent naturally-occurring inhibitor of platelet aggregation known. Weksler and associates (1977, 1978) subsequently demonstrated prostacyclin synthetase activity in cultured human and bovine endothelial cells, and found that PGI$_2$ production was stimulated by thrombin.

Prostacyclin appears to be the major metabolite of arachidonic acid in the walls of arteries and veins in several species, including man. It is a physiological antagonist of the pro-aggregatory vasoconstrictor, thromboxane A_2, that is formed in platelets from prostaglandin endoperoxides (Hamberg et al. 1974). Based on these findings, Moncada and Vane (1979) have hypothesized that the capacity of the endothelial lining to produce PGI_2 is the fundamental mechanism underlying vascular thromboresistance. According to this theory, deficiencies in PGI_2 production, resulting from endothelial injury or metabolic dysfunction would tend to promote platelet-vessel wall interactions and thrombosis. Although recent in vitro studies (Curwen et al. 1980) indicate that the primary adherence of platelets to normal endothelial surfaces may not be sensitive to PGI_2, this endothelial product clearly can influence other aspects of platelet function, including the release of vasoactive mediators and growth factors.

Thus, the study of endothelial blood-compatibility has revealed an intricate, highly evolved homeostatic mechanism. No longer can the endothelium be considered as simply a passive, inert membrane, insulating the blood from thrombogenic connective tissues. Although continuity of the endothelial lining is essential to its "container function," certain forms of metabolic dysfunction also may be important in atherogenesis, and its thrombotic complications.

Endothelial Injury and Repair

Any form of arterial injury that is sufficient to cause endothelial cell death or desquamation can evoke a complicated "wound-healing" response in the vascular wall. Depending upon the severity and duration of the injurious stimulus, and the rate of subsequent endothelial regeneration, varying degrees of intimal hyperplasia typically result. In terms of its cellular and biochemical components, this reparative/inflammatory reaction of the intima bears important similarities to naturally occurring or dietary-induced atherosclerotic lesions in man and certain experimental animals. The association of intimal fibromuscular hyperplasia with endothelial injury thus forms a central part of the current "Response-to-Injury Hypothesis" of atherogenesis. Therefore, there has been considerable interest in factors which can initiate or promote endothelial injury, and the mechanisms of endothelial repair.

A variety of experimental models have been devised to study the acute and chronic consequences of endothelial injury. Mechanistically, they are diverse, and include: focal mechanical abrasion of the intima (Björkerud and Bondjers 1971; Moore 1973), extensive balloon-catheter denudation (Baumgartner 1974; Stemerman and Ross 1972; Spaet et al. 1975), dessication (Fishman et al. 1975); chemically-induced injury, e.g., homocystinemia (Harker et al. 1976) or endotoxinemia (Gaynor et al. 1970; Gerrity et al. 1976); dietary-induced chronic hyperlipidemia, alone or in combination with mechanical injury (Ross and Harker 1976); experimentally altered hemodynamics (Stehbens 1974); and immune-mediated mechanisms (Alonso et al. 1977). In general, most of these "injury models" share in common varying amounts of endothelial desquamation, which is associated with a basically similar histological pattern of intimal reaction. None, however, are totally selective for endothelial cells (Thorgeirsson and Robertson 1978), and with certain mechanical methods (e.g., balloon-catheterization), disruption of the intimal lining is more abrupt and extensive than could occur naturally.

Several studies of dietary-induced atherosclerosis in rabbits (Weber et al. 1974; Nelson et al. 1976; Goode et al. 1977; Reidy and Bowyer 1978), swine (Nelson et al. 1976; Gerrity et al. 1979), and subhuman primates (Ross and Harker 1976), as well as spontaneously occurring atherosclerosis in pigeons

(Lewis and Kottke 1977), have suggested that alterations in the integrity of the endothelial lining are associated with, and in some instances appear to precede, the appearance of lipid-containing intimal plaques. However some workers (Davies et al. 1976; Goode et al. 1977) have noted altered endothelial morphology, without frank desquamation, in the area of intimal lesions, and have emphasized the potential for artifacts in the processing of lipid-containing vascular specimens for scanning electron microscopy.

Focal areas of increased permeability and endothelial cell turnover have been observed to occur in normocholesterolemic animals in regions of the arterial vasculature which are subjected to increased turbulence or wall shear stress (Caplan and Schwartz 1973). Similarly, alterations in aortic endothelial morphology, permeability and cell turnover also have been observed with hypertension (Schwartz and Benditt 1977). Further study is needed of the occurrence and nature of endothelial injury in association with other risk factors. Hopefully, with increasing knowledge of endothelial biology, "injury" will be assessible by a broader spectrum of functional criteria than currently are available.

Following desquamative injury, new endothelial cells are derived from existing endothelium, through a process of cellular migration and division (Poole et al. 1958; Schwartz et al. 1975; Schwartz et al. 1978). Upon reconstitution of an intact monolayer, this reparative process abruptly ceases, and endothelial cell turnover returns to its normal slow rate (Wright 1970; Schwartz and Benditt 1973). In vivo studies have well documented the morphological sequence of events in this orderly process, but have not provided much information about its regulation.

Postconfluent endothelial cultures appear to provide a useful in vitro analog to large vessel endothelium for studies of growth control and regeneration (Gimbrone et al. 1974; Gimbrone 1976). Using this model system, the following basic features of endothelial growth have been established: 1) Endothelial cells appear to be fundamentally different than vascular smooth muscle in their response to growth-promoting substances. For example, platelet-derived growth factor, which is a potent stimulator of vascular smooth muscle proliferation in vitro (Ross et al. 1974), appears to have essentially no effect on endothelial cell growth (Wall et al. 1978; Thorgeirsson and Robertson 1978). In addition, confluent endothelial monolayers are remarkably insensitive to various other growth factors present in plasma or serum (Gimbrone et al. 1974; Haudenschild et al. 1976). 2) Extensive healing of small mechanical "wounds" in endothelial monolayers can occur, in the absence of cell division, through a process of cell migration (Sholley et al. 1977). Factors influencing cellular migration, thus, may be relevant to the problem of endothelial regeneration (Thorgeirsson et al. 1979; Selden and Schwartz 1979). 3) Endothelial growth can be stimulated by products released by activated macrophages (Polverini et al. 1977; Martin et al. 1979), and inhibited by substances isolated from the aortic wall (Eisenstein et al. 1979). Through the use of endothelial cell cultures as in vitro bioassay systems, further isolation and characterization of these putative endothelial growth regulators should be possible. 4) Replicating or regenerating endothelial cells in vitro exhibit more fluid endocytosis (Davies and Ross 1978), receptor-mediated uptake of low-density lipoproteins (Vlodavsky et al. 1978), and lipoprotein degradation (Coetzee et al. 1979) than quiescent, contact-inhibited endothelial cells. Such growth-related alterations in cell function may have important implications for the role of regenerating endothelium in the accumulation of lipid in the injured artery wall (Minick et al. 1977).

In view of the vast amount of experimental data implicating endothelial injury in the pathogenesis of atherosclerosis, the mechanisms of endothelial regeneration clearly warrant further study. Many basic questions remain to

be answered. For example, does regenerative capacity decline with aging?
And, do certain of the recognized risk factors in atherogenesis operate
through inhibition of normal reparative mechanisms?

Endothelial Dysfunction and the Response-to-Injury Hypothesis

As has been emphasized by the other speakers at this symposium, an important
mechanistic link between endothelial injury and intimal fibromuscular hyperplasia appears to be the interaction of platelets with the injured vascular
wall. Focal desquamation of the endothelial lining results in the adhesion
of platelets to exposed subendothelial connective tissues; adherent platelets generate thromboxanes and release dense granule components, such as
adenosine diphosphate, which serve to recruit more platelets at the injury
site. During this accretion process, release of alpha granule components
also occurs, presumably resulting in the delivery of a concentrated bolus
of platelet-derived substances into the vascular wall. Platelet growth
factor, together with low-density lipoproteins and other plasma factors,
stimulate medial smooth muscle cell migration into the intima, where cellular proliferation and connective tissue synthesis result in the development
of a hyperplastic fibromuscular lesion.

The above formulation of the "Response-to-Injury Hypothesis" (Ross and
Glomset 1976) has stimulated much fruitful research into the biology of
platelets, smooth muscle, and endothelium, and their potential interactions
in the context of vascular injury. However, much of the experimental animal modeling, to date, has emphasized the production, or detection, of frank
desquamative injury in the intimal lining. As the above review of its selective permeability and blood compatibility functions indicates, the classic picture of endothelium as a passive, anatomical barrier recently has
undergone considerable revision. Clearly, our working concept of endothelial "injury" similarly must be broadened to include endothelial "dysfunction". For example, in contrast to normal endothelial cells, the surfaces
of chemically mutagenized (Zetter et al. 1978), or virally transformed
(Curwen et al. 1980), endothelial cells are highly reactive with platelets
in vitro. Transient interactions of circulating platelets with analogously
(viz., chemically, virally, immunologically) "altered", or "dysfunctional",
endothelial cells, in vivo, conceivably could result in a localized release
of platelet products into the vessel wall, in the absence of a frank desquamative lesion. Another example comes from the recent observations of Minick
et al. (1977) on the topographical pattern of intimal changes in the rabbit
aorta, following extensive endothelial cell loss. Intimal thickening and
lipid accumulation were more marked in those areas covered by regenerating
endothelium than in denuded areas. Thus, the functional status of the
endothelial lining appears to be more important than its physical presence
or absence.

In conclusion, there is much experimental data indicating that endothelial
integrity, in both the anatomical and functional sense, is essential for
the health of the arterial wall. Further insights into the pathogenesis
of atherosclerosis may come from a broader understanding of the causes of
various forms of endothelial dysfunction and their pathophysiologic consequences.

References

Alonso DR, Starek PK, Minick CR (1977) Studies on the pathogenesis of athero-arteriosclerosis induced in rabbit cardiac allografts by the synergy of graft rejection and hypercholesterolemia. Amer J Pathol 87: 415

Baumgartner HR (1974) In: Deutsch E, Brinkhous KM, Lechner K, Hinnom S (eds) Thrombosis: Pathogenesis and Clinical Trials. Schattauer-Verlag, Stuttgart (p 91)

Becker CG, Harpel PC (1976) Alpha$_2$-macroglobulin on human vascular endothelium. J Exp Med 144: 1

Björkerud S, Bondjers G (1971) Arterial repair and atherosclerosis after mechanical injury. I. Permeability and light microscopic characteristics of endothelium in non-atherosclerotic and atherosclerotic lesions. Atherosclerosis 13: 355

Birdwell CR, Gospodarowicz D, Nicolson GL (1978) Identification, localization, and role of fibronectin in cultured bovine endothelial cells. Proc Natl Acad Sci USA 75: 3273

Booyse FM, Quarfoot AJ, Bell S, Fass DN, Lewis JC, Mann KG, Bowie EJW (1977) Cultured aortic endothelial cells from pigs with von Willebrand disease: In vitro model for studying the molecular defect(s) of the disease. Proc Natl Acad Sci USA 74: 5702

Buonassisi V, Root M (1975) Enzymatic degradation of heparin related mucopolysaccharides from the surface of endothelial cell cultures. Biochim Biophys Acta 383: 1

Caplan BA, Schwartz CJ (1973) Increased endothelial cell turnover in areas of in vivo evans blue uptake in the pig aorta. Atherosclerosis 17: 401

Coetzee GA, Stein O, Stein Y (1979) Uptake and degradation of low density lipoproteins (LDL) by confluent, contact-inhibited bovine and human endothelial cells exposed to physiological concentrations of LDL. Atherosclerosis 33: 425

Curwen KD, Gimbrone MA, Jr, Handin RI (1979) In vitro studies of thromboresistance: The role of prostacyclin (PGI$_2$) in platelet adhesion to cultured normal and virally transformed human vascular endothelial cells. Lab Invest (in press)

Curwen K, Smith S (1977) Aortic glycosaminoglycans in atherosclerosis susceptible and resistant pigeons. Exp Mol Pathol 27: 121

Davies PF, Reidy MA, Goode TB, Bowyer DE (1976) Scanning electron microscopy in the evaluation of endothelial integrity of the fatty lesion in atherosclerosis. Atherosclerosis 25: 125

Davies PF, Ross R (1978) Mediation of pinocytosis in cultured arterial smooth muscle and endothelial cells by platelet-derived growth factor. J Cell Biol 79: 663

DeForrest JM, Hollis TM (1978) Shear stress and aortic histamine synthesis. Amer J Physiol 234(6): H701

Dicorleto PE, Zilversmit DB (1975) Lipoprotein lipase activity in bovine aorta. Proc Soc Exp Biol Med 148: 1101

Eisenstein R, Schumacher B, Matijevitch B (1979) Intrinsic regulators of arterial cell growth. Fed Proc 38(3): 1075

Fishman JA, Ryan FB, Karnovsky MJ (1975) Endothelial regeneration in the rat carotid artery and the significance of endothelial denudation in the pathogenesis of myointimal thickening. Lab Invest 32: 339

Fuster V, Bowie EJW, Lewis JC, Fass DN, Owen CA, Jr, Brown AL (1978) Resistance to arteriosclerosis in pigs with von Willebrand's disease. J Clin Invest 61: 722

Gamse G, Fromme HG, Kresse H (1978) Metabolism of sulfated glycosaminoglycans in cultured endothelial cells and smooth muscle cells from bovine aorta. Biochim Biophys Acta 544: 514

Gaynor E, Bouvier CA, Spaet TH (1970) Vascular lesions: possible pathogenetic basis of the generalized Shartzman reaction. Science 170: 986

Gerrity RG, Naito HK, Richardson M, Schwartz CJ (1979) Dietary induced atherogenesis in swine: Morphology of the intima in prelesion stages. Amer J Pathol 95: 775

Gerrity RG, Richardson M, Caplan BA, Cade JF, Hirsh J, Schwartz CJ (1976) Endotoxin-induced vascular endothelial injury and repair II. Focal injury, en face morphology, ^{3}H thymidine uptake and circulating endothelial cells in the dog. Exp Mol Pathol 24: 59

Gimbrone MA, Jr (1976) Culture of vascular endothelium. In: Spaet TH (ed) Progress in hemostasis and thrombosis Vol. III. Grune & Stratton, New York

Gimbrone MA, Jr (1977) Culture of vascular endothelium and atherosclerosis. In: Brinkley BR, Porter KR (eds) International cell biology 1976-1977. The Rockefeller University Press

Gimbrone MA, Jr (1980) Vascular endothelium and atherosclerosis. In: Moore S (ed) Arteriosclerosis. Marcel Dekker, New York (in press)

Gimbrone MA, Jr. Alexander RW (1977) Prostaglandin production by vascular endothelial and smooth muscle cells in culture. In: Silver MJ, Kocsis JJ (eds) Prostaglandins in hematology. Sprectrum Publications, New York

Gimbrone MA, Jr, Cotran RS, Folkman J (1974) Human vascular endothelial cells in culture: Growth and DNA synthesis, J Cell Biol Biol 60: 673

Goode TB, Davies PF, Reidy MA, Bowyer DE (1977) Aortic endothelial cell morphology observed in situ by scanning electron microscopy during atherogenesis in the rabbit. Atherosclerosis 27: 235

Habliston DL, Ryan US, Ryan JW (1978) Endothelial cells degrade adenosine-5'-diphosphate. J Cell Biol 78: 206a

Hamberg M, Svensson J, Samuelsson B (1974) Prostaglandin endoperoxides. A new concept concerning the mode of action and release of prostaglandins. Proc Natl Acad Sci USA 71: 3824

Harker LA, Ross R, Slichter SJ, Scott CR (1976) Homocystine-induced arteriosclerosis: The role of endothelial cell injury and platelet response in its genesis. J Clin Invest 58: 731

Haudenschild CC, Zahniser D, Folkman J, Klagsbrun M (1976) Human vascular endothelial cells in culture: Lack of response to serum growth factors. Exp Cell Res 98: 175

Hial V, Gimbrone,MA, Jr, Peyton MP, Wilcox GM, Pisano JJ (1979) Angiotensin metabolism by cultured human vascular endothelial and smooth muscle cells. Microvascular Res 17: 314

Hollis TM, Rosen LA (1972) Histidine decarboxylase activity of bovine aortic endothelium and intima-media. Proc Soc Exp Biol Med 141: 978

Howard VV, Macarak EJ, Gunson D, Kefalides NA (1976) Characterization of the collagen synthesized by endothelial cells in culture. Proc Natl Acad Sci USA 73: 2361

Iverius PH (1972) The interaction between human and plasma lipoproteins and connective tissue glycosaminoglycans. J Biol Chem 247: 2607

Jaffe EA, Minick CR, Adelman B, Becker CG, Nachman R (1976) Synthesis of basement collagen by cultured human endothelial cells. J Exp Med 144: 209

Jaffe EA, Mosher DF (1978) Synthesis of fibronectin by cultured human endothelial cells. J Exp Med 147: 1779

Jaffe EA, Hoyer LW, Nachman RL (1974) Synthesis of von Willebrand factor by cultured human endothelial cells. Proc Natl Acad Sci USA 71: 1906

Johnson AR, Erdos EG (1977) Metabolism of vasoactive peptides by human endothelial cells in culture. J Clin Invest 59: 684

Lewis JC, Kottke BA (1977) Endothelial damage and thrombocyte adhesion in pigeon atherosclerosis. Science 196: 1007

Loskutoff DJ, Edgington TS (1977) Synthesis of a fibrolytic activator and inhibitor by endothelial cells. Proc Natl Acad Sci USA 74: 3903

Macarak EJ, Kirby E, Kirk T, Kefalides NA (1978) Synthesis of cold-insoluble globulin by cultured calf endothelial cells. Proc Natl Acad Sci USA 75: 2621

Majno G (1965) Ultrastructure of the vascular membrane. Chapter 64 In: Hamilton WF, Dow P (eds) Handbook of physiology, Section 2: Circulation

Vol II. American Physiological Society, Washington, D.C.

Majno G, Joris I (1978) Endothelium 1977: A review. In: Chandler AB et al (eds) The thrombotic process in atherogenesis. Plenum Press, New York

Martin BM, Baldwin WM, Gimbrone MA, Jr, Unanue ER, Cotran RS (1979) Macrophage factor(s): stimulation of cell growth in vitro and new blood vessels in vivo. J Cell Biol 83: 376a

Maynard JR, Heckman CA, Pitlick FA, Nemerson Y (1975) Association of tissue factor activity with the surface of cultured cells. J Clin Invest 55: 814

Minick CR, Stemerman MB, Insull W, Jr (1977) Effect of regenerated endothelium on lipid accumulation in the arterial wall. Proc Natl Acad Sci USA 74(4): 1742

Moncada S, Gryglewski R, Bunting S, Vane JR (1976) An enzyme isolated from arteries transforms prostaglandin endoperoxides to an unstable substance that inhibits platelet aggregation. Nature 263: 663

Moncada S, Vane JR (1979) Arachidonic acid metabolites and the interactions between platelets and blood-vessel walls. N Engl J Med 300: 1142

Moore S (1973) Thromboatherosclerosis in normolipemic rabbits: A result of continued endothelial damage. Lab Invest 29: 478

Nelson E, Gertz GD, Forbes MS, Rennels ML, Heald FP, Kahn MA, Farber TM, Miller E, Husain MM, Earl FL (1976) Endothelial lesions in the aorta of egg yolk-fed miniature swine: A study by scanning and transmission electron microscopy. Exp Mol Pathol 25: 208

Olivecrona T, Bengtsson G, Hook M, Luidohl U (1976) Physiologic implications of the interaction between lipoprotein lipase and some sulfated glycosaminoglycans. In: Greten H (ed) Lipoprotein metabolism. Springer, Berlin

Pearson JD, Gordon JL (1979) Vascular endothelial and smooth muscle cells in culture selectively release adenine nucleotides. Nature 281: 384

Pelikan P, Gimbrone MA, Jr, Cotran RS (1979) Distribution and movement of anionic cell surface sites in cultured human vascular endothelial cells. Atherosclerosis 32: 69

Polverini PJ, Cotran RS, Gimbrone MA, Jr, Unanue ER (1977) Activated macrophages induce vascular proliferation. Nature 269: 804

Poole JCF, Sanders AG, Florey HM (1958) The regenration of aortic endothelium. J Pathol Bacteriol 75: 133

Reidy MA, Bowyer DE (1978) Distortion of endothelial repair. The effect of hypercholesterolaemia on regeneration of aortic endothelium following injury by endotoxin. Atherosclerosis 29: 459

Ross R, Glomset JA (1976) Medical Progress: The pathogenesis of atherosclerosis. N Engl J Med 295: 369

Ross R, Glomset J, Kariya B, Harker L (1974) A platelet-dependent serum factor that stimulates the proliferation of arterial smooth muscle cells in vitro. Proc Natl Acad Sci USA 71: 1207

Ross R, Harker L (1976) Hyperlipidemia and atherosclerosis: Chronic hyperlipidemia initiates and maintains lesions by endothelial cell desquamation and lipid accumulation. Science 193: 1094

Sakariassen KS, Bolhuis PA, Sixma JJ (1979) Human blood platelet adhesion to artery subendothelium is mediated by factor VIII - von Willebrand factor bound to the subendothelium. Nature 279: 636

Schwartz SM, Benditt EP (1973) Cell replication in the aortic endothelium: A new method for study of the problem. Lab Invest 28: 699

Schwartz SM, Benditt EP (1977) Aortic endothelial cell replication I. Effects of age and hypertension in the rat. Circ Res 41: 248

Schwartz SM, Haudenschild CC, Eddy EM (1978) Endothelial regeneration I. Quantitative analysis of intial stages of endothelial regeneration in rat aortic intima. Lab Invest 38: 568

Schwartz SM, Stemerman MB, Benditt EP (1975) The aortic intima II. Repair of the aortic lining after mechanical denudation. Amer J Pathol 81: 15

Scow RO, Blanchette-Mackie EJ, Smith LC (1976) Role of capillary endothelium in the clearnace of chylomicrons. A model for lipid transport from blood by lateral diffusion in cell membranes. Circ Res 39: 149

Selden SC, III, Schwartz SM (1979) Cytochalasin B inhibition of endothelial proliferation at wound edges in vitro. J Cell Biol 81: 348

Sholley MM, Gimbrone MA, Jr, Cotran RS (1977) Cellular migration and replication in endothelial regeneration: A study using irradiated endothelial cultures. Lab Invest 36: 18

Spaet TH, Stemerman MB, Veith FJ, Lejnieks I (1975) Intimal injury and regrowth in the rabbit aorta: Medial smooth muscle cells as a source of neointima. Circ Res 36: 58

Skutelsky E, Rudich Z, Danon D (1975) Surface charge properties of the luminal front of blood vessel walls: an electron microscopical analysis. Thromb Res 7: 623

Srinivasan SR, Dola P, Radhakrishuamunthy B, Pargonkar PS, Berenson GS (1975) Lipoprotein-acid mucopolysaccharide complexes of human atherosclerotic lesion. Biochim Biophys Acta 388: 58

Stehbens WE (1974) Haemodynamic production of lipid deposition, intimal tears, mural dissection and thrombosis in the blood vessel wall. Proc R Soc Lond (Biol) 185: 357

Stemerman MB, Ross R (1972) Experimental arteriosclerosis. I. Fibrous plaque formation in primates, an electron microscope study. J Exp Med 136: 769

Stevens RL, Colombo M, Gonzales JJ, Hollander W, Schmid K (1976) The glycosaminoglycans of the human artery and their changes in atherosclerosis. J Clin Invest 58: 470

Thorgeirsson G, Robertson AL, Jr (1978) The vascular endothelium - pathobiologic significance. Amer J Pathol 93: 803

Thorgeirsson G, Robertson AL, Jr (1978) Platelet factors and the human vascular wall: Variations in growth response between endothelial and medial smooth muscle cells. Atherosclerosis 30: 67

Vlodavsky I, Fielding PE, Fielding CJ, Gospodarowicz D (1978) Role of contact inhibition in the regulation of receptor-mediated uptake of low density lipoprotein in cultured vascular endothelial cells. Proc Natl Acad Sci USA 75(1): 356

Wall RT, Harker LA, Quadracci LJ, Striker GE (1978) Factors influencing endothelial cell proliferation in vitro. J Cell Physiol 96: 203

Weber G, Fabbrini P, Resi L (1974) Scanning and transmission electron microscopy observations on the surface lining of aortic intimal plaques in rabbits on a hypercholesterolic diet. Virchows Arch A Pathol Anat Histol 364: 325

Weksler BB, Ley CW, Jaffe EA (1978) Stimulation of endothelial cell prostacyclin production by thrombin, trypsin, and the ionophore A 23187. J Clin Invest 62: 923

Weksler BB, Marcus AM, Jaffe EA (1977) Synthesis of prostaglandin I_2 (prostacyclin) by cultured human and bovine endothelial cells. Proc Natl Acad Sci USA 74: 3922

Wight TN, Ross R (1975) Proteoglycan in primate arteries. I. Ultrastructural localization and distribution in the intima. J Cell Biol 67: 660

Wright HP (1970) Endothelial turnover. In: Koller F, Brinkhous KM, Biggs R, Rodman NF, Hinnom S (eds) Vascular factors and thrombosis. Schattauer Verlag, New York

Zetter BR, Johnson LK, Shuman MA, Gospodarowicz D (1978) The isolation of vascular endothelial cell lines with altered cell surface and platelet-binding properties. Cell 14: 501

Prostacyclin and Thromboxane A₂ in Platelet Vessel Wall Interactions

Salvador Moncada

Prostacyclin was originally found as a product of the conversion of prostaglandin endoperoxides by a microsomal enzyme from blood vessels. It was described as an unstable substance which is a potent vasodilator and an inhibitor of platelet aggregation (Moncada et al. 1976a). This compound, originally called PGX (Bunting et al. 1976; Gryglewski et al. 1976; Moncada et al. 1976b), was later chemically identified by Johnson et al. (1976) as an intermediate in the formation of 6-oxo-$PGF_{1\alpha}$, a compound already known (Dawson et al. 1976; Pace-Asciak 1976). PGX was then renamed prostacyclin and given the abbreviation of PGI_2.

Prostacyclin is formed by vascular tissues from all species so far tested (Bunting et al. 1976; Dusting et al. 1977; Moncada et al. 1977a) and is the main metabolic product of arachidonic acid in vascular tissue (Johnson et al. 1976; Salmon et al. 1978). Prostacyclin is the most potent endogenous inhibitor of platelet aggregation yet discovered. It is 30-40 times more potent than PGE_1 (Moncada & Vane 1977) and more than 1000 times more active than adenosine (Born 1962). In vivo, prostacyclin applied locally in low concentrations inhibits thrombus formation due to ADP in the microcirculation of the hamster cheek pouch (Higgs et al. 1977), and given systemically to the rabbit it prevents electrically induced thrombus formation in the carotid artery and increases bleeding time (Ubatuba et al. 1979). The duration of these effects in vivo is short, disappearing within 30 min of administration. Prostacyclin disaggregates platelets in vitro (Moncada et al. 1976b; Ubatuba et al. 1979) in extracorporeal circuits where platelet clumps have formed on collagen strips (Gryglewski et al. 1978a, 1978b) and in the circulation of man (Szczeklik et al. 1978a). Moreover, it has also been shown that it inhibits thrombus formation in a coronary artery model in the dog when given locally or systemically (Aiken et al. 1979) and protects against sudden death induced by intravenous arachidonic acid in rabbits (Bayer et al. 1979).

Prostacyclin is unstable and its activity disappears within 15 s on boiling or within 10 min at 22^OC at neutral pH. In blood at 37^OC, prostacyclin has a half-life of 2-3 min (Moncada et al. 1976a). Basic pH increases the stability of prostacyclin (Johnson et al. 1976) so that at pH 10.5 at 25^OC, it has a half-life of 100 h.

In platelets, arachidonic acid or prostaglandin endoperoxides are converted via the cyclo-oxygenase enzyme to the powerful vasoconstrictor and pro-aggregating agent thromboxane A_2 (TXA_2). However, vessel microsomes in the absence of cofactors can utilise prostaglandin endoperoxides but not arachidonic acid to synthesise prostacyclin (Moncada et al. 1976a). Fresh vascular tissue can utilise both precursors although it was far more effective in utilising prostaglandin endoperoxides (Bunting et al. 1976). Moreover, vessel microsomes, fresh vascular rings or endothelial cells treated with indomethacin can, when incubated with platelets, generate a prostacyclin-like anti-aggregating activity (Bunting et al. 1976, 1977; Gryglewski et al. 1976). The release of this substance is inhibited by 15-hydroperoxy arachidonic acid (15-HPAA), a selective inhibitor of prostacyclin formation (Gryglewski et al. 1976; Moncada et al. 1976b). From all these results it was concluded that the vessel wall can synthesise prostacyclin from its own endogenous precursors, but that it can also utilise prostaglandin endoperoxides released by the platelets, thus suggesting a biochemical cooperation between platelets and vessel wall (Moncada & Vane 1978, 1979).

This latter hypothesis has proved to be controversial. Needleman and associates demonstrated that while arachidonic acid was rapidly converted to prostacyclin by perfused rabbit hearts and kidneys, PGH_2 was not readily used. The authors concluded that some degree of vascular damage is necessary for the endoperoxide to be utilised by the prostacyclin synthetase (Needleman et al. 1978). On the other hand, incubation of PRP with fresh indomethacin-treated arterial tissue leads to an increase in platelet cAMP which parallels the inhibition of the aggregation (Best et al. 1977) and which can be abolished by previous treatment of the vascular tissue with tranylcypromine, a less active inhibitor of prostacyclin formation (Gryglewski et al. 1976). Additionally, Tansik et al. (1978) showed that lysed aortic smooth muscle cells could be fed prostaglandin endoperoxides by lysed human platelets, and Nordoy et al. (1978a) have demonstrated that endothelial cells can be fed with endoperoxides released from platelets during collagen-induced aggregation. Further, undisturbed endothelial cell monolayers readily utilise PGH_2 to transform it into prostacyclin (Marcus et al. 1978).

In contrast, work by Needleman et al. (1979) and Hornstra et al. (1979) using vessel microsomes and fresh vascular tissue, suggests that the feeding of endoperoxides from platelets does not take place under their experimental circumstances. However, Needleman et al. (1979) made the observation that when platelets were treated with a TXA_2 synthetase inhibitor then endoperoxides were available for utilisation by the vessel wall. Interestingly, in the presence of a thromboxane synthetase inhibitor, arachidonic acid or collagen added to blood in vitro lead to the formation of 6-oxo-$PGF_{1\alpha}$ rather than TXB_2, showing that some cell other than platelets has synthesised prostacyclin (Blackwell et al. 1978). These results support our suggestion that thromboxane synthetase inhibitors might have a superior antithrombotic effect to simple cyclo-oxygenase inhibitors (Moncada & Vane 1977, 1978). It is important to realize at this stage however, that all these observations have been made in in vitro systems and that in vivo experiments are necessary in order to clarify further the nature of the interaction between platelets and normal or damaged vessel wall.

In the vasculature, the enzyme which metabolises prostaglandin endoperoxides to prostacyclin (prostacyclin synthetase) is most highly concentrated in the intimal surface and progressively decreases in activity towards the adventitial surface (Moncada et al. 1977b). Production of prostacyclin by cultured cells from vessel walls also shows that endothelial cells are the most active producers of prostacyclin (Harker et al. 1977; MacIntyre et al. 1978; Weksler et al. 1977a); moreover, this production persists after numerous sub-cultures in vitro (Christofinis et al. 1979).

Generation of prostacyclin is an active mechanism by which the vessel wall could be protected from deposition of platelet aggregates. Thus, prostacyclin formation provides an explanation of the long recognised fact that contact with healthy vascular endothelium is not a stimulus for platelet clumping.

Vascular damage leads to platelet adhesion but not necessarily to thrombus formation. When the injury is minor, platelet thrombi are formed which break away from the vessel wall and are washed away by the circulation. The degree of injury is an important determinant, and there is general agreement that for the development of thrombosis, severe damage or physical detachment of the endothelium must occur. All these observations are in accord with the distribution of prostacyclin synthetase, for it is abundant in the intima and progressively decreases in concentration from the intima to the adventitia. Moreover, the pro-aggregating elements increase from the sub-endothelium to the adventitia. These two opposing tendencies render the endothelial lining anti-aggregatory and the outer layers of the vessel wall thrombogenic (Moncada et al. 1977b).

The ability of the vascular wall actively to prevent aggregation has been postulated before (Saba & Mason 1974). For instance, the presence of an ADP-ase in the vessel wall has led to the suggestion that this enzyme, by breaking down ADP, limits platelet aggregation (Heyns et al. 1974; Lieberman et al. 1977). We have confirmed the presence of an ADP-ase in the vascular wall. However, the anti-aggregating activity of the vascular wall is mainly related to the release of prostacyclin, for 15-HPAA or 13-hydroperoxy linoleic acid (13-HPLA), two inhibitors of prostacyclin formation which have no activity on the ADP-ase system, abolish most if not all of the anti-aggregatory activity of vascular endothelial cells (Bunting et al. 1977). Similar results have been obtained using an antiserum which cross-reacts with and neutralises prostacyclin in vitro (Bunting et al. 1978). Endothelial cells pretreated with this antiserum lose the ability to inhibit ADP-induced aggregation (Bunting et al. 1978; Christofinis et al. 1979). It is not yet clear whether or not prostacyclin is responsible for all the thromboresistant properties of the vascular endothelium. However, work by Czervionke et al. (1979) with endothelial cell cultures has demonstrated that platelet adherence in the presence of thrombin increases from 4% to 44% after treatment with l mM aspirin. This increase was parallelled by a decrease in 6-oxo-PGF$_{1\alpha}$ formation from 107 nM to < 3 nM and could be reversed by addition of 25 nM of exogenous PGI$_2$. This work suggests that prostacyclin, although probably not responsible for all the thromboresistant properties of vascular endothelium, plays a very important role in the control of platelet aggregability.

The fact that prostacyclin inhibits platelet aggregation (platelet-platelet interaction) at much lower concentrations than those needed to inhibit adhesion (platelet-collagen interaction) (Higgs et al. 1978a) suggests that, indeed, prostacyclin allows platelets to stick to vascular tissue and to interact with it, while at the same time preventing or limiting thrombus formation. Certainly, platelets adhering to a site where prostacyclin synthetase is present could well feed the enzyme with endoperoxide, thereby producing prostacyclin and preventing other platelets from clumping onto the adhering platelets, limiting the cells to a monolayer. Recently, Weiss and Turitto (1979) have observed some degree of inhibition of platelet-subendothelium interactions with low concentrations of prostacyclin at high shear rates, but at none of the concentrations used could they observe total inhibition of platelet adhesion.

It is also possible that formed elements of blood such as the white cells, which produce endoperoxides and TXA$_2$ (Davison et al. 1978; Goldstein et al. 1977; Higgs et al. 1976), interact with the vessel wall to allow formation of prostacyclin, as do the platelets. This suggestion, coupled with the fact that prostacyclin may modulate white cell behaviour (Higgs et al. 1978b; Weksler et al. 1977b) could well mean that prostacyclin plays a role in the control of white cell migration during the inflammatory response (see below).

Unlike other prostaglandins, such as PGE$_1$ and PGF$_{2\alpha}$, prostacyclin is not inactivated on a passage through the pulmonary circulation (Dusting et al. 1978), and this is probably due to the fact that prostacyclin, although a good substrate for lung PGDH, is not a substrate for the uptake mechanism responsible for transport from the circulation to the intracellular enzyme (Hawkins et al. 1978). Indeed, the lung can constantly release small amounts of prostacyclin into the circulation (Gryglewski et al. 1978a; Moncada et al. 1978). The concentrations of prostacyclin are higher in arterial than in venous blood due to overall inactivation of about 50% in one circulation through peripheral tissues (Dusting et al. 1978). Thus, platelet aggregability in vivo is modulated by circulating prostacyclin which will reinforce the actions of locally produced prostacyclin throughout the vasculature. The possibility that other organs also release PGI_2 into the circulation as a result of a specific stimulus, such as bradykinin, has been recently suggested (Mullane et al. 1979).

Mechanism of Action

Prostacyclin inhibits platelet aggregation by stimulating adenylate cyclase, leading to an increase in cAMP levels in the platelets (Gorman et al. 1977; Tateson et al. 1977). In this respect prostacyclin is much more potent than either PGE_1 or PGD_2 (Tateson et al. 1977). 6-oxo-$PGF_{1\alpha}$ has very weak anti-aggregating activity and is almost devoid of activity on platelet cAMP (Ubatuba et al. 1979).

Prostacyclin is not only more potent than PGE_1 in elevating cAMP but the elevation persists longer. The elevation induced by PGE_1 starts falling after 30 s, while prostacyclin stimulation is not maximal until after 30 s and is maintained for 2 min after which it gradually wanes over 30 minutes (Gorman et al. 1977). Prostacyclin is also a strong direct stimulator of adenylate cyclase in isolated membrane preparations (Gorman et al. 1977).

Prostacyclin, as well as the less active PGE_1 and PGD_2, seems to increase adenylate cyclase activity by acting on two separate receptors on the platelet membrane (Miller & Gorman 1979; Whittle et al. 1978). PGE_1 and prostacyclin act on one, whereas PGD_2 acts on another. This is shown both by differences in activity in different species (Williams & Downing 1977) and by the use of a prostaglandin antagonist (Eakins et al. 1976) which selectively prevents the inhibition of platelet aggregation induced by PGD_2, but not that induced by prostacyclin or PGE_1 (Whittle et al. 1978). Moreover, studies of agonist-specific sensitisation of cAMP accumulation in platelets show that PGE_1 or PGE_2 can desensitise for subsequent PGE_1 or prostacyclin activation and that subthreshold concentrations of prostacyclin desensitise PGE_1 stimulation. PGD_2, however, desensitises to a further dose of PGD_2 but not to PGE_1 or prostacyclin (Miller & Gorman 1979). These results suggest (Miller & Gorman 1979; Whittle et al. 1978) that the previously recognised PGE_1 receptor in platelets (Minkes et al. 1977) might be in fact a prostacyclin receptor.

There have not been many detailed studies on the mechanism of action of prostacyclin. In contrast to TXA_2 it enhances Ca^{++} sequestration (Kazer-Glanzman et al. 1977). Moreover, an inhibitory effect on platelet phospholipase (Lapetina et al. 1977; Minkes et al. 1977) and platelet cyclo-oxygenase have been described (Malmsten et al. 1976). All these effects are related to its ability to increase cAMP in platelets. Moreover, prostacyclin inhibits endoperoxide-induced aggregation suggesting additional sites of action, still undefined, but dependent on the cAMP effect (Minkes et al. 1977). These observations have extended and given important biological significance to the original observation of Vargaftig and Chignard (1975), who demonstrated that substances that increase cAMP such as PGE_1 inhibit the release of TXA_2 (measured as Rabbit aorta contracting substance; RCS) in platelets. Prostacyclin, by inhibiting several steps in the activation of the arachidonic acid metabolic cascade, exerts an overall control of platelet aggregability in vivo.

The fact that prostacyclin increases cAMP levels in cells other than platelets (Gorman et al. 1979; Hopkins et al. 1978), and the possibility that in those cells an interaction with the thromboxane system could lead to a similar control of cell behaviour to that observed in platelets, suggests that the PGI_2/TXA_2 system has wider biological significance in cell regulation.

Prostacyclin, Thromboxane A_2 - Thrombosis and Haemostasis

In vivo, prostaglandin endoperoxides are at the crossroads of arachidonic acid metabolism, for they are precursors of substances with opposing biological properties. On the one hand, TXA_2 produced by the platelets is a strong contractor of large blood vessels and induces platelet aggregation. On the other hand, prostacyclin produced by the vessel wall is a strong vasodilator and the most potent inhibitor of platelet aggregation known. Each substance has opposing effects on cAMP concentrations, thereby giving a balanced control mechanism which will, therefore, affect thrombus and haemostatic plug formation. Selective inhibition of the formation of TXA_2 should lead to an increased bleeding time and inhibition of thrombus formation, whereas inhibition of prostacyclin formation should be propitious for a "pro-thrombotic state". The amount of control exerted by this system can be tested, for selective inhibitors of each pathway have been described (Moncada & Vane 1978; Nijkamp et al. 1977).

The utilisation of aspirin as a pharmacological tool to investigate the interaction between these two substances has been fruitful. Aspirin is highly active against platelet cyclo-oxygenase in vivo and in vitro. Moreover, this effect is long lasting because aspirin acetylates the active site of the enzyme leading to irreversible inhibition (Roth & Majerus 1975; Roth and Siok 1978). Platelets are unable to synthesise new protein (Marcus 1978) and cannot replace the cyclo-oxygenase. Therefore, the inhibition will only be overcome by new platelets coming into the circulation after the block of cyclo-oxygenase in megakaryocytes has worn off (Burch et al. 1978). Interestingly, the cyclo-oxygenase of vessel walls is much less sensitive to aspirin than that of platelets (Baenziger et al. 1977). It has also been suggested that endothelial cells in vitro and in vivo recover from aspirin inhibition by regeneration of the cyclo-oxygenase (Czervionke et al. 1978; Kelton et al. 1978). This has been reinforced by the observation that the recovery of the endothelial cell synthetase in cell cultures can be prevented by treatment with the protein synthesis inhibitor, cycloheximide (Czervionke et al. 1979).

Studies in rabbits (Amezcua et al. 1978; Korbut & Moncada 1978) suggest that low doses of aspirin reduce TXA_2 formation to a greater extent than prostacyclin formation. These experiments also showed that inhibition of TXA_2 formation is longer lasting than that of prostacyclin. Indeed, infusions of arachidonic acid into rabbits and cats, lead to an anti-thrombotic effect and to an increase in bleeding time which can be potentiated by low doses of aspirin and blocked by larger doses (which would inhibit prostacyclin and TXA_2 formation) (Amezcua et al. 1978; Korbut & Moncada 1978).

Any anti-thrombotic activity of dipyridamole can also be linked with the prostacyclin system, for this substance is an inhibitor of phosphodiesterase and thus amplifies the effects of the increase in cAMP induced by circulating prostacyclin (Moncada & Korbut 1978). Dipyridamole is most effective when there is a favourable PGI_2/TXA_2 ratio, after a small dose of aspirin or more than 24 h after a high dose. These experiments have provided the explanation for the well recognised synergism of small doses of aspirin and dipyridamole in experimental models or in clinical experience (Harker & Slichter 1972; Honour et al. 1977). A selective inhibitor of thromboxane formation and a phosphodiesterase inhibitor should now be tested for anti-thrombotic efficacy, since theoretically this provides an advantage over aspirin in leaving endoperoxides from platelets available for the vessel walls or other cells to synthesise prostacyclin.

These results also suggest that, when aspirin is used, a small daily dose or a large dose at weekly intervals, alone or in combination with a phosphodiesterase inhibitor such as dipyridamole, would be a useful therapeutic combination. Clearly, it is important not to use too high a dose of aspirin, for that will neutralise the whole system including prostacyclin formation and might lead to deleterious effects.

Until the discovery of prostacyclin, the use of aspirin as an anti-thrombotic, based on its effects on platelets, looked very clear (Majerus 1976). Now, however, the situation needs further clarification, especially with respect to the optimal dose of aspirin. Aspirin in high doses (200 mg/kg) increases thrombus formation in a model of venous thrombosis in the rabbit (Kelton et al. 1978), and in vitro treatment of endothelial cells with aspirin enhances thrombin-induced platelet adherence to them (Czervionke et al. 1978). In addition, there is an inverse correlation between platelet adhesion and aggregation and the amount of prostacyclin produced by the tissue. Moreover, aspirin treatment of arterial tissue in vitro increases its thrombogenicity (H. Baumgartner personal communication).

In humans, O'Grady and Moncada (1978) showed that a low single dose of aspirin (0.3 g) increased bleeding time 2 h after ingestion, whereas a high dose (3.9 g) had no effect. Some workers have confirmed these results (Rajah et al. 1978), but others have been unable to do so (Godal et al. 1979). Recent work suggests that the cutaneous bleeding time decreases with age probably due to a progressive decrease in the synthesis of prostacyclin and a predominance of the thromboxane A_2 generation. As a result of this the response to aspirin varies, being paradoxical between low and high doses in the young and both doses leading to an increase in the old (Jorgensen et al. 1979). Moreover, after a single high dose of aspirin (3.9 g) platelet aggregation and TXA_2 formation is blocked 2 h after aspirin. The bleeding time is unchanged at that time but 24 and 72 h after aspirin it is increased and slowly recovers toward pretreatment levels over a period of 168 h, in a manner which is a mirror image of the recovery of TXA_2 formation and platelet aggregability (Amezcua et al. 1979). An extension of the concept comes from the demonstration that tranylcypromine, an inhibitor of prostacyclin formation, enhances platelet aggregation in an experimental model of thrombosis in the microcirculation of the brain of the mouse (Rosenblum & El-Sabban 1978). All these results clearly demonstrate that the balance between TXA_2/PGI_2 is an important mechanism of control of platelet aggregability in vivo. Clearly, manipulation of this control mechanism might lead to pro- or anti-thrombotic states of clinical relevance. In this context it is interesting that Mustard's group has shown that hydrocortisone treatment of normal or thrombocytopenic rats blocks prostacyclin formation in the vessel wall and decreases the bleeding time (Blajchman et al. 1979), a result which would be expected from the interference with arachidonic acid release induced by steroids (Flower 1978). The authors (Blajchman et al. 1979) mention that for years it has been the clinical impression that steroids decrease the bleeding time in thrombocytopenic patients without increasing the platelet count.

Whether other drugs exert their antithrombotic effect by acting on the prostacyclin/thromboxane system mechanism is not yet known but studies using sulphinpyrazone in cultured endothelial cells (Gordon & Pearson 1978) and ticlopidine given orally to rats (Ashida & Abiko 1978) suggest that these compounds have little or no effect on prostacyclin formation at concentrations at which they affect platelet behaviour.   A compound which might stimulate prostacyclin formation in humans after oral ingestion has also been described (Vermylen et al. 1979).

Fatty Acids and Thrombosis

Before the discovery of prostacyclin, it was suggested that the use of dietary dihomo-γ-linolenic acid, the precursor of the E_1 series of prostaglandins, could be an approach to the prevention of thrombosis, for PGG_1 and TXA_1 are not pro-aggregegating and PGE_1 is anti-aggregating. Other reports tend to agree with this proposal but there is some controversy, for feeding rabbits with dihomo-γ-linolenic acid leads to increased tissue content of this acid without change in platelet responsiveness, at least to ADP.   The main criticism of all this work, including that on human platelets is that the conclusions are based on studies performed in vitro in which platelets are studied as isolated cells without contact with vessel walls (Moncada & Vane 1978, 1979).

It is now evident that the use of dihomo-γ-linolenic acid to direct the synthetic machinery of the platelets is not the most rational approach for prevention of thrombosis. This is because the endoperoxides PGG_1 and PGH_1 are not substrates for the formation of prostacyclin or because their precursor might adversely affect the prostacyclin protective mechanism.

Man has the enzymes to elongate and desaturate linoleic acid (C18:2ω6) to arachidonic acid (C20:4ω6).   We also obtain preformed arachidonic acid from the meat of land animals. Eicosapentaenoic acid (C20:5ω3) comes from marine animals and is the precursor of a different series of prostaglandins.   It can be used to generate an anti-aggregating agent in the vessel wall which is probably a prostacyclin (Dyerberg et al. 1978). However, if a thromboxane is formed by platelets, it does not induce their aggregation (Raz et al. 1977).   The consumption of this fatty acid then, could afford a dietary protection against intra-vascular thrombosis, for it would swing the balance towards the anti-thrombotic side of the system. Indeed, the low incidence of myocardial infarction in Eskimos and their increased tendency to bleed is probably due to the high eicosapentaenoic acid and low linoleic and arachidonic acid content of their marine diet and, therefore, of their tissues (Dyerberg et al. 1978). It has been known for some years that this is associated with a lowered blood cholesterol.

In a well controlled cross-over study von Lossonczy et al. (1978) measured the effects of the addition of fish (to give 8 g daily of 3 fats) or cheese to a lacto-ovo-vegetarian diet in men and women. Serum cholesterol and triglycerides were lowered and high density lipoprotein was increased by the fish diet as compared with the cheese diet.   There was also a strong decrease in the very low density lipoprotein.   Each of these changes is thought to lower the risk of arterial disease.

All these results, taken together with the findings that the balance of the prostacyclin/thromboxane system can also be changed by consumption of fish oils, lend great importance to future research into the effects of specific rather than general polyunsaturated fats in the diet. The "polyunsaturated" fats as a group may well have less relevance to the prevention of cardiovascular disease than those that can lead to prostacyclins, especially eicosapentaenoic acid.

As a source of eicosapentaenoic acid, cod liver oil contains 10% but to imitate an Eskimo's intake would mean drinking 700 calories worth of oil a day. Indeed, the fats of most common fish contain 8-12% eicosapentaenoic acid. The fats of the more exotic sea foods, such as scallops, oysters and red caviare, contain more than 20%! Interestingly, Dyerberg and Bang (1979) have recently published studies which demonstrate that Eskimos in norther Greenland have decreased ex vivo platelet aggregation and increased bleeding time.

γ-Linolenic acid (C18:3ω3) is the vegetable oil which, if elongated and desaturated, would lead to eicosapentaenoic acid. Whether this occurs in man appears to be uncertain, but Sanders et al. (1977) made an important comparison of the fatty acid composition of plasma choline phosphoglycerides and red cell lipids in vegans and omnivores. The only striking differences were in the ω3 series and, as far as eicosapentaenoic acid was concerned, the vegans had only 12-15% of the levels of omnivores. Clearly, it is important to establish whether man converts sufficient linolenic acid to eicosapentaenoic acid, for the latter is found especially as a constituent of brain cell lipids.

What bearing does all this have on the continuing debate about dietary polyunsaturates? Margarines contain anything from 9-48% of linoleic acid, depending on the brand. The rest of the fats are C16:0 (7-18%), C18:0 (1.5-14%), C18:1 (8-53%) and C18:3 (0.1-5%) (Weihrauch et al. 1977). Of these fatty acids, only C18:2 can act (when in the cis form) as a precursor (when elongated) for prostacyclin. However, a substantial and variable proportion of the linoleic acid in margarine is in the trans form (Weihrauch et al. 1977). Certainly, to choose a margarine with a high content of C18:2ω6 in the cis form needs more information than is provided on the label, and none exists with a high content of C20:5ω3, which may be preferable.

Thus, as providers of precursors for prostacyclin and other prostaglandins, many of the "polyunsaturated" fats in margarine are unimportant and could even have a deleterious effect if the non-precursor fats are peroxidised, for lipid peroxides inhibit prostacyclin production. Polyunsaturated fatty acids are easily auto-oxidized or enzymically converted to the corresponding linear hydroperoxy fatty acids. Peroxides of fatty acids, including arachidonic, dihomo-γ-linolenic, α-linolenic and γ-linolenic acids, inhibit prostacyclin synthetase when incubated with this enzyme at low concentrations (between 1-2 μM). Interestingly, in the absence of vitamin E, which is a natural anti-oxidant, polyunsaturated fatty acid-rich diet fed to pigs causes endothelial damage and subsequent thrombosis (Nafstad 1974).

Selective inhibition of prostacyclin formation by lipid peroxides could also lead to a condition in which platelet aggregation is increased and this could play a role in the development of atherosclerosis. Indeed, lipid peroxidation takes place in plasma as a non-enzymic reaction (Harman & Piette 1966) and it is known to occur in certain pathological conditions (Slater 1972). Hence, lipid peroxides present in these conditions could be shifting the balance of the system in favour of TXA_2 and predispose to thrombus formation. In this context it is interesting that Gryglewski's group (Dembinska-Kiec et al. 1977) has found that there is a strong reduction in prostacyclin formation by hearts or vessel walls of rabbits made atherosclerotic. Similarly, there have been reports that human atherosclerotic tissue does not produce prostacyclin, whereas tissue obtained from a nearby normal vessel does (Angelo et al. 1978; Sinzinger et al. 1979).

The role of lipid peroxides in the development of atherosclerosis has been debated for the last 25 years since Glavind et al. (1952) described the presence of lipid peroxides in human atherosclerotic aortae. They found the peroxide content in diseased arteries to be directly proportional to the severity of the atherosclerosis.

Subsequent investigations by Woodford et al. (1965) suggested Glavind's findings were artifactual, ascribing the presence of lipid peroxides to their formation during the preparative procedure (Woodford et al. 1965). Despite this, the presence of conjugated diene hydroperoxides in lipids of human atheroma has again been reported (Fukazumi 1965; Fukazumi and Iwata 1963) and lipid peroxides have been found in atherosclerotic rabbit aortae (Iwakami 1965), subjected to an extraction procedure which avoids lipid peroxidation in vitro. Some authors (Brooks et al. 1971; Harland et al. 1971) favour the suggestion that lipid peroxides are present in atherosclerotic plaques, whether or not these peroxides act by inhibiting prostacyclin formation and as a consequence reduce the wall's defence mechanism. This theory is of interest, especially since other substances related to atherosclerosis such as the cholesterol carriers, low density lipoproteins (LDL), have also been shown to inhibit prostacyclin formation in endothelial cell cultures (Nordoy et al. 1978b). Interestingly, it has recently been shown that hydroperoxide-mediated inactivation of prostacyclin synthetase seems to be related to the generation of a hydroxyl radical (Weiss et al. 1979). In addition, PGI_2 synthetase is highly sensitive to the destruction by an oxidant released during chemical reduction of hydroperoxy fatty acids. Thromboxane synthetase on the contrary is completely resistant to this effect (Ham et al. 1979). A decrease in prostacyclin formation by lipid peroxidation with a consequent increase in platelet reactivity with the vessel wall as an important factor in the origin and development of atherosclerosis is an interesting proposal which incorporates comprehensibly the fundamental facts of the two previously opposed theories of atherosclerosis, the thrombogenic or encrustation theory, and the lipid theory. This new hypothesis is especially attractive since it has been shown that even early atherosclerotic lesions, the "fatty streaks", lead to a decrease of PGI_2 synthesis in the vascular tissue (Sinzinger et al. 1979).

Prostacyclin and Therapeutics

Prostacyclin or chemical analogues may find a use as a "hormone replacement" therapy in conditions such as acute myocardial infarction or "crescendo angina" and other states in which excessive platelet aggregation takes place in the circulation. Moreover, we have suggested its use in extracorporeal circulation systems such as cardiopulmonary bypass and renal dialysis (Moncada & Vane 1979). In these systems the main problems are platelet loss with the formation of micro-aggregates which, when returning to the patient, are responsible for the cerebral and renal impairment observed after bypass (Abel et al. 1976; Branthwaite 1972). In addition, there are side effects associated with the chronic use of heparin, especially the development of osteoporosis (Griffith et al. 1965).

Several anti-platelet drugs have been suggested to deal with these two problems and some have been used with moderate success. PGE_1 has been reported to be beneficial during cardiopulmonary bypass (Balanowski et al. 1977). However, prostaglandins of the E type induce diarrhoea (Main & Whittle 1975), an effect not shared by prostacyclin (Robert et al. 1979; Ubatuba et al. 1979). Therefore prostacyclin is not only more potent but more specific in achieving platelet protection. Prostacyclin has now been beneficially used in several systems of extracorporeal circulation in experimental animals, including renal dialysis, cardiopulmonary bypass and charcoal haemoperfusion (Bunting et al. 1979; Coppe et al. 1979; Longmore et al. 1979; Woods et al. 1978). In one of these systems (renal dialysis), prostacyclin can replace heparin altogether (Woods et al. 1978). In charcoal haemoperfusion, heparin is also necessary since charcoal particles seem to activate directly the clotting cascade (Bunting et al. 1979). Following reports that PGE_1 has been used successfully in the treatment of peripheral vascular disease

(Carlson and Olsson 1976) prostacyclin has been shown to have a similar effect, producing a long lasting increase in muscle blood flow, disappearance of ischemic pain and healing of throphic ulcers after an intra-arterial infusion to the affected limb for 3 days (Szczeklik et al. 1979).

Thromboxane A$_2$ and Prostacyclin Imbalance in Other Pathological States

Increased production of prostaglandin endoperoxides or TXA$_2$ in vitro by platelets has been found in patients with arterial thrombosis, deep venous thrombosis or recurrent venous thrombosis (Lagarde & Dechavanne 1977). These conditions are associated with a shortened platelet survival time (Lagarde & Dechavanne 1977). In addition, increased sensitivity to aggregating agents and increased release of RCS has been described in rabbits made atherosclerotic by diet (Shimamoto et al. 1978) and in patients who have survived myocardial infarction (Szczeklik et al. 1978b). Moreover, platelets from rats made diabetic release more TXA$_2$ (Harrison et al. 1978; Johnson et al. 1979). Diseases associated with changes in prostacyclin production have been described. An increased production has been suggested in uraemic patients to explain their haemostatic defect (Remuzzi et al. 1977). On the other hand, a lack of prostacyclin production has been suggested in patients with idiopathic thrombocytopaenic purpura (Remuzzi et al. 1978). Both diseases are linked by the accumulation during uraemia or the lack of production during idiopathic thrombocytopaenia purpura of an ill-defined "plasma factor" which stimulates prostacyclin synthesis (MacIntyre et al. 1978).

More recently, a decreased production of prostacyclin by the blood vessels of rats made diabetic has also been described (Harrison et al. 1978; Johnson et al. 1979); this decreased production can be corrected by chronic treatment with insulin (Harrison et al. 1978). Finally, increased prostacyclin production has been described in blood vessels of spontaneously hypertensive rats (Pace-Asciak et al. 1978).

As yet, a clear relationship between different diseases and the PGI$_2$/TXA$_2$ balance is not established. However, it seems that conditions which favour the development of thrombosis are associated with an increase in TXA$_2$ and a decrease in prostacyclin formation, whereas an increased prostacyclin formation plus decreased TXA$_2$ is present in some conditions associated with an increased bleeding tendency. These are, however, wide generalisations which need much more experimental and clinical evidence.

References

Abel RM, Buckley MJ, Austen WG, Barnett GO, Beck CH, Fischer JE (1976) Etiology, incidence and prognosis of a prospective analysis of 500 consecutive patients. J Thorac Surg 71: 323-333

Aiken JW, Gorman RR, Shebuski RJ (1979) Prevention of blockage of partially obstructed coronary arteries with prostacyclin correlates with inhibition of platelet aggregation. Prostaglandins 17: 483-494

Amezcua J-L, Parsons M, Moncada S (1978) Unstable metabolites of arachidonic acid, aspirin and the formation of the haemostatic plug. Thromb Res 13: 477-488

Amezcua J-L, O'Grady J, Salmon JA, Moncada S (1979) Prolonged paradoxical effect of aspirin on platelet behaviour and bleeding time in man. Thromb Res 16: 69-79

Angelo VD, Villa S, Myskiewiec M, Donati MB, de Gaetano G (1978) Defective fibrinolytic and prostacyclin-like activity in human atheromatous plaques. Thromb Haem 39: 535-536

Ashida S-I, Abiko Y (1978) Effect of ticlopidine and acetylsalicylic acid on generation of prostaglandin I_2 like substance in rat arterial tissue. Thromb Res 13: 901-908

Baenziger NL, Dillender MJ, Majerus PW (1977) Cultured human skin fibroblasts and arterial cells produce a labile platelet-inhibitory prostaglandin. Biochem Biophys Res Commun 78: 294-301

Balanowski PJP, Bauer J, Machiedo G, Neville WE (1977) Prostaglandin influence on pulmonary intravascular leukocytic aggregation during cardiopulmonary bypass. J Thorac Cardiovasc Surg 73: 221-224

Bayer B-L, Blass K-E, Forster W (1979) Anti-aggregatory effect of prostacyclin (PGI_2) in vivo. Br J Pharmac 66:10-12

Best LC, Martin TJ, Russell RGG and Preston FE (1977) Prostacyclin increases cyclic AMP levels and adenylate cyclase activity in platelets. Nature (Lond) 267:850-851

Blackwell GJ, Flower RJ, Russell-Smith N, Salmon JA, Thorogood PB and Vane JR (1978) 1-n-Butylimidazole: a potent and selective inhibitor of "Thromboxane Synthetase". Br J Pharmac 64:436P

Blajchman MA, Senyi AF, Hirsh J, Surya Y, Buchanan M and Mustard JF (1979) Shortening of the bleeding time in rabbits by hydrocortisone caused by inhibition of prostacyclin generation by the vessel wall. J Clin Invest 63:1026-1035

Born GVR (1962) Aggregation of blood platelets by adenosine diphosphate and its reversal. Nature (Lond) 194:927-929

Branthwaite MA (1972) Neurological damage related to open heart surgery. Thorax 27:748-753

Brooks CJW, Steel G, Gilbert JD and Harland WA (1971) Lipids of human atheroma. Part 4. Characteristics of a new group of polar sterol esters from human atherosclerotic plaques. Atherosclerosis 13:223-237

Bunting S, Gryglewski R, Moncada S and Vane JR (1976) Arterial walls generate from prostaglandin endoperoxides a substance (prostaglandin X) which relaxes strips of mesenteric and coeliac arteries and inhibits platelet aggregation. Prostaglandins 12:897-913

Bunting S, Moncada S and Vane JR (1977) Antithrombotic properties of vascular endothelium. Lancet ii:1075-1076

Bunting S, Moncada S, Reed P, Salmon JA and Vane JR (1978) An antiserum to 5,6-dihydro prostacyclin (PGI_2) which also binds prostacyclin. Prostaglandins 15:565-574

Bunting S, Moncada S, Vane JR, Woods HF and Weston MJ (1979) Prostacyclin improves hemocompatibility during charcoal hemoperfusion. In: Bergstrom S, Vane JR (eds) Prostacyclin. Raven Press, New York, pp 361-369

Burch JW, Stanford N, Majerus PW (1978) Inhibition of platelet prostaglandin synthetase by oral aspirin. J Clin Invest 61: 314-319

Carlson LA, Olsson AG (1976) Intravenous prostaglandin E_1 in severe peripheral vascular disease. Lancet ii: 810p

Christofinis GJ, Moncada S, MacCormick C, Bunting S, Vane JR (1979) Prostacyclin (PGI_2) release by rabbit aorta and human umbilical vein endothelial cells after prolonged subculture. In: Vane JR, Bergstrom S (eds) Prostacyclin. Raven Press, New York, pp 77-84

Coppe D, Wonders T, Snider M, Salzman EW (1979) Preservation of platelet number and function during extracorporeal membrane oxygenation (ECMO) by regional infusion of prostacyclin. In: Vane JR, Bergstrom S (eds) Prostacyclin. Raven Press, New York, pp 371-383

Czervionke RL, Hoak JC, Fry GL (1978) Effect of aspirin on thrombin-induced adherence of platelets to cultured cells from the blood vessel walls. J Clin Invest 62: 847-856

Czervionke RL, Smith JB, Fry GL, Hoak JC (1979) Inhibition of prostacyclin by treatment of endothelium with aspirin. J Clin Invest 63: 1089-1092

Davison EM, Ford-Hutchinson AW, Smith MJH, Walker JR (1978) The release of thromboxane B_2 by rabbit peritoneal polymorphonuclear leukocytes. Br J Pharmac 63: 407P

Dawson W, Boot JR, Cockerill AF, Mallen DNB, Osborne DJ (1976) Release of novel prostaglandins and thromboxanes after immunological challenge of guinea pig lung. Nature (Lond) 262: 699-702

Dembinska-Kiec A, Gryglewska T, Zmuda A, Gryglewski RJ (1977) The generation of prostacyclin by arteries and by the coronary vascular bed is reduced in experimental atherosclerosis in rabbit. Prostaglandins 14: 1025-1034

Dusting GJ, Moncada S, Vane JR (1977) Prostacyclin (PGX) is the endogenous metabolite responsible for relaxation of coronary arteries induced by arachidonic acid. Prostaglandins 13: 3-15

Dusting GJ, Moncada S, Vane JR (1978) Recirculation of prostacyclin (PGI_2) in the dog. Br J Pharmac 64: 315-320

Dyerberg J, Bang HO (1979) Haemostatic function and platelet polyunsaturated fatty acids in Eskimos. Lancet ii: 433-435

Dyerberg J, Bang HO, Stoffersen E, Moncada S, Vane JR (1978) Polyunsaturated fatty acids, atherosclerosis and thrombosis. Lancet ii: 117-119

Eakins KE, Rajadhyaksha V, Schroer R (1976) Prostaglandin antagonism by sodium p-benzyl-4-(1-oxo-2-(4-chlorobenzyl)-3-phenylpropyl) phenyl phosphonate (N-0164). Br J Pharmac 58: 333-339

Flower RJ (1978) Steroidal anti-inflammatory drugs as inhibitors of phospholipase A_2. In: Paoletti R, Samuelsson B (eds) Advances in Prostaglandin and Thromboxane Research, Academic Press, New York, Vol. 3 pp 105-112

Fukazumi K (1965) Lipids of the atherosclerotic artery. III A hypothesis on the cause of atherosclerosis from the viewpoint of fat chemistry. Yukagaku 14: 119-122

Fukazumi K, Iwata Y (1963) Lipids of atherosclerotic artery. II. Dialysis of lipids of abdominal aorta and lipids in lipid protein complexes existing in the aorta. Yukagaku 12: 93-97

Glavind J, Hartmann S, Clemmesen J, Jessen KE, Dam H (1952) Studies on the role of lipoperoxides in human pathology. II. The presence of peroxidized lipids in the atherosclerotic aorta. Acta Pathol Microbiol Scand 30: 1

Godal HC, Eika C, Dybdahl JH, Daae L, Larsen S (1979) Aspirin and bleeding time. Lancet i: 1236

Goldstein IM, Malmsten CL, Kaplan HB, Kindahl H, Samuelsson B and Weissman G (1977) Thromboxane generation by stimulated human granulocytes: Inhibition by glucocorticoids and superoxide dismutase. Clin Res 25: 518A

Gordon JL, Pearson JD (1978) Effects of sulphinpyrazone and aspirin on prostaglandin I_2 (prostacyclin) synthesis by endothelial cells. Br J Pharmac 64: 481-483

Gorman RR, Bunting S, Miller OV (1977) Modulation of human platelet adenylate cyclase by prostacyclin (PGX). Prostaglandins 13: 377-388

Gorman RR, Hamilton RD, Hopkins NK (1979) Stimulation of human foreskin fibroblast adenosine 3':5'-cyclic monophosphate levels by prostacyclin (prostaglandin I_2). J Biol Chem 254: 1671-1676

Griffith GC, Nichols G, Asher JD, Flanagan B (1965) Heparin osteoporosis. J Am Med Ass 193: 91-94

Gryglewski RJ, Bunting S, Moncada S, Flower RJ, Vane JR (1976) Arterial walls are protected against deposition of platelet thrombi by a substance (Prostaglandin X) which they make from prostaglandin endoperoxides. Prostaglandins 12: 685-714

Gryglewski RJ, Korbut R, Ocetkiewicz, AC (1978a) Generation of prostacyclin by lungs in vivo and its release into the arterial circulation. Nature (Lond) 273: 765-767

Gryglewski RJ, Korbut R, Ocetkiewicz AC (1978b) De-aggregatory action of prostacyclin in vivo and its enhancement by theophylline. Prostaglandins 15: 637-644

Ham EA, Egan RW, Soderman DD, Gale PH, Kuehl FA Jr (1979) Peroxidase-dependent deactivation of prostacyclin synthetase. J Biol Chem 254: 2191-2194

Harker LA, Joy N, Wall RT, Quadracci L, Striker G (1977) Inhibition of platelet reactivity by endothelial cells. Thromb Haem (Abstract) 38: 137

Harker LA, Slichter SJ (1972) Platelet and fibrinogen consumption in man. N Eng J Med 287: 999-1005

Harland WA, Gilbert JD, Steel G, Brooks CJW (1971) Lipids of human atheroma. Part 5. The occurrence of a new group of polar sterol esters in various stages of human atherosclerosis. Atherosclerosis 13: 239-246

Harman D, Piette LH (1966) Free radical theory of ageing: free radical reaction in serum. J Gerontol 21: 560-565

Harrison HE, Reece AH, Johnson M (1978) Decreased vascular prostacyclin in experimental diabetes. Life Sci 23: 351-356

Hawkins HJ, Smith BJ, Nicolaou KC, Eling TE (1978) Studies of the mechanisms involved in the fate of prostacyclin (PGI$_2$) and 6-keto-PGF$_{1\alpha}$ in the pulmonary circulation. Prostaglandins 16: 871-884

Heyns AduP, van den Berg, DJ, Potgieter GM, Retief FP (1974) The inhibition of platelet aggregation by an aorta intima extract. Thromb Diath Haemorrh 32: 417-431

Higgs EA, Moncada S, Vane JR, Caen JP, Michel H, Tobelem G (1978a) Effect of prostacyclin (PGI$_2$) on platelet adhesion to rabbit arterial subendothelium. Prostaglandins 16: 17-22

Higgs GA, Bunting S, Moncada S, Vane JR (1976) Polymorphonuclear leukocytes produce thromboxane A$_2$-like activity during phagocytosis. Prostaglandins 12:749-757

Higgs GA, Moncada S, Vane JR (1977) Prostacyclin (PGI$_2$) inhibits the formation of platelet thrombi induced by adenosine diphosphate (ADP) in vivo. Br J Pharmac 61: 137p

Higgs GA, Moncada S, Vane JR (1978b) Prostacyclin (PGI$_2$) reduces the number of "slow moving" leukocytes in hamster cheek pouch venules. J Physiol 280: 55-56P

Honour AJ, Hockaday TDR, Mann JI (1977) The synergistic effect of aspirin and dipyridamole upon platelet thrombi in living blood vessels. Br J Exp Path 58: 268-272

Hopkins NK, Sun FF, Gorman RR (1978) Thromboxane A$_2$ biosynthesis in human lung fibroblasts, W1-38. Biochem Biophys Res Commun 85: 827-836

Hornstra G, Haddeman E, Don JA (1979) Blood platelets do not provide endoperoxides for vascular prostacyclin production. Nature 279: 66-68

Iwakami M (1965) Peroxides as a factor of atherosclerosis. Nagoya J Med Sci 28: 50-66

Johnson M, Reece AH, Harrison HE (1979) Decreased vascular prostacyclin in experimental diabetes. Advances in Pharmacology & Therapeutics 4: 865p

Johnson RA, Morton DR, Kinner JH, Gorman RR, McGuire JC, Sun FF, Whittaker N, Bunting S, Salmon J, Moncada S, Vane JR (1976) The chemical structure of prostaglandin X (prostacyclin). Prostaglandins 12: 915-928

Jorgensen KA, Olesen AS, Dyerberg J, Stoffersen E (1979) Aspirin and bleeding time: Dependency of Age. Lancet ii: 302

Kazer-Glanzman R, Jakabova M, George J, Luscher E (1977) Stimulation of calcium uptake in platelet membrane vesicles by adenosine 3',5'-cyclic monophosphate and protein kinase. Biochim Biophys Acta 466: 429-440

Kelton JG, Hirsch J, Carter CJ, Buchanan MR (1978) Thrombogenic effect of high dose aspirin in rabbits; relationship to inhibition of vessel wall synthesis of prostaglandin I_2 like activity. J Clin Invest 62: 892-895

Korbut R, Moncada S (1978) Prostacyclin (PGI_2) and thromboxane A_2 interaction in vivo. Regulation by aspirin and relationship with anti-thrombotic therapy. Thromb Res 13: 489-500

Lagarde M, Dechavanne M (1977) Increase of platelet prostaglandin cyclic endoperoxides in thrombosis. Lancet i: 88

Lapetina EG, Schmitges CJ, Chandrabose K, Cuatrecasas P (1977) Cyclic adenosine 3',5'-monophosphate and prostacyclin inhibit membrane phospholipase activity in platelets. Biochem Biophys Res Commun 76: 828-835

Lieberman GE, Lewis GP, Peters TJ (1977) A membrane-bound enzyme in rabbit aorta capable of inhibiting adenosine-diphosphate-induced platelet aggregation. Lancet ii: 330-332

Longmore DB, Bennett G, Gueirrara D, Smith M, Bunting S, Reed P, Moncada S, Read NG, Vane JR (1979) Prostacyclin: A solution to some problems of extracorporeal circulation. Lancet i:1002-1005

MacIntyre DE, Pearson JD, Gordon JL (1978) Localisation and stimulation of prostacyclin production in vascular cells. Nature 271: 549-551

Main IHM, Whittle BJR (1975) Potency and selectivity of methyl analogues of prostaglandin E_2 on rat gastrointestinal function. Br J Pharmac 54: 309-317

Majerus PW (1976) Why aspirin? Circulation 54: 357-359

Malmsten C, Granstrom E, Samuelsson B (1976) Cyclic AMP inhibits synthesis of prostaglandin endoperoxide (PGG_2) in human platelets. Biochem Biophys Res Commun 68: 569-576

Marcus AJ (1978) The role of lipids in platelet function with particular reference to the arachidonic acid pathway. J Lipid Res 19: 793-826

Marcus AJ, Weksler BB, Jaffe EA (1978) Enzymatic conversion of prostaglandin endoperoxide H_2 and arachidonic acid to prostacyclin by cultured human endothelial cells. J Biol Chem 253: 7138-7141

Miller OV, Gorman RR (1979) Evidence for distinct PGI_2 and PGD_2 receptors in human platelets. J Pharm Exp Ther, in press

Minkes M, Stanford M, Chi M, Roth G, Raz A, Needleman P, Majerus P (1977) Cyclic adenosine 3',5'-monophosphate inhibits the availability of arachidonate to prostaglandin synthetase in human platelet suspensions. J Clin Invest 59: 449-454

Moncada S, Korbut R (1978) Dipyridamole and other phosphodiesterase inhibitors act as anti-thrombotic agents through potentiating endogenous prostacyclin. Lancet i: 1286-1289

Moncada S, Vane JR (1977) The discovery of prostacyclin - a fresh insight into arachidonic acid metabolism. In: Kharasch N, Fried J (eds), Academic Press, New York, San Francisco, London, pp 155-177

Moncada S, Vane JR (1978) Unstable metabolites of arachidonic acid and their role in haemostasis and thrombosis. Br Med Bull 34: 129-135

Moncada S, Vane JR (1979) Arachidonic acid metabolites and the interactions between platelets and blood vessel walls. New Eng J Med 300: 1142-1147

Moncada S, Gryglewski RJ, Bunting S, Vane JR (1976a) An enzyme isolated from arteries transforms prostaglandin endoperoxides to an unstable substance that inhibits platelet aggregation. Nature (Lond) 263: 663-665

Moncada S, Gryglewski RJ, Bunting S, Vane JR (1976b) A lipid peroxide inhibits the enzyme in blood vessel microsomes that generates from prostaglandin endoperoxides the substance (Prostaglandin X) which prevents platelet aggregation. Prostaglandins 12: 715-733

Moncada S, Higgs EA, Vane JR, (1977a) Human arterial and venous tissues generate prostacyclin (prostaglandin X) a potent inhibitor of platelet aggregation. Lancet i:18-21

Moncada S, Herman AG, Higgs EA, Vane JR (1977b) Differential formation of prostacyclin (PGX or PGI$_2$) by layers of the arterial wall. An explanation for the anti-thrombotic properties of vascular endothelium. Thromb Res 11: 323-344

Moncada S, Korbut R, Bunting S, Vane JR (1978) Prostacyclin is a circulating hormone. Nature (Lond) 273: 767-768

Mullane KM, Moncada S, Vane JR (1979) Prostacyclin release induced by bradykinin may contribute to the anti-hypertensive action of angiotensin converting enzyme inhibitors. 4th Int Prost Cong, Washington, Raven Press, New York, in press

Nafstad I (1974) Endothelial damage and platelet thrombosis associated with PUFA-rich, vitamin E deficient diet fed to pig. Thromb Res 5: 25

Needleman P, Bronson, SD, Wyche A, Sivakoff M, Nicolaou KC (1978) Cardiac and renal prostaglandin I$_2$. J Clin Invest 61: 839-849

Needleman P, Wyche A, Raz A (1979) Platelet and blood vessel arachidonate metabolism and interactions. J Clin Invest 63: 345-349

Nijkamp FP, Moncada S, White HL, Vane JR (1977) Diversion of prostaglandin endoperoxide metabolism by selective inhibition of thromboxane A$_2$ biosynthesis in lung, spleen or platelets. Eur J Pharmac 44: 179-187

Nordoy A, Svensson B, Hoak JC (1978a) The inhibitory effect of human endothelial cell monolayers on platelet reactions and its inhibition by aspirin. Thromb Res 12: 597-608

Nordoy A, Svensson B, Wiebe D, Hoak JC (1978b) Lipoproteins and the inhibitory effect of human endothelial cells on platelet function. Circ Res 43: 527-534

O'Grady J, Moncada S (1978) Aspirin: A paradoxical effect on bleeding time. Lancet ii: 780

Pace-Asciak C (1976) Isolation, structure and biosynthesis of 6-keto prostaglandin F$_{1\alpha}$ in the rat stomach. J Am Chem Soc 98: 2348-2349

Pace-Asciak CR, Carrara MC, Rangaraj G, Nicolaou KG (1978) Enhanced formation of PGI$_2$, a potent hypotensive substance, by aortic rings and homogenates of the spontaneously hypertensive rat. Prostaglandins 15: 1005-1012

Rajah SM, Penny S, Kester R (1978) Aspirin and bleeding time. Lancet ii: 1104

Raz A, Minkes MS, Needleman P (1977) Endoperoxides and thromboxanes. Structural determinants for platelet aggregation and vasoconstriction. Biochim Biophys Acta 488: 305-311

Remuzzi G, Cavenaghi AE, Mecca G, Donati MB, de Gaetano G (1977) Prostacyclin (PGI$_2$) and bleeding time in uremic patients. Thromb Res 11: 919-920

Remuzzi G, Misiani R, Marchesi D, Livio M, Mecca G, de Gaetano G, Donati MB (1978) Haemolytic-uraemic syndrome: deficiency of plasma factor(s) regulating prostacyclin activity. Lancet ii: 871-872

Robert A, Hanchar AJ, Lancaster C, Nezamis JE (1979) Prostacyclin inhibits enteropooling and diarrhea. In: Vane JR, Bergstrom S (eds) Prostacyclin, Raven Press, New York, pp 147-158

Rosenblum WI, El-Sabban F (1978) Enhancement of platelet aggregation by tranylcyprominne in mouse cerebral microvessels. Circ Res 43: 238-241

Roth GJ, Majerus PW (1975) The mechanism of the effect of aspirin on human platelets. I. Acetylation of a particular fraction protein. J Clin Invest 56: 624-632

Roth GJ, Siok CJ (1978) Acetylation of the NH$_2$-terminal serine of prostaglandin synthetase by aspirin. J Biol Chem 253: 3782-3784

Saba SR, Mason RG (1974) Studies of an activity from endothelial cells that inhibits platelet aggregation, serotonin release and clot retraction. Thromb Res 5: 747-757

Salmon JA, Smith DR, Flower RJ, Moncada S, Vane JR (1978) Further studies on the enzymatic conversion of prostaglandin endoperoxide into prostacyclin by porcine aorta microsomes. Biochim Biophys Acta 523: 250-262

Sanders TAB, Ellis FR, Dickerson JWT (1977) Polyunsaturated fatty acids and the brain. Lancet i: 751

Shimamoto T, Kobayashi M, Takahashi T, Takashima Y, Sakamoto M, Morooka S (1978) An observation of thromboxane A_2 in arterial blood after cholesterol feeding in rabbits. Jap Heart J 19: 748-753

Sinzinger H, Feigl W, Silberbauer K (1979) Prostacyclin generation in atherosclerotic arteries. Lancet ii:469

Slater TF (1972) Free radical mechanisms in tissue injury. Pion Ltd., London

Szczeklik A, Gryglewski RJ, Nizankowski R, Musial J, Pieton R, Mruk J (1978a) Circulatory and antiplatelet effects of intravenous prostacyclin in healthy man. Pharm Res Commun 10: 545-556

Szczeklik A, Gryglewski RJ, Musial J, Grodzinska L, Serwonska M, Marcinkiewicz E (1978b) Thromboxane generation and platelet aggregation in survivals of myocardial infarction. Thromb Haem 40: 66-74

Szczeklik A, Nizankowski R, Skawinski S, Szczeklik J, Gluszko P, Gryglewski RJ (1979) Successful therapy of advanced arteriosclerosis obliterans with prostacyclin. Lancet i: 1111-1114

Tansik RL, Namm DH, White HL (1978) Synthesis of prostaglandin 6-keto $F_{1\alpha}$ by cultured aortic smooth muscle cells and stimulation of its formation in a coupled system with platelet lysates. Prostaglandins 15: 399-408

Tateson JE, Moncada S, Vane JR (1977) Effects of prostacyclin (PGX) on cyclic AMP concentrations in human platelets. Prostaglandins 13: 389-399

Ubatuba FB, Moncada S, Vane JR (1979) The effect of prostacyclin (PGI_2) on platelet behaviour, thrombus formation in vivo and bleeding time. Thromb Haem 41: 425-434

Vargaftig BB, Chignard M (1975) Substancces that increase the cyclic AMP content prevent platelet aggregation and concurrent release of pharmacologically active substances evoked by arachidonic acid. Agents and Actions 5: 137-144

Vermylen J, Chamone DAF, Verstraete M (1979) Stimulation of prostacyclin release from vessel wall by BAYg6575, an antithrombotic compound. Lancet i:518-520

Von Lossonczy TO, Ruiter A, Bronsgeest-Schoute HC, van Gent CM, Hermus RJJ (1978) The effect of a fish diet on serum lipids in healthy human subjects. Am J Clin Nutr 31: 1340

Weihrauch JL, Brignoli CA, Reeves JB, Iverson JL (1977) Fatty acid composition of margarines, processed fats and oils. Food Technology 31: 80

Weiss HJ, Turitto VT (1979) Prostacyclin (prostaglandin I_2, PGI_2) inhibits platelet adhesion and thrombus formation on subendothelium. Blood 53: 244-250

Weiss SJ, Turk J, Needleman P (1979) A mechanism for the hydroperoxide-mediated inactivation of prostacyclin synthetase. Blood 53: 1191-1196

Weksler BB, Marcus AJ, Jaffe EA (1977a) Synthesis of prostaglandin I_2 (prostacyclin) by cultured human and bovine endothelial cells. Proc Natl Acad Sci USA 74: 3922-3926

Weksler BB, Knapp JM, Jaffe EA (1977b) Prostacyclin (PGI_2) synthesized by cultured endothelial cells modulates polymorphonuclear leukocyte function. Blood 50(5): Suppl 1. p287

Whittle BJR, Moncada S, Vane JR (1978) Comparison of the effects of prostacyclin (PGI_2), prostaglandin E_1 and D_2 on platelet aggregation in different species. Prostaglandins 16: 373-388

Williams KI, Downing I I (1977) Prostaglandin and thromboxane production by rat decidual microsomes. Prostaglandins 14: 813-817

Woodford FP, Bottcher, CJF, Oette K, Ahrens EH Jr. (1965) The artifactual nature of lipid peroxides detected in extracts of human aorta. J Atheroscler Res 5: 311-316

Woods HF, Ash G, Weston MJ, Bunting S, Moncada S, Vane JR (1978) Prostacyclin can replace heparin in haemodialysis in dogs. Lancet ii: 1075-1077

The Platelet-Derived Growth Factor[1]

Russell Ross, Arthur Vogel, Elaine Raines, and Beverly Kariya

Introduction

The platelet is well known for its importance in the process of blood coagulation and hemostasis. However, only in recent years has it become apparent
that this cell also plays an important role in the process of inflammation
and in the stimulation of cell proliferation. It is in this latter context
that the platelet may play a vital role in the process of atherogenesis (Ross
and Glomset 1976; Ross and Harker 1976). The discovery that platelets are
important in cell proliferation was made as a result of the observation that
serum derived from cell-free plasma lacked the capacity to induce DNA synthesis in cells in culture (Ross et al. 1974). At the same time, however,
such plasma-derived serum retains the capacity to sustain many diploid cells
in culture in a quiescent and well-nourished state for periods as long as six
to eight weeks. Re-addition of whole blood serum to quiescent cultures of
cells such as 3T3 or smooth muscle in plasma-derived serum initiates proliferation in these cell populations (Ross et al. 1978) (Figure 1).

Platelets were shown to be the principal source of mitogenic activity in whole
blood serum in experiments in which platelet extracts were added to cells made
quiescent in cell-free, plasma-derived serum. Frozen-thawed platelets or the
supernatant from thrombin-released platelets restored growth-promoting activity to plasma-derived serum. The platelet-derived growth factor stimulates
smooth muscle (Ross et al. 1974), fibroblasts (Rutherford and Ross 1976),
3T3 cells (Kohler and Lipton 1974), and glial cells (Westermark and Wasteson
1976). If cells are cultured in the presence of 5% cell-free, plasma-derived
serum, less than 3% of the cells will incorporate thymidine into DNA and go
on to divide (Rutherford and Ross 1976). Exposure of such quiescent cells
to the platelet-derived growth factor causes initiation of DNA synthesis
within 12 to 18 hours, and is maximal at approximately 24 hours. The cells
can be exposed to the platelet-derived growth factor for as little as one
hour, followed by thorough washing, and a population of cells that are in the
appropriate position in the cell cycle will be committed to undergo a cell
doubling if sufficient plasma is present.

Characteristics of the Platelet-Derived Growth Factor

Several laboratories are in the process of purifying and characterizing the
platelet-derived growth factor. Most approaches have utilized frozen-thawed,
outdated human platelet-rich plasma. The platelets are concentrated, and
supernatant material obtained after freeze-thawing and centrifugation is chromatographed through a series of steps including Carboxymethyl Sephadex, gel

[1] This research was supported in part by grants from the USPHS, no. AM 13970,
HL 18645, AG-00299 and RR-00166.

442

filtration, and various combinations of isoelectric focusing, affinity chromatography, and SDS preparative gel electrophoresis.

In our laboratory we have used the steps denoted in Table 1 for the separation of the molecule. The series of chromatographic steps used in this approach has provided relatively large yields at each step. We anticipate that this approach with further refinement will provide a homogeneous protein and can be used as a large-scale preparatory procedure. The data thus far demonstrate that the platelet-derived growth factor is a highly stable, cationic protein (pI 9.5-10.3). The molecule is stable after exposure to denaturing agents such as guanidine hydrochloride, urea and SDS. It is also stable at 56°C for 30 minutes or 100°C for 2 to 10 minutes. Its stability is also retained over a wide pH range (2-10).

There is some disagreement as to the molecular weight of the nascent protein as determined by SDS gel electrophoresis. Molecular weights have been reported of both ∿30,000 (Heldin et al. 1979; Ross et al. 1979) and 35,000 (Antoniades 1979) after elution from SDS gels. The method is in general subject to question as an absolute reference. The platelet-derived growth factor, being extremely basic, would bind presumably the same amount of SDS as reference proteins, but its overall net charge would not be as acidic as the references. In addition, since reduction destroys the biological activity (Antoniades et al. 1979; Heldin et al. 1979; Ross et al. 1979), the gels are run under non-reducing conditions and thus the disulfide bonds would prevent formation of the ideal rod-like particles and may also prevent maximal binding

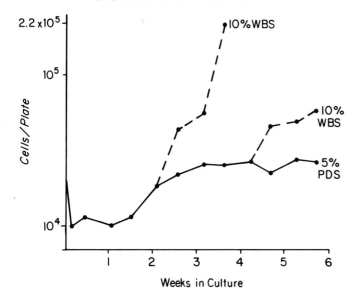

MI26THA
T_2, 4/4/78

Maintenance of Smooth Muscle Cells in 5% PDS

FIG. 1. Arterial smooth muscle cells from <u>Macaca</u> <u>nemestrina</u> were plated in DME containing 5% pooled homologous cell-free, plasma-derived serum. They were maintained in this medium for 6 weeks and were fed three times weekly. At 2 and 4 weeks, subgroups were changed to 10% pooled homologous whole blood serum.

Table 1. Platelet-Derived Growth Factor

Fraction	Specific Activity μg/ml Media	Units of Growth-Promoting Activity Per mg	% Recovery of Growth-Promoting Activity From Starting Material	For Individual Steps
*5% Calf Serum Standard Conditions	3250	1.0		
Human Platelet-Rich Plasma frozen-thawed, defibrinogenated	1075	3.0	100	
CM-Sephadex, fraction III eluted 0.1 M(NH$_4$)$_2$CO$_3$, pH 8.9	3.0	1083	42	42
Biogel Filtration, fraction II mw range 10-40,000 in 1.0 N acetic acid	0.79	4167	30	71
DEAE-Sephadex, fraction I flow thru in 50mM Tris, pH 8.9	0.52	6250	19	64
Phenyl-Sepharose, fraction III 50mM Tris, 3M GuHCl, pH 8.9	0.15	21667	15	79

* All values normalized to growth response of additional 5% calf serum. Growth-promoting activity assayed on Balb 3T3 cells grown to confluence in 5% calf serum in either 35mm plates or 16mm wells (4-5 x 10^4 cells/cm^2). Values represent an average of 2 to 5 experiments. Protein concentrations were estimated from A$_{280}$ or folin.

of SDS. Other methods of analysis will be necessary to ascertain the molecular weight of the nascent protein.

There also is a difference of opinion as to the molecular weight once the platelet-derived growth factor is reduced with values of 13,000 (Antoniades et al. 1979) and two distinct peaks of 13,000 and 17,000 (Heldin et al. 1979). In the former case the platelet-derived growth factor was treated with fluorescamine and in the latter it was labeled with ^{125}I, and this difference in treatment may account for the molecular weight differences. There is agreement, however, that reduction of the platelet-derived growth factor destroys most of the biological activity (Antoniades et al. 1979; Heldin et al. 1979; Ross et al. 1979), with the degree of activity reduction proportional to the efficiency of the reduction.

Antoniades et al. (1975) earlier isolated a serum-derived growth factor by similar methods of ion exchange chromatography. Antibodies to this factor cross-react with material present in the platelets, suggesting that they are one and the same (Antoniades and Scher 1977). In addition, these same investigators have utilized this antibody to develop a radioimmunoassay for the serum-derived growth factor and have found that serum derived from whole blood contains approximately 770 pg of the growth factor per milligram of protein, whereas serum derived from platelet-poor blood contains approximately 112 pg of the factor per milligram of protein. With the material purified from platelets in the studies of Antoniades et al. (1979), they have demonstrated that 1 to 2 ng of the growth factor stimulates confluent 3T3 cells to replicate in culture.

Platelet-Derived Growth Factor Acts Coordinately with Plasma

Vogel et al. (1978) and Pledger et al. (1977) have shown that both plasma and the platelet-derived growth factor are necessary to induce both DNA synthesis and cell cycle traverse by cells in culture that are responsive to serum. Pledger et al. (1977) suggest that the platelet-derived growth factor appears to commit cells to progress from G_0 to G_1 and to enter the S phase of the cell cycle. They have suggested that the platelet-derived growth factor commits the cells to synthesize DNA and that they will not traverse further into the cycle without plasma constituents. Stiles et al. (1979) have suggested that one of the molecules in plasma necessary for cell cycle traverse is somatomedin C.

Vogel et al. (1978) have shown that both the platelet-derived growth factor and plasma are required for cell proliferation in vitro. The amount of each in the culture medium will control the amount of proliferation of cells such as 3T3 cells. The platelet-derived growth factor acts to recruit quiescent cells into cell cycle traverse in a dose-dependent fashion in the presence of optimal amounts of plasma. In the presence of limiting concentrations of platelet factor and optimal amounts of plasma, only a small fraction of the cells synthesize DNA and go on to divide. For cells such as 3T3 to undergo multiple rounds of division in the presence of high concentrations of the platelet-derived growth factor, plasma must also be present. When the plasma is limiting (0.5% or less) and the amount of platelet factor is optimal, some or all of the cells will undergo one round of cell division and then cease to divide. Further addition of optimal amounts of plasma will then permit multiple cell doublings. Thus, in the absence of adequate amounts of plasma the cells are unable to utilize the platelet-derived growth factor that is present to undergo more than one round of division.

In studies to determine the role of the platelet-derived growth factor in density-dependent inhibition of proliferation in 3T3 cells, Vogel et al. (1979) have demonstrated that the level of platelet-derived growth factor is the limiting entity that determines the final cell density in cultures grown in whole blood serum (Figure 2). In addition, the amount of platelet-derived growth factor per cell needed to stimulate proliferation increases with increasing cell density so that at high density the amount of platelet-derived growth factor in the medium is not sufficient to stimulate cell growth. Addition of plasma-derived serum at this point has no effect upon such density-inhibited cultures (Figure 2).

Other Effects of the Platelet-Derived Growth Factor

The platelet-derived growth factor has been shown to have several different effects upon cells such as 3T3 or smooth muscle. Exposure of quiescent cells to the platelet-derived growth factor induces a marked enhancement of pinocytosis. Davies and Ross (1978) demonstrated that endocytosis of ^{14}C-sucrose and of horseradish peroxidase was increased several-fold upon exposure of cells to the platelet-derived growth factor. Habenicht et al. (1979) observed that the platelet-derived growth factor increases cholesterol synthesis in cultured monkey arterial smooth muscle cells. In addition, this growth factor increases phospholipase A_2 activity in 3T3 cells in culture (Shier 1979).

Burke and Ross (1977) have also shown that collagen synthesis is markedly stimulated as a result of general stimulation of protein synthesis by exposure of smooth muscle cells or fibroblasts to whole blood serum versus plasma-derived serum, presumably as a result of the action of the platelet-derived growth factor. Wight (personal communication) has observed in a preliminary series of studies that glycosaminoglycan formation is enhanced by the factor as well.

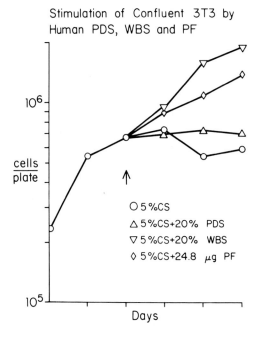

Stimulation of Confluent 3T3 by Human PDS, WBS and PF

10^6

cells / plate

○ 5% CS
△ 5% CS + 20% PDS
▽ 5% CS + 20% WBS
◇ 5% CS + 24.8 μg PF

10^5

Days

FIG. 2. 3T3 cells were plated at 2×10^5 cells/plate in 35 mm dishes containing 1.5 ml of 5% calf serum-supplemented medium. Three days later, when the cells had become quiescent, platelet factor, human PDS or whole blood serum was added. ^3H-Tdr (2.5 μCi/ml, 6.17 Ci/mmol) was added at the time of addition of growth factors. Plates were processed for autoradiography and determination of cell number at the indicated times. Platelet factor was partially purified by carboxymethyl Sephadex chromatography.

Thus, the biological effects of the platelet-derived growth factor cover a broad spectrum of effects, some of which may be due to factors other than the growth factor, since several of these studies were performed with a crude extract derived from platelets. It remains to be determined whether all of the effects that have been shown are due to the actions of the same molecule or to several different molecules derived from the thrombocyte.

The Role of the Platelet in Atherogenesis

Numerous investigations have demonstrated that intact platelet function is a necessary prerequisite for induction of the intimal smooth muscle proliferative lesions of experimental atherosclerosis. Harker et al. (1976) observed that platelet survival was markedly decreased in baboons made chronically homocystinemic. Associated with this decrease in platelet survival was evidence of injury to approximately 10% of the endothelium of the aorta. After being homocystinemic for three months, the baboons had early proliferative fibrous plaques. Harker et al. (1976) were able to inhibit the intimal smooth muscle proliferative response in these lesions by treatment of the baboons with dipyridamole. Dipyridamole specifically inhibited platelet adherence and release and normalized platelet survival. Under these circumstances the amount of endothelial injury remained unchanged; however, no intimal proliferative lesions were present. Therefore, interference with platelet function appears to be important in inhibition of intimal smooth muscle proliferation.

In a similar series of experiments, Harker et al. (unpublished data) have studied the same model of chronic homocystinemia in the baboon by treating the animals with sulfinpyrazone. Sulfinpyrazone also normalized platelet survival in these animals; however, in this instance the sulfinpyrazone somehow appears to protect the endothelium, since the amount of "injured" endothelium was markedly decreased. It is presumed that by protecting the endothelium platelet interaction at the sites of endothelial injury is prevented; thus, platelet survival is normal and platelet release is interfered with. Under these circumstances they again observed that the intimal smooth muscle proliferative lesions of homocysteine-induced atherosclerosis were inhibited.

In a different series of studies, Moore et al. (1976) and Friedman et al. (1977) used intra-arterial catheters to abrade and remove the endothelium in a series of rabbits that subsequently developed atherosclerotic plaques. If the rabbits were made thrombocytopenic with an anti-platelet serum, then no intimal proliferative lesions resulted from the injury to the endothelium.

In a series of studies of swine with von Willebrand's disease, Fuster and his colleagues (1978) also observed that the platelet plays an important role in experimental atherogenesis. They studied normal swine and von Willebrand swine, both made equally hyperlipemic with a high-fat diet. The normal swine on the high-fat diet developed extensive lesions of atherosclerosis, whereas the fat-fed von Willebrand swine had fatty infiltrates but very few, if any, proliferative lesions. In swine homozygous for von Willebrand's disease, factor VIII antigen is missing and platelets are apparently unable to adhere and undergo the release reaction.

All of these in vivo studies strongly support the notion that the platelet plays a key role in inducing intimal smooth muscle proliferation in experimental atherogenesis. One key question remains to be answered. Is the platelet-derived growth factor the specific agent responsible for this intimal smooth muscle proliferative response when platelet activation occurs? The answer to this question will help to close the chasm of evidence in relation to understanding this phenomenon.

447

Summary

The platelet can be shown to be the repository of an extremely potent growth
factor that plays the role as the principal mitogen in serum that induces
cell proliferation in culture. In addition, intact platelet function is a
necessary prerequisite to inducing the intimal smooth muscle proliferative
lesions of experimental atherogenesis. Much work remains to be done to
further characterize this growth factor, to determine its role _in vivo_ in
atherosclerosis and to understand its mode of action at the cellular and
molecular levels.

Acknowledgment

The authors would like to gratefully acknowledge the expert technical assistance of Mary Jane Rivest and M. Patricia Beckmann.

References

Antoniades HN, Scher CD (1977) Radioimmunoassay of a human serum growth factor
    for Balb/c-3T3 cells: derivation from platelets. Proc Natl Acad Sci USA
    74: 1973-1977
Antoniades HN, Stathakos D, Scher CD (1975) Isolation of a cationic poly-
    peptide from human serum that stimulates proliferation of 3T3 cells.
    Proc Natl Acad Sci USA 72: 2635-2639
Antoniades HN, Scher CD, Stiles CD (1979) Purification of the human platelet-
    derived growth factor. Proc Natl Acad Sci USA 76: 1809-1813
Burke J, Ross R (1977) Collagen synthesis by monkey arterial smooth muscle
    cells during proliferation and quiescence in culture. Exp Cell Res 107:
    387-395
Davies PF, Ross R (1978) Mediation of pinocytosis in cultured arterial smooth
    muscle and endothelial cells by platelet-derived growth factor. J Cell
    Biol 79: 663-671
Friedman RJ, Stemerman MB, Wenz B, Moore S, Gauldie J, Gent M, Tiell ML,
    Spaet TH (1977) The effect of thrombocytopenia on experimental arterio-
    sclerotic lesion formation in rabbits. Smooth muscle proliferation and
    reendothelialization. J Clin Invest 60: 1191-1201
Fuster V, Bowie EJW, Lewis JC, Fass DN, Owen CA Jr, Brown AL (1978) Resistance
    to arteriosclerosis in pigs with von Willebrand's disease. J Clin Invest
    61: 722-730
Habenicht A, Glomset J, Ross R (1979) Platelet growth factor increases choles-
    terol synthesis in cultured monkey smooth muscle cells. Abstract No. 230,
    5th International Symposium on Atherosclerosis, Houston, Texas, November
    6-9, 1979
Harker L, Ross R, Slichter S, Scott C (1976) Homocystine-induced arterio-
    sclerosis: the role of endothelial cell injury and platelet response in
    its genesis. J Clin Invest 58: 731-741
Heldin CH, Westermark B, Wasteson A (1979) Platelet derived growth factor:
    purification and partial characterization. Proc Natl Acad Sci USA 76:
    3722-3726
Kohler N, Lipton A (1974) Platelets as a source of fibroblast growth-promoting
    activity. Exp Cell Res 87: 297-301
Moore S, Friedman RJ, Singal DP, Gauldie J, Blajchman M (1976) Inhibition of
    injury induced thromboatherosclerotic lesions by antiplatelet serum in
    rabbits. Thromb Diath Haemorrh 35: 70-81

Pledger WJ, Stiles CD, Antoniades HN, Scher CD (1977) Induction of DNA synthesis in BALB/c 3T3 cells by serum components: reevaluation of the commitment process. Proc Natl Acad Sci USA 74: 4481–4485

Ross R, Glomset J (1976) The pathogenesis of atherosclerosis. N Engl J Med 295: 369–377, 420–425

Ross R, Harker L (1976) Hyperlipidemia and atherosclerosis. Science 193: 1094–1100

Ross R, Glomset J, Kariya B, Harker L (1974) A platelet-dependent serum factor that stimulates the proliferation of arterial smooth muscle cells in vitro. Proc Natl Acad Sci USA 71: 1207–1210

Ross R, Nist C, Kariya B, Rivest M, Raines E, Callis J (1978) Physiological quiescence in plasma-derived serum: influence of platelet-derived growth factor on cell growth in culture. J Cell Physiol 97: 497–508

Ross R, Vogel A, Davies P, Raines E, Kariya B, Rivest M, Gustafson C, Glomset J (1979) The platelet-derived growth factor and plasma control cell proliferation. In: Hormones and cell culture. Cold Spring Harbor, NY (Sixth Cold Spring Harbor Conference, pp 3–16)

Rutherford RB, Ross R (1976) Platelet factors stimulate fibroblasts and smooth muscle cells quiescent in plasma serum to proliferate. J Cell Biol 69: 196–203

Shier WT (1979) Serum stimulation of phospholipase A_2 and prostaglandin release in 3T3 cells is associated with platelet-derived growth promoting activity. Proc Natl Acad Sci USA (in press)

Stiles CD, Capone GT, Scher CD, Antoniades HN, Van Wyck JJ, Pledger WJ (1979) Dual control of cell growth by somatomedins and platelet derived growth factor. Proc Natl Acad Sci USA 76: 1279–1283

Vogel A, Raines E, Kariya B, Rivest M, Ross R (1978) Coordinate control of 3T3 cell proliferation by platelet-derived growth factor and plasma components. Proc Natl Acad Sci USA 75: 2810–2814

Westermark B, Wasteson A (1976) A platelet factor stimulating human normal glial cells. Exp Cell Res 98: 170–174

Portacaval Shunt for Type II Hyperlipidemia[1]

Thomas E. Starzl, Lawrence Koep, and Richard Weil, III

Amelioration of Type 2 hyperlipidemia by completely diverting portacaval shunt was first reported in 1973 (Starzl et al). Since then, 5 additional patients have been similarly treated by us and others have been treated elsewhere. The compiled first cases have been published (Starzl, Putnam and Koep 1978) and, doubtless more will be added by Stein in his review later today. My remarks today will be confined to a brief description of 6 patients treated at the University of Colorado from one month to 6 1/2 years ago.

Case Material

All 6 patients had Type 2 hyperlipidemia. Familial studies always were obtained to determine the probability of the homozygous or heterozygous state. The conclusions were compatible with tissue culture analysis of cholesterol synthesis. Five children had homozygous disease. A 52 year old man was heterozygous.

The 6 patients had been followed in established lipid centers during long periods of study and treatment. The referring physicians were H.P. Chase of Denver (Case 1), D.W. Bilheimer, J.L. Goldstein, and M.S. Brown of Dallas (Case 2), N.B. Javitt of New York and J. Rey of Paris (Case 3), E.H. Ahrens of New York (Cases 4 and 6), and E.J. Schaefer of Bethesda (Case 5). By collaborating with authorities in the field, three objectives were met. First, the patients were assured accurate diagnosis as well as trials with the most advanced methods of non-surgical treatment including (Cases 3 and 5) plasma exchange. Second, sophisticated studies of cholesterol and/or bile acid metabolism at the referring institution were obtained before and after the brief (one to two weeks) admission to Colorado General Hospital for surgical care. Finally, the aftercare and conclusions about the clinical results were the purview of objective observers who were not notable proponents of a surgical approach. Data and photographs were provided by the referring physicians, of whom some have published separate investigations.

The preoperative cardiovascular status of the patients was variable. In addition to aortic stenosis, (gradient 56 mmHg) Patient 1 had had a myocardial infarction 1 1/2 months before portacaval shunt, leading to a large left ventricular aneurysm. Patient 6 had had a myocardial infarction treated 5 years earlier with a triple coronary artery bypass; the diseased residual vessels were not susceptible to further reconstruction. Patients 2 and 5 had continuous angina pectoris and multiple coronary artery lesions, and in

[1]This work was supported by research grants from the Veterans Administration; by grant numbers AM-17260 and AM-07772 from the National Institutes of Health; and by grant numbers RR-00051 and RR-00069 from the General Clinical Research Centers Program of the Division of Research Resources, National Institute of Health.

addition Patient 2 had a large intraluminal plaque occupying two thirds of the ascending aortic lumen. Patient 3 had large asymptomatic intraaortic plaques in the chest and abdomen. Patient 4 had aortic stenosis with a gradient of 35 mmHg during a cardiac output of 5 1/min. Tendinocutaneous xanthomas were present in each case, and were exceptionally prominent in Patients 1, 2 and 5. The average serum cholesterol concentrations before portacaval shunt are shown in Table 1. These values usually were obtained during a low cholesterol diet and in spite of medicinal therapy. All 6 patients had normal liver function tests.

Results

There was no operative mortality nor any surgical complications. Five of the 6 patients are still alive. The first patient died suddenly 18 1/2 months after operation, probably from a cardiac arrhythmia.

Effect of serum cholesterol

A fall in serum cholesterol concentrations was already identifiable within a few postoperative weeks, and by August and September 1979, were at the levels shown in Table 1. In some patients, slow declines continued for a year or longer after operation. Late secondary rises of serum cholesterol concentrations were not seen. Low density lipoprotein (LDL) falls paralleled those of cholesterol.

Effect on xanthomas

In Cases 1-5, there was a remarkable involution of the tendinocutaneous xanthomas which was evident within a month or two by a softening of these lesions and by the development of redundant overlying skin folds. Complete disappearance in the oldest cases required one to 3 years. Patient 6 who had minimal xanthomas has been followed for too short a time to see a definite change.

Cardiovascular disease

During the first 16 months postoperatively, the aortic valve gradient in Patient 1 fell from 56 to 10 mmHg, but she had a large ventricular aneurysm and residual stenoses of the right, left main, and circumflex coronary arteries. An error was made at that time by deciding against coronary revascularization since the patient's death 2 1/2 months later was apparently due to a cardiac arrhythmia.

Patient 2 had myocardial ischemia and persistent angina. Ultimately, she underwent aortic and mitral valve replacement and double coronary artery bypass. She is now 5 years postoperative and asymptomatic under treatment with a low cholesterol diet, cholestyramine, and Atromid-S. Patients 3-6 have not had follow up angiographic studies.

The effect on the liver

Standard liver function tests have not been perturbed except for minor and generally persistent increases in alkaline phosphatase and serum transaminases. Patient 3 has had slightly elevated blood ammonia concentrations. None of the patients have had encephalopathy nor have they experienced pyschological disturbances.

Patient 1 had a liver biopsy at the time of and 6 months after portacaval shunt. The liver was examined again after her death at 18 1/2 months. The findings in the second 2 specimens included hepatocyte atrophy, depletion of rough endoplasmic reticulum, deglycogenation, and fatty infiltration. These same hepatic changes have been documented after complete portal diversion in all species so far studied including rats, dogs, swine, subhuman primates and humans (Putnam, Porter and Starzl, 1976).

Physique

The growth and development of the children have been uninterrupted or in some instances somewhat more rapid than preoperatively. Growth spurts were not seen of the magnitude of those following portacaval shunt for glycogen storage disease.

Discussion

Most of the reported patients with Type 2 hyperlipidemia treated with portal diversion have had reductions in serum cholesterol although the degree has been variable (Starzl, Putnam and Koep 1977). Thrombosis of the portacaval shunt with restoration by collaterals of hepatopetal splanchnic flow has been a well documented cause of failure.

The antilipidemic effect of portacaval shunt has not been satisfactorily examined. It does not depend upon the prior existence of high serum lipids. A fall in serum cholesterol and often in triglycerides and phospholipids can be produced with this procedure in normal rats, dogs, pigs and monkeys as reviewed by Starzl, Putnam and Koep (1978). The penalty is damage to the liver which is striking by histopathological criteria but which is more subtle as measured by liver function. The eventual consequence in pigs, dogs, and monkeys is hepatic encephalopathy and death within a few months. In rats and humans, portacaval shunt is compatible with long survival inspite of the fact that the morphologic changes produced in the liver are no less severe. The antilipidemic effect is probably due in part to reduced hepatic cholesterol synthesis by the altered liver (Starzl, Putnam and Koep 1978), but other mechanisms may play a significant role.

Appreciation of the potential hepatic and cerebral complications of portacaval shunt dictated our earlier policy of treating only patients with homozygous disease who were refractory to medical therapy and who seemed to have a grim short term prognosis. The fact that our first 5 patients were children may have contributed to their resistance to encephalopathy. The fate of our heterozygous adult patient will be a matter of great interest in assessing broader applicability of portal diversion for the treatment of hyperlipidemia.

The hope that vascular disease might be controlled or even regress has been supported by observations such as those in Case 1. However, a complete reversal of vascular lesions which possess a fibrotic component is often not a realistic hope even though there is dramatic resolution of the visible peripheral xanthomas and objective evidence that the same can occur within the heart valves and blood vessels. An aggressive surgical approach such as that taken in Case 2 might have saved our first patient. The combination of coronary revascularization plus portacaval shunt used in Cases 2 and 6 deserves further trials.

Table 1. Patients with type II hyperlipidemia treated with portal diversion at the University of Colorado Health Sciences Center.

No.	Age/Sex		Date Shunt	Cholesterol (mg%)		Clinical State
				Before	After*	
1	12	F	3/1/73	770	290 (38%)	Died after 18 1/2 months
2	7	F	10/4/74	1000	400 (40%)	Excellent
3	8	M	8/5/75	1000	510 (51%)	Excellent
4	5	M	12/14/78	800	515 (64%)	Excellent
5	14	M	6/19/79	880	600 (68%)	Excellent
6	52	M	8/7/79	575	390 (68%)	Too soon to evaluate

*Last values for living patients in late August and early September, 1979. Percentages are those of preoperative values.

References

Putnam CW, Porter KA, Starzl TE (1976) Hepatic encephalopathy and light and electron micrographic changes of the baboon liver after portal diversion. Ann Surg 184: 155-161

Starzl TE, Chase HP, Putnam CW, Porter KA (1973) Portacaval shunt for the treatment of hyperlipoproteinemia. Lancet 2: 940-944

Starzl TE, Putnam CW, Koep LJ (1978) Portacaval shunt and hyperlipidemia. Arch Surg 113: 71-74

Combined Medico-Surgical Strategy for Severe Familial Hypercholesterolaemia

Gilbert Thompson, Nicolas Myant, Celia Oakley, Robert Steiner, and Ralph Sapsford

The term severe is used here in the context of familial hypercholesterolaemia (FH) to encompass homozygotes and heterozygotes with coronary heart disease (CHD). The preceding papers have dealt with the various non-pharmacological methods used to lower serum cholesterol levels and we wish to describe how we have combined such measures, especially plasma exchange (Thompson et al. 1975), with surgical procedures aimed at correcting the cardiovascular complications of severe FH. The presence of such complications can often be suspected by non-invasive diagnostic methods but delineation of their severity necessitates angiographic and haemodynamic assessment.

Angiographic Features of FH

Florid but localised atheroma of the supravalvular part of the aorta is a well-described feature of homozygous FH which causes a characteristic narrowing of the aortic root at angiography (Stanley et al. 1965). Atheromatous involvement of the aorta spreads downwards into the sinuses of Valsalva and encroaches on the coronary ostia, causing ostial stenosis. Although these features can occur in a milder form in heterozygotes the latter differ in one important respect in that they do not develop lesions of the aortic valve (Roberts et al. 1973). Thickening and fibrosis of the valve cusps leading to aortic stenosis (Cook et al. 1947) seems to be restricted to homozygotes and it is this lesion, rather than the supravalvular narrowing, which is responsible for the development of a left ventricular-aortic pressure gradient. One other angiographic feature of note is the frequency with which disease of the main stem of the left coronary artery occurs in both homozygotes and heterozygotes (Bloch et al. 1976). Unless treated surgically such lesions are known to be associated with a high risk of sudden death.

Management of Homozygotes

During the past 5 years 6 homozygotes have been investigated and treated, as shown in Table 1. We regard the presence of a haemodynamically significant gradient across the aortic valve as an indication for surgical intervention. One approach is to enlarge the aortic annulus, using the Konno operation (Konno et al. 1975), and replace the aortic valve with a Bjork-Shiley prosthesis, simultaneously inserting triple coronary artery bypass graphs (CABG) obtained from the saphenous vein; this was done successfully in A.R. and N.E. In neither of these patients nor in P.A., who died immediately after a CABG operation, had effective control of hypercholesterolaemia been achieved during the preceding years. However, it should be possible to achieve this postoperatively by means of plasma exchange, via an arteriovenous fistula if necessary. In the other 3 homozygotes, whose hypercholesterolaemia has been effectively controlled by regular plasma exchange, aortic gradients and angiographic abnormalities have remained unchanged, as illustrated in Table 1 and Fig. 1.

Table 1. Left ventricular-aortic systolic pressure gradients in FH homozygotes studied at Hammersmith Hospital, 1974-1979

Patient	Sex	Current Age	Date	Gradient (mm of Hg)	Treatment		
					Pre-op	Operation	Post-op
P.A.	F	(23)	9/74	35	PE	CABG	Died
			11/76	75			
A.R.	F	29	1/75	34	PE,	B-S valve	PE via
			11/78	130	P-C shunt	& CABG	A-VF
R.W.	M	26	10/75	40			
			6/77	30	PE	–	–
			5/78	50			
D.L.	M	16	1/77	19			
			1/78	0	PE	–	–
			10/78	20			
M.M.	M	15	12/78	0	PE via A-VF	–	–
N.E.	M	19	4/79	80	No PE	B-S valve & CABG	PE planned

Abbreviations:-
PE: plasma exchange
P-C: portacaval
B-S: Bjork-Shiley
CABG: coronary artery bypass graft
A-VF: arterio-venous fistula

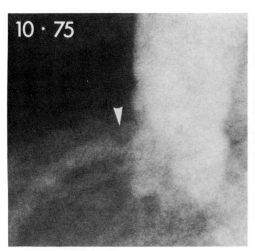
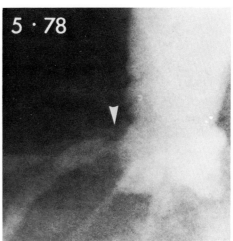

FIG. 1. Aortagrams (lateral view) in a homozygote (R.W.) before and after 2½ years of plasma exchange, showing non-progression of aortic root lesion and right coronary ostial stenosis (arrowed).

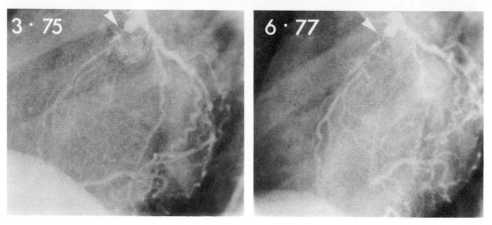

FIG. 2. Lack of improvement in severe stricture (arrowed) of anterior descending branch of left coronary artery in a heterozygote after 21 months of plasma exchange (left anterior oblique view).

Management of Heterozygotes

Four heterozygotes with angina have been studied in a similar manner. All had advanced triple vessel disease on angiography but none showed any narrowing of the aortic root nor any aortic gradient. One patient, who was found to have severe left ventricular dyskinesia, died suddenly after 5 months but the other 3 completed 14-23 months of plasma exchange. Two subsequently underwent CABG operations, one for clinical reasons the other because angiography revealed no improvement following plasma exchange (Fig. 2). The remaining patient showed sufficient symptomatic and angiographic improvement with plasma exchange (Fig. 3) to obviate the need for CABG. The hypercholesterolaemia in these 3 heterozygotes is currently being controlled by conventional means alone.

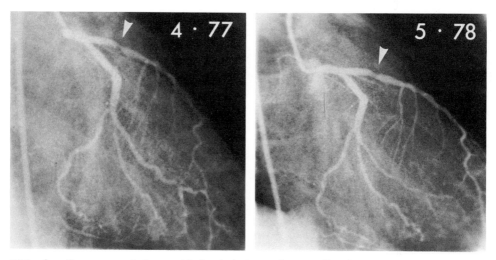

FIG. 3. Improvement in partial stricture (arrowed) of anterior descending branch of left coronary artery in a heterozygote after 13 months of plasma exchange (right anterior oblique view).

Conclusions

Intensive application of effective cholesterol-lowering measures may prevent progression of aorto-coronary atheroma in homozygotes and possibly induce regression in heterozygotes. Certain lesions are irreversible however, presumably due to their fibrotic nature, and require surgical relief. These include advanced strictures of the ostia and major branches of the coronary arteries and aortic valve stenosis, the latter affecting only homozygotes. Post-operatively hypercholesterolaemia is probably best controlled by twice-monthly plasma exchange in homozygotes, and by conventional therapy or ileal bypass in heterozygotes.

References

Bloch A, Dinsmore RE, Lees RS (1976) Coronary angiographic findings in Type II and Type IV hyperlipoproteinaemia. Lancet 1: 928-930

Cook CD, Smith HL, Giesen CW, Berdez GL (1947) Xanthoma tuberosum, aortic stenosis, coronary sclerosis and angina pectoris. Amer J Dis Child 73: 326-333

Konno S, Yasuharu I, Yoshinao I, Nakajima M, Tatsuno K (1975) A new method for prosthetic valve replacement in congenital aortic stenosis associated with hypoplasia of the aortic valve ring. J Thorac Cardiovasc Surg 70: 909-917

Roberts WC, Ferrans WJ, Levy RI, Fredrickson DS (1973) Cardiovascular pathology in hyperlipoproteinemia. Amer J Cardiol 31: 557-570

Stanley P, Chartrand C, Davignon A (1965) Acquired aortic stenosis in a twelve-year old girl with xanthomatosis. New Engl J Med 273: 1378-1380

Thompson GR, Lowenthal R, Myant NB (1975) Plasma exchange in the management of homozygous familial hypercholesterolaemia. Lancet 1: 1208-1211

Plasma Exchange in the Treatment of Familial Hypercholesterolemia[1]

G. Michael B. Berger, François Bonnici, Hymie S. Joffe, and Daniel W. Dubovsky

Introduction

Homozygous familial hypercholesterolemia does not readily respond to conventional forms of lipid-lowering therapy. Nicotinic acid has achieved significant lowering of plasma cholesterol levels (Lux 1972), but in practice
compliance is difficult to maintain and side-effects may be unpleasant and
severe. More heroic measures include: portacaval shunt, partial ileal bypass, hyperalimentation, biliary diversion and plasma exchange (Berger et
al. 1978). Extracorporeal removal of LDL-cholesterol by means of affinity
chromatography has been described (Lupien et al. 1976). Though all forms
of therapy can be faulted on one or more grounds plasma exchange appears to
be the most desirable in its ability to lower plasma cholesterol and its
relative safety and feasibility. We report our experience using repeated
plasma exchange in 3 homozygous patients and in one heterozygote with familial hypercholesterolemia and assess its role in the treatment of this disorder.

Case Reports

Case 1, a 17 year-old white male, previously reported (Berger et al. 1978),
suffers from homozygous familial hypercholesterolemia based upon standard
clinical and biochemical criteria. Despite conventional therapy the patient's
cholesterol remained high (724 mg/100ml) and angina of effort, relieved by
glyceryl trinitrate, developed by the age of 10 years. Immediately prior to
the introduction of plasma exchange an ECG showed ST plane segment depression
of 2.0 mm in leads 2, 3, aVF and V_4-V_6. On coronary angiography a 40-60%
stenosis near the origin of the left anterior descending coronary artery was
noted. Numerous planar, cutaneous xanthomata were present and his Achilles
tendons were thickened. He has received 69 plasma exchanges over a period
of 3 years and 4 months. Cholestyramine (24 g/day) and clofibrate (1.5 g/
day) were administered initially but these were stopped after 31 exchanges
the patient remaining, however, on a cholesterol-lowering diet.

Case 2, a 9 year-old white female has also been reported previously (Berger
et al. 1978). On the basis of accepted clinical and biochemical criteria
she was diagnosed as a case of homozygous familial hypercholesterolemia
complicated by a severe supra-valvular aortic stenosis. A portacaval shunt
performed at another hospital one year prior to the present study did not
elicit a fall in plasma cholesterol (FIG. 1a). Plasma exchange was attempted in order to reduce possible atherosclerotic deposits contributing to the

---

[1] We wish to thank the Cape Provincial Administration, the Medical Research
Council (SA), the Beryl Cronwright Burger Bequest, and the Harry Crossley
Foundation for financial support.

severe aortic stenosis. Chest pain recurred and surgical intervention was undertaken with the removal of the fibrous supra-valvular aortic ring and the insertion of a Dacron® patch. The patient was discharged to her home town on conventional lipid-lowering therapy, digoxin, and propranolol.

Case 3, also a 9 year-old white girl, presented at the age of $2\frac{1}{2}$ years with xanthomata, thickened Achilles tendons and a cholesterol level of 597 mg/100ml. Both parents were hypercholesterolemic and the diagnosis of homozygous familial hypercholesterolemia was made. She remained free of clinical disease until November 1978 when severe and increasing angina on effort developed. Her ECG showed suspicious ST segment depression in lead 1 and coronary angiography revealed a critical narrowing of the left mainstem coronary artery, the remainder of the coronary tree being apparently free of significant disease. Plasma exchange was attempted but angina recurred at rest and a reversed, autogenous, saphenous vein bypass graft from the aorta to the proximal left anterior descending coronary artery was inserted. At operation widespread atheromatous disease of the coronary vessels was present as well as marked swelling of the aortic intima with obliteration of the coronary ostia. A regular schedule of plasma exchange was started shortly after discharge.

Case 4, a 30 year-old white female, presented 5 years earlier with severe fatigue and angina on effort. Her cholesterol and triglyceride plasma levels were raised. Despite widespread xanthomata and the early death of her father following myocardial infarction, the patient has been diagnosed as a case of heterozygous familial hypercholesterolemia since her mother is normocholesterolemic. Coronary angiography revealed severe, diffuse, triple vessel disease and her effort ECG was strongly positive. This patient has received 8 plasma exchanges in 4 months.

Experimental

Plasma exchange was performed throughout using vein-to-vein extracorporeal circulation through an IBM Continuous-Flow Blood Cell Separator. Antecubital veins were utilised where possible but in Case 3 an arterio-venous fistula was necessary. Plasma was replaced with a 4 g/100ml, cholesterol-free, human albumin solution so as to transiently lower total plasma cholesterol values by approximately 50%. The intervals between exchanges varied from 1-3 weeks. Patients have all been maintained on a cholesterol lowering diet but specific drug therapy was inconsistent. Laboratory analyses were carried out using well established standard techniques. Equilibrium cholesterol values refer to measurements done immediately prior to each exchange whereas steady-state refers to levels observed prior to the use of plasma exchange.

Results

Lipid and lipoprotein levels

In all 4 patients, repeated plasma exchange reduced equilibrium plasma cholesterol levels relative to the steady-state values obtained prior to this study. The reduction achieved was greater the shorter the interval between exchanges (FIG. 1a). HDL-cholesterol levels were relatively unaffected or possibly increased with repeated plasma exchange but the LDL-cholesterol shared the fate of total plasma cholesterol. Withdrawal of

cholestyramine and clofibrate in Case 1 did not effect his equilibrium
lipid and lipoprotein values.

Return of perturbed cholesterol towards equilibrium was followed in 3 of
the 4 patients (FIG. 1b). The rate of increase after exchange was greatest
in Case 1. This curve reflects observations made after a number of exchanges
in the early part of the study while the values in Cases 2 and 4 were obtained immediately following the first exchange in each instance. The 1°
rate constant of cholesterol clearance in Case 1, calculated according to
the model used by Apstein et al (1978), was 0.35. This figure yields an
extrapolated steady-state synthetic rate of 179 mg/kg per day. These
figures are considerably in excess of previous reports on cholesterol turnover in homozygotes (Apstein et al. 1978; Bilheimer et al. 1975).

Clinical and Cardiological

Case 1 provides the best test of clinical and cardiological response to
plasma exchange in our series. A marked and steady increase in exercise
tolerance occurred to the point where he currently participates successfully in 8 kilometer road races. Coronary angiography performed 18 months
after the start of plasma exchange showed an equivocal widening of the 40-
60% stenosis present originally. The pre-exchange ECG evidence of ischemia
at rest disappeared after 18 months and during an effort ECG the patient
achieved a pulse rate of 192/minute with no ischemic changes observed though
he complained of pain. The patient's xanthomata disappeared after 18 months
of treatment and have not recurred. Case 3 was re-assessed at periodic
intervals following her bypass graft. During an effort ECG she achieved a
pulse rate of 156/minute without pain or evidence of ischemia. Her exercise

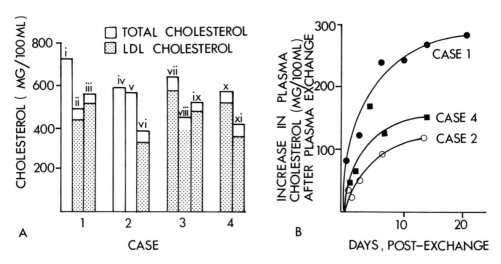

FIG. 1a and b. Effect of plasma exchange on cholesterol values (a) Comparison of steady-state and equilibrium total- and LDL cholesterol values
in Cases 1-4. i steady-state; ii equilibrium (2-weekly exchange); iii
equilibrium (3-weekly exchange); iv steady-state before portacaval shunt;
v steady-state after portacaval shunt; vi equilibrium (2-weekly exchange);
vii steady-state; viii equilibrium (8 d interval); ix equilibrium
(15 d interval); x steady-state; xi equilibrium (2-weekly exchange).
(b) Return of plasma cholesterol to equilibrium level post-exchange.

tolerance is much improved despite the creation of an arterio-venous shunt and a BP of $90/40$ mmHg. Substantial regression of her xanthomata have occurred in this time. After 8 exchanges and despite a substantial lowering of her plasma cholesterol Case 4 has noticed little alteration in her exercise tolerance or regression of her xanthomata. An objective cardiological re-assessment has not been undertaken to date.

Comment

Plasma exchange must be considered in relation to alternative forms of treatment and in the context of an intractable and progressive disorder. Our experience and that of others (Thompson et al. 1978; Apstein et al. 1978), shows that plasma exchange can substantially reduce plasma cholesterol, the extent depending on the amount exchanged, the frequency, and concomitant therapy. The use of a protein-containing replacement solution to avoid reactive hyperlipidemia due to reduced colloid osmotic pressure (Lundsgaard-Hansen 1977), is mandatory. The clinical response has been excellent in Case 1 and acceptable in Case 3 considering the relatively short period of treatment. These findings confirm the larger series reported by Thompson et al (1978) and suggest that regression of atherosclerosis can occur. We have also argued earlier that clinical improvement may not depend solely upon reversal of atherosclerosis (Berger et al. 1978).

The marked transient fall in plasma cholesterol may have beneficial effects per se. It has been suggested that plasma exchange is followed by an efflux of cholesterol from tissue pools (Thompson et al. 1977; Simons et al. 1978). Furthermore, by depleting the plasma of 'aged' LDL particles susceptible to rapid uptake by macrophages, cholesterol clearance from plasma into the tissues may be significantly retarded for a period following exchange. These and other questions deserve further study.

References

Apstein CS, Zilversmit DB, Lees RS, George PK (1978) Effect of intensive plasmapheresis on the plasma cholesterol concentration with familial hypercholesterolemia. Atherosclerosis 31: 105-115

Berger GMB, Miller JL, Bonnici F, Joffe HS, Dubovsky DW (1978) Continuous-flow plasma exchange in the treatment of homozygous familial hypercholesterolemia. Am J Med 65: 243-251

Bilheimer DW, Goldstein JL, Grundy SM, Brown MS (1975) Reduction in cholesterol and low density lipoprotein synthesis after portacaval shunt surgery in a patient with homozygous familial hypercholesterolemia. J Clin Invest 56: 1420-1430

Lundsgaard-Hansen P (1977) Intensive plasmapheresis as a risk factor for arteriosclerotic cardiovascular disease. Vox Sang 33: 1-4

Lupien PJ, Moorjani S, Awad J (1976) A new approach to the management of familial hypercholesterolemia: removal of plasma cholesterol based on the principle of affinity chromatography. Lancet i: 1261-1265

Lux SE (1972) In: Dietary and drug treatment of primary hyperlipoproteinemia. Ann Intern Med 77: 267-292

Simons LA, Gibson JC, Isbister JP, Biggs JC (1978) The effects of plasma exchange on cholesterol metabolism. Atherosclerosis 31: 195-204

Thompson GR, Kilpatrick D, Raphael M, Oakley C, Myant NB (1977) Use of plasma exchange to induce regression of atheroma in familial hypercholesterolemia. Eur J Clin Invest 7: 233

Thompson GR, Kilpatrick D, Oakley C, Steiner R, Myant NB (1978) Reversal of cholesterol accummulation in familial hypercholesterolemia by long-term plasma exchange. Circulation 58: II-171

Partial Ileal Bypass: A Test of the Lipid-Atherosclerosis Hypothesis[1]

Henry Buchwald, Richard B. Moore, and Richard L. Varco

In 1962, we postulated that a partial ileal bypass operation should result
in a significant cholesterol reduction by a 2-fold mode of action: (1) interference with the enterohepatic cholesterol cycle and, thereby, a direct drain
on the body cholesterol pool; and (2) interference with the enterohepatic
bile acid cycle, resulting in a marked increase in bile acid synthesis from
the cholesterol pool and, thereby, an indirect drain of the body cholesterol
pool. The original laboratory assessment of this hypothesis was carried out
in the rabbit and the pig (Buchwald 1963a, 1963b, 1964; Buchwald and Gebhard
1964, 1968, 1974; Gebhard and Buchwald 1970), and was confirmed in the rabbit
(Okuboye et al. 1968), the dog (Scott et al. 1966), the Rhesus monkey (Scott
et al. 1977), and the white Carneau pigeon (Gomes et al. 1971). The first
partial ileal bypass operation in humans specifically for circulating cholesterol concentration reduction was performed in May of 1963. Since then our
series has grown to approximately 250 patients and reports of other series
have been published from both sides of the Atlantic.

The partial ileal bypass must, of course, not be confused with the 90% jejuno-
ileal bypass for the management of morbid obesity. In essence, the technique
for partial ileal bypass consists of transection of the ileum 200 cm from the
ileocecal valve, or 1/3 the length of the small bowel, whichever is longer;
anastomosis of the upper small intestine, end-to-side, to the cecum on the
anterior taenia just above the inverted appendiceal stump; closure of the
upper end of the bypassed distal bowel with tacking to the anterior taenia
of the cecum, between the anastomosis and the appendiceal stump, to prevent
future intussusception; and careful closure of the small divisional and the
large rotational mesenteric defects.

Certain metabolic studies in patients have further confirmed the mechanism
of action of the partial ileal bypass operation. Cholesterol absorption is
reduced by an average 60%; fecal steroid excretion is increased 3.8-fold
(4.9-fold increase in bile acids and 2.7-fold increase of neutral sterols);
cholesterol synthesis is increased 4.5-fold; cholesterol turnover is increased
3-fold; and the miscible body cholesterol pools are reduced 35%, with a relatively greater decrease in the less freely miscible pool than in the freely
miscible pool (Buchwald and Varco 1967; Moore et al. 1969, 1970). These metabolic data have been confirmed by Miettinen and Lempinen (1977), among others.

Clinical Results

In our initial series, the average plasma cholesterol reduction after partial
ileal bypass, from the preoperative but post-dietary baseline, was 41.4%
Comparable cholesterol reductions occurred in all of the lipoprotein pheno-

[1]Supported by NHLBI grant HL 11901 and HL 15265, the Minnesota Medical Foundation, the Graduate School of the University of Minnesota, and a Special
Legislative Appropriation of the State of Minnesota.

types (Buchwald et al. 1974). The effect of the bypass procedure has been lasting. Both Miettinen and ourselves have found that the response, or lack of response, to cholestyramine is not predictive of the response of the patient to a partial ileal bypass operation.

We have reported (Buchwald et al. 1968) a study of 24 heterozygous type II patients with an average pre-treatment plasma cholesterol concentration of 423 mg%. After three months of a fairly stringent low cholesterol, low saturated fat diet, an average circulating cholesterol reduction of 11% was achieved. The average plasma cholesterol level of this cohort, one year following a subsequent partial ileal bypass, was 224 mg%, representing an additional 42% average plasma cholesterol lowering. Thus, dietary measures and partial ileal bypass management act synergistically and can in concert achieve, essentially, a halving of the cholesterol concentration.

Our results in the homozygous type IIA patients have been disappointing, though reductions of approximately 20% of the circulating plasma cholesterol concentrations have been achieved.

Partial ileal bypass is a safe operative procedure, with an operative mortality less than 0.5%, despite the presence of marked coronary artery disease in the majority of patients operated upon. Early and long-term operative morbidity has been minimal.

Following this procedure, patients experience transient diarrhea, with a gradual return to normal stools after one year. As a rule, approximately 90% of patients no longer require even mild bowel-controlling drugs at one year or longer after the procedure. No long-term weight changes are engendered by the partial ileal bypass. There have been no abnormalities in serum electrolytes, including the calcium and potassium levels, in our experience. Prophylactically, vitamin B_{12} parenterally is prescribed (1,000 micrograms intramuscularly at 2 month intervals).

We, as well as others (Helsinger and Rootwelt 1969), have noted a decrease in size and the disappearance of peri-orbital xanthelasma, subcutaneous xanthomata, and even tendon xanthomata following partial ileal bypass. It has been documented by at least four other teams of investigators (Clot et al. 1971; Fritz and Walker 1966; Swan and McGowen 1968; Streuter - personal communication), as well as ourselves, that certain partial ileal bypass patients, within weeks of the operation, volunteer that their symptoms of angina pectoris have decreased in frequency and severity, or are completely absent, often in association with an increase in exercise capacity. We believe this to be a real finding and we suspect that the marked reduction in blood cholesterol may enhance oxygen diffusion through the RBC membrane.

Our associates in radiology have assessed the serial coronary arteriograms in our patients and in comparable sets of angiograms in 22 patients, with an average interval between arteriograms of 36.5 months, they have read progression in 22.7%, no change in 54.5%, questionable angiographic improvement in 9.1%, and apparent angiographic improvement in 13.6% (Baltaxe et al. 1969; Knight et al. 1972).

Program on Surgical Control of the Hyperlipidemias (POSCH)

Though the exponential association of the risk of atherosclerotic cardiovascular disease with the plasma cholesterol concentration has been proven, the converse of that statement has not. It has not been shown by randomized clinical trial that lowering cholesterol will engender a positive effect on cardiovascular prognosis. The 20 or so completed trials to-date have been negative in their conclusions or, at best, inconclusive. Possibly, these disappointing results have been due to the less than 10% cholesterol reduction obtained in the drug trials and the 14-18% cholesterol lowering in the best of the diet studies.

Currently, there are two NHLBI funded primary intervention studies — the Lipid Research Clinics Primary Intervention Trial and the Multiple Risk Factor Intervention Trial — and one secondary intervention trial — the Program on Surgical Control of the Hyperlipidemias (POSCH). The POSCH study utilizes partial ileal bypass as the method of intervention.

It is reasonable to state that an ideal method of intervention for a clinical trial should have maximum cholesterol lowering capability, be lasting in its effect, be safe, and provide obligatory adherence, all with a known mechanism of action. The partial ileal bypass satisfies these criteria. We have every expectation, therefore, that the POSCH will provide a definitive test of the lipid-atherosclerosis hypothesis.

The lipid results of the POSCH are not considered to be masked data, since this is not a trial of the method but of the hypothesis. At two years in this trial, there has been a 30% total plasma cholesterol reduction; with a 42% lowering of the LDL-cholesterol (46% differential between control and bypass patients); and, as yet, an unexplained 6% increase in the differential in the HDL-cholesterol (11% at one year). An 83% increase in the HDL/LDL ratio has ensued. These data are associated with a greater than 60% hypothetical reduction in risk by analyses based on the Cornfield equation (Cornfield 1962), and the Castelli HDL/LDL ratio curve (Kannel 1978). Time and the completion of the POSCH trial will confirm, or deny, these speculations.

References

Baltaxe H, Amplatz K, Varco RL, Buchwald H (1969) Coronary arteriography in hypercholesterolemic patients. Am J Roentgenol 105:784
Buchwald H (1963a) Localization of cholesterol absorption. Circulation 28: 649
Buchwald H (1963b) Surgical operation to lower circulating cholesterol. Circulation 28(II):649
Buchwald H (1964) Lowering of cholesterol absorption and blood levels by ileal exclusion: Experimental basis and preliminary clinical report. Circulation 29:713
Buchwald H, Gebhard RL (1964) Effect of intestinal bypass on cholesterol absorption and blood levels in the rabbit. Am J Physiol 207:567
Buchwald H, Gebhard RL (1968) Localization of bile salt absorption in vivo in the rabbit. Ann Surg 167:191
Buchwald H, Gebhard RL (1974) Relative secretion of cholesterol-4-C^{14} in the bile and upper and lower small intestinal washings of the bile fistula in rabbit. Surgery 75:266
Buchwald H, Moore RB, Lee GB, Frantz ID Jr, Varco RL (1968) Combined dietary, surgical and bile salt binding resin therapy in the treatment of hypercholesterolemia. Arch Surg 97:275
Buchwald H, Moore RB, Varco RL (1974) Surgical treatment of hyperlipidemias: Part I – Apologia; Part II – The laboratory experience; Part III – Clinical status of the partial ileal bypass operation. Circulation 49(I):1
Buchward H, Varco RL (1967) Partial ileal bypass for hypercholesterolemia and atherosclerosis. Surg Gyn and Ob 124:1231

Clot JP, Rouffy J, Loeper J, Mercadier M (1971) Derivation ileale, therapeutique, chirurgicale des hypercholesterolemies pures majeures (a propos de deux observations). Chirurgie 97:57

Cornfield J (1962) Joint dependence of risk of coronary heart disease on serum cholesterol and systolic blood pressure: A discriminate function analysis. Fed Proc 21:58

Fritz SH, Walker WJ (1966) Ileal bypass in the control of intractable hypercholesterolemia. Am Surg 32:691

Gebhard RL, Buchwald H (1970) Cholesterol absorption after reversal of the upper and lower halves of the small intestine. Surgery 67:474

Gomes MM, Kottke BA, Bernatz P, Titus JL (1971) Effect of ileal bypass on aortic atherosclerosis of white Carneau pigeons. Surgery 70:353

Helsinger N Jr, Rootwelt K (1969) Partial ileal bypass for surgical treatment of hypercholesterolemia. Nord Med 82:1409

Kannel WB (1978) Coronary risk handbook using HDL-cholesterol for persons over 50; from the Framingham Study. Am Ht Assoc Publ, May

Knight L, Scheibel R, Amplatz K, Varco RL, Buchwald H (1972) Radiographic appraisal of the Minnesota partial ileal bypass study. Surg Forum 23:141

Miettinen TA, Lempinen M (1977) Cholestyramine and ileal bypass in the treatment of familial hypercholesterolaemia. Europ J Clin Invest 7:509

Moore RB, Frantz ID Jr, Buchwald H (1969) Changes in cholesterol pool size, turnover rate, and fecal bile acid and sterol excretion after partial ileal bypass in hypercholesterolemic patients. Surgery 65:98

Moore RB, Frantz ID Jr, Varco RL, Buchwald H (1970) Cholesterol dynamics after partial ileal bypass. In: Jones RJ (ed) Atherosclerosis II. Springer-Verlag, New York, pp 295

Okuboye JA, Ferguson CC, Wyatt JP (1968) The effect of ileal bypass on dietary induced atherosclerosis in the rabbit. Can J Surg 11:69

Scott HW Jr, Stephenson SE Jr, Hayes CW, Younger RK (1967) Effects of bypass of the distal fourth of small intestine on experimental hypercholesterolemia and atherosclerosis rhesus monkeys. Surg Gyn Ob 125:3

Scott HW Jr, Stephenson SE Jr, Younger RK, Carlisle RB, Turney SW (1966) Prevention of experimental atherosclerosis by ileal bypass: Twenty percent cholesterol diet and ^{131}I-induced hypothyroidism in dogs. Ann Surg 163:795

Swann DM, McGowan JM (1968) Ileal bypass in hypercholesterolemia associated with heart disease. Am J Surg 116:81

Selective Removal of Low Density Lipoproteins from Blood by Affinity Chromatography

Paul-J. Lupien, Sital Moorjani, and Madeleine Lou

Lowering of plasma low density lipoproteins (LDL) is considered desirable in patients with familial hypercholesterolemia (FH) due to higher risk of morbidity and mortality attributed to early development of coronary artery disease in these patients (Slack 1978). Several forms of therapies have been used to lower plasma cholesterol levels in these subjects and they have been reviewed recently by Thompson (1978). We have described a new approach (Lupien et al. 1976; Moorjani et al. 1977; Awad et al. 1977) to lower selectively the concentration of very low density lipoproteins (VLDL) and LDL, without affecting the levels of high density lipoproteins (HDL). This treatment procedure therefore, has a definite therapeutic advantage, for it removes LDL from circulation (which has defective catabolism in FH and is considered as atherogenic), without affecting the concentration of HDL, (presumably antiatherogenic).

The treatment procedure is based on the principle of affinity chromatography. Heparin prepared from porcine intestinal mucosa (Sigma Chemical Company, MO) is covalently linked to beaded agarose (Biogel A5M, Bio-Rad Laboratories, CA) by the procedure of Iverius (1971) as described previously by Moorjani et al. (1977). The heparin-agarose (H-A) washed in 0.003 M Tris-HCl buffer, pH 7.4, containing 0.15 M NaCl is used in *in vitro* studies and its sterile apyrogenic preparation in 0.154 M NaCl is used in *in vivo* studies.

In vitro Studies

These experiments were carried out to study the binding of plasma lipoproteins to H-A at various concentrations of VLDL, LDL and HDL. Furthermore, the effect of addition of calcium at non-physiological concentration (0.02 M) was studied on the binding of various lipoproteins to H-A as well as its effect on the final levels of serum calcium.

Pooled serum samples were prepared by mixing sera from normal and hyperlipidemic patients (with the exception of grossly lipemic and icteric sera) to obtain desirable levels of serum lipoprotein concentration. The pooled serum samples were incubated with ethanolamine-treated agarose gel (E-A) and H-A in the presence and absence of calcium ions. The incubations were carried out at room temperature in plastic tubes as described previously by Moorjani et al. (1977). The tubes were centrifuged and the supernatant serum was decanted for the isolation of various lipoprotein fractions by ultracentrifugation as described by Havel et al. (1955). Lipoproteins were analysed for cholesterol on Auto-Analyser II (Technicon, Terrytown, NY) after extraction by the method of Folch et al. (1957).

The results shown in table 1 indicate that both VLDL and LDL bind to H-A, but the LDL has higher affinity for H-A than the VLDL. The binding of both VLDL and LDL is stimulated in the presence of calcium ions but again the binding of LDL is much higher than that of VLDL. It is interesting to note that under the same conditions HDL virtually does not bind to H-A in both experiments. The addition of calcium at a concentration of 0.02 M, which is 8 times the normal serum calcium concentration, has no effect on the final levels of serum calcium as previously described by Moorjani et al. (1977).

Table 1. *In vitro* Interaction of heparin-agarose (H-A) and ethanolamine-agarose (E-A) with plasma lipoproteins: effect of calcium ions.

	VLDL	LDL	HDL	Calcium
	Cholesterol in supernatant (mg/dl)			(mg/dl)
Experiment 1				
Serum + E-A	15	204	31	9.4
Serum + H-A	12(20)[a]	93(54)	30(3)	–
Serum + H-A + Ca^{2+}	10(34)	19(91)	30(3)	9.5
Experiment 2				
Serum + E-A	174	80	9	–
Serum + H-A	156(10)	45(44)	9	–
Serum + H-A + Ca^{2+}	138(21)	15(81)	9	–

[a]Values in parentheses are percentage of cholesterol bound to H-A.

In vivo Studies

Two patients with FH underwent treatment with heparin-agarose: patient 1 is an 18 year-old male with homozygous FH whereas patient 2 is a 39 year-old female with heterozygous FH. Their initial plasma cholesterol levels were 671 and 417 mg per dl, respectively. Patient 1 has undergone 51 treatments and patient 2 has received 20 treatments. At each treatment a total of 1,800 ml of blood was treated with H-A as described previously (Lupien et al. 1976; Lupien et al. 1979) representing 43 and 48 percent of the total blood volume in each patient. Despite chronic treatment no adverse side effects have been noticed in both patients as judged from routine laboratory tests and physical examination; on the contrary a diminution in the size of tuberous xanthomas has been observed in patient 1 and relief from angina in patient 2, however the latter finding is subjective and will require further investigation.

Table 2. Effect of extracorporeal treatment of blood with heparin-agarose on the levels of plasma lipids and serum calcium in two patients with familial hypercholesterolemia.

	Cholesterol	Triglycerides	Phospholipids	Calcium
	.....................mg per dl.....................			
Patient 1				
Pre-Treatment	488 ± 65[a]	135 ± 60	340 ± 47	9.9 ± 0.4
Post-Treatment	398 ± 54	41 ± 16	284 ± 45	9.6 ± 0.6
	(18)[b]	(70)	(16)	
p	< 0.01	< 0.001	< 0.02	NS
Patient 2				
Pre-Treatment	284 ± 12	99 ± 8	254 ± 14	8.7 ± 0.2
Post-Treatment	229 ± 12	46 ± 9	214 ± 8	8.6 ± 0.1
	(19)	(54)	(16)	
p	< 0.001	< 0.001	< 0.001	NS

[a]Values are mean ± SD for 12 treatments in patient 1 and 8 treatments in patient 2.
[b]Values in parentheses are percentage decrease from the pre-treatment value.

Table 3. Effect of extracorporeal treatment of blood with heparin-agarose on the levels of plasma lipoproteins and apolipoproteins in two patients with familial hypercholesterolemia.

	VLDL-C	LDL-C	HDL-C	Apo-B	Apo-A
	...................mg per dl....................				
Patient 1					
Pre-Treatment	17 ± 11[a]	441 ± 59	30 ± 3	220 ± 18	150 ± 6
Post-Treatment	2 ± 1	367 ± 55	29 ± 3	175 ± 22	148 ± 6
	(88)[b]	(17)	(3)	(20)	(1)
p	< 0.001	< 0.02	NS	< 0.01	NS
Patient 2					
Pre-Treatment	11 ± 4	240 ± 12	33 ± 4	133 ± 4	208 ± 30
Post-Treatment	2 ± 1	197 ± 11	32 ± 2	104 ± 5	210 ± 28
	(82)	(18)	(3)	(22)	(0)
p	< 0.001	< 0.001	NS	< 0.001	NS

[a]Values are mean ± SD for 12 treatments in patient 1 and 8 treatments in patient 2.
[b]Values in parentheses are percentage decrease from the pre-treatment value.

Plasma cholesterol and triglycerides were analysed after extraction with isopropanol on Auto-Analyseur II (Technicon, Terrytown, NY). Plasma phospholipid phosphorous was determined after TCA precipitation (Zilversmit and Davis (1950) by the method of Fiske and Subbarow (1925). The cholesterol content of lipoprotein fractions was determined by analysing the density fraction < 1.006 and the density fraction > 1.006, before and after precipitation with heparin (412 USP units per ml) and manganese chloride (0.095 M). The concentration of apoproteins A and B was measured by electroimmunoassay as described by Laurell (1972).

The data shown in table 2 indicates that, treatment of 1,800 ml of blood results in an average decrease of 18 and 16 percent in plasma cholesterol and phospholipid concentration respectively, in both patients. A similar decrease was noticed in two heterozygous patients for one single treatment (Lupien et al. 1976). The average reduction in plasma cholesterol pool was 2.4 g for patient 1 and 1.3 g for patient 2. The lowering of plasma cholesterol is mainly due to decrease of LDL cholesterol (table 3), since the concentration of HDL cholesterol is virtually unaffected by the treatment. Although VLDL cholesterol is greatly reduced during the treatment, its contribution to over all reduction of plasma cholesterol is not appreciable due to low cholesterol content of this fraction. In fact, the decrease in VLDL cholesterol (table 3) as well as plasma triglycerides (table 2) is due to hydrolysis of VLDL by lipoprotein lipase released in the circulation by heparin used as anticoagulant. However, some VLDL and intermediary lipoprotein particles may also be removed by heparin-agarose which may also explain a higher decrease noted for apoprotein-B (table 3) as compared to LDL cholesterol in both patients. Apoprotein-A levels did not vary with the treatment, further confirming that HDL is not removed from circulation by H-A.

As seen in *in vitro* studies (table 1) the circulating levels of calcium were not affected by the treatment with heparin-agarose (table 2) although calcium was added at a 0.02 M concentration for the selective removal of LDL from the circulation. This is due to ability of heparin-agarose beads to retain excess calcium through high affinity binding to ionized sulfate groups of heparin covalently linked to agarose beads (Moorjani, unpublished data).

468

References

Awad J, Lupien PJ, Moorjani S, Cloutier R (1977) A simple method for the removal of undesirable substances from the blood: Removal of plasma cholesterol. Curr Ther Res 21:525-536

Fiske CH, Subbarow Y (1925) The colorimetric determination of phosphorous. J Biol Chem 66: 375-400

Folch J, Lees M, Sloane-Stanley GH (1957) A simple method for the isolation and purification of total lipids from animal tissues. J Biol Chem 226: 497-501

Havel RJ, Eder HA, Bragdon JH (1955) The distribution and chemical composition of ultracentrifugally separated lipoproteins in human serum. J Clin Invest 34:1345-1353

Iverius PH (1971) Coupling of glycosaminoglycans to agarose beads (Sepharose 4 B). Biochem J 124:677-683

Laurell CB (1972) Electroimmunoassay. Scand J Clin Lab Invest 29, Suppl 124: 21-37

Lupien PJ, Moorjani S, Awad J (1976) A new approach to the management of familial hypercholesterolemia: Removal of plasma cholesterol based on the principle of affinity chromatography. Lancet 1:1261-1265

Lupien PJ, Moorjani S, Lou M, Brun D, Gagne C (1979) Removal of cholesterol from blood by affinity binding to heparin-agarose: Evaluation of treatment in homozygous familial hypercholesterolemia. Pediat Res, in press

Moorjani S, Lupien PJ, Awad J (1977) Extracorporeal removal of plasma lipoproteins by affinity binding to heparin-agarose. Clin Chim Acta 77:21-31

Slack J (1978) Inheritance of familial hypercholesterolemia. In: Paoletti R, Gotto AM (eds) Atherosclerosis Reviews. Raven Press, New York, pp 35-66

Thompson GR (1978) Management of familial hypercholesterolemia and new approaches to the treatment of atherosclerosis. In: Paoletti R, Gotto AM (eds) Atherosclerosis Reviews. Raven Press, New York, pp 67-90

Zilversmit DB, Davis AK (1951) Microdetermination of plasma phospholipids by trichloroacetic acid precipitation. J Lab Clin Med 35:155-160

Comparison of Cholestyramine, Ileal By-Pass and Portacaval Shunt in the Treatment of Familial Hypercholesterolemia

Tatu A. Miettinen[1]

Since familial hypercholesterolemia is known to be associated with enhanced development of ischemic heart disease (Stone et al. 1974), a long term reduction of the serum cholesterol level is felt to be an important preventive procedure. Dietary hypocholesterolemic measures alone are insufficient in the long term and therefore either drugs or surgical procedures should be included in the treatment to achieve a maximal serum cholesterol reduction. Even though the latter is used as a marker of the efficacy of these measures their ultimate benefit should be demonstrated by a reduced coronary morbidity and/or mortality. The present paper compares the effects of ion exchangers, partial ileal exclusion, and portacaval shunt on serum cholesterol and on some other measures of cholesterol metabolism in familial hypercholesterolemia.

Ion Exchangers and Ileal By-Pass

Ion exchangers and an ileal by-pass operation effectively reduce serum cholesterol in cases heterozygous for familial hypercholesterolemia. A comparison can be made between the two measures mainly on the basis of different series of patients. Evidence has accumulated to indicate that cholestyramine and colestipol reduce serum cholesterol in short term and intermediate term studies by 20-25% but therapeutic failures can occur in longer term treatment (Grundy 1972; Witters et al. 1976; Miettinen 1979). In a large series of a controlled 3-year trial on a nonclassified material the effect of colestipol on serum cholesterol was clearly less (Dorr et al. 1978). Long term results following the ileal by-pass operation, in which according to Buchwald 200 cm or more of the terminal ileum is by-passed, have indicated a permanent, above 30% decrease in serum cholesterol (Buchwald et al. 1974; Miettinen 1978). Table 1 reveals that a continuous supervision in the lipid clinic gives surprisingly good long term results in patients started with cholestyramine, even though after the 10-year follow-up only one third were still on ion exchanger; the mean serum cholesterol reduction (24%) was significantly less in the cholestyramine group than in the ileal by-pass group (38%). The ultimate results could have been poorer in the cholestyramine group if the values of the cases no longer visiting the lipid clinic were available.

The two hypocholesterolemic measures have been compared in two studies on the same patients. A fairly short ileal exclusion decreases serum cholesterol and increases fecal steroids quite similarly to cholestyramine (Grundy et al. 1971). However, a longer ileal by-pass lowered serum cholesterol, stimulated cholesterol elimination as bile acids, and increased markers of cholesterol synthesis clearly more strongly than large doses (32 g/day) of cholestyramine (Miettinen and Lempinen 1977). The response to the ileal by-pass was detectable also in cases quite resistant to the resin. It was interesting to note that cholestyramine potentiated the effects of the ileal by-pass (Miettinen 1978), the overall decrease in serum cholesterol being 45% with the combined

[1]Supported by the National Council for Medical Sciences, Finland.

treatment. The data available at the moment indicate that the ileal by-pass operation is superior to ion exchangers in reducing the serum cholesterol level. It has also been reported to reduce tissue cholesterol pools (Buchwald et al. 1974), an observation not made during the ion exchanger treatment. Economical reasons, dietary restrictions, constipation and convenience frequently limit the long term use of the bile acid sequestering resins, while these factors become less important after the ileal by-pass procedure. However, diarrhea can be annoying after the operation. In fact, one third of the cases with ileal by-pass in Table 1 have learned to use ion exchangers, periodically at least, for management of diarrheal bouts but none would like to have intestinal continuity restored. Some evidence has been presented that colestipol reduces coronary mortality in a nonclassified hypercholesterolemic material (Dorr et al. 1978). No evidence is available as yet that a similar effect could be obtained with ion exchangers or ileal by-pass in patients heterozygous for familial hypercholesterolemia.

Bile acid sequestering resins alone are usually ineffective even in the short term in patients homozygous for familial hypercholesterolemia and occasionally the serum cholesterol may even increase (Khachadurian 1968; Grundy et al. 1971; Miettinen 1979). Ileal by-pass can decrease serum cholesterol to some extent (Buchwald et al. 1971), but a beneficial effect in the long term is questionable (Table 2). Since, moreover, even complete biliary diversion is quite ineffective in those patients (Deckelbaum et al. 1977), serum cholesterol lowering appears to fail by interruption of enterohepatic circulation of bile acids alone.

Table 1. A ten-year follow-up of patients with familial hypercholesterolemia treated with cholestyramine and ileal by-pass.

Period	No. of subjects	Age, years	Body weight, kg	Serum lipids, mmol/1 Cholesterol	Triglycerides
			Cholestyramine		
Initial	32	39±1	69±2	13.8±0.5	1.54±0.12
Final	32	49±1	70±2	10.5±0.3	1.72±0.30
Change	32	±10±1[x]	+1±1	−3.3±0.5[x]	+0.18±0.16
			Ileal by-pass		
Initial	27	36±2	69±4	15.0±0.5	2.10±0.21[*]
Final	27	45±2	64±2	9.3±0.4[*]	2.02±0.28
Change	27	9±1[x]	−5±3	−5.7±0.4[**]	−0.08±0.31

[*]Statistically significant ($p<0.05$ at least) difference between the groups.
[x]Statistically significant ($p<0.05$ at least) change from the initial values.
Of the 52 case controls selected (matched for age, initial body weight and initial serum cholesterol) from the lipid clinic material of the Outpatient Department of Medicine (University of Helsinki) 32 had visited the clinic at a rate comparable to 27 subjects with ileal by-pass and were included in the cholestyramine study; the remaining 20 patients had discontinued their lipid clinic visits and no follow-up data were available. The initial values are mostly those obtained when the patients were admitted to the clinic on their usual home diet. Thereafter dietary treatment was started and trials with different drugs, including ion exchangers, were performed in both groups. Ileal by-pass operation was performed after a mean follow-up of 2 years, the postoperative follow-up being 7 years. At the end of the 10-year follow-up 34% of patients in the cholestyramine group were still on that drug, 9% had died and the remainder were on various medication. Four patients with ileal by-pass had died (15%).

Table 2.   Effects of cholestyramine, ileal by-pass and portacaval shunt in two children homozygous for familial hypercholesterolemia. Mean±SE.

Treatment	Age range, years	Mean weight, kg	Serum lipids, mmol/l Cholest.	Triglyc.	DMS, µg/dl	Fecal steroids, mg/day Acidic	Neutral	Total
			Case 1					
None	5	15	30.9	2.06	23	26	263	289
Resin	5	15	31.1	2.00	77	532	297	828
IB-P	6	16	23.9	2.05	66	741	236	977
IB-P	6-8	19	24.1±2.4	2.16±0.22	70	705	584	1289
IB-P	9-11	28	29.6±2.3	3.11±1.47	105	1013±57	430±26	1443±39
IB-P+PCS	11-12	31	15.8±0.7	0.97±0.06	15	790±93	264±25	1054±77
IB-P+PCS	13-15	47	11.9±0.3	0.71±0.04	19	805	290	1095
			Case 2					
None	5	19	26.7±0.5	1.00±0.10	56	133	370	503
Resin	5	19	24.4±0.5	1.52±0.04	149	1305±13	534±23	1839±36
PCS	5 1/2	19	21.5	0.50	30	79	180	259
PCS	6	21	19.0	0.80	9	128	196	324
PCS+IB-P	6 1/2	23	16.8	0.94	83	664	198	861

IB-P = ileal by-pass; PCS = portacaval shunt; Resin = cholestyramine 24 and 16 g/day for 12-14 days. Ileal by-pass and portacaval shunt were performed at the age of 6 and 11 years, respectively, in case 1, and 7 and 6 years, respectively, in case 2. Correlation of the serum dimethyl sterol (DMS = cholesterol percursor) level with the fecal total steroid output (mg/kg; almost equal to cholesterol synthesis since dietary cholesterol was 1-2 mg/kg/day) was statistically significant in both case 1 ($r = 0.776$) and case 2 ($r = 0.960$). Cholesterol absorption was 38% before and 28-50% after the portacaval shunt in case 1; combined with fecal neutral steroids this means that biliary cholesterol secretion was clearly reduced by PCS.

Portacaval Shunt and Ileal By-Pass

At the moment portacaval shunt is the only reliable measure to reduce serum cholesterol in patients homozygous for familial hypercholesterolemia (Starzl et al. 1978). At present at least 27 subjects have been operated on and during an up to 5-year follow-up the average decrease in serum cholesterol has been 40%, range 20-60% (SC Mitchell 1979, NIH Registry, personal communication). Reduced synthesis of lipoproteins and cholesterol appears to be the major hypocholesterolemic mechanism of this procedure (Bilheimer et al. 1975). Ion exchangers or ileal by-pass can be considered to potentiate the hypocholesterolemic effect of portacaval shunt provided the latter significantly inhibits cholesterol synthesis. We have combined portacaval shunt with ileal by-pass in two homozygous children (Table 2). Elimination of cholesterol as fecal bile acids and neutral sterols, and the serum concentration of cholesterol precursors indicated that portacaval shunt actually suppresses to some extent the marked increase in cholesterol synthesis caused by the ileal by-pass to compensate for enhanced elimination of cholesterol as fecal bile acids. This appears to have a favorable effect on serum cholesterol, too.

Conclusions

The ileal by-pass operation is a more effective hypocholesterolemic measure than the use of ion exchange resins and it can be recommended for the treatment of patients heterozygous for familial hypercholesterolemia. Ion exchangers potentiate the hypocholesterolemic action of ileal by-pass and improve diarrheal bouts occasionally provoked by the ileal exclusion. Portacaval shunt is superior to ileal by-pass in reducing serum cholesterol and it is an effective hypocholesterolemic measure in patients homozygous for familial hypercholesterolemia. Trials combining ion exchangers or even the ileal by-pass with the portacaval shunt are worth while.

References

Bilheimer DW, Goldstein JL, Grundy SM, Brown MS (1975) Reduction in cholesterol and low density lipoprotein synthesis after portacaval shunt surgery in a patient with homozygous familial hypercholesterolemia. J Clin Invest 56: 1420

Buchwald H, Moore RB, Varco RL (1974) Surgical treatment of hyperlipidemia. Circulation 49: suppl 1: 1

Deckelbaum RJ, Lees RS, Small DM, Hedberg SE, Grundy SM (1977) Failure of complete bile diversion and oral bile acid therapy in the treatment of homozygous familial hypercholesterolemia. N Engl J Med 296: 465

Dorr AE, Gundersen K, Schneider JC Jr, Spencer TW, Martin WB (1978) Colestipol hydrochloride in hypercholesterolemic patients - Effect on serum cholesterol and mortality. J Chron Dis 31: 5

Grundy SM (1972) Treatment of hypercholesterolemia by interference with bile acid metabolism. Arch Int Med 130: 638

Grundy SM, Ahrens EH Jr, Salen G (1971) Interruption of the enterohepatic circulation of bile acids in man: comparative effects of cholestyramine and ileal exclusion on cholesterol metabolism. J Lab Clin Med 78: 94

Khachadurian AK (1968) Cholestyramine therapy in patients homozygous for familial hypercholesterolemia. J Atheroscler Res 8: 177

Miettinen TA (1978) New insights into cholesterol dynamics. Arch Surg 113: 45

Miettinen TA (1979) Effects of hypolipidemic drugs on bile acid metabolism in man. In: Kritchevsky D, Paoletti R (eds) Advances in lipid research. In press

Miettinen TA, Lempinen M (1977) Cholestyramine and ileal by-pass in the treatment of familial hypercholesterolaemia. Eur J Clin Invest 7: 509

Starzl TE, Putman CW, Koep LJ (1978) Portacaval shunt and hyperlipidemia. Arch Surg 113: 71

Stone NJ, Levy RI, Fredrickson DS, Verter J (1974) Coronary artery disease in 116 kindred with familial type II hypercholesterolemia. Circulation 49: 476

Witters LA, Herbert PN, Shulman RS, Krauss RM, Levy RI (1976) Therapeutic failure in familial type II hyperlipoproteinemia. Metabolism 25: 1017

Homozygous Hypercholesterolemia; Treatment by Portacaval Shunt

Evan A. Stein and Charles J. Glueck

As recently as 1973, the prognosis for patients suffering from homozygous hypercholesterolemia was regarded as hopeless, with death from myocardial infarction invariably occurring prior to age 20. In the intervening six years since that time, two new and different forms of therapy have emerged which offer considerable promise. Diversion of portal blood via a porta-caval shunt, originally performed for this disease by Starzl et al. (1973), has now been reported from a number of centers (Cywes et al. 1976; Stein et al. 1975; Farriaux et al. 1976; Russell et al. 1976) with generally favorable results. The second approach of repeated plasma exchange was first used for the treatment of homozygous hypercholesterolemia by Thompson et al. (1975). The procedure had been previously used (Turnberg et al. 1972) with success in reducing plasma lipids and severe xanthoma in patients suffering from xanthomatous neuropathy as a result of primary biliary cirrhosis. Like the portacaval shunt procedure, the use of plasma exchange in the treatment of homozygous hypercholesterolemia has also been carried out in a number of centers (Berger et al. 1978; Stein et al. 1978).

Although an informal registry was started in 1974 at the National Heart and Lung Institute (Mitchell and Levy 1974), in order to facilitate collection and disbursement of information relevant to portacaval shunts, the registry is no longer current with the last recorded entry in 1978. The task force formed at the same time to collect information about both the medical and surgical management of homozygous hypercholesterolemia is still active (SC Mitchell 1979, personal communication) and is due to release a comprehensive updated report in the near future.

There are now known to be at least 34 patients who have undergone portacaval shunt although the true number may be well in excess of this number. Although the operation was originally proposed for the therapy of homozygous hypercholesterolemia, it is probable that at least one patient with the heterozygous form of the disease has had a portacaval shunt (Weglicki et al. 1977). The largest group of patients has been reported from Johannesburg (JDL Hansen 1978, personal communication) where 11 have undergone portal diversion. The patients range in age from 2 to 28 years at time of operation and include both sexes.

Biochemical Changes

Pre-operative total cholesterols have varied from approximately 500 mg/dl to 1500 mg/dl. The results following portal diversion have been variable, with an average decrease of approximately 40%. No patients have achieved age and sex adjusted "normal" values. A number of patients have experienced no reduction in plasma lipid and lipoprotein concentrations; in 3 patients the lack of post-operative response appears to be related to thrombosis of the shunt and the rapid development of collaterals. In one of these patients, a repeat operation with diversion of the collateral portal blood into the systemic circulation resulted in the subsequent reduction in serum cholesterol (SC Mitchell 1979, personal communication).

The reduction in total cholesterol is due almost entirely to decreases in the low density lipoprotein (LDL) fraction. Alterations in high density lipoprotein (HDL) values have not been consistently reported. However, HDL cholesterol levels are invariably low in the homozygous hypercholesterolemic patient. Plasma triglyceride concentrations, although not a feature of the disease, have been reported to decrease after portal diversion in patients who had elevated triglycerides pre-operatively.

Clinical Results

Clinically, the results of portacaval shunting have been variable. Four patients are known to have died following the operation, 3 of cardiac related deaths and the fourth from a cerebral infarction (RI Levy 1976, personal communication; Faergeman et al. 1978. The time of death after portacaval shunt has ranged from 3 days to 18½ months (S.C. Mitchell, 1979, personal communication). A number of patients have done remarkably well considering that the disease was previously considered totally irreversible despite intensive and long-term diet and drug therapy. Although the majority of patients operated on have not yet been reported in detail, it would appear at this stage that approximately one third of patients operated on have experienced clinical improvement. A number of patients have experienced reductions in size and number of xanthoma (Starzl et al. 1974; Krogh and Wickens 1974; Stein et al. 1975; Weglicki et al. 1977). Almost all patients who experienced angina prior to portacaval shunt have reported reduction in frequency and severity following the operation and most had encouraging improvements in their levels of exercise tolerance and quality of life. One child is now even reported to be a long distance runner (SC Mitchell 1979, personal communication). Whether the improvement in cardiac status is related solely to reduction in circulating LDL and reversal of previous atherosclerotic lesions as a consequence of a portacaval shunt is complicated in a number of patients by combining the operation with coronary artery bypass surgery (Weglicki et al. 1977; Starzl et al. 1978). Improvements in arterial and cardiac blood flow has been recorded in a number of patients ranging from a "semi-objective" decrease in intensity of aortic and femoral bruits (Krogh and Wickens 1974) to more solid evidence such as a diminution of the aortic valve gradient from 56 to 10 mm Hg (Starzl et al. 1974). The younger patients operated on have nearly all returned to regular schooling and a number of adults have resumed their previous occupations (SC Mitchell 1979, personal communication; Weglicki et al. 1977). As mentioned previously, results between and even within various centers have varied considerably, with some centers (Starzl et al. 1978) reporting consistently good clinical results while other centers have experienced little or no success with the operation (R Lees 1978, personal communication). One significant and fairly striking difference does seem to emerge in predicting outcome, and that is the age at which the shunt is performed and perhaps more importantly, the severity of pre-existing cardiovascular disease. It would also appear from the data so far accumulated that patients who respond with significant reductions in LDL cholesterol during intervenous hyperalimentation prior to portacaval shunting are more likely to have better clinical results following the operation (Stein et al. 1975).

Overall, approximately one third of patients experienced clinical benefit. Of the remaining patients, about one half remained clinically unchanged, despite the at times significant reductions in circulating lipids. The remaining subjects continue to show clinical deterioration, with or without reductions in plasma cholesterol.

Complications

Complications have been surprisingly few. The initial concern about portal systemic encephalopathy has so far not been substantiated and both normal mental and physical growth have been reported in children and adolescents following portacaval shunt. There have as yet been no reports of liver dysfunction, or tumors. Two side effects not widely appreciated have been recorded and should perhaps be further explored. The first is the increase in platelet aggregation (Faergeman et al. 1976) which may be of importance in increasing the risk of venous, and especially portal vein thrombosis. The second side effect, reported by the Johannesburg group (JDL Hansen 1978, personal communication) appears to be infertility in two of the female patients following portal diversion. As reported by Hansen "this may be fine eugenically, but it is causing great distress to the ladies concerned".

Mechanism of Action

The exact mechanism by which total diversion of portal blood into the systemic circulation causes a reduction in circulating lipids and lipoproteins is not entirely known. It has been suggested by Starzl et al. (1975), based on dog and baboon studies, that the reduction is mainly due to diversion of the hormone-rich venous return from the upper splanchnic organs with resultant reduction in hepatic cholesterol or LDL synthesis. It is also suggested that the bypassing of the liver by blood rich in nutrients may play a secondary role. The reduction in LDL synthesis is supported by studies done by Bilheimer et al. (1975) on a patient following portacaval shunt. A number of less well supported theories have also been advanced, including enhanced oxygen tension in the liver as a cause of decreased hepatic cholesterol synthesis (Stender et al. 1975) and increased cholesterol catabolism to bile salts and increased bile salt secretion and excretion (Butzow et al. 1978).

The results of portacaval shunt for homozygous hypercholesterolemia are so far promising in that in a previously disfiguring, debilitating, lethal and untreatable disease, at least a third of patients have been reported to experience early and so far sustained clinical improvement, despite discontinuance of diet and drug therapies. Whether these benefits continue and an increase in duration of life results from the portacaval shunt remains to be determined. It will also be necessary to evaluate in some form of controlled study the results obtained by portacaval shunting with those of plasma exchange.

Acknowledgement

We are grateful to Drs. Sheila Mitchell and John Hansen for their assistance in gathering much of the data in this report.

References

Berger GMB, Miller JL, Binnici F et al. (1978) Continuous flow plasma exchange in the treatment of homozygous familial hypercholesterolemia. Am J Med 65: 243

Bilheimer DW, Goldstein JL, Grundy SM et al. (1975) Reduction in cholesterol and low density lipoprotein synthesis after portacaval shunt surgery in a patient with homozygous familial hypercholesterolemia. J Clin Invest 56: 1420

Butzow GH, Dammann HG, Czok G (1978) Effect of portacaval shunt on biliary cholesterol and bile salt secretion in normal rats. European J Clin Invest 8: 411

Cywes S, Davies MRQ, Louw JH et al.(1976) Portacaval shunt in two patients with homozygous type II hyperlipoproteinemia. South Afr Med J 50: 239

Faergeman O, Gormsen J, Meinertz H (1976) Anti-platelet drugs and porta-caval anastomosis for homozygous hypercholesterolemia. (Letter) Lancet 2: 1416

Farriaux JP, Ribet M, Bertrand M et al.(1976) Treatment of Type II familial hypercholesterolemia through portacaval anastomosis. Arch Fr Pediatr 33: 745

Krogh L, Wickens JT (1974) Portacaval shunt for hypercholesterolemia. (Letter) South Afr Med J 48: 2302

Mitchell SC, Levy RI (1974) Portacaval shunt in familial hypercholesterolemia. (Letter) Lancet 2: 1263

Russell D, Heimann KW, Levin SE et al.(1976) Portacaval shunt for homozy-gous hypercholesterolemia. (Letter) Lancet 2: 1205

Starzl TE, Chase HP, Putnam CW et al.(1973) Portacaval shunt in hyperlipo-proteinaemia. Lancet 2: 940

Starzl TE, Chase HP, Putnam CW et al.(1974) Follow up of patient with porta-caval shunt for the treatment of hyperlipidemia. (Letter) Lancet 2: 714

Starzl TE, Lee IY, Porter KA et al.(1975) The influence of portal blood upon lipid metabolism in normal and diabetic dogs and baboons. Surg Gynecol Obstet 140: 381

Starzl TE, Putnam CW, Koep LJ (1978) Portacaval shunt and hyperlipidemia. Arch Surg 113: 71

Stein EA, Levine R, Glueck CJ et al.(1979) Repetitive plasmapheresis for severe primary and secondary hypercholesterolemia. (Abstract) Clin Res 27: 377A

Stein EA, Pettifor J, Mieny C et al.(1975) Portacaval shunt for homozygous hypercholesterolemia. South Afr Med J 48: 2302

Stender S, Astrup P, Damgaard-Peders F (1975) Enhanced oxygen tension in the liver and serum cholesterol lowering effect of portacaval shunt in hyperlipidemia. (Letter) Lancet 2: 776

Thompson GR, Lowenthal R, Myant NB (1975) Plasma exchange in the manage-ment of homozygous familial hypercholesterolemia. Lancet 1: 1208

Turnberg LA, Mahoney MP, Gleeson MH et al.(1972) Plasmaphoresis and plasma exchange in the treatment of hyperlipidemia and xanthomatous neuropathy in patients with primary biliary cirrhosis. Gut 13: 976

Weglicki WB, Ganda OP, Soeldner JS et al.(1977) Portacaval diversion for severe hypercholesterolemia. Arch Surg 112: 634

High Density Lipoproteins: An Overview

William P. Castelli

The reports on High Density Lipoproteins (HDL) presented at this conference seem to be unanimous about the fact that the higher these lipoproteins go the better the subject seems to do, at least as regards coronary
heart disease (CHD) in particular and atherosclerosis in general. Both
Tavia Gordon and NE Miller have described the long history of this knowledge; it seems that HDL was discovered by David Barr and his associates
(1951) and rediscovered about every three years since then. The latest
discovery for which NE and G Miller deserve a lot of credit looks like it
may gain a permanent place for HDL in medical practice.

As the reader will recognize, not all HDL measures are the same. Some
just measure the cholesterol carried in HDL (the HDL cholesterol) as a
measure of HDL. Some measure different kinds of HDL in the ultracentrifuge
and talk of HDL_2 and HDL_3. Others measure other constituents of HDL like
apo A1 or apo A2.

Most of the large clinical and epidemiological studies have measured HDL-
cholesterol and as Tavia Gordon has described, this measure of HDL is a
powerful, independent assessor of coronary heart disease in all its varied
clinical presentations. Whether some subfraction such as HDL_2, but not
HDL_3, will be an even better test - taking into account such mundane things
as cost - remains to be seen. Of course, irrespective of cost, one might
learn even greater detail about the comings and goings of cholesterol in
our body. As NE Miller points out, HDL_2 correlates better with the mass
of slowly exchangeable cholesterol (Pool B) than that of the rapidly exchangeable Pool A. Others such as Mahley (1974) have described an even
different kind of HDL which appears in animals and humans after atherogenic diets whose true significance remains to be known.

Dr. Glueck has further broadened our horizons with the different levels of
HDL found in various races, ages, sexes, as well as the difference in different cultures. I have been intrigued by the generally lower HDL cholesterols found in South Americans; it seems a paradox when one recognizes
that they have much lower coronary rates. The world epidemiological data
suggests that countries with the highest total cholesterols have the highest HDL cholesterols. Even in Framingham there is a small but positive
correlation of HDL cholesterol with total cholesterol. Dr. Epstein has
really alluded to this problem by letting us look at the interaction of
total cholesterol, reflecting really the levels of LDL cholesterol - the
most atherogenic cholesterol and HDL cholesterol in CHD case production.
The worst category to be in is to have high LDL (or total cholesterol) and
low HDL. Not long ago I looked at as many countries as I could get data
from, and found that instead of looking at absolute values of HDL cholesterol and risk, I looked at the ratio of total to HDL. When one does this,
low risk countries with low absolute HDL cholesterol (but much lower total
cholesterol) actually tend to have a better ratio (lower) of total cholesterol to HDL cholesterol. If one applies such considerations to the American population as Dr. Epstein has, it suggests that we have a gigantic
task. If one forgets that a ratio of 3.5 would be best and picks a more

practical value such as 4.5, we need to lower LDL cholesterols to bring them into line with HDL cholesterols in over half the women and more than half the men in America.

In any event, if HDL is so good for us, or at least if a major fraction of it is, how does it work? There have been several theories put forth to explain the mechanisms and since science in our country seems largely deductive, it is well for all of us to pick a few theories to follow just to see how the data collected and to be collected will support or defeat them.

HDL is secreted primarily by the liver (Figure 1), but some comes from the gut and some may be pinched off from chylomicrons. Hamilton and his colleagues (1976) have proposed that the initial HDL which is secreted into serum is a flat disc resembling a slice of the cell membrane. This nascent HDL is thus a simple bilamellar structure of mostly lecithin and free cholesterol. Whether this is the HDL_3 of the ultracentrifuge studies is still a matter of some debate. In any event, it would appear that this nascent HDL is converted to a spherical HDL by the enzyme Lecithin Cholesterol Acyl Transferase (LCAT). The main purpose of this enzyme is to transfer an acyl group to free cholesterol to make it into cholesterol ester. Since cholesterol-ester is not a polar lipid it cannot stay in a water-lipid interface environment and so it goes inside filling up the center of these flat HDL discs, converting them into spheres containing a center full of cholesterol-ester. Apparently LCAT won't work if apo Al is not around in abundance. Is this spherical HDL really HDL_2?

One of the major roles of HDL seems to derive from this activated LCAT it carries as Glomset has demonstrated (1973). For 25 years (Figure 2) it has been known that free cholesterol moves very rapidly across cell membranes and exchanges with free cholesterol in the outer crusts of any lipoprotein particle which happens by but no net exchange occurs until HDL comes by where LCAT esterifies this free cholesterol and tucks it inside as cholesterol-ester. Cholesterol-ester cannot bounce back readily into cells and so a net flux of cholesterol out of cells is effected. From there it has been postulated that HDL initiates the transport of cholesterol back to the liver where 95% of the cholesterol we excrete per day is excreted. As NE Miller has shown HDL is inversely related to total body cholesterol (1976), and this could well fit this role of HDL as the heart of the reverse cholesterol transport system.

In addition, another theory about how HDL may benefit us comes from a consideration of what may be the major cellular lesion of atherosclerosis, the so-called fat cell syndrome postulated by deDuve (1975) (Figure 3). deDuve is saying that LDL is internalized into cells into vacuoles which are then digested by fusion with a sack of enzymes known as the lysosomes. These lysosomes must keep up with an enormous flux of LDL in North American societies. Brown and Goldstein (1959) estimate that we have perhaps more than four to five times as much LDL as we need to control cellular cholesterol production and supply cholesterol to cells for proper function. What happens when the lysosomes cannot keep up with LDL digestion - particularly digesting cholesterol-ester to free cholesterol which can easily diffuse out of these vacuoles? The cell fills with cholesterol-ester fat droplets and may eventually die.

Two very rare diseases underline the importance of lysosomal lipase to effect this digestion: Wolman's disease (Patrick AD, Lake BD 1969) where babies are born without lysosomal lipase and die at 14 months from the fat cell syndrome - even though LDL pressures at these ages are extremely low; Cholesteryl Ester Storage disease (Fredrickson DS, Ferrans V 1978) where the subjects have less than 10% of the normal lysosomal activity and so

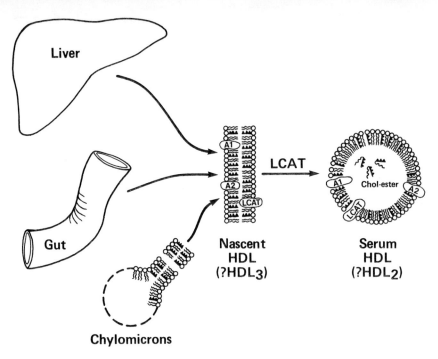

FIG. 1. Sites of production of high density lipoproteins.
Adapted from the work of Tall and Small and, Hamilton et al. (1976).

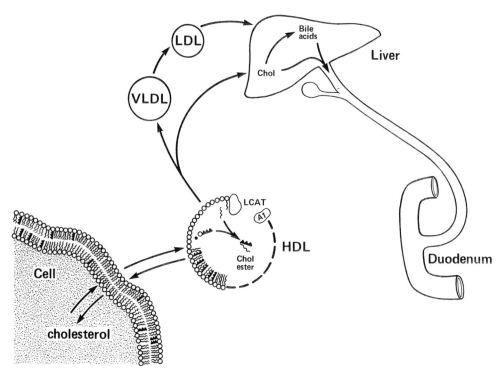

FIG. 2. Reverse cholesterol transport system. Adapted from Glomset and
Norun (1973).

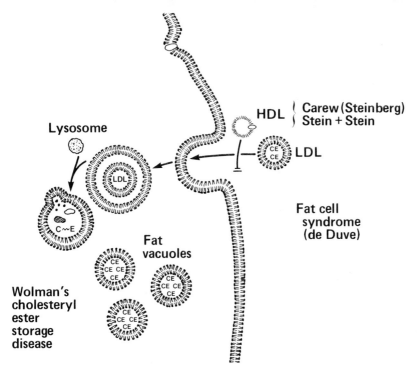

FIG. 3. Fat cell syndrome and possible interactions of HDL and LDL (CE = cholesterol ester).

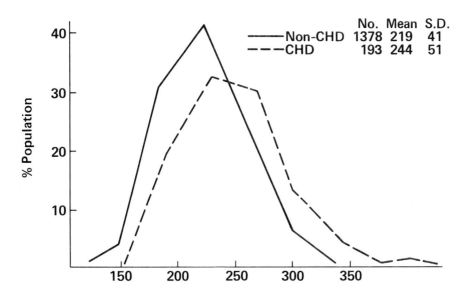

	No.	Mean	S.D.
Non-CHD	1378	219	41
CHD	193	244	51

FIG. 4. Distribution of serum cholesterol in subjects free of coronary heart disease versus those developing CHD in 16 years. Men 30–49 years of age at entry, Framingham.

badly defend themselves against the onslaught of LDL getting into grave medical trouble by the third decade.

Of course, deDuve is speculating that perhaps all of us whose cholesterols range in the 200's and who have four to five times too much LDL cholesterol are in trouble early and often but mostly certainly by the late middle age. It is here, however, that work by Carew (1976) and Stein and Stein (1976) showing that HDL blocks internalization of LDL that we see the potential for another very important role of HDL. Indeed, after such a schema we are the outcome of this battle between HDL and LDL at our cellular membrane level. The higher our HDL the less LDL will penetrate to strain our cellular digestion mechanisms.

Finally, how do we translate all this body of knowledge to our clinical colleagues who are still trying to do all their lipid predictions with the total cholesterol? The dilemma they face is best portrayed in Figure 4. It shows the distributions of total cholesterol in people who stayed free of CHD and who developed CHD in 16 years at Framingham. Notice the enormous overlap. One of our problems in the public epidemic of CHD is that far too many lipid specialists will only act on a serum cholesterol which is 300 or over. While these people frequently have severe genetic (familial) disorders of lipoprotein metabolism they account at best for only about 25% of the coronary heart disease. The other 75% are generally ignored in this country because their cholesterols fall between 150 and 300 mg %. Is there a really safe cholesterol? The answer is probably yes and it may be one below 150 mg %. The real problem in terms of cholesterol, however, is how does one tell where they stand or really on which curve do they fall if their cholesterol is between 150 and 300 mg %? One great step in this direction would be to do the HDL cholesterol. At any given total cholesterol, one is in trouble if their HDL cholesterol is low but primarily if the ratio of total to HDL cholesterol is 4.5 or higher, since this is getting too close to the average ratios of CHD victims in Framingham which range from 4.8 to 5.7. Since 4.5 is the average ratio of our women we come back to our former statement that half the women and more than half the men have something concrete to do about their lipids.

What path should they take is also open to speculation. Frankly, I side with Dr. Epstein that they need to lower their LDL cholesterol to bring it into line, but I will admit with Dr. Glueck that there may be some pleasant surprises for those who raise HDL to improve the "ratio" from the other side. Finally, the potential role of HDL to remove cholesterols from deposits (? pool B) begs on the larger question of whether atherosclerosis is reversible and whether we have overlooked a grand potential for medical therapy because of our lackadaisical management of cholesterol to levels of 200, 220 or 270 have produced such scanty clinical results. A study of the natural history of this disease suggests that such levels are very atherogenic and that we all need to lower our cholesterols to the "world" average which may be just over 160 mg % so as to enhance the potential of HDL to undo the accumulated lesions of a lifetime of sloth and gluttony.

References

Barr DP, Russ EM, Eder HA (1951) Protein-lipid relationships in human plasma. Am J Med 11:480-493

Carew TE, Koschinsky T, Hayes SB, Steinberg D (1976) A mechanism by which high density lipoproteins may slow the atherogenic process. Lancet 1: 1315-1317 deDuve C (1975) Subcellular events in atherosclerosis. Circ 52:II-2

Fredrickson DS, Ferrans V (1978) Acid cholesteryl ester hydrolase deficiency (Wolman's Disease and Cholesteryl Ester Storage Disease) in the Metabolic Basis of Inherited Disease. Ed. by Stantury JP, Wyngaarden JB, and Fredrickson DS. McGraw-Hill Book Company, pp. 670-687, New York

Glomset JA, Norun KR (1973) The metabolic role of lecithin; cholesterol acyltransferase: perspectives from pathology. Adv Lipid Res 23: 535-547

Goldstein JL, Brown MS (1959) The origin of cholesterol in liver, small intestine, adrenal gland, and testes of the rat: dietary versus endogenous contributions. J Biol Chem 234:1095

Hamilton RL, Williams MC, Fielding CJ et al (1976) Discoidal bilayer structure of nascent high density lipoproteins from perfused rat liver. J Clin Invest 58:667-680

Mahley RW, Weisgraber KH, Innerarity T (1974) Canine lipoproteins and atherosclerosis. II. Characterization of the plasma lipoproteins associated with atherogenic and non-atherogenic hyperlipidemia. Circulation Research 35:722-733

Miller NE, Nestel PJ, Clifton-Bligh (1976) Relationships between plasma lipoprotein cholesterol concentrations and the pool size and metabolism of cholesterol in man. Atherosclerosis 23:535-547

Patrick AD, Lake BD (1969) Deficiency of an acid lipase in Wolman's Disease. Nature 222:1067

Stein O, Stein Y (1976) High density lipoproteins reduce the uptake of low density lipoproteins by human endothelial cells in culture. Biochem Biophys Acta 43:363-368

Role of HDL in Individual Prediction and Community Prevention of Coronary Heart Disease

Frederick H. Epstein

It is likely, depending on age and still limited information, that high-density lipoprotein (HDL) levels predict coronary heart disease (CHD) risk probably as well and possibly better than total serum cholesterol (TSC) and, certainly, that their combination permits more powerful prediction than either measurement alone (Kannel et al. 1979). The correlation between TSC and low-density lipoprotein (LDL) is very high so that TSC level measures the atherogenic potential of LDL. Since there is also much evidence that HDL is causally related to atherosclerosis as a protective factor, the balance of LDL and HDL as reflected by their serum levels is likely to be a key element in atherosclerosis prevention.

Based on such reasoning, there is a current tendency to conclude that TSC has lost its usefulness unless HDL levels are also known. This is true for the optimal prediction of risk in an individual. At the same time, however, it must be remembered that the marked rise of mean TSC with age, which is in all likehood one of the main, if not the main single reason for the high frequency of CHD in industrialized societies, is almost totally due to a rise in LDL, leading to an increasingly unfavourable TSC/HDL-C ratio with rising age well into the fifties. From the point of view of prevention, therefore, the first aim must be to prevent or slow this rise in TSC and, by implication, LDL. If, concurrently, average HDL levels could be raised, this would be an added advantage. The first emphasis is still on lowering LDL since the need for as much HDL as possible arises from the overabundance of LDL in societies with certain faulty nutritional habits. The lower the LDL, the less HDL is required to dispose of it! Indeed, in cultures with low TSC, HDL levels also tend to be low (Connor et al. 1978).

CHD Risk and Preventability of CHD in the Community

For the assessment of individual risk, it is apparent from the Framingham data (Coronary Risk Handbook, 1978) that a higher HDL-C (cholesterol contained in HDL) level reduces CHD risk at any level of LDL and, presumably, TSC. In order to assess risk on the community level, however, it is necessary to know not only the relative risks associated with different combinations of HDL and LDL or TSC, but also the frequency with which they occur in the population. No such cross-tabulations have been published so far but were supplied through the courtesy of the Framingham Group (W.P. Castelli, M.C. Hjortland and P. Sorlie, personal communication). The data are based on 1024 men among whom 117 CHD events occured over 8 years (Table 1). The categories in the original tables have been reduced for greater clarity and to increase the numbers in each cell. Around half of the men have TSC over 220 (46%) or HDL-C under 45 dl% (49%). In these two categories, 49 and 63% of the new CHD events occur, respectively, Clearly, HDL-C performs better in concentrating a higher percentage of events in the higher risk group; similarly, the risk gradient is steeper for HDL-C than for TSC. In evaluating these findings, it must be realized that the predictive power of serum cholesterol decreases with age and, in these data, is markedly lower than in the Pooling Project data (1978) under age 55. Since HDL-C remains or becomes even more predictive beyond age 50, its value is of necessity enhanced in this set of data which applies to older men. Taking the data at face value, it is possible to calculate for the population the risk attributable to levels of TSC above 220 and HDL-C below 45. If all the men included had TSC levels under 220, total events would be reduced only from 117 to 108, if all had HDL-C over 45, events would now number 85 instead of 117 but a combination of both, resulting in a population which in all men had TSC levels under 220 and HDL-C over 45, could be expected to reduce events by 40% from 117 to 68, assuming a totally causal relationship. Such reductions would be a measure of the preventive effect which might result from a shift in the distribution of TSC (and LDL), as well as HDL in the community.

Table 1: Eight-year Incidence of CHD - Framingham men

TSC (mg/dl)	Men in Risk Category (%)			Events in Risk Category (%)			Incidence (%)		
	HDL-C (mg/dl)			HDL-C (mg/dl)			HDL-C (mg/dl)		
	45	45+	Total	45	45+	Total	45	45+	Total
220	28	26	54	32	19	51	12.7	8.1	10.5
220-259	14	16	30	20	14	34	16.7	10.1	13.2
260+	7	9	16	11	4	15	18.3	5.8	11.5
Total	49	51	100	63	37	100	14.6	8.3	11.4

Levels of TSC and HDL-C in the Population

At the present time, only 26% of men in middle-age and beyond have risk factor levels which are relatively low in TSC (220) and high (45+) in HDL (Table 1). It would seem entirely unrealistic to think that most of the remaining three quarters of the men are prepared to change their living habits to an extent which will bring them into the favourable range. It is, however, not at all unreasonable to hope that a new generation will grow up in which LDL shows less rise with age and HDL will be higher on account of less obesity and more exercise. It is now thought (W.P. Castelli, personal communication) that a TSC/HDL-C ratio of 3.5 or lower should be the aim for men, corresponding to about half of the standard CHD risk prevailing to-day. Mean TSC may now be as low as 180 mg/dl (Rifkind et al. 1979) among men in the twenties, with HDL-C around 45 mg/dl, giving an average ratio of 4, being still somewhat above 3.5. This simple consideration gives an idea of the magnitude of needed prevention measures. Almost a quarter of men in their twenties have HDL-C levels below 40 (Lipid Research Clinics Program, unpublished data), - a level below which CHD risk is about 20% or more higher than the standard value at 45 mg/dl (Kannel et al. 1979); the detailed data upon which Table 1 is based, indicate that as many as close to half of the new events occur at HDL-C levels under 40.

This rather unfavourable assessment of the current risk factor status of men is supported by data from a subset of the Lipid Research Clinics Program (D.R. Jacobs and H. Blackburn, personal communication), raising the question how many men with elevated TSC carry enough HDL-C to give them a reasonable degree of protection. At ages 20-39, a fifth of the men have TSC levels over 234 mg/dl; only a third of them have HDL-C over 47 mg/dl. At ages 40-59, the lower cutting point of the top quintile lies at 270 mg/dl; only about 30% of these men have HDL-C levels over 47 mg/dl. While it is true that an elevated serum cholesterol level does not necessarily indicate a high risk, depending on the concurrent HDL-C level, about two-thirds of American high-risk men are not protected in these terms.

The same subset of data can also be looked upon in another way, taking as a base not high-risk men but the whole population. In this fashion, a more encouraging picture is obtained. If levels of TSC below 193 mg/dl or of HDL-C over 47 mg/dl can be considered as being reasonably protective, then 62% of men aged 20-39 have either a total serum cholesterol below or an HDL cholesterol above these cutting points. This is probably a reflection of the fact that TSC levels have declined in the United States in recent years (Proceedings of the Conf. on the Decline of CHD Mortality 1979), parallel with a decline in CHD mortality. The present position, therefore, would be that the risk factor status of American men with regard to lipoproteins is generally unsatisfactory, even though there are indications for recent changes in the desirable direction.

Have TSC Measurements become Outdated?

Prevention has both clinical and community aspects (Epstein 1973). From the clinical point of view, it has now become clear that CHD risk may differ greatly for two people with the same TSC level, depending on the proportion of cholesterol carried in HDL. Thus, a person with a relatively low TSC may be at considerable CHD risk and require preventive measures. In such a person, there is a particular need to take care of coexistent risk factors and, to be sure, since HDL-C in this situation is low, further lowering of LDL - even though it is already in the lower range - would only be advantageous. Conversely, if TSC is relatively high, with a low TSC/HDL-C ratio, the risk can presumably be further lowered by reducing the ambient LDL level. Therefore, in either situation, TSC - to the extent it still reflects LDL - has not become redundant!

On the community level, the position is much more clearcut. The evidence is overwhelming that the average serum cholesterol level in adulthood in a population is highly correlated with the frequency of coronary heart disease. There is nothing to suggest, based on the admittedly limited current information available, that these population risks are influenced to a major extent by the prevailing distribution of HDL-C. This is not to say that HDL-C may not play a role in determining community risk in addition to TSC. Thus, the proportionately higher HDL-C levels in American black adults (Tyroler et al. 1975) and children Srinivasan et al. 1976) may affect their CHD risk. Likewise, on the community level, one of the main pillars of the lipid theory remains the almost universal demonstration that CHD risk rises with increasing TSC. It is true that, within the same population, a test of future risk based on a measure which includes HDL-C is more sensitive and specific than measuring TSC alone (W.P. Castelli, unpublished data). So far, this demonstration is based only on the Tromsø and Israeli studies besides Framingham. Beyond remaining uncertainties, it is still true that populations, like individuals, with lower ranges of TSC show a lower CHD frequency, implying that reducing TSC or, even better, preventing its rise will very probably contribute to preventing premature CHD. The statement just made is in no way contradicted by the fact that there are populations which differ in CHD frequency at similar TSC levels (Epstein, in press). Any such populations would nevertheless still benefit from shifting the TSC distribution curve to the left, remembering that a lower overall risk in one population compared with another does not, in industrialized societies, mean a low risk.

Summary and Conclusion

Total serum cholesterol (TSC) and HDL-C predict the risk of coronary heart disease (CHD) better than either measurement alone for the individual. Likewise, the combined impact of lowering TSC and raising HDL-C on reducing CHD risk in the community will be greater than either measurement alone. At present, the distribution of TSC and HDL-C is not favourable in the American population inasmuch as few men have TSC/HDL-C ratios close to 3.5 or lower. The new findings regarding the protective effect of HDL in no way change the view that a shift in the distribution of TSC and, therefore LDL, must remain a cornerstone of CHD prevention in the community.

References

Coronary Risk Handbook using HDL-Cholesterol for Persons over 50. From the Framingham Study: W.B. Kannel, M.D., Director, May 1978

Epstein FH (1973) Coronary heart disease epidemiology revisited: clinical and community aspects. Circulation 48:185-194

Epstein FH (in press) Myocardial infarction in Europe. In: International Meeting on Myocardial Infarction (G.G. Neri Serneri, ed.) Excerpta Medica Publ., Amsterdam

Kannel WB, Castelli WP and Gordon T (1979) Cholesterol in the prediction of atherosclerotic disease. Ann Int Med 90:85-91

Pooling Project Research Group (1978) Relationship of blood pressure, serum cholesterol, smoking habit, relative weight and ECG abnormalities to incidence of major coronary events. J Chronic Dis 31:201-306

Proceedings of the Conference on the Decline in Coronary Heart Disease Mortality (1979) (RJ Havlik and M Feinleib eds) US Dept of HEW, Public Health Service, Nat.Inst. of Health, NIH Publ. No. 79-1610

Rifkind BM, Tamir I, Heiss G, Wallace RB and Tyroler HA (1979) Distribution of high density and other lipoproteins in selected LRC prevalence study populations: a brief survey. Lipids 14:105-112

Srinivasan SR, Frerichs RR, Webber LS and Berenson GS (1979) Serum lipid profile in children from a biracial community. Circulation 54:309-318

Tyroler HA, Hames CG, Krishan I, Heyden S, Cooper G and Cassel JC (1975) Black-white differences in serum lipids and lipoproteins in Evans County. Prevent Med 4:541-549

Cross-Cultural, Ethnic, Demographic, and Environmental Factors Affecting High Density Lipoprotein Cholesterol and Their Mutual Interrelationships with Coronary Heart Disease

Charles J. Glueck,[1] John A. Morrison, Peter S. Gartside, Peter Laskarzewski, Kathe A. Kelly, and Soaira Mendoza

High Density Lipoprotein Cholesterol, a Negative CHD Risk Factor

Population studies in diverse geographical areas including the United States (Gordon et al. 1977), Norway (Miller et al. 1977), Hawaii (Rhoads et al. 1976), and Israel (Goldbourt et al. 1979) have revealed that C-HDL is an independent risk factor inversely associated with coronary heart disease (CHD) risk. Detailed kindred studies have shown that familial elevations of high density lipoprotein cholesterol are associated with reduced CHD morbidity and mortality and with decreased longevity (Glueck et al. 1975, 1976). Studies of cohorts selected by extraordinary age (octo- and nonagenarians [Glueck et al. 1977; Nicholson et al. 1979]) identify many subjects having relatively high levels of C-HDL, some with familial hyperalpha-lipoproteinemia, and many having relatively low levels of the major atherogenic lipoprotein cholesterol, low density lipoprotein cholesterol, C-LDL. Because of the uniformity and consistency of these findings both in populations and in kindred studies, attention has been focused upon factors which may affect high density lipoprotein cholesterol levels, with the ultimate aim of better understanding HDL physiology, and pathophysiology, and ultimately to devise methods to consistently, safely, and effectively raise C-HDL levels.

Studies of cross-cultural, ethnic, and demographic factors relating to high density lipoprotein cholesterol levels

As summarized in Figure 1, for adult males and females, when matched by age and total plasma cholesterol, blacks have significantly higher HDL cholesterol than whites (Morrison et al. 1979). Moreover, black school-children of both sexes, ages 7-12 and 13-18 years, have higher HDL choles-terol levels than whites, Figure 1, (Morrison et al. 1978). These black-white differences cannot be explained by systematic differences in relative obesity, since similar high C-HDL in blacks was observed after covariance adjustment for Quetelet index, (Morrison et al. 1978, 1979). However, as summarized in Figure 1, there are no significant black-white differences in cord blood high density lipoprotein cholesterol (Glueck et al. 1977). Moreover, no significant black-white differences in C-HDL were noted by the Bogalusa study group in preschool children, ages 2 1/2 to 5 1/2, (Berenson et al. 1978). Hence, although black-white C-HDL differences are similar and consistent in school age children and adults, they do not appear until age seven. Whether this reflects delayed phenotypic expression of genetic differences or acquired differences which are not reflected in neonates and early childhood remains to be determined.

---

[1] From the Lipid Research Clinic and General Clinical Research Center, University of Cincinnati, College of Medicine, Cincinnati, Ohio, and from the Pathophysiology Department, School of Medicine, University of Los Andes (ULA) and Hormone Laboratory, University Hospital, Merida, Venezuela

Comparative studies of Russian and American adult males, ages 40-49 and 50-59 years (Figure 3), have revealed significantly higher HDL cholesterol levels in Russians (US-USSR Steering Committee 1977). However, in comparative studies of Russian and American male neonates, Figure 2, C-HDL distribution curves are almost superimposable, with American males having slightly higher C-HDL levels. Again, as was the pattern for blacks, (Figure 1), highly significant differences were observed in adults, but none in neonates. Whether this reflects a simple lack of expression of a "genetic" factor in cord blood or differential acquisition of acquired environmental factors in adults remains speculative.

Unlike the age-related C-HDL dichotomies noted in white-black and Russian-American comparisons, Figures 1 and 2, Venezuelan-American cross-cultural studies present a consistent pattern, Figure 3. Adult Venezuelan Mestizo males and females had significantly lower HDL cholesterol and higher triglyceride and C-VLDL than did American adults, Figure 3, (Mendoza et al. 1979). Similar Venezuelan-American differences were replicated in studies of both 7-12 and 13-18 year old Venezuelan and American children, Figure 3. Both male and female American children had significantly higher HDL cholesterol throughout the entire distribution, Figure 3 (Mendoza et al. 1979). Moreover, male and female Venezuelan neonates have appreciably lower HDL cholesterol levels than American neonates, Figure 3, (Mendoza et al. 1979, personal communication). The consistency of these Venezuelan-American C-HDL differences with age suggests, in part, a genetic effect, whose metabolic foundations have yet to be understood, but may provide important information pertinent to HDL metabolism and pathophysiology.

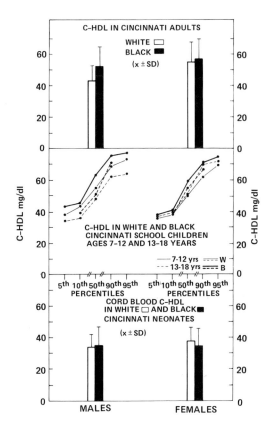

FIG. 1. Black-white differences in C-HDL.

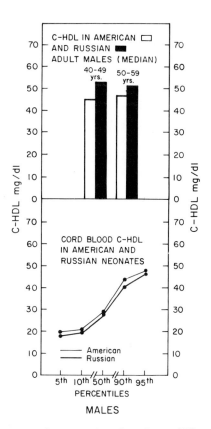

FIG. 2. Russian-American differences in C-HDL.

489

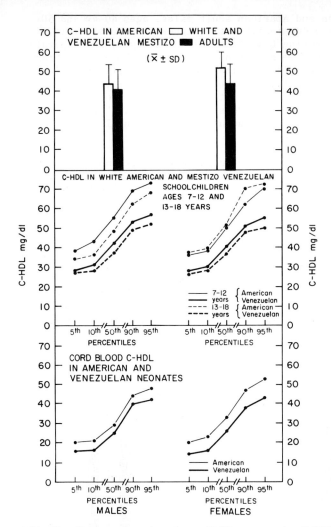

FIG. 3. Venezuelan-American differences in C-HDL.

Changes in high density lipoprotein cholesterol with age

As can be seen in Figures 1 and 3, at birth, mean HDL cholesterol levels
for males and females of both races in Cincinnati population groups are
about 75% of adult values. This is also congruent with the findings in
Russian neonates, Figure 2, and Venezuelan neonates, Figure 3. By age 1,
however, HDL values in female American black and white children more nearly
approximate those observed in adult American females (Tsang et al.1979).
Moreover, as summarized in Figures 1 and 3, prior to adolescence (ages 7-12),
males have higher HDL cholesterol than females. However, in 13-18 year old
males, the entire HDL cholesterol distribution shifts downward, (probably
due to testosterone release), so that by the end of adolescence, females
have higher HDL than males (Morrison et al.1979). After conclusion of
adolescence, in white males and females, there is a moderate increase in
C-HDL up to ages 55-65, followed by relatively constant levels after age 70
(Rifkind et al.1970).

Table 1. Factors associated with high density lipoprotein cholesterol levels.

	Higher levels of C-HDL	Lower levels of C-HDL
Age[a]	Prepuberty, both races and sexes	Cord blood, both races and sexes
Sex[b,c,d,e]	Males prior to adolescence	Females prior to adolescence
Race[b,f]	Black schoolchildren of both sexes	White schoolchildren of both sexes
	Black adults of both sexes	White adults of both sexes
Culture[g]	Russian adult males	American adult males
	American adults, both sexes	Venezuelan adults, both sexes
Obesity[h]	Low Quetelet indices	High Quetelet indices
Cigarette smoking[i]	Nonsmokers	Smokers
Alcohol intake[j]	Moderate drinkers	Nondrinkers
Chlorinated hydrocarbon pesticide exposure[k,l]	DDT exposure	PCB exposure
Habitual exercise[m]	Marathon runners	No consistent exercise pattern
Disease states	Dilantin[n]	Uremia[o]
Drugs	Estrogens[s]	Poorly controlled diabetes[p]
	Pregnancy 1st trimester[t]	Thiazide antihypertensives[q]
		High level corticosteroids[o]
		Androgenic steroids[r]
Genetic factors	Familial hyperlipoproteinemia[u]	An alpha-lipoproteinemia[v]
	Major gene inheritance for familial hyperlipoproteinemia[w]	Familial types I, V hyperlipoproteinemia[x]
	Major gene for apo AI inheritance[y]	Familial type II hyperlipoproteinemia[z]
Sucrose intake	Low sucrose, high fat diets	High sucrose, low fat diets
Polyunsaturated fat[zz]	Higher saturates, lower poly	Higher poly, lower saturates

[a]Klimov et al. (1979)
[b]Morrison et al. (1978)
[c]Morrison et al. (1979)
[d]Rifkind et al. (1979)
[e]Carlson et al. (1977)
[f]Morrison et al. (1979)
[g]US-USSR Steering Committee (1979)
[h]Goldbourt et al. (1977)
[i]Garrison et al. (1977)
[j]Castelli et al. (1977)
[k]Carlson et al. (1972)
[l]Baker et al. (1979)
[m]Wood et al. (1976)
[n]Nikkila et al. (1978)
[o]Curtis et al. (1978)
[p]Calvert et al. (1978)
[q]Hegeland et al. (1978)
[r]Nikkila (1978)
[s]Bradley et al. (1978)
[t]Tsang et al. (1978)
[u]Glueck et al. (1975)
[v]Fredrickson et al. (1972)
[w]Siervogel et al. (1979)
[x]Glueck et al. (1977)
[y]Berg et al. (1978)
[z]Kwiterovitch et al. (1974)
[zz]Shepherd et al. (1978)

Genetic and environmental factors associated with HDL cholesterol

That both genetic and environmental factors are associated with C-HDL levels is a functional truism. Table I summarizes factors known to be associated with C-HDL levels. Effects of age, sex, culture-geographical group, and race have been detailed in Figures 1-3. As summarized by Table 1, C-HDL levels are also affected by obesity, cigarette smoking, alcohol intake, exposure to chlorinated hydrocarbon pesticides, habitual exercise levels, multiple disease states and drugs, and by known monogenic dyslipoproteine-mias. Nutritional intake may also affect HDL metabolism. What is not currently known are the mechanisms of action by which these factors affect HDL metabolism, and how they concurrently affect CHD risk. Table 1 is presented to stimulate development of hypotheses relative to biochemical etiologies, with an ultimate aim of developing regimens designed to safely and effectively raise HDL cholesterol levels.

References

Baker EL, Landrigan PJ, Glueck CJ, Zack MM, Liddle JA, Burse VW, Housworth W, Bayse DD, Needham LL (1979) Metabolic consequences of population exposure to polychlorinated biphenyls. Am J Epidem, in press

Berenson GS, Foster TA, Frank GC, Frerichs RR, Srinivasan SR, Voors AW, Webber LS (1978) Cardiovascular disease risk factors variables at preschool age: The Bogalusa Heart Study. Circulation 57:603-612

Berg K (1978) Genetic influence on variation in serum high density lipoprotein. In: Gotto AM, Miller NE, Oliver MF (eds) High Density Lipoproteins and Atherosclerosis. Elsevier-North Holland Biomedical Press, pp 207-211

Bradley DD, Wingerd J, Petitti DB, Krauss RM, Ramchara S (1978) Serum high density lipoprotein cholesterol in women using oral contra-ceptives, estrogens, and progestins. New Engl J Med 299:17-20

Calvert GD, Graham JJ, Mannik T, Wise PH, Yeates RA (1978) Effects of therapy on plasma high density lipoprotein cholesterol concentration in diabetes mellitus. Lancet 8:66-68

Carlson LA, Kolmodin-Hedman B (1972) Hyperalpha-lipoproteinemia in men exposed to chlorinated hydrocarbon pesticides. Acta Med Scand 192: 29-32

Carlson LA, Hardell LI (1977) Sex differences in serum lipids and lipoproteins at birth. Eur J Clin Invest 7:133-135

Castelli WP, Doyle JT, Gordon T (1977) Alcohol and blood lipids. Lancet 2:153-155

Curtis JJ, Galla JH, Woodford SY, Rees ED, Luke R (1978) Effects of renal transplantation on hyperlipidemia and high density lipoprotein cholesterol, HDL. Transplantation 26:364-366

Fredrickson DS, Levy RI (1972) Familial hyperlipoproteinemias. In: Stanbury JB, Wyngaarden JB, Fredrickson DS (eds) The Metabolic Basis of Inherited Disease. 3rd edn. McGraw-Hill, New York

Garrison RJ, Kannel WB, Feinleib M, Castelli WP, McNamara PM, Padgett SJ (1977) Cigarette smoking and HDL cholesterol: The Framingham Study. Circulation Suppl III:55-56:III-44

Glueck CJ, Fallat RW, Millett F, Gartside PS, Elston RC, Go RCP (1975) Familial hyperalpha-lipoproteinemia: studies in 18 kindreds. Metab 24:1243-1265

Glueck CJ, Gartside PS, Fallat RW, Sielski J, Steiner PM (1976) Longevity syndromes: familial hypobeta- and familial hyperalpha-lipoproteinemia. J Lab Clin Med 88:941-957

Glueck CJ, Gartside PS, Steiner PM, Miller L, Todhunter T, Haaf J, Pucke M, Terrana M, Fallat RW, Kashyap ML (1977) Hyperalpha- and hypobeta-lipoproteinemia in octogenarian kindreds. Atherosclerosis 27:387-406

Goldbourt U, Medalie JH (1977) Characteristics of smokers, nonsmokers, and exsmokers among 10,000 adult males in Israel. Am J Epidem 105: 75-86

Goldbourt U, Medalie JH (1979) High density lipoprotein cholesterol and incidence of coronary heart disease - the Israeli Ischemic Heart Disease Study. Am J Epidem 109:296-308

Gordon T, Castelli WP, Hjortland MC, Kannel W, Dawber TR (1977) High density lipoprotein as a protective factor against coronary heart disease: Framingham Study. Am J Med 62:707-714

Helgeland A, Hjermann I, Leren P, Enger S, Holme I (1978) High density lipoprotein cholesterol and antihypertensive drugs: The Oslo study. Br Med J 2:403

Klimov AN, Glueck CJ, Gartside PS, JaMagracheva E, JaLivtchak M, Shestov DB, Anderson DW, Tsang RC, Stein EA, Steiner PM (1979) Cord blood high density lipoproteins: Leningrad and Cincinnati. Ped Res 13: 208-210

Kwiterovich PO, Jr., Fredrickson DS, Levy RI (1974) Familial hyper-cholesterolemia (one form of familial type II hyperlipoproteinemia): A study of its biochemical, genetic, and clinical presentation in childhood. J Clin Invest 53:1236-1249

Mendoza S, Contreras G, Ineichen E, Fernandez M, Nucete H, Morrison JA, Gartside PS, Glueck CJ (1979) Lipids and lipoproteins in Venezuelan and American Schoolchildren: within and cross-cultural comparisons. Ped Res, in press.

Mendoza S, Nucete H, Ineichen E, Salazar E, Zerpa A, Glueck CJ (1979) Lipids and lipoproteins in subjects at 3,500 and 1,000 meters altitude. Arch Environ Health, in press.

Miller NE, Forde OH, Thelle DS, Mjos OD (1977) The Tromso Heart Study. High density lipoprotein and coronary heart disease: a prospective case-control study. Lancet 1:965-968

Morrison JA, deGroot I, Edwards BK, Kelly KA, Mellies MJ, Khoury P, Glueck CJ (1978) Lipids and lipoproteins in 927 schoolchildren, ages 6-17 years. Pediatrics 62:990-995

Morrison JA, deGroot I, Kelly KA, Mellies MJ, Khoury P, Edwards BK, Lewis D, Lewis A, Fiorelli M, Heiss G, Tyroler HA, Glueck CJ (1979) Black-white differences in plasma lipids and lipoproteins in adults-The Cincinnati Lipid Research Clinic Population Study. Prev Med 7: 34-39

Morrison JA, Laskarzewski PM, Rauh JL, Brookman R, Mellies MJ, Frazer M, Khoury P, deGroot I, Kelly K, Glueck CJ (1979) Lipids, lipoproteins, and sexual maturation during adolescence: The Princeton Maturation Study. Metabolism 28:641-649

Nicholson J, Gartside PS, Siegel M, Spencer W, Steiner PM, Glueck CJ (1979) Lipid and lipoprotein distributions in octo- and nonagenarians. Metabolism 28:51-55

Nikkila EA (1978) Metabolic regulation of plasma high density lipoprotein concentrations. Eur J Clin Invest 8:111-113

Nikkila EA, Kaste M, Ehnholm C, Viikari J (1978) Elevation of high density lipoprotein in epileptic patients treated with phenyltoin. Acta Med Scand 204:517-520

Rhoads GG, Gulbrandsen CL, Kagan A (1976) Serum lipoproteins and coronary heart disease in a population study of Hawaii-Japanese men. New Engl J Med 294:293-298

Rifkind BM, Tamir I, Heiss G (1979) Preliminary high density lipoprotein findings: The Lipid Research Clinic Program. International Proceedings of the International Symposium on High Density Lipoprotein, in press

Shepherd J, Packard CJ, Patsch JR, Gotto AM, Taunton OD (1978) Effects of dietary polyunsaturated and saturated fat on properties of high density lipoproteins and metabolism of apolipoprotein A-I. J Clin Invest 61:1582-1592

Siervogel RM, Morrison JA, Kelly K, Mellies MJ, Gartside PS, Glueck CJ (1979) Familial hyperalpha-lipoproteinemia in 26 kindreds. Clin Genetics in press

Tsang RC, Glueck CJ (1979) Atherosclerosis: a pediatric perspective: In: Glueck L (ed) Current problems in Pediatrics. Yearbook Medical Publishers Vol. IX #3, 1-38

Tsang RC, Glueck CJ, McLain C, Russel P, Joyce T, Bove K, Mellies MJ, Steiner PM (1978) Pregnancy, parturition and lactation in familial homozygous hypercholesterolemia. Metabolism 27:823-829

US-USSR Steering Committee for Problem Area #1: The Pathogenesis of Atherosclerosis. Collaborative US-USSR study on the prevalence of dyslipoproteinemias and ischemic heart disease in American and Soviet populations. Am J Cardiol 40:260-268

Wood PD, Haskell W, Kelin H, Lewis S, Stern MP, Farquhar JW (1976) The distribution of plasma lipoproteins in middle aged male runners. Metab 25:1249-1257

Epidemiology and High Density Lipoproteins

Tavia Gordon

While there is now a fairly firm concensus that high density lipoproteins (HDL) are inversely related to the risk of coronary heart disease (CHD), it was not a consensus that came easily. Its history provides a vivid illustration of the vagaries and faddishness that sometimes characterizes scientific development and the difficulty a new finding may encounter when it is outside the main line of investigation.

As early as 1951 it had been noted (Barr et al. 1951) that alpha lipoprotein concentrations were lower and beta lipoprotein concentrations were higher in persons who had developed clinical evidence of atherosclerosis (chiefly in the form of myocardial infarction) than in normal controls. In this series alpha was a stronger risk factor than beta, but Barr et al. did not feel a need to choose between the two findings, considering them both to be important. They concluded by emphasizing the desirability of exploring protein-lipid relationships in order "to clarify the pathogenesis of atherosclerosis and to assist in its early detection." (It may be, and indeed probably is, true that the alpha and beta lipoproteins are related to myocardial infarction in large part through their impact on atherosclerosis, but of course they--like epidemiologists generally--collected only data on clinical events).

Several points should be noted here. The laboratory technique they used was a quantitative overlay on a qualitative procedure. While it was apparently a good technique in their hands, it was difficult and not easily standardized. The study itself used the case-control method. Such methods are always open to skepticism, since they are sensitive to the choice of controls and the contrast between cases and controls may be an artifact of selection bias. Despite these problems, their work was followed by a number of confirmatory case-control studies (Nikkila 1953, Jencks et al. 1956, Brunner et al. 1962). Finally, in 1966, the first prospective confirmation was reported (Gofman et al. 1966). Thus by 1966 there was a solid body of evidence that the level of HDL was inversely related to the risk of CHD. Despite this, interest in HDL remained low and there was little epidemiological, clinical or laboratory work undertaken to clarify this interesting finding. Not until another decade had passed was the subject revived. Why the delay?

Several factors may have contributed to the initial response. One was the setting in which the earlier discoveries appeared. It had been known for some time that total blood cholesterol (Total-C) was positively associated with the risk of CHD. A large and varied body of epidemiological evidence supported that conclusion. Measurement of Total-C was included in the procedures of most serious studies of cardiovascular epidemiology. Moreover, there was good evidence that it was possible to alter blood cholesterol levels by altering the diet. The evidence was so persuasive and the potential for preventive medicine so great that it is fair to say that information bearing on that set of relations was of greater interest than other evidence on lipid-CHD relations. Beta (LDL) lipoprotein carried the largest part of Total-C and thus was the lipoprotein of greatest interest. The most urgent methodological question appeared to be whether it was necessary to measure beta lipoprotein separately or whether it was sufficient to measure Total-C, which was simpler to do, cheaper and more reliable. The facts seemed to favor Total-C (Gofman et al. 1956).

Another, more subtle, factor may have been the unusual character of a negative risk factor--a protecive factor, so to speak. There is a quite pervasive notion that CHD is the consequence of excess, almost of some sort of moral failure. This vague puritanical theme runs through a good deal of the discussion of the causes and cures for CHD and may be more influential in our thinking than we would like to believe.

A third factor may have been simply technical. The quantitative ultracentrifuge, which is the most precise instrument for measuring the lipoproteins, was initially used to measure the LDL and VLDL spectrum, and the HDL portion was eliminated in the specimen preparation. While HDL-C can be separated by preparative ultracentrifuge and measured directly, the usual concentration in this portion is so low that it requires an unusually competent laboratory to measure it reliably. Thus, the techniques for measuring HDL or HDL-C were somewhat complicated for epidemiological uses, which are best served by simple, sturdy procedures.

The re-introduction of HDL into cardiovascular epidemiology in recent years was based on a new technical development, used initially in the study of lipoprotein phenotypes (Fredrickson et al. 1967). The primary interest lay in the roles of LDL and VLDL, but the procedure used involved the separate measurement of HDL-C. When a number of epidemiological studies undertook a cooperative lipoprotein phenotyping study (Castelli et al. 1975), measurements of HDL-C became available for a large series of CHD cases and controls. The investigators had no a priori interest in these. However, a routine examination of the study data revealed that in almost every instance, whether the data were looked at by age, race or sex, the concentration of HDL-C was on the average lower for the CHD cases than the controls. This relationship was at least as strong as the opposite relationship of LDL-C with CHD. Multivariate analysis demonstrated that neither was explained by the other.

This serendipitous finding happened to coincide with new and promising work in the metabolism of the lipoproteins (Miller and Miller 1975, Carew et al. 1976), in which the special role of the high density component was becoming of increasing interest. The synergistic effect of this concurrence is evident in the research done since then and in the belated concession of the importance of HDL as a factor in the development of CHD.

What, briefly, is the character of the epidemiological evidence respecting the relation of HDL to CHD? While the initial findings came from case-control studies, they have now been confirmed by several prospective studies (Gofman et al. 1966, Gordon et al. 1977, Goldbourt and Medalie 1979). In the study by Gordon et al. (1977) Framingham men and women free of CHD, ages 50-80, were followed for four years after their HDL-C levels were determined. In that series the inverse relation of HDL-C to CHD was the strongest lipid-CHD relation in evidence. Surprisingly, the LDL-C was also predictive of CHD at these older ages, despite earlier suggestions that neither Total-C nor LDL-C was predictive of CHD at advanced ages.

Since all of the lipoproteins are intercorrelated, the question naturally arises whether the predictive value of one fraction reflects the predictive value of another. Furthermore, where the correlation is fairly high, the question has to be asked which fraction is the one of primary interest for prediction. The word prediction is emphasized to make it clear that these are not questions about the atherogenic process (which are not well studied by static measurements, anyhow), but rather that they refer to a statistical question: What is the probability that a person with certain characteristics will subsequently manifest CHD?

The correlation between HDL and LDL cholesterol in the Framingham Study series was quite low (-0.04 for men, -0.16 for women). Thus, there was little reason to be concerned that the concentration of one was a reflection of the concentration of the other. On the other hand, the correlation of HDL-C with total triglycerides was somewhat stronger (-0.35 for men, -0.44 for women). (For convenience, it is customary to measure total triglycerides rather than VLDL-C, since the two are highly correlated and total triglycerides can be measured more reliably than the very small amount of cholesterol in VLDL.) The question as to which was the more useful predictor of CHD was investigated by two methods, by cross-classification and by multivariate logistic regression. The answer from both was unequivocal: the power of HDL concentration to predict CHD was unimpaired if triglyceride concentration was taken into account, whereas the predictive power of triglyceride concentration disappeared if HDL concentration was considered.

How does the HDL affect the risk of CHD? Unpublished data seem to indicate an inverse association between HDL-C concentration and coronary artery occlusion. Such data, because they are obtained from persons symptomatic of CHD, are bound to be somewhat biased. They are, however, consistent with the various metabolic studies, as they are presently reported and interpreted.

The epidemiological data also tend to confirm the hypothesis that HDL is related to CHD, at least in part, by way of its role in atherogenesis. Even in the early case-control studies (Nikkila 1953), the inverse association between HDL levels and CHD risk was evident both for myocardial infarction and angina pectoris. In the prospective data from the Framingham Study, the association was manifest both for coronary attacks (i.e., myocardial infarction, coronary insufficiency and CHD death) and for angina pectoris without any previous or concurrent coronary attack. It was evident both for fatal and non-fatal CHD. Such consistency tends to implicate coronary atherosclerosis as the central mechanism by which low HDL levels increase the risk of CHD. It might be added that the Framingham Study has also found an inverse relation between HDL-C levels and one of the major consequences of CHD, namely, congestive heart failures.

What determines HDL levels? Can they be modified? Is it desirable to do so? For illustrative purposes, two factors might be considered--alcohol and estrogens. Both raise HDL levels (Miller and Miller 1975, Castelli et al. 1977). Higher HDL levels are associated with lower CHD risk. Are either alcohol or estrogens, therefore, useful in preventing CHD?

Data from a number of sources, some unpublished, indicate that a greater alcohol consumption tends to be associated with a lower CHD risk, particularly the risk of coronary atacks (Yano et al. 1977, Klatsky et al. 1974, Barboriak et al. 1977). In all likelihood, alcohol will eventually join the roster of generally recognized CHD risk factors. It is even possible that it will eventually be found that the chief modality by which alcohol affects CHD risk is through its effect on HDL concentrations. But there is a considerable price to be paid for alcohol consumption. The social costs are substantial, as is generally recognized. But there are also other costs--a greater risk of certain cancers, cirrhosis of the liver, hypertension and stroke. More generally, I know of no persuasive evidence that total mortality is reduced by alcohol consumption and some evidence that it may be increased. Thus, this appears to be an instance where in the process of reducing one risk we increase others--always a hazard when intervention is undertaken.

Estrogen is an even more dramatic case. Estrogens raise HDL levels. Women have higher levels than men. Women have lower CHD risk than men. Ipso facto, why not the administration of estrogens as a CHD preventive?

Such efforts have been made, both in men and women. The effect in men was disastrous (The Coronary Drug Project Research Group 1973). Not only did the drug have unpleasant side effects but it tended to raise mortality. The effect on women appears to be the same. Estrogens are administered for contraceptive purposes and to alleviate post-menopausal symptoms. In both cases there is reason to believe that rather than lowering CHD risk they raise it (Mann 1978).

Whatever its role in causing or preventing CHD, HDL is clearly useful in predicting CHD. CHD is a multifactorial disease, but even when the other major factors are considered in a multivariate analysis, HDL is important in prediction (Gordon et al. 1977). There is no longer any serious question of that.

References

Barboriak JJ, Rimm AA, Anderson AJ et al. (1977) Coronary artery occlusion and alcohol intake. Br Heart J 39: 289-293
Barr DP, Russ Em, Eder HA (1951) Protein-lipid relationships in human plasma. Am J Med 11: 480-493
Brunner D, Altman S, Lobl K, Schwartz S (1962) Alpha-cholesterol percentages in coronary patients with and without increased total serum cholesterol
levels and in healthy controls. J Atheroscler Res 2: 424-437
Carew TE, Koschinsky T, Hayes S, Steinberg D (1976) A mechanism by which high-density lipoproteins may slow the atherogenic process. Lancet 1: 1315-1317
Castelli WP, Doyle JT, Gordon T et al. (1975) HDL cholesterol levels (HDLC) in coronary heart disease (CHD): a cooperative lipoprotein phenotyping study. Circulation 52: 11-97
Castelli WP, Doyle JT, Gordon T et al. (1977) Alcohol and blood lipids: the cooperative lipoprotein phenotyping study. Lancet 2:153-155
Fredrickson DS, Levy RI, Lees RS (1967) Fat transport and lipoproteins--an integrated approach to mechanisms and disorders. N Eng J Med 276:32-44
Gofman JW, Hanig M, Jones HM et al. (1956) Evaluation of serum lipoprotein and cholesterol measurements as predictors of clinical complications of atherosclerosis. Circulation 14: 691-742
Gofman JW, Young W, Tandy R (1966) Ischemic heart disease, atherosclerosis and longevity. Circulation 34: 679-697
Goldbourt U, Medalie JH (1979) High density lipoprotein cholesterol and incidence of coronary heart disease--The Israeli Ischemic Heart Disease Study. Am J Epid 109: 296-308
Gordon T, Castelli WP, Hjortland MC et al. (1977) High density lipoprotein as a protective factor against coronary heart disease: The Framingham Study. Am J Med 62: 707-714
Jencks WP, Hyatt MR, Jetton MR et al. (1956) A study of serum lipoproteins in normal and atherosclerotic patients by paper electrophoretic techniques. J Clin Invest 9: 980-990
Klatsky AL, Friedman GD, Siegelaub AB (1974) Alcohol consumption before myocardial infarction: results from the Kaiser-Permanente epidemiologic study of myocardial infarction. Ann Intern Med 81: 294-301
Mann JI (1978) Oral contraceptives and the cardiovascular risk. In Oliver MF (ed) Coronary heart disease in young women. Churchill Livingstone, Edinburgh, pp 184-194

Miller GJ, Miller NE (1975) Plasma-high-density-lipoprotein concentration and development of ischemic heart disease. Lancet 1: 16-20

Nikkila E (1953) Studies on the lipid-protein relationship in normal and pathologic sera and the effect of heparin on serum lipoproteins. Scand J Clin Lab Invest 5 (Suppl 8)

The Coronary Drug Project Research Group (1973) Findings leading to the discontinuation of the 2.5 mg/day estrogen group. JAMA 226: 652-657

Yano K, Rhoads GG, Kagan A (1977) Coffee, alcohol and risk of coronary heart disease among Japanese men living in Hawaii. N Eng J Med 297: 405-409

HDL Cholesterol, Tissue Cholesterol and Coronary Atherosclerosis: Epidemiological Correlations

N.E. Miller

Evidence that susceptibility to clinical coronary heart disease (CHD) varies inversely with the plasma high density lipoprotein cholesterol (HDL-C) concentration has been provided by case-control comparisons, prevalence studies, and prospective studies.

It has been apparent since the early 1950's that patients with clinically evident CHD have a low mean HDL-C level. Miller and Miller (1975) re-analysed some of these early data, and obtained evidence that the low HDL-C in CHD victims was independent of the plasma very low density (VLDL) and low density (LDL) lipoprotein levels. Subsequent case-control comparisons supported this contention (eg, Albers et al. 1978).

The Honolulu Heart Study (Rhoads et al. 1976) and the Cooperative Lipoprotein Phenotyping Study (Castelli et al. 1977) extended these observations by demonstrating that clinical CHD prevalence in middle-aged subjects was a negative function of HDL-C, independently of VLDL and LDL. This was true for each of five cohorts, for both sexes and for both myocardial infarction and angina pectoris. More recently Streja et al. (1978) reported a similar correlation in a large kindred with familial hypercholesterolaemia. The only significant difference between heterozygotes of similar age with and without clinical CHD was a lower HDL-C concentration in the former.

Evidence that the relationship of CHD to HDL-C concentration precedes its clinical manifestation was provided by the Framingham Study (Gordon et al. 1977), the Tromsø Heart Study (Miller et al. 1977) and the Israeli Ischaemic Heart Disease Study (Goldbourt and Medalie. 1979). In each survey HDL-C and LDL-C (or total plasma cholesterol) emerged as independent predictors of clinical events.

That the relationship of HDL-C to clinical events reflects an underlying relationship to coronary atherosclerosis has been demonstrated in three recent investigations (Jenkins et al. 1978; Pearson et al. 1979; Moore et al. 1979). In each of these studies the severity of disease, as quantified by coronary angiography, was negatively correlated with HDL-C, independently of VLDL and LDL.

Cholesterol is only one component of HDL, and it is pertinent to examine the relationships of coronary disease to other components. Present information indicates that the plasma concentration of the major proteins of HDL, apo AI and apo AII, are also reduced in coronary victims (Berg et al. 1976; Albers et al. 1978), but perhaps to a lesser degree than the HDL-C concentration (Albers et al. 1978). Prospective data suggest that the apo AI concentration is a weaker predictor of clinical events than is HDL-C (Ishikawa et al. 1978).

The HDL fraction is composed of two major subclasses of differing composition, HDL_2 and HDL_3, the former having a greater cholesterol/protein ratio. In 1966 Gofman et al. documented low HDL_2 concentrations, measured by analytical ultracentrifugation, in 38 men aged 20-66 yrs who subsequently developed clinical CHD during 10 years of follow-up. The HDL_3 concentration was also reduced, but to a lesser degree, resulting in a reduced HDL_2/HDL_3 mass ratio.

We have recently examined the relationship of coronary atherosclerosis, quantified by 'blind' scoring of coronary angiograms, to the concentrations of lipids in different lipoprotein fractions (separated by preparative ultracentrifugation) in subjects undergoing investigation of chest pain. Preliminary findings suggest that increasing coronary artery score is associated with a decrease in HDL_2 cholesterol, but not in HDL_3 cholesterol, resulting in a reduction of the HDL_2/HDL_3 cholesterol ratio (Table 1).

Table 1. High density lipoprotein subfractions in relation to angiographically defined coronary atherosclerosis (mean values).

Coronary artery score*	HDL_2 Cholesterol (mg/dl)	HDL_3 Cholesterol (mg/dl)	HDL_2/HDL_3 ratio
0-10	17.9	21.1	0.85
11-20	14.0	28.1	0.50
21-30	14.0	31.6	0.44
> 30	8.6	30.8	0.28

* Computed from the number, length and degree of stenoses in major segments of the coronary vasculature.

Preliminary findings in 32 men. Data from Hammett et al. (1979).

What is the significance of these observations in relation to atherogenesis? Do they reflect a causal relationship, and, if so, by what mechanism? The answers to these questions are not yet available. It is noteworthy, however, that body cholesterol pool size, measured by isotope dilution, has also been found to be inversely related to the plasma HDL-C concentration. This correlation was originally demonstrated in a group of hyperlipidaemic subjects, whose HDL-C levels ranged from 27 to 58 mg/dl (Miller et al. 1976). This observation has now been extended by our finding that the mass of slowly exchangeable cholesterol (pool B), but not that of rapidly exchangeable cholesterol (pool A), was significantly lower in five subjects with hyperalphalipoproteinaemia (mean HDL-C, 100 mg/dl) than in age-matched controls with normal HDL-C levels (mean, 55 mg/dl) (Table 2). Subjects with familial hyperalphalipoproteinaemia are known to have a virtual absence of clinical CHD (Glueck et al. 1976).

Table 2. Body cholesterol pool sizes in subjects with
hyperalphalipoproteinaemia (mean values).

	Pool A* (g/70 kg body wt)	Pool B+ (g/70 kg body wt)
Controls (n = 4)	18.5	51.5
Hyperalphalipo- proteinaemia (n = 5)	13.1	21.5
P	NS	< 0.01

* Minus plasma cholesterol pool.
+ Assuming no synthesis in pool B.

Data from P.J. Nestel and N.E. Miller (unpublished observations).

Summary.

The currently available data from clinical and epidemiological
studies indicate the following:
1) The plasma HDL-C concentration is a negative risk factor for
   clinical CHD, independently of the VLDL and LDL concentrations,
   in men and women of western societies.
2) This largely reflects an underlying negative correlation
   between the concentration of the HDL_2 subfraction and the
   severity of coronary atherosclerosis.
3) The size of the slowly exchanging pool of tissue cholesterol
   (to which most of atheroma cholesterol belongs) in man is
   also a negative function of the plasma HDL-C concentration
   over a wide range of concentrations.
4) The postulated causal relationship between disordered HDL
   metabolism and coronary atherosclerosis, mediated by augmented tissue cholesterol deposition, remains to be established.

References.

Albers JJ, Cheung MC, Hazzard WR (1978) High-density lipoproteins
    in myocardial infarction survivors. Metabolism 27: 479-485
Berg K, Børresen MH, Dahlen G (1976) Serum high density lipo-
    protein and atherosclerotic heart disease. Lancet 1: 499-501
Castelli WP, Doyle JT, Gordon T, Hames CG, Hjortland MC, Hulley
    SB, Kagan A, Zukel WJ (1977) HDL cholesterol and other
    lipids in coronary heart disease. The Cooperative Lipo-
    protein Phenotyping Study. Circulation 55: 767-772
Glueck CJ, Gartside P, Fallat RW, Sielski J, Steiner PM (1976)
    Longevity syndromes - familial hypobeta and familial hyper-
    alphalipoproteinemia. J Lab Clin Med 88: 941-957
Gofman JW, Young W, Tandy R (1966) Ischemic heart disease,
    atherosclerosis and longevity. Circulation 34: 679-697
Goldbourt U, Medalie JH (1979) High density lipoprotein cho-
    lesterol and incidence of coronary heart disease - the
    Israeli Ischaemic Heart Disease Study. Am J Epid 109:
    296-308

Gordon T, Castelli WP, Hjortland MC, Kannel WB, Dawber TR (1977) High density lipoprotein as a protective factor against coronary heart disease. The Framingham Study. Am J Med 62: 707-714

Ishikawa T, Fidge N, Thelle DS, Førde OH, Miller NE (1978) The Tromsø Heart Study: serum apolipoprotein AI concentration in relation to future coronary heart disease. Europ J Clin Invest 8: 179-182

Hammett F, Saltissi S, Miller N, Rao S, Van-Zeller H, Coltart J, Lewis B (1979) Relationship of coronary atherosclerosis to plasma lipoproteins. Circulation (In press) Abstr.

Jenkins PJ, Harper RW, Nestel PJ (1978) Severity of coronary atherosclerosis related to lipoprotein concentration. Br Med J 2: 386-391

Miller GJ, Miller NE (1975) Plasma high density lipoprotein concentration and development of ischaemic heart disease. Lancet 1: 16-19

Miller NE, Førde OH, Thelle DS, Mjøs OD (1977) The Tromsø Heart Study. High density lipoprotein and coronary heart disease: a prospective case-control study. Lancet 1: 965-968

Miller NE, Nestel PJ, Clifton-Bligh P (1976) Relationships between plasma lipoprotein cholesterol concentrations and the pool size and metabolism of cholesterol in man. Atherosclerosis 23: 535-547

Moore RB, Long JM, Matts JP, Amplatz K, Varco RL, Buchwald H, et al (1979) Plasma lipoproteins and coronary arteriography in subjects in the program on the surgical control of the hyperlipidemias. Atherosclerosis 32: 101-119

Pearson TA, Bulkley BH, Achuff SC, Kwiterovich PO, Gordis L (1979) The association of low levels of HDL cholesterol and arteriographically defined coronary artery disease. Am J Epid 109: 285-295

Rhoads GG, Gulbrandsen CL, Kagan A (1976) Serum lipoproteins and coronary heart disease in a population study of Hawaii Japanese men. New Engl J Med 294: 293-298

Streja D, Steiner G, Kwiterovich PO (1978) Plasma high-density lipoproteins and ischemic heart disease. Studies in a large kindred with familial hypercholesterolemia. Ann Intern Med 89: 871-880

The Multiple Risk Factor Intervention Trial[1]

Prepared for The Multiple Risk Factor Intervention Trial Group[2] by William L. Holmes

The Multiple Risk Factor Intervention Trial is a multicenter, collaborative, randomized, non-double blind clinical trial of the efficacy of multiple risk factor modification for the reduction of coronary heart disease (CHD) mortality. Of the several identified risk factors for CHD three -- elevated blood cholesterol, elevated blood pressure, and cigarette smoking -- stand out as major ones and appear to offer the greatest potential for modification.

The primary objective of the MRFIT is to determine whether for a group of men at increased risk of death from CHD, a special intervention program directed simultaneously toward three risk variables will result in a significant reduction in CHD mortality. Secondary objectives include assessing the effects of intervention on the incidence of myocardial infarction, all cardiovascular disease mortality, and total mortality. For identification of specific goals having a reasonable chance of attainment, the following general specifications of risk factor modification expressed as average change were made: 1) a 10% reduction from baseline in serum cholesterol for those with serum levels ≥ 220 mg/dl; 2) a 10% reduction from baseline in diastolic blood pressure if equal to or greater than 90 mm Hg; 3) a 20, 30, or 40% net reduction in amount of cigarette smoking for heavy, moderate, and light cigarette smokers, respectively.

Although methods used for selection of participants for the trial, and intervention techniques have been described previously (see references) they will be reviewed briefly in this report followed by a discussion of some of the results of risk factor modification observed in the SI group at the 12 and 24 month recall visits.

Methods

Recruitment

Twenty-two centers in various areas of the United States screened men between the ages of 35 and 57 and determined their history of smoking, blood pressure, and serum cholesterol. Men who were in the upper 15 and later 10 percent of risk of heart attack based on a risk function derived from the Multiple Logistic Equation applied to the Framingham Study population, and who were not excluded for history of myocardial infarction, treatment of diabetes mellitus, or exceptionally high risk due to serum cholesterol ≥ 350 mg/dl or a diastolic blood pressure ≥ 115 mm Hg were invited to return for a second visit. The second screen consisted of a physical examination, measurement of height, weight and BP, urinalysis, resting ECG, PA chest x-ray, pulmonary function test, one-hour glucose tolerance and a battery of clinical chemistry tests including lipoprotein phenotyping. Participants re-

---

[1] This work was supported by MRFIT contract NHLBI - N01-HV 33110
[2] See Appendix

maining eligible were invited to a third screen. At this visit BP was taken again, a baseline and treadmill-exercise test were performed, nutritional, smoking, and other social-behavioral data were obtained. After the nature of the trial was fully explained and consent to participate was received each participant was randomized into either the Special Intervention Group (SI) or the Usual Care Group (UC). The latter were referred to their usual source of medical care for the management of their risk factors.

Intervention

The SI Group attended eight to ten integrated intervention sessions of approximately 2 hours each at weekly intervals. Each group was comprised of 6 to 12 participants and their spouses. In order to standardize intervention techniques among centers the Steering Committee devoted an intensive effort to the preparation of a common protocol and to the selection and preparation of educational materials appropriate for the trial. The strategies of these sessions combined lectures, selected principles from the disciplines of behavior modification and group dynamics, and the use of group process to facilitate change in a supportive atmosphere.

Emphasis in nutrition was on the use of an overall balanced diet low in saturated fat and cholesterol. The basic diet was planned to provide less than 35% of calories in the form of fat, less than 10% from saturated fatty acids and 10-13% from polyunsaturated fatty acids, approximately 250 mg of cholesterol per day, and modification of carbohydrates as required. A step-care program of weight reduction followed by appropriate drugs, if necessary, was selected for the management of hypertension. The smoking modality emphasized complete cessation using a variety of techniques, special supporting materials, and audiovisual aids.

Upon completion of the intensive intervention phase, all SI participants are seen regularly at intervals of four months. The UC participants return annually for a medical history, physical examination, and laboratory studies. Those SI participants who attained risk factor modification goals are entered into a maintenance program. Those not attaining goals are placed in an extended intervention program. This includes frequent visits for management of hypertension, monthly or bimonthly visits for nutrition counseling and determination of serum cholesterol for those having difficulty in reducing their cholesterol level, and other special counseling sessions either individually or in small focal groups for weight control or smoking intervention.

Results

A total of 361,629 first screen visits were completed on men in the age range 35-57 years. A group of 12,866 men, representing approximately 50% of those found to be risk eligible at the initial screen, were enrolled in the study; 6,428 were assigned to the SI group and 6,438 to the UC group.

Table 1 summarizes the reported dietary fat and cholesterol intake for 5,094 participants who attended both the third screen and 24 month visit. The data for the 12 month recall for a cohort of 5,901 participants are essentially the same hence they are not presented here. It is evident that the reported total daily calories are reduced by some 22 percent, reported total and saturated fat and cholesterol intake are at goal and reported consumption of polyunsaturated fat although increased is still slightly below recommended levels.

Table 1. Mean reported dietary fat intake (percent of total calories) SI participants at third screen and 24 months, N=5094.

	Recom- mended	Third screen	24 months	Difference S_3-24 months
Total calories/day	–	2513	1915	597
Total fat	<35	38.3	33.8	4.5
Saturated fat	<10	13.9	10.1	3.8
Polyunsaturated fat	>10	6.6	8.7	−2.1
Cholesterol mg/day	≤250	458	255	203

Table 2. Mean serum cholesterol at first screen and 12 and 24 months for SI participants.

	Cholesterol mg/dl		
	First screen	Mean at visit	Decrease from screen I
12 Mos. N=6063	253.9	238.3	15.6
24 Mos. N=5985	254.1	238.2	15.9

Table 3. Relationship of weight loss to decrease in blood-cholesterol, SI participants screen 2 to 2 years.

Weight loss (lbs)	Percent change in cholesterol			
	Total	LDL	VLDL	HDL
0.5 – 4.5	−5.2	−2.5	+6.0	+2.5
4.5 – 9.5	−6.2	−4.5	–	+4.5
>9.5	−9.6	−6.1	−15.0	+8.9

Table 4. Effect of hypertension intervention on SI participants with goal blood pressure determined.

	No. Goal determined	Baseline DBP	Mean DBP at visit	Percent	
				≤Goal	<90 mm Hg
12 months	2836	95.6	85.4	52.6	73.0
24 months	3429	95.0	83.2	63.8	81.8

Examination of serum cholesterol results (Table 2) shows a decrease of 15.6 and 15.9 mg/dl (6.1%; includes presence of regression to the mean) from the first screen to the 12 and 24 month visits, respectively. An investigation of plasma total and lipoprotein cholesterol at second screen and 24 months showed a mean decrease in cholesterol level of 14.2 mg/dl of which 11.2 mg/dl was accounted for by a decrease in LDL; there was very little overall change in VLDL and HDL cholesterol except when dietary change was accompanied by weight loss (Table 3).

Initially no special emphasis was placed on weight loss except for borderline hypertensives. As the project developed an association between weight loss and cholesterol lowering became apparent (Table 3). A comparison of these data with predicted weight loss based on the Keys equation indicated that this loss adds a substantial increment to the decrease in serum cholesterol

Table 5. Reported cessation rates at twelve and twenty-four months by initial smoking group

Cigarettes/day	Number of men		% reporting cessation	
	12 Mos.	24 Mos.	12 Mos.	24 Mos.
1-19	417	412	70.5	69.9
20-39	1759	1715	45.4	47.5
>40	1651	1608	33.7	33.9
All Smokers	3827	3735	43.1	44.1

over and above the effect of change in dietary lipid intake. Examination of lipoprotein cholesterol suggests that a modest weight loss of 4.5 pounds or more results in desirable changes in all fractions.

Goal blood pressure is based on the DBP taken at the visit at which drug therapy is initiated and is defined for all SI participants as DBP of 89 mm Hg, or 10 mm Hg less than the average DBP at that visit, whichever is lower. At 12 months goal blood pressure had been determined for 2836 participants (Table 4), mean DBP had decreased 10.2 mm Hg, 52.6% were at goal and 73.0% had a DBP <90 mm Hg. The number with goal determined increased to 3429 by 24 months of which 63.8% had attained goal and 81.8% had DBP <90 mm Hg.

The number of men who reported smoking at first screen and who were seen at both the 12 and 24 month visits are shown in Table 5 together with the percentage who reported smoking cessation. The reported quit rates of 43 and 44% at 12 and 24 months considerably exceeded both our expectations and the results of most other comparable programs. The cessation results for each group of smokers, light, moderate and heavy are in the direction that might be anticipated, i.e., a greater incidence of cessation among light smokers as compared to heavy smokers.

In summary, one of the major accomplishments of the MRFIT Trial is the demonstration of the feasibility of enlisting and retaining large numbers of healthy individuals in such a public health program as evidenced by attendance at the 24 month visit (UC-93%; SI-94%). The long-term results of hypertension and smoking intervention have been most gratifying and have certainly exceeded expectations. The overall average reduction in serum cholesterol has been somewhat less than predicted. The MRFIT baseline data suggest that one reason for falling short of prediction is that many Americans had already made significant dietary changes in the direction recommended by MRFIT which might affect the magnitude of their response to the new eating pattern. Also a sizeable group of poor dietary adherers has been identified which undoubtedly has had an impact on the overall results. Despite these problems a substantial subgroup, estimated at 55 percent of the SI participants have shown an excellent response to nutrition intervention; the mean serum cholesterol lowering being 13 percent (range 5 to 42%).

References

The Multiple Risk Factor Intervention Trial Group (1976) A national study of primary prevention of coronary heart disease. JAMA 235:825-827
The Multiple Risk Factor Intervention Trial Group (1977) Statistical design considerations in the NHLBI Multiple Risk Factor Intervention Trial (MRFIT). J Chron Dis 30:261-275
The Multiple Risk Factor Intervention Trial Group (1978) The Multiple Risk Factor Intervention Trial. Ann NY Acad Sci 304:293-308

The Multiple Risk Factor Intervention Trial Group:
from the American Health Foundation, C.B. Arnold[*], E.L. Wynder[**], R.Mandriota, J. Eisenbach, R. Ames, S. Goldstein; from Boston University, H.E.Thomas,Jr.[*], W.B. Kannel[**], F.N. Brand, L.K. Smith, P. Greene, H. Lewis, J. Connors; from Cox Heart Institute, P. Kezdi[*], E.L. Stanley, F.A. Ernst, W.L. Black, F. Paris; from Dade County Department of Public Health, G. Christakis[*], J.Burr[**], T. Gerace, M.E. Wilcox; from Dalhousie University, P.M. Rautaharju[*], H.Wolf; from Harvard University, R. Benfari[*], K. McIntyre[**], O. Paul[**], J. Ockene, D. Dousch, J. Stoll; from the Kaiser Foundation Research Institute(Portland), J.B. Wild[*], M. Greenlick[**], J. Grover[**], S. Lamb, J. Bailey, J. Dyer, E. Brokop, W. Wiest, R. Worthington, V. Stevens; from Lankenau Hospital, W. Holmes[*], J.E. Pickering, G. Rubel, J. Allaire, B. Feinstein, D. Fellon; from the National Center for Disease Control, G.R. Cooper[*], from New Jersey Medical School (Newark), N. Lasser[*], N. Hymowitz[**], E.D. Munves; from Northwestern University, J. Stamler[*], R. Cooper, A. Dyer, G. Greene, D. Moss, V. Persky, E. Robinson, K. Shannon, L. VanHorn, M. Voracheck; from University of Chicago, L. Cohen[*], J. Morgan[**], G. Grundmann, L. Slowie; from St. Joseph Hospital, D.M. Berkson[*], G. Lauger, S. Grujic, D. Obradovic, E. Pardo; from the Institutes of Medical Sciences–University of California at San Francisco & Berkeley, J. Billings[**], S.B. Hulley[**], W.M. Smith[**], S.L. Syme[**], R.Cohen, L. Dzvonik, J. Appelbaum, M. Woolley, S. Gordon, A. Geissler, D. Davies; from the Institutes of Medical Sciences, San Francisco Central Lab, G.M. Widdowson[**], G.Z. Williams[**], S.B. Hulley[**], from Rush Presbyterian-St. Luke's, J.A. Schoenberger[*], R.B. Shekelle, J. Schoenenberger, G. Neri; T. Dolecek, Y. Hall; from Rutgers Medical School, N.H. Wright[*], S.A. Kopel[**], M. Schorin, K.R. Suckerman; from St. Louis Heart Association, N. Simon[*], J.D. Cohen[**], E. Bunkers; from University of Alabama in Birmingham, H.W. Schnaper[*], G.H. Hughes[**], A. Oberman, C.C. Hill; from University of California at Davis, N.O. Borhani[*], C. Sugars, K. Kirkpatrick; from University of Maryland, R. Sherwin[*], M.S. Sexton[**], P. Dischinger; from University of Minnesota, H. Blackburn[*], R. Crow[**], M. Mittelmark[**], R. Grimm, A.S. Leon, E. Rotman, D. West, K. Lenz, W. Thorp, D. Jacobs; from University of Minnesota ECG Coding Center, R.J. Prineas[*], D. Brasseur, R. Crow, from the University of Minnesota Coordinating Center, M.O. Kjelsberg[*], G.E. Bartsch, J. Neaton, P. Ashman, A. DuChene, S. Broste; from University of Pittsburgh, L. Kuller[*], R. McDonald, E. Meilahn, A. Caggiula, L. Falvo-Gerard; from University of South Carolina, W.K. Giese[*], J.F. Martin[**], S. Blair; from University of Southern California, J. Marmorston[*], E. Fishman, R. Johnson; from the Policy Advisory Board, W. Insull, Jr.[*], J.C. Cassel (deceased), J. Farquhar, C.D. Jenkins, D.J. Thompson, P.W. Willis, C.M. Young(deceased), W.J. Zukel, J. Cornfield(deceased), W.T.Friedewald; from the National Heart, Lung, & Blood Institute Staff, M. Farrand, W. Friedewald, E. Furberg, T. Gordon, C. Kaelber, J. Tillotson, E. Passamani, P. Dern, K. Eberlein

---

[*]   Principal Investigator
[**]   Co-Principal Investigator

Test of the Lipid Hypothesis: The Coronary Primary Prevention Trial (CPPT) of the Lipid Research Clinics Program[1]

Robert H. Knopp[2]

Since the lipid hypothesis was formulated (Anitschkow and Chalatow 1913), a vast quantity of data has accumulated to confirm that hypercholesterolemia is a "risk factor" for heart attack (see Kannel et al. 1979). While diet does lower blood cholesterol (See Hazzard and Knopp 1976 for review) and is considered the most readily available treatment for hypercholesterolemia, dietary cholesterol intake is not uniformly associated with accelerated atherosclerosis (Kannel and Gordon 1970) and dietary attempts to prevent arteriosclerotic heart disease have not met with unequivocal benefit. For instance, primary prevention studies employing diet as the sole treatment show a favorable reduction in heart disease mortality without statistically significant reduction in mortality overall (Dayton et al. 1969; Miettinen et al. 1972; Frantz et al. 1975; see Hazzard and Knopp 1976 for review). Therefore, there is still skepticism that cholesterol lowering reduces heart disease mortality at all or enough to justify the effort and expense.

Criticisms of these previous attempts to answer the lipid-heart disease question form the basis for a new therapeutic trial embodied in the Lipid Research Clinics (LRC) Program (see Lippel et al. 1977; The Lipid Research Clinics Program Epidemiology Committee 1979; Rifkind et al. 1979 for overviews of this program). The major features of the LRC Coronary Primary Prevention Trial (CPPT) are presented in Table 1 opposite the criticisms of previous heart disease prevention trials. The experimental design of the CPPT has been recently described in detail (Lipid Research Clinics Program 1979).

Sample size calculations. The number of subjects required is based on the following assumptions: cholesterol will be lowered 24% with cholestyramine and 4% with diet, subjects will discontinue medication at a rate of 5% per year, the interval from initiation of intervention to maximum effect is 3 years, and the expected incidence of heart attack is equal to that of subjects in the top 5% of the Framingham distribution of serum cholesterol. The probability of concluding that a difference exists between the two groups when it does not (alpha error) is set at 0.01 (i.e., significance level). The probability that a difference does not exist between the two groups when it does (beta error) is set to 0.10 (i.e., power of the study). Using the normal approximation of the binomial (Halperin et al. 1968), the number of subjects required is 3,550.

Subject recruitment. The number of subjects actually recruited is 3,810 from the 12 collaborating North American clinics. The middle age range, 35-59, is specified because lipid associated heart disease risk is greater

---

[1]This study is supported by NHLBI contracts HV1-2156-L, HV1-2160-L, HV1-1914-L, HV3-2931-L, HV3-0010-L, HV2-2913-L, HV1-2158-L, HV1-2161-L, HV2-2915-L, HV2-2932-L, HV2-2917-L, HV2-2916-L, HV1-2157-L, HV1-2243-L, HV1-2159-L, HV3-2961-L, and HV6-2941-L.
[2]Collaborators in this 12-clinic project are listed at the end of this chapter.

Table 1. Criticisms of trials of heart disease prevention vs CPPT design.

Critique	CPPT Design
Subjects	
Too few	3,810
Cholesterol not a risk factor	Hypercholesterolemic men, ages 35–59
High risk for non CVD mortality	Healthy, free living
Already have heart disease	No overt heart disease or angina
Not randomized	Stratified and randomized
Treatment	
Not double blind	Placebo control, double blind
Multiple not single intervention	Cholestyramine (C) is the sole intervention
No diet control	All subjects on diet
Cholesterol lowering insufficient	C lowers cholesterol 15–30%
Adherence suboptimal	Adherence counselling is a priority
Duration insufficient	Seven yr follow-up
Drug toxic	No evidence of toxicity
Follow-up infrequent	Bimonthly visits
Endpoint identification weak	Aggressive endpoint verification
Study stopped prematurely	Termination date predetermined

in this group than in older subjects. Study subjects were recruited from approximately 500,000 primary screens in industries, blood banks, entertainment events and shopping centers of the respective communities. An initial casual cholesterol $\geq$ 265 mg/dl was the basis for further testing which required a low density lipoprotein (LDL) cholesterol of $\geq$190 mg/dl after a 12-14 hour fast (approximately the 95th percentile) (Rifkind et al. 1978). A diet consisting of a P/S ratio of 0.6-1.0 and a daily cholesterol intake of 400 mg was then taught and the response judged at the next two clinic visits. If LDL cholesterols fell below 175 mg/dl $\geq$ 90th percentile) on either of these visits, subjects were excluded, leaving those individuals with a presumably constitutional basis for hypercholesterolemia remaining in the trial.

Subjects were further excluded if they had: cardiovascular disease, diabetes or hypertension requiring medication, blood pressures exceeding 150/100 mm Hg on 3 visits, a mean of 3 plasma triglyceride measurements exceeding 300 mg/dl, floating β lipoprotein, a history of myocardial infarction, angina pectoris by history or exercise test to 90% of maximum effort, or conditions causative of secondary hyperlipidemia. Subjects were repeatedly instructed in the exigencies of the trial and encouraged to withdraw if they had misgivings about successfully adhering to the drug regimen.

Randomization. To assure a successful randomization to cholestyramine or control groups, subjects were allocated to cells based on stratification according to three prognostic factors: 1) LDL cholesterol above or below 215 mg/dl (97.5 percentile of males aged 35-59 in the LRC prevalence study) (Rifkind et al. 1978), 2) ST segment depression on graded exercise testing greater than 0.1 mV at the J junction or 80 m-sec thereafter with reversion at rest, 3) a multiple logistic risk function based on diastolic blood pressure, smoking, and age. Randomization was begun November 13, 1973 and completed July 31, 1976. The success of randomization is illustrated in Table 2 where selected baseline characteristics at the second prerandomization visit match closely.

Drug regimen. Subjects were instructed in the taking of study medicine beginning with 2 packets or 8 grams twice daily, then raising to 3 packets

Table 2. CPPT Randomization Quality.

		Placebo	Cholestyramine
Total cholesterol	(mg/dl)	291.8	291.4
LDL Cholesterol	(mg/dl)	216.2	215.6
HDL Cholesterol	(mg/dl)	44.0	44.0
Triglyceride	(mg/dl)	158.5	159.8
Systolic BP	(mm)	120.6	120.7
BMI (x10^3)	(Kg/cm^2)	2.65	2.69
Smokers	(%)	36.7	38.4

or 12 grams twice daily after 2 weeks. Dose adjustment was required, particularly in those subjects experiencing constipation, a symptom best relieved with temporary dose reductions, Metamucil, Hydrocil, or occasionally Colace. About half of the men experienced symptoms of constipation, abdominal fullness, or indigestion but for the most part reached optimal symptomatic baseline within 6 months to 1 year. Adherence to drug and dietary regimens is enhanced by the monitoring each subject receives at the bimonthly visits, careful training of physicians, nurses, and dietitians and other professionals in counseling skills, and individualized assessment of each subject's psychosocial adaptation to the trial. Perhaps the most powerful adherence tool is a sense of trust and personal friendship that exists between staff and study participants.

Monitoring. Medical and diet history and screening clinical chemistries are obtained bimonthly, cardiovascular system and xanthoma exam and resting EKG are performed every 6 months, and complete physical exam and graded exercise tests are done yearly. Study participants maintain contact with a private physician to whom all matters of medical treatment are referred.

Endpoint determination. The primary endpoints in the CPPT are coronary heart disease death and definite non-fatal myocardial infarction. All data are collected using standardized procedures and forms across all 12 clinics. Major cardiovascular endpoints are reviewed by a panel of LRC cardiologists for accuracy of classification and adequacy of data. If data collection is not ideal, further data collection efforts are made.

Trial safety and determination. A Safety and Data Monitoring Board consisting of cardiovascular disease, epidemiology, and clinical trial experts not directly involved in the daily conduct of the trial reviews quarterly reports and convenes on at least a 6-month basis to review the complete statistical analysis of the trial including potential benefits and toxicity. At this writing, the trial has been in progress for 3-1/2 years. No toxic reactions to cholestyramine have been announced indicating the safety of this drug. The trial is expected to last about 7 years with an estimated completion date of July 1983. Hopefully then we will have a definite answer to the question: can cholesterol lowering prevent heart disease.

Acknowledgments

The following have contributed to the coronary primary prevention trial: Program Office. R. Levy, B. Rifkind, G. Nelson, C. Blum, G. Morrison, R. Havlik, A. Seplowitz, D. Gordon, K. Lippel, V. Keating. Central Patient Registry. D. Williams, E. Davis. Lipid Research Clinic Directors. F. Abboud, E. Bierman, R. Bradford, V. Brown, W. Connor, G. Cooper, J. Farquhar, I. Frantz, C. Glueck, A. Gotto, W. Hazzard, W. Insull, R. Knopp, P. Kwiterovich, J. LaRosa, A. Little, F. Mattson, M. Mishkel, G. Schonfeld, D. Steinberg. CPPT Directors. W. Benedict, R. Bradford, M. Ezekowitz, R.

Fallat, R. Gross, D. Hunninghake, M. Kashyap, R. Knopp, J. LaRosa, R. Lee,
T. Maneatis, M. Mishkel, J. Ogilvie, J. Probstfeld, H. Schrott, E. Stein,
G. Steiner, M. Stern, D. Taunton, T. Whayne, E. Wittels, J.
Witztum, L. Wyndham. <u>LRC Support Facilities</u>. S. Agras, G. Cooper,
J. Dunbar, V. Grambsch, S. Irving, T. Sheffield, S. Zifferblatt.

References

Anitschkow N, Chalatow S (1913) Ueber experimentelle cholesterin-steatase
    und ihre Bedeutung fur die Enstehung einiger pathologischer Prozesse. Zel
    tralbl Allg Pathol Pathol Anat 24: 1-9
Dayton S, Pearce ML, Hashimoto S, Dixon WJ, Tomiyasu U (1969) A controlled
    clinical trial of a diet high in unsaturated fat in preventing complications
    of atherosclerosis. Circulation 40 (Suppl II): 1-63
Frantz ID Jr, Dawson EA, Kuba K, Brewer ER, Gatewood LC, Bartsch GE (1975)
    The Minnesota coronary survey: effect of diet on cardiovascular events
    and deaths.
Halperin M, Rogot E, Gurian J, Ederer F (1968) Sample sizes for medical
    trials with special reference to long-term therapy. J Chron Dis 21: 13-24
Hazzard WR, Knopp RH (1976) Aging and atherosclerosis. Interactions with
    diet, heredity, and associated risk factors. In: Rockstein M, Sussman
    ML (eds) Nutrition, Longevity, and Aging. Academic Press, New York,
    pp 143-195
Kannel WB, Castelli WP, Gordon T (1979) Cholesterol in the prediction of
    atherosclerotic disease. Ann Int Med 90: 85-91
Kannel WB, Gordon T (eds) (1970) The Framingham Study. An epidemiological
    investigation of cardiovascular disease. Section 24: the Framingham diet
    study: diet and the regulation of serum cholesterol. U.S. Government
    Printing Office, Washington
Lipid Research Clinics Program (1979) The coronary primary prevention trial:
    design and implementation. J Chron Dis 32: 609-631
Lipid Research Clinics Program Epidemiology Committee (1979) Plasma lipid
    distributions in selected North American populations: The Lipid Research
    Clinics Program prevalence study. Circulation 60: 427-439, 1979
Lippell K, Ahmed S, Albers JJ, Bachorik P, Cooper G, Helms R, Williams J
    (1977) Analytical performance and comparability of the determination of
    cholesterol by 12 Lipid-Research Clinics. Clin Chem 23: 1744-1752
Miettinen M, Turpeinen O, Karvonen MJ, Elosuo R, Paavilainen E (1972) Effect
    of cholesterol-lowering diet on mortality from coronary heart disease and
    other causes; a twelve-year clinical trial in men and women. Lancet 2:
    835-838
Rifkind BM, Tamir I, Heiss G, Wallace RB, Tyroler HA (1979) Distribution of
    high density and other lipoproteins in selected LRC prevalence study popu-
    lations: a brief survey. Lipids 14: 105-112

The Chicago Heart Health Curriculum Program[1]

James A. Schoenberger, Albert J. Sunseri, Joan Kruc, and Leonard Bickman

The program I will describe cannot be considered a clinical trial in the usual sense, but in the opinion of the moderators of this workshop and myself, it represents a new direction for research into the prevention of atherosclerosis. I am pleased to have this opportunity to present the program even though it is only in its early stages of implementation and no results can be reported.

The Chicago Heart Health Curriculum Project is a logical evolutionary step in the long history of the Chicago Heart Association, whose programs have been directed at primary prevention and early detection of heart disease. In times past, this Heart Association Affiliate has made significant contributions to the control of beta hemolytic streptococcal infection and heart sound screening. As rheumatic fever ebbed, studies of the problem of the detection of those at high risk for coronary heart disease became a major concern. These studies revealed that a significant proportion of the adult population is at high risk for the development of coronary heart disease, that the majority of these high risk individuals are unaware of their risk and that they are not benefiting from the potential for prevention. From these and other studies has come the impetus to confirm by traditional clinical trials the value of intervention. Unfortunately, human behavior in adults in regard to diet and smoking has been found to be quite resistant to change. Further, many of the clinical trials have failed to show any benefit from lowering cholsterol levels by diet or controlling hypertension by drugs in the adult population.

Other studies had demonstrated that atherosclerosis had an early onset since young Americans killed in battle already showed significant, but subclinical, degrees of atherosclerosis of the coronary vessels. Further, there are an appreciable number of young children who already are a above-average risk according to adult standards. The American Way of Life can be dangerous to health, and the danger apparently begins earlier in life than had been supposed.

Thus, in the Muscatine Study, mean serum cholesterol was 182 mg/dl for children of all ages from 6 to 18 years and for both sexes. As shown in Figure 1, it can be seen that there is no apparent increase in cholesterol levels within the ages under study. The lowest 5% of these children had levels of 140 mg/dl or below. In contrast, 24% had levels of 200 mg/dl or greater, 9% had levels of at least 220 mg/dl and 5% at least 230 mg/dl. These relationships are seen in Figure 2. Although levels of cholesterol in children follow a unimodal distribution, there appears to be skewing to the right. The values are considerably higher than those seen in other cultures an above the levels considered to be safe based on animal studies in subhuman primates.

Blood pressure in these children, on the other hand, rose with age as shown in Table 1. In the age range 6-9 years virtually none of the children

---

[1]Supported by NHLBI grant HL 21892-02.

Table 1. Muscatine Study: Blood pressures.

Systolic (mmHg)	Systolic Blood Pressures				Diastolic (mmHg)	Diastolic Blood Pressures			
	6–9 yr (% total)	10–13 yr (% total)	14–18 yr (% total)	6–18 yr (% total)		6–9 yr (% total)	10–13 yr (% total)	14–18 yr (% total)	6–18 yr (% total)
At least 160	0.1	0.4	1.3	0.5	At least 110	0.0	0.2	0.3	0.2
150–159	0.1	1.2	1.8	0.9	100–109	0.1	0.5	1.6	0.6
140–149	0.3	2.8	5.8	2.7	90–99	1.1	6.3	10.2	5.4
130–139	0.9	9.7	17.2	8.4	80–89	16.3	27.4	43.1	27.4
120–129	7.3	18.5	27.0	16.6	70–79	37.3	41.4	35.8	38.3
110–119	22.6	30.7	26.7	26.6	60–69	31.9	19.5	7.5	21.0
100–109	35.9	25.8	16.2	27.0	50–59	12.3	4.2	1.2	6.5
Under 100	32.9	10.9	3.9	17.4	40–49	1.1	0.4	0.2	0.6
N	1,845	1,669	1,315	4,829	N	1,845	1,669	1,315	4,829

514

Table 2. Estimates of the percentage of current, regular cigarette smokers, teenagers, aged 12 to 18, United States, 1968-1974.

Year	Ages 12-14		Ages 15-16		Ages 17-18		Ages 12-18	
	Male	Female	Male	Female	Male	Female	Male	Female
1968	2.9	0.6	17.0	9.6	30.2	18.6	14.7	8.4
1970	5.7	3.0	19.5	14.4	37.3	22.8	18.5	11.9
1972	4.6	2.8	17.8	16.3	30.2	25.3	15.7	13.3
1974	4.2	4.9	18.1	20.2	31.0	25.9	15.8	15.3

exceeded levels of 140 and/or 90 mmHg. With increasing age, levels of blood pressure considered to be hypertensive were seen with increasing frequency. By the age of 14-18 years, 8.9% had systolic levels of 140 mmHg or higher and 12.1% had diastolic levels of greater than 90 mmHg. These relationships are shown in Figure 3 for selected percentiles.

Finally, cigarette smoking has become an increasing problem in the United States for youngsters aged 12-18 as shown in Table 2. For the period reported, cigarette smoking rose in all age groups of girls over the years, reaching an alarming 25.9% in girls aged 17-18. For boys the peak prevalence appears to have been reached in 1970, but still, 31% of boys

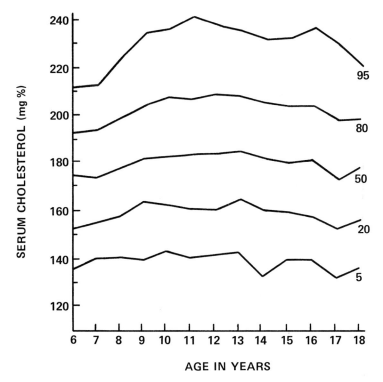

FIG. 1. Selected percentiles of serum cholesterol levels for boys and girls aged 6-18 years. N indicates the number of children measured in each age group. There was little difference between the levels of cholesterol in boys and girls (Lauer et al. 1975). Permission granted by the Journal of Pediatrics and the authors.

aged 17-18 were regular smokers in 1974.

It is little wonder, then, with the higher than ideal mean levels of serum cholesterol, the significant prevalence of cigarette smoking and the not inconsiderable numbers of hypertensives in these younger people, that many have come to consider atherosclerosis to be a pediatric problem. Eating styles and cigarette smoking have become deeply ingrained habits of living in adults, highly resistant to change. It is the thesis of this program that achieving healthier habits of living and prevention of cigarette smoking can be more successfully achieved in youngsters and that the greatest hope for successful prevention of coronary heart disease lies in effective intervention in the young.

Education, the basis for this program, has in the past relied heavily on imparting information with little or no concern for the impact of the knowledge acquired on attitudes or behavior. Programs have been evaluated on the basis of short term assessment of cognitive retention. The Chicago Heart Health Curriculum differs from previous educational efforts, not only because of the philosophical basis of the educational approach, but also because of the attempts to quantitate changes in attitude and behavior as a result of the educational program. These studies will be carried out within the context of true experimental designs. For this presentation, I would like to describe the concept of humanistic education on which the program rests, the broad outline of the program and the methods of evaluation. I believe that research in education of this sort is unique and may lead to invaluable insights for improving the process in the future. The not unrealistic hope that the epidemic of coronary heart disease can be controlled lies in beginning the process of successful intervention at ever younger ages.

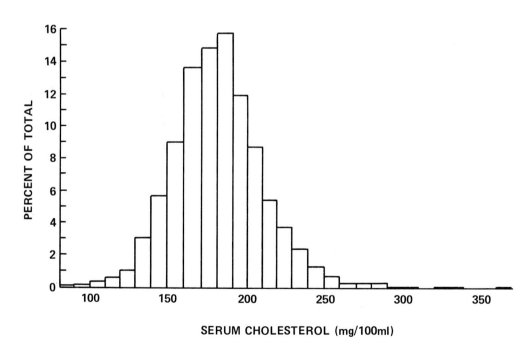

FIG. 2. Histogram of serum cholesterol levels of Muscatine children ages 6-18 years (Lauer et al. 1975). Permission granted by the Journal of Pediatrics and the authors.

Humanistic education is based on the concept that values, attitudes and beliefs play a critical role in health related decisions. The major dimensions of this model include the following concepts:

1. Indeterminism: the learner is an active and responsible chooser in selection of those attitudes which control behavior
2. Holism: the learner is more than a sum of the separate parts and behavior is not determined by any one element alone
3. Phenomenalism: the learner makes conclusions based on selective perceptions of the information to which he is exposed

These philosophic dimensions are expressed in humanistic eductional theory in the following manner:

1. Decision making: development of judgement, self-regulation, independence and cooperation will lead to responsible life-enhancing choices
2. Confluence: both cognitive and affective aspects of learning must flow together
3. Awareness: the fact that cognitive information has a personal meaning to the learner and the new information can be applied to problem-solving

These concepts are utilized in the application to health problems in the

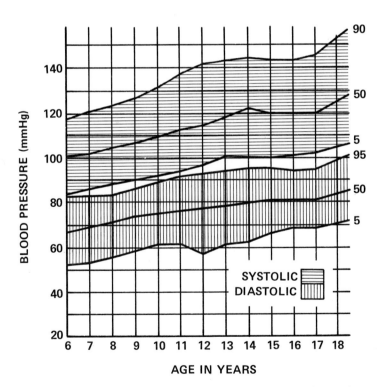

FIG. 3. Selected percentiles of systolic and diastolic blood pressure in children 6-18 years. There was little difference between boys and girls. N indicates the number measured at each age level (Lauer et al. 1975). Permission granted by the Journal of Pediatrics and the authors.

following skill areas:

1. Personal: the learner can achieve problem solving skills which will enhance the quality of his life
2. Interpersonal: these skills can have a positive effect on other individuals
3. Extrapersonal: these skills can have a significant bearing on society at large

In sum, the goals and objectives of the program are the development of skills in solving health problems with the expectation that these skills will modify behavior in the direction of more healthful life styles which will then be maintained throughout life.

The Chicago Heart Health Curriculum

The program has been designed for the sixth grade level of Chicago schools. Five specific learning objectives and health problem skills are included in the program: 1) students will understand the importance of feelings and emotions in relation to health; 2) students will learn the importance of good nutrition and modify personal eating habits to conform; 3) students will establish a personal exercise program for cardiovascular fitness; 4) students will relate personal health practices to the prevention of cardiovascular diseases; 5) students will decide that cigarette smoking is not compatible with healthful living and choose not to smoke.

The program is divided into five modules. Unique materials such as activity sheets, a personal health log, films, film-strips and video tapes have been developed. All are specific for the age group under study and have been field tested and refined so as to be highly appealing and interesting to sixth grade students.

Volunteer teachers will be trained in workshops in the use of the materials and will have available an extensive teachers manual for guidance in implementing the program. Workshop training of teachers is ongoing at the present time and the program will be carried out from January through May of 1980. The content of teaching by each participating teacher will be monitored by weekly reports of materials used and subjects covered and by at least two visits during program implementation by project staff.

The program has recruited 200 volunteer teachers of sixth grade classes in the Chicago school system. The program will be implemented by random selection in 100 of these classes. The other 100 classes will serve as controls. They will be matched for socioeconomic variables and reading level. Fifty teachers in each group will undergo a simple cardiovascular risk assessment (height, weight, skinfold thickness, blood pressure, cholesterol, and carbon monoxide breath analysis) in addition to a smoking questionnaire and a dietitian supervised three-day food recall. These examinations will be repeated at the end of the school year to evaluate the changes made by the teachers in their own behavior.

In subsequent years a cross-over design will utilize control teachers from the first year in an enriched program based on formative evaluation of the first years experience and involvement of a parental component. Longitudinal follow-up of students from the first year's program will be carried out.

All aspects of the program will be studied by an external evaluation conducted by the Westinghouse Evaluation Institute. Health knowledge will be tested by field tested and validated cognitive instruments developed both for teachers and students. Teacher and student attitudes will be tested by a modified Likert Scale, a Health Locus of Control Scale and by a Behavior Consequences instrument based on the Fishbein Intention to Behave Model. According to the Fishbein theory, a person's intentions to behave in a certain way are determined in part by attitudes toward the behavior, which are in turn determined by the expected value of the consequences of the behavior and the probability of the behavior leading to these consequences. Since long term observation of actual behavior by students or teachers is impractical, the use of this instrument should prove to be of great value in supplementing self-reported behavior.

Appropriate pre- and post-testing of teachers and students will be carried out with a Solomon four group design to allow examination of the data for possible reactivity of the pre-test and for interactions between the treatments and pre-tests.

Direct observations of behavior will also be carried out to confirm the data obtained from the attitudinal instruments. Unobtrusive data collection will be utilized. This will include observation of food choices made in the lunch room to evaluate the impact of the program on eating habits. Ability of students to withstand peer pressure to smoke will be tested in an Asch-type conformity study.

The impact of the program on teachers' own health behavior will be studied in the risk factor screening component. An attempt will be made to determine if these teachers who reduce their own personal risk of coronary disease serve as more effective role models and teachers than those who make no reduction in risk after exposure to the program.

Summary

The Chicago Heart Health Curriculum hopes to influence the affective and cognitive skills of the learner to the end that more appropriate health behaviors will be adopted. Using the humanistic approach should assist in the comprehension and assimilation of new knowledge, attitudes and behaviors leading to healthy life styles in this group of youngsters. If the program is successful it should be made available widely to classrooms throughout the nation.

Reference

Lauer RM, Connor WE, Leaverton PE, Reiter MA, Clarke WR (1975) Coronary heart disease risk factors in school children: The Muscatine Study. J Pediatrics 86:697-706

Summary of Concepts Concerning the Arterial Wall and Its Atherosclerotic Lesions[1]

Donald M. Small

Since the original observation made over 100 years ago that cholesterol accumulates in the arterial wall in atherosclerosis, great interest has been placed on the histology, chemistry, biochemistry, cytochemistry and physical chemistry of the arterial wall. I wish to briefly bring together some facts concerning the lipids of the arterial wall and the changes that occur during the development of the advanced atherosclerotic plaque.

The major lipids accumulating in atherosclerosis include: free cholesterol, cholesterol esters, and phospholipids. The same three lipids are the major constituents of low and high density lipoproteins. The lipid composition of the arterial wall and its different lesions is expressed on triangular coordinates in Figure 1. The figure also demonstrates the phase behavior of these lipid classes in aqueous systems as previously described by Small and Shipley (1974). The plots of lipid compositions of normal arterial wall of children (Smith et al. 1967; Day and Wahlquist 1970) are very different from the various arterial lesions. These differences in the chemical composition predict changes in the physical chemistry of the lipids involved. Thus, one would expect all of the lipids in the childs arterial wall to exist in the single phospholipid-rich phase consisting of the membranes and cellular or-ganelles of the cells of the intima. Other lesions of atherosclerosis how-ever involve the formation of new lipid phases within the arterial intima. In fact the atherosclerotic plaque has at least three such separate indi-vidual phases (Small and Shipley 1974; Katz et al 1976). Many investigators have studied the lipids and lipoproteins of the arterial wall and have found a variety of loosely or tightly bound particles or aggregates. I will at-tempt to relate these findings to the physical-chemical characterization of the different atherosclerotic lesions.

Normal intima of children. Normal intima of children from 1 to 5 years of age appears to contain only a single lipid phase. By light and electron microscopy the lipids appear to be part of the membranes and organelles of the cells of the intima. No separated oil phases are seen. The composition of children's intima is representative of cellular lipid compositions from other peripheral tissues such as muscle. The free cholesterol content does not appear to saturate the phospholipid system and this may reflect that many of the cell organelles usually have a much lower cholesterol-phospho-lipid ratio than do plasma membranes (Small 1977). The cholesterol ester content is very low. Nothing is known of the LDL content of such intima, but the fact that cholesterol ester content is low mitigates against high LDL concentrations in these intimas. These intimas should be considered the normal state of the human intima.

"Normal" intima from adults. The early studies of Smith et al. (1965, 1967) indicated that small droplets of extra cellular lipid were present along the elastic and collagen fibrils. These lipids had cholesterol ester compo-sitions similar to LDL and because they could be seen by microscope were

[1]Supported by U.S. Public Health Service Grants HL-18673, HL-13272 and Training Grant HL-07291.

The Average Lipid Composition of Normal Intima and the Different Lesions of Atherosclerosis

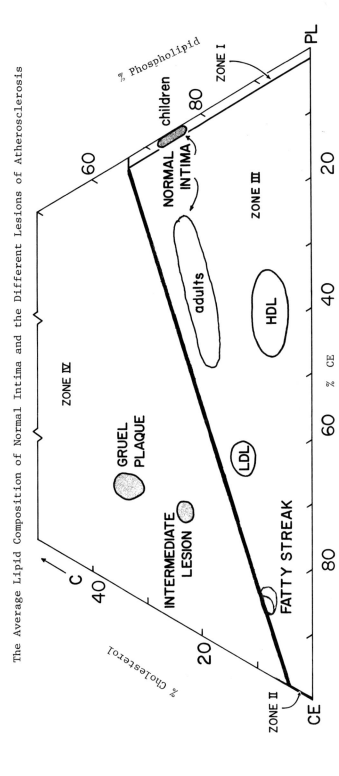

FIG. 1. The compositions are plotted on triangular coordinates representing the physical behavior of the major lipid components of atherosclerotic lesions and low density lipoprotein (see Small 1977a). Zone I is a single phase made up of lipid bilayers analagous to membranes. About 33% cholesterol and 2% cholesterol ester can be incorporated into this zone. Zone II is made up of an oil or liquid crystalline phase of cholesterol esters into which a small amount of free cholesterol can dissolve. Zone III is a two-phase zone containing both the phospholipid bilayer phase and a cholesterol ester-oil phase. Zone IV is a zone which contains three phases: a phospholipid bilayer phase, the cholesterol ester phase, and free cholesterol monohydrate crystals. The composition of normal intima of children and adults and different lesions of atherosclerosis are plotted. For comparison the composition of LDL and HDL are also given.

The development of atherosclerosis shows a progressive change from normal intima of children (which is apparently a single phase made up of membrane-like elements) to the gruel plaque which contains at least 3 separate lipid phases.

clearly larger than LDL. These were called perifibrinous lipid. It is not clear from the original studies whether droplets were artifacts of fixation and staining. Recent studies by Smith (1980) show that there is a very high concentration of LDL immunological activity in the intima. The level appears to drop off precipitously in the underlying media. Furthermore the LDL activity appears to be proportional to the serum concentration of LDL and appears to be retained more than other protein molecules of similar size. Hoff (1980) has confirmed that there are large quantities of easily removed LDL-like material in the "normal" intima of adults, but that it is probably not true LDL. The amino acid analyses of the protein are somewhat different than normal LDL and the electrophoretic mobility is more negative. Furthermore, we found that these particles appear to be somewhat more heterogeneous in size than native LDL. Other larger particles having flotation characteristics of VLDL have also been isolated (Hollander et al. 1979). These particles are very heterogeneous in size and could represent some of the material which stains to give the appearance of perifibrinous lipid. The overall lipid composition of the smaller particles is similar to LDL but the larger particles contain too much cholesterol ester and too little triglyceride to be plasma VLDL. Thus, the normal adult intima have a high concentration of material of density and size similar to LDL and VLDL which have LDL immuno reactivity but which are not native LDL. They may represent different stages of denatured, aggregated or fused LDL.

Fatty streak lesions. The lipid in fatty streak lesions is largely intracellular. Histologically these lesions consist of surprisingly healthy appearing foam cells filled with droplets of lipid. No cholesterol crystals were noted and none would be expected since the overall composition appears to be less than saturated with cholesterol (Katz et al. 1976). However, Katz et al. (1976a) found that the individual cells contain droplets with somewhat different melting temperatures, suggesting different pools of cholesterol ester within a given cell. Further there was a wide range of melting temperatures between individual fatty streak cells, suggesting different stages of cellular metabolism. Therefore, while the overall composition gives an average view of the physical state, the individual physical state may vary from cell to cell and from organelle to organelle within a given cell. Hoff (1980) found that little LDL could be extracted from these lesions whereas large droplets have been isolated after tissue homogenization (Lang and Insull 1970; Hata and Insull 1973; Katz et al. 1976). Presumably these large droplets represent the intracellular accumulations of both lysosomal (membrane bound) and stored (non-membrane bound) cholesterol esters. This lesion is characterized by an increase in cells which apparently have an ability to phagocytose particles and store the cholesterol as cholesteryl oleate-rich droplets. It is not known if the source of cholesterol is the high intimal concentration or the somewhat abnormal LDL and larger particles present in the normal adult intima. The various biochemical pathways of cellular cholesterol metabolism and the blocks which could result in this lesion have been outlined previously (Small 1977a).

The intermediate lesions. Histologic observations have indicated that there may be lesions intermediate between fatty streaks and more advanced fibrous plaques. Katz et al. (1976) found a lesion which appeared grossly as a fatty streak but which contained an excessive amount of free cholesterol and had an intermediate chemical composition between the advanced atherosclerotic plaque and the ordinary fatty streak. They called it the intermediate lesion. These lesions (Figure 1) fall in Zone IV and thus should have contained cholesterol crystals. However, very few of the lesions actually contained crystals and only small amounts of necrotic cells were noted. We suggested that these lesions represent fatty streaks which had become supersaturated with free cholesterol and that they therefore could serve as precursors of plaques. Crystallization of the excess cholesterol from such lesions could lead to necrosis and produce a necrotic core characteristic of the fibrous plaque. Since the composition of these lesions is clearly very different from either low density lipoproteins or ordinary fatty streaks, one must ask where the excess free cholesterol comes from. A change in the relative concentration of free cholesterol could arise from the hydrolysis of LDL cholesterol esters into free cholesterol. If such cholesterol could not leave the lysosome (the site of the hydrolysis) it would accumulate and ultimately precipitate. Studies by Fowler et al. (personal communication 1979) have suggested that lysosomes in fatty streak-like lesions in cholesterol-fed rabbits contain excessive amounts of free cholesterol possibly in crystalline form. This would indicate that there is a block in the movement of free cholesterol across the lysosomal membranes in such cells. The crystallization of cholesterol within lysosomes could disrupt the lysosomes and lead to necrosis and the development of the necrotic part of the atherosclerotic plaque.

Fibrous plaques. These lesions are larger, often contain more than 30% lipid by dry weight and have a necrotic center and a fibrous cap. The region between the necrotic center and the fibrous cap often contains lipid laden cells in different degrees of degeneration and necrosis (Smith and Slater 1972).

The fibrous cap is apparently chemically similar to the adult intima (Smith et al.1972). The intermediate area between the fibrous cap and the core contains cells whose lipid composition and cholesterol ester fatty acids appear to be very similar to that of the intermediate lesion (Small and Shipley 1974; Katz et al.1976). The fact that necrosis of cells often occurs near the core zone suggests that these cells are in part responsible for generating the lipid which deposits in the core. The core contains almost no viable cells. It consists of altered connective tissue proteins and a vast variety of different sized and shaped globules of lipid. Material which floats like VLDL, LDL and HDL have been described (Hollander et al.1979), but these should not be considered equivalent to their plasma namesakes nor are they necessarily derived directly from plasma lipoproteins. Hoff has found very little easily extractable immunoactivity for apoB, however more tightly bound lipid can be extracted by Triton-X100. An important characteristic of the fibrous plaque is that they contain, almost without exception, crystalline cholesterol monohydrate in rather large plate-like crystals (Katz et al.1976).

References

Day AJ, Wahlquist ML (1970) Cholesterol ester and phospholipid composition of normal aortas and of atherosclerotic lesions in children. Exp Mol Pathol 13:199-216
Hata Y, Insull Jr, W (1973) Significance of cholesterol esters as liquid crystal in human atherosclerosis. Jpn Circ J 37:269-275
Hoff HF, Heideman CL, Gaubatz JW (1980) Low density lipoproteins in the aorta: Relation to atherosclerosis. This volume
Hollander W, Paddock J, Colombo M (1979) Lipoproteins in human atherosclerotic vessels. Exp Mol Path 30:144-171
Katz SS, Shipley GG, Small DM (1976) Physical chemistry of the lipids of human atherosclerotic lesions. Demonstrations of a lesion intermediate between fatty streaks and advance plaques. J Clin Invest 58:200-211
Katz SS, Small DM, Brooks JG et al. (1976a) The physical state of lipids in foam cells of Tangier disease and human atherosclerotic plaques. Circulation 53,54: Suppl 2:II-180
Lang PD, Insull Jr W (1970) Lipid droplets in atherosclerotid fatty streaks of human aorta. J Clin Invest 49:1479-1488
Small DM, Shipley GG (1974) Physical-chemical basis of lipid deposition in atherosclerosis. Science 185:222-229

Small DM (1977) Liquid crystals in living and dying systems. J Colloid and Interface Sci 58:581-602

Small DM (1977a) Cellular mechanisms for lipid deposition in atherosclerosis. NEJM (Seminars in Medicine) 297:873-877 & 924-929

Smith EB (1965) The influence of age and atherosclerosis on the chemistry of aortic intima. Part I. The lipids. Atheroscler Res 5:224-240

Smith EB, Evans PH, Downham MD (1967) Lipid in the aortic intima. The correlation of morphological and chemical characteristics. J Atheroscler Res 7:171-186

Smith EB, Slater RS (1972) The microdissection of large atherosclerotic plaques to give morphologically and topographically defined fractions for analysis. Part I. The lipids in the isolated fractions. Atheroscl 15:37-56

Smith EB (1980) Transport of macromolecules across the artery wall. This volume

Transport of Macromolecules Across the Artery Wall

Elspeth B. Smith[1]

Unlike most organs, arteries have two distinct characteristics: they are
tubes that are subjected to external haemodynamic stresses and pulsatile
bombardment with plasma constituents under pressure, and they are also met-
abolizing tissues that may face special problems in the supply of nutrients
and oxygen and in changes in cellular environment resulting from accumulation of abnormal quantities of plasma macromolecules. In this workshop we
have experts in both these areas, and I hope that this will lead to a stimulating interchange of ideas. I would like to start the discussion by considering some of the information available on transport of plasma proteins
and lipoproteins into and across arterial wall.

Concentration of Plasma Macromolecules in Intima and Media

There is extensive evidence from immunofluorescent microscopy and immunoelectrophoresis that low density lipoprotein (LDL), fibrinogen and most other
plasma proteins are present in normal adult human arterial intima and in
atherosclerotic lesions (reviewed in Smith 1974). After the fourth decade
the concentration of LDL in normal intima is virtually the same as its concentration in plasma, and is highly correlated with it (Smith and Slater
1972; Hoff et al. 1977).

In preliminary studies on LDL, α_2-macroglobulin, high density lipoprotein
(HDL) and albumin the concentration in intima appeared to be a function of
the concentration in plasma and molecular weight, so that the relation between
plasma and intimal concentrations differed for each protein (Smith and Crothers 1975). These observations have now been extended to 17 samples of intima that appeared normal and free of fragmentary elastic laminae by light
microscopy, which were obtained from patients from whom a blood sample was
available during the week before death; the results are summarized in Table
1. The intimal macromolecules were measured by quantitative immunoelectrophoresis both in terms of the patients' own plasma and a standardized plasma.
From the patient's plasma we can calculate the retention of different proteins
as % of LDL retention with automatic correction for variation in plasma concentration, and from the standard plasma we can calculate the absolute concentrations in both intima and the patient's plasma. The results confirm
the linear regression of retention on molecular weight that was found previously. Calculation of the concentrations in intima and plasma illustrate
the resultant change in composition (Table 1).

What is the mechanism for this striking enrichment of the largest molecules
and depletion of smaller molecules? It is the reverse of the change between
plasma and lymph. It seems unlikely that LDL crosses arterial endothelium
six times faster than albumin; our previous finding that the volume of the

---

[1]The author's research is supported by a grant from the Medical Research
Council.

Table 1. Plasma macromolecules in normal aortic intima from 13 men and 4 women aged 27-68 (average age 51).

| | Percent of LDL Retention | Concentrations | |
		Intima: mg/100cc	Patients plasma: mg/100 ml
LDL	100	367 ± 80[a]	363 ± 38
α_2-macroglobulin	43.3 ± 3.2[a]	86 ± 28	204 ± 10
fibrinogen	31.1 ± 1.8	168 ± 48	511 ± 63
HDL	21.4 ± 4.5	58 ± 19	258 ± 67
Albumin	16.3 ± 2.2	329 ± 71	$2,907 \pm 303$

[a] Mean $\pm$ SEM

patient's plasma from which the intimal LDL is derived remains rather constant (Smith and Slater 1973) suggested that a package of whole plasma crosses endothelium and the equilibrium concentrations are determined by rates of egress from the intima.

To study this egress we have examined the relative concentrations in successive layers across normal human aortic wall. In 8 aortas the intima was subdivided into inner (luminal) and outer layers, and the concentrations of LDL and other plasma proteins measured in each layer. For all proteins the concentration in the outer layer was approximately half the concentration in the inner layer. In paired t-tests between LDL and α_2-macroglobulin, fibrinogen, transferrin, HDL and albumin there were no significant differences in the changes in concentration. Thus there appears to be no selective molecular sieving within the intima.

In 15 aortas normal intima was accurately stripped on the internal elastic lamina (IEL) which was clearly defined and appeared to be mainly intact by light microscopy; the media was divided into an inner layer immediately below the IEL (layer 2), middle (layer 3) and outer layers (layer 4), but the outermost 15% was rejected. Figure 1A shows the concentrations of LDL and other plasma proteins in each medial layer expressed as percentage of the concentration in intima (layer 1). The IEL was penetrated by less than 4% of LDL (MW = 20-30 x 10^5), by 15-20% of the intermediate group of proteins (MW range 2-8 x 10^5) and by 25-30% of albumin and α_1-antitrypsin (MW = 0.68 and 0.52 x 10^5). In 9 of the aortas LDL concentration in layer 2 was less than 1% of intimal LDL; in this sub-group from subjects aged 31-69 years (average 49) the IEL appears to be "functionally" intact, and the results are presented separately in Figure 1B. In this group α_2-macroglobulin (MW = 7.2 x 10^5) separates from fibrinogen, transferrin and HDL.

Thus, surprisingly, in normal areas of adult human aorta the IEL presents an almost impassable barrier for LDL, whereas penetration by smaller plasma proteins is an inverse function of molecular weight. This differential egress through the media seems, however, to account for only half the differences between intimal and plasma concentrations. This suggests that the endothelium must also play a significant role by selective uptake of large molecules, or by allowing more rapid escape of small ones. Finkelstein et al. (1976) concluded from kinetic analyses in rabbits that both these mechanisms may be operative.

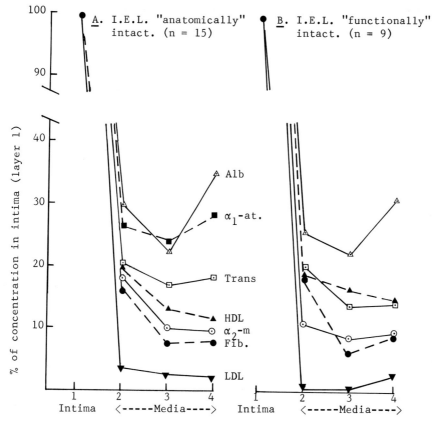

Fig. 1A and B. The concentration of plasma proteins in inner (2), middle (3) and outer (4) layers of the media expressed as percentage of the concentration in intima.   (A)   All samples in which the IEL appeared intact by light microscopy.   (B)   Samples in which there was less than 1% LDL in layer 2.   Albumin ▲ ; α_1-antitrypsin ■ ;   transferrin ▣ ;   HDL ▲ ; α_2-macroglobulin ⊙ ;   fibrinogen ● ;   LDL ▼ .

Comparison with Experimental Studies

Studies on the passage of labelled proteins across arterial wall in experimental animals have been discussed by Colton (1979).   The results of these dynamic studies are entirely compatible with the equilibrium concentration studies reported here.   Although the outermost 15% of media (containing most of the vasa vasorum) was rejected we found (Fig. 1) the marked kick-up in albumin concentration in outer media described by Adams et al. (1968). In normal animals the intima is only one or two cells thick ($<10\mu$M) and in most experimental studies the innermost layer analysed must have contained a substantial proportion of media.   Impermeability of the IEL explains the discrepancy between the high concentrations of LDL found in isolated human aortic intima and the low concentrations reported in the mainly medial preparations used in experimental studies.   In inner and middle media we found the LDL concentration was 0.3% of the concentrations in intima and plasma (Fig. 1B), and this is similar to the concentrations found by Bratzler et al. (1977) in rabbit media 4-24 hours after administration of protein-labelled LDL.

Conclusions

Thus LDL appears to be trapped between endothelium and the IEL, but we do not understand the role of endothelium in its preferential accumulation; this is an area that requires further investigation. Our ignorance of the role of endothelium is highlighted by the studies of Minick et al. (1977) who found greater lipid accumulation in areas with endothelial regeneration than in areas denuded of endothelium, and by our own recent findings of very low concentrations of LDL in arterial graft pseudo-intimas and mural thrombi that were not endothelialized (Smith et al. 1979).

References

Adams CWM, Virag S, Morgan RS, Orton CC (1968) Dissociation of (3-H) cholesterol and 125-I-labelled plasma protein influx in normal and atheromatous rabbit aorta. J Atheroscler Res 8:679

Bratzler RL, Chisholm GM, Colton CK, Smith KA, Lees RS (1977) The distribution of labelled low-density lipoproteins across the rabbit thoracic aorta in vivo. Atherosclerosis 28:289

Colton CK (1979) Transport of protein and lipid into the arterial wall. In: Wolf S, Werthessen NT (eds) Dynamics of arterial flow. Advan Exp Med Biol 115:299

Finkelstein JN, Ghosh S, Schweppe JS (1976) Kinetic analysis of in vivo lipoprotein flux in the normal rabbit aorta. Artery 2:161

Hoff HF, Heideman CL, Gotto AM, Gaubatz JW (1977) Apolipoprotein B retention in the grossly normal and atherosclerotic human aorta. Circ Res 41:684

Minick CR, Stemerman MB, Insull W (1977) Effect of regenerated endothelium on lipid accumulation in the arterial wall. Proc Natl Acad Sci USA 74:1724

Smith EB (1974) The relationship between plasma and tissue lipids in human atherosclerosis. Advan Lipid Res 12:1

Smith EB, Crothers DC (1975) Interaction between plasma proteins and the intercellular matrix. In: Peeters H (ed) Protides of the Biological Fluids 22:315 (Pergamon Press, Oxford)

Smith EB, Slater RS (1972) Relationship between low density lipoprotein in aortic intima and serum lipid levels. Lancet i:463

Smith EB, Slater RS (1973) Lipids and low density lipoproteins in intima in relation to its morphological characteristics. In: Atherogenesis: Initiating factors. Ciba Foundation Symposium (New Series) 12:39

Smith EB, Staples EM, Dietz HS, Smith RH (1979) Role of endothelium in sequestration of lipoprotein and fibrinogen in aortic lesions, thrombi and graft pseudo-intimas. Lancet ii:812

Cholesteryl Ester-Rich Lipid Inclusions in the Development of Experimental Atherosclerosis in Rabbits[1]

Yoshiya Hata, Hiroshi Shigematsu, Kazuo Aihara, Minoru Yamamoto, Yoshio Yamauchi, and Takamitsu Oikawa

The fundamental cellular and biochemical processes that occur in human and experimental atherosclerosis are proliferation of smooth muscle cells, accumulation of intra- and extracellular lipids, and deposition of such intercellular ground substances as collagen, elastin and proteoglycans (Ross and Glomset 1973). Of these changes, we focus our attention on the arterial wall lipids, since they are of particular importance in initiation and development of atherosclerosis for the following seven reasons; (i) the arterial wall is a catabolic site of serum low density lipoproteins (LDL) carrying the major portion of cholesteryl esters, (ii) the derangement of catabolic process of LDL in arterial tissue leads to accumulation of lipids in situ, (iii) the arterial lipid contents are related to both the serum lipid level and the severity of lesions, (iv) in experimental animals atherosclerosis can be induced by cholesterol feeding, (v) it regresses when serum cholesterol is lowered both in man and animals, (vi) the other risk factors alone can not produce atherosclerosis without hypercholesterolemia and (vii) there is no atherosclerosis without accumulation of lipids in arterial tissues.

We have studied the lipids in normal and atherosclerotic lesions of man by several methods in which the arterial specimens are neither exposed to organic solvent for dehydration nor embedded in resin materials (Insull et al. 1971, Hata and Insull 1973, Hata et al. 1974, Insull et al. 1974), and classified them into five forms (Hata and Ishii 1978). They are (I) lipids in the form of membrane matrix and those bound to intercellular substances of the tissue, called structural lipids, (II) lipids incorporated into arterial tissue in a particulate form solubilized in cytosol and intercellular fluid of the tissue, designated as lipoprotein lipids, (III) lipids in the form of anisotropic spheres of liquid crystal, (IV) those in the form of isotropic spheres in liquid state and (V) lipids in the form of solid crystal (Figure 1). Among these five forms of lipids in normal and atherosclerotic tissue of arteries, we consider the lipid inclusions as the most important in initiation and progression of atherosclerosis. To confirm the role of the inclusions in pathogenesis of atherosclerosis, we have produced experimental atherosclerosis in rabbits and analyzed the accumulated lipids from the viewpoint of the classification in five forms of atheromatous lipids.

Material and Method

Twenty eight albino rabbits (body weight 3,241±489g) were fed with the daily ration of 150g laboratory chew with 0.67% cholesterol added, and their serum cholesterol checked every three weeks, then sacrificed at third, sixth and ninth month, while 33 rabbits (3,000±693 g) served as the control. The aortic specimen was prepared by removing adventitial adipose tissue and opening

[1]This work was partly supported by a grant-in-aid for scientific research (C-357312) Ministry of Education, Science and Culture, Japan (1978), and the grants-in-aid for research from Keio Health Counseling Center, Tokyo (1978).

529

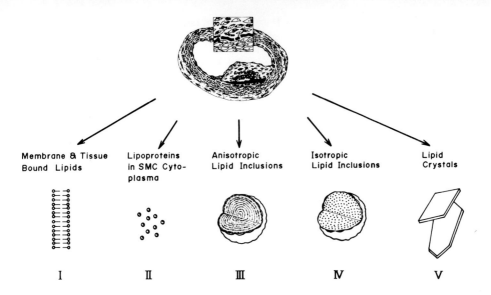

FIG 1. Classification of atheromatous lipids into five forms; (I) structural lipids, (II) lipoprotein lipids, (III) anisotropic lipid inclusions (IV) isotropic lipid inclusions, and (V) crystal lipids.

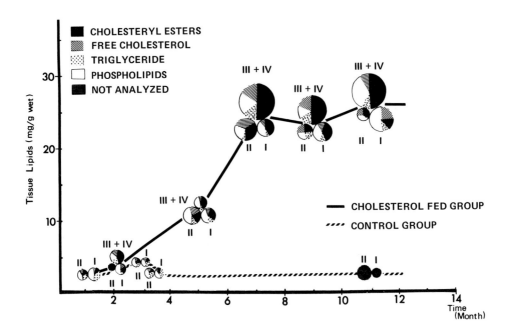

FIG. 2. The contents and the composition of normal and atherosclerotic tissue of the aorta in rabbits.

longitudinally along the anterior wall. The intimal surface was assessed
for atherosclerotic lesions by xerox method (Hata et al. 1978), then a portion
of unfixed lesion was examined for optical and crystallographic properties
of lipid inclusions by polarizing light microscopy (Hata et al. 1974). The
rest of the tissue was homogenized and the homogenate was fractionated into
three fractions of inclusions, supernatant and residue by centrifugation at
3,800 G for 45 minutes. The chemical analyses of these three fractions were
performed by quantitative thin layer chromatography (Lang and Insull 1970).

Results and Discussion

By feeding rabbits with 0.67% cholesterol for 3 to 5 months, atheromatous
lesions evolved in the intima starting from the arch to the thoracic aorta
covering the surface of 5-35% of the total aorta. Atheromatous lesions
appeared as lightly elevated, yet soft, opaque yellow lesions with irregular
boundaries. Histological specimen of the lesion revealed accumulation of

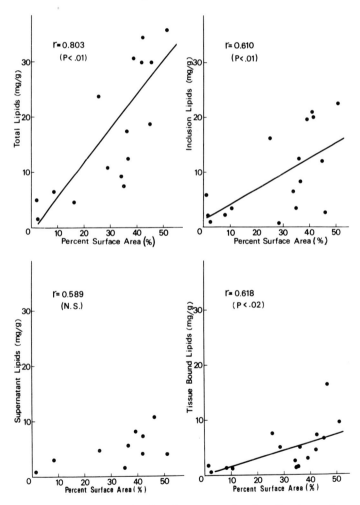

FIG 3.   The correlation between the involved surface area and the three
fractions of atheromatous lipids.

531

lipids stained red with Oil Red-O, localized mostly in the intima, often penetrating into the media.

The lipid contents and the chemical compositions of the inclusion, supernatant and residue fractions are shown in Figure 2. As the lesion developed, the lipid contents in arterial tissue increased from the level of 5mg/g wet weight tissue to 25mg/g and this increase was caused mainly by the increment in the fraction of lipid inclusions, amounting to about 50% of the increased total lipids and characteristically rich in cholesteryl oleate (Figure 2). The correlation between these three fractions of accumulated lipids and the surface area involved in atheromatous lesion was shown in Figure 3. Among three fractions of lipids, the closest correlation was seen between the amount of lipid inclusions and the involved surface area ($r=0.610$, $p<0.01$).

Optical and crystallographic characteristics of the lipid inclusions are similar or even identical with those of humans. The black Formee cross image and the pattern of interference colors indicated that the longer axis of the constituent molecules of cholesteryl esters were oriented in radial symmetry to form a concentric lamellar structure, definitive as lyotropic smectic mesophase. Physical properties of the inclusions such as resilience, lyotropy and swelling were also similar to those of humans (Hata et al. 1978).

Thus, the lipid inclusions in the macromolecular form of cholesteryl esters act as a molecular entity of the formation of foam cells, and the foam cells constitute a cellular entity to develop the lesion in arterial tissues.

References

Hata, Y. and Insull, W. (1973) Significance of cholesterol esters as liquid crystal in human atherosclerosis. Jap Circ J 37: 269-273

Hata, Y., Hower, J. and Insull, W. (1974) Cholesteryl ester-rich inclusions from human aortic fatty streak and fibrous plaque lesions of atherosclerosis. I. Crystalline properties, size and internal structure. Am J Pathol 75: 423-456

Hata, Y., Shigematsu, H., Tsushima, M., Aihara, K. and Miyazaki, K.(1978) A xerographic method for the quantitative assessment of atherosclerotic lesions. Atherosclerosis 29: 251-258

Hata, Y., Shigematsu, H., Tsushima, M., Aihara, K. and Miyazaki, K. (1978) Similarity of lipid inclusions in experimental atherosclerosis of rabbits to those of humans. Acta Histochem Cytochem 11: 369-383

Hata, Y. and Ishii, T.(1978) The lipids in human atherosclerosis - Morphological demonstration of five forms of atheroma lipids - Adv Exp Biol Med 109: 129-143

Insull, W., Hata, Y., Meakin, J.D. and Marchant, L.(1971) Morphology of lipid rich organelles in tissue of man and rat. In: Johari, O., and Corvin, I.(eds) Scanning Electron Microscopy 1971, IIT Research Institute, Chicago, pp. 337-344

Insull, W., Hata, Y., Meakin, J.D., Marchant, L., Andrews, C.W. and Buzek, B. (1974) Morphology of cholesteryl ester-rich inclusions in lesions of atherosclerosis in man. Atherosclerosis 19: 555-560

Lang, P.D. and Insull, W. (1970) Lipid droplets in atherosclerotic fatty streaks of human aorta. J Clin Invest 49: 1479-1488

Ross, R. and Glomset, J.A. (1973) Atherosclerosis and the arterial smooth muscle cell. Science 180: 1332-1339

Low Density Lipoproteins in the Aorta: Relation to Atherosclerosis[1]

Henry F. Hoff, Carol L. Heideman, and John W. Gaubatz

A link between plasma low density lipoproteins (LDL) and the atherosclerotic process has been suggested from both clinical-correlative studies in man (Kannel et al. 1964) and diet-fed experimental animal models (St. Clair 1976). LDL is the major carrier of cholesterol into the arterial wall and the deposition of cholesterol is the hallmark of the atherosclerotic process (St. Clair 1976). However the details surrounding the transport and deposition of cholesterol are not completely understood. LDL could transit the entire vessel wall and enter the lymphatics. It could be metabolized following uptake by arterial smooth muscle cells as was shown in cultured fibroblasts (Goldstein and Brown 1977). In a non-human primate model as much as 25% of total LDL entering the aorta became TCA-soluble, suggesting breakdown of the protein moiety (Hollander et al. 1977). Finally some LDL could be selectively retained in the arterial intima. A retention of this lipoprotein in the intimal lining of major arteries has been demonstrated by numerous immuno-fluorescence studies from our laboratory (Hoff et al. 1974, 1975a,b).

In this report we will summarize the data obtained in this laboratory on the quantitation and localization of apo B-containing lipoproteins in the tunica intima of the human aorta. We used a quantitative immunochemical procedure (electroimmunoassay)(Hoff et al. 1977a,b) directed against apo B, the protein moiety of LDL, to measure the amount of LDL in the grossly normal intima, fatty streaks, and fatty-fibrous plaques, from the human aorta obtained at autopsy. Following tissue homogenization we demonstrated that arterial LDL could be isolated into two operationally defined fractions, one extracted with a conventional buffer (Hoff et al. 1977a,b) and one containing the detergent, Triton X-100 (Hoff et al. 1978a).

Grossly normal aortic intima contained buffer-soluble apo B, presumed to represent LDL, at a greater concentration than the LDL present in plasma of normolipemics (Hoff et al. 1978a), i.e., 1 mg/cm^3 of tissue or 5 µg/mg tissue dry weight. The high level of LDL in grossly normal intima suggests selective retention to this tissue, since apo B values in other organs, such as heart, kidney, lung, were at least one order of magnitude lower than that in the intima, and the adjacent tunica media did not contain measurable apo B. By contrast, intimal content of human serum albumin was only a fifth of the plasma concentration.

The LDL content per unit dry weight in grossly normal intima increased slightly with age. It also correlated negatively with the DNA content of the intima (Hoff et al. 1977c), suggesting that the increased cellularity of the normal intima might result in greater uptake and degradation of LDL by the intimal smooth muscle cells resulting in less intact LDL in the extracellular space. This is consistent with the breakdown of LDL following uptake by cultured fibroblasts (Goldstein and Brown 1977).

----

[1]Supported in part by USPH Grants HL 17269 and NS 09287, and a Grant-in-Aid from the American Heart Association. Henry F. Hoff is an Established Investigator of the American Heart Association.

We also correlated the amount of LDL in the normal intima with the plasma cholesterol level from the same case and found a significant positive correlation between arterial and plasma LDL levels (Hoff et al. 1977a), as was previously observed by Smith and Slater (1972), suggesting the LDL pools in plasma and aortic intima to be in equilibrium.

The amount of buffer-extractable apo B per unit weight showed a negative correlation with increasing lesion development, i.e., from normal intima to fatty streak to fibrous plaque (Hoff et al. 1978d). On the other hand, the Triton-extractable or tightly-bound lipoprotein correlated positively with lesion progression. Normal intima had the lowest value, followed by the fatty streak and then by fibrous plaque. The differences between each of the lesions were statistically significant.

The tightly-bound fraction extractable with Triton could also be released in part from pellets of plaque homogenates by treatment with a number of different hydrolytic enzymes, such as elastase and collagenase. We were able to demonstrate that approximately 50% of the Triton-extracted fraction was extractable with elastase and therefore measurable in a buffer-soluble form (Hoff and Gaubatz 1979). Hollander (1977) also extracted a residual fraction of LDL from plaques following extraction with 1.6 M saline. Likewise, Srinivasan et al. (1978) found that following initial extraction of minces with saline, a residual fraction could be removed with collagenase, and the released lipoprotein was associated with sulfated glycosaminoglycans. Smith et al. (1976) found that following electrophoresis of minces of plaques in a gel containing anti-apo B, a residual fraction of LDL, at least one-half of the initial amount could be released by digesting the minces with plasmin.

In grossly normal intima most LDL as measured by apo B content was present in a loosely-bound form and extractable with a conventional buffer (Hoff et al. 1977a,b,c). By contrast, in the fatty streak lesion up to 25% of the total LDL found in this lesion could be extracted only with Triton X-100. This increased to approximately 50% in fatty-fibrous plaques. In microdissected fibrotic caps of fatty-fibrous plaques most apo B was buffer-soluble, while in microdissected necrotic cores of these plaques most apo B was extractable only with Triton (Hoff et al. 1978c).

Quantitation of LDL was generally consistent with the localization pattern of LDL in arteries. The normal intima demonstrated a localization which at times was diffuse and at other times more localized to connective tissue fibers (Hoff et al. 1974,1975a,b,1977a). A similar diffuse localization was found in fatty streak lesions, in which some foam cells also demonstrated localization of LDL. In fatty-fibrous plaques the localization was found predominantly in the lipid-filled necrotic core at the base of plaques, as well as to larger bands of collagen fibers and some elastica. Although localization was frequently very widespread and intense in plaques, there were large regions, particularly in the fibrotic cap, that were negative for LDL (Hoff et al. 1974,1975a,b), thus explaining the lower LDL content of plaques on a dry weight basis as compared to that of normal intima. However, on a surface area basis plaques still contained much more apo B than normal intima. On the ultrastructural level using an immunoperoxidase technique, apo B was associated with spheres in the size range of LDL and VLDL, mainly in the necrotic core of plaques (Hoff and Gaubatz 1977). These spheres were both freely dispersed as well as associated with collagen and elastic fibers.

To evaluate the percent of cholesterol present as an LDL particle in the intima, we converted the total apo B content (buffer- plus Triton-extractable) in aortic intima to LDL-cholesterol and compared that value to a total tissue cholesterol value. Assuming all apo B to be in an LDL particle, in normal intima nearly all the tissue cholesterol could be accounted for by the presence of accumulated intact LDL (Hoff et al. 1979b). In fatty streaks 16%

of the tissue cholesterol could be present theoretically in LDL particles, while in fibrous plaques this figure was 11%. In some plaques up to 20% of the total tissue cholesterol could be theoretically in the form of an intact LDL particle. If one-fifth of the lipid in a plaque core were still within a lipoprotein, it is possible that this fraction could be mobilized during regression.

Although these immunochemical studies indicated the presence of LDL within the aortic wall, we still needed to show that the apo B was present within a lipoprotein similar to LDL. A study was therefore initiated to characterize the apo B-containing material in the grossly normal intima and plaques of the human aorta. The supernatant fraction of buffer extracts was subjected to differential ultracentrifugation to isolate a d 1.006-1.063 gm/ml density fraction depicting the classical density fraction of plasma LDL. By electron microscopy following negative staining with phosphotungstic acid, particles in the size range of LDL were found in both normal and plaque isolates (Hoff et al. 1979a). However, some larger-sized material was also present in isolates from plaque. When these isolates from normal and plaque were subjected to protein and lipid analysis, the lipid composition resembled that of plasma LDL, with the exception that in plaque isolates the free cholesterol level was higher and the cholesterol ester fraction lower than that of plasma LDL. Moreover, the fatty acid pattern of the cholesterol ester fraction from isolates of both normal intima and plaque differed from that of plasma LDL. In particular, the ratio of linoleate to oleate was lower in the isolates from aorta compared to plasma. There were also certain differences in the amino acid analyses of the isolates from arteries compared to that of LDL. Arterial isolates showed relative increases in glutamic acid, proline, glycine, alanine, valine and arginine, and decreases in serine, isoleucine, and tryosine compared to plasma LDL (Hoff et al. 1979, unpublished data). Furthermore, LDL extracted from both normal intima and plaques showed greater electronegative mobility than the corresponding plasma LDL (Hoff et al. 1979a). Similar results were recently obtained by Hollander et al. (1979).

Further purification of the isolates by gel filtration separated the larger particles from the LDL-sized material (Hoff et al. 1979, unpublished data). The lipid composition of the purified LDL-sized particles from plaque isolates was essentially identical to that of plasma LDL. The material in the void volume of the column was rich in free cholesterol, suggesting that this material was probably not plasma LDL. Yet, in the LDL fraction changes in surface charge and amino acid composition persisted.

Our studies have demonstrated the presence of substantial amounts of material closely resembling plasma LDL in the arterial wall of both the grossly normal intima and raised fatty-fibrous atherosclerotic lesions. By a combination of immunochemical, histochemical, physical, and chemical procedures, we have identified this material as LDL, but with some structural alterations. Future studies will show whether the changes are a result of enzymatic alteration within the arterial wall or of a preferential retention by the arterial wall of a subclass of plasma LDL.

References

Goldstein JL, Brown MS (1977) Atherosclerosis: The low-density lipoprotein receptor hypothesis. Metabolism 26: 1257
Hoff HF, Gaubatz JW (1977) Ultrastructural localization of apolipoprotein B in human aortic and coronary atherosclerotic plaques. Exp Mol Path 26:214
Hoff HF, Gaubatz JW (1979) Residual apo B in aortic plaques: Comparison of amounts extracted with hydrolytic enzymes and with Triton X-100. Artery (in press)
Hoff HF, Jackson RL, Mao JT, Gotto AM (1974) Localization of low density lipoproteins in arterial lesions from normolipemics employing a purified

fluorescent labeled antibody. Biochim Biophys Acta 351: 407

Hoff HF, Heideman CL, Jackson RL, Bayardo RJ, Kim HS, Gotto AM (1975a) The localization patterns of plasma apo-lipoproteins in human atherosclerotic lesions. Circ Res 37: 72

Hoff HF, Lie JT, Titus JL, Jackson RL, DeBakey ME, Bayardo R, Gotto AM (1975b) Lipoproteins in atherosclerotic lesions. Localization by immunofluorescence of apo-low density lipoproteins in human atherosclerotic arteries from normal hyperlipoproteinemics. Arch Path 99: 253

Hoff HF, Heideman CL, Gaubatz JW, Gotto AM, Erickson EE, Jackson RL (1977a) Quantitation of apolipoprotein B (apoB) in grossly normal human aorta. Cir Res 40: 56

Hoff HF, Heideman CL, Gotto AM, Gaubatz JW (1977b) Apolipoprotein (apoB) retention in the grossly normal and atherosclerotic human aorta. Circ Res 41: 684

Hoff HF, Heideman CL, Gaubatz JW (1977c) Relationship between retention of buffer-extracted apo B and components of the human aortic intima. Artery 3: 379

Hoff HF, Gaubatz JW, Gotto AM (1978a) Apo B concentration in the normal human aorta. Biochem Biophys Res Comm 85: 1424

Hoff HF, Heideman CL, Gaubatz JW, Gotto AM, Scott DW (1978b) Detergent extraction of tightly-bound apo B from extracts of normal aortic intima and plaques. Exp Mol Path 28: 290

Hoff HF, Heideman CL, Gaubatz JW, Scott D, Titus JL, Gotto AM (1978c) Correlation of apolipoprotein B retention with the structure of atherosclerotic plaques from human aortas. Lab Invest 38: 560

Hoff HF, Heideman CL, Gaubatz JW, Titus JL, Gotto AM (1978d) Quantitation of apo B in human aortic fatty streaks: A comparison with grossly normal intima and fibrous plaques. Atherosclerosis 30: 263

Hoff HF, Bradley WA, Heideman CL, Gaubatz JW, Karagas MD, Gotto AM (1979a) Characterization of an LDL-like particle in the human aorta from grossly normal and atherosclerotic regions. Biochim Biophys Acta 573: 361

Hoff HF, Karagas M, Heideman CL, Gaubatz JW, Gotto AM (1979b) Correlation in the human aorta of apo B fractions with tissue cholesterol and collagen content. Atherosclerosis 32: 259

Hollander W (1976) Unified concept on the role of acid mucopolysaccharides and connective tissue proteins in the accumulation of lipids, lipoproteins and calcium in the atherosclerotic plaque. Exp Mol Path 25: 106

Hollander W, Paddock J, Colombo MA (1977) Arterial uptake and synthesis of low density lipoproteins. Prog Biochem Pharmacol 13: 123

Hollander W, Paddock J, Colombo M (1979) Lipoproteins in human atherosclerotic vessels.I.Biochemical properties of arterial low density lipoproteins, very low density lipoproteins, and high density lipoproteins. Exp Mol Path 30: 144

Kannel WB, Dawber TR, Friedman CD (1964) Risk factors in coronary heart disease: An evaluation of several serum lipids as predictors of coronary heart disease. Am Intern Med 61: 888

Smith EB, Slater RS (1972) Relationship between low-density lipoprotein in aortic intima and serum-lipid levels. Lancet 1: 463

Smith EB, Massie IB, Alexander KM (1976) The release of an immobilized lipoprotein fraction from atherosclerotic lesions by incubation with plasmin. Atherosclerosis 25: 71

Srinivasan SR, Radhakrishnamurthy B, Dalferes ER, Berenson GS (1978) Interactions of lipoproteins and connective tissue components in human atherosclerotic plaques. In: Intl Conf on Atherosclerosis, Raven Press, p. 585

St. Clair R, Lofland H, Clarkson T (1976) Influence of duration of cholesterol feeding on esterification of fatty acids by cell-free preparation of pigeon aorta: Studies on the mechanism of cholesterol esterification. Circ Res 27: 213

Cyclic Nucleotides and Atherosclerosis[1]

Fujio Numano

Since the discovery of cyclic AMP by Sutherland (1958), the cyclic nucleotides have been extensively studied as to their function and relation to
cell metabolism (Sutherland 1971; Greengard 1972). Increasing attention
has been given cyclic GMP and the role of this substance in the pathophysiology of organs and specific tissues (Ashman 1963; Goldberg 1973). Our
group has for many years focussed attention on the role of the nucleotides
in the vessel wall, the relation to vascular injury and the progression and
regression of atherosclerosis (Numano 1976a, 1978b, 1979).

To measure the levels of cyclic AMP and GMP in samples of only 500 µg dry
weight of tissue, we combined Lowry's quantitative histochemical method
with radioimmunoassay, with certain modifications (Lowry 1972; Numano 1973,
1976b). This approach enables the separate estimation of the levels of
cyclic nucleotides in the intima and media of the arterial wall and comparisons can be made to histological changes in the tissues. Four samples
from different areas of each rabbit aorta were obtained and in each sample,
cyclic AMP and GMP were measured in triplicate. Thus, a total of twelve
measurements were made from each aorta and the average was taken to be representative of the levels of cyclic nucleotides.

Vascular Injury and Cyclic Nucleotides

Vascular injury initiates and accelerates atherosclerosis (Shimamoto 1963;
Numano 1977, 1978a). We studied changes in levels of cyclic nucleotides in
the aortic wall following induced chemical and mechanical injuries (Numano
1978b).

A single dose of cholesterol (1 g/kg p.o.) or angiotensin II (10 µg/kg i.v.)
resulted in edemetous changes in the intima and the upper layer of the media of the aorta in rabbits. These challenges were repeated once daily ×14.
The edemetous changed intima revealed a statistically significant decrease
in the levels of cyclic AMP and GMP, as compared with findings in normal
rabbits ($p < 0.05$). However, a two weeks' challenge resulted in a restoration of cyclic AMP levels and a statistically significant increase in cyclic GMP levels, as compared to findings in the control tissues. Histological studies showed the existence of a small amount of droplets of fatty
substances in the smooth muscle tissue of the subendothelial layers. Levels of cyclic AMP and GMP in the media revealed no statistically significant change in these animals.

Thromboxane A_2 and growth factors are released from platelets adhering to
the vessel wall (Ross 1976; Samuelsson 1978). In research on their role in
relation to cyclic nucleotides, a Fogarty catheter(4F) was passed to the
aorta through the femoral artery, inflated(0.4cc of water) and propelled

[1]Supported by Grants for scientific research from the Ministry of Education,
Science and Culture, and from the Japan Atherosclerosis Research Foundation.

537

along the aorta to denude the endothelial cells. The animals were sacrificed 6, 24, 48 and 72 hours after the denudation. SEM photos revealed a gradual increase of accumulation of platelets on the denuded surface of the aortic wall. An almost complete covering of the surface with platelets was frequently seen in rabbits sacrificed over 48 hours after the denudation. Here, the platelet counts had recovered to the level seen before the denudation. Plasma thromboxane B_2 levels revealed a statistically high level between 30 min and 2 hours and 24 hours after denudation. Levels of cyclic AMP and GMP revealed a statistically significant decrease in the aortic wall of rabbits sacrificed 6 hours after the denudation ($p < 0.01$), however, in the animals sacrificed over 24 and 48 hours, there was remarkable increase in the levels of cyclic GMP in the aorta ($p < 0.01$). Here evidence of repair was statistically confirmed.

Atherosclerosis and Cyclic Nucleotide Levels with Cholesterol Feeding

In previous work, we determined the levels of cyclic AMP in intima and atherosclerotic lesions of rabbit aorta (Numano 1976a,b). The animals had been fed a diet high in cholesterol for various weeks. The intima of animals on the diet for 2 weeks exhibited a higher content of cyclic AMP than in the normal controls. The level then gradually decreased and a statistically significant decrease was confirmed in the atherosclerotic lesions of rabbits on the diet for more than 9 weeks. Changes in levels of cyclic GMP were then studied and the findings compared with data on the levels of cyclic AMP.

Fifteen rabbits were fed a diet containing one percent cholesterol. Three rabbits each were sacrificed at 3, 6, 9, 12, 15 weeks after being on this diet. The average levels of cyclic AMP and cyclic GMP in intima of aorta taken from 3 age-matched control rabbits were 1.03 ± 0.16 and 0.40 ± 0.04 pmoles/mg protein, respectively, and in the media exhibited 0.78 ± 0.10 and 0.16 ± 0.02 pmoles/mg protein. Here also, levels of cyclic AMP in the intima showed a statistically significant increase in rabbits fed the cholesterol containing diet for 3 weeks and then a gradual decrease followed by a statistically significant decrease was found in animals fed the diet for over 9 weeks, as compared to the controls. On the other hand, in the media, the level of cyclic AMP showed no remarkable change, except in groups so fed for 15 weeks. The level of cyclic GMP in the intima of the aorta of rabbits fed the diet for 3 weeks increased to twice the levels seen in the controls.

However, the other groups showed a statistically significant decrease in cyclic GMP levels, as compared to the controls. In the media, a statistically significant increase was observed in rabbits fed the diet for 3 weeks. The other groups showed no changes in the level of cyclic GMP (Table 1).

Histological examination revealed thickening in the intima of the aorta in the rabbits fed the diet for 3 weeks. Accumulated typical foam cells appeared in atherosclerotic lesions in the animals fed the diet for over 6 weeks.

These comparative studies on the histological features of initiation and progression of atherosclerosis and changes in levels of nucleotides revealed the close relationship between intimal changes characterized by proliferation of smooth muscles, formation of foam cells and production of connective tissues and increased levels of cyclic nucleotides.

The levels of cyclic AMP and cyclic GMP were usually altered in parallel, not reversely as suggested by the "Ying-Yang Theory" (Goldberg 1973). However, they exhibited characteristic changes in accordance with progression of the atherosclerosis. The level of cyclic GMP increased characteristical-

Table 1. The level of cyclic nucleotides in intima, atherosclerotic lesion or media of aorta in cholesterol-fed rabbits.

Cyclic Nucleotides	Aortic Site	Cholesterol feeding for[a]					
		before	3 weeks	6 weeks	9 weeks	12 weeks	15 weeks
cAMP	intima or lesion	1.03 ±0.16	1.39[b] ±0.34	1.08 ±0.12	0.81[b] ±0.16	0.68[c] ±0.12	0.78[c] ±0.08
cAMP	media	0.78 ±0.10	1.20 ±0.21	0.81 ±0.22	0.84 ±0.19	0.62 ±0.24	0.51[b] ±0.161
cGMP	intima or lesion	0.40 ±0.04	0.81[d] ±0.21	0.13[d] ±0.02	0.12[d] ±0.01	0.16[d] ±0.01	0.18[d] ±0.01
cGMP	media	0.16 ±0.02	0.23[d] ±0.02	0.12 ±0.01	0.13 ±0.01	0.14 ±0.03	0.18 ±0.01

[a] Values are pmoles/mg protein.
[b] $p < 0.01$; cAMP:before vs cholesterol feeding.
[c] $p < 0.05$; cAMP:before vs cholesterol feeding.
[d] $p < 0.01$; cGMP:before vs cholesterol feeding.

ly after 48 hours after denudation or in the case of a short term of cholesterol feeding. These results may reflect the proliferation of smooth muscle in the intima. Tissue cultures using endothelial cells and smooth muscles of cow and rabbit aorta showed positive results in support of the present data and growth factors may enhance the increase in cyclic GMP thus resulting in a proliferation of smooth muscle in the intima. The level of cyclic AMP showed a remarkable decrease in the late stages of progression of atherosclerosis as characterized by formation of foam cells and production of connective tissue. Decrease in the levels of cyclic AMP led to phagocytosis of these smooth muscle cells in the intima and foam cells were produced.

References

Ashman DF, Lipton R, Melicow MM, Price TD (1963) Isolation of adenosine 3',5'-monophosphate and guanosine 3',5'- monophosphate from rat urine. Biochem Biophy Res Comm 11: 330-334

Goldberg ND, O'Dea RF, Haddox MK (1973) Cyclic GMP. In: Greengard P, Robison GA (eds) Advances in Cyclic Nucleotide Research. Raven Press, New York, Vol 3, pp 155-223

Greengard P, Paoletti R, Robison GA (eds) (1972) Advances in Cyclic Nucleotides Research Vol.1 Physiology and Pharmacology of Cyclic AMP. Raven Press, New York

Lowry OH, Passonneau JV (eds) (1972) A Flexible System of Enzymatic Analysis. Academic Press, New York

Numano F, Sagara A, Takenobu M, Yamazawa S, Shimamoto T (1973) Microbiochemical analysis of the arterial wall. Atherosclerosis 17: 333-343

Numano F, Maezawa H, Shimamoto T, Adachi K (1976a) Changes of cyclic AMP and cyclic AMPphosphodiesterase in the progression and regression of experimental atherosclerosis. Ann N.Y. Acad Sci 275: 311-320

Numano F, Watanabe Y, Takeno K, Takano T, Arita M, Numano F, Maezawa H, Shimamoto T, Adachi K (1976b) Microassay of cyclic nucleotides in vessel wall. I. Cyclic AMP. Exp Mol Path 25: 172-181

Numano F (1977) Progression and regression of atherosclerosis. Asian Med J 20: 626-644

Numano F, Shimamoto T (1978a) Prevention and regression of atherosclerosis. In: Carlson LA, Paoletti R, Weber G (eds) International Conference on Atherosclerosis. Raven Press, New York, pp 631-636

Numano F, Kuroiwa T, Takeno K, Takano T, Watanabe Y, Maezawa H, Moriya K, Shimamoto T (1978b) The effect of vascular injury caused by angiotensin II or cholesterol and epinephrine in phosphofructokinase, glycose-6-phosphate dehydrogenase activity and cyclic nucleotides in the rabbits aorta. Artery 4: 322-329

Numano F (1979) Cyclic nucleotides and atherosclerosis. In: Cehovic G, Robison GA (eds) Cyclic Nucleotides and Therapeutic Perspectives. Pergamon Press, Oxford, pp 137-146

Ross R, Glomset JA (1976) The pathogenesis of atherosclerosis. New Eng J Med 295: 420-425

Samuelsson B, Folco G, Granstrom E, Kindahl H, Malmsten C (1978) Prostaglandin and thromboxanes. In: Coceani F, Olley PM (eds) Advances in Prostaglandin and Thromboxane Research. Raven Press, New York, Vol 4, pp 1-36
New York).

Shimamoto T (1963) The relationship of edematous reaction in arteries to atherosclerosis and thrombosis. J Atheroscler Res 3: 87-102

Sutherland EW, Rall TW (1958) Fractionation and characterization of a cyclic adenine ribonucleotide formed by tissue particles. J Biol Chem 232: 1077-1091

Sutherland EW (1971) An introduction. In: Robison GA, Butcher RW, Sutherland EW (eds) Cyclic AMP. Academic Press, New York, third edition, pp 5-16

Differences in the Metabolism of Abnormal Atherogenic Low Density Lipoproteins from ○-Cholesterol-Fed Nonhuman Primates by Cells in Culture[1]

Richard W. St. Clair

Hypercholesterolemia is a well recognized risk factor for development of atherosclerosis. In nonhuman primates and other animal models, the hyper-cholesterolemia resulting from consumption ot dietary cholesterol is associ-ated with marked changes in the content and composition of the plasma lipo-proteins. In most nonhuman primate species, greater than 80% of this excess cholesterol is transported as LDL (Rudel et al. 1979). This LDL is markedly different from the LDL of noncholesterol-fed animals in that it contains sig-nificantly more cholesterol (mainly as cholesteryl esters) per LDL particle, resulting in an increased particle size as determined by molecular weight. In addition, a highly significant, positive correlation has been shown be-tween LDL molecular weight and severity of coronary artery atherosclerosis in at least two species of nonhuman primates (Pitts et al. 1976; Leathers et al. 1978). When serum from animals with diet-induced hypercholesterolemia is added to smooth muscle cells and skin fibroblasts in culture (St. Clair and Leight 1978) or to organ cultures of arterial tissue (St. Clair and Har-pold 1975), it is more effective in stimulating cholesterol accumulation and cholesterol esterification than is an equivalent amount of cholesterol as normal serum. Much of this enhanced ability of hypercholesterolemic serum to promote cholesterol accumulation is due to the presence of the large mo-lecular weight hypercholesterolemic LDL. Thus, the increased atherogenicity of the hypercholesterolemic LDL correlates with its enhanced ability to pro-mote cholesterol accumulation and esterification in vitro. The purpose of the present study was to determine the mechanism(s) whereby hypercholester-olemic LDL enhances the accumulation of cholesterol in cells in culture.

Methods

Aortic smooth muscle cells and skin fibroblasts from rhesus monkeys were grown from explants as described previously (St. Clair and Leight 1978). After the cells had reached confluency they were incubated for 48-72 hours with lipoprotein-deficient medium in order to deplete them of cholesterol prior to the addition of normal or hypercholesterolemic LDL. The lipopro-teins used in these studies were isolated by agarose-column chromatography (Rudel et al. 1974) from fasted normal or diet-induced hypercholesterolemic rhesus (Macaca mulatta) of cynomolgus macaques (M. fascicularis).

Results

As shown in Figure 1, cells incubated with hypercholesterolemic LDL accumu-lated significantly more cholesterol than those incubated with normal LDL. This was most apparent for accumulation of cholesteryl esters. The magnitude of the cholesteryl ester accumulation varied with the individual cell line but was consistently greater for skin fibroblasts than smooth muscle cells. Associated with the greater accumulation of cholesteryl esters was a 30-50% enhancement of cholesterol esterification in cells incubated with hypercho-

[1]Supported by Grant HL 14164 from the National Heart, Lung, and Blood Insti-tute.

lesterolemic LDL (Figure 1). The extent of the stimulation in cholesterol esterification also correlated with the enhanced ability of skin fibroblasts to accumulate cholesteryl esters.

In order to evaluate whether differences in the metabolism of hypercholesterolemic LDL could explain these differences in cholesterol accumulation we incubated cells with ^{125}I-labeled normal or hypercholesterolemic LDL (St. Clair et al. 1979). As shown in Figure 2, over twice as many particles of normal LDL were bound, internalized, and degraded than hypercholesterolemic LDL. Scatchard analysis of specific binding data indicated that the affinity for binding of hypercholesterolemic LDL was about twice that of normal LDL (2.63 µg protein/ml of hypercholesterolemic LDL required to achieve half-maximum binding [K_d] versus 4.35 µg protein/ml for normal LDL); yet, at maximum binding capacity only about 50% as many particles of hypercholesterolemic LDL were able to bind to the receptor compared to normal LDL.

To determine whether normal and hypercholesterolemic LDL bound to the same receptor and whether the difference in binding affinity was a result of the larger amount of cholesteryl ester per LDL particle we compared the ability of native and partially delipidated normal and hypercholesterolemic LDL to compete for LDL receptors with ^{125}I-normal LDL (Figure 3). Results from this and other experiments using several different cell lines indicated that both normal and hypercholesterolemic LDL bind to the same LDL receptor. At equivalent concentrations, native hypercholesterolemic LDL was more effective than normal LDL in competing for binding, internalization, and degradation, consistent with the conclusion that hypercholesterolemic LDL has a greater affinity for binding. Partial delipidation of the LDL (Gustafson 1965) resulted

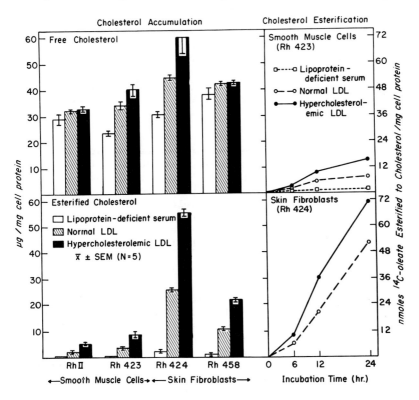

FIG. 1. Cholesterol accumulation and esterification in cells incubated at 37°C with normal or hypercholesterolemic LDL (50 µg protein/ml). For accumulation studies, cells were incubated for 24 hours with the indicated LDL.

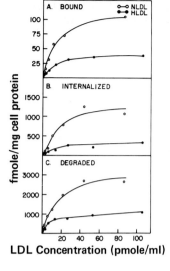

FIG. 2. Metabolism of normal and hypercholesterolemic LDL by rhesus monkey smooth muscle cells. Cells were incubated for 5 hours at 37°C with ^{125}I-labeled normal (NLDL) or hypercholesterolemic LDL (HLDL). Bound LDL was removed with heparin. Results are the mean of duplicate cultures.

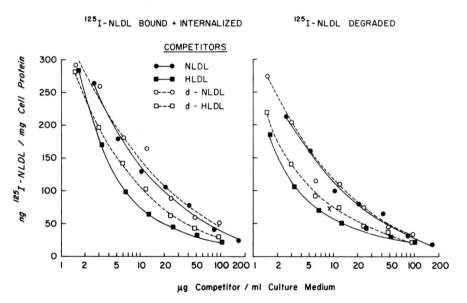

FIG. 3. Competition of native (NLDL, HLDL) and partially delipidated normal and hypercholesterolemic LDL (d-NLDL, d-HLDL) for ^{125}I-NLDL binding to LDL receptors. Rhesus monkey skin fibroblasts were incubated for 4 hours at 37°C with 0.89 µg of ^{125}I-normal LDL and the indicated concentrations of unlabeled LDL. Results are the mean of duplicate determinations.

in complete removal of cholesterol, cholesteryl esters, and triglycerides and approximately 30% of the phospholipids in both LDL preparations, but did not eliminate the enhanced binding affinity of the hypercholesterolemic LDL.

Having identified these differences in binding affinity and capacity of hypercholesterolemic LDL, we investigated whether differences in LDL metabolism could explain the enhanced accumulation of cholesterol. For this, cells were incubated with ^{125}I-labeled normal or hypercholesterolemic LDL for 24 hours and the total amount of LDL metabolized (bound + internalized + degraded) was measured along with the net amount of cholesterol that accumulated. From the ratio of protein to cholesterol in the LDL it was possible to calculate the amount of cholesterol that would have been delivered to the cells by the metabolism of a known amount of LDL protein. This calculated value was compared with the actual net amount of cholesterol that accumulated (Figure 4). The total amount of cellular cholesterol accounted for by the metabolism of LDL ranged from 33-96%. In all cell lines, a greater percentage of the accumulated cholesterol was accounted for by the metabolism of normal LDL than for hypercholesterolemic LDL, and only 14-27% of the difference in the cholesterol that accumulated with hypercholesterolemic LDL, relative to normal LDL, could be explained by differences in LDL metabolism.

Conclusion

These studies indicate that both normal and hypercholesterolemic LDL bind to the same surface LDL receptor with high affinity and are internalized and degraded by mechanisms that appear identical to those described by Goldstein and Brown (1977) for human LDL. However, only about one-half as many hypercholesterolemic LDL particles bind relative to normal LDL, but do so with approximately twice the affinity of normal LDL. This enhanced binding affinity appears primarily to be a function of the apoproteins since complete removal of the LDL core lipids (cholesteryl esters and triglycerides) as well as free cholesterol did not eliminate the enhanced binding. We have been unable, thus far, to identify consistent differences in the composition of the apolipoproteins of hypercholesterolemic LDL that could explain this effect. It is possible that relatively minor changes in the content of an apo-

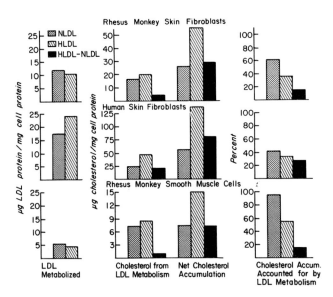

FIG. 4. Cholesterol accumulation accounted for by metabolism of normal or hypercholesterolemic LDL. Cells were incubated for 24 hours at 37°C with 50 µg protein/ml of ^{125}I-normal (NLDL) or hypercholesterolemic LDL (HLDL) and LDL metabolized was calculated from the sum of bound + internalized + degraded LDL. The cholesterol from LDL metabolism was calculated from the known ratio of cholesterol/protein in the LDL. Results are the mean of five separate experiments with triplicate dishes for each assay.

protein with high affinity for the LDL receptor, such as apo-E, (Pitas et al. 1979) could be responsible for the enhanced binding. It is also possible that the enhanced binding could be secondary to differences in the confirmation of the major apoprotein of LDL (apo-B) on the surface of these abnormal LDL particles. The mechanism of decreased binding capacity of the hypercholesterolemic LDL is also incompletely understood. Some of this difference may be the result of the larger particle size preventing the same number of hypercholesterolemic LDL particles from occupying the same area of LDL receptors as normal LDL. Size alone, does not appear to be able to account completely for this effect (St. Clair et al.1979). Even with these differences in binding affinity and capacity, differences in the metabolism of LDL were unable to explain the enhanced accumulation of cholesterol in cells incubated with hypercholesterolemic LDL. This suggests that some free or esterified cholesterol may enter cells independent of the uptake of the intact LDL particle, and that the independent entry of cholesterol is greater from the hypercholesterolemic LDL than from normal LDL. Such a mechanism could provide an explanation for the enhanced atherogenicity of the hypercholesterolemic LDL since there would be no control over the pathologic accumulation of cholesterol if cholesterol entered cells of the arterial wall by circumventing the highly regulated LDL receptor mechanism.

References

Goldstein JL, Brown MS (1977) The low density lipoprotein pathway and its relation to atherosclerosis. Ann Rev Biochem 46: 897-930

Gustafson A (1965) New method for partial delipidation of serum lipoproteins. J Lipid Res 6: 512-517

Leathers CW, Bond MG, Rudel LL (1978) Effects of ethanol on dyslipoproteinemia and coronary artery atherosclerosis in nonhuman primates. Circulation 58: 296

Pitas RW, Innerarity TL, Arnold KS, Mahley RW (1979) Rate and equilibrium constants for binding of apo-E HDL_c (a cholesterol-induced lipoprotein) and low density lipoproteins to human fibroblasts: Evidence for multiple receptor binding of apo-E HDL_c. Proc Natl Acad Sci 76: 2311-2315

Pitts LL, Rudel LL, Bullock BC, Clarkson TB (1976) Sex differences in the relationship of low density lipoproteins to coronary atherosclerosis in Macaca fascicularis. Fed Proc 35: 293

Rudel LL, Lee JA, Morris MD, Felts JM (1974) Characterization of plasma lipoproteins separated and purified by agarose-column chromatography. Biochem J 139: 89-95

Rudel LL, Shah R, Green DG (1979) Studies of the atherogenic dyslipoproteinemia induced by dietary cholesterol in rhesus monkeys (Macaca mulatta). J Lipid Res 20: 55-65

St Clair RW, Harpold GJ (1975) Stimulation of cholesterol esterification in vitro in organ culture of normal pigeon aorta. Exptl Molec Path 22: 207-219

St Clair RW, Leight ML (1978) Differential effects of isolated lipoproteins from normal and hypercholesterolemic rhesus monkeys on cholesterol esterification and accumulation in arterial smooth muscle cells in culture. Biochim Biophys Acta 530: 279-291

St Clair RW, Mitschelen JJ, Leight M (1979) Metabolism by cells in culture of low density lipoproteins of abnormal composition from nonhuman primates with diet-induced hypercholesterolemia. Biochim Biophys Acta (in press)

Factor VIII/Willebrand Factor and the Interaction of Blood Platelets with Subendothelium

Hans R. Baumgartner and Thomas B. Tschopp

Factor VIII/Willebrand factor (FVIII/WF) is synthesized by vascular endothelium and is part of the FVIII complex in plasma (Jaffe et al. 1974). Plasma of patients with von Willebrand's disease (VWD), an inherited bleeding disorder, is deficient of FVIII/WF. The plasma of these patients contains decreased amounts of factor VIII procoagulant activity (VIII/C) and their platelets release and aggregate normally upon stimulation with adenosinediphosphate in vitro. However, agglutination induced by the antibiotic ristocetin and platelet retention in glass bead columns are impaired in VWD (Weiss 1975). The combination of clinical and laboratory findings was suggestive of a platelet disorder and it has long been speculated that a defect in platelet adhesion to vascular structures might cause the prolonged bleeding time in VWD. Tschopp et al. (1974) were the first to demonstrate in a quantitative assay that this is indeed the case. In this paper the evidence which lends support to the concept that FVIII/WF acts as a cofactor for platelet adhesion, especially under blood flow conditions with high wall shear rates, is summarized and some recent observations in rabbits are reported for the first time.

Annular Perfusion Chamber

The device used to investigate platelet interaction with subendothelium is an annular chamber on whose core everted segments of deendothelialized rabbit aorta are mounted (Baumgartner et al.1976).Native or anticoagulated blood is circulated through the annular space around the vessel by a pump. A wide range of wall shear rates (50 - 10,000 s^{-1}) is obtained by varying the blood flow rate and/or the effective diameter of the perfusion chamber. The following parameters of platelet surface interactions are determined in cross sections by stereological techniques: surface coverage with contact (C) and spread (S) platelets (C+S = adhesion); surface coverage with platelet microthrombi (T); aggregation (100 T/S); thrombus volume per surface area; thrombus height distribution and maximum thrombus height (Baumgartner et al. 1976, 1980).

Interaction of Human Platelets with Rabbit Aorta Subendothelium

Experiments with blood of normal subjects. In citrated blood platelet adhesion to subendothelium increased with exposure time until 100 % surface coverage was attained. Platelet thrombi were transient, reaching a maximum between 5 and 10 min and eventually disappearing at longer exposure times. Rates of adhesion increased with wall shear rate to 650 s^{-1}; at higher values of shear no significant increase was observed and the rate of adhesion remained at approx. 12 %/min. No platelet thrombi formed below wall shear rates of 350 s^{-1}, but they increased continuously as shear rate increased to 10,000 s^{-1} (Turitto et al. 1980). The thrombi observed after native blood perfusion were larger and higher and thus probably more stable than those which formed in citrated blood (Baumgartner et al. 1980).

Experiments with blood of patients with VWD. A significant reduction of platelet adhesion to subendothelium was observed with citrated VWD-blood at 800 s^{-1} shear rate. Thrombi were reduced as well, however, when expressed per surface covered with spread platelets, aggregation (100 T/S) was normal (Tschopp et al. 1974). The rate of adhesion decreased with increasing shear rate when either citrated or native blood of patients with VWD was perfused. Thus the magnitude of the adhesion defect in VWD increased with increasing shear rate (Weiss et al. 1978a). Addition of FVIII/WF containing fractions from chromatographed cryoprecipitate to VWD-blood corrected the adhesion defect (Weiss et al. 1978b).

Antibody-induced inhibition of adhesion. Antibodies raised in rabbits against human FVIII/WF (Meyer et al. 1973), as well as a homologous antibody to FVIII/WF from a patient with severe VWD (Shoa'i et al. 1977), when added to blood of control subjects, inhibited platelet adhesion to subendothelium in a shear rate dependent manner. Thus, adhesion was reduced by 38 and 99 % at 650 and 5200 s^{-1} shear rate, respectively. In contrast, antibodies to VIII/C had no effect (Baumgartner et al. 1979).

Speculation. In flowing blood, platelet adhesion to a surface is governed by two mechanisms: transport of platelets to the surface and reaction of platelets with the surface. The former increases with shear rate and has been discussed extensively (Turitto et al. 1977; Turitto and Baumgartner 1979). The latter involves a number of steps including the initial attachment and firm binding of a platelet at the surface and subsequent spreading, release and aggregation. The initial events including spreading are a prerequisite for the secondary reaction which, in turn, may influence the first steps. The above evidence indicates that FVIII/WF is essential for the reactions of a platelet with a surface at least at high wall shear rates (as observed in small arteries and the microvasculature), i.e. when the residence time of a platelet at the reactive surface is short. Sakariassen et al. (1979) suggested that binding of FVIII/WF to subendothelium is important for platelet adhesion. However, additional results are needed to eventually elucidate the role of FVIII/WF in the mechanisms of platelet-vessel wall interaction.

Interaction of Rabbit Platelets with Rabbit Aorta Subendothelium

The interaction of rabbit platelets with rabbit aorta subendothelium and its dependence on wall shear rate in the annular perfusion chambers is qualitatively very similar to the interaction of human platelets described above. However, antibodies against human FVIII/WF do not precipitate with rabbit FVIII complex, and ristocetin does not agglutinate rabbit platelets. If FVIII/WF is of physiologic importance for platelet adhesion, its depletion should nevertheless inhibit platelet adhesion in another species as well. We therefore tested the effect of an antibody raised in guinea pigs against rabbit FVIII complex. This antibody was kindly provided by Dr. Dominique Meyer. The results are shown in table 1.

The anti FVIII complex antiserum inhibited adhesion and thrombi. The inhibitory effect on adhesion was highly shear rate dependent. Thus, adhesion was inhibited by 43, 55 and 93 % at 200, 650 and 2600 s^{-1} shear rate, respectively. Aggregation on subendothelium was abolished by the addition to rabbit FVIII complex (Table 1). On the other hand the same antiserum had no effect on ADP-induced aggregation in platelet-rich plasma, but inhibited collagen-induced aggregation. These observations correspond to those made with citrated human blood and platelet-rich plasma to which antibodies against human FVIII/WF were added (Baumgartner et al. 1979).

Table 1. Effect of an Antiserum raised in Guinea Pigs against Rabbit FVIII Complex on the Interaction of Rabbit Platelets with Subendothelium of Rabbit Aorta.

Condition of blood perfusion		Addition to citrated blood of rabbits			
		Guinea pig serum (10µl/ml)		Antiserum to rabbit FVIII complex (10µl/ml)	
shear rate (s^{-1})	exposure time (min)	Adhesion $(C+S)^a$	Thrombi $(T)^b$	Adhesion $(C+S)^a$	Thrombi $(T)^b$
200	3	$14\pm3(9)^c$	0	$8\pm2(9)$ns	0
650	5	$72\pm4(7)$	5 ± 4	$32\pm4(7)$***	0
2600	3	$56\pm7(10)$	14 ± 5	$4\pm1(10)$***	0

a   percent coverage of the subendothelial surface with contact (C) and spread (S) platelets

b   percent coverage of the subendothelial surface with platelet microthrombi >5µm in height

c   mean $\pm$ SE (number of experiments)

*** $2p < 0.001$ as compared to corresponding control (Student's t-test)

Conclusion. Our new observations lend further support to the view that FVIII complex plays an important role as cofactor for platelet adhesion to subendothelium, especially under blood flow conditions with high wall shear rates. Ristocetin is widely used to measure FVIII/WF concentrations in plasma, an activity which was more correctly termed ristocetin cofactor activity (VIIIR/RCo). Although the adhesion promoting activity of human plasma seems to be related to VIIIR/RCo, no correlation in indivudual VWD patients between the extent of platelet adhesion and VIIIR/RCo in plasma was found (Weiss et al. 1978a). Ristocetin does not agglutinate rabbit platelets, nevertheless depletion of FVIII complex in this species was associated with impaired adhesion. We thus conclude that the activity in plasma which promotes adhesion (FVIII/WF) is not identical with VIIIR/RCo.

Possible Implications for the Pathogenesis of Arteriosclerosis

Platelet adhesion to subendothelium is followed by migration and proliferation of smooth muscle cells (Ross and Glomset 1976, Baumgartner and Studer, 1977), a process which might be initiated by a platelet-derived growth factor (PDGF) known to stimulate proliferation of smooth muscle and other cells in vitro (Ross and Glomset 1976). Antoniades et al. (1979) have highly purified PDGF in the meantime. It is conceivable that less PDGF would reach the smooth muscle cells in a condition with impaired platelet adhesion and thus less smooth muscle cell proliferation and consecutive connective tissue synthesis would occur. Fuster et al. (1978) have demonstrated that pigs with VWD develop fewer raised lesions in their aorta than normal pigs, a finding which is in favour of the above hypothesis. Our findings show that the magnitude of the adhesion defect increased with the blood shear rate at the vessel wall. Shear rates higher than those in the aorta are found in smaller arteries and in the microvasculature (Copley and King 1976). Studies investigating the formation of arteriosclerotic lesions in VWD should therefore not concentrate on the aorta but include smaller arteries as well.

REFERENCES

Antoniades HN, Scher ChD, Stiles ChD (1979)   Purification of human platelet-derived growth factor. Proc Nat Acad Sci US 76: 1809-1813

Baumgartner HR, Muggli R, Tschopp ThB, Turitto VT (1976) Platelet adhesion, release and aggregation in flowing blood: effects of surface properties and platelet function. Thrombos Haemostas 35: 124-138

Baumgartner HR, Studer A (1977) Platelet factors and the proliferation of vascular smooth muscle cells. In: Atherosclerosis IV, Schettler G, Goto Y, Hata Y, Klose G (eds). Springer, Heidelberg

Baumgartner HR, Tschopp ThB, Meyer D (1979) Shear rate dependent inhibition of platelet adhesion and aggregation on collagenous surfaces by antibodies to human factor VIII/von Willebrand factor. Brit J Haematol (in press)

Baumgartner HR, Turitto VT, Weiss HJ (1980) Effect of shear rate on platelet interaction with subendothelium in citrated and native blood. II Relationships among platelet adhesion, thrombus dimensions and fibrin formation. J Lab Clin Med (in press)

Copley AL, King RG (1976) Polymolecular layers of fibrinogen systems and the genesis of thrombosis. Thromb Res, Suppl II, 8: 393-408

Fuster K, Bowie EJW, Lewis JC, Fass DN, Owen ChA Jr, Brown AL (1978) Resistance to arteriosclerosis in pigs with von Willebrand's disease. J Clin Invest 61: 722-730

Jaffe EA, Hoyer LW, Nachman RL (1974) Synthesis of von Willebrand factor by cultured human endothelial cells. Proc Nat Acad Sci US 71: 1906-1909

Meyer D, Jenkins CSP, Dreyfus MD, Larrieu MJ (1973) An experimental model for von Willebrand's disease. Nature 243: 293-294

Ross R, Glomset JA (1976) The pathogenesis of atherosclerosis. N Engl J Med 295: 369-377 and 420-425

Sakariassen KS, Bolhuis PA, Sixma JJ (1979) Human blood platelet adhesion to artery subendothelium is mediated by factor VIII-von Willebrand factor bound to the subendothelium. Nature 279: 636-637

Shoa'i I, Lavergne JM, Ardaillou N, Obert B, Ala F, Meyer D (1977) Heterogeneity of von Willebrand's disease: study of 40 Iranian cases. Brit J Haematol 37: 67-83

Tschopp ThB, Weiss HJ, Baumgartner HR (1974) Decreased adhesion of platelets to subendothelium in von Willebrand's desease. J Lab Clin Med 83: 296-300

Turitto VT, Baumgartner HR (1979) Platelet interaction with subendothelium in flowing rabbit blood: effect of blood shear rate. Microvasc Res 17: 38-54

Turitto VT, Muggli R, Baumgartner HR (1977) Physical factors influencing platelet deposition on subendothelium: importance of blood shear rate. Ann NY Acad Sci 283: 284-292

Turitto VT, Weiss HJ, Baumgartner HR (1980) The effect of shear rate on platelet interaction with subendothelium exposed to citrated human blood. (unpublished data)

Weiss HJ (1975) Platelet physiology and abnormalities of platelet function. N Engl J Med 293: 531-541 and 580-588

Weiss HJ, Turitto VT, Baumgartner HR (1978a) Effect of shear rate on platelet interaction with subendothelium in citrated and native blood. J Lab Clin Med 92: 750-764

Weiss HJ, Baumgartner HR, Tschopp ThB, Cohen D (1978b) Correction by factor VIII of the impaired platelet adhesion to subendothelium in von Willebrand's disease. Blood 51: 267-279

Do Platelets Contribute to Atherogenesis?

G.V.R. Born[1]

The pathogenesis of atherosclerosis is still uncertain (see Schettler et
al. 1977). The old thrombogenic hypothesis of atherosclerosis (von
Rokitansky 1841; Duguid 1948) has reappeared in modern costume as claims
that platelets contribute to atherogenesis in three ways. First, through
damaging arterial endothelial cells by releasing injurious agents,
presumably where circulating platelets adhere (Mustard et al. 1977).
Secondly, through the release in such situations of a factor responsible
for smooth muscle proliferation in the arterial wall (Ross and Glomset
1973). Thirdly, through the formation of persistent mural thrombi which
are organized into intimal thickenings (see, e.g., Mustard and Packham
1975). The evidence for these propositions is circumstantial and none has
been established as relevant to atherosclerosis in animals or man (see
Walton 1975). Underlying all three is the assumption that a proportion of
normal, circulating platelets settle on arterial walls for long enough to
release some of their contents. There is not observational basis for this
assumption in normal arteries. Therefore it is assumed further that
arterial endothelium is continuously subject to damage or injury of some
kind as a precondition for the adherence of platelets. So far there is
little evidence for this generalisation which could be relevant to man.
The only experimental basis which could conceivably apply to human arteries
is the higher replacement rate of endothelium around the openings of
branches than elsewhere in guinea pig aorta (Payling Wright and Born 1971)
most simply explained by assuming a dependence of endothelial turnover on,
inter alia, haemodynamic effects due to non-laminar blood-flow over such
areas. But this should be thought of more correctly as a
quasi-physiological effect and, even there, platelets are rarely if ever
seen adhering to the walls.

Instead, these observations make more sense for explaining why these are
the areas where the first lesions of atherosclerosis appear in the form of
accumulation of lipids. Such slowly increasing accumulations can be
accounted for most simply by postulating that the rate of influx of
lipoproteins from the plasma is greater than their efflux and breakdown
(see Born 1979). As these fluxes are continuous throughout life, the
difference in their rates need be only very small indeed. Within a
population both rates are presumably subject to biological variation which
depends on many factors. However, some movement of lipoprotein from plasma
to vessel wall is presumably inevitable. Now, the predilection of lipids
for wall areas immediately around arterial branch-points can be explained
on the basis of the physiological effect represented by the higher turnover
rate of endothelium on these areas (Payling Wright and Born 1971). Between
dividing but not between resting endothelial cells there are gaps (Stehbens
1965). As endothelium constitutes the main barrier against the diffusion
of plasma lipoproteins into arterial walls (Caro 1977) a higher frequency
of gaps could account for greater influx of lipoproteins. The influx will

___
[1] I wish to thank the Fritz Thyssen Foundation and the Minna-James-Heineman
Foundation for financial support for the research referred to in this contribution.

be slowed by lowering the lipoprotein concentration in the blood to slow down or even reverse the progress of atherosclerosis and, to a limited extent, this can be achieved by appropriate diet and drugs (see Wissler and Vesselinovitch 1976). Rigorous evidence for this in man has so far been limited to some patients with hyperlipidaemia (Barndt et al. 1977). The incidence of thrombosis could then by expected to diminish roughly in proportion.

The turnover rate of endothelium is increased in experimental hypertension (Payling Wright 1972). This is compatible with hypertension as a "risk factor" for coronary heart disease. It seems more likely that this is because of an accelerating effect on plasma lipoprotein accumulation through inter-endothelial gaps (Stehbens 1965; Caro 1977) than due to an increase in the indiscriminate or even selective deposition of platelets on arterial walls. Indeed, there are other ways in which hypertension could accelerate atherosclerosis (see Caro 1977).

The barrier function of endothelium against plasma lipoproteins, and its quasi-physiological defectiveness just considered, has become more significant still through the discovery of highly specific cell membrane receptors for the low-density lipoproteins (LDL) of plasma (Goldstein and Brown 1977). These receptors mediate the breakdown of LDL, and their relevance to atherogenesis is strongly supported by the observation that the receptors are absent in patients suffering from the homozygous form of familial hypercholesterolaemia.

Recent observations on the distribution of LDL receptors between different cell types provide support for our earlier conclusion (Payling Wright and Born 1971) that the main control over the movement of lipoproteins from blood into arterial walls is exerted by the endothelium. LDL receptors have been demonstrated on aortic smooth muscle cells and fibroblasts (Goldstein and Brown 1976). Although vascular endothelial cells possess the receptors (Vlodavsky et al. 1978) LDL is not taken up as long as the cells are confluent, indicating that close mutual contact inhibits the receptor mechanism. When something breaks contact between cells, e.g., mechanical damage, lipoproteins are rapidly taken up into cells immediately around the injury site, but not elsewhere. These observations provide independent support for our conclusions that the initial accumulation of lipid, e.g., as "butterfly lesions" around aortic branches, can be explained by interendothelial gaps over these sites.

If this reasoning is substantiated with more evidence, the next crucial question is whether differences in turnover rate of endothelium depend on differences in flow properties of the blood. This proposition is being investigated experimentally.

Do platelets also adhere to these physiological interendothelial gaps, and, if so, for long enough to affect the vessel wall, e.g., through the release of "injurious" or stimulating agents? That is part of the wider question of whether or not platelets can be shown to adhere intravascularly under any conditions relevant to atherogenesis and for sufficient time to affect the vessel wall? That this is so is an assumption implicit in the proposition (see above) that platelets contribute to atherogenesis.

Current investigations of ours may begin to provide experimental answers to these questions. Platelets from platelet-rich plasma of hamsters were labeled by incubation with fluoroisothiocyanate in Ringer-citrate-dextrose solution (Wesselman et al. 1979). Labeled platelets were reinjected into a tail vein of hamsters previously prepared for vital-microscopic observation of the mesenteric vasculature. Using a low-level-light camera, labeled platelets could be observed by a fluorescence technique as distinct luminescent particles moving with the blood stream, and their flow behaviour could be observed.

Our first observations (Kortenhaus and Born 1979) have been made with venules where the flow velocities are less than in arterioles and quantification is therefore easier. A small proportion of single platelets stuck temporarily to apparently normal vessel walls but almost all of them for only very short times (less than 1 second). About 20% were arrested for up to two minutes, and about 3% for longer. There was no correlation with the adhesion of granulocytes.

Planned extensions of these experiments to arterioles and small arteries, normal and after exposure to different possible atherogenic agents, should provide evidence for or against the proposition that agents released from platelets contribute towards the pathogenesis of the lesions.

Far more progress has been made with support for the hypothesis (Born et al. 1977; Born 1979) that the thrombogenic adhesion of platelets to vessel walls depends indirectly on the haemodynamic properties of the blood as it flows through arteries narrowed by atherosclerosis.

Gross and histological appearances of arterial thrombi establish that their central mass consists mainly of aggregated platelets. What, therefore, is the mechanism responsible for rapid and extensive platelet aggregation in an artery as an apparently random event in time? Close serial sectioning of obstructed coronary arteries established some time ago that the platelet thrombus responsible is invariably associated with recent haemorrhage into an underlying atherosclerotic plaque (Friedman and Byers 1965; Constantinides 1966). The haemorrhages occur through fissures or fractures in the plaque; and it is a reasonable assumption that the sudden appearance of such a fissure or fracture is the random, individually unpredictable event affecting coronary arteries that has to be assumed to account for the clinical onset of acute myocardial infarction (Born 1979). Why such a defect should develop at a particular moment is uncertain. Perhaps it is analogous to the sudden appearance of fine cracks in the wings of jet aircraft which can be ascribed to nothing more precise than the cumulative effects of variable stresses on metal known as metal fatigue. The chance event of plaque fissure can in principle be prevented only by preventing atherosclerosis which is, as we know, still very problematical. Fortunately the subsequent thrombotic process due to platelet aggregation is now understood to the extent that it may before long become preventable by drugs.

How does this haemorrhage into a ruptured plaque start off platelet thrombogenesis? This can be regarded as part of the general question of how platelets are caused to aggregate through haemorrhage, most effectively from arteries? An explanation commonly put forward is that the process is initiated by platelets adhering to collagen which is exposed where damaged vessel walls are denuded of endothelium. Adhering platelets then release other agents including thromboxane A_2 and ADP which in turn are responsible for the adhesion of more platelets as growing aggregates. This explanation is unlikely to be correct for the following reasons. First, haemostatic and thrombotic aggregates of platelets grow without delay and very rapidly (Hugues 1979). When an arteriol 200 µm in diameter is cut into laterally, the rate of accession of platelets to the haemostatic plug is of the order of 10^4 per second (Born and Richardson, unpublished data). In contrast, although the adhesion of platelets to collagen is almost instantaneous the subsequent aggregation of platelets begins, even under optimal conditions for rapid reactivity, only after a delay or lag period of at least 15 to 30 sec (Wilner et al. 1969). Secondly, platelets tend to aggregate as mural thrombi when anti-coagulated blood flows through the plastic vessels of artificial organs such as oxygenators or dialyzers (Richardson et al. 1976) which contain no collagen nor anything else capable of activating platelets similarly. This implies that there are conditions under which platelets are activated in the blood by something other than collagen or other constituents of the walls of living vessels. The plaque on which a thrombus grows has usually narrowed the arterial lumen. At constant blood pressure the flow of blood is faster through the constriction than elsewhere in the artery. Therefore, high flow and wall shear rates are no hindrance to the aggregation of platelets as thrombi (Born 1977). Indeed the question arises of whether the activation of platelets which precedes their aggregation depends in some way on such abnormal haemodynamic conditions.

Measurements of the haemodynamic forces required to activate platelets directly (Hellums and Brown 1977) indicated that the blood flow over atherosclerotic lesions in vivo is unable to do so (Colantuoni et al. 1977). Therefore, the activation must be indirect. Now it has been known for many years that platelets can be activated by at least one agent, namely ADP, derived from the red cells which outnumber and surround the platelets in the blood. Clear evidence of increased platelet adhesiveness brought about by the operation of flow-mechanical factors on erythrocytes was provided by experiments in which blood was made to flow through branching channels in extra-corporeal shunts (Rowntree and Shionya 1927; Mustard et al. 1962). Deposits of platelets formed consistently on the shoulders of a bifurcation in the flow chamber but nowhere else in the channels. When the chambers were perfused not with blood but with platelet-rich plasma no deposit was formed, showing that red cells were somehow essential.

The increased deposition of platelets from flowing blood associated with the presence of the red cells could be caused by physical or chemical mechanisms or, of course, by both acting synergistically. A physical mechanism would depend essentially on an increase in the diffusivity of platelets caused by the flow behaviour of the erythrocytes. Indeed, the diffusivity of platelets in flowing blood has been estimated to be two orders of magnitude greater than that calculated for platelets diffusing in plasma (Turitto et al. 1972; Turitto and Baumgartner 1975). This is consistent with the enhanced radial fluctuations of erythrocytes and latex microspheres (2 μm in diameter) in flowing suspensions of red cell ghosts (Goldsmith 1971). High platelet diffusivity is required also to explain the growth of mural thrombi. This must depend on successful platelet-to-platelet collisions, the rate of which between platelets following streamlines near the walls would hardly be sufficietly high to account for the rapidity of growth observed in vivo (Begent and Born 1970; Richardson 1973).

There is increasing evidence for a chemical mechanism in the increased adhesiveness of platelets in the presence of red cells, i.e., through their ADP. The concentrations of ADP required for activating platelets are small (10^{-6} M or less) so that its direct demonstration in plasma is difficult.

It has recently become possible to demonstrate the appearance of free ADP in blood directly in concentrations sufficiently high to activate platelets (Schmid-Schönbein et al. 1979). In specially designed apparatus whole blood or resuspended red cells are exposed to controlled, different shear stresses for known time periods. The apparatus is designed to cover the range of these variables presumed to be relevant to the in vivo situations. The experiments show that ADP appears in the plasma in concentrations required for platelet activation (0.1 to 1.0 μM) but in direct proportion to free haemoglobin, indicating that platelet activation can result from small degrees of haemolysis due to haemodynamic stresses such as occur during haemorrhage, whether external or through a plaque fissure. It seems, moreover, that the appearance of free ADP is rapid enough to account for in vivo aggregation. This process is much faster than the release of ADP from the platelets themselves or of thromboxane A_2 produced by them which, in any case, induces aggregation via ADP (B Samuelsson and A Marcus, personal communication).

Any hypothesis for arterial thrombosis must be able to account for the following facts: (1) thrombi do not form in normal arteries; (2) thrombi form in atherosclerotic arteries; (3) arterial thrombi consist primarily of aggregated platelets; (4) atherosclerosis increases slowly, whereas thrombosis occurs rapidly and is individually unpredictable; therefore, atherosclerotic arteries must be subject to sudden, unpredictable events capable of initiating platelet aggregation; and (5) occlusive arterial thrombi are always associated with fissures in underlying atheromatous plaques.

The erythrocyte-haemodynamics hypothesis (Born 1979) proposes that the sudden unpredictable event that starts arterial (typically coronary) thrombosis is plaque fissure; haemorhage through the fissure is associated with increased haemodynamic stress causing red cell ADP (and other adenine nucleotides) to appear in the plasma; and this ADP is principally responsible for activating platelets and their aggregation as mural thrombi.

Evidence in support of this hypothesis includes the following: (1) in atherosclerotic arteries platelet thrombi form only when blood flow is sufficiently abnormal, i.e., as a result of haemorrhage into a fissure, or in tortuous and or stenotic regions; (2) In artificial blood vessels mural thrombi of platelets grow where, and only where flow is non-laminar; (3) in artificial vessels the formation of platelet thrombi in non-laminar flow depends on the presence of red cells; (4) adhesion and aggregation of platelets on artificial surfaces increase with red cell concentration and are abolished by ADP-removing enzymes; (5) the haemodynamic stress associated with experimental haemorrhage is insufficient in duration and magnitude to activate platelets directly, but sufficient in both to induce release of red cell ADP (Born and Wehmeier 1979).

References

Barndt R, Blankenhorn DH, Crawford DW, Brooks SH (1977) Regression and progression of early femoral atherosclerosis in treated hyperlipoproteinemic patients. Ann Int Med 86:139-146
Begent NA, Born GVR (1970) Growth rate in vivo of platelet thrombi, produced by iontophoresis of ADP, as a function of mean blood flow velocity. Nature 227:926-930
Born GVR (1977) Fluid-mechanical and biochemical interactions in haemostasis. Br Med Bull 33:193-197
Born GVR (1979) Arterial thrombosis and its prevention. Plenary lecture to VIII World Congress of Cardiology, Tokyo. Amsterdam, Excerpta Medica
Born GVR, Bergqvist D, Arfors KE (1976) Evidence for inhibition of platelet activation in blood by a drug effect of erythrocytes. Nature 259:233-235
Born GVR, Wehmeier A (1979) Inhibition of platelet thrombus formation by chlorpromazine acting to diminish haemodynamically induced haemolysis. Nature, in press
Caro CG (1977) Mechanical factors in atherogenesis. In Hwang NH, Norman NA (eds) Cardiovascular flow dynamics and measurements. University Park Press, Baltimore, pp 473-487

Colantuoni G, Hellums JD, Moake JL, Alfrey CP Jr (1977) The response of human platelets to shear stress at short exposure times. Tran Am Soc Artif
Intern Organs 23:626-631
Constantinides P (1966) Plaque fissures in human coronary thrombosis. J Atherosclerosis Res 6:1-17
Duguid JB (1948) Thrombosis as a factor in the pathogenesis of aortic atherosclerosis. J Path Bact 60:57
Friedman M, Byers SO (1965) Induction of thrombi upon pre-existing arterial
plaques. Amer J Path 46:567-575
Goldstein JL, Brown MS (1976) The LDL pathway in human fibroblasts: A recep-
tor-mediated mechanism for the regulation of cholesterol metabolism. Cur-
rent Topics in Cellular Regulation 11:147-181
Horecker BL, Stadtman ER (eds) Academic Press, New York, Vol 2
Goldstein JL, Brown MS (1977) Atherosclerosis: The low-density lipoprotein re-
ceptor hypothesis. Metabolism 26:1257-1275
Hellums JD, Brown CH (1977) Blood cell damage by mechanical forces. In: Hwang
NH, Normann NA (eds) Cardiovascular flow dynamics and measurements. Uni-
versity Park Press, Baltimore
Hugues J (1959) Thromb Diath Haemorrh 3:177
Kortenhaus H, Born GVR (1979) Quantification of platelet adhesion in vivo.
In: Thrombos Haemostas (VII Int Congr Thromb Haemostas) Abstract 1175.
Stuttgart
Mustard JF, Moore S, Packham MA, Linlough-Rathbone RL (1977) Platelets, throm-
bosis and atherosclerosis. Prog Biochem Pharmacol 13:312-325
Mustard JF, Murphy EA, Rowsell HC, Downie HG (1962) Factors influencing throm-
bus formation in vivo. Amer J Med 33:621
Mustard JF, Packham MA (1975) The role of blood and platelets in atherosclero-
sis and the complications of atherosclerosis. Thromb Diath Haemorrh 33:
444-456
Payling Wright H (1972) Atherosclerosis 15:93
Payling Wright H, Born GVR (1971) In: Hartert H and Copley AL (eds) Theoreti-
cal and Clinical Haemorrheology. Springer-Verlag, Berlin, pp 220-226
Richardson PD (1973) Effect of blood flow velocity on growth rate of platelet
thrombi (letter). Nature 245:103-104
Richardson PD, Galletti PM, Born GVR (1976) Regional administration of drugs
to control thrombosis in artificial organs. Trans Am Soc Artif Intern
Organs 22:22-29
Rokitansky C von (1841-1846) Handbuch er pathologischen Anatomie. Braumuller
and Seidel, Vienna
Ross R, Glomset JA (1973) Atherosclerosis and the arterial smooth muscle
cell: Proliferation of smooth muscle is a key event in the genesis of the
lesions of atherosclerosis. Science 180:1332-1339
Rowntree LG, Shionoya T (1927) J Exp Med 46:7
Schettler G, Goto Y, Hata Y, Klose G (1977) Atherosclerosis IV. Springer-
Verlag, Heidelberg
Schmid-Schönbein H, Rohling-Windel I, Blasberg P, Jungling E, Wehmeier A,
Born GVR, Richardson PD (1979) Release of ADP from erythrocytes under
high shear stressed in tube flow. In: Thrombos Haemostas (VII Int Congr
Thromb Haemostas) Abstract 0835. Stuttgart
Stehbens WE (1965) Endothelial cell mitosis and permeability. Quart J Exp
Physiol 50:90-92
Turitto VT, Baumgartner HR (1975) Platelet interaction with subendothelium
in a perfusion system: Physical role of red blood cells. Microvasc Res
9:335-344
Turitto VT, Benis AM, Leonard EF (1972) Platelet diffusion in slowing blood.
Indust Eng Chem Fund 11:216
Vlodavsky I, Fielding P, Fielding CJ, Gospodarowicz D (1978) Role of contact
inhibition in the regulation of receptor-mediated uptake of low density
lipoprotein in cultured vascular endothelial cells. Proc Natl Acad Sci
USA 75:356-360
Walton KW (1975) Amer J Cardiol 35:542

Wesselman G, Kortenhaus H, Schröer H (1979) Vital microscopic observation of fluorescent labeled platelets. In: Thrombos Haemostass (VII Int Congr Thromb Haem) Abstract 0635. Stuttgart

Wilner GD, Nossel HL, LeRoy EC, (1968) Aggregation of platelets by collagen. J Clin Invest 47:2616–2621

Wissler RW, Vesselinovitch D (1976) Studies of regression of advanced atherosclerosis in experimental animals and man. Ann NY Acad Sci 275:363–378

Platelet and Endothelial Alterations in Experimental Arteriosclerosis[1]

Laurence A. Harker

Despite the established importance of lipids in atherogenesis the mechanism whereby hyperlipidemia induces atherosclerosis remains unclear (National Heart and Lung Institute Task Force on Arteriosclerosis, 1971; Paoletti and Gotto 1978; Ross and Glomset 1976). While the effect could simply involve an alteration in the transport of lipid into the vessel wall (Bell et al. 1975; Davies and Ross 1978; French 1966), a large number of studies using hyperlipidemic animals have concluded that the endothelium itself is "injured" as reflected by changes in permeability, altered ultrastructure, actual denudation and changes in platelet kinetics and function (Lewis and Kottke 1977; Nelson et al. 1976; Ross and Harker 1976; Still 1974; Svendsen and Gorgensen 1976; Weber et al. 1974). The findings of deendothelialization and platelet utilization are of particular interest in view of the evidence linking a platelet released growth factor to the smooth muscle cell proliferation of arteriosclerosis (Baumgartner et al. 1971; Bjorkerud and Bondjers 1971; Clowes and Karnovsky 1977; Friedman et al. 1977; Fuster et al. 1978; Harker et al. 1976; Minnick and Murphy 1973; Moore et al. 1976; Stemerman and Ross 1972). Baumgartner and coworkers (1971) showed intimal thickening in rabbits when the aortic endothelium was removed by a balloon catheter. Similar observations have also been reported by others following removal of the aortic endothelium (Bjorkerd and Bondjers 1971). This work was applied to nonhuman primates by Stemerman and Ross (1972). Interest in the role of the platelet in this process stemmed from the obvious platelet reaction on the denuded surface together with the demonstration that platelets release a factor that has been shown in vitro to stimulate both the proliferation and migration of medial smooth muscle cells (Clowes and Karnovsky 1977; Friedman et al 1977; Fuster et al. 1978; Harker et al 1976; Minnick and Murphy 1973; Moore and Friedman 1976; Ross et al. 1974).

In studies using experimental homocystinemia (Harker et al. 1976) patchy endothelial injury was manifest as desquamation using perfusion fixation with silver nitrate which comprised about 10% of the aortic surface. Neither endothelial cell loss nor regeneration was changed significantly by dipyridamole. This homocysteine-induced vascular deendothelialization was associated with a threefold increase in platelet consumption that was interrupted by dipyridamole. Homocystinemic animals also developed typical arteriosclerotic intimal lesions composed of proliferating smooth muscle cells averaging 10-15 cell layers surrounded by large amounts of collagen, elastic fibers, glycosaminoglycans and sometimes lipid. Intimal lesion formation was prevented by dipyridamole therapy (80 µmol/kg body weight /day). In contrast to dipyridamole, which showed no protective effect on the endothelium, oral sulfin-pyrazone (250 µmol/kg body weight/day in three divided doses) in seven homo-cystinemic animals (0.14mM $\pm$ 0.04) decreased markedly the extent of aortic endothelial desquamation and normalized platelet survival measurements. This agent also prevented intimal lesion formation when compared with 15 untreated homo-cystinemic animals.

The capacity of pharmacological agents to protect the endothelium from injury was also studied in vitro, using a cytotoxicity assay with cultured ^{51}Cr-labeled human

[1] This work was supported in part by research grants HL-18645; HL-11775 and RR-0016 from the U.S. Public Health Service

557

endothelial cells. In vitro specific release of ^{51}Cr from prelabeled confluent human umbilical vein endothelial cells was induced by rabbit antibody prepared against human endothelial cells or homocysteine in a dose dependent manner. Sulfinpyrazone reduced specific ^{51}Cr-release induced by either immune or sulfhydryl mediated endothelial injury in a concentration related fashion between 10^{-4} and 10^{-6}M. Dipyridamole and acetylsalicylic acid did not measurably modify specific ^{51}Cr release induced immunologically or chemically. These studies suggest that endothelial cell protection from injury in vitro may predict in vivo prevention of endothelial cell desquamation and its consequences and that pharmacologic protection of the endothelium may be therapeutically important in the prevention of arteriosclerotic vascular disease.

Experiments were performed in a series of normolipidemic monkeys to correlate the loss of endothelium with the amount of platelet utilization. A known amount of endothelium was removed from each of a series of animals (M. nemestrina) with a balloon catheter, and platelet survival and turnover were measured serially (Harker 1978; Ross and Harker 1976). A direct correlation was observed between the amount of endothelium removed and the extent of the decrease in platelet survival. Platelet survival was measured in six hyperlipidemic monkeys (maintained on the lipid-rich diet for longer than twelve months), and compared with eight control animals. Platelet survival in the animals that were hyperlipidemic for more than six months averaged 5.8 days, compared to 8.0 days in the control animals (p < 0.01). Matched cross-over platelet survival experiments were also carried out between six normolipidemic and six hyperlipidemic monkeys. Donor platelets were labeled with ^{51}Cr and their survival in the respective recipient was determined. Platelets from hyperlipidemic monkeys survived normally after infusion into normolipidemic animals. In contrast, platelets from normolipidemic animals infused into hyperlipidemic animals had a decreased survival time comparable with that of autologous platelets (Ross and Harker 1976). Chronically hyperlipidemic animals were assessed for endothelial integrity by examining the entire aorta and iliac arteries after perfusion in vivo with silver nitrate. In these preparations of the hyperlipidemic animals there was focal loss of endothelial cells amounting to 5% of the aortic surface. These data were consistent with the proposition that the mechanism of hyperlipidemia-induced experimental atherosclerosis involved platelet utilization by exposed subendothelium. While there is reason to believe that the extent of denudation in the hyperlipidemic animals was overestimated as discused later the evidence for the role of platelets and endothelial "injury" in experimental atherosclerosis is rather compelling.

While these results establish that some form of endothelial "injury" and platelet interaction is involved in hyperlipidemia, the concept of endothelial "injury" needs further definition. Recently Davies et al. (1976), Riedy and Bowyer (1977) and Taylor et al. (1978) reported on the scanning electron microscopy of the endothelium of animals in the early stages of hyperlipidemia. In these studies the endothelium remained intact until after intimal lesions were already present. These studies obviously contradicted earlier studies (Nelson et al. 1976; Still 1974; Weber et al. 1974), including our own (Ross and Harker 1976). The differences appear to result largely from the development of methods for fixation. Using improved methods of fixation, and in preliminary studies in the monkey (M. nemestrina) we have confirmed the earlier observations in rabbits that endothelial denudation appears primarily after lesions have formed. It is important to point out, however, that the absence of denuded areas does not imply that the endothelium is uninjured. Endothelial injury may represent a functional change without loss of cells, or cells may be lost and replaced sufficiently rapidly that no denuded areas appear. As noted earlier, studies have reported not only morphologic evidence of endothelial injury but functional changes as well (Bell et al. 1975; Davies and Ross 1978).

Recently, hyperlipidemic and sulfinpyrazone treated hyperlipidemic animals have been compared using improved in vivo pressure fixation with glutaraldehyde combined with silver staining in vitro. Examination of en face whole mount preparations of the aorta comparing control and experimental animals that have been post-stained with silver nitrate have demonstrated the following changes in the appearance of the endothelium in hyperlipidemic monkeys: (a) missing endothelial cells; (b) gaps betwen endothelial cells, presumably due to sites where junctions appear to be "altered"; (c) "streams" of narrow, elongated endothelial cells with increased cell density, localized particularly to outflow tracts and behind raised lesions; (d) "rounded" or unusually shaped endothelial cells; (e) heavily silver stained endothelial cells. Actual endothelial denudation was observed over lesions but was less than 1.0% of the luminal surface. Sulfinpyrazone markedly reduced the amount of altered endothelial morphology as well as the extent of intimal lesion formation. Studies using human endothelial cells in vitro have also failed to show a level of injury that is detectable when utilizing endothelial detachment or ^{51}Cr release as measures of injury (R. Wall et al. unpublished observations). In these in vitro studies, sera from patients with the classical patterns of hyperlipoprotenemia were incubated for up to 72 and 24 hours and the cells were assessed with respect to both detachment and ^{51}Cr release tests.

Studies in cell culture have permitted a number of endothelial cell functions to be identified that could be potentially important in the development of vascular disease and its complications, such as functions related to lipoprotein metabolism, functions related to platelet thromboresistance, prostaglandin metabolism, or functions related to smooth muscle cell-endothelial cell interaction, such as the production of endothelial cell derived growth factor, glycosaminoglycans or collagen synthesis. It has also become clear that endothelial cells can be lost from the surface without measureable denudation. This depends upon the ability of the endothelial cells to repair by migration and regeneration rapidly enough to replace lost cells and maintain continuity. This concept is of particular interest in view of evidence demonstrating maintenance of endothelial integrity despite increased cell turnover (Florentin et al. 1969). Furthermore, studies of cells in culture as well as studies of the intact animal suggest that regenerating cells may be functionally altered in endocytosis and, possibly, in proteoglycan production (Davies and Ross 1978; Davies et al. 1979; Vlodavsky et al. 1978).

In considering non-denuding injuries, it is important to ask whether or not platelet factor might be released at injury sites where the subendothelium is either not exposed or exposed only briefly. Studies have shown, in vitro, that smooth muscle cells are stimulated to divide by exposure to the platelet factor for as little as 1 hour (Rutherford and Ross 1976). These findings emphasize the need to characterize and measure precisely the various types of endothelial injury in hyperlipidemia in relationship to platelet activation in vivo. Since platelet survival is shortened in hyperlipidemic animals and preliminary results show increased plasma levels of PF4 and TG in these animals, the endothelium may transport platelet derived factors to the subendothelium and thereby mediate smooth muscle cell proliferative lesions in hyperlipidemia. Another possibility is based upon the observations that hyperlipidemic LDL is mitogenic to smooth muscle cells (Fischer-Dzoga et al. 1976). A third possibility is that the endothelial cell may be stimulated by hyperlipidemia to synthesize and release endothelial cell derived growth factor that may contribute to intimal lesion formation (Fass et al. 1978; Gajdusek et al. 1979).

One of the basic functional characteristics of intact, normal endothelium is its nonreactivity to platelets, leukocytes, or coagulation systems. The surface properties conferring this thromboresistant state may be a consequence of certain cell surface glycoproteins, or the surface charge produced by these cell surface components. Moncada, Higgs, and Vane described the synthesis of prostaglandin I_2 (PGI_2) by blood vessel rings (1977) and observed that this prostaglandin inhibited platelet aggregation, and at high concentrations, platelet adhesion. Moreover modulation of PGI_2 production by injury factors including activated clotting enzymes serves to limit locally any hemostatic response (Weksler et al. 1978). The capacity of endothelium to regulate PGI_2 production is thought to be one mechanism contributing to the nonthrombogenic properties of intact vascular endothelium. Studies of PGI_2 release from arterial segments using vessels from diabetic and atherosclerotic animals have shown impaired synthesis of PGI_2-like activity compared with the control vessels, and this defect may in part contribute to the thrombooclusive complications associated with these disorders (Masotti et al. 1979; Stilberbauer et al. 1979). Baumgartner has also shown an inverse relationship between PGI_2 synthesis by deendothelialized arterial segments and the platelet thrombus forming capability of those segments (Baumgartner and Tschopp 1979). Recent work in vitro suggests that hyperlipidemia might be expected to impair the synthesis of PGI_2 by affected vessels (Weiss et al. 1979).

The recently developed technology for the in vitro study of the biologic properties of vessel wall cells in isolation has greatly contributed to our understanding of the interaction of platelets, plasma coagulation factors, and the endothelium (Gimbrone 1976; Ross and Glomset 1976). Cultured endothelium, but also cultured vascular smooth muscle cells and to a lesser degree fibroblasts, can be stimulated to synthesize PGI_2 from endogenous arachidonate (Baenziger et al. 1979; Weksler et al. 1977). Exposure of endothelium to arachidonic acid, trypsin, thrombin, and possibly other factors increases the rate of PGI_2 synthesis by cultured endothelial cells (Weksler et al. 1978). Production of thrombin at a site of vascular injury could, by increasing the production of PGI_2 by endothelial cells adjacent to the area of injury localize thrombus formation. Moreover enhanced PGI_2 synthesis might serve as an indicator of sublethal endothelial injury. There are a number of components of the blood that may modify the response of the vessel to endothelial injury. These include hormones such as insulin, vasoactive peptides, substances released by blood cells that may manifest an altered endothelial function.

Since platelets appear to be important in both the thrombotic complications of atherosclerotic vascular disease and the atherogenic process, platelet survival has been used previously to detect in vivo platelet involvement in thrombus formation but this measurement is neither sensitive nor specific (Harker 1978). Moreover platelet viability may not be affected by some types of activation in vivo as shown by the observation that platelets subjected to in vitro release of dense granules survive normally in vivo (Riemers et al. 1976). PF4 and βTG, platelet specific proteins present in the α granule, have been shown to be readily released from platelets both in vitro and in vivo. There is great interest in the possibility that plasma levels of these proteins may be indicators of platelet activation in vivo (Bolton et al. 1976; Kaplan et al. 1978; Levine and Krentz 1977; Witte et al. 1978).

References

Baenziger NL, Becherer PR, Majerus PW (1979) Characterization of prostacyclin synthesis in cultured human arterial smooth muscle cells, venous endothelial cells and skin fibroblasts. Cell 16: 967

Baumgartner HR, Stemerman MB, Spaet TH (1971) Adhesion of blood platelets to subendothelial surface: distinct adhesion to collagen. Experientia 27: 283.

Baumgartner H, Tschopp TB (1979) Platelet interaction and aortic subendothelium in vitro: locally produced PGI_2 inhibits adhesion and formation of mural thrombi in flowing blood. Thromb and Haemostas 42: 6

Bell FP, Day AJ, Gent M, Schwartz CJ (1975) Differing patterns of cholesterol accumulation and ^{3}H-cholesterol of influx in areas of the cholesterol-fed pig aorta identified by Evans Blue dye. Exp Mol Pathol 22: 366

Bjorkerud S, Bondjers G (1971) Arterial repair and atherosclerosis after mechanical injury: L Permeability and light microscopic characteristics of endothelium in nonatherosclerotic and atherosclerotic lesions. Atherosclerosis 13: 355

Bolton AE, Ludlam CA, Petter DS, Moore J, Cash JD (1976) A radioimmunoassay for platelet factor 4. Thromb Res 8: 51

Clowes AW, Karnovsky MJ (1977) Failure of certain antiplatelet drugs to affect myointimal thickening following arterial endothelial injury in the rat. Lab Invest 36: 452

Davies PF, Reidy MA, Goode TB, Bowyer DE (1976) Scanning electron microscopy in the evaluation of endothelial integrity of the fatty lesion in atherosclerosis. Atherosclerosis 25: 125

Davies PF, Ross R (1978) Mediation of pinocytosis in cultured arterial smooth-muscle and endothelial cells by platelet-derived growth factor. J Cell Biol 79:663

Davies PF, Seldon SC, Schwartz SM (in press) Enhanced rates of fluid pinocytosis during exponential growth and monolayer regeneration by cultured arterial endothelial cells. J Cell Phys

Fass DN, Dawning MR, Meyers P, Bowie EJ, Widde LD (1978) Cell growth stimulation by normal and von Willebrand's porcine platelets and endothelial cells. Blood 51: 181

Fischer-Dzoga K, Fraser R, Wissler RW (1976) Stimulation of proliferation in stationary primary cultures in monkey and rabbit aortic smooth muscle cells. I. Effects of lipoprotein fractions of hyperlipemic serum and lymph. Exp Mol Pathol 24: 346

Florentin RA, Nam SC, Lee KT, Thomas WA (1969) Increased ^{3}H-thymidine incorporation into endothelial cells of swine fed cholesterol for 3 days. Exp Mol Path 10: 250

French JE (1966) Atherosclerosis in relation to the structure and function of the arterial intima, with special reference to the endothelium. Int Rev Exp Path 5: 253

Friedman RJ, Stemerman MB, Wenz B, Moore S, Gauldie J, Gent M, Tiell ML, Spaet TH (1977) The effect of thrombocytopenia on experimental arteriosclerotic lesion formation in rabbits. Smooth muscle cell proliferation and re-endothelialization. J Clin Invest 60: 1191

Fuster V, Bowie EJ, Lewis JC, Fass DN, Owen Jr, CA (1978) Resistance to arteriosclerosis in pigs with von Willebrand's disease. Spontaneous and high cholesterol diet-induced arteriosclerosis. J Clin Invest 61: 722

Gajdusek C, Schwartz S, DiCorleto, Ross R (1979) Endothelial cell derived mitogenic activity. Fed Proc (Abst) 38: 1075 (part II)

Gimbrone MA, Jr. (1976) Culture of Vascular Endothelium. In: Spaet TH (ed) Progress in Hemostasis and Thrombosis Volume 3. Grune and Stratton, New York 4: 1

Harker LA (1978) Platelet survival time: Its measurement and use. In: Spaet TH (ed) Progress in Hemostasis and Thrombosis, Vol. IV. Grune and Stratton, New York pp. 321

Harker LA, Ross R, Slichter SJ, Scott CR (1976) Homocystine-induced arteriosclerosis: The role of endothelial cell injury and platelet response in its genesis. J Clin Invest 58: 731

Kaplan KL, Nossel HL, Drillings M, Lesnik G (1978) Radioimmunoassay of platelet factor 4 and B-thromboglobulin: development and application to studies of platelet release in relation to fibrinopeptide A generation. Br J Hematol: 39, 129

Levine SP, Krentz LS (1977) Development of a radioimmunoassay for human platelet factor 4. Thromb Res 11: 673

Lewis JC, Kottke BA (1977) Endothelial damage and thrombocyte adhesion in pigeon atherosclerosis. Science 196: 1007

Moncada S, Higgs EA, Vane JR (1977) Human arterial and venous tissues generate prostacyclin (prostaglandin X), a potent inhibitor of platelet aggregation. Lancet 1: 18

Masotti G, Galanti G, Poggesi L, Curcio A, Neri Serneri GG (1979) Early changes of the endothelial antithrombotic properties in cholesterol fed rabbits. Decreased PGI$_2$ production by aortic wall. Thromb and Haemostas 42(1): 423

Minnick CR, Murphy GE (1973) Experimental induction of athero-arteriosclerosis by the synergy of allergic injury to arteries and lipid rich diet. II. Effect of repeatedly injected foreign protein in rabbits fed a lipid-rich, cholesterol-poor diet. Am J Pathol 73: 265

Moore R, Friedman RJ, Singal DP, Gauldie J, Blajchman NH (1976) Inhibition of injury induced thromboatherosclerotic lesions by antiplatelet serum in rabbits. Thromb Haemostas (Stuttg) 35: 70

National Heart and Lung Institute Task Force on Arteriosclerosis. Arteriosclerosis. June 1971. Department of Health, Education and Welfare Publ. No. 72-219. National Institutes of Health, Bethesda, Md. 2: 4-27.

Nelson E, Gertz SD, Forbes MS, Rennels ML, Heald FP, Kahn MA, Farber TM, Miller E, Husain MM, Earl FL (1976) Endothelial lesions in the aorta of egg yolk-fed miniature swine. Exp Mol Pathol 25:208

Paoletti R, Gotto AM (1978) Atherosclerosis Reviews, Vol 3. Raven Press, New York

Reidy MA, Bowyer DE (1977) Scanning electron microscopy of aortic endothelium following injury by endotoxin and during subsequent repair. Atherosclerosis 26: 319

Reimers HJ, Cazenave JP, Senyi AF, Hirsh J, Kinlough-Rathbone RL, Packham MA, Mustard JF (1976) In vitro and in vivo functions of thrombin-treated platelets. Thromb Haemostas 35: 151

Ross R, Glomset JA (1976) The pathogenesis of atherosclerosis. N Engl J Med 295 (7): 369; 420.

Ross R, Glomset J, Kariya B, Harker LA (1974) A platelet-dependent serum factor that stimulates the proliferation of arterial smooth cells in vitro. Proc Natl Acad Sci USA 71: 1207

Ross R, Harker LA (1976) Hyperlipidemia and atherosclerosis. Science 193: 1094

Rutherford RB, Ross R (1976) Platelet factors stimulate fibroblasts and smooth muscle cells quiescent in plasma serum to proliferate. J Cell Biol 69: 196

Stemerman MB, Ross R (1972) Experimental arteriosclerosis. I. Fibrous plaque formation in primates, an electron microscope study. J Exp Med 136: 769

Stilberbauer K, Schernthaver G, Sinzinger H, Clopath P, Piza-Katzer H, Winter M (1979) Diminished prostacyclin generation in human and experimentally induced diabetes mellitus. Thromb and Haemostas 42(1): 334

Still WIS (1974) The topography of cholesterol-induced fatty streaks. Exp Mol Path 20:374

Svendsen E, Jorgensen L (1976) Loss of endothelial cells in rabbit aorta following short-term cholesterol feeding. In: Schettler G, Goto Y, Hata Y, Klose G (eds) Atherosclerosis IV. Springer-Verlag, New York p 289

Taylor K, Glagov S, Lamberti J, Vesselinovitch D, Schaffner T (1978) Surface configuration of early atheromatous lesions in controlled-pressure perfusion-fixed monkey aortas. Scanning Electron Microscopy II: 449

Vlodavsky I, Fielding PE, Fielding CJ, Gospodarowicz D (1978) Role of contact inhibition in the regulation of receptor mediated intake of LDL in cultured vascular endothelial cells. Proc Natl Acad Sci USA 75:2810

Weber G, Fabbrini P, Resi L (1974) Scanning and transmission electron microscopy observations on the surface lining of aortic plaques in rabbits on a hyper-cholesterolic diet. Virchows Arch (Pathol Anat) 364: 325

Weiss SJ, Turk J, Needleman P (1979) A mechanism for the hydrogen peroxide-mediated inactivation of prostacyclin synthetase. Blood 53: 1191

Weksler BB, Lwy CW, Jaffe EA (1978) Stimulation of endothelial cell prostacyclin production by thrombin, trypsin, and ionophore A 23187. J Clin Invest 62: 923.

Weksler BB, Marcus AJ, Jaffe EA (1977) Synthesis of prostaglandin I_2 (prostacyclin) by cultured human and bovine endothelial cells. Proc Natl Acad Sci USA 74:3922.

Witte LD, Kaplan LL, Nossel HL, Lages BA, Weiss HJ, Goodman DS (1978) Studies of the release from human platelets of the growth factor for cultured human arterial smooth muscle cells. Circ Res 42: 402

Endothelium in Experimental Atherosclerosis

C. Richard Minick, Domenick J. Falcone, and David P. Hajjar[1]

Endothelium acts as a thromboresistant surface and limits entry of large macromolecules such as lipoproteins and immune complexes to the underlying wall (Thorgeirsson and Robertson, 1978). Following loss of endothelium, primary hemostasis may be initiated at the surface of the artery and increased quantities of macromolecules may gain access to the wall of the artery. Although these events may initially be considered protective, eventually they may be important in the genesis of arterial disease.

There is clinicopathologic and experimental evidence to indicate that arterial injury and the subsequent reactive changes may favor the accumulation of lipid at the site of injury and lead to atherosclerosis (Minick, 1976; Ross and Glomset, 1976). In this regard, it has been suggested that endothelial injury is the initiating event in arterial disease following several seemingly disparate types of arterial injury including mechanical, immunological, and chemical injury. Following endothelial injury, mitogenic stimuli derived from factor (s) released by platelet interaction with the vessel surface and low density lipoproteins may induce proliferation of medial smooth cells and lead to intimal thickening (Fischer-Dzoga, et al. 1974; Ross, et al. 1974). If the absence of endothelium persists, the continued influx of lipoproteins into the arterial intima may lead to lipid accumulation and atherosclerosis.

The following evidence supports this endothelial injury hypothesis of atherogenesis:

1. Factor (s) from platelets and low-density lipoproteins derived from hyperlipemic serum have been found to lead to proliferation of vascular smooth muscle cells in vitro (Fischer-Dzoga, et al. 1974; Ross, et al. 1974).
2. Endothelial injury and/or denudation have been shown to be a significant and early feature of arterial disease resulting from mechanical, chemical, and immunologic arterial injury (Ross and Glomset, 1976).
3. Severe thrombocytopenia induced by antiplatelet serum inhibits the intimal thickening that usually follows endothelial denudation (Friedman, et al. 1977).
4. Diet-induced hypercholesterolemia will lead to intimal thickening even in animals made thrombocytopenic prior to injury (Friedman, et al. 1978).
5. Pigs with von Willebrand's disease do not develop atherosclerosis. In this disease, platelets do not react normally with the exposed vessel surface (Fuster et al. 1978).

In experiments summarized here, we tested the hypothesis that endothelial loss will predispose to intimal thickening and lipid accumulation. In

[1] The authors' personal research cited was supported by Grants HL-01803, and HL-18828 from the National Heart, Lung and Blood Institute of the National Institutes of Health and by The Cross Foundation.

these experiments aortas of rabbits were de-endothelialized with a balloon-catheter and rabbits were then continued on a lipid-poor diet to allow endothelial regeneration and intimal thickening to occur. Subsequently, some rabbits were fed cholesterol supplemented diets or semi-synthetic lipid-rich diets in order to test the effect of diet-induced hypercholesterolemia on re-endothelialized and de-endothelialized neointima. Control rabbits were continued on the lipid-poor diet. The extent of atherosclerotic change in de-endothelialized and re-endothelialized areas was assessed by measuring the degree of intimal thickening and evaluating the amount of lipid accumulation morphometrically and chemically. Results of our experiments indicate the following:

1. Arterial injury led to intimal thickening. However, in both normocholesterolemic and hypercholesterolemic rabbits the intima was significantly thicker in the re-endothelialized areas as compared to adjacent de-endothelialized areas. Serum cholesterol concentrations exceeding 350 mg/100ml accentuated intimal thickening in re-endothelialized areas but not in adjacent de-endothelialized areas (Minick et al. 1979).

2. There was significantly more oil red O staining material in arterial intima lined by regenerated endothelium as compared to adjacent intima lacking an endothelial lining (Minick, et al. 1977, 1979).

3. Of five lipid classes, i.e. nonesterfied cholesterol, cholesteryl ester, nonesterfied fatty acids, triacylglycerols, and squalene, only nonesterfied cholesterol and cholesteryl ester differed significantly in re-endothelialized and de-endothelialized areas (Falcone, et al. 1979; Falcone, et al. unpublished observations).

4. In normocholesterolemic rabbits, there was approximately a three-fold increase in cholesteryl ester in re-endothelialized areas as compared to de-endothelialized areas. In hypercholesterolemic rabbits, re-endothelialized areas contained a significant increase in both nonesterfied cholesterol and cholesteryl ester as compared to de-endothelialized areas (Falcone, et al. 1979; Falcone, et al. unpublished observations).

5. There was a significant correlation between serum cholesterol concentration and total aortic cholesterol in re-endothelialized areas but not in adjacent de-endothelialized areas (Falcone, et al. unpublished observations).

6. Taken together, these findings indicate that the extent of atherosclerosis as assessed by intimal thickening and intimal lipid accumulation is greater in re-endothelialized areas than in adjacent de-endothelialized areas. Thus, these findings do not support the hypothesis that the persistent absence of endothelium enhances atherogenesis. Rather, they indicate that the extent of atherosclerosis is greater in intima covered by regenerated endothelium.

The pathogenesis of this increased intimal thickness and lipid accumulation in re-endothelialized areas is unclear. Increased lipid accumulation in these areas could result from one or more of the following: increased transport of lipid or lipoprotein into re-endothelialized areas as compared to adjacent de-endothelialized areas, decreased efflux of lipid from re-endothelialized areas, metabolic differences in re-endothelialized and de-endothelialized intima and/or structural differences in re-endothelialized and de-endothelialized neointima.

Preliminary results of recent experiments suggest that there are differences in metabolism of glycosaminoglycans and cholesteryl esters in re-endothelialized as compared to de-endothelialized neointima that are expressed as structural differences. Preliminary findings of experiments of Minick, et al.(1977) and Wight, et al. (1979) indicate that in both normocholesterolemic and hypercholesterolemic rabbits there are increased quantities of glycosaminoglycans in the neointima covered by endothelium as compared to adjacent de-endothelialized intima. Results of experiments of Wight, et al. (1979) indicate that this increase is composed primarily of heparitin sulfate. These findings may be important in atherogenesis. Sulfated glycosaminoglycans have been found to inhibit lysosomal enzymes in leukocytes (Avila, 1978) spleen (Robinson and Stirling, 1978) and liver (Kint et al. 1973). Glycosaminoglycans have also been shown to bind to low-density lipoprotein (Iverius, 1972). Thus, glycosaminoglycans could lead to increased accumulation of lipid either by inhibiting cholesteryl ester hydrolase or binding to lipoproteins.

Findings of recent experiments also suggest that there are differences in cholesteryl ester metabolism in re-endothelialized areas of aorta. In normocholesterolemic rabbits, there is a selective increase of cholesteryl ester, nonesterfied fatty acids and squalene in re-endothelialized aorta as compared to uninjured aorta (Falcone, et al. unpublished observations). Preliminary findings of Hajjar, et al. (unpublished observations) suggest that there is significantly less cholesteryl ester hydrolase activity in re-endothelialized as compared to the de-endothelialized aortic wall.

In summary, results of our experiments do not support the hypothesis that the continued absence of endothelium enhances atherogenesis. Rather, results indicate that the presence of regenerated endothelium increases intimal lipid accumulation and by this or other means enhances intimal thickening. We believe these findings are important since they indicate that endothelium has an active role in influencing intimal thickening and intimal lipid accumulation and that atherosclerosis is not simply a result of passive transport of increased quantities of lipid into the arterial wall.

References

Avila JL (1978) The influence of the type of sulphate bond and degree of sulfation of glycosaminoglycans on their interaction with lysosomal enzymes. Biochem J 171:489-491

Falcone DJ, Hajjar DP, Minick CR (1979) Role of endothelium in intimal lipid accumulation. Fed Proc 38:1346

Fischer-Dzoga K, Chen R, Wissler RW (1974) Effects of serum lipoproteins on the morphology, growth, and metabolism of arterial smooth muscle cells. Adv Exp Med Biol 43:299-311

Friedman RJ, Stemerman MB, Wenz B, Moore S, Gauldie J, Gent R, Tiell ML, Spaet TH (1977) The effect of thrombocytopenia on experimental arteriosclerotic lesion formation in rabbits I. Smooth muscle cell proliferation and re-endothelialization. J Clin Invest 60:1191-1201

Friedman RJ, Tiell ML, Sussman LL, Minick CR, Eder H, Stemerman MB, Spaet TH (1978) The role of hyperlipemia on smooth muscle cell proliferation following intimal injury in thrombocytopenic rabbits. Fed Proc 37: 930

Fuster V, Bowie EJ, Lewis JC, Fass PN, Owen CA, Brown AL (1978) Resistance to arteriosclerosis in pigs with von Willebrand's Disease. J Clin Invest 61:722-730

Iverius PH (1972) The interaction between human plasma lipoproteins and connective tissue glycosaminoglycans. J Biol Chem 247:2607-2613

Kint JA, Dacremont G, Carton D, Orye E, Hooft C (1973) Mucopolysaccharidosis: secondarily induced abnormal distribution of lysosomal isoenzymes. Science 181:352-354

Minick CR (1976) Immunologic arterial injury in atherogenesis. Proceedings of 1st International Symposium on Atherogenesis. Ann NY Acad Sci 275: 210-227

Minick CR, Alonso DR, Litrenta MM, Silane MF, Stemerman MB (1977) Regenerated endothelium and intimal proteoglycan accumulation. Circulation 42, Suppl III, 144

Minick CR, Litrenta MM, Alonso DR, Silane MF, Stemerman MB (1977) Further studies on the effect of regenerated endothelium on intimal lipid accumulation. Prog Biochem Pharm 14:115-122

Minick CR, Stemerman MB, Insull W, Jr (1979) Role of endothelium and hypercholesterolemia in intimal thickening and lipid accumulation. Am J Pathol 95:131-158

Robinson D, Stirling JL (1978) N-acetyl-B glucosaminodases in human spleen. Biochem J 107:321-327

Ross R, Glomset JA, Kariya B, Harker LA (1974) A platelet-dependent serum factor that stimulates proliferation of arterial smooth muscle cells in vitro. Proc Natl Acad Sci (USA) 71:1207-1210

Ross R, Glomset JA (1976) The pathogenesis of atherosclerosis. N Eng J Med 295:369-377

Thorgeirsson G, Robertson AL, Jr (1978) The vascular endothelium – Pathobiologic significance. A review. Am J Pathol 93:803-848

Wight TN, Curwen KD, Homan WP, Minick CR (1979) Effect of regenerated endothelium in glycosaminoglycan accumulation in the arterial wall. Fed Proc 38:1075

Smooth Muscle Cell Kinetics in Vivo: A Comparative Study[1]

Michael B. Stemerman, Itzhak D. Goldberg, Ruth T. Gardner, and Robert L. Fuhro

Introduction

The importance of the vascular smooth muscle cell (SMC) in atherogenesis has been well established (Wissler 1973; Ross and Glomset 1973). As a result, these cells have come under intense scrutiny for their synthetic and growth capacities; many of these studies have been carried out in tissue culture. Some studies have been performed in vivo, but have been hampered by the difficulty in obtaining quantitative data other than by performing autoradiography or morphometry. These latter techniques are time-consuming and require large experimental populations to provide accurate measurements. We have recently developed a quantitative assay for SMC growth kinetics in vivo by measuring SMC DNA specific activity (Goldberg et al. 1979). This assay provides an accurate and rapid assessment of SMC growth following endothelial removal. We have applied this assay to both the rabbit and rat to determine differences in SMC growth kinetics among the different animals.

Methods

DNA measurements and specific activity of thymidine incorporation have been recently reported (Goldberg et al. 1979). All animals were stripped of their endothelium using a modification of the Baumgartner balloon catheter technique (Baumgartner 1963; Stemerman 1973). Completeness of endothelial removal was assessed by injecting Evans Blue 1/2 hr prior to sacrifice (Stemerman et al. 1977). At various periods of time after balloon de-endothelialization, ranging from 0 to 28 days, animals were sacrificed as follows. Each animal was given an intravenous injection of 0.5 µCi/kg of tritiated thymidine (20 mCi/mMole, New England Nuclear) one hour before sacrifice, and Evans blue was given 1/2 hr after the tritiated thymidine. The animals were anesthetized with ether and exsanguinated via cardiac puncture and the thoracic aortas were removed. The area from the 1st to 3rd intercostals was fixed in 2% gluteraldehyde, 0.1 M cacodylate, pH 7.4, room temperature, and the aorta from the 3rd to the 12th intercostal was immediately frozen. All fixed specimens were processed for light and electron microscopy (Stemerman 1973), and all frozen sections were assayed for the specific activity of the incorporation of thymidine into SMC DNA (Goldberg et al. 1979). One micron sections for light microscopy were further processed for autoradiography and were also used for quantitation of intimal cells (Goldberg et al. 1979).

[1]This work was supported by NIH grants HL 21429, HL 11414 and HL 22602.

Results

Growth curves for rats and rabbits SMC are seen in Figure 1. Following balloon injury, there was a latent period of 24 hours. Little tritiated thymidine was incorporated in this time period.

Specific activity levels in the two animals showed a general similarity in behavior, but the levels and duration of synthetic activity differed. Rat specific activity levels began to rise at 24 hours and quickly peaked to a level of about 50 DPM/μgm DNA at 48 hours. This activity abruptly dropped and returned to baseline by day three and was at baseline levels by day 14.

In contrast, the level of specific activity of DNA in the rabbit is higher and persists longer than the rat. Again, the latent period of 24 hours after injury is shared with the rat, but the specific activity is greater, and the duration of the effect, instead of returning to baseline levels by the third day, persists until the fourth day. The specific activity levels were compared with autoradiography (Goldberg et al. 1979). The coefficient of correlations between DNA specific activity and autoradiography was r = .89. Intimal cell growth was quantitated and was shown to be reflective of the DNA specific activity levels (Goldberg et al. 1979).

Discussion

Smooth muscle cell proliferation is considered by many to be a central event in the formation of the atherosclerotic plaque. Much investigation has centered on the growth characteristics of these cells in tissue culture. Although this methodology has and will continue to provide a background of information on the cellular biology of SMC's, plating of SMC in tissue culture readily produces alterations in their metabolism (Fowler et al. 1977). This

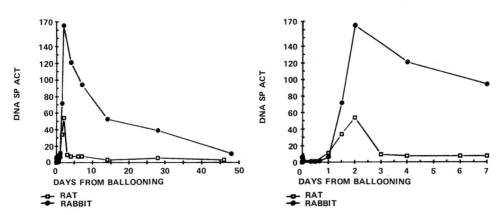

FIG. 1A and B. Rabbit thoracic vs. rat thoracic specific activity. This compares the DNA specific activity of rat and rabbit vascular smooth muscle cells. Each point represents the mean value of a minimum of 5 animals. Specific activity of DNA (expressed as disintegrations per minute per microgram of DNA) are plotted as a function of time. Figure 1A shows the period from time 0 to 48 days while Figure 1B is a closer look at days 0-7. At each day after the first 24 hours, 2.5 - 3.0 kg New Zealand white male rabbits' specific activity continued to be greater than that in 400 grams male Sprague-Dawley rats.

is not unexpected since these cells are now exposed to a static medium quite different from their normal mileau. This difference in environment ranges from a change in pressure and pulsation experienced in the vessel wall as well as the manner and concentration of the fluid bathing the tissue. The aim of these studies is to apply a new system which provides detailed information on the growth characteristics of these cells in vivo. It is the further objective to add to the detailed knowledge gained from tissue culture by studying the course of the growth patterns seen in vivo using this assay.

The difference in SMC growth kinetics seen between rat and rabbit after endothelial removal is a possible reflection of differences in the degree of injury sustained by the vessel wall in each animal. There is no control which can clearly remove this possibility; however, rabbits deendothelialized with a high pressure balloon have the same pattern of H^3-thymidine incorporation as rabbits injured with low pressure balloons. It is therefore likely that different types of animal SMC's will respond differently to similar stimuli. Although the method of SMC proliferation in our present study was the mechanical removal of endothelium, other stimuli might produce a desparity of response between species, i.e. hypercholesterolemia. A method is now available for the study of SMC growth in vivo. The use of this new assay should provide fresh insight into mechanisms of SMC growth kinetics.

References

Baumgartner HR (1963) Eine neue methode zur erzeugung von thromben durch gezielte uberdehnung der gefasswand. Z Ges Exp Med 137:227-236

Fowler S, Shio H, Wolinsky H (1977) Subcellular fractionation and morphology of calf aortic smooth muscle cells. Studies on whole aorta, aortic explants and subculture grown under different conditions. J Cell Biol 75: 166-184

Goldberg ID, Stemerman MB, Schnipper LE, Ransil BJ, Crooks GW, Fuhro RL (1979) Vascular smooth muscle cell kinetics: A new assay for studying patterns of cellular proliferation in vivo. Science 205:920-922

Ross R, and Glomset JA (1973) Atherosclerosis and the arterial smooth muscle cell. Science 180:1332-1339

Stemerman MB (1973) Thrombogenesis of the rabbit arterial plaque: An electron microscopic study. Am J Path 73:7-26

Stemerman MB, Spaet TH, Pitlick FA, Cintron S, Lejnieks I, Tiell ML (1977) Intimal healing: The pattern of re-endothelialization and intimal thickening. Am J Path 87:125-137

Wissler RW (1973) Development of the atherosclerotic plaque. Hosp Prac 8:3: 61-72

Turnover and Metabolism of Body Cholesterol in Humans[1]

DeWitt S. Goodman, Frank R. Smith, Alan H. Seplowitz, Rajasekhar Ramakrishnan, and Ralph B. Dell

During the past few years, kinetic studies have provided a considerable amount of information about cholesterol turnover and metabolism in intact humans. These studies have generally involved analysis of the turnover of plasma cholesterol following injection of radioactively labeled cholesterol, in experiments of about 10-12 weeks duration (Goodman and Noble 1968; Nestel et al. 1969; Goodman et al. 1973a), or of much longer duration (Samuel and Perl 1970; Goodman et al. 1973b; Samuel and Lieberman 1973; Smith et al. 1976). In 1976, we reported the results of long-term studies (32-49 weeks) of the turnover of plasma cholesterol in 8 normal and 16 hyperlipidemic subjects (Smith et al. 1976). We now report the results of similar long-term studies carried out in a total population of 54 subjects.

Subjects studied. The characteristics of the subjects studied are summarized in Table I. Fifteen subjects were normal. Ten subjects had hypercholesterolemia with normal triglyceride levels, and 21 had hypertriglyceridemia with normal cholesterol levels. Eight subjects had both hypercholesterolemia and hypertriglyceridemia (mixed hyperlipidemia). Twenty-one of the 39 hyperlipidemic subjects had a familial form of hyperlipidemia, and the presence or absence of a familial lipid disorder was indeterminate in 11 of the other hyperlipidemic subjects.

Turnover studies and compartmental model. $4\text{-}^{14}C$-Cholesterol, complexed with the subject's own lipoproteins, was injected intravenously, and the specific radioactivity of serum total cholesterol was determined in samples collected serially thereafter, as described in detail previously (Goodman et al. 1973b; Smith et al. 1976). For most of the subjects, 36-46 samples were collected during study periods of from 38 to 46 weeks.

The specific radioactivity data were analyzed by a weighted, least-squares technique (Goodman et al. 1973b; Dell et al. 1973), to determine the parameters of a three-pool mammillary model which would provide the best fit. The model used has been described in detail (Goodman et al. 1973b; Smith et al. 1976). The fitting process yields 6 unique model parameters: PR (cholesterol production rate in g/day), M_1 (size of pool 1 in g), and the constants k_{12}, k_{21}, k_{13}, and k_{31} (rate constants for transfer between pool 2 or 3 and pool 1 in days $^{-1}$). In addition, minimum and maximum values for the sizes of pools 2 and 3 (that is, for M_2 and M_3) can be determined.

As described above, the study population was quite heterogeneous. Even with this heterogeneity, however, the three-pool model provided the best fit to the long-term turnover data in every subject. Thus, this model seems to be generally valid for the study of cholesterol turnover in intact humans, and for comparison of hyperlipidemic patients with normals and with each other.

---

[1]This work was supported by Arteriosclerosis SCOR Grant HL 21006 from the National Heart, Lung and Blood Institute.

570

Table 1. Characteristics of the subjects studied.

Group[a]	n	Number familial	Serum lipid level[b] (mg/dl) Cholesterol	Triglyceride
Normal	15	–	199 ± 33	103 ± 35
Hypercholesterolemia	10	7	406 ± 105	131 ± 28
Hypertriglyceridemia	21	9	223 ± 27	421 ± 182
Mixed hyperlipidemia	8	5	368 ± 91	361 ± 175
Total	54	21	272 ± 104	270 ± 197

[a]Hypercholesterolemia was arbitraily defined as serum cholesterol
>275 mg/dl, and hypertriglyceridemia as serum triglyceride >200 mg/dl.
[b]Mean ± S.D.

Some information is available about the anatomic localization of the cholesterol molecules that comprise the three pools of the mathematical model.
Pool 1 mainly consists of cholesterol in plasma, blood cells, liver and in-
testines. Pool 2 consists of cholesterol which equilibrates at an intermediate rate with plasma cholesterol, and probably includes some of the
cholesterol in viscera and in peripheral tissues. Pool 3, the most slowly
miscible pool, includes cholesterol in adipose cells (Schreibman and Dell
1975), and in such slowly exchanging tissue sites as connective tissue and
arterial walls.

Data analysis. The principal aim of this work was to delineate relationships that may exist between the model parameters of whole body cholesterol
turnover and various physiological variables that were measured in each subject. In other words, our aim was to try to relate the model parameters to
such physiological variables as plasma lipid levels and measurements of body
size, plus age and sex.

A goal such as this is usually approached by taking each model parameter
and performing a stepwise multiple regression analysis for that parameter
as a function of the independent physiologic variables. One difficulty with
such a procedure is that only a limited number of linear relationships are
usually examined.

Our approach instead has been to conduct an extensive search for correlations between many different forms of the model parameters as dependent
variables, and many different forms of the physiological variables as independent variables. For the model parameters, we used the parameters themselves, three different estimates each for the size of pools 2 and 3, turnover times (which are the reciprocals of the rate constants), turnover rates
expressed as mass flow rates, and other expressions as well. In all, 50
different forms of the model parameters were used as dependent variables.

Seven physiological variables were determined in each subject: age, sex,
height, weight, frame size, serum cholesterol and serum triglyceride concentrations. From some of these (see Smith et al. 1976) we calculated surface
area, percent of ideal body weight, and excess weight (defined as total body
weight minus ideal body weight). The latter two variables were used as indices of adiposity, whereas total body weight and surface area were used as
indices of overall body size. In addition to the physiological variables
themselves, several nonlinear transformations (e.g., the logarithm of the
triglyceride concentration), and many cross-product terms (e.g., the product of serum cholesterol concentration times body weight) were also used
as independent variables. In all, we used 53 different independent vari-

ables in the data analysis. Thus, a wide range of both linear and non-linear relationships was explored, as well as possible relationships involving interactions between pairs of variables.

When one conducts an enormous search for statistically significant relationships, one will find false significance at the level at which the search is carried out. Thus, if 100,000 regression equations are examined, 1,000 of them would appear to be statistically significant at the 1% level by chance alone. Hence, a method needs to be used to guard against declaring significance when, in fact, none is present. The method used in the present study was to divide the total study population of 54 into two matched groups, one of which (hypothesis generating group, 36 subjects) would be used to find the most significant of the relationships to be considered, and the other group (hypothesis testing group, 18 subjects) for testing the significance of these relationships.

All possible multiple regression equations were computed in the hypothesis generating group for each of the 50 forms of the model parameters as a function of the 53 forms of the physiological variables. A BMDP-9R computer program, entitled All Possible Subsets Regression and written at UCLA (Dixon and Brown 1977) was used for the computations, which were performed on the IBM 360-75/91 computer system at Columbia University. For each of the 50 forms of the model parameters, the program considered more than 100,000 regression equations and selected a relatively small number that comprised the best regression equations for that model parameter. After applying rigid statistical criteria and physiological considerations, 21 regression equations were found that were highly significant and that contained interesting physiological relationships for 4 model parameters and functions thereof.

Confirmed, predictive equations. The 21 regression relationships were then tested for significance in the hypothesis-testing group of 18 subjects. In this analysis, the significance of each independent variable in each of the 21 regression equations was tested separately. Eighteen of the 21 equations were found to be significant in the testing group. From these, we selected, as independent and confirmed, 6 equations that related physiological variables with the 4 model parameters for which equations were found (PR, and the sizes of pool 1, pool 3, and total exchangeable body cholesterol). These relationships were both physiologically meaningful and provided a set of physiological variables that predicted the 4 model parameters quite well. In contrast, no significant relationships were found for any of the estimates of the size of pool 2 (M_2), or for any of the 4 intercompartmental rate constants.

The final values for the confirmed, predictive equations are given in Table II. All of the multiple correlation coefficients shown are 0.73 or higher, so that the sets of physiological variables shown can account (as r^2) for 55 to 75% of the observed variation in the 4 model parameters listed.

Body weight entered into the equations for all four model parameters. Serum cholesterol level entered into equations for cholesterol mass, i.e., for the sizes of pool 1, pool 3, and total exchangeable body cholesterol. Age influenced significantly the size of pool 3. Serum triglyceride level only had an effect on the size of pool 1, and this was best shown by a discontinuous transformation of the serum triglyceride concentration.

The major determinant of cholesterol PR was body weight alone ($r = 0.80$). No function of serum lipid levels significantly influenced PR. Thus, body size accounts for about two-thirds of the observed variation in PR amongst people, and serum lipid levels add no further information.

Table 2. Confirmed equations for production rate, M_1, M_3 (minimum), and total M (minimum).[a]

Dependent Variable	Independent Variable and Regression Coefficient[b]			Intercept	Multiple r
PR	0.024 Wt			−0.580	0.80
M_1	0.287 Wt	+ 0.0358 Chol	− 2.40 TGGP	−1.72	0.87
M_3 min	0.622 Wt	+ 0.0500 Chol	+ 0.550 Age	−49.57	0.78
	0.842 EWt	+ 0.480 Age		7.77	0.73
M_{tot} min	0.884 Wt	+ 0.0991 Chol		−11.88	0.83
	0.831 EWt	+ 0.00118 Chol·Wt		51.48	0.83

[a]The coefficients listed were determined for the entire study population of 54 subjects.
[b]Wt = total body weight (kg); EWt = excess body weight (observed weight minus ideal weight, in kg); Chol = serum cholesterol concentration (mg/dl); TGGP = variable equal to 1, 2, or 3 depending on serum triglyceride concentration (<200, 200–300, or >300); Age (years); Chol·Wt = serum cholesterol concentration times body weight.

Two equations were found for the minimum value of M_3. These showed that M_3 min is significantly related to body size, age, and (in one equation) the serum cholesterol level. These findings suggest that with time cholesterol deposition occurs in certain tissues and increases as cholesterol level increases. The relationship with age may in part reflect changes in body composition (particularly relative increases in fat tissue) which occur with increasing age. This relationship is also consistent with the increase in cholesterol in connective tissue with age reported by Crouse et al. (1972). These tissues (adipose and connective tissue) represent important components of pool 3. The finding of a relationship between M_3 min and the serum cholesterol level suggests (see also Smith et al. 1976) that the kinetic analysis as used here may be able to provide a method for estimating the size of pathological accumulations of cholesterol in slowly equilibrating tissue sites (presumably including arteries) in patients with hypercholesterolemia.

Lipoprotein relationships. In 30 of the most recently studied patients in the total study population (54 subjects), measurements of HDL cholesterol level (23 subjects) and of the levels of apolipoprotein A-I and A-II (30 patients) were also carried out. The latter (apoprotein) assays were conducted by Dr. Conrad Blum by radial immunodiffusion assay on samples of plasma that had been stored frozen at −20°C. In this smaller, mainly hypertriglyceridemic group of subjects, there was no significant association of plasma HDL cholesterol, apo A-I, or apo A-II levels with the size of kinetically defined pools of exchangeable body cholesterol. Weak negative correlations (p<0.05) were found between HDL cholesterol and apoprotein levels and estimates of the relative size of the side pools (pools 2 and 3) as compared to pool 1. The possible significance of these weak relationships requires further study for confirmation and clarification.

Simplified sampling schedule. Studies have also been conducted to try to assess the optimal sampling times and the minimal sampling frequency needed to estimate the parameters of the three-pool model. In the usual procedure, 35-40 blood samples are collected over a 10 month period. This schedule requires frequent clinic visits and is inconvenient, reducing patient compliance. For the three-pool model, only 6 accurate points, at critical times, are required to estimate the model parameters. Accuracy can be achieved by replicating the specific activity analyses at each critical sampling time. The first 3 critical times are 1, 7, and 24 days. The last 3 times must be chosen for each subject individually, from the results of the first 3 samples and prior information. This 6-point schedule was compared with the usual schedule (36-points) in 19 subjects. From residual error analyses, the total error of 5.2% was found to be about half analytical error and half biological variation. The mean values for production rate (in g/day) and pool sizes (in g), and the coefficients of variation (C.V.) between the 2 schedules were:

	PR	M_1	M_2 min	M_3 min	M_{tot} min
36-point	1.47	25.2	18.8	41.1	85.0
6-point	1.47	24.6	16.7	43.2	84.5
C.V. (%)	1.4	4.1	36.0	13.0	4.8

Thus, the simplified schedule yields parameter estimates that are close to, although more variable (less precise) than, those obtained with the usual strategy. The simplified schedule should be particularly useful for population studies, such as studies comparing two or more groups of patients.

Conclusions. In conclusion, we have obtained a confirmed set of predictive equations which describe some of the major body cholesterol kinetic parameters. These equations were generated in one subgroup of the total study population and tested in another subgroup, thereby giving us confidence in the validity and soundness of the equations. These equations account for a great deal of the variation found between people in the model parameters of production rate, M_1, and the minimal values of M_3 and of total body exchangeable cholesterol. In future work, these verified equations can be used both to predict these parameters of total body cholesterol metabolism in intact humans, and as the basis for studies of abnormalities in selected families and patients. The development of a simplified sampling schedule may be of considerable value in the conduct of such future work.

References

Crouse JR, Grundy SM, Ahrens, Jr. EH (1972) Cholesterol distribution in the bulk tissues of man: variation with age. J Clin Invest 51: 1292-1296

Dell RB, Sciacca R, Lieberman K, Case DB, Cannon PJ (1973) A weighted least-squares technique for the analysis of kinetic data and its application to the study of renal [133]Xenon washout in dogs and man. Circ Res 32: 71-84

Dixon WJ, Brown MB (1977) BMDP-77 Biomedical Computer Programs P-Series. Univ. of California Press

Goodman DS, Noble RP (1968) Turnover of plasma cholesterol in man. J Clin Invest 47: 231-241

Goodman DS, Noble RP, Dell RB (1973a) The effects of colestipol resin and of colestipol plus clofibrate on the turnover of plasma cholesterol in man. J Clin Invest 52: 2646-2655

Goodman DS, Noble RP, Dell RB (1973b) Three-pool model of the long-term turnover of plasma cholesterol in man. J Lipid Res 14: 178-188

Nestel PJ, Whyte HM, Goodman DS (1969) Distribution and turnover of cholesterol in humans. J Clin Invest 48: 982-991

Samuel P, Lieberman S (1973) Improved estimation of body masses and turnover of cholesterol by computerized input-output analysis. J Lipid Res 14: 189-196

Samuel P, Perl W (1970) Long-term decay of serum cholesterol radioactivity: body cholesterol metabolism in normals and in patients with hyperlipoproteinemia and atherosclerosis. J Clin Invest 49: 346–357

Schreibman PH, Dell RB (1975) Human adipocyte cholesterol. Concentration, localization, synthesis, and turnover. J Clin Invest 55: 986–993

Smith FR, Dell RB, Noble RP, Goodman DS (1976) Parameters of the three-pool model of the turnover of plasma cholesterol in normal and hyperlipidemic humans. J Clin Invest 57: 137–148

Turnover of Very Low Density Lipoprotein Proteins

Paul J. Nestel and Noel H. Fidge

Measurements of the rate of synthesis and removal, and of the distribution of VLDL within body pools have been derived from analysis of specific radioactivity-time curves after intravenous injections of VLDL radio-labelled in the lipid or protein moieties. Of the lipid constituents, triglyceride and to a lesser extent cholesteryl esters have been intensively studied but will be considered in this review only as part of an overall discussion of VLDL turnover.

Plasma VLDL proteins comprise at least six apoproteins: apo-B is the major structural protein, the absence of which, as in abetalipoproteinaemia, precludes VLDL secretion; the other major apoproteins are the C group and apo-E. Estimates of the turnover of each of these proteins require either specific radiolabelling of individual proteins or the isolation of each protein from plasma VLDL after the injection of generally labelled VLDL. Recently published studies have used the latter approach.

VLDL B-apoprotein can be studied more readily than the other VLDL apoproteins, because apo-B is easily isolated by precipitation or column chromatography. Initial reports of VLDL-B turnover in a single subject had suggested (Phair et al. 1972) as with previous studies with VLDL-triglyceride (Barter and Nestel 1972) sequential delipidations of VLDL leading to a cascade of progressively smaller particles, ending with the formation of a small LDL. Sigurdsson et al. (1975) showed that in man, LDL was almost entirely derived from VLDL catabolism; furthermore, measurements of flux rates of simultaneously injected VLDL-B and LDL-B suggested that VLDL was mostly converted to LDL. They had however omitted to isolate and study the IDL fraction separately which may be critical in the study of some hyperlipoproteinaemic subjects since two-thirds of IDL catabolism might occur through direct removal from the circulation. The latter pathway resembles that seen in the rat in which more than 90% of VLDL-B apoprotein is removed in the liver at the stage of an IDL particle, a pathway that has also been established through the study of the cholesteryl ester moiety of rat VLDL (Faergeman et al. 1975).

We have determined the relative importance of the two pathways of VLDL catabolism in a study of 15 normal and hyperlipidaemic subjects (Reardon et al. 1978). The simultaneous quantification of apo-B flux through VLDL, IDL and LDL demonstrated that virtually all VLDL was converted successively to IDL and then to LDL in normolipidaemic subjects (Table 1). However, in hypertriglyceridaemic individuals, in whom the total transport of VLDL-B was substantially higher than in normal subjects, the excess VLDL flux was cleared from the circulation at the stage of IDL formation (shown to be in the Sf 20-60 range of particle size). Two possibilities exist for this "shunt" pathway: since LDL-B flux was similar in normal and hypertriglyceridaemic subjects (also reported by Sigurdsson et al. [1976]), conceivably LDL-B transport cannot be readily increased to accommodate a higher flux of VLDL-B; alternatively, the VLDL, and hence IDL, secreted in hypertriglyceridaemia are structurally or functionally different from normal VLDL and IDL, leading to alternative routes of catabolism. Support for the latter possibility derives from in vitro studies of the metabolism of VLDL by fibroblasts and lymphocytes: the uptake into these cells and the intra-cellular metabolic sequelae are not uniform for all populations of VLDL (Gianturco et al. 1978; Poyser and Nestel, unpublished). The in vivo diversion of IDL to alternative sites of catabolism may therefore reflect recognition and removal by specific cells of particles secreted by hyper-triglyceridaemic subjects.

Table 1. Simultaneously measured VLDL, IDL and LDL B-apoprotein transport rates.

Lipoprotein Phenotype	Daily transport (mg/kg)		
	VLDL(Sf 60–400)	IDL(Sf 20–60)	LDL(Sf 12–20)
Normal	12.5	13	12
Familial Hypercholesterolaemia	16.5	16	17
Hypertriglyceridaemia	28	25.5	11
Combined Hyperlipoproteinaemia	19	17.5	15

Although earlier studies had suggested single-pool kinetics for plasma VLDL-B catabolism, resembling that proposed initially for VLDL-triglyceride, more detailed analysis has revealed multicompartmental metabolism. Reardon et al. (1978) demonstrated the presence of at least two pools, the faster and larger of the two extending beyond the plasma. The two-pool model is consistent with the secretion of more than one population of particles as suggested by the nature of the VLDL-IDL relationship (the IDL specific activity curve peaking after crossing the VLDL curve). The two-pool model of VLDL-B metabolism might also reflect heterogeneity of catabolic processes, as discussed above.

The more detailed, computer assisted analyses of Berman and colleagues (1978) clearly document the two potential pathways for VLDL-B catabolism, particularly in subjects with Type 3 hyperlipoproteinaemia who show both independent entry and exit of IDL-like particles through the plasma pool. Their model requires at least 4 compartments along the delipidation pathway in normal subjects plus the slow delipidation path in Type 3 subjects.

Although overproduction of VLDL-B (as well as VLDL-triglyceride and VLDL-cholesteryl esters) occurs in hypertriglyceridaemia, the question arises whether the expanded pool of VLDL-B denotes also inefficiency in clearance. Since turnover studies require steady-state conditions, increased input and expanded pool size must give rise to reduced fractional clearance. However, recently published studies (Nestel et al. 1979a) demonstrate that impaired clearance may act independently of increased input to induce hyperlipo-proteinaemia. Analysis of VLDL-B apoprotein studies in 28 subjects showed that overweight gave rise to expanded VLDL-B pools by affecting removal and not production. Additional studies in which VLDL-B pool sizes were altered by high sucrose diets, also showed that both expansion and contraction of pool size were much more closely related to changes in removal rate than in production. In short-term sucrose feeding studies, subjects who showed increases in VLDL-B pools also showed reduced fractional clearance rates for reinjected VLDL-B; by contrast higher clearance rates were found in two subjects in whom the pool sizes actually fell (Nestel et al. 1979b). This is of additional interest in view of the converse findings when VLDL-triglyceride turnover is studied: increases in triglyceride pool size aris-ing from overweight (Grundy et al. 1979) or sucrose-rich diets (Nestel 1973) are related mainly to increased production. Factors that stimulate VLDL triglyceride secretion need not simultaneously affect VLDL-B protein production; the greater load of triglyceride can be transported through the formation of larger VLDL. Although the flux of VLDL triglyceride and that of VLDL-B tend to be correlated significantly (+0.67 in one comparison) (Chait et al. 1977) the two are not invariably linked. This is also seen in the higher than normal VLDL triglyceride production rate reported for familial hypertriglyceridaemia but not for familial combined hyperlipo-proteinaemia (Chait et al. 1979); by contrast Nestel et al. (1979a) and Chait et al. (1979) have shown similar, albeit higher than normal, product-ion rates for VLDL-B protein in both forms of hyperlipoproteinaemia (Table 2). It would appear that both groups of hyperlipoproteinaemic subjects have increased VLDL secretion but only those with familial hypertriglyceridaemia also show raised triglyceride production.

Table 2. VLDL-B kinetics[a] in hyperlipoproteinaemia (+1 SE)[b]

Group of subjects (n)	Pool size (mg)	Flux (mg/d)	Removal rate (hr^{-1})
Normolipidaemia (8)	286± 84	1177±185	0.41±0.07
Hypertriglyceridaemia (10)	1066±228	2125±245	0.17±0.03
Combined hyperlipoproteinaemia (8)	629±113	1862±266	0.24±0.03

[a] Data refer to rapidly exchangeable pool

[b] Nestel et al. (1979a)

The lower than normal fractional clearance of VLDL-B, also observed in these hyperlipidaemic individuals, may reflect the longer transit in plasma of partially catabolized VLDL particles due to the length of time required to delipidate the greater load of triglyceride. The findings in Type 3 hyper-lipoproteinaemia are less consistent; whereas it is generally agreed from studies of VLDL-B protein and VLDL-triglyceride kinetics that conversion of IDL to LDL is delayed or aberrant, there is disagreement as to whether prod-uction is also raised (Berman et al. 1978; Chait et al. 1978).

The metabolism of VLDL associated C-apoproteins has received less attention than that of apo-B, mainly for technical reasons. The C-apoproteins comprise, in man, at least 4 proteins, CI, CII, $CIII_1$ and $CIII_2$, though recent separation by isoelectric focusing has revealed additional minor proteins (Catapano et al. 1978). In VLDL the C-apoproteins comprise about half the total protein. Precise metabolic data can be derived only from the study of isolated proteins. We have recently carried out such studies. Human VLDL have been radioiodinated and reinjected and the VLDL isolated from samples of plasma obtained over periods of 48 hours. After removing apo-B by precipitation, the remaining proteins were separated by isoelectric focusing and the specific radioactivity calculated for each of CII, $CIII_1$ and $CIII_2$. The removal of these three apoproteins occurred in parallel and the curves could be resolved into two exponential functions. The half-life of the first component averaged 1.5 hours and that of the second component 30 hours in normal subjects. The half-lives were longer in hypertriglycer-idaemic subjects. The catabolic rates of the C-apoproteins are therefore considerably slower than that of apo-B, since the C-apoproteins recycle between VLDL and HDL, and between VLDL undergoing catabolism and VLDL newly entering the plasma. Additional studies, in which the specific radioactiv-ity of the C-apoproteins of HDL were also determined, showed rapid equil-ibration between the corresponding C-apoproteins of VLDL and HDL.

The values for transport, fractional catabolic rate and pool size for each C-apoprotein are presented elsewhere in this book by Fidge et al. It is worth noting here that in hypertriglyceridaemic subjects, the pool sizes of

C-apoproteins were larger than normal, the fractional removal rates less than normal but mass transport was not significantly different from normal. Berman et al. (1978) have published a study of C-apoprotein kinetics derived from computer assisted analyses of total C-apoprotein radioactivity in VLDL. The multicompartmental model constructed by Berman et al. (1978) required entry of apo-C within HDL, bidirectional transfer of protein between HDL and nascent VLDL, with return of apo-C from each of the catabolic products, including IDL, derived from the sequential delipidation of VLDL. The model resembles that constructed for VLDL apo-B metabolism, with 4 normal delipidation compartments (representing sequentially diminishing VLDL particles), a slowly catabolized additional pathway for direct removal of a fraction of VLDL in type 3 hyperlipoproteinaemia, an IDL compartment and intravascular and extravascular HDL-apo-C compartments.

References

Barter PJ, Nestel PJ (1972) Precursor-product relationship between pools of very low density lipoprotein triglyceride. J Clin Invest 51:174–180

Berman M, Hall M, Levy RI, Eisenberg S, Bilheimer DW, Phair RD, Goebel RH (1978) Metabolism of apoB and apoC lipoproteins in man: Kinetic studies in normal and hyperlipoproteinemic subjects. J Lipid Res 19:38–56

Catapano AL, Jackson RL, Gilliam EB, Gotto AM Jr, Smith LC (1978) Quantification of apoC-II and apoC-III of human very low density lipoproteins by analytical isoelectric focusing. J Lipid Res 19:1047–1052

Chait A, Albers JJ, Brunzell JD (1977) Comparison of methods of plasma triglyceride turnover. In: Schettler G, Goto Y, Hata Y, Klose G (eds) Atherosclerosis IV. Springer-Verlag, Heidelberg, pp 132–137

Chait A, Hazzard WR, Albers JJ, Kushwaha RP, Brunzell JD (1978) Impaired very low density lipoprotein and triglyceride removal in broad beta disease: Comparison with endogenous hypertriglyceridemia. Metabolism 27:1055–1066

Chait A, Albers JJ, Brunzell JD (1979) Very low density lipoprotein overproduction in genetic forms of hypertriglyceridemia. Clin Res 27:363A

Faergeman O, Sata T, Kane JP, Havel RJ (1975) Metabolism of apoprotein B of plasma very low density lipoproteins in the rat. J Clin Invest 56:1396–1403

Gianturco SH, Gotto AM, Jackson RL, Patsch JR, Sybers HD, Taunton OD, Yeshurun DL, Smith LC (1978) Control of 3-hydroxy-3-methylglutaryl-CoA reductase activity in cultured human fibroblasts by very low density lipoproteins of subjects with hypertriglyceridemia. J Clin Invest 61:320–328

Grundy SM, Mok H, Zech L, Steinberg D, Berman M (1979) Transport of very low density lipoprotein triglycerides in varying degrees of obesity and hypertriglyceridemia. J Clin Invest 63:1274–1283

Nestel PJ (1973) Triglyceride turnover in man. Prog Biochem Pharmacol 8:125–160

Nestel PJ, Reardon MF, Fidge NH (1979a) Sucrose-induced changes in VLDL- and LDL-B apoprotein removal rates. Metabolism 28:531–535

Nestel PJ, Reardon MF, Fidge NH (1979b) Very low density lipoprotein B-apoprotein kinetics in human subjects. Circ Res 45:35–40

Phair RD, Hammond MG, Bowden JA, Fried M, Berman M, Fisher WR (1972) Kinetic studies of human lipoprotein metabolism in type IV hyperlipoproteinemia. Fed Proc 31:421

Reardon MF, Fidge NH, Nestel PJ (1978) Catabolism of very low density lipoprotein B apoprotein in man. J Clin Invest 61:850–860

Sigurdson G, Nicoll A, Lewis B (1975) Conversion of very low density lipoprotein to low density lipoprotein. A metabolic study of apolipoprotein B kinetics in human subjects. J Clin Invest 56:1481–1490

Sigurdson G, Nicoll A, Lewis B (1976) The metabolism of low density lipoprotein in endogenous hypertriglyceridemia. Europ J Clin Invest 6:151–158

Low Density Lipoprotein Metabolism in Familial Hypercholesterolemia

David W. Bilheimer[1]

The study of Low Density Lipoprotein (LDL) metabolism in patients with Familial Hypercholesterolemia has provided important information concerning the factors responsible for maintaining the plasma LDL concentration. Familial Hypercholesterolemia (FH) is a common inherited disorder of lipoprotein metabolism characterized by increased LDL concentrations in the plasma (Goldstein and Brown 1978; Fredrickson et al. 1978). FH is inherited as an autosomal dominant trait and homozygotes for the condition exist. The homozygotes, who have two doses of the mutant gene, exhibit higher LDL levels and a more severe clinical syndrome than do the heterozygotes who have only one dose of the mutant gene (Goldstein and Brown 1978; Fredrickson et al. 1978). Thus the influence of one or two doses of the mutant gene on the parameters of LDL metabolism can be investigated in individuals with this disease. Moreover, the interpretation of LDL turnover studies is facilitated by knowing that the genetic defect in FH involves the gene encoding a cell surface receptor for LDL.

Studies in tissue culture have demonstrated that this receptor normally facilitates the cellular uptake and degradation of plasma LDL, supplying cholesterol to body cells and simultaneously suppressing their endogenous cholesterol synthesis (Goldstein and Brown 1974, 1977). Fibroblasts from FH heterozygotes express half the normal number of LDL receptors and degrade LDL at half the normal rate (Goldstein and Brown 1977). Fibroblasts from FH homozygotes express an absence or near-absence of LDL receptor activity and therefore show no high affinity degradation of LDL (Goldstein and Brown 1974, 1977). Furthermore, patients with FH can have any of at least three different mutations at the LDL receptor locus. One of these, termed (R^{b°) specifies a receptor that does not bind LDL in detectable amounts (Goldstein and Brown 1974). Another allele (R^{b-}) specifies a receptor that can bind up to 10% of the normal amount of LDL (Goldstein et al. 1975). The third allele (R^{b+,i°) specifies a receptor that can bind but not transport LDL into cells for degradation (Brown and Goldstein 1976a; Goldstein et al. 1977).

Early studies of ^{125}I-LDL turnover in FH heterozygotes indicated that the FCR for LDL was reduced but the LDL synthetic rate was the same as that in normal subjects (Langer et al. 1972). Later studies of ^{125}I-LDL turnover in FH homozygotes indicated that these patients exhibited not only a reduced FCR but also significant overproduction of LDL as compared to normal controls (Reichl et al. 1974; Simons et al. 1975; Bilheimer et al. 1975). These previous studies involved FH heterozygotes and homozygotes studied in different laboratories and were conducted before the three abnormal alleles at the LDL receptor locus were discovered. In the present investigation, we compared ^{125}I-LDL metabolism in a series of intact subjects with well-defined types of FH in an attempt to learn how the receptor abnormality in tissue culture translated into a two- to three-fold elevation in plasma LDL levels in FH heterozygotes and a four- to eight-fold elevation in FH homozygotes.

[1] This research was supported by a grant from the National Institutes of Health (HL15949).

Methods and Results

The study group consisted of 6 normal volunteers, 6 patients with heterozygous FH and 7 patients with homozygous FH (Bilheimer et al. 1979). All subjects were housed on a metabolic ward and were fed diets low in cholesterol content. After steady state conditions were achieved, an LDL turnover study was performed in each subject. To initiate the turnover study, ^{125}I-LDL was injected intravenously and its disappearance from the plasma compartment was measured over time. LDL turnover parameters were calculated from the plasma die-away curve for ^{125}I-LDL using a 2-pool kinetic model (Langer et al. 1972; Bilheimer et al. 1975).

LDL turnover in normal subjects (Table 1): The mean age for the normal group was 26.2 years and their mean weight was 66.4 ± 11.6 kg. The mean plasma LDL cholesterol in this group was 76 ± 11 mg/dl. The mean Fractional Catabolic Rate (FCR) calculated from the plasma die-away curve using the 2-pool model was 0.450 ±0.072/day and the absolute rate of synthesis of apoLDL standardized for body weight was 8.0 ± 0.7 mg/kg per day.

LDL turnover in FH heterozygotes (Table 1): The mean age for this group was 31 yr and did not differ significantly from that of the normal group. None of the subjects was obese and their mean weight was 57.7 ± 7.4 kg. Four of the six heterozygotes were members of the same pedigree with FH (Bilheimer et al. 1978) and the other two were obligate heterozygotes in that they were mothers of FH homozygotes. The mean plasma LDL cholesterol level in this group was 230 ± 25 mg/dl. The mean FCR for apoLDL was significantly reduced from normal to 0.287 ± 0.040/day and confirms the findings of previous reports (Langer et al. 1972; Bilheimer et al. 1975; Packard et al. 1976). The mean value for apoLDL synthesis was 1.7-fold greater than normal in the heterozygotes (13.8 ± 3.6 mg/kg per day), a value significantly different from that in the normal controls.

Table 1. Kinetic Parameters for ^{125}I-LDL turnover studies in normals and FH heterozygotes.[¶]

Patient	Age (yr)	Sex	Weight (kg)	Plasma LDL Cholesterol* (mg/dl)	FCR[+] day^{-1}	Rate of Synthesis and Catabolism of apoLDL (mg/kg/day)
Normal						
J.Ch	22	M	52.4	58	0.541	8.1
R.P.	24	M	85.5	85	0.381	7.6
J.W.	26	F	64.9	77	0.437	8.9
P.D.	26	F	58.8	89	0.393	8.3
I.K.	27	M	72.8	79	0.409	6.9
D.A.	28	F	64.1	69	0.537	8.2
Mean±SD	26±2		66.4±11.6	76±11	0.450±0.072	8.0±0.7
Heterozygotes						
R.M.	22	F	50.9	233	0.307	17.1
B.O.	28	F	55.3	202	0.237	7.9
J.C.	30	F	59.6	199	0.334	17.6
M.M.	31	F	49.0	239	0.237	12.3
M.B.	31	M	63.7	238	0.304	13.4
C.C.	44	F	67.9	266	0.301	14.7
Mean±SD	31±7		57.7±7.4	230±25[‡]	0.287±0.040[+]	13.8±3.6[‡]

[+]Fractional catabolic rate.
*Mean values during the turnover study.
[‡]Significantly different from normal (p < 0.05).
[¶]Adapted from Bilheimer et al. (1979).

LDL turnover in FH homozygotes (Table 2): The FH homozygotes were younger (mean age = 11.7 ± 5.9 yr) and smaller (mean weight = 44.8 ± 28.1 kg) than members of the other two study groups but the shortened lifespan in this form of the disease precludes the study of older patients. All of the patients had cutaneous xanthomas to varying degrees and all but one had clinical evidence of atherosclerotic cardiovascular disease. With regard to receptor status, three were receptor-negative, three were receptor-defective and one exhibited the internalization defect (Table 2). The plasma LDL cholesterol level in this group was markedly increased to 568 ± 180 mg/dl.

The key kinetic parameters for ^{125}I-LDL turnover in this group are listed in Table 2 and the most striking abnormalities were found in the FCR and the apoLDL synthetic rate. The mean FCR was about one-third of normal and the apoLDL synthetic rate was significantly increased when compared to either the heterozygotes or normals. Of note, the homozygotes with different genotypes could not be distinguished clinically or by plasma lipoprotein levels manifested during the metabolic studies. With one exception (D.R.), the values for the FCR were remarkably similar and fell within a narrow range (0.144-0.179/day) (Table 2). The patient, D.R., who exhibited the highest FCR also exhibited the highest number of LDL receptors on her cultured skin fibroblasts (15-20% of normal). Except for the value in D.R., the FCR did not differ significantly among the genotypes and the same was true for the apoLDL synthetic rate (Table 2).

When the relationship between the apoLDL synthetic rate and the plasma apoLDL concentration in the homozygotes was investigated, a high degree of correlation was observed (r = 0.943), indicating that the FCR is not the only major determinant of pool size in these patients. A similar high degree of correlation was found between these two variables in FH heterozygotes (r = 0.86).

Table 2. Kinetic parameters for ^{125}I-LDL turnover studies in FH homozygotes.[¶]

Patient	Receptor Status[+]	Age (yr)	Sex	Plasma LDL Cholesterol[*] (mg/dl)	FCR[‡] day^{-1}	Rate of Synthesis and Catabolism of apoLDL (mg/kg/day)
M.C.	N	7	F	801	0.153	41.6
F.W.	N	13	F	386	0.153	15.6
B.H.	N	21	M	535	0.173	17.8
J.M.	D	5	M	508	0.179	21.4
S.W.	D	6	F	843	0.144	38.6
D.R.	D	15	F	432	0.250	25.9
J.D.	ID	15	M	472	0.178	24.0
Mean ± SD				568 ± 180°	0.176 ± .040°	26.4 ± 10.0°

+ N = receptor-negative; D = receptor-defective; ID = Internalization defect.
* Mean values during the turnover study.
‡ Fractional Catabolic Rate for apoLDL.
° $p < 0.05$.
¶ Adapted from Bilheimer et al. (1979).

Discussion

The investigation of these well-characterized patients with either heterozygous or homozygous FH was undertaken to evaluate the gene-dosage effect on certain parameters of lipoprotein metabolism in vivo. The results can be summarized as follows: homozygotes with FH exhibited a three-fold increase in apoLDL synthesis, whereas the fractional catabolic rate for the apoprotein is only about one-third of normal (tables 1 and 2). Heterozygotes, with one dose of the mutant FH gene, exhibit intermediate values for both parameters:

their synthetic rate for apoLDL is 1.7-fold above normal and their fractional catabolic rate for apoLDL is about two-thirds of normal (tables 1 and 2).

Among the FH homozygotes, these defects appeared equally severe whether the subjects belonged to the receptor-negative class, the receptor-defective class, or the internalization-defective class. Similar results in FH homozygotes have been reported previously (Reichl et al. 1974; Simons et al. 1975; Bilheimer et al. 1975) as has the reduced FCR in FH heterozygotes (Langer et al. 1972; Bilheimer et al. 1975; Packard et al. 1976). Overproduction of apoLDL in FH heterozygotes has not been consistently found (Langer et al. 1972) but a trend toward overproduction was noted in affected members of a family with FH who were studied as outpatients (Packard et al. 1976).

Several lines of evidence indicate that the reduced FCR in this disease results from altered clearance of apoLDL caused by abnormal receptor activity rather than from saturation of normal catabolic pathways. First, the FCR for LDL appears to be fixed in FH homozygotes at $\cong$ 17%/day. Thus, among FH homozygotes whose plasma LDL cholesterol levels varied from 432 to 843 mg/dl, the FCR showed little variation from the mean of 17%/day, whereas the absolute synthetic and degradative rate for apoLDL varied nearly three-fold (15.6-41.6 mg/kg per day), indicating that the variation in plasma LDL levels observed in these patients is caused by the variation in the plasma apoLDL synthetic rates. Second, a similar phenomenon was seen in FH heterozygotes in whom the values for apoLDL synthetic rates varied widely. Third, observations that portacaval shunt surgery (Bilheimer et al. 1975) and plasmapheresis (Thompson et al. 1977) in FH homozygotes lower the plasma apoLDL level without affecting the FCR for apoLDL are also consistent with the interpretation that the diminished FCR is a consequence of the genetic defect in FH.

Considered together, the available data indicate that the primary genetic defect in FH produces two distinct abnormalities of LDL metabolism: an increase in the synthetic rate for apoLDL, and a decrease in the efficiency of apoLDL catabolism. The reduced FCR, which is lower in FH homozygotes then in heterozygotes, correlates directly with the number of functional cellular LDL receptors which are reduced in heterozygotes and nearly or completely absent in homozygotes. The mechanism by which an LDL receptor deficiency causes overproduction of LDL has not been defined. It has been postulated that an LDL receptor may normally exist on liver cells and that one of its functions is to monitor the plasma LDL level and to suppress production of that lipoprotein (Simons et al. 1975; Brown and Goldstein 1976; Bilheimer 1977) or its precursor, very low-density lipoprotein (VLDL). The absence of such an LDL receptor on liver cells of FH homozygotes would cause the liver to sense a deficiency of LDL in plasma and thereby secrete the lipoprotein directly into plasma (Simons et al. 1975; Brown and Goldstein 1976b; Bilheimer 1977). In support of this concept, recent studies have shown that in FH homozygotes, in contrast to normal subjects, a considerable portion of LDL is secreted directly into plasma without passing through VLDL (Soutar et al. 1977).

Acknowledgement: Dr. Michael S. Brown and Dr. Joseph L. Goldstein performed the tissue culture studies on these patients.

REFERENCES

Bilheimer DW, Goldstein JL, Grundy SM, Brown MS (1975) Reduction in cholesterol and low density lipoprotein synthesis after portacaval shunt surgery in a patient with homozygous familial hypercholesterolemia. J Clin Invest 56: 1420-1430

Bilheimer DW (1977) Needed: new therapy for hypercholesterolemia. N Eng J Med 296: 508-509

Bilheimer DW, Ho YK, Brown MS, Anderson RGW, Goldstein JL (1978) Genetics of the low density lipoprotein receptor: diminished receptor activity in lymphocytes from heterozygotes with familial hypercholesterolemia. J Clin Invest 61: 678-696

Bilheimer DW, Stone NJ, Grundy SM (1979) Metabolic studies in familial hypercholesterolemia: evidence for a gene-dosage effect in vivo. J Clin Invest 64:524-533

Brown MS, Goldstein JL (1975) Familial Hypercholesterolemia: genetic biochemical, and pathophysiologic considerations. Adv Intern Med 20: 273-296

Brown MS, Goldstein JL (1976a) Analysis of a mutant strain of human fibroblasts with a defect in the internalization of receptor-bound low density lipoprotein. Cell 9: 663-674

Brown MS, Goldstein JL (1976b) Familial Hypercholesterolemia: a genetic defect in the low density lipoprotein receptor. N Eng J Med 294: 1386-1390

Fredrickson DS, Goldstein JL, Brown MS (1978) The familial hyperlipoproteinemias. In: Stanbury JB, Wyngaarden JB, Fredrickson DS (eds) The metabolic basis of inherited disease. McGraw-Hill, New York

Goldstein JL, Brown MS (1974) Binding and degradation of low density lipoproteins by cultured human fibroblasts: comparison of cells from a normal subject and from a patient with homozygous familial hypercholesterolemia. J Biol Chem 249: 5153-5162

Goldstein JL, Dana SE, Brunschede GY, Brown MS (1975) Genetic heterogeneity in familial hypercholesterolemia: evidence for two different mutations affecting functions of low density lipoprotein receptor. Proc Natl Acad Sci USA 72: 1092-1096

Goldstein JL, Stone NJ, Brown MS (1977) Genetics of the LDL receptor: evidence that the mutations affecting binding and internalization are allelic. Cell 12: 629-641

Goldstein JL, Brown MS (1977) The low density lipoprotein pathway and its relation to atherosclerosis. Annu Rev Biochem 46: 897-930

Langer T, Strober W, Levy RI (1972) The metabolism of low density lipoprotein in familial type II hyperlipoproteinemia. J Clin Invest 51: 1528-1536

Packard CJ, Third JLHC, Shepherd J, Loumer AR, Morgan HG, Lawrie TDV (1976) Low density lipoprotein metabolism in a family of familial hypercholesterolemia patients. Metabolism Clin Exp 25: 995-1006

Reichl D, Simons LA, Myant NB (1974) The metabolism of low-density lipoprotein in a patient with familial hyperbetalipoproteinemia. Clin Sci Mol Med 47: 635-638

Simons LA, Reichl D, Myant NB, Mancini M (1975) The metabolism of the apoprotein of plasma low density lipoprotein in familial hyperbetalipoproteinemia in the homozygous form. Atherosclerosis 21: 283-298

Soutar AK, Myant NB, Thompson GR (1977) Simultaneous measurement of apolipoprotein B turnover in very-low- and low-density lipoproteins in familial hypercholesterolemia. Atherosclerosis 28: 247-256

Thompson GR, Spinks T, Ranicar A, Myant NB (1977) Non-steady-state studies of low-density-lipoprotein turnover in familial hypercholesterolemia. Clin Sci Mol Med 52: 361-369

Metabolism of Very Low Density Lipoprotein-Triglyceride in Man[1]

Scott M. Grundy

Several methods have been used for estimating turnover of triglycerides (TG) in very low density lipoproteins (VLDL) of man. One technique has been to inject labelled precursors of TG and to analyze the resulting specific radioactivity curves of plasma VLDL-TG. Precursors have included labelled fatty acids and glycerol. The use of ^{3}H-glycerol was developed by Farquhar et al. (1965) and has been used extensively for estimating VLDL-TG flux. In most previous studies estimations of VLDL-TG transport have been made by single-exponential analysis. This was based on the observation that shortly after the injection of ^{3}H-glycerol there is an initial build-up in specific activity of VLDL-TG followed by a single-exponential decay for several hours thereafter. The rate of this decay was assumed to represent the fractional catabolic rate (FCR) of VLDL-TG. However, in studies carried out for longer periods it has been noted that the fall in specific activity is not log-linear to zero, but after several hours the rate of decay declines producing a tail on the curve. During the past several years we have examined this latter phenomenon in some detail in conjunction with Drs. Loren Zech and Mones Berman at the National Institutes of Health. During the course of these studies a multi-compartmental model has been developed for analysis of VLDL-TG kinetics (Zech et al. 1979), and this method has been employed to examine these kinetics in a large group of subjects of normal and increased weight with and without hypertriglyceridemia (Grundy et al. 1979). In the following discussion, the major questions examined in these studies will be reviewed.

What are the components of the specific activity curve of VLDL-TG after injection of ^{3}H-glycerol?

In all cases the specific activity curve of VLDL-TG was found to have 4 components: 1) an early-rising phase, 2) a flatness at the top, 3) a rapidly-decaying phase up to 12-18 hrs, and 4) a more slowly-decaying curve producing a "tail" to the curve out to 48 hours. In some patients a fifth component, a "hump" in the decay curve at 12-30 hours was noted.

What model best fits the VLDL-TG specific activity curve?

The model which was developed to account for the various components described above had the following compartments: (1) a glycerol subsystem in the plasma, (2) a delay compartment in the synthetic pathway that was needed to account for delay in the initial upswing of radioactive glycerol, (3) two synthetic pathways: one of these pathways was designated "fast" to account for the rapid phase of the curve, and the other was called "slow" to explain the tail of the curve, (4) a 4-step pathway in degradation of VLDL in the plasma to explain the flatness at the top of the curve, and

----

[1] This research was supported by the Veterans Administration and NIH Grant HL-14197.

(5) a recycling pathway for ^{3}H-glycerol to return to the synthetic compartments after hydrolysis of VLDL-TG in the plasma. Sensitivity testing showed that this latter pathway is insignificant because less than 5% of ^{3}H-glycerol is reused for new VLDL-TG synthesis. The model described above is consistent not only with the known metabolism of VLDL-TG but also with VLDL-apoprotein metabolism as described by Phair et al. (1976).

What factors contribute to the tail of the curve?

Although a slow synthesis pathway was considered the predominant cause of the tail of the curve, other possibilities were examined. For example, it is possible that VLDL could exchange with extra-plasma sources, or the TG in VLDL might exchange with non-VLDL lipoproteins in plasma. The former seems unlikely because several workers have been unable to identify appreciable VLDL in extra vascular compartments. The latter mechanism, that is, back transfer of labelled TG from LDL or HDL seems improbable because of the relatively small sizes of their TG pools; although some back exchange may occur, our calculations indicated that its magnitude would be too small to account for the tail of the curve. A more likely cause of the tail could be a slowly metabolized species of VLDL, such as found in patients with dysbetalipoproteinemia (Type III phenotype). Indeed, it has been demonstrated that the decay curve following injection of VLDL-apo B-^{125}I has a tail that is best explained by a slowly-metabolized VLDL (beta-VLDL). Nevertheless, several considerations make it unlikely that beta-VLDL can account for most of the tail in normal subjects or those with hypertriglyceridemia (other than Type III). These are as follows: (1) Studies of kinetics of VLDL-apo B in patients with normotriglyceridemia and Type IV patterns revealed that the slow component was usually less than 5% of the peak of the curve which presumably indicated a paucity of beta-VLDL in these patients; in contrast, for VLDL-TG studies, the magnitude of the tail (frequently 30-50% of the peak of the curve) was much greater than that seen with apo B turnover. Indeed, considering the slow turnover of TG in beta-VLDL and the large size of the tail, the quantity of beta-VLDL-TG in the plasma would have to represent 50-70% of the total TG mass in VLDL. This obviously cannot be the case because this value even exceeds the quantity of beta-VLDL in patients with the Type III phenotype. Additional evidence for a low quantity of beta-VLDL in non-Type III patients is derived from cholesterol: triglyceride ratios in VLDL. Since beta-VLDL is known to have a high ratio ($\sim$0.83), the low ratios normally found in VLDL (0.15-0.30) excludes the possibility of large amounts of beta-VLDL in this fraction. Using this ratio, we have proposed a method for estimating the amount of beta-VLDL-TG in VLDL and for subtracting this quantity from the tail of the curve.

The above discussion reveals that except for the slow-synthesis pathway, none of the possibilities can account for the high tail found in most VLDL-TG curves. Thus by exclusion we arrived at the conclusion that a slow-synthesis pathway was the predominant cause of the tail. This conclusion was bolstered by a series of dual-isotope studies using ^{3}H-glycerol, ^{14}C-glycerol, and ^{14}C-palmatic acid.

Does single-exponential analysis give an adequate representation of VLDL-TG kinetics?

Because of the magnitude of the tail of the specific activity curves, we considered it unlikely that single exponential analysis using only the phase of rapid decay would provide an accurate estimate of VLDL-TG transport. Indeed, studies in 59 patients showed a poor correlation between transport rates determined by our multicompartmental analysis and single-exponential analysis ($r = 0.46$), and this was not improved by segregating patients according to degree of obesity or hyperlipidemia. Furthermore, there were no consistent trends in the differences between the two methods so that a "correction factor" cannot be added to the results of single-exponential analysis to approximate that obtained by using multicompartmental analysis.

How should VLDL-TG data be expressed?

Since patients vary in height and weight, some method of normalization is required to obtain a meaningful comparison between groups. A common method for comparison is to normalize data for total body weight, that is, to express VLDL-TG transport as mg/hr/kg. When this is done for obese subjects, however, values for transport are misleadingly low; in other words, dividing outputs by a large mass of adipose tissue could obscure real increases in production of VLDL-TG, a process presumably confined to the liver and adipose tissue. For this reason, we suggest that it would be better to normalize results to ideal weight, and we showed that this normalization gives much better correlation with absolute transport rates than does correction for total body weight.

What are normal values for VLDL-TG turnover?

Five groups of patients were studied for VLDL-TG kinetics as shown in Table 1. The patients in these studies had varying levels of body weight and triglyceride concentrations. Group I consisted of 18 patients of normal weight and triglyceride levels. Their mean transport rate was 11 ± 1 mg/hr/kg ideal weight (IW), and their average fractional catabolic rate (FCR) was 0.193 ± 0.02/hr. These values for VLDL-TG transport correspond closely to those obtained by Havel et al. (1970) who carried out direct measurements of VLDL-TG production by hepatic vein catheterization.

What are the causes of hypertriglyceridemia in patients of normal weight?

As shown for normal-weight subjects with hypertriglyceridemia (Group II) (Table 1) mean transport of VLDL-TG was significantly higher than normal (23 ± 2 mg/hr/kg) and the average FCR was only slightly decreased (0.129/hr). This suggests that overproduction of VLDL-TG is the major cause of hypertriglyceridemia in this group. Two of 10 patients had only marginally-elevated production of VLDL-TG and the dominant factor for raising plasma TG in them appeared to be a low catabolic rate. In the remaining 8 patients, overproduction was the major factor.

What are the effects of obesity on VLDL-TG transport?

Group III was composed of 10 markedly obese patients (mean 163 ± 4% ideal weight) who had normotriglyceridemia. On the average these patients had a striking overproduction of VLDL-TG (mean transport = 20 ± 3 mg/hr/kg IW). They were able to maintain a normal plasma TG by increasing their rate of clearance (mean FCR = 0.316/hr). Thus obesity per se would appear to cause an overproduction of VLDL-TG even when plasma TG are not elevated. Although a few patients with marked obesity did not show increased production, others had extremely elevated values.

What are the causes of hypertriglyceridemia in obese subjects?

Groups IV and V included patients with mild and marked obesity, respectively, and in both groups, VLDL-TG concentrations were elevated. Again, production rates were generally elevated which must have contributed to their hypertriglyceridemia. In contrast to Group III, however, the FCR's in these groups were generally lower. The net result was a higher level of TG in Groups IV and V. These data suggest that while obesity usually

Table 1. Values for VLDL-TG Transport in Five Groups of Patients[a]

Group	No.	% IW[b]	Plasma TG	VLDL-TG Conc.	VLDL-TG Transport	VLDL-TG FCR
			mg/dl	mg/dl	mg/hr/kg IW	hr^{-1}
I	18	103± 3	166± 10	134± 9	11±1	0.193±0.02
II	10	109± 2	491± 61	426±57	23±2	0.129±0.01
III	10	163± 4	152± 13	127±15	20±3	0.316±0.06
IV	11	126± 1	348± 51	294±51	18±2	0.140±0.01
V	8	176±15	471±105	387±83	27±6	0.162±0.04

[a]All values are expressed as means ± SEM.

[b]IW = ideal weight.

causes overproduction of VLDL-TG, the resulting plasma concentration is a function of clearance capacity. In those patients who can increase their clearance, hypertriglyceridemia does not result, but in those without this capacity, an elevation in triglycerides is inevitable.

These findings imply that hypertriglyceridemia in normal weight patients usually results from an unexplained overproduction of VLDL-TG. In obese patients, on the other hand, hypertriglyceridemia can be considered to be related primarily to a removal defect; this is to say, a "normal" obese subject can increase clearance of VLDL-TG to compensate for his overproduction.

What factors affect the relative proportions of fast and slow synthetic pathways?

Table 2 shows the fraction of VLDL-TG synthesis in fast and slow pathways. In normal subjects, about 67% occurred in the fast path. The slow path was more dominant in the other 4 groups. In the latter groups total synthesis was elevated. Thus, with increased VLDL-TG production more TG went via the slow path. This difference could reflect the size of the TG pool in synthetic compartments. For instance, an increased synthesis might produce a greater TG pool at synthetic sites. In turn labelled VLDL-TG could enter plasma more slowly from a large pool; consequently, the slow path would be increased.

Table 2. Percent of VLDL-TG synthesis in fast and slow synthesis pathways.

Group	Synthesis Path Fast %	Synthesis Path Slow %
I	67±4[a]	33±4
II	44±4	56±4
III	57±4	43±4
IV	50±7	50±7
V	45±7	55±7

[a]Values = mean ± SEM

References

Farquhar JW, Gross RC, Wagner RM, Reaven GM (1965) Validation of an incompletely coupled two-compartment nonrecycling catenary model for turnover of liver and plasma triglyceride in man. J Lipid Res 6: 119-134

Grundy SM, Mok HYI, Zech L, Steinberg D, Berman M (1979) Transport of very low density lipoprotein triglycerides in varying degrees of obesity and hypertriglyceridemia. J Clin Invest 63: 1274-1283

Havel RJ, Kane JP, Balasse EO, Segel N, Basso LV (1970) Splanchnic metabolism of free fatty acids and production of triglycerides of very low density lipoproteins in normotriglyceridemic and hypertriglyceridemic humans. J Clin Invest 49: 2017-2035

Phair RD, Hall M, Bilheimer DW, Levy RI, Goebel RH, Berman M (1976) Modeling lipoprotein metabolism in man. In: Proceedings of the 1976 Summer Computer Simulation Conference, Washington, D.C. Simulation Councils, Inc., La Jolla, Calif. 486-492

Zech LA, Grundy SM, Steinberg D, Berman M (1979) Kinetic model for production and metabolism of very low density lipoprotein triglycerides. J Clin Invest 63: 1262-1273

Effect of Drugs on High Density Lipoprotein Metabolism[1]

James Shepherd and Christopher J. Packard

Human plasma high density lipoprotein (HDL) consists of a spectrum of particles in the density range 1.063 - 1.210 g/ml which are separable into two major subfractions (HDL_2, d = 1.063 - 1.125 g/ml; HDL_3, d = 1.125 - 1.210 g/ml) by rate zonal ultracentrifugation (Patsch et al., 1974). Although the lipoprotein appears to confer protection against coronary heart disease (Miller and Miller 1975; Rhoads et al. 1976; Gordon et al. 1977), the role played by each subfraction in this regard is not clear. Circumstantial evidence suggests that HDL_2 may be the major antiatherogenic component. For example, Gofman et al. (1966) have shown that in many subjects who develop coronary artery disease, the reduction in HDL mass primarily involves HDL_2. Moreover, premenopausal females (who are generally resistant to atherosclerosis) have a higher HDL_2 level than age-matched males (Gofman et al. 1954; Barclay et al. 1963), while the levels of HDL_3 in both sexes are not significantly different. The increase in HDL_2 associated apolipoprotein A-I and cholesterol in females (Figure 1) produces the higher concentration of these components in the plasma of that sex (Cheung and Albers 1977). These findings suggest that the influence of putative antiatherogenic drugs on the HDL subfraction distribution may constitute an important biochemical indicator of their efficacy. Consequently we have examined the effect of two widely employed hypolipidaemic agents - cholestyramine and nicotinic acid - on HDL subfraction distribution and apolipoprotein A metabolism.

Cholestyramine and HDL Metabolism

Cholestyramine is a sequestering agent which binds bile acids in the intestinal lumen and increases their faecal excretion (Hashim and Van Itallie 1965). It effectively lowers circulating LDL cholesterol levels but its effect on HDL has

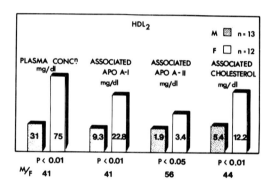

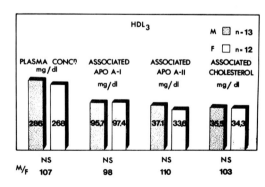

FIG. 1. HDL subfraction concentrations in men and women.

[1]This work was supported by a grant (K/MRS/50/C113) from the Scottish Home and Health Department. Bristol Laboratories, a division of Bristol-Meyers Co. (GB) supplied cholestyramine (Questran) resin and NAPP Laboratories Ltd. provided controlled-release nicotinic acid.

591

not been studied in detail. We have examined the influence of the drug (16 g/day) on the metabolism and subfraction distribution of HDL in four type II hyperlipoproteinaemic subjects (Shepherd et al. 1979a). The results (Table 1) show that although the drug lowered plasma (ie LDL) cholesterol, it did not alter significantly the level of that lipid in HDL. However, it did increase substantially (by 84%) the concentration of HDL_2 without affecting that of HDL_3. These changes were accompanied by a 12% rise in plasma apolipoprotein A-I due to an increase in its synthesis. The level of apolipoprotein A-II was unaffected by treatment, possibly reflecting the association of this protein primarily with HDL_3 (Cheung and Albers 1977; Shepherd et al. 1979b).

These results are remarkable in light of the fact that cholestyramine is not absorbed systemically and hence its action on HDL must be mediated by changes in cholesterol metabolism secondary to intestinal bile salt sequestration. Glomset and Norum (1973) have suggested that HDL may act as a transport vehicle for cholesterol from the periphery to the liver. Mobilisation of this lipid from peripheral tissues appears in part to be mediated by lecithin:cholesterol acyltransferase (LCAT). The changes in HDL metabolism which we observed during cholestyramine therapy may derive from stimulation of this transport mechanism. Apolipoprotein A-I activates LCAT (Fielding et al. 1972). The cholestyramine induced increase in plasma apolipoprotein A-I may promote the activity of this enzyme and stimulate the conversion of "nascent" HDL to HDL_2 (Menzel et al. 1978). This provides a tentative explanation (Figure 2) for the observed increase in plasma HDL_2 during treatment.

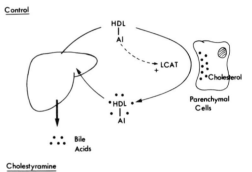

Nicotinic Acid and HDL Metabolism

Nicotinic acid in pharmacologic doses reduces plasma cholesterol and is effective in the treatment of hyperlipidaemia. Its mechanism of action is complex, reflected in the variable response of the plasma lipoprotein classes in the different hyperlipoproteinaemic phenotypes (Carlson et al. 1977). One major effect of the drug is to inhibit free fatty acid release from adipose tissue, causing a reduction in its flux to the liver and lowering VLDL synthesis (Kissebah et al. 1974). The response of LDL is variable (Carlson et al. 1977) while HDL cholesterol and the HDL_2/HDL_3 ratio are significantly raised by treatment (Blum et al. 1977). We have

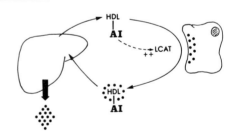

FIG. 2. Postulated effect of cholestyramine on HDL metabolism.

examined the effects of nicotinic acid therapy on the composition and metabolism of HDL in normal (Shepherd et al. 1979b), type II (a and b) and type IV hyperlipoproteinaemic subjects. The treatment effectively reduced plasma cholesterol and triglyceride and raised HDL cholesterol in all but the type IIb patients (Table 2).

All subjects in our series showed an increase in total HDL concentration during nicotinic acid therapy, but the effect of the drug on the HDL subfraction distribution varied according to the initial plasma triglyceride level. In normotriglyceridaemic subjects, including the type IIa patients, treatment produced a large increase in HDL_2 with a fall in HDL_3. On the other hand,

Table 1. Effects of cholestyramine on plasma HDL metabolism in four type IIa hyperlipoproteinaemic subjects.

Plasma Cholesterol (mg/dl)		Plasma Triglyceride (mg/dl)		HDL Cholesterol (mg/dl)		§HDL$_2$ (mg/dl)		Plasma concentration of §HDL$_3$ (mg/dl)		ApoA-I (mg/dl)		ApoA-II (mg/dl)	
*C	T	C	T	C	T	C	T	C	T	C	T	C	T
395	267+	136	140	54	50	31	57+	317	332	136	152+	32	33

Table 2. Effects of nicotinic acid on plasma HDL metabolism.

Phenotype	Plasma Cholesterol (mg/dl)		Plasma Triglyceride (mg/dl)		HDL Cholesterol (mg/dl)		§HDL$_2$ (mg/dl)		Plasma concentration of §HDL$_3$ (mg/dl)		ApoA-I (mg/dl)		ApoA-II (mg/dl)	
	*C	T	C	T	C	T	C	T	C	T	C	T	C	T
Normal (n = 5)	163	139+	79	58¶	52	64+	50#	323#	392#	209¶	135	145+	29	25+
Type IIa (n = 3)	414	326	132	89	37	52	31	141	227	170	120	.123	41	33
Type IIb (n = 3)	480	482	334	294	36	36	27	26	256	308	105	110	36	37
Type IV (n = 4)	262	194¶	614	233+	31	42+	13	39+	190	240+	108	125¶	32	31

§ determined from zonal elution profiles using specific extinction coefficients for HDL2 and HDL3 of 0.6 and 0.86 mg protein/A280nm and compositional data.

* C, control; T, drug treatment

HDL subfraction concentrations obtained by calculation (Shepherd et al., 1979b)

¶ C vs T, p <0.05   + C vs T, p <0.01

the increment in total HDL seen in nicotinic acid treated hypertriglyceridaemic subjects (including the type IIb group) resulted primarily from a rise
in HDL_3. These changes in the HDL_2/HDL_3 ratio were parallelled by similar
alterations in the plasma apoA-I/apoA-II ratio. The different responses of
the normo- and hypertriglyceridaemic subjects may derive from a differential
effect of the drug on triglyceride (VLDL) metabolism in the two groups, in
keeping with the observations that, both in vitro (Patsch et al. 1978) and
in vivo (Eisenberg et al. 1973) HDL subfraction redistribution is linked to
VLDL lipolysis.

If we accept that HDL_2 is protective against atherosclerosis, then both of
these drugs should, by raising the level of this subfraction in the plasma,
be beneficial to the recipients.

Acknowledgments:

We acknowledge the expert technical assistance of Mrs J. M. Stewart and the
secretarial help of Ms Sheena M. Brownlie.

REFERENCES

Barclay M, Barclay RK, Skipski FP (1963) High density lipoprotein concentrations in men and women. Nature 200: 362

Blum CB, Levy RI, Eisenberg S, Hall M, Goebel RH, Berman M (1977) High density
lipoprotein metabolism in man. J Clin Invest 60: 795

Carlson LA, Olson AG, Ballantyne D (1977) On the rise in low density and high
density lipoproteins in response to the treatment of hypertriglyceridaemia
in type IV and type V hyperlipoproteinaemias. Atherosclerosis 26: 603

Carlson LA, Oro L, Ostman J (1968) Effects of nicotinic acid on plasma lipids
in patients with hyperlipoproteinaemia during the first week of treatment.
J Atheroscler Res 8: 667

Cheung MC, Albers JJ (1977) The measurement of apolipoprotein A-I and A-II
levels in men and women by immunoassay. J Clin Invest 60: 43

Eisenberg S, Bilheimer DW, Levy RI, Lindgren FT (1973) On the metabolic conversion of human plasma very low density lipoprotein to low density lipoprotein. Biochim Biophys Acta 326: 361

Fielding CJ, Shore VC, Fielding PE (1972) A protein cofactor of lecithin:
cholesterol acyltransferase. Biochem Biophys Res Commun 46: 1493

Glomset JA, Norum KR (1973) The metabolic role of lecithin:cholesterol acyltransferase - perspectives from pathology. Adv Lipid Res 11: 1

Gofman JW, De Lalla O, Glazier F, Freeman NK, Lindgren FT, Nichols AV,
Strisower B, Tamplin AR (1954) The serum lipoprotein transport system in
health, metabolic disorders, atherosclerosis and coronary artery disease.
Plasma 2: 413

Gofman JW, Young W, Tandy R (1966) Ischaemic disease, atherosclerosis and
longevity. Circulation 34:679

Gordon T, Castelli WP, Hjortland MC, Kannel WB, Dawber TR (1977) High density lipoprotein as a protective factor against coronary heart disease. Am J Med 62: 707

Hashim SA, Van Itallie TB (1965) Cholestyramine resin therapy for hypercholesterolemia. JAMA 192:289

Kissebah AH, Adams PW, Harrigan P, Wynn V (1974) The mechanism of action of clofibrate and tetranicotinylfructose on the kinetics of plasma free fatty acid and triglyceride transport in type IV and type V hypertriglyceridaemia. Europ J Clin Invest 4: 163

Menzel HJ, Deiker P, Utermann G (1978) In vitro substitution of LCAT[+] - deficiency serum. In: Protides of Biological Fluids, Vol 25, Pergamon Press New York pp 217

Miller GJ, Miller NE (1975) Plasma high density lipoprotein concentration and development of ischaemic heart disease. Lancet i: 16

Patsch JR, Gotto AM, Olivecrona T, Eisenberg S (1978) Formation of high density lipoprotein$_2$ - like particles during lipolysis of very low density lipoproteins in vitro. Proc Natl Acad Sci US 75: 4519

Patsch JR, Sailer S, Kostner G, Sandhofer F, Holasek A, Braunsteiner H (1974) Separation of the main lipoprotein classes of human plasma by rate zonal ultracentrifugation. J Lipid Res 15: 356

Rhoads GG, Gulbrandsen CL, Kagan A (1976) Serum lipoproteins and coronary heart disease in a population study of Hawaii Japanese men. New Engl J Med 294: 293

Shepherd J, Packard CJ, Morgan HG, Third JLHC, Stewart JM, Lawrie TDV (1979a) The effects of cholestyramine on high density lipoprotein metabolism. Atherosclerosis, in press.

Shepherd J, Packard CJ, Patsch JR, Gotto AM, Taunton OD (1979b) Effects of nicotinic acid therapy on plasma high density lipoprotein subfraction distribution and composition and on apolipoprotein A metabolism. J Clin Invest 63: 858

Liver and Cholesteryl Ester Transfer Amongst Lipoprotein—One Suggested Model

Allan Sniderman and Babie Teng[1]

Recently, cholesteryl ester uptake from apparently intact LDL has been demonstrated across the splanchnic bed of man (Sniderman et al. 1978a); as well, protein-mediated exchange and transfer of cholesteryl esters amongst plasma lipoproteins has been repeatedly observed using in vitro models (Zilversmit et al. 1975; Chajek and Fielding 1978; Sniderman et al. 1978b; Barter and Lally 1978). To provide a possible physiologic rationale for these observations, this paper suggests the following hypothesis: in man, plasma LDL and/or HDL, while in an extravascular hepatic pool, transfer cholesteryl esters to nascent VLDL and HDL; the movement of cholesteryl esters amongst lipoproteins is protein mediated and may account for the cholesteryl ester composition of plasma VLDL. If so, it proceeds at a rate related principally to VLDL production.

Cholesteryl esters could be produced either by ACAT in liver and intestine or in plasma by the LCAT system. In the rat, the former appears to account for VLDL cholesteryl ester, whereas in man, the latter mechanism is more likely (Havel et al. 1979). To be sure, ACAT does appear to be present in small amounts in human liver (Balasubramanian et al. 1979), but the fatty acid composition of human VLDL cholesterol esters is consistent with derivation from LCAT, not ACAT (Glomset and Norum 1973). (The converse is of course, true for the rat (Gidez et al. 1965).) It is also clear that sufficient cholesteryl esters could be synthesized by human LCAT - about 1800 mg/day (Barter 1974) - to account for cholesteryl esters irreversibly lost from plasma in LDL (1100 mg/day) and HDL (165 mg/day) (Havel et al. 1979).

If LCAT is the source of lipoprotein cholesteryl ester and HDL, its prime substrate, then transfer of this lipid moiety must occur to VLDL and LDL. A non-enzymatic transfer of cholesteryl ester in return for triglyceride was first suggested by the results of Nichols and Smith (1965). That cholesteryl ester exchange was dependent on a specific plasma protein was first demonstrated by Zilversmit et al. (1975). This group, using an in vitro system, has demonstrated only exchange, not net transfer between HDL, VLDL, and LDL. In contrast, Chajek and Fielding (1978), Marcil et al. (1979), and Barter and Lally (1978), while confirming that cholesteryl exchange occurs between HDL and LDL, have demonstrated net transfer between plasma HDL and VLDL. Chajek and Fielding (1978) also observed net transfer of cholesteryl ester between HDL and LDL. However, for the present considerations, the major point is that rapid transfer (or exchange) of cholesteryl esters has been repeatedly demonstrated between human plasma lipoproteins.

At this point, one other concept should be introduced. Kinetic analysis of LDL B protein turnover in swine and man is consistent with a biexponential model (Langer et al. 1972; Sniderman et al. 1975); such a model points to the existence of an extravascular pool of LDL in rapid equilibrium with the plasma pool. In the swine, this model has been verified by screening and tissue

---

[1] This work was supported by grants from the Medical Research Council of Canada (MA 5480).

distribution experiments and the liver was shown to be the major site of this extravascular pool. That is, these studies indicated that from plasma, each LDL molecule enters an extravascular space in the liver and then reenters plasma. Although equilibration is rapid, each LDL particle does spend a substantial period of time in this hepatic extravascular pool. A similar pool may exist for HDL, but has not been directly shown.

There is unfortunately, no direct evidence of an important element in our hypothesis which is that nascent human VLDL and HDL contain little cholesteryl ester. Nevertheless, we think this deduction likely based on the evidence previously noted that lipoprotein cholesteryl esters are produced principally by the action of LCAT.

Two potential sites are available for cholesteryl ester transfer to nascent lipoproteins; these are plasma and the extravascular hepatic space. Nascent lipoproteins would, upon secretion, encounter a large extracellular extravascular hepatic pool of LDL, and possibly HDL. The fenestrated hepatic capillary endothelium should allow transfer protein to also enter this extravascular space. Thus, cholesteryl ester rich lipoproteins - plasma LDL and HDL - would be in close approximation to cholesteryl ester poor lipoproteins - nascent VLDL and HDL - in the presence of transfer protein. Two predictions result from this scheme: first, there would be depletion of cholesterol ester from either LDL or HDL; and second, the extent of this depletion would be related to simultaneous VLDL and HDL production.

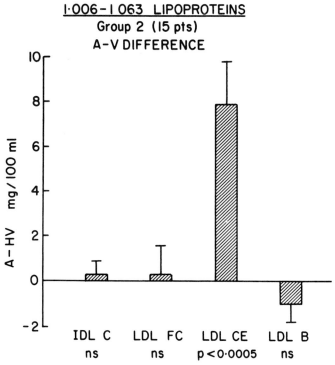

FIG. 1. The AV difference for cholesterol (C) in IDL and LDL is shown for 15 patients studied. Only for LDL cholesteryl ester (CE) is the difference significant. A-HV aortic-hepatic vein, FC, free cholesterol. Reprinted with permission of Journal of Clinical Investigation.

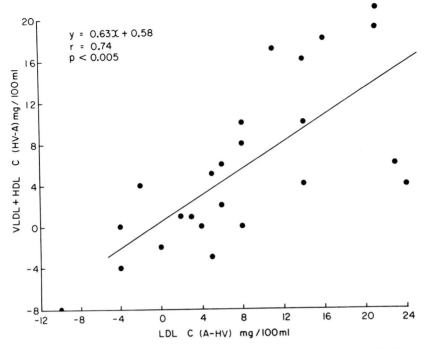

FIG. 2. The LDL cholesterol (C) AV difference for each of 24 patients is plotted on the abscissa, the corresponding net VA (i.e. hepatic vein - aorta) difference for VLDL and HDL cholesterol is on the ordinate. The significant linear relation between these is shown. A-HV, aorta- hepatic vein. Reprinted with permission of Journal of Clinical Investigation.

When lipoprotein composition was examined across the human splanchnic bed, results were obtained that confirm - or at least are consistent with - both predictions (Sniderman et al. 1978a). Plasma was obtained simultaneously from both an arterial site (femoral artery or aorta) and hepatic vein in patients undergoing cardiac catherization. Lipoproteins were separated by preparative ultracentrifugation and arteriovenous gradients calculated for VLDL, LDL and HDL. The principal findings are summarized in Figures 1 and 2. No significant difference across the splanchnic bed was found for total cholesterol, LDL free cholesterol or LDL B protein. There was, however, a significant decrease in the LDL cholesteryl ester concentration between artery and hepatic vein. The findings demonstrated in Figure 2 are of particular interest. In 24 patients, the apparent cholesterol uptake from LDL is plotted against the output of cholesterol from the splanchnic bed in VLDL and HDL. A significant linear relationship results, confirming the predictions made.

VLDL contains (by dry weight) 55% triglyceride and 12% cholesterol esters. Although VLDL triglyceride turnover is usually 15 gm/day, it can rise under certain conditions to as much as 100 gm/day (Wolfe and Ahuja 1977). Using the minimum estimate per day, about 3,600 mg cholesterol esters would be cycled through VLDL. This amount is too large for an LCAT source and thus, it seems likely that cholesterol ester must recycle through VLDL entering newly synthesized VLDL. The arguments made earlier suggest the cholesterol ester source may be LDL, the site of transfer may be the hepatic extravascular space and the mechanism of transfer is likely protein mediated. At present, this scheme is at best only consistent with experimental observations and its validity must still be established by more direct observations.

Acknowledgement

The authors wish to acknowledge the suggestions of Dr. Richard Havel, which were valuable in formulating this hypothesis.

References

Balasubramaniam KA, Metropoulous KA, Myant NB, Mancini M, Postiglione A (1979) Acyl-coenzyme A-cholesterol acyltransferase activity in human liver. Clin Science 56: 373-375

Barter PJ (1974) Production of plasma esterified cholesterol in lean normo-triglyceridemic humans. J Lipid Res 15: 234-242

Barter PJ, Lally JI (1973) The activity of an esterified cholesterol trans-ferring factor in human and rat serum. Biochem Acta 531: 233-236

Chajek T, Fielding CJ (1978) Isolation and characterization of a human serum cholesteryl transfer protein. Proc Natl Acad Sci USA 75: 3445-3449

Gidez LI, Roheim PS, Eder HA (1965) Effect of diet on the cholesterol ester composition of liver and plasma lipoproteins in the rat. J Lipid Res 6: 377-382

Glomset JA, Norum KR (1973) The metabolic role of lecithin-cholesterol acyl transferase: perspectives from pathology. Adv Lip Res 11:1-65

Havel RJ, Goldstein JL, Brown MS (1979) Lipoproteins and lipid transport. In: Bondy PK, Rosenberg LE (eds) Metabolic Control and Disease. 8th Edition W.B. Saunders, Philadelphia, in press

Marcil YL, Vezina C, Teng B, Sniderman AD (1979) Transfer of cholesterol esters between human high density lipoproteins and triglyceride-rich lipoproteins controlled by a plasma protein factor. Atherosclerosis, in press

Nichols AV, Smith L (1965) Effect of very low-density lipoproteins on lipid transfer in incubated serum. J Lipid Res 6: 206-210

Sniderman AD, Carew TW, Steinberg D (1975) Turnover and tissue distribution of ^{125}I labelled low density lipoprotein in swine and dogs. J Lipid Res 16: 293-299

Sniderman AD, Thomas D, Marpole DG, Teng B (1978a) Low density lipoprotein - A metabolic pathway for return of cholesterol to the splanchnic bed. J Clin Invest 61: 867-873.

Sniderman AD, Teng B, Vezina C, Marcel YL (1978b) Cholesterol ester exchange between human plasma high and low density lipoproteins mediated by a plasma protein factor. Atherosclerosis 31: 327-333.

Wolfe BM, Ahuja SD (1977) Effects of intravenously administered fructose and glucose on splanchnic secretion. Metab Clin Exp 26: 963-978

Zilversmit DB, Hughes LB, Bulmer J (1975) Stimulation of cholesterol ester exchange by lipoprotein-free rabbit plasma. Biochim Biophys Acta 409: 393-398

Role of Chylomicrons in Atherogenesis[1]

Donald B. Zilversmit[2]

Among the biochemical factors in plasma that are most often cited as signals
for atherogenesis and future clinical manifestations of atherosclerosis are
high levels of fasting serum cholesterol and low density lipoproteins, and
low levels of high density lipoproteins (Fredrickson et al. 1978; Miller and
Miller 1975). Even those investigators who rank serum triglyceride concentrations as independent risk factors usually think in terms of fasting serum
triglyceride levels (Carlson and Böttiger 1972; Dolder and Oliver 1975;
Carlson et al. 1975). Elsewhere I have proposed that postprandial lipemia
in people on relatively high cholesterol diets is an important contributor
to atherogenesis (Zilversmit 1973, 1976, 1979). This view is based largely
on recently developed insights into the metabolic fate of chylomicrons.

Transport of Chylomicrons

Dietary fat, absorbed from the intestinal lumen, is packaged into finely
divided droplets (chylomicrons) which are composed of a liquid core of triglyceride and cholesterol ester and a "skin", or monolayer, of phospholipid,
unesterified cholesterol and several apolipoproteins. Upon entry into the
bloodstream by way of the thoracic duct, these chylomicrons are rapidly adsorbed to endothelial cells of blood capillaries. Lipoprotein lipase, probably located on the surface of endothelial cells hydrolyzes most of the triglyceride. While the triglyceride breakdown products diffuse through the
capillary walls and are taken up by muscle cells or adipocytes, most of the
nondigestible residues, the chylomicron remnants, are returned to the circulating blood. At this point the fate of the remnant depends on the circumstances. In a rat the circulating remnant is rapidly removed by the liver
(Redgrave 1970). In a rabbit the remnant also disappears rapidly from the
bloodstream if little or no cholesterol is present in the diet. However,
even after a single meal of cholesterol, remnant removal from the circulation is greatly impaired (Ross and Zilversmit 1977). It is not yet known
whether or not the increased cholesterol ester content of the remnant is
responsible for the slowed removal process or whether dietary cholesterol
alters the remnant composition in other ways or somehow reduces the capacity
of liver cells to ingest chylomicron remnants.

Hypercholesterolemia Due to Remnants

Cholesterol-fed rabbits develop massive hypercholesterolemia followed by
cholesterol-containing lipid plaques in their arteries. We have recently
shown, by the use of labeled retinol, that by far the largest fraction of
the serum cholesterol in very low density and intermediate density lipo-

---

[1]Supported by HL 10933 from the National Heart, Lung and Blood Institute,
National Institutes of Health, United States Public Health Service.
[2]Career Investigator of the American Heart Association.

proteins represent chylomicron remnants (Ross and Zilversmit 1977). These remnants can be recognized by their high content of cholesteryl ester and of apolipoprotein E (or arginine-rich apolipoprotein), by a retarded mobility during agarose electrophoresis compared to the normal very low density lipoproteins, as well as by their ability to transport vitamin A esters. It seems likely that one can extrapolate these findings to other animal species because lipoproteins with similar properties also accumulate in the plasma of cholesterol-fed dogs, rats, pigs, and various types of monkeys (Mahley et al. 1974, 1976; Mahley and Holcombe 1977; Mahley et al. 1975; Hill and Silbernick 1975, Fless et al. 1976).

The situation in humans is less clear. Patients with Type III hyperlipoproteinemia show evidence of premature peripheral vascular and coronary heart disease and have, even in the fasting state, high levels of intermediate density lipoproteins with the properties of chylomicron remnants (Hazzard and Bierman 1976). There are essentially no data, however, on the prevalence of transient accumulations of remnants in the hours following high-fat, high-cholesterol meals. It seems likely that among so-called "normal" individuals a wide spectrum of remnant clearance rates may prevail. Given the observation that chylomicron remnants are avidly internalized by human arterial smooth muscle cells in vitro (Albers and Bierman 1976), it is reasonable to assume that high levels of cholesterol-enriched circulating remnants contribute to atherogenesis.

Arterial Lipoprotein Lipase and Atherogenesis

Even in people who do not show transient elevations of remnant levels, there is an additional mechanism whereby cholesterol-containing chylomicrons could be atherogenic. In analogy with the degradation of chylomicrons on the capillary surfaces by lipoprotein lipase, I have proposed that these lipid droplets can be converted to remnants upon contact with the intimal surface of large arteries, which have been shown to contain lipoprotein lipase (Zilversmit 1973, 1979). Aortas of cholesterol-fed rabbits appear to contain amounts of lipoprotein lipase in proportion to the degree of atheromatosis (Corey and Zilversmit 1977). The enzymatic pathway required for the conversion of chylomicrons to remnants is present in both the intima and media of large arteries (DiCorleto and Zilversmit 1975) and it seems likely that some chylomicrons, upon entry into the circulation, may be directly adsorbed to the normal or injured aortic surface, degraded by lipoprotein lipase, and then be transported by filtration or endocytosis to become a source for arterial lipid deposits. The argument that patients with chylomicronemia rarely show signs of premature atherosclerosis has been advanced to discard the notion that chylomicrons are atherogenic. However, such patients appear to be deficient in lipoprotein lipase activity and may therefore not be subjected to excessive formation of circulating or arterial chylomicron remnants (Hazzard et al. 1970).

Relative Atherogenicity of Chylomicron Remnants and Low Density Lipoproteins

In support of the foregoing arguments it is of interest that cholesterol-fed rabbits, with elevated plasma chylomicron remnant concentrations, develop atheromatosis to the same extent and severity as hypercholesterolemic animals fed a cholesterol-free, low-fat, casein-sucrose diet (Ross et al. 1978); the latter develop primarily high concentrations of low density lipoproteins. Apparently, at equal plasma cholesterol concentrations, hypercholesterolemia primarily due to chylomicron remnants is as atherogenic as that due to endogenously synthesized cholesterol in the form of very low density and low density lipoproteins.

601

Conclusions

Dietary fat and cholesterol are transported initially as chylomicrons which are then degraded to chylomicron remnants by lipoprotein lipase. Retinyl ester in d<1.019 lipoproteins appears to be a marker for chylomicron and remnant transport. Experiments in rabbits show that the rate at which serum cholesterol is taken up by the aorta parallels both the concentration of circulating (chylomicron remnant) cholesterol, and the amount of arterial lipoprotein lipase. Dietary cholesterol, which is present in plasma primarily as chylomicron remnants, and endogenously synthesized cholesterol, which is present in very low and low-density lipoproteins, appear to be equally atherogenic.

References

Albers JJ, Bierman EL (1976) The influence of lipoprotein composition on binding, uptake and degradation of different lipoprotein fractions by cultured human arterial smooth muscle cells. Artery 2: 337–348

Carlson LA, Böttiger LE (1972) Ischaemic heart-disease in relation to fasting values of plasma triglycerides and cholesterol. Lancet 1: 865–868

Carlson LA, Ekelund LG, Olsson AG (1975) Frequency of ischaemic exercise E.C.G. changes in symptom-free mew with various forms of primary hyperlipaemia. Lancet 2: 1–8

Corey JE, Zilversmit DB (1977) Effect of cholesterol feeding on arterial lipolytic activity in the rabbit. Atherosclerosis 27: 201–212

DiCorleto PE, Zilversmit DB (1975) Lipoprotein lipase activity in bovine aorta. Proc Soc Exp Biol Med 148: 1101–1105

Dolder MA, Oliver MF (1975) Myocardial infarction in young men. Study of risk factors in nine countries. Br Heart J 37: 493–503

Fless GM, Wissler RW, Scanu AM (1976) Study of abnormal plasma low-density lipoprotein in Rhesus Monkeys with diet-induced hyperlipidemia. Biochemistry 15: 5799–5805

Fredrickson DS, Goldstein JL, Brown MS (1978) The familial hyperlipoproteinemias. In: Stanbury JB, Wyngaarden JB, Fredrickson DS (eds) The metabolic basis of inherited disease, 4th edition. McGraw Hill, New York

Hazzard WR, Bierman EL (1976) Delayed clearance of chylomicron remnants following vitamin-A-containing oral fat loads in broad-β disease (Type III hyperlipoproteinemia). Metabolism 25: 777–801

Hazzard WR, Porte D Jr, Bierman EL (1970) Abnormal lipid composition of chylomicrons in broad-β disease (Type III hyperlipoproteinemia). J Clin Invest 49: 1853–1858

Hill EG, Silbernick CL (1975) Development of hyperbetalipoproteinemia in pigs fed atherogenic diet. Lipids 10: 41–43

Mahley RW, Holcombe KS (1977) Alterations of the plasma lipoproteins and apoproteins following cholesterol feeding in the rat. J Lipid Res 18: 314–324

Mahley RW, Weisgraber KH, Innerarity T (1974) Canine lipoproteins and atherosclerosis II. Characterization of the plasma lipoproteins associated with atherogenic and nonatherogenic hyperlipidemia. Circ Res 35: 722–733

Mahley RW, Weisgraber KH, Innerarity T (1976) Atherogenic hyperlipoproteinemia induced by cholesterol feeding in the Patas Monkey. Biochemistry 15: 2979–2985

Mahley RW, Weisgraber KH, Innerarity T, Brewer HB Jr, Assmann G (1975) Swine lipoproteins and atherosclerosis. Changes in the plasma lipoproteins and apoproteins induced by cholesterol feeding. Biochemistry 14: 2817–2823

Miller GJ, Miller NE (1975) Plasma-high-density-lipoprotein concentration and development of ischaemic heart-disease. Lancet 1: 16–19

Redgrave TG (1970) Formation of cholesteryl ester-rich particulate lipid during metabolism of chylomicrons. J Clin Invest 49: 465–471

Ross AC, Zilversmit DB (1977) Chylomicron remnant cholesteryl esters as the major constituent of very low density lipoproteins in plasma of cholesterol-fed rabbits. J Lipid Res 18: 169–181

Ross AC, Minick CR, Zilversmit DB (1978) Equal atherosclerosis in rabbits fed cholesterol-free, low-fat diet or cholesterol-supplemented diet. Atherosclerosis 29: 301–315

Zilversmit DB (1973) A proposal linking atherogenesis to the interaction of endothelial lipoprotein lipase with triglyceride-rich lipoproteins. Circ Res 33: 633–638

Zilversmit DB (1976) Role of triglyceride-rich lipoproteins in atherogenesis. Ann NY Acad Sci 275: 138–144

Zilversmit DB (1979) Atherogenesis: A postprandial phenomenon. Circulation: 60:473–485

Contributions of Invited Speakers

Plenary Session: Plasma Lipids, Lipoproteins and Atherosclerosis

Co-Chairpersons: Angelo M. Scanu and Daniel Steinberg
Speakers: Antonio M. Gotto, Jr.
   Heiner Greten
   Robert W. Mahley
   Yechezkiel Stein

Workshop: Mutants Affecting Lipoproteins and Apoproteins

Co-Chairpersons: Gerd Assmann and J. Alick Little
Speakers: W.C. Breckenridge
   H. Bryan Brewer
   Peter N. Herbert
   Gerd Utermann

Workshop: Hypertension

Chairperson: John M. Laragh
Speakers: Aram V. Chobanian
   Yuichiro Goto
   Richard Lovell
   Philippe Meyer

Workshop: Regression

Co-Chairpersons: David H. Blankenhorn and Jack P. Strong
Speakers: Mark L. Armstrong
   Henry Buchwald
   Thomas B. Clarkson
   Assaad S. Daoud
   Herbert C. Stary
   Robert W. Wissler

Workshop: The Inter-relationship Between Lipid and Prostaglandin Metabolism

Speakers: Ryszard J. Gryglewski
   Kafait U. Malik
   Rodolfo Paoletti
   Bengt Samuelsson

Workshop: Cellular Metabolism of Lipoproteins

Chairperson: Edwin L. Bierman
Speakers: Alan M. Fogelman
    George Rothblat
    Olga Stein
    Daniel Steinberg

Workshop: Apoprotein Quantification

Co-Chairpersons: Petar Alaupovic and Dietrich Seidel
Speakers: M.C. Cheung
    Pietro Avogaro
    Noel Fidge
    Gustav Schonfeld

Relationship Between the Properties of the Apo B Containing Low-Density Lipoproteins (LDL) of Normolipidemic Rhesus Monkeys and their Mitogenic Action on Arterial Smooth Muscle Cells Grown In Vitro[1]

Gunther M. Fless, Tomas Kirchhausen, Katti Fischer-Dzoga, Robert W. Wissler, and Angelo M. Scanu

Introduction

The heterogeneity of the low-density lipoproteins (LDL) of rhesus monkeys (M. mulatta) has recently been the subject of intensive investigation (Hill et al. 1975; Nelson and Morris 1976; Rudel et al. 1977; Fless and Scanu 1979). In our laboratory, we have concentrated on the physico-chemical characterization of the multiple species of LDL from normolipemic monkeys with the goal in mind of discovering the structural and functional basis for the diversity of these particles (Fless and Scanu 1979). The need of having pure homogeneous lipoprotein fractions prompted us to devise suitable methodology for the isolation of the various LDL species, namely, a combination of isopycnic and rate zonal density gradient ultracentrifugations in swinging bucket rotors. The purpose of this report is to describe the physico-chemical properties of four LDL species isolated from normolipidemic rhesus monkeys and their effect on arterial smooth muscle cells grown in vitro.

Physico-Chemical Properties of LDL Subspecies

LDL-I, LDL-II, and LDL-III. Heterogeneity of rhesus LDL was demonstrated by centrifuging either plasma or the total lipoproteins isolated at d 1.21 g/ml on a 0 to 10% NaCl or NaBr gradient (Fig. 1a and b). The representative LDL profiles from two different monkeys illustrate the heterogeneity within each animal and also the differences among animals. We have designated the fractions floating at d 1.027, 1.036, and 1.050 g/ml, LDL-I, LDL-II, and LDL-III, respectively. LDL-I and LDL-II were found in 28 out of 30 male monkeys tested (Fig. 1a and b) and LDL-III was present in 15 of them (Fig. 1a). LDL-I and LDL-II could not be completely resolved by density gradient ultracentrifugation because of their overlapping buoyant densities, but LDL-III was easily separated from the less dense LDLs although small amounts of HDL were present.

At first we removed the HDL by gel filtration on either Sepharose 4B or 6B; however, because of poor recoveries of LDL-III, we subsequently utilized rate zonal density gradient ultracentrifugation. This technique is usually used to separate proteins on the basis of their sedimentation rates in density gradients but applies equally well to flotation studies. Since LDL-III is an order of magnitude larger than HDL, it also has a proportionally higher flotation rate in high salt solutions and can be separated from HDL

[1]This work was supported in part by HL-15062 and HL-18577 from the U.S. Public Health Service and A-77-19 from the Chicago Heart Association. T.K. was supported by NIH National Research Service Award T-32 HL-7237 from the National Heart, Lung and Blood Institute.

607

after centrifugation for 3 to 4 hours at 35,000 rpm or 16 hours at 20,000 rpm in the SW-40 rotor on a 7.5% to 30% NaBr gradient (Fig. 2).

Equilibrium ultracentrifugation in the analytical centrifuge revealed that LDL-III, with a mean buoyant density of 1.050 g/ml, had an unexpectedly large molecular weight of 3.47×10^6 when compared to 3.32×10^6 for LDL-I and 2.75×10^6 for LDL-II which had densities of 1.027 and 1.036 g/ml, respectively (Table 1). Thus, LDL-III did not obey the usual negative size-density correlation described for human LDLs. Frictional ratios calculated from the corresponding diffusion coefficients and molecular weights showed that LDL-III had significantly higher values than those of LDL-I and LDL-II. This is attributable in all likelihood to a greater degree of hydration of LDL-III over LDL-I or LDL-II since electron microscopy suggested that the particles were spherical and not asymmetric.

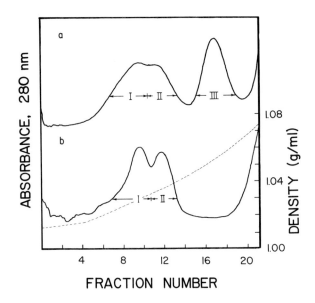

FIG. 1a and b. Density gradient ultracentrifugation of rhesus low-density lipoproteins. Fractions I, II, and III have mean buoyant densities of 1.027, 1.036, and 1.050 g/ml and are called LDL-I, LDL-II, and LDL-III, respectively. The arrows define the fractions that were pooled for analysis.

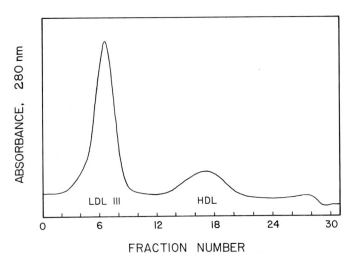

FIG. 2. Rate zonal separation of LDL-III from HDL contaminant of similar buoyant density. Data from Fless and Scanu (1979).

Table 1. Physical parameters of rhesus LDL.

		LDL-I	LDL-II	LDL-III
Molecular weight	–	3.32×10^6	2.75×10^6	3.47×10^6
Buoyant density	ml/g	1.027	1.036	1.050
Diffusion coefficient	cm/S^2	1.78×10^{-7}	2.00×10^{-7}	1.59×10^{-7}
Frictional ratio	–	1.07	1.04	1.20
Hydration	$g\ H_2O/g\ LDL$	0.22	0.12	0.69

The unusual physical properties of LDL-III appear to be due to its large protein moiety which consists only of apo B but contains more galactose and three times more sialic acid than apo LDL-I or apo LDL-II. By radioimmunoassay, LDL-III was only 46% as reactive as LDL-I or LDL-II to antibodies raised against LDL-II. In addition, LDL-III moved slower than LDL-I or LDL-II by electrophoresis in 4% agarose gels, which was probably due to increased electroendosmosis (Fig. 3).

Further clarification of these differences was achieved through a compositional analysis of these rhesus LDLs and their comparison to human lipoproteins. Knowing the chemical composition and molecular weight for each LDL, we calculated the number of components per particle (Table 2). This table shows that each component of LDL-II was smaller in number relative to LDL-I or LDL-III, which had remarkably similar contents of phospholipid, free cholesterol, and cholesteryl ester. However, the protein content of LDL-III was much greater than that of LDL-I or LDL-II, which explains its different buoyant density.

By calculating the volume and the surface area of the hydrophobic core of each of the rhesus LDL, we found that they showed the same relationships

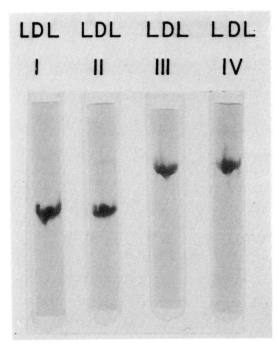

FIG. 3. Gel electrophoresis of rhesus LDL on 4% agarose. The gels were stained with Coomassie blue.

609

Table 2. Number of components per lipoprotein particle.[a]

	H-LDL[b]	LDL-I[c]	LDL-II[c]	LDL-III[c]
Molecular weight	3.52×10^6	3.32×10^6	2.75×10^6	3.47×10^6
Amino acid	6230	6142	5720	8328
Phospholipid	1090	1118	898	1133
Triglyceride	47	336	246	249
Free cholesterol	846	695	554	664
Cholesterol esters	2588	1915	1578	1847
Total cholesterol	3434	2610	2132	2511

[a] The following molecular weights were used for the calculations: amino acids, 100; phospholipid, 775; cholesterol, 387; cholesterol ester, 650; triglyceride, 850.

[b] H-LDL refers to the LDL from diet-induced hyperlipidemic rhesus monkeys isolated from the density interval 1.019 to 1.050 g/ml. Data taken from Fless and Scanu (1976); amino acid content was corrected for the different chromogenicity of apo-LDL relative to bovine serum albumin in the Lowry method for protein as in c.

[c] Data taken from Fless and Scanu (1979).

observed with human lipoproteins. On the other hand, the packing of the protein at the lipoprotein surface of LDL-I, LDL-II, and particularly LDL-III, indicated a deviation from the one calculated for human lipoproteins (Fig. 4). From the Y intercepts of the lines, we calculated the molecular area per amino acid for LDL-I and LDL-II to be 13 Å^2 as opposed to 9 Å^2 for LDL-III. These results may be taken to indicate that the apo protein of rhesus LDL and particularly LDL-III is packed more tightly on the surface because the protein moieties of human lipoproteins appear to occupy a molecular area of 15.6 Å^2 per amino acid. In the case of LDL-III, the

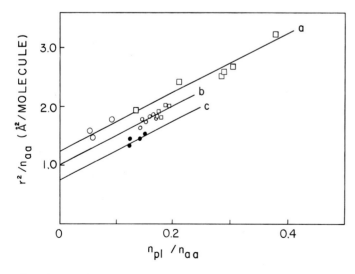

FIG. 4. Packing of protein and phospholipids at the lipoprotein-water interface. Data from Fless and Scanu (1979).

apparent tight packing of the protein at the surface could be explained if one assumes that only a fraction of its protein moiety is packed with a density similar to LDL-I or LDL-II and that the rest of the apoprotein has more contact with the solution than the interface.

LDL-IV. Recently, we discovered a fourth LDL fraction in rhesus plasma, which we call LDL-IV, with a mean buoyant density of 1.061 g/ml. This LDL was obscured by HDL on the 10% NaCl or NaBr gradients and was seen only after the previous removal of HDL. We obtain now the complete LDL profile from LDL-I through LDL-IV by eliminating the HDL from the total lipoproteins floating at d 1.21 g/ml with a short rate zonal ultracentrifugation and then centrifuging the total LDL to isopycnic equilibrium on a 0 to 12% NaBr density gradient (Fig. 5). In contrast to LDL-I, LDL-II, and LDL-III, equilibrium ultracentrifugation of LDL-IV yielded curved plots of log c versus the square of the distance from the center of rotation that gave molecular weights ranging from 3 to 5 x 10^6. This was true for the relatively homogeneous LDL-IV (Fig. 5B) and also for the heterogenous LDL-IV fraction even after the latter was subfractionated (Fig. 5A).

In order to establish the frequency of LDL-IV, we obtained sera from 40 normolipemic male and female rhesus monkeys and determined their LDL profiles. This led to the observation that LDL from male and female monkeys exhibits a similar degree of LDL heterogeneity; nearly all monkeys contained LDL-IV, although usually in amounts substantially smaller than the other three LDLs. Subsequent studies revealed that LDL-IV is related to LDL-III in that both particles possess the same electrophoretic mobility on 4% agarose gels (Fig. 3), and their apoproteins, which had the same amino acid composition, ran similarly on 4% agarose gels containing SDS. Furthermore, both apo LDL-III and apo LDL-IV have the same carbohydrate composition which differs with those of apo LDL-I and apo LDL-II. Also, the circular dichroic spectra of LDL-III and LDL-IV are analogous and differ from those of LDL-I and LDL-II. The percentage of protein is higher in LDL-IV than in LDL-III, which is consistent with its higher buoyant density (Table 3). Both LDL-III and LDL-IV cross react with antisera directed to human Lp(a)

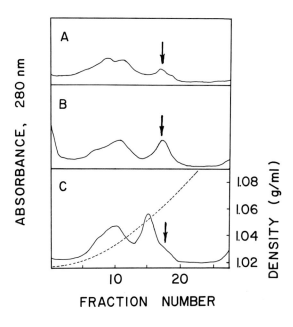

FIG. 5. Density gradient ultracentrifugation of the total rhesus low-density lipoproteins. A: LDL profile of same rhesus monkey as in Fig. 1b, now showing the presence of LDL-IV floating at d = 1.061 g/ml upon the removal of the HDL fraction. B: Typical pattern from another animal also showing the presence of LDL-IV. C: LDL profile of another rhesus monkey. There is a prominent LDL-III peak with a shoulder due to LDL-IV that illustrates the position of LDL-III on the gradient in relation to LDL-IV. The arrow designates the position of LDL-IV.

Table 3. Percent chemical composition of rhesus LDL-III and LDL-IV.

Component	LDL-III Weight (%)	LDL-IV[a] Weight (%)
Protein	24.0	27.4
Protein-bond carbohydrate	2.6	2.9
Phospholipid	25.3	26.3
Free cholesterol	7.4	8.1
Cholesteryl ester	34.6	32.6
Triglyceride	6.1	2.9

[a]D. Barbeau, G. Fless, and A.M. Scanu, unpublished observations.

whereas neither LDL-I nor LDL-II are reactive. Thus the serum of normo-lipemic monkeys contains two Lp(a)[+] particles which differ in composition and density. The relationship between these two particles is unknown at present but further work on this problem is now in progress.

Mitogenic Effect of LDL Sub-Fractions on
Rhesus Monkey Arterial Smooth Muscle Cells Grown in vitro

This work was prompted by the previous observation that the serum LDL de-rived from diet-induced hyperlipidemic rhesus monkeys induces stimulation of cell growth of optimally nourished primary cultures of smooth muscle cells which are in the stationary phase (Fischer-Dzoga et al. 1973, 1976). This response was not observed when either the serum or the whole LDL frac-tion of normolipidemic rhesus monkeys was used. In view of the microhetero-geneity discussed in the previous section, it appeared of interest to deter-mine whether one or more of the LDL subspecies could trigger the prolifera-tive response of the tissue culture system. For this purpose, we utilized primary explants of medial smooth muscle cells from the thoracic aorta of normolipidemic rhesus monkeys according to the technique of Fischer-Dzoga et al. (1973, 1976). Each 2-mm-diameter explant was placed in a 30 ml Falcon plastic tissue culture flask and incubated at 37°C with 5% CO_2 in 95% air. The growth medium consisted of Eagle's Basal Medium (BME) with Hank's balanced salt solution, supplemented with 10% calf serum. The ex-periments were initiated about 8 weeks after explantation, when the cultures had reached the stationary growth phase and consisted of circular colonies exhibiting the characteristic pattern of mono and multilayers. Groups of three to six cultures of comparable size were treated for 7 days by replac-ing half of the calf serum in the medium with the lipoprotein to be tested to a final concentration of 250 µg cholesterol/ml. Prior to their use, the different lipoproteins were extensively dialyzed against BME. Each experi-ment included as controls calf serum as well as normolipidemic and hyper-lipidemic rhesus monkey sera (5%). Cellular proliferation was evaluated by measuring the diameter of the circular cell colonies on two perpendicular axes and expressed as surface area. This was confirmed by autoradiography: the cultures were labeled with ^{3}H-thymidine (1 µCi/flask; spec. activity, 6.7 Ci/mM) and the number of labeled nuclei determined on autoradiographic preparations (Fischer-Dzoga et al. 1976). The proliferative response was studied for fractions LDL-I, LDL-II, and LDL-III and compared with the LDL fraction (H-LDL) isolated from the serum of monkeys fed a diet containing

Table 4. Stimulation of growth of primary cultures of aortic medial smooth muscle cells.

Additions to culture medium (BME plus 5% calf serum)	Increase in surface area $(mm^2 \pm SEM)$[a]
Calf serum	7.7 ± 2.7
Normolipidemic monkey serum	21.3 ± 5.9
Hyperlipidemic monkey serum	97.3 ± 9.1[b]
H-LDL	93.0 ± 23.9[b]
LDL-I	105.6 ± 22.2[b]
LDL-II	3.7 ± 3.7
LDL-III	13.1 ± 6.5
Sialidase treated LDL-III	72.4 ± 14.9[b]

[a]Net increase in surface area calculated for each culture and averaged for each group $(mm^2 \pm SEM)$ after 7 days of incubation with the different samples.

[b]The increment in the surface area was compared to the corresponding 10% calf serum control and found to be significantly higher; $P < 0.005$ (Student T-test for paired values).

25% coconut oil and 2% cholesterol that consists of essentially one LDL-I-like component. Fraction LDL-IV from normolipidemic monkeys was not studied because it is as yet insufficiently characterized.

Of the LDL species examined, LDL-I exhibited a marked proliferative response which was comparable to that exhibited by H-LDL when measured by the significant increase in the area of the colonies (Table 4) and in the number of ^{3}H-thymidine labeled nuclei as compared to control cultures exposed to calf serum. This observation was interesting in that LDL-I is the lipoprotein particle from normal monkeys most similar in size and density to H-LDL and also has a relatively large total cholesterol content (Table 2). In contrast, neither LDL-II, which was smallest in size and had the fewest number of lipid components per particle, nor LDL-III proved to have a proliferative effect. The result with LDL-III was unexpected, since in size and number of lipid components this particle was comparable to LDL-I. With the knowledge that LDL-III had an unusually high sialic acid content, we treated LDL-III with neuraminidase (C. perfringens sialidase, E.C. 3.2.1.18) at low ionic strength in 0.01 M Tris-acetate buffer, pH 6.8 (1 mg/ml LDL protein incubated at 37°C for 4 hours with 0.1 unit/mg of enzyme/LDL proteins). Under the experimental conditions used, LDL-III was deprived of the whole of its sialic acid content. This sialic acid-free particle stimulated cell proliferation to a similar extent as LDL-I and H-LDL (Table 4). It is apparent, therefore, that both size and lipid mass of the LDL particles and their surface content of sialic acid can influence the proliferation of stationary cultures of aortic medial smooth muscle cells in vitro.

Discussion

The results of the current studies have shown that the LDL class isolated from the serum of normolipidemic rhesus monkeys is composed of at least four species, all containing apo B but differing by one or more of these factors: size, density, electrophoretic mobility, and carbohydrate content. Two of them, LDL-III and LDL-IV, were reactive to human Lp(a) antisera and had also the high sialic acid content reported for Lp(a) particles (Ehnholm et al. 1972). The structural relationship between Lp(a)$^+$ and Lp(a)$^-$ particles and their metabolic regulation is unclear at this time; it appears that LDL-I and LDL-II, on the one hand, and LDL-III and LDL IV on the other are related due to their similar protein and carbohydrate moieties.

A most noteworthy feature of this work was the observed correlation between the structure of the LDL species and their capacity to stimulate the proliferation of arterial smooth muscle cells grown in culture. Those particles having the largest size and lipid mass, namely, LDL-I and H-LDL, were also the ones having mitogenic properties (Tables 2 and 4). This also applied to LDL-III once its sialic acid moiety was removed by digestion with sialidase. It is evident, therefore, that normolipidemic rhesus monkey serum contains lipoproteins which have a mitogenic action similar to that exhibeted by LDL from hyperlipidemic animals. The only difference is quantitative in that in hyperlipidemia the LDL particles are essentially all mitogenic, whereas in normolipidemia the LDL-I particles are a relatively smaller sample of the LDL population. Could the proliferative effect on cultured smooth muscle cells be equated to atherogenicity? This is a hypothesis which needs experimental testing, and therefore the importance of defining the heterogeneity of the LDL class in normolipidemia becomes apparent. This consideration also applies to man, since studies from this laboratory have shown that some control subjects contain LDL particles with mitogenic activity (unpublished observation).

As to the mechanism whereby LDL particles of relatively large size and mass exhibit mitogenic activity, we are only allowed speculations. A plausible hypothesis is that mitogenic LDL, by having a relatively high mass in lipid and particularly cholesteryl esters, on becoming internalized may raise the level of free cholesterol in the cell. This process could lead to changes in cellular cholesterol homeostasis which may, in turn, affect the physicochemical state of membranes in areas of the cell capable of modulating the synthesis of nucleic acid leading to cellular proliferation.

At this time, we have no experimental facts to support this hypothesis. It is clear, however, that our results call for a detailed investigation on the relationship between cholesterol and nucleic acid metabolism within the cells.

References

Ehnholm C, Garoff H, Renkonen O, Simons K (1972) Protein and carbohydrate composition of Lp(a) lipoprotein from human plasma. Biochemistry 11: 3229–3232
Fischer-Dzoga K, Fraser R, Wissler RW (1976) Stimulation of proliferation in stationary primary cultures of monkey and rabbit aortic smooth muscle cells. Exp Mol Pathol 24: 346–359
Fischer-Dzoga K, Jones RM, Vesselinovitch D, Wissler RW (1973) Ultrastructural and immunohistochemical studies of primary cultures of aortic medial cells. Exp Mol Pathol 18: 162–176
Fless GM, Scanu AM (1979) Isolation and characterization of the three major low density lipoproteins from normolipidemic rhesus monkeys (Macaca mulatta). J Biol Chem 254: 8653–8661

Fless GM, Wissler RW, Scanu AM (1976) Study of abnormal plasma low-density lipoprotein in rhesus monkeys with diet-induced hyperlipidemia. Biochemistry 15: 5799–5805

Hill P, Martin WG, Douglas JF (1975) Comparison of the lipoprotein profiles and the effect of N-phenylpropyl-N-benzyloxy acetamide in primates. Proc Soc Exp Biol Med 148: 41–49

Nelson CA, Morris MD (1976) A new serum lipoprotein found in many rhesus monkeys. Biochem Biophys Res Commun 71: 438–444

Rudel LL, Greene DG, Shah R (1977) Separation and characterization of plasma lipoproteins of rhesus monkeys (Macaca mulatta). J Lipid Res 18: 734–744

Lipoprotein Structure and Metabolism: Inhomogeneity, Variability and Species Specificity

Daniel Steinberg[1]

Recent years have seen accelerating progress in our understanding of lipoprotein structure and metabolism. The system grows ever more complex and
all of us are striving to find the simplest possible scheme within which to
understand and account for all of the observed phenomena. This is as it
should be. Our goal in science is to find the broadest general principles
that can be applied. The danger, however, is that in seeking simplification
and generalization we may be tempted to overlook exceptions that are possibly
awkward (sometimes even irritating!) but nevertheless important. The purpose
of these opening remarks, then, is to sound a cautionary note to all of us
who are students of lipoprotein structure and metabolism. I will cite three
general areas in which the early bloom of enthusiasm for simplicity and gen-
erality has faded with the accumulation of new information.

I. Structural Heterogeneity of Lipoprotein Classes

A variety of methods can be used to isolate and define classes of lipoproteins (e.g. preparative ultracentrifugation; zonal ultracentrifugation; electrophoresis in various media; gel chromatography; selective precipitation).
However, the final fractions isolated seldom (if ever!) represent collections
of truly identical macromolecules. For example, the human high density lipoprotein (HDL) fraction isolated by preparative ultracentrifugation and classically defined as those molecules with density between 1.063 and 1.21 is now
known to consist of at least three subclasses (HDL_{2a}, HDL_{2b}, and HDL_3) (Anderson et al. 1978).

Whether or not the heterogeneity in a given lipoprotein fraction is important
depends on the experimental question being addressed. Let us take human low
density lipoprotein (LDL) as an example. If one isolates an LDL fraction
containing exclusively apoprotein B and if one is studying the interactions
of LDL with its specific cell-surface receptor (Goldstein and Brown 1977),
then it probably makes little difference that there is microheterogeneity
with respect to lipid composition. By that I mean small differences in
lipid content and composition that account for the spectrum of densities
found in even the purest LDL preparations. Available evidence suggests that
LDL interaction with the receptor is determined almost exclusively by the
apoprotein B and that changes in lipid content do not affect this very much.
To cite an extreme example, studies in our laboratory (Steinberg et al. 1978)
have shown that extraction of all the nonpolar lipids from human LDL has little effect on its binding and rate of catabolism by human skin fibroblasts
even though molecular size and shape are radically altered.

In contrast, if the biological question is different, then the heterogeneity
even in highly purified LDL fractions can be of great importance. For example,

[1]The original research from the author's laboratory cited was supported by
NIH Research Grant HL-14197 awarded by the National Heart, Lung and Blood
Institute, PHS/DHEW.

616

Curtiss and Edgington (1976) have demonstrated the presence in "pure" LDL preparations of a quantitatively minor subfraction (probably less than 4 to 7% of the total) with a striking biological activity. This subfraction inhibits the in vitro stimulation of human lymphocytes by mitogens. They have designated it the LDL inhibitory fraction (LDL-In). This subfraction interacts with a lymphocyte receptor distinct from the Brown and Goldstein LDL receptor.

Mahley and Innerarity (1978) have reviewed the striking heterogeneity — functionally significant heterogeneity — in the lipoproteins of animals fed large amounts of cholesterol. An unusual category of lipid-rich HDL (HDL$_C$) accumulates, characterized best by its enrichment in apoprotein E. It contains no apoprotein B. The lipid content varies considerably and thus HDL$_C$ can appear in the LDL density class (d 1.019–1.063) and even at lower densities. The metabolism of these HDL$_C$ particles is unique because of their apoprotein E content. A small fraction of HDL$_C$ molecules in dogs contains only apoprotein E and this fraction is removed from the plasma with an extremely short half-life. Obviously kinetic studies of an "LDL" fraction isolated from cholesterol-fed animals and not further subfractionated could give confusing and misleading results!

Scientists are sometimes categorized either as "lumpers" — those who seek to bring order through synthesis — or "splitters" — those who seek to subclassify and further fractionate concepts. With respect to definition of lipoprotein classes we would all be well advised for now to lean toward the "splitter" category.

II. Variability in the Pathways of Lipoprotein Metabolism

Each of us has a "road map" in his slide collection that schematically represents the current major pathways of lipoprotein metabolism. The La Jolla "road map" for 1979 is shown in Fig. 1. We shall not review this scheme in

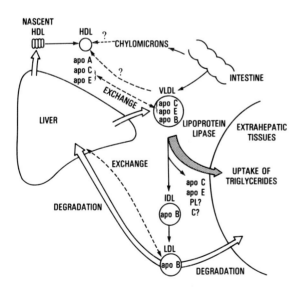

FIG 1. Schematic summary of the major pathways of lipoprotein metabolism.

617

any detail in this introduction. We show it only to make the point that it is incomplete, as are most such schemes. There are a number of side roads and detours that don't usually show on these maps. For purposes of overview it is certainly legitimate to neglect alternative and minor pathways. However, they become important in some circumstances and they must not be forgotten. Let us use the conversion of VLDL to LDL as an example.

The "road map" depicts VLDL as the sole precursor of LDL, the conversion being effected by the action of lipoprotein lipase and other catabolic enzymes. The apoproteins other than apo B are lost but all of the apo B goes on to LDL. The latter is then degraded, as we now know, both in the liver and in extrahepatic tissues (Pittman et al. 1979). But the map is sometimes wrong. Soutar et al. (1977) first showed that the turnover of apo B in the LDL fraction of patients with familial hypercholesterolemia is much greater than that of apo B in their VLDL fraction. There must be an alternative source of LDL, probably by direct secretion from the liver. Evidence for some degree of direct LDL secretion both in patients with hyperlipoproteinemia and in experimental animals has been obtained in several laboratories (Illingworth, 1975; Phair et al. 1975; Nakaya et al. 1977; Fainaru et al. 1977; Fidge and Poulis, 1978).

The standard "road map" shows all of the apo B from VLDL going on to LDL and that is at least close to the truth in normal man (Sigurdsson et al. 1975). But it is certainly not true in the normal rat. In fact most of the VLDL apo B in the rat is removed with remnants by the liver without ever appearing in the LDL fraction (Faergman et al. 1975). Nor is it true in patients with some forms of hyperlipoproteinemia (Janus et al. 1977; Melish et al. 1977). In those cases there is a significant alternative route, a VLDL "shunt", by which apo B-containing particles exit the plasma prior to LDL formation.

A revised and more complete "road map" for the VLDL-LDL system is shown in Fig. 2, adding direct LDL synthesis (r_4) and the VLDL "shunt" pathway (r_5) to the classical "straight-through" pathway of VLDL synthesis (r_1), VLDL-LDL conversion (r_2) and LDL degradation (r_3). In one sense this multiplication of alternative routes makes matters irritatingly complex. But in another

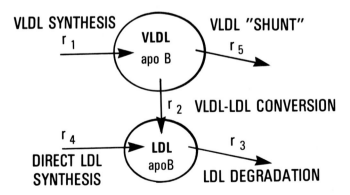

FIG 2. Schematic summary of VLDL and LDL metabolism including alternative pathways as discussed in the text.

sense it opens the way to a better understanding of the kinds of metabolic
perturbations that can lead to various patterns of hyperlipoproteinemia.
For example, it has been puzzling as to why some patients have high VLDL
apo B levels and yet have normal LDL apo B levels. A relative increase in
the VLDL "shunt" (r_5) accompanying an increase in VLDL synthesis (r_1) could
easily account for such a pattern. (A high VLDL triglyceride level due to
synthesis of VLDL particles with a normal apo B content poses no problems
since apo B delivery to LDL need not be increased as pointed out by Melish
et al. [1977]). Overproduction of VLDL without an increase in the "shunt"
would be expected to cause increases in both VLDL and LDL levels as in some
cases of familial combined hyperlipoproteinemia. With five variables to
manipulate instead of three it is easy to see that a given pattern of hyperlipoproteinemia could arise in several ways. Reciprocally, a basic underlying
metabolic error might be expressed in different ways depending on the pattern
of compensatory changes (Steinberg 1979).

III. Species Specificity

For several decades the "lumpers" in biochemistry and cell biology have held
the field. We are all impressed by the degree of conservation during evolution that allows us to study even bacteria and often obtain results that
apply to much more complex organisms. However, real limitations are already
apparent with regard to this kind of "lumping", especially in the area of
gene regulation. In the field of lipoprotein metabolism, the "lumpers" are
already getting their lumps because there are significant species differences.
We have already cited the example of the fate of VLDL apo B. In the rat it
is mostly taken up by the liver; in man it mostly goes on to LDL. In man
the HDL fraction contains only a small amount of apo E while rat HDL is much
richer in apo E, a difference with metabolic significance as we shall see in
a moment.

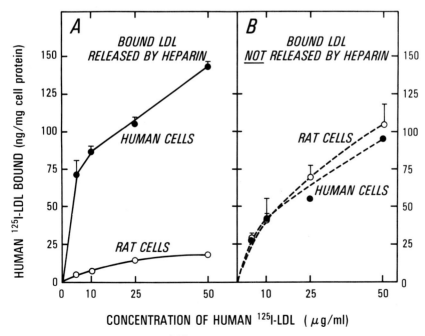

FIG 3. Binding of human ^{125}I-LDL to human and to rat
skin fibroblasts.

Another sort of species difference relates to the specificity of receptors. Many laboratories, including our own, have used human lipoprotein to investigate lipoprotein metabolism by cells from other species. This is tempting because its so much easier to obtain enough pure lipoprotein for such studies from human plasma than, say, rat plasma. However, this mixing instead of matching may give erroneous results, at least quantitatively and sometimes even qualitatively. In closing we present some recent studies from our laboratory done in collaboration with Dr. Christian A. Drevon, Mr. Alan Attie and Ms. Sharon Pangburn. These studies, using rat lipoproteins to study rat cells suggest an unexpected function for rat HDL that would have been overlooked if only human HDL had been used.

We first compared the binding at 4°C of human ^{125}I-LDL to cultured human skin fibroblasts and to rat skin fibroblasts previously incubated 48 h in lipoprotein-deficient medium. As shown in Fig. 3, Panel A, the LDL bound to human cells and released by heparin (Goldstein et al. 1976) was 5 to 10 times that bound to rat cells. Moreover, the binding curve for human cells was clearly biphasic, as expected, indicating both a high-affinity and a low-affinity component in the binding process. In the case of the rat cells, high-affinity binding was minimal. Bound LDL not released by heparin (Panel B) was comparable in the two cell types. As shown in Fig. 4, degradation of the human ^{125}I-LDL was also much greater in human cells than in rat cells. Prior incubation of human fibroblasts in the presence of unlabeled human LDL reduced the rate of degradation of ^{125}I-LDL by more than 80%, in agreement with the findings of Brown and Goldstein (1975), showing that the number of high-affinity receptors is reduced when LDL cholesterol is delivered to the cell. In contrast, prior incubation with LDL had no effect at all on LDL degradation by rat fibroblasts. These results show a striking species difference. Either the rat fibroblast has few if any high-affinity LDL receptors or, if it has, these receptors do not recognize human LDL.

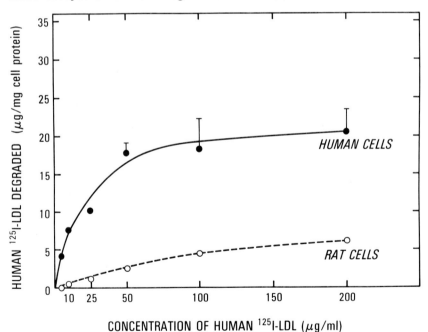

FIG. 4. Degradation of human ^{125}I-LDL by human and by rat skin fibroblasts as a function of LDL concentration. Cells were preincubated 24 h in lipoprotein-deficient medium and than 20 h with ^{125}I-LDL. TCA-soluble, noniodide ^{125}I in the medium was measured. Data points represent mean ± standard deviation for three separate dishes.

Table 1. Effects of homologous and heterologous LDL and HDL on HMGCoA
reductase activity in human and rat skin fibroblasts.[a]

Additions to medium	Enzyme activity relative to control (=100)	
	Human cells	Rat cells
Human LDL (50 µg/ml)	6.3±1.1 (7)[b]	80.0±8.8 (7)
Rat (50 µg/ml)	5.9±2.3 (2)	28.3±6.3 (4)
Human HDL (600 µg/ml)	136±18.8 (4)	167±14.4 (6)
Rat (600 µg/ml)	19.8±9.8 (4)	26.6±3.7 (5)

[a]Cells were first incubated 24 h in medium containing lipoprotein-deficient
serum (5 mg protein/ml) and then 20 h in the presence of LDL (d 1.02–1.05)
or HDL (d 1.09–1.21). Reductase activity was measured in cell-free extracts
as described by Brown et al. (1973).
[b]Data represent mean ± standard error; number of experiments given in parentheses.

When homologous LDL was incubated with rat fibroblasts, the curve relating
degradation rate to LDL concentration was biphasic (Fig. 5) suggesting that
rat cells do have a high-affinity receptor that recognizes rat LDL (d 1.02–
1.045). Degradation of heterologous (human) LDL by the rat cells was less
than that of homologous (rat) LDL.

Uptake of LDL by the high-affinity receptor mechanism is associated with inhibition of beta-hydroxy-beta-methylglutaryl coenzyme A(HMGCoA) reductase
while uptake by low-affinity mechanisms is not (Goldstein and Brown 1977).
As shown in Table I, human LDL suppressed HMGCoA reductase in human cells,
as expected, but had only a minimal effect on reductase in rat cells. On
the other hand rat LDL lowered reductase activity in rat cells by 72%. Taken
together these data indicate that rat skin fibroblasts have receptors functionally analogous to the LDL receptor in human fibroblasts. However, the rat
LDL receptor binds and takes up homologous LDL much more readily than it does
human LDL. In part this may reflect species differences in apo B structure,
difference in receptor structure or both. A second possibility is that the
LDL density class in rats may include enough apo E to contribute to the observed preferential binding of the homologous LDL. Innerarity and Mahley
(1978) have shown that apo E-containing lipoproteins may have as much as 10-
to 100-fold greater affinity for the receptor than apoB-containing lipoproteins.

Finally, rat and human HDL metabolism were compared in the two cell lines.
As shown in Fig. 5 rat HDL was degraded by rat cells more rapidly than was
human HDL (both fractions d 1.09–1.21). We then examined the effects on
HMGCoA reductase. Human HDL does not inhibit HMGCoA reductase in human fibroblasts even at very high concentrations (Goldstein and Brown 1977). As shown
in Table I, we found that human HDL at 600 µg protein/ml (a level approaching
that in human plasma) caused if anything a slight increase in reductase activity in human cells and a somewhat greater increase in rat cells. In striking contrast, rat HDL at the same concentrations decreased reductase activity
by 70-80% in both cell lines. It also enhanced acyl CoA:cholesterol acyltransferase activity (ACAT) 2- to 3-fold (data not shown).

The basis for the very different behavior of rat and human HDL is not yet
established but probably relates to differences in their apoproteins. Rat
HDL contains more apo E than does human HDL. Rat HDL contains apoprotein
A-IV as a major component while human HDL contains predominantly A-I and
A-II. Whatever the molecular basis for the difference may be, the present
findings point up a potentially important difference in function in vivo.
The inhibition of HMGCoA reductase and stimulation of ACAT activity implies
that rat HDL is delivering cholesterol to the fibroblast. We suggest that
in the rat the HDL fraction, rather than or in addition to the LDL fraction

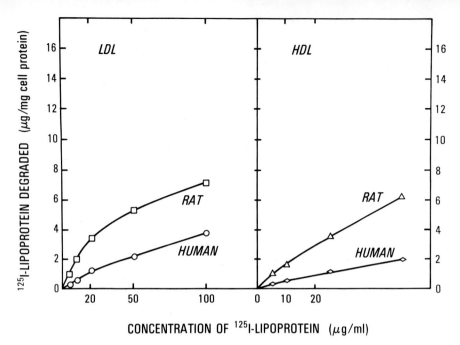

FIG. 5. Degradation of homologous and heterologous ^{125}I-LDL by human and by rat skin fibroblasts as a function of LDL concentration. Conditions as in legend to FIG. 4.

plays a major role in the delivery of cholesterol to extrahepatic tissues. Anderson and Dietschy (1976) have shown that HDL does deliver cholesterol to at least one tissue, the adrenal cortex. In the rat, HDL may serve functions analogous to those served by LDL in man.

IV. Summary

We have reviewed three areas in which problems can be and have been encountered when we try to generalize prematurely or too broadly. With the application of increasingly sophisticated methods for fractionation, lipoprotein classes, however defined, may split and yield structural and functional subclasses! The best way to avoid confusion is to define our preparations operationally and characterize them as much as possible so that experimental results as reported can be reevaluated in the light of later findings.

The pathways of lipoprotein metabolism grow ever more complex — tortured and torturing. The multiple exchange processes now demonstrated, involving almost all of the component proteins and lipids, make it very difficult indeed to come up with a comprehensive, meaningful "road map". We need to be aware that the maps are different for different species. The maps include alternative routes within a given species and thus may vary under different circumstances even in a given animal.

While related in a number of ways, the apoproteins in different species are not necessarily identical. The cell receptors in different species do not necessarily recognize heterologous apoproteins in the same way they recognize their homologous apoproteins. Mixing instead of matching can lead to quantitative and even qualitative misinterpretations. The contrast between rat HDL and human HDL may be only one example of many.

References

Anderson DW, Nichols AV, Pan SS, Lindgren FT (1978) High density lipoprotein distribution. Atherosclerosis 29: 161-179

Brown MS, Dana SE, Goldstein JL (1973) Regulations of 3-hydroxy-3-methly-glutaryl coenzyme A reductase activity in human fibroblasts by lipoproteins. Proc Nat Acad Sci (USA) 70: 2162-2166

Brown MS, Goldstein JL (1975) Regulation of the activity of the low density lipoprotein receptor in human fibroblasts. Cell 6: 307-316

Curtiss LK, Edgington TS (1976) Regulatory serum lipoproteins: regulation of lymphocyte stimulation by a species of low density lipoproteins. J Immunol 116: 1452-1458

Faergeman O, Sata T, Kane JP, Havel RJ (1975) Metabolism of apoprotein B of plasma very low density lipoproteins in the rat. J Clin Invest 56: 1396-1403

Fainaru M, Felker TE, Hamilton RL, Havel RJ (1977) Evidence that a separate particle containing B-apoprotein is present in high-density lipoproteins from perfused rat liver. Metabolism 26: 999-1004

Fidge NH, Poulis P (1978) Metabolic heterogeneity in the formation of low density lipoprotein from very low density lipoprotein in the rat: evience for the independent production of a low density lipoprotein subfraction. J Lipid Res 19: 324-349

Goldstein JL, Basu SK, Brunschede GY, and Brown MS (1976) Release of low density lipoprotein from its cell surface receptor by sulfated glycosaminoglycans. Cell 7: 85-95

Goldstein JL, Brown MS (1977) The low-density lipoprotein pathway and its relation to atherosclerosis. Am Rev Biochem 46: 897-930

Illingworth DR (1975) Metabolism of lipoproteins in nonhuman primates. Studies on the origin of low density lipoprotein apoproteins in the plasma of the squirrel monkey. Biochim Biophys Acta 388: 38-51

Innerarity TL, Mahley RW (1978) Enhanced binding by cultured human fibroblasts of apo E-containing lipoproteins as compared with low denisty lipoproteins. Biochemistry 17: 1440-1447

Janus E, Wootton R, Nicoll A, Turner P, Lewis B (1977) Quantitation of very low density (VLDL) to low density lipoprotein (LDL) in normal and hyperlipidaemic man. Circulation 56: III-21

Mahley RW, Innerarity TL (1978) Properties of lipoproteins responsible for high affinity binding to cell surface receptors of fibroblasts and smooth muscle cells. Adv Exptl Med Biol 109: 99-127

Melish J, Le NA, Ginsberg H, Brown WV, Steinberg D (1977) Effect of high carbohydrate diet on very low density lipoprotein apoprotein-B and triglyceride production. Circulation 56: III-5

Nahaya N, Chung BH, Patsch JR, Tauton OD (1977) Synthesis and release of low density lipoproteins by the isolated perfused pig liver. J Biol Chem 252: 7530-7533

Phair RD, Hammond MG, Bowden JA, Fried M, Fisher WR, Berman M (1975) A preliminary model for human lipoprotein metabolism in hyperlipoproteinemia. Fed Proc Fed Am Socs exp Biol 34: 2263

Pittman RC, Attie AD, Carew TE, Steinberg D (1979) Tissue sites of degradation of low density lipoprotein: Application of a new general method for determining the fate of plasma proteins. Proc Nat Acad Sci 76: 5345-5349

Sigurdsson G, Nicoll A, Lewis B (1975) Conversion of very low density lipoprotein to low density lipoprotein: a metabolic study of apolipoprotein B kinetics in human subjects. J Clin Invest 56: 1481-1490

Soutar AK, Myant NB, Thompson GR (1977) Simultaneous measurements of apolipoprotein B turnover in very low— and low-density lipoproteins in familial hypercholesterolaemia. Atherosclerosis 28: 247-256

Steinberg D, Nestel PJ, Weinstein DB, Remaut-Desmeth M, Chang CM (1978) Interactions of native and modified human low density lipoproteins with human skin fibroblasts. Biochim Biophys Acta 528: 199-212

Steinberg D (1979) Origin, turnover and fate of plasma low-density lipoprotein. Prog biochem Pharmacol 15: 166-199

Structure and Function of the Human Plasma Apolipoproteins[1]

Henry J. Pownall,[2] James T. Sparrow,[2] Louis C. Smith, and Antonio M. Gotto, Jr.

Introduction

Studies of the role of the human plasma lipoproteins in this laboratory have emphasized the correlations between lipoprotein structure and physiologic function. It is a common biochemical hypothesis that a given physiologic determinant can be localized to specific regions of individual macromolecules. In plasma lipoproteins, a determinant can even be localized to specific sequences or segments of an apoprotein component of a lipoprotein. Some fragments of native apolipoproteins derived from chemical cleavage contain a physiologic determinant. Many times this is not the case and an alternative method for obtaining other fragments must be used. Solid phase peptide synthesis has emerged as a powerful tool that can be combined with other physical and biochemical procedures to produce structure-function correlations which could not otherwise be formulated. Using this strategy, we have been able to correlate apoprotein structure with enzyme activation, lipophilicity and antigenicity. This correlation has been achieved with the major soluble proteins of plasma lipoproteins apoA-I (244 residues), apoA-II (a dimer of identical 77 residue chains), apoC-I(57 residues), apoC-II(78 residues) and apoC-III(79 residues).

Enzyme Activation

Lecithin:cholesterol acyltransferase (LCAT), a plasma enzyme secreted by the liver catalyzes the conversion of cholesterol and lecithin to cholesteryl ester and lysolecithin. The reaction rate is enhanced by apoA-I from high density lipoproteins (HDL) and apoC-I from HDL or very low density lipoproteins (VLDL). ApoA-I is a polypeptide of known sequence which can be fragmented into 4 smaller peptides by treatment with cyanogen bromide (CNBr). The first localization of an enzyme activating determinant in a native apolipoprotein is that of Soutar et al. (1975) who have found that two of the cyanogen bromide fragments of apoA-I retain part of the LCAT activating determinant. Compared to apoA-I only the longer fragments corresponding to residues 1-89 and 151-244 exhibit activation that is comparable (40-50%) to that of the native protein. Neither of the CNBr fragments of apoC-I activate LCAT. More recently, Sigler et al. (1976) have shown that a synthetic peptide, corresponding to apoC-I and fragment

[1] Support for this work was provided by the National Heart and Blood Vessel Research and Demonstration Center, Baylor College of Medicine, a grant supported research project of the National Heart, Lung and Blood Institute (HL-17269) and National Institutes of Health Grants (HL-19459) and (HL-15648) and the American Heart Association.

[2] HJP and JTS are Established Investigators of the American Heart Association.

624

17-57 activates LCAT to the same extent as the native protein. Fragments corresponding to residues 24-57 and 32-57 gave 50% of the activation of that of native apoC-I; shorter fragments did not activate.

Identification of an enzyme-activating determinant has also been achieved with apoC-II, which stimulates the activity of lipoprotein lipase (LPL). Kinnunen et al. (1977) have tested the potency of both native (CNBr) and synthetic fragments of apoC-II as activators of LPL catalyzed hydrolysis of triglyceride. CNBr fragments corresponding to residues 1-9 and 10-59 do not activate; the native and synthetic fragments corresponding to residues 60-78 produce about 50% of the activation achieved by apoC-II. Synthetic fragments 50-78 and 55-78 give activation comparable to that of the native protein, whereas synthetic fragment 66-78 does not activate. Removal of the carboxyl-terminal residues, Gly-Glu-Glu, decreases activation by 95%. These results suggest that the minimal LPL-activating determinant of apoC-II is contained in residues 55-78. We anticipate that the LCAT and LPL activating determinants can be further localized by the judicious selection of other peptides obtained by solid phase synthesis.

Lipid-Protein Association

The affinity of an amphiphilic substance for lipids is operationally defined as lipophilicity. Though the search for the lipophilic determinant in the plasma apolipoproteins is still ongoing, considerable progress has been made in the past 10 years. Much of the theoretical formalism for lipophilicity derives from the descriptive work of Segrest et al. (1974) who have proposed that a good lipid-associating peptide will have the polar and non-polar residues distributed through the sequence such that, when placed in an α-helix, the polar residues will appear on one face of the helix and the non-polar residues will appear on the opposite side. Hypothetically, the axis of the helix would be tangential to the surface of a lipoprotein so that the non-polar side would penetrate part way into the hydrocarbon region of the putative phospholipid monolayer and the polar side would lie at the surface nearly coplanar with the phospholipid polar head groups.

ApoA and apoC have been studied by a variety of physical methods, many of which have been summarized by Morrisett et al. (1977). The following experimental criteria for a lipid-associating peptide have been established:

1) an increase in the α-helical content of the protein upon association with lipid;
2) a blue-shift in the intrinsic tryptophan fluorescence of the lipid-bound protein compared to that of the free species;
3) clarification of liposomal turbidity due to the formation of complexes that are much smaller than the wavelength of visible light; and
4) isolation of a lipid-protein complex by ultracentrifugation in a density gradient or by molecular permeation chromatography.

The following studies using these criteria have provided the basis on which to refine the original and amphipathic theory.

Morrisett et al. (1973,1974) have demonstrated that apoC-III spontaneously associates with egg lecithin vesicles to form an isolable complex that retains the essential vesicular structure. In contrast, when apoC-III is mixed with saturated lecithins such as dimyristoyl-(DMPC) and dipalmitoyl phosphatidylcholine, a smaller micellar complex is formed (Novosad et al.

1976). In a more detailed study, Pownall et al. (1974) found that at or above the gel → liquid crystalline phase transition of DMPC, T = 24 , (Mabrey and Sturtevant, 1976) the association of apoC-III with the lipid was the most rapid.

The first localization of a lipid-binding determinant in apoC-III was provided by Sparrow et al. (1973,1977) who synthesized a series of peptides corresponding to residues 41-79, 48-79, 55-79, and 61-79 of the native apoC-III. Only the longest fragment satisfied all of the criteria for a good lipid associating peptide. Thrombin cleavage of apoC-III gives a pair of peptides corresponding to residues 1-40 (C-III-A) and 41-79 (C-III-B) (Sparrow et al. 1977). C-III-B has a higher calculated hydrophobicity (-839 cal/residue) than C-III-A (-609 cal/residue); C-III-A, however, has a slightly higher helical content in solution than has C-III-B. Since the latter binds phospholipid and the former does not, we propose that a lipid-associating peptide must have a high hydrophobicity. It also appears that helical content in solution is not an important lipid-binding determinant, although, in the lipid-protein complex the helicity should be high. Moreover, helix formation during complex formation, and not the helicity of the free peptide, is the important driving force for lipid-protein association. Massey et al. (1979) found that each mole of residues of apoA-II and apoC-III converted from a random coil to an α-helix contributes about -1.3 kcal of enthalpy to the free energy of lipid-protein association. Therefore, a large increase in the helical content of an apoprotein upon binding lipid will provide a commensurately large increase in the stability of the complex. This finding is quantitative support for the view that helical potential is more important than helical content in a lipid-associating protein.

Sparrow et al. (1977) have designed and tested a series of model peptides based upon the amphipathic helical model of apolipoproteins. The sequences of some of these peptides are given below.

I. Val-Ser-Ser-Leu-Lys-Glu-Tyr-Trp-Ser-Ser-Leu-Lys-Glu-Ser-Phe-Ser

II. Val-Ser-Ser-Leu-Lys-Glu-Ala-Ala-Ser-Ser-Leu-Lys-Glu-Ser-Phe-Ser

III. Val-Ser-Ser-Leu-Lys-Glu-Ala-Trp-Ser-Ser-Leu-Lys-Glu-Ser-Phe-Ser

IV. Val-Ser-Ser-Leu-Leu-Ser-Ser-Leu-Lys-Glu-Tyr-Trp-Ser-Ser-Leu-Lys-
Glu-Ser-Phe-Ser

Only peptide IV exhibits lipid-binding behavior comparable to that of the native apolipoproteins. In fact, when combined with phospholipid, peptide IV gives some of the most dramatic spectral changes that we have observed; these include an increase in the calculated helical content from 10 to 90%; the fluorescence maximum is shifted from 352 nm to 330 nm; the turbidity of liposomes of DMPC in a lipid-peptide molar ratio of 20 is completely clarified in a few minutes after mixing. Although all three of these model peptides have a relatively high hydrophobicity, only the 20-residue analog (IV) binds to phospholipid. Therefore, a certain minimal length of a peptide is required to produce a lipid-protein complex.

It is usually assumed that the hydrophobic effect is also an important driving force for the association of apolipoproteins with phospholipid. There are some formidable barriers to measuring the magnitude of that term. The hydrophobic effect is produced through an entropy driven process in

626

which ordered water adjacent to exposed hydrophobic non-polar amino acid side chains is transferred to the bulk aqueous phase. In the association of an apolipoprotein with phospholipids the hydrophobic groups would, presumably, be buried part way into the hydrocarbon region of the lipid. The hydrophobic term in the free energy of association of an apoprotein with lipid can be calcuated by summing the free energy of transfer of individual amino acid side chains located in lipid-binding regions of the apolipoprotein. For apoA-II these regions have been identified (Chen et al. 1979; Mao et al. 1977). For apoA-II the calculated free energy of transfer of non-polar amino acid side chains of the lipid-binding region from water to hydrocarbon, based on the values of Bull and Breese (1974), is -98 kcal/mole., i.e., the $T\Delta S$ term of the free energy change, ΔG, is on the order of the strength of a covalent bond. To measure equilibria with a value of even -20 kcal is very difficult so that verification of the importance of the hydrophobic effect in excess of -20 kcal requires an indirect method.

Massey et al. (1980, unpublished results) have studied the enthalpy of association of apoA-II with DMPC as a function of temperature. In that study they observe spontaneous association of the lipid and protein above and below the transition temperature of the lipid. Although the association is exothermic at or above T_c, below T_c the enthalpy is endothermic; i.e. $\Delta H = +90$ kcal. Since the reaction is spontaneous, the free energy of association, ΔG, must be negative. Furthermore,

$$\Delta G = \Delta H - T\Delta S$$

$$\therefore\ T\Delta S > \Delta H$$

i.e. the entropic ($T\Delta S$) or hydrophobic term must be greater than 90 kcal to compensate for the unfavorable enthalpy of association. A value on the order of $T\Delta S = 100$ kcal is consistent with our experimental observations and in good agreement with the theoretical value. It is of interest that this kind of measurement cannot be made with physiological lecithins because their T_c's are very low. Thus, molecular information obtained from recombinants of apoproteins with nonphysiologic synthetic lecithins is otherwise inaccessible and illustrates the value of these lipids in studies of lipoprotein structure and function.

Collective consideration of our results allows us to formulate a number of rules to identify the properties of a lipid-binding protein. These are:

1. The peptide need not have an α-helical structure in solution but must have the potential to form a helix.
2. The peptide must have a certain length, designated as the critical amphipathic length, of approximately 20 residues.
3. The peptide must have a high hydrophobicity.
4. When the peptide assumes a helical structure, hydrophobic residues appear on one face of the helix which, presumably, would penetrate the lipid matrix; the polar residues would be on the opposite side of the helix exposed to water at a depth that is nearly coplanar with the polar head groups of the phospholipid.

The calorimetric studies show that the helical contribution to the free energy of lipid-protein association can be measured and that the hydrophobic contribution can be estimated. It is anticipated that the combination of chemical synthesis of model peptides and physicochemical testing of their properties will continue to be a productive combination of techniques that will eventually provide a clear view of how lipids and proteins associate.

Following the landmark work of Atassi (1975) who located the antigenic sites on whale myoglobin, other investigators have attempted to extend that work to other systems. It might be particularly useful to locate the antigenic sites in the apolipoproteins to determine whether those regions are masked or exposed in native and reassembled lipoproteins.

Mao et al. (1975,1979) have obtained the first localization of the antigenic sites of an apolipoprotein in their work on the native and synthetic fragments of apoA-II. Using a specific radioimmunoassay for apoA-II, Mao et al. (1975) found that the carboxyl-terminal (residues 27-77) CNBr fragment was more reactive than the amino terminal (residues 1-26) region; the respective amino- and carboxyl-terminal fragments contained 30% and 70% of the immunoreactivity of native apoA-II. This work has been further refined by Mao et al. (1979) who obtained a better localization of the antigenic site by studying the immunoreactivity of tryptic and synthetic fragments of apoA-II. Immunoreactivity is assessed from the competitive inhibition of the binding of $[^{125}I]$apoA-II to its antisera. Tryptic fragments containing residues 4-23 (disulfide at Cys-6 intact), 31-39, and 56-77 give 28, 10 and 25% inhibition, respectively. A synthetic fragment corresponding to residues 40-46 gave 10% inhibition. Glycine ethyl ester was coupled to Glu-59 and Glu-69 of the 56-77 tryptic fragment; the modified peptide does not form an immunoprecipitant line with anti-apoA-II. Since the 60-77 fragment gave an immunoprecipitate of complete identity to fragment 56-77, we conclude that a major antigenic determinant is contained in residues 60 and 77 and that Glu-69 is a part of that determinant. Peptides corresponding to residues 1-26 and 56-77 do not associate with phospholipid. Therefore, the antigenic sites of apoA-II are localized to regions of the peptide that are distinct from those involved in lipid-protein association. This finding is consistent with the high immunoreactvity of apoA-II in high density lipoproteins.

Lipid Exchange

It is clear that the plasma apolipoproteins are much more than carriers of lipids. They function also as regulators of the metabolism of the lipids with which they are associated. On the basis of the amphipathic helical model, the charged amino acid residues of an apolipoprotein are predicted to be on the surface of a lipoprotein, thereby controlling the surface charge of the lipoprotein and perhaps the structure of water at the water-lipoprotein interface. One important but poorly understood phenomenon influenced by the interfacial water layer is that of lipid exchange. Smith and co-workers have sudied the rate of exchange of fluorescent lipid analogues in lipoproteins and simple model system. All of these lipid analogues contain pyrene as a covalently bound fluorescent label. A useful property of pyrene is that its fluorescence intensity at 475 nm decreases upon dilution. Therefore, transfer of a pyrene labeled lipid from one lipoprotein to another unlabeled lipoprotein results in a decrease in fluorescence at 475 nm. The rate of decrease reflects the rate of lipid transfer or exchange. Using a stopped-flow unit the rates of transfer of a number of pyrene labeled lipids have been measured (Kao et al. 1977; Doody et al. 1980; Charlton et al. 1976, 1979). The rates vary greatly, depending on the lipid. The half-times for transfer from HDL to HDL are as follows: sterol, 75 sec; fatty acid, 40 msec(pH 4); 2.5 sec(pH 7); lecithin, 60 min; diglyceride, 150 msec, and hydrocarbon, 4 msec. One important finding emerging from these studies is that there is an interfacial barrier to the transfer of lipids out of a phospholipid vesicle. This discovery suggests that the apoproteins could effect the rate of transfer through modification of the interfacial barrier. This regulatory role can be added to the growing list of functions of the plasma apolipoproteins.

Overview

Until recently, the plasma apolipoproteins were viewed as little more than lipid-binding proteins; it is now clear that they contribute to the regulation of lipid metabolism in both plasma and in the cells of the arterial wall. It is probable that the list of metabolic functions assigned to plasma apolipoprotiens will continue to grow as new metabolic processes are identified. Furthermore, the structure-function correlations obtained by combining physical methods, enzymology and peptide synthesis will certainly continue as an important component of studies that contribute to a better understanding of lipid metabolism.

REFERENCES

Atassi MZ (1975) Antigenic structure of myoglobin: The complete immunochemical anatomy of a protein and conclusions relating to antigenic structures of proteins. Immunochem 12: 423–429
Bull HB, Breese K (1974) Surface tension of amino acid solutions: A hydrophobicity scale of the amino acid residues. Arch Biochem Biophys 161: 665–670
Charlton SC, Olson JS, Hong K-Y, Pownall HJ, Louie DD, Smith LC (1976) Stopped flow kinetics of pyrene transfer between human high density lipoproteins. J Biol Chem 251: 7952–7955
Charlton SC, Hong K-Y, Smith LC (1978) Kinetics of rac-1-Oleyl-2-[4-(3-pyrenyl)butanoyl] glycerol transfer between high density lipoproteins. Biochemistry 17: 3304–3309
Chen TC, Sparrow JT, Gotto AM Jr, Morrisett JD (1979) Apolipoprotein A-II: Chemical synthesis and biophysical properties of three peptides corresponding to fragments in the amino-terminal half. Biochemistry 18: 1617–1622
Doody MC, Pownall HJ, Kao YJ, Smith LC (1980) Mechanism and kinetics of transfer of a fluorescent fatty acid between single walled phosphatidylcholine vesicles. Biochemistry, in press
Kao YJ, Charlton, SC, Smith LC (1977) Cholesterol Transfer to High Density Lipoproteins. Fed Proc 36: 936–941.
Kinnunen PKJ, Jackson RL, Smith LC, Gotto AM Jr, Sparrow JT (1977) Activation of lipoprotein lipase by native and synthetic fragments of human plasma apolipoprotein C-II. Proc Natl Acad Sci USA 73: 4848–4851
Mabrey S, Sturtevant JM (1976) Investigation of phase transition of lipids and lipid mixtures by high sensitivity differential scanning calorimetry. Proc Natl Acad Sci USA 73: 3862–3866
Mao SJT, Gotto AM Jr, Jackson RL (1975) Immunochemistry of human plasma high density lipoproteins. Radioimmunoassay of apolipoprotein A-II. Biochemistry 14: 4127–4131
Mao SJT, Sparrow JT, Gilliam EB, Gotto AM Jr, Jackson RL (1977) Mechanism of lipid-protein interaction in the plasma lipoproteins: Lipid-binding properties of synthetic fragments of apolipoprotein A-II. Biochemistry 16: 4150–4156
Mao SJT, Sparrow JT, Gotto AM Jr, Jackson RL (1979) Mechanism of

lipid-protein interaction in the plasma lipoproteins: Relationship of lipid-binding sites in apolipoprotein A-II. Biochemistry 18: 3984-3988

Massey JB, Gotto AM Jr, Pownall HJ (1979) Contribution of α-helix formation in human plasma apolipoproteins to their enthalpy of association with phospholipids. J Biol Chem 254: 9359-9361

Morrisett JF, David JSK, Pownall HJ, Gotto AM Jr (1973) Interaction of apolipoprotein (ApoLP-Alanine) with phosphatidylcholine. Biochemistry 12: 1290-1299

Morrisett JD, Gallagher JG, Aune KC, Gotto AM Jr (1974) Structure of the major complex formed by interaction of phosphatidylcholine bilamellar vesicles and apolipoprotein-alanine (apoC-III). Biochemistry 13: 4765-4771

Morrisett JD, Jackson RL, Gotto AM Jr (1977) Lipid protein interactions in the plasma lipoproteins. Biochim Biophys Acta 474: 93-133

Novosad Z, Knapp RD, Gotto AM Jr, Pownall HJ, Morrisett JD (1976) Structure of an apolipoprotein-phospholipid complex: ApoC-III induced changes in the physical properties of dimyristoyl-phosphatidylcholine. Biochemistry 15: 3176-3183

Pownall HJ, Morrisett JD, Sparrow JT, Gotto AM Jr (1974) The requirement for lipid fluidity in the formation and structure of lipoproteins: Thermotropic analysis of apolipoprotein-alanine binding to dimyristoylphosphatidylcholine. Biochem Biophys Res Commun 60: 779-786

Segrest JP, Jackson RL, Morrisett JD, Gotto AM Jr (1974) A molecular theory of lipid-protein interractions in the plasma lipoproteins. FEBS Lett 38: 247-253

Sigler GF, Soutar AK, Smith LC, Gotto AM Jr, Sparrow JT (1976) The solid phase synthesis of a protein activator for lecithin: cholesterol acyltransferase corresponding to human plasma apoC-I. Proc Natl Acad Sci USA 73: 1422-1426

Soutar AK, Garner GW, Baker HN, Sparrow JT, Jackson RL, Gotto AM Jr, Smith LC (1975) Effect of the human plasma apolipoproteins and phosphatidylcholine acyl donor on the activity of lecithin: cholesterol acyltransferase. Biochemistry 14: 3057-3064

Sparrow JT, Jackson RL, Morrisett JD (1973) Chemical synthesis and biochemical properties of peptide fragments of apolipoprotein-alanine. Proc Natl Acad Sci USA 70: 2124-2128

Sparrow JT, Pownall HJ, Hsu F-J, Blumenthal LD, Culwell AR, Gotto AM Jr, (1977) Lipid binding by fragments of apolipoprotein C-III-1 obtained by thrombin cleavage. Biochemistry 16: 5427-5432

Enzymatic Regulation of Lipoprotein Catabolism

Heiner Greten, Jochen Grosser, Isolde Becht, Otto Schrecker, Klaus Preissner, and Gerald Klose

Introduction

Chylomicron and VLDL-metabolism occur through multiple interactions with various enzymes, hydrolysis of triglycerides, transfer of fatty acids and decrease of the core volume. During this process the core of these particles changes from a more triglyceride-rich to a predominant cholesteryl-ester-rich one. Apo C molecules are progressively removed from VLDL to be associated with HDL until they recirculate to newly formed VLDL or chylomicrons which enter the circulation. This transfer only occurs when VLDL-triglycerides are catabolized. Thus HDL are looked upon as a reservoir for the physiologically most important molecules which, apart from their function as lipid carriers, regulate the lipolytic action of various enzymes. Plasma-LDL which contain all of the apo B molecules present in VLDL-particles then regulate intracellular HMG-Co A-reductase.

A molecular mechanism by which HDL precursors can be produced from the surface of chylomicrons or VLDL during their catabolism in peripheral tissue has recently been suggested (Tall and Small 1978). LPL at the capillary endothelium hydrolyzes chylomicron triglycerides. As triglycerides are removed the core shrinks and the surface constituents form lipid bilayer folds projecting from the chylomicron. These sheets then form vesicles, a more stable form of the bilayer, which offer an excellent substrate for LCAT if apo AI is present. Though there is no evidence that LCAT acts directly on either chylomicrons or VLDL or on remnants, action of LCAT on HDL can indirectly lead to removal of surface lipid from VLDL. This mechanism may be the basis for various clinical observations in which impaired peripheral catabolism of TG-rich lipoproteins was shown to cause a partial block in HDL function.

The three plasma enzymes, LPL, H-TGL and LCAT, thus catalyze a cascade of reactions including the hydrolysis of phospholipids at the surface of VLDL lipoproteins, the breakdown of triglycerides in the core and the transfer of free cholesterol to cholesteryl esters to form spherical HDL. The exact sequence of events is not known and many of these assumptions are still hypothetical. Especially the exact role of LPL and H-TGL during delipidation of VLDL and chylomicrons remains to be established.

In this presentation today I would like to focus on the physiological role and the molecular properties of the two enzymes lipoprotein lipase and hepatic triglyceride lipase. They are both glycoproteins with molecular weights of about 60.000 with differences in carbohydrate and amino acid composition. They have different antigenic determinants. There is a requirement of lipoprotein lipase for apo CII as cofactor. Both enzymes show different sensitivities to changes in ionic strength, and there are differences by kinetic criteria and differences in genetically determined diseases and various clinical disorders (Augustin and Greten 1979, 1979).

In this presentation I will try to cover the following aspects which, I hope, will shed some light on the functions and role of both H-TGL and LPL in normal plasma lipoprotein metabolism as well as in diseased states. We will begin with experiments performed in our laboratory with the aim to evaluate the particular function of hepatic triglyceride lipase. I will then briefly report on experiments dealing with the purification of plasma lipoprotein lipase and finally discuss the mechanism of lipoprotein lipase activation by apoprotein CII. The process was studied in two ways - kinetic parameters for triolein hydrolysis by lipoprotein lipase with substrates consisting of well-defined apoprotein-triolein complexes were determined. Secondly, the question was persued if there is any region of the apoprotein CII molecule which preferentially sticks into the aqueous layer and could thus come into contact with the enzyme molecule. And finally, lipo-protein lipase and hepatic triglyceride lipase activity was analyzed in various metabolic disorders. Again, the results of these studies may help to better un-derstand the physiological role of LPL and H-TGL in normal and abnormal plasma lipoprotein metabolism.

Function of H-TGL

The aim of this investigation was to verify that specific inhibition of hepatic triglyceride lipase in the plasma compartment with an anti-H-TGL serum would indeed affect triglyceride removal. Hepatic triglyceride lipase was purified from rat liver tissue by heparin sepharose affinity chromatography. Disc gel electrophoresis of the purified enzyme in the presence of sodium dodecylsulfate exhibited a single major component. The purified rat H-TGL then exhibited the properties previously described for this enzyme. The material obtained through this purification procedure was then used for antibody production in rabbit. Rabbits were immunized several times with rat H-TGL. The immunization sched-ule consisted of a bi-weekly to monthly injection of 100 to 200 µg of enzyme protein in the scapular regions of rabbits over a period of several months. Anti-serum was obtained and gamma globulins were isolated. These gamma globulins were further purified by means of immunadsorption on sepharose with covalently linked purified rat H-TGL which contained specific antirat H-TGL rabbit gamma globulin. For the present studies, sera from one single rabbit were utilized. The inhibition of rat H-TGL with antibodies was both studied in vitro and in vivo. Increasing amounts of antirat H-TGL were incubated with rat liver homo-genate. After incubation the tubes were centrifuged and enzymatic activity was determined in the supernatant. As shown on Fig. 1 almost total inhibition of rat liver lipase could be demonstrated.

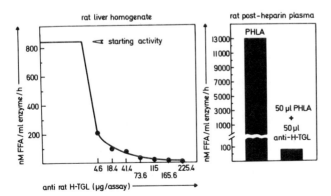

Fig. 1. Inhibition of rat H-TGL with antibodies in vitro.

Similar experiments were performed with rat postheparin plasma. The addition of 50 μl of anti-H-TGL to 50 μl of PHLA led to the inhibition of plasma H-TGL, the remaining activity being lipoprotein lipase activity. It should be pointed out at this time that rats fed with a normal diet only show little lipoprotein lipase activity while the majority of lipases is due to hepatic lipase. The selective inhibition of the postheparin plasma lipase activity with our antibodies could again be shown by the addition of increasing amounts of antibodies which caused almost complete inhibition of hepatic lipase while lipoprotein lipase essentially remained constant. Parallel incubations were carried out with control rabbit gamma globulins which had no effect on either H-TGL or LPL activity.

The following experimental design was used to study the effect of antibody injection in vivo. Two catheters were placed in the femoral vein and artery of a rat. The catheters were then inserted under the skin of the rodent so that the rat could not bite the polyethylene catheters for the long-term experiment. Animals were fasted 14 hours before the experiment. Anti-H-TGL was injected and blood was drawn at various time intervals for determination of triglycerides, cholesterol and phospholipids in both whole serum and isolated lipoproteins. The administration of anti-H-TGL gamma globulins resulted in a dramatic rise in total plasma triglycerides with a peak at about 4 hrs. after the injection. A constant fall of triglyceride concentration was observed and even after 36 hrs. plasma triglycerides still remained significantly increased. Both cholesterol and phospholipids also gradually increased (Fig. 2).

There was almost no change in cholesterol and phospholipids in VLDL while there was an increase in triglyceride concentration after anti-H-TGL injection due to an increase in VLDL-triglycerides. There was a slight but yet significant increase of the triglyceride moiety in low density lipoproteins with the concurrent peak after 4 hours. One might speculate that this represents some form of an intermediate breakdown product of VLDL - again caused by inhibition of H-TGL in vivo. An interesting effect of HDL composition could be demonstrated with almost no change in HDL-triglyceride composition but a perpetual increase of HDL-phospholipid concentration rather late in the course of the experiment was observed.

A similar observation has recently been made by Kuusi et al. (1979) and we would like to assume that this increase in HDL-phospholipid concentration is due to the block of phospholipase activity which has constantly been shown to be associated with hepatic triglyceride lipase both in man and in animals (Augustin et al. 1978). The same changes in lipoprotein composition following inhibition

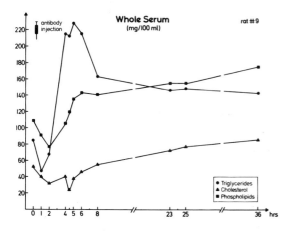

Fig. 2.   Inhibition of H-TGL in vivo.

of hepatic lipase in vivo can be visualized by looking at the lipoprotein pattern on agarose gel electrophoresis. With a peak at about 4 to 4 1/2 hours, the pre-beta lipoproteins dramatically increased and returned only slowly to normal concentrations after 25 to 36 hours. An increase in the lipid staining of alpha-lipoproteins is seen rather late during the course of the experiments with a peak at about 25 to 36 hours.

This study documents the ability of liver tissue lipase to induce antibodies in rabbit. The inhibition of triglyceride removal in vivo by antiserum prepared against hepatic triglyceride lipase demonstrates that this enzyme together with lipoprotein lipase is responsible in vivo for the catabolism of VLDL triglyceride. The blocking of triglyeride removal, which did not occur instantaneously, may lead to various speculations with regard to the site of action of hepatic lipase either in tissue or the plasma compartment. With an intact lipoprotein lipase enzyme in these in vivo systems, probably triglyceride hydrolysis begins in a normal fashion. The blockage of hepatic lipase then leads to an increase of plasma triglycerides later in the VLDL-IDL-LDL pathway probably not in plasma but in the liver. Further analyses, specially of the apoprotein composition of these particles are certainly required and are presently performed in our laboratory.

Purification of LPL

I would now like to report on experiments carried out in our laboratory aimed at the further purification of plasma lipoprotein lipase. Augustin and Brown (1978) have reported that amino acid composition, terminal amino acids and tryptide peptide mapping are similar for LPL and H-TGL with the main differences being in the carbohydrate moiety. Östlund-Lindqvist (1978) (personal communication), however, have recently demonstrated significant differences in amino acid composition between H-TGL and LPL. The purification procedure in their experiments included affinity chromatography on heparin sepharose with low affinity for antithrombin and SDS-polyacrylamide gel electrophoresis. Antithrombin was shown to be a major contamination in all lipoprotein lipase purification procedures. Experiments therefore were carried out in our laboratory to find a method which allows separation of antithrombin III from the enzyme after the usual heparin sepharose affinity chromatography and to stabilize the purified enzyme in a way to allow enzymatic measurement in the final purified stage. Lipoprotein lipase purification from postheparin plasma was started in the usual way by applying heparin sepharose affinity chromatography. The eluate from this column was then concentrated by pressure dialysis in the presence of 0.1 % Triton X-100 . The addition of this non-ionic detergent at this precise concentration stabilized the enzyme. As an additional purification procedure gel filtration on Biogel A-5M was introduced. A typical elution pattern is shown on Fig. 3.

LPL eluted with a sharp peak immediately after the void volume and could thus be easily separated from antithrombin III. This can be seen by gel electrophoresis with different systems either in Tris glycin buffer or in an SDS gel system. The advantage of the Tris glycin buffer system without SDS was to allow enzymatic measurement after gel electrophoresis. The gel reveals that contaminating proteins migrate near the top of the gel, and it also shows that the yield of purified lipoprotein lipase is extremely low. We would estimate that we can probably isolate about 10 μg of purified lipase from 1 l of postheparin plasma. In terms of protein measurement postheparin plasma at least in humans contains much more hepatic triglyceride lipase than lipoprotein lipase. Experiments therefore aimed to compare H-TGL and LPL with regard to their amino acid or carbohydrate composition are exceedingly difficult to perform if one starts with

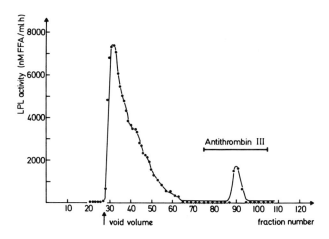

Fig. 3. Gel filtration on biogel A-5-m (buffer: 5mM Na-barbital, 0.1% Triton X 100).

postheparin plasma as enzyme source. The question of the protein identity or non-identity of these two plasma enzymes therefore still remains unresolved.

CII Activation

One of most interesting differences between the two enzymes certainly is the fact that lipoprotein lipase requires a protein as cofactor for full activity whereas hepatic triglyceride lipase does not. The mechanism of CII-activation for LPL therefore is of particular interest and may help to evaluate the precise functional role of these enzymes in triglyceride catabolism. In order to study this interaction we prepared highly purified C-apoproteins and plasma lipoprotein lipase as just outlined. Human plasma VLDL apolipoproteins CI, CII and CIII were recombined in vitro with triolein in the absence of phospholipids or detergents. The lipid protein complexes were analyzed by ultracentrifugal floation, agarose gel electrophoresis, immunoelectrophoresis, and electron microscopy. I will now focus exclusively on the CII-triolein complexes. On agarose gel electrophoresis the apoprotein-triolein complexes migrated in alpha-position faster than chylomicrons, VLDL and even the free C-apoproteins. Apo CII-triolein complexes tested against antiapo CII by immunelectrophoresis show a precipitation line in the same position. Electronmicrographs of negatively stained apo CII-triolein emulsion exhibited spherical particles. Their diameters varied between 200 and 2,000 Å. The distribution of the particle size seem to depend on the time of sonication, the apoprotein-triolein ratios as well as the apoprotein species. With high protein-triglyceride ratios relatively homogeneous lipoprotein populations were obtained rather similar to normal VLDL.

Two sets of experiments were performed in order to evaluate the particular CII-LPL activating mechanisms. First the question was asked if there is any region on the apoprotein CII molecule which preferentially sticks into the aqueous layer and could thus come into contact with the enzyme molecule. If this question would be answered positively, it should be possible to form cross-links between the enzyme and the apoproteins within the complex. Secondly, kinetics of triolein hydrolysis were studied using these artificial lipoprotein substrates with different apoprotein-triolein ratios. The analyses of the kinetic parameters V_{max} and K_m then should also provide information as to the particular mechanism of CII-LPL activation.

CII Structure

In analogy to previous experiments performed by Stoffel and Preissner (1979) for reconstituted apolipoprotein AII with phosphatidylcholine and lysophosphatidylcholine, which was covalently linked to the imidoester groups of a polystyrene resin, similar experiments were performed employing these artificial CII-triolein complexes. In order to bind only those lysine residues of apoprotein CII protruding from the surface of the lipoprotein complex, the reactive imidoester groups of the solid phase resin should not extend too far from the solid phase matrix. The imidoester resin and the reconstituted apo CII particles were allowed to react and the products were then delipidated with chloroform-methanol. Thermolysine hydrolysis removed long parts of the apo CII sequence except for those peptides linked to the resin. These peptides were cleaved from the resin and separated by fingerprint analysis. Parallel experiments were performed with apo CIII. The fingerprint analysis revealed four peptides which were eluted and analyzed for their amino acid composition. These correspond to positions No. 1-3, 22-30, 74-76 and 71-76 in the sequence of apo CII. The cross-linked lysine residues were those in position 29 and 75. Peptide No. 1 corresponded to the amino terminal group of apo CII. In accord with experiments performed by Dr. Gotto's group here in Houston we would like to interpret our results as follows: As has been shown previously apo CII contains different sites for lipid binding and enzyme interaction. The analysis of resin-bound peptides leads to the assumption that the protein chain regions around the assigned lysine residues are protruding from the surface of the lipoprotein complex. Lysine No. 29 and the amino terminal end was found in a region where phospholipid binding with apo CII has been postulated. However, lysine No. 75 was found in a region where CII enzyme interaction had previously been expected to occur (Fig. 4).

Kinetics

We then used another approach to understand apo CII-activation of lipoprotein lipase. Kinetics of triolein hydrolysis by purified plasma lipoprotein lipase was studied with the artificial apo CII-triolein complex with different apoprotein-triolein ratios. Sonication of the triolein substrate together with albumin in the

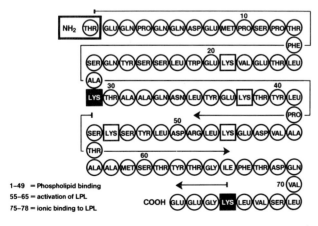

1-49 = Phospholipid binding
55-65 = activation of LPL
75-78 = ionic binding to LPL

Fig. 4. Functional regions on apo CII.

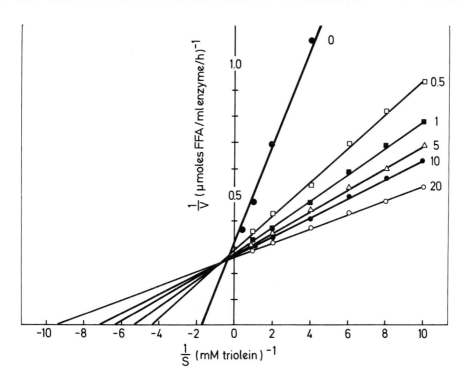

Fig. 5.

absence of apo CII resulted in near complete inhibition of triglyceride lipase activity. Double reciprocal plots, $\frac{1}{v}$ versus $\frac{1}{s}$, resulted in straight lines indicating that the hydrolytic reaction followed Michaelis-Menten's kinetics. The kinetic parameters V_{max} and apparrent K_m were calculated from the axial intercepts of the Lineweaver-Burke plot. The apparent K_m decreased significantly with increasing apo CII-triolein ratios with almost no change in V_{max} (Fig. 5).

When substrates containing apo CII were incubated with anti-apo CII rabbit gamma globulins prior to the hydrolysis by LPL the decreasing effect on the apparent K_m was reversed. Digestion with trypsin also reversed apparent K_m.

Based on these experiments we would like to propose the following molecular mechanism for apo CII-triolein-lipoprotein lipase interaction. We would suggest that the affinity of lipoprotein lipase with the lipid-water interface is increased by its cofactor. Apo CII may not only have binding sites for triglycerides and phospholipids but also sites which interact with the enzyme protein thus supporting the proper orientation of the enzyme. Apo CII may act as a specific receptor for chylomicrons and VLDL for lipoprotein lipase at the capillary endothelium (Schrecker and Greten 1979).

Clinical Studies

In the remaining part of this lecture I would like to report on clinical studies. In these studies the analysis of lipoprotein lipase and hepatic lipase activities was performed in various metabolic disorders and following drug treatment. With methods available to distinguish between LPL and H-TGL based on enzyme antibody precipitation, interesting results have been obtained which suggest possible specificity of function of these enzymes in lipoprotein metabolism. When specific measurement of these enzymes was applied to the study of hypertriglyceridemia it was found that patients with type I lipoprotein pattern have extremely low LPL levels with normal values for H-TGL. Many of the patients with a type V lipoprotein pattern also have extremely low LPL levels with normal H-TGL-activity which may suggest a common pathogenetic mechanism for these two groups of patients; it also implies heterogeneity among patients with type V hyperlipidemia. Normal heparin released lipases were found in patients with floating beta-lipoproteinemia as they were in patients with familial LCAT-deficiency. To investigate the pathogenesis of hypertriglyceridemia in patients with renal disease, we measured plasma lipoprotein composition as well as hepatic triglyceride- and lipoprotein lipase in three groups with renal disease namely conservatively treated chronic uremia, patients undergoing maintenance hemodialysis and in renal allograft recipients. A selective decrease of hepatic triglyceride lipase with normal lipoprotein lipase was found in conservatively treated uremia and in patients undergoing hemodialysis (Mordasini et al. 1977). These patients also had elevated levels of VLDL and increased triglycerides in LDL. In contrast, hepatic TGL and LPL were both normal in patients after renal transplantation when they actually tend to show hypercholesterolemia with increased LDL-cholesterol and decreased HDL-cholesterol. It is tempting to speculate that the accumulation of triglyceride-rich LDL, as observed in the majority of patients with renal failure, is a consequence of the demonstrated low H-TGL-activity in these patients. The demonstration of normal extrahepatic lipoprotein lipase in these patients may then imply that the conversion of intermediate lipoproteins to LDL occurs in the liver (Klose et al. 1977). Hypertriglyceridemia occurring in patients with liver disease has also been studied by measuring H-TGL and plasma LPL together with the determination of lecithin-cholesterol-acyltransferase. In general it is seen that total PHLA decreases with the severity of liver dysfunction. This decrease is mainly due to low H-TGL and only to some degree to low LPL-activity. H-TGL-activity in patients with different forms of liver disease, namely acute hepatitis, chronic hepatitis and cirrhosis of the liver was low both for men and women these values are low compared to normal controls. Recently a large study was initiated in our clinic to evaluate the relationship between pancreatitis and hypertriglyceridemia. A prospective clinical trial with more than 30 patients was begun. Normal healthy volunteers as well as heavy alcohol drinkers who had not yet abnormal liver function tests or any symptoms of pancreatitis served as controls. Without elaborating on the details of the design some of the more interesting results of this clinical trial should be mentioned. Lipoprotein composition and lipolytic measurement in pancreatitis and after heavy alcohol abuse were as follows: Most of the patients who were admitted to the hospital because of acute and relapsing pancreatitis showed an elevation of VLDL-triglyceride. This was also true for most of the alcoholics. However triglycerides in LDL were usually normal in alcoholics contrary to those with pancreatitis. Another noteworthy finding was the decreased HDL-cholesterol and decreased apo AI concentration in all patients with pancreatitis. While this was a consistent finding in all our patients with pancreatitis, heavy alcohol drinkers either had normal or slightly elevated HDL-cholesterol levels while their apo AI concentration usually were normal. The possible cause, at least for the observed hypertriglyceridemia in pancreatitis, were low H-TGL and LPL in the majority of patients, while both enzymes were normal in the group of alcoholics. If one looks at the change of lipoprotein abnormalities and plasma enzymes from admission to recovery, it can be seen that most of the abnormalities returned to normal with a decrease of triglycerides in VLDL, an increase in HDL-cholesterol and apo AI concentration in patients with pancreatitis and the normalization of both lipolytic enzymes (Fig. 6).

Differences in LPL and H-TGL activity in other clinical disorders have been reported by other investigators, and diverse effects of various hormones and drugs on human H-TGL and LPL have also been reported. In summary these clinical and pharmacological studies performed in our laboratory as well as in

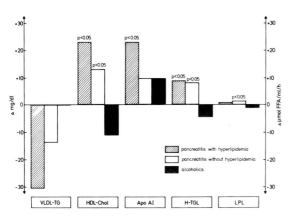

Fig. 6. Change of lipoprotein abnormalities and plasma lipolytic enzymes from admission to recovery.

others have demonstrated selective deficiency of either hepatic lipase or lipoprotein lipase in parallel with increased lipoprotein triglyceride concentration.

Summary

The pathogenesis of lipid disorders accompanied by hypertriglyceridemia or
hypercholesterolemia has not been completely elucidated yet. The clinical
relevance of these metabolic diseases to coronary heart disease, peripheral
occlusive atherosclerotic disease, cerebral vascular disease and gastroentero-
logic manifestations has been documented. The purpose of this lecture was to
summarize new information available both on the molecular properties and the
clinical relevance of plasma lipolytic enzymes. I tried to cover four distinct
aspects of enzyme research which were of particular interest to us. These were
the functional role of hepatic lipase. We used specific antibody injection in
animal experiments to learn more about the precise role of this enzyme in vivo.
I briefly covered some of the problems that are encountered when purifying lipoprotein lipase from human postheparin plasma. I reported on experiments relating to the mechanism of apo CII activation of LPL involving both structural analysis of apo CII as well as kinetic analysis of the enzyme reaction. And I summarized some of the clinical studies that we performed recently.

References

Augustin J, Greten H (1979) The role of lipoprotein lipase – molecular properties and clinical relevance. Atherosclerosis Rev 5: 91–124

Augustin J., Greten H (1979) Hepatic triglyceride in tissue and plasma.
Prog biochem Pharmacol 15: 5–40

Augustin J, Freeze H, Tejada P, Brown WV (1978) A comparison of molecular
properties of hepatic triglyceride lipase and lipoprotein lipase from human
postheparin plasma. J Biol Chem 253: 2912–2920

Klose G, Windelband J, Weizel A, Greten H (1977) Secondary hypertri-glyceridaemia in patients with parenchymal liver disease. Europ J Clin Invest 7: 557–652

Kuusi T, Kinnunen PKJ, Nikkilä E (1979) Hepatic endothelium lipase antiserum influences rat plasma low and high density lipoproteins in vivo. FEBS Letters 104,2: 384–388

Mordasini R, Frey F, Flury W, Klose G, Greten H (1977) Selective deficiency of hepatic triglyceride lipase in uremic patients. New Engl J Med 297: 1362–1366

Schrecker O, Greten H (1979) Activation and inhibition of lipoprotein lipase – Studies with artificial lipoproteins. Biochim Biophys Acta 572: 244–256

Stoffel W, Preissner K (1979) Surface localisation of apolipoprotein AII in lipoprotein complexes. Hoppe-Seyler's Z Phys Chem 360: 685–690

Tall AR, Small DM (1978) Plasma high density lipoprotein. New Engl J Med 299: 1232–1236

Cholesterol Feeding: Effects on Lipoprotein Structure and Metabolism

Robert W. Mahley

The consumption of diets high in cholesterol and fat produces marked changes in plasma lipoproteins. Comparative studies of a variety of species have revealed that certain of these changes in lipoproteins are consistent among the species (for review, see Mahley 1978). Alterations in canine lipoproteins are the most dramatic changes induced in any species and highlight changes which span a spectrum of other species, including man (Mahley et al. 1974, 1975, 1976b, 1977b, 1978a; Mahley and Holcombe 1977). It is the purpose of this paper to describe the cholesterol-induced changes in canine lipoproteins and to describe how these lipoproteins interact, in vitro and in vivo, with a variety of cells which are potentially important in the development of accelerated atherosclerosis.

Alterations in Plasma Lipoproteins Associated with Atherosclerosis

Canine plasma lipoproteins and the changes induced by high fat, high cholesterol diets can be appreciated by comparing the lipoprotein electrophoretic patterns (FIG. 1). The electrophoretic pattern of the lipoproteins (top pattern) of a control, chow-fed dog with a plasma cholesterol level of 120 mg/dl is contrasted with the patterns for 4 cholesterol-fed dogs (the cholesterol levels for the hypercholesterolemic dogs are indicated on the individual electrophoretograms in FIG. 1). Before the lipoproteins are described, a few comments regarding canine atherosclerosis are appropriate. Dogs do not spontaneously or naturally develop any proliferative or lipid-laden arterial lesions which could be called atherosclerosis. Canine atherosclerosis develops only if the plasma cholesterol levels are maintained at levels in excess of 750 mg/dl for longer than 4 months (Mahley et al. 1974, 1977b). Such animals develop extensive and severe atherosclerosis and are referred to as hyperresponders (hyper, FIG. 1). Hyporesponders, with plasma cholesterol levels of 350 – 650 mg/dl, do not develop atherosclerosis even after 1 or 2 years at these high cholesterol levels (hypo, FIG. 1).

In an attempt to understand why plasma cholesterol levels of less than 750 mg/dl are non-atherogenic whereas levels in excess of 750 mg/dl are atherogenic, we studied in detail the changes in the plasma lipoproteins. The lipoproteins of a normal dog include the low density lipoproteins (LDL), which are similar to LDL in man, and two α-migrating lipoproteins referred to as high density lipoproteins (HDL_1 and HDL_2)(FIG. 1). The HDL_2 are similar to the 80 – 100 Å, A-I/A-II apoprotein-rich HDL of man. The HDL_1 and HDL_2 are referred to as high density lipoproteins, regardless of the actual density at which they float, because they contain the A-I apoprotein and lack the B apoprotein (Mahley and Weisgraber 1974; Mahley et al. 1978b). Lipoproteins equivalent to canine HDL_1 and HDL_2 have been described in rats (Weisgraber et al. 1977), swine (Reitman and Mahley 1979), and man (Mahley et al. 1978b; Innerarity et al. 1978). Dogs also have very low density lipoproteins (VLDL) but they are present in such low concentrations that they are not seen on the electrophoretic patterns.

When the plasma cholesterol is elevated to the 350 – 650 mg/dl range (hypore-sponders with non-atherogenic hyperlipidemia), the increased plasma choles-terol is transported by α_2-migrating lipoproteins similar to the HDL_1 of control dogs (FIG. 1). Since some of their properties change with cholesterol feeding, the lipoproteins have been referred to as HDL_c (the subscript c indicating that they are cholesterol-induced) to distinguish them from the HDL_1 of dogs on control diets (Mahley 1978; Mahley et al. 1974, 1977b). The cholesterol-induced HDL_c become more cholesterol-rich, float at lower densi-ties, and develop altered apoprotein contents. At progressively higher levels of plasma cholesterol, the HDL_c contain less apo-A-I and more of the arginine-rich apoprotein (apo-E). In fact, in dogs with plasma cholesterol levels in excess of 700 – 800 mg/dl, a subclass of HDL_c which contains only the apo-E can be isolated (Mahley et al. 1977b). In addition, the LDL of the hyporesponders increase as the plasma cholesterol increases.

The dogs which develop atherosclerosis (hyperresponders with plasma choles-terol levels greater than 750 mg/dl) have more complicated electrophoretic patterns which are characterized by the presence of a broad β band (hyper, FIG. 1). The prominence of the β band is accounted for by an increase in LDL and by the appearance of a β-migrating lipoprotein in the d < 1.006 ultra-centrifugal fraction, a fraction that normally contains only pre-β VLDL (Mah-ley et al. 1974, 1977b). This β-migrating lipoprotein, B-VLDL, is similar to a lipoprotein found in patients with Type III hyperlipoproteinemia. A notable characteristic of the B-VLDL both of Type III patients (Havel and Kane 1973) and of cholesterol-fed dogs (Mahley et al. 1977b) is a prominence of the arginine-rich apoprotein, along with apo-B, and a high cholesteryl ester content. The electrophoretic patterns of the hyperresponders also show that the HDL_c remain prominent and typical HDL (HDL_2) decrease. However, the major difference between non-atherogenic and atherogenic hypercholesterolemia is the occurrence of B-VLDL. We will return to this point later.

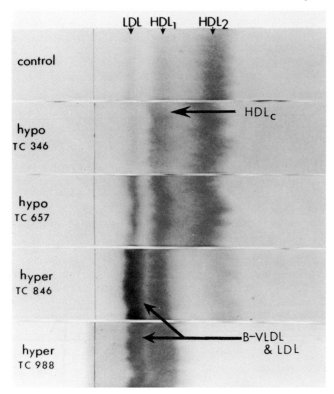

FIG. 1. Paper electro-phoretograms of the plasma lipoproteins of a control dog (top strip) and four different cho-lesterol-fed dogs with variable degrees of hy-percholesterolemia (TC = total plasma cholesterol in mg/dl). Canine hyper-cholesterolemia is pro-duced by feeding a semi-synthetic diet contain-ing coconut oil and cho-lesterol (Mahley et al. 1977b) or by feeding a high fat, high choles-terol diet to a thyroid-ectomized animal (Mahley et al. 1974). Similar results are obtained with either protocol. Reproduced with permis-sion of the American Heart Association, Inc. from Mahley et al., 1974.

The distribution of the plasma cholesterol among the various lipoproteins reflects the striking differences between non-atherogenic and atherogenic hypercholesterolemia (Mahley et al. 1974). In the control dog, >70% of the total plasma cholesterol is carried by typical HDL (HDL_2). In hyporesponders with non-atherogenic hypercholesterolemia, usually >50% of the plasma cholesterol is in the d = 1.006 – 1.063 ultracentrifugal fraction containing the LDL and HDL_c. By contrast, in hyperresponders with atherogenic hypercholesterolemia, as much as 50 to 70% of the total plasma cholesterol is carried by the d < 1.006 ultracentrifugal fraction (Mahley et al. 1974). This fraction contains principally the B-VLDL (∼90% B-VLDL, 10% pre-β VLDL).

Similar changes in the plasma lipoproteins following high cholesterol, high fat diets occur to a greater or lesser extent in other animals, including rats (Mahley and Holcombe 1977), swine (Mahley et al. 1975) and Patas monkeys (Mahley et al. 1976b). The changes include the occurrence of B-VLDL, an increase in LDL, and the appearance of HDL_c. Recently, we have demonstrated that HDL_c also occur in man after the consumption of high cholesterol diets (Mahley et al. 1978a). Thus, the changes in the canine lipoproteins resemble those of higher species more closely than previously realized.

Canine atherosclerosis likewise resembles human atherosclerosis in certain aspects (for review, see Mahley 1979). The terminal abdominal aorta and coronary arteries of the hyperresponders are often severely involved with complicated atherosclerosis. Small peripheral arteries are also involved under certain dietary conditions (Mahley et al. 1976a, 1977b; Mahley 1979). In some locations, such as the terminal aorta, the atherosclerosis is histologically very similar to human atherosclerosis. There is a marked intimal proliferative reaction with a fibrous cap, and deposits of intracellular and extracellular lipid can be extensive (FIG. 2a). The cells which accumulate the lipid, principally cholesterol, are difficult to identify and may be

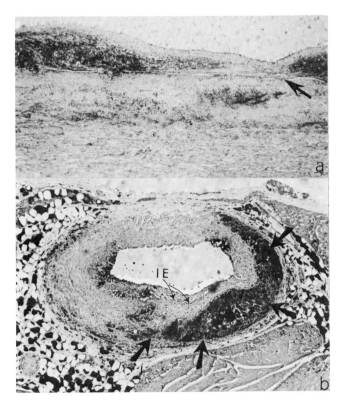

FIG. 2a and 2b. (a) Section of the ventral abdominal aorta from a coconut oil cholesterol-fed dog (top). This demonstrates an intimal proliferative atherosclerotic lesion with lipid deposition. The internal elastica is indicated by an arrow (oil red O stained, X 70). (b) Cross section of the anterior descending coronary artery from the same animal (bottom). Note the extensive medial deposition of lipid on the right side of the vessel (arrows). The internal elastica is indicated (IE). An intimal proliferative lesion occurs on the left (oil red O stained, X 55). Reproduced with permission from Mahley et al. 1977.

smooth muscle cells or mononuclear foam cells such as macrophages. In other sites, the atherosclerosis is unlike the typical human disease in that the media of the artery is severely involved, with little or no intimal reaction (FIG. 2b). The medial disease is characterized by accumulation of large amounts of intracellular lipid in mononuclear foam cells. Many of these cells may be monocytes or macrophages (Mahley 1979; Mahley et al. 1977b). Previously, Geer (1965) described the histologic characteristics of canine atherosclerosis and stressed the probable role of monocytes in lipid accumulation.

Consideration of the types of lipoproteins associated with accelerated atherosclerosis and the types of cells which might accumulate the cholesterol led us to study how two different cells - smooth muscle cells and macrophages in culture - responded to the various lipoproteins. With respect to the binding, internalization, and degradation of the lipoproteins, we have found that smooth muscle cells and fibroblasts behave similarly. For that reason, most of the studies to be reported were actually performed in detail with cultured human fibroblasts and confirmed in smooth muscle cells.

Plasma Lipoprotein Interaction with Smooth Muscle Cells and Fibroblasts

A few years ago, the eloquent work of Drs. Goldstein, Brown, and coworkers established that there was a specific high affinity receptor site for LDL on the cell surface of cultured fibroblasts (Brown et al. 1976; Goldstein and Brown 1977; Brown and Goldstein 1979). They showed that the binding of LDL initiates a series of intracellular events including internalization of the LDL, degradation of the lipoprotein, and regulation of intracellular cholesterol metabolism. Cholesterol synthesis is inhibited by suppression of HMG-CoA reductase activity, and cholesteryl ester synthesis is increased by stimulation of the acyl-CoA:cholesterol acyltransferase activity. The number of cell surface receptors is regulated by the requirement of the cell for more or less cellular cholesterol.

Our studies were designed to determine how these cells respond to the various cholesterol-induced lipoproteins and to gain an understanding of the properties of the lipoproteins responsible for their interaction with the receptors. We found that the apo-B-containing lipoproteins (LDL, B-VLDL) and the apo-E-containing lipoproteins (HDL_1, HDL_c) both bind to the same cell surface receptors and regulate intracellular cholesterol metabolism in fibroblasts (Mahley et al. 1977a; Innerarity and Mahley 1978; Mahley and Innerarity 1978; Weisgraber et al. 1978). Comparing the metabolism of the apo-B-containing LDL and apo-E HDL_c proved highly useful in establishing the validity of the above-mentioned conclusions.

The LDL and HDL_c are approximately the same size (200 Å in diameter) and are both cholesteryl ester-rich. However, they are distinctly different with respect to their protein contents. The LDL contain primarily or exclusively the B apoprotein. The HDL_c lack the B apoprotein and contain the A-I and the arginine-rich (E) apoproteins. In some cases, HDL_c contain only the E apoprotein (referred to as apo-E HDL_c). With these lipoproteins, it was possible to establish that the determinants responsible for binding were the protein moieties and that either B- or E-containing lipoproteins could bind to the cell surface receptors (the apo-B,E receptors) (Mahley and Innerarity 1978;

644

Mahley et al. 1977a; Weisgraber et al. 1978). Lipoproteins which lack the B or E apoprotein (such as HDL$_3$ of man) do not bind to the high affinity receptor site.

These conclusions have been supported by our use of selective chemical modifications of specific amino acid residues of apo-E or apo-B. Modification of a limited number of arginine (Mahley et al. 1977a) or lysine (Weisgraber et al. 1978) residues totally prevents the LDL or HDL$_c$ from interacting with the cell surface receptors of fibroblasts. Arginine residues were modified with 1,2 - cyclohexanedione, a useful procedure because it is very mild and can be quantitatively reversed. Lysine residues were modified by a variety of procedures including acetoacetylation, carbamylation, and reductive methylation. For example, modification of 20% or more of the lysine residues of LDL by reductive methylation prevented the binding, internalization, and degradation of the LDL by fibroblasts (Weisgraber et al. 1978) or smooth muscle cells (Mahley et al. unpublished data).

The selective modifications were helpful not only in determining the roles of apo-B and apo-E in the receptor interaction, but also in establishing a functional role for the cell surface receptors in lipoprotein metabolism in vivo. Our hypothesis was that if a modification prevented the LDL from interacting with the cell surface receptors in vitro, then a retarded clearance of modified LDL from the plasma after intravenous injection would reflect an interference in the receptor-mediated catabolism of LDL in vivo. As predicted, when reductively methylated LDL were injected into rats or monkeys, the clearance of these lipoproteins from the plasma was retarded (Mahley et al. 1979). As shown in FIG. 3., when rat LDL were injected into rats, the t$_{\frac{1}{2}}$ for the reductively methylated LDL was 7 hr vs. 4.7 hr for control LDL. Likewise, the methylated LDL had a smaller fractional catabolic rate than control LDL (0.133 vs. 0.256). If it is correct to postulate that methylation interferes with the receptor-mediated process, as in the in vitro studies, then one can conclude that ∿50% of LDL clearance in the rat occurs by this receptor-mediated uptake process, in vivo.

The situation is the same for the monkey. The clearance of reductively methylated human LDL from the plasma of rhesus monkeys was retarded (FIG. 4). As in the rat, approximately 50% of the LDL appeared to be cleared by the receptor-mediated uptake process (Mahley et al. 1979).

The studies with fibroblasts and smooth muscle cells have provided important information. Lipoproteins containing the B or E apoproteins are bound, internalized, and degraded via the same receptor-mediated process. All the cholesterol-rich lipoproteins -- B-VLDL, LDL, and HDL$_c$ -- interact with the cell surface receptors and regulate intracellular metabolism. Furthermore, support for the physiologic significance of the receptor-mediated process in vivo was obtained using the methylated LDL. Nonetheless, it is difficult to explain atherosclerosis on the basis of these results. The receptor-mediated uptake process is subject to feedback control. Fibroblasts and smooth muscle cells will accumulate only a limited amount of cholesterol before receptor synthesis is inhibited. The existence of a cell type or subpopulation of cells capable of unregulated uptake or accumulation of cholesterol-rich lipoproteins is necessary to explain foam cell formation. Such a role has been postulated for a "scavenger cell system" (Goldstein and Brown 1977). A possible mechanism whereby unregulated cholesterol accumulation may occur in smooth muscle cells will be discussed below (see Summary).

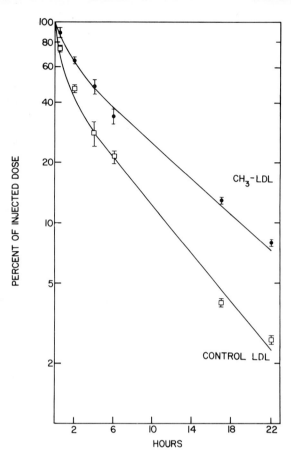

FIG. 3. Percent of the total injected dose of control rat ^{131}I-LDL (□) and reductively methylated rat ^{125}I-LDL (CH$_3$-LDL, ●) which remained in the plasma after intravenous injection into rats. The means ± SD (bar) represent values obtained in 3 rats by dual isotope counting at each time point. Approximately 95% of the lysine residues of the LDL were modified. Each rat received 20 μg of control and methylated LDL protein. Modified from Mahley et al. (1979c).

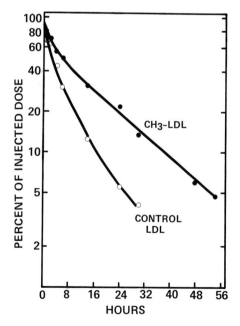

FIG. 4. Percent of the total injected dose of control human ^{131}I-LDL (o) and methylated human ^{125}I-LDL (CH$_3$-LDL, ●) which remained in the plasma of a Rhesus monkey after 500 μg of each lipoprotein had been simultaneously injected. The methylated LDL had 90% of the total lysine residues modified. Modified from Mahley et al. (1979c).

646

The possibility that the foam cells (at least in canine atherosclerosis) are macrophages prompted us to determine the types of lipoproteins taken up and degraded by macrophages. We had observed that acetoacetylation of a limited number of lysine residues of LDL caused these lipoproteins to be rapidly cleared from the plasma (Mahley et al. 1979a, 1979b). Within 5 to 10 minutes after intravenous injection of the acetoacetylated LDL into rats (Mahley et al. 1979b) or dogs (Mahley et al. 1979a), 90 to 95% of the modified LDL is removed from the plasma and approximately 90% is accounted for in the liver. It has been established that the reticuloendothelial cells of the liver (Kupffer cells) are responsible for the uptake and degradation of the modified LDL (Mahley et al. 1979b). Furthermore, when the acetoacetylated LDL are incubated with canine peritoneal macrophages, they are taken up and degraded (Mahley et al. 1979a). As shown in FIG. 5., several-fold more acetoacetylated LDL than normal LDL are degraded by macrophages. Normal LDL are only very minimally degraded. These data agree with the recent studies reported by Goldstein et al. (1979) who demonstrated that mouse peritoneal macrophages are capable of taking up and degrading acetylated human LDL. They presented evidence which indicates that macrophages have receptor sites for the acetylated LDL but not for normal LDL. It is important to consider whether such a mechanism could ever be responsible for clearance of lipoproteins, and whether modifications such as acetoacetylation occur in the plasma or in the artery wall and trigger uptake of modified lipoproteins by tissue macrophages. Such a hypothesis remains to be tested.

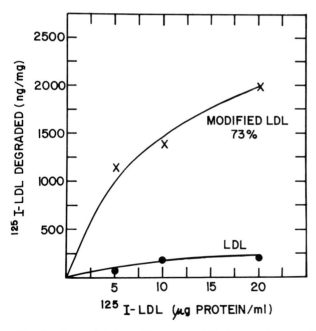

FIG. 5. Degradation of canine LDL by canine peritoneal macrophages. Control ^{125}I-LDL (●) were compared with acetoacetoacetylated ^{125}I-LDL (x, 73% of the lysine residues modified). From Mahley et al. (1979a).

In collaborative studies conducted with Drs. Goldstein, Ho, and Brown, we have investigated the possibility that there are naturally occurring lipoproteins in normal or cholesterol-fed animals which are taken up and degraded by peritoneal macrophages (Goldstein et al. 1980). We have found that the synthesis and accumulation of cholesteryl esters by macrophages is stimulated 20 - to 160 - fold by B-VLDL from cholesterol-fed dogs. Other lipoproteins from normal or cholesterol-fed dogs, including LDL and HDL$_c$, had little or no effect on cholesteryl ester synthesis or content in macrophages.

Macrophages have been shown to possess a high affinity receptor that recognizes B-VLDL. Receptor-mediated uptake of these lipoproteins leads to cholesteryl ester accumulation in the macrophages (Goldstein et al. 1980). Incubation of the macrophages at 37°C for 21 hr with up to 350 μg/ml of d < 1.006 lipoprotein cholesterol in the media results in a progressive accumulation of cellular cholesteryl esters up to 141 μg of sterol/mg of cell protein (Table 1). By contrast, incubation of canine and swine smooth muscle cells (Mahley et al. 1977b) or human fibroblasts (Brown et al. 1975) with high levels of lipoprotein cholesterol do not result in the accumulation of cholesteryl esters in excess of 50 μg of sterol/mg of protein.

Table 1. Accumulation of cholesteryl esters by macrophages incubated with d < 1.006 (B-VLDL) lipoproteins from a hypercholesterolemic dog.[a]

Prior Treatment	Concentration of Lipoprotein (μg chol/ml)	Cellular Content (μg sterol/mg protein)
None	0	1.0
B-VLDL	35	6.8
B-VLDL	105	51.0
B-VLDL	305	141.0

[a]Each monolayer was incubated at 37°C for 21 hr with B-VLDL or without addition of lipoprotein for measurement of esterified cholesterol content.

FIG. 6 compares the ability of normal canine VLDL and the ability of hypercholesterolemic d < 1.006 (containing primarily B-VLDL) to stimulate cholesteryl ester formation in monolayers of mouse peritoneal macrophages. The hypercholesterolemic d < 1.006 (B-VLDL) fraction is much more potent. Oleate incorporation into cellular cholesteryl esters is a measure of the lipoprotein cholesterol which is re-esterified after the uptake and degradation of the B-VLDL (Goldstein et al. 1980).

The B-VLDL and the pre-β migrating VLDL from the hypercholesterolemic dog can be isolated by Geon-Pevikon block electrophoresis. The B-VLDL and the cholesterol-rich VLDL are both potent (FIG. 7). Note that the LDL and HDL$_c$ do not significantly stimulate cholesteryl ester synthesis.

The question arises as to whether the cholesteryl ester deposition observed in vitro in macrophages with canine B-VLDL bears any relation to the atherosclerosis induced by cholesterol feeding in dogs. The foam cells that characterize canine atherosclerosis develop only when the plasma cholesterol level exceeds 750 mg/dl, and a major alteration in the plasma lipoprotein pattern which occurs at this cholesterol level is the appearance of B-VLDL as a major cholesterol-carrying lipoprotein. Whether the B-VLDL actually produce the cholesteryl ester deposition in macrophages in the arterial wall remains to be determined.

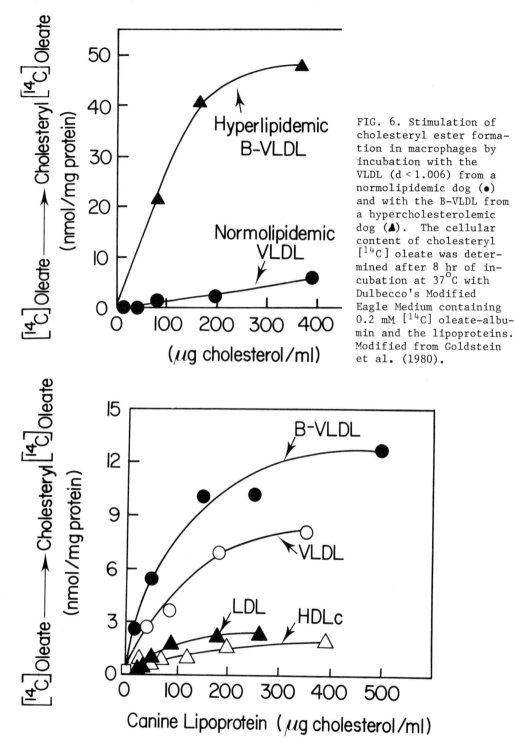

FIG. 6. Stimulation of cholesteryl ester formation in macrophages by incubation with the VLDL (d < 1.006) from a normolipidemic dog (●) and with the B-VLDL from a hypercholesterolemic dog (▲). The cellular content of cholesteryl [^{14}C] oleate was determined after 8 hr of incubation at 37°C with Dulbecco's Modified Eagle Medium containing 0.2 mM [^{14}C] oleate-albumin and the lipoproteins. Modified from Goldstein et al. (1980).

FIG. 7. Stimulation of cholesteryl ester formation in macrophages incubated for 10 hr at 37°C with varying concentrations of lipoproteins from a hyperlipidemic dog. The hypercholesterolemic B-VLDL and VLDL were isolated by block electrophoresis from the d< 1.006 fraction. Modified from Goldstein et al. (1980).

Summary

The roles of the various cholesterol-induced lipoproteins in stimulating cholesteryl ester accumulation in fibroblasts, smooth muscle cells, and macrophages have been reveiwed. It appears that the feedback control of the receptor-mediated uptake process in fibroblasts and smooth muscle cells would prevent conversion of these cells to typical foam cells. However, it can be speculated that arterial wall smooth muscle cells behave differently and are not strictly regulated. It is also possible that the arterial smooth muscle cells develop altered properties (macrophage-like activity) under the stimulus of high levels or abnormal types of lipoproteins. On the other hand, the lipoproteins in the arterial wall may be altered in such a way as to stimulate unregulated cholesterol accumulation. Cationized LDL have been shown to cause the accumulation of cholesteryl esters in cultured smooth muscle cells (Goldstein et al. 1977).

It is intriguing that the macrophage does accumulate large amounts of cholesteryl ester when presented with chemically-modified LDL. Subtle changes in the lipoprotein protein, as occur with acetoacetylation of lysine residues of LDL, profoundly alter the in vitro and in vivo metabolism of these lipoproteins. It remains to be determined if metabolically significant chemical modification of lipoproteins occurs in the plasma or artery wall. The observation that the naturally occurring B-VLDL of cholesterol-fed dogs cause cholesteryl ester accumulation in macrophages may be of potential importance in elucidating the role of the macrophage in atherosclerosis. However, the relative contribution of smooth muscle cells and macrophages to foam cell production in human atherosclerosis remains to be determined.

References

Brown MS, Goldstein JL (1979) Familial hypercholesterolemia: Model for genetic receptor disease. The Harvey Lectures (1977-1978) 73: 163-201

Brown MS, Faust JR, Goldstein JL (1975) Role of the low-density lipoprotein receptor in regulating the content of free and esterified cholesterol in human fibroblasts. J Clin Invest 55: 783-793

Brown MS, Ho YK, Goldstein JL (1976) The low-density lipoprotein pathway in human fibroblasts: Relation between cell surface receptor binding and endocytosis of low-density lipoprotein. Ann NY Acad Sci 275: 244-257

Geer JC (1965) Fine structure of canine experimental atherosclerosis. Am J Pathol 47: 241-269

Goldstein JL, Brown MS (1977) The low-density lipoprotein pathway and its relation to atherosclerosis. Annu Rev Biochem 46: 897-930

Goldstein JL, Anderson RGW, Buja LM, Basu SK, Brown MS (1977) Overloading human aortic smooth muscle cells with low-density lipoprotein cholesteryl esters reproduces features of atherosclerosis in vitro. J Clin Invest 59: 1196-1202

Goldstein JL, Ho YK, Basu SK, Brown MS (1979) A binding site on macrophages that mediates the uptake and degradation of acetylated low-density lipoprotein, producing massive cholesterol deposition. Proc Natl Acad Sci USA 76: 333-337

Goldstein JL, Ho YK, Brown MS, Innerarity TL, Mahley RW (1980) Cholesteryl ester accumulation in macrophages resulting from receptor-mediated uptake and degradation of hypercholesterolemic canine B - very low density lipoproteins. J Biol Chem, in press

Havel RJ, Kane JP (1973) Primary dysbetalipoproteinemia: predominance of a specific apoprotein species in triglyceride-rich lipoproteins. Proc Natl Acad Sci USA 70: 2015-2019

Innerarity TL, Mahley RW (1978) Enhanced binding by cultured human fibroblasts of apo-E-containing lipoproteins as compared to low density lipoproteins. Biochemistry 17: 1440-1447

Innerarity TL, Mahley RW, Weisgraber KH, Bersot TP (1978) Apoprotein (E-A-II) complex of human plasma lipoproteins. II. Receptor binding activity of a high-density lipoprotein subfraction modulated by apo (E-A-II) complex. J Biol Chem 253: 6289-6295

Mahley RW (1978) Alterations in plasma lipoproteins induced by cholesterol feeding in animals including man. In: Dietschy JM, Gotto AM, Jr, Ontko JA (eds) Disturbances in lipid and lipoprotein metabolism. American Physiological Society, Bethesda, MD pp 181-197

Mahley RW (1979) Dietary fat, cholesterol, and accelerated atherosclerosis. In: Paoletti R, Gotto AM, Jr (eds) Atherosclerosis Reviews. Raven Press, New York Vol 5, pp 1-35

Mahley RW, Holcombe KS (1977) Alterations of the plasma lipoproteins and apoproteins following cholesterol feeding in the rat. J Lipid Res 18: 314-324

Mahley RW, Innerarity TL (1978) Properties of lipoproteins responsible for high affinity binding to cell surface receptors. In: Kritchevsky D, Paoletti R, Holmes WL (eds) Advances in experimental medicine and biology, Sixth international symposium on drugs affecting lipid metabolism. Plenum Press, New York Vol 109, pp 99-127

Mahley RW, Weisgraber KH (1974) Canine lipoproteins and atherosclerosis. I. Isolation and characterization of plasma lipoproteins from control dogs. Circ Res 35: 713-721

Mahley RW, Weisgraber KH, Innerarity T (1974) Canine lipoproteins and atherosclerosis. II. Characterization of the plasma lipoproteins associated with atherogenic and non-atherogenic hyperlipidemia. Circ Res 35: 722-733

Mahley RW, Weisgraber KH, Innerarity T, Brewer HB, Jr, Assmann G (1975) Swine lipoproteins and atherosclerosis. Changes in the plasma lipoproteins and apoproteins induced by cholesterol feeding. Biochemistry 14: 2817-2823

Mahley RW, Nelson AW, Ferrans VJ, Fry DL (1976a) Thrombosis in association with atherosclerosis induced by dietary perturbations in dogs. Science 192: 1139-1141

Mahley RW, Weisgraber KH, Innerarity TL (1976b) Atherogenic hyperlipoproteinemia induced by cholesterol feeding in the patas monkey. Biochemistry 15: 2979-2985

Mahley RW, Innerarity TL, Pitas RE, Weisgraber KH, Brown JH, Gross E (1977a) Inhibition of lipoprotein binding to cell surface receptors of fibroblasts following selective modification of arginyl residues in arginine-rich and B apoproteins. J Biol Chem 252: 7279-7287

Mahley RW, Innerarity TL, Weisgraber KH, Fry DL (1977b) Canine hyperlipoproteinemia and atherosclerosis. Accumulation of lipid by aortic medial cells in vivo and in vitro. Am J Pathol 87: 205-225

Mahley RW, Innerarity TL, Bersot TP, Lipson A, Margolis S (1978a) Alterations in human high-density lipoproteins, with or without increased plasma-cholesterol, induced by diets high in cholesterol. Lancet II: 807-809

Mahley RW, Weisgraber KH, Bersot TP, Innerarity TL (1978b) Effects of cholesterol feeding on human and animal high-density lipoproteins. In: Gotto AM, Jr, Miller NE, Oliver MF (eds) High-density lipoproteins and atherosclerosis. Elsevier/North-Holland, New York pp 149-176

Mahley RW, Innerarity TL, Weisgraber KH, Oh SY (1979a) Altered metabolism (in vivo and in vitro) of plasma lipoproteins after selective chemical modification of lysine residues of the apoproteins. J Clin Invest 64: 743-750

Mahley RW, Weisgraber KH, Innerarity TL, Windmueller HG (1979b) Accelerated clearance of low-density and high-density lipoproteins and retarded clearance of E apoprotein-containing lipoproteins from the plasma of rats after modification of lysine residues. Proc Natl Acad Sci USA 76: 1746–1750

Mahley RW, Weisgraber KH, Melchior GW, Innerarity TL, Holcombe KS (1979c) Inhibition of receptor-mediated clearance of lysine- and arginine-modified lipoproteins from the plasma of rats and monkeys. Proc Natl Acad Sci USA, in press

Reitman JS, Mahley RW (1979) Yucatan miniature swine lipoproteins: Changes induced by cholesterol feeding. Biochim Biophys Acta, in press

Weisgraber KH, Mahley RW, Assmann G (1977) The rat arginine-rich apoprotein and its redistribution following injection of iodinated lipoproteins into normal and hypercholesterolemic rats. Atherosclerosis 28: 121–140

Weisgraber KH, Innerarity TL, Mahley RW (1978) Role of the lysine residues of plasma lipoproteins in high affinity binding to cell surface receptors on human fibroblasts. J Biol Chem 253: 9053–9062

Metabolism of Plasma Lipoproteins[1]

Yechezkiel Stein and Olga Stein

This review will attempt to survey some of the progress made in the study of chylomicron and very low density lipoprotein (VLDL) metabolism since the last International Symposium on Atherosclerosis in Tokyo, 1976. Emphasis will be given to the differences in the metabolic fate of these lipoproteins in the human and smaller experimental animals. Because of these considerations as well as space limitation, the review will be selective but not exhaustive.

Stages of chylomicron metabolism

The metabolism of chylomicrons can be subdivided into several phases which are represented in a schematic form in Fig. 1. These include the intracellular events occurring during the synthesis and secretion of the chylomicrons; the changes in apoprotein and lipid composition which take place in the lymph and plasma and the fate of the various components of the chylomicrons produced during hydrolysis of the triglyceride core.

Chylomicron synthesis and secretion. Ingestion of dietary lipid initiates intensive metabolic activity in the absorptive cells of the small intestine which culminate in the secretion of chylomicrons. The intracellular events which lead to the formation and secretion of chylomicrons (Strauss 1968) parallel those occurring in the liver (Stein and Stein 1967) during secretion of VLDL. Intestinal secretion of triglyceride (TG) rich particles differs from hepatic secretion of VLDL in three major aspects: 1) the much larger size of the chylomicrons, especially after fat feeding; 2) a more restricted synthesis of some apolipoproteins, and 3) the intermediary phase of transport in lymph. The ability of the intestine to secrete TG-rich lipoproteins 3 times larger in diameter than those secreted by the liver seems to be a more economical process with respect to conservation of apolipoprotein B, which is mandatory for chylomicron secretion. The particle which emerges into the lymph consists mainly of triglycerides and contains its full complement of esterified cholesterol, formed by the ACAT reaction (Imaizumi et al. 1978a). The presence of apolipoprotein B in Golgi derived rat chylomicrons was ascertained by Mahley et al. (1971). More recent studies on biopsies of human intestinal mucosa provide evidence for the synthesis and secretion of apolipoprotein B, A-I and A-II (Rachmilewitz et al. 1978; Rachmilewitz and Fainaru 1979). Analysis of rat lymph has shown that intestinal secretion can account for more than 90% of chylomicron associated protein A-I (Imaizumi et al. 1978b). The contribution of the rat intestine to the total amount of plasma apolipoprotein A-I has been estimated to be 56% (Wu and Windmueller 1979). A similar figure was derived also for the human based on the study of two patients with mesenteric-lymphatic-urinary fistulae (Green et al. 1979).

---

[1] This investigation was supported in part by a grant from the United States-Israel Binational Science Foundation and from the Delegation Generale a la Recherche Scientifique et Technique of the French Government. Dr. O. Stein and Dr. Y. Stein are Established Investigators of the Ministry of Health.

653

Apolipoprotein A-IV is apparently a major protein component of human and rat chylomicrons (Green et al. 1979; Imaizumi et al. 1978a) and was shown to be derived from intestinal synthesis (Wu and Windmueller 1979), which in the rat contributes towards 59% of total plasma content of A-IV. As noted above the intestinal particles emerge from the cell with an amount of apolipoprotein B which is much lower than that of liver VLDL when related to their triglyceride content (ApoB : TG is about 1 : 200 in chylomicrons and 1 : 20 in hepatic VLDL). This explains why the total contribution of the intestine towards plasma apoprotein B is not more than 16% in the rat and apparently less in the human. In analogy, the intestine seems to deliver only about 5% of the apolipoproteins C, and less than 1% of apolipoprotein E (Wu and Windmueller 1979; Imaizumi et al. 1978b).

Transfer of lipids and apolipoproteins in lymph and plasma. Following secretion into chyle and subsequent transfer into plasma, the "nascent" chylomicrons undergo very rapid and extensive changes of surface components, i.e., phospholipids, unesterified cholesterol and certain apoproteins. The changes in the surface lipid components of rat chylomicrons have been well documented by Minari and Zilversmit (1963) and were recently confirmed by Imaizumi et al. (1978a). Loss of lecithin from the chylomicrons and an enrichment in unesterified cholesterol were shown to occur upon incubation of chylomicrons with whole plasma or d > 1.006 infranate of plasma also at 4° and thus are not dependent on enzymic activity. The major donors of the unesterified cholesterol or recipients of the phospholipids are high density lipoproteins. Concomitantly with the transfer of the lipid surface components there is a change in the apoprotein content of the chylomicrons (Imaizumi et al. 1978a; Green et al. 1979). The total protein content of both human and rat chylomicrons isolated from the plasma is about three times higher than that of the chyle chylomicrons. The most prominent change is due to an increase in apolipoproteins C and E which amount to 56-75% and 11-15% of the total chylomicron

STAGES OF CHYLOMICRON METABOLISM

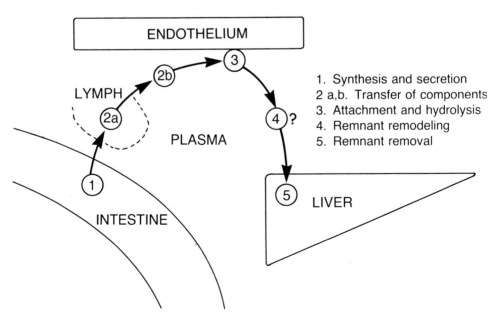

1. Synthesis and secretion
2. a,b. Transfer of components
3. Attachment and hydrolysis
4. Remnant remodeling
5. Remnant removal

FIG. 1. Outline of phases of chylomicron metabolism.

Table 1. Change in apoprotein composition of chylomicrons isolated from lymph or plasma.

	Rat[a]		Human[b]	
	Chyle	Plasma	Chyle	Plasma
	mg protein/g chylomicron			
Total protein	7.7	25.6	13.3	38.7
Apoprotein B	0.6	0.6	0.3	0.4
Apoprotein A-I	2.4	0.9	2.0	1.0
Apoprotein A-IV	0.6	-		1.3
Apoprotein E	0.3	2.7	0.6	5.4
Apoprotein C	2.9	19.2	6.3	22.0

[a]From Imaizumi et al. (1978a).   [b]From Green et al. (1979).

Stage 3
ATTACHMENT TO ENDOTHELIUM

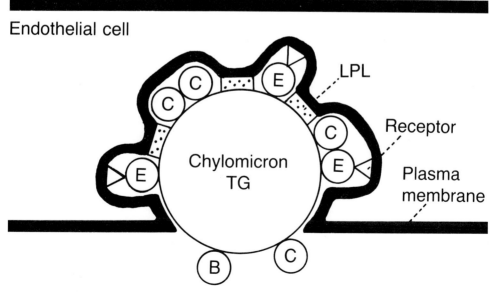

FIG. 2. Attachment of the chylomicron to endothelium. (B, C and E = apolipoproteins; TG = triglyceride; LPL (stippled) = lipoprotein lipase.

protein respectively. At the same time there is a loss of apolipoprotein A-I
(Table 1) (Imaizumi et al. 1978a; Green et al. 1979).

Attachment of the chylomicron to the endothelial surface and hydrolysis of
the triglyceride core. The enzyme responsible for the hydrolysis of chylomicron triglyceride is lipoprotein lipase (LPL) which acts at the luminal surface of vascular endothelium. Studies in perfused rat heart (Fielding and
Higgins 1974) have provided evidence that lipoprotein lipase is a membrane-
supported enzyme, and in the experiments with cultured rat heart cells it became evident that no enzymic activity is detached from the cell surface during
interaction with TG-rich particles (Chajek et al. 1978). These considerations
in addition to ultrastructural evidence of close contact between the endothelial cell surface and the chylomicron (Schoefl and French 1968), suggest
that prior to hydrolysis there is an attachment of the chylomicron to the
endothelial cell surface. The attachment could occur to the enzyme, but one
might consider also the possibility of an additional but not obligatory binding to endothelial apolipoprotein receptors. Such a possibility is presented
schematically in Fig. 2 in which in addition to the contact between LPL and
the chylomicron surface there is a possible anchoring of the particle through
the apolipoprotein E receptor. In the presence of apolipoprotein C-II hydrolysis of the triglyceride proceeds, and the liberated fatty acids are transported to the various tissues. During the stage of triglyceride hydrolysis
there is also a progressive loss of surface components, i.e., unesterified
cholesterol, phospholipid and apoprotein C (Mjøs et al. 1975; Redgrave and
Small 1979). The loss of the core lipid results in a partial collapse of
the particle (Fig. 3) and when more than 90% of the triglyceride is hydrolyzed
the loss of phospholipid is about 75% (Redgrave and Small 1979). This collapse

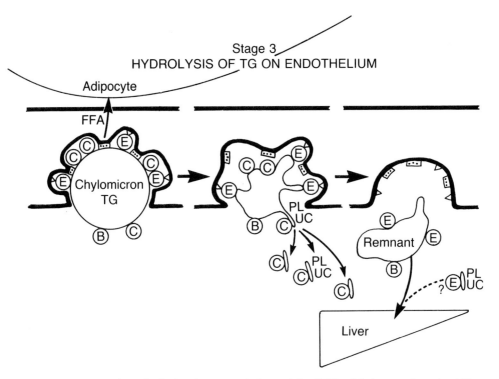

FIG. 3. Hydrolysis of chylomicron triglyceride (TG) which results in liberation of free fatty acid (FFA) is accompanied by a loss of apoprotein C
unesterified cholesterol (UC), phospholipid (PL) and formation of a core
remnant particle which delivers its cholesterol ester to the liver.

will promote detachment of the remnant particle and indeed such particles can be isolated from the plasma of hepatectomized rats which had been injected with chylomicrons (Redgrave 1970; Mjøs et al. 1975; Redgrave and Small 1979). These studies as well as the finding of cholesterol ester in the liver after injection of labeled chylomicrons (Stein et al. 1969) provided evidence that in the rat the hepatocytes are the main site of chylomicron remnant catabolism. One can speculate only that the same may be true also in the human, but so far no direct experimental evidence is available.

Stages of VLDL metabolism

In analogy to the section on chylomicrons the metabolism of VLDL will be subdivided into stages (Fig. 4) and the similarities and differences between chylomicron and VLDL metabolism will be discussed.

Synthesis and secretion of hepatic VLDL. The sites of synthesis of the various components of plasma VLDL as well as their transport from the endoplasmic reticulum through the Golgi apparatus to the sinusoidal cell surface have been well characterized in rat liver (Stein and Stein 1967; Stein et al. 1974) and one might assume that a similar pathway occurs in human liver. However, the nascent VLDL secreted from rat liver differs from human VLDL in its lipid composition, i.e., while rat VLDL is secreted with its full complement of esterified cholesterol, human VLDL acquires most of its cholesterol ester in the circulation (Glomset, 1979). In that aspect the human hepatic VLDL differs from the intestinal chylomicron, which emerges also with most of its cholesterol ester. Another major difference between hepatic VLDL and intestinal chylomicrons lies in their apoprotein composition. The liver is the main source of apolipoprotein E (Windmueller et al. 1973; Marsh 1976; Felker et al. 1977; Wu and Windmueller 1979), and thus apoprotein E is a component of nascent hepatic VLDL (Felker et al. 1977) but the chylomicrons

STAGES OF VLDL METABOLISM

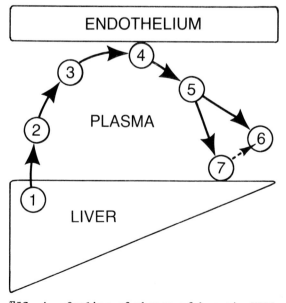

1. Synthesis and secretion
2. Transfer of apoproteins
3. Transfer of EC
4. Attachment and hydrolysis
5. Remnant remodeling
6. LDL formation
7. Remnant removal

FIG. 4. Outline of phases of hepatic VLDL metabolism.

acquire the apolipoprotein E only in the circulation. The same is true also for the apoproteins C, even though the hepatic VLDL secreted from the perfused liver or from cultured hepatocytes is relatively poor in apo C (Hamilton 1972; Davis et al. 1979). Another difference between hepatic VLDL and chylomicrons is the much higher apo B to triglyceride ratio in the former and a high content of apo A-I in the latter.

Transfer of apolipoproteins and lipids. The nascent hepatic VLDL is undergoing a series of changes prior to and during the fulfillment of its metabolic role, i.e., delivery of FFA to extrahepatic tissues. Upon entry into circulation hepatic VLDL becomes highly enriched in apolipoproteins C which constitute the major apoprotein fraction of plasma VLDL (Schaefer et al. 1978). The source of the C apolipoproteins is plasma HDL (Eisenberg 1979) and it seems relevant to digress here and discuss the apparent discrepancy between the low amounts of apolipoproteins C which are secreted by the liver and the finding of their being major components of plasma VLDL and chylomicrons. This apparent discrepancy is a result of conservation of apolipoproteins C in the circulation (see next section) as during lipolysis, the C apolipoproteins are transferred from VLDL and chylomicrons, which are particles with short half lives (minutes for chylomicrons, hours for VLDL), to HDL (Eisenberg 1979), a family of particles with a long half-life of about 5 days (Blum et al. 1977). Another modulation which takes place upon the entry of nascent VLDL into the plasma is transfer of apolipoprotein E from the HDL density range to VLDL. Information concerning this process is derived mainly from studies of plasma from LCAT-deficient patients. These studies have shown that an extensive transfer of apolipoprotein E from HDL to VLDL occurs upon the addition of LCAT to the enzyme deficient plasma (Glomset 1979). Concomitantly with the change in apolipoproteins, the nascent VLDL is transformed from a particle poor in esterified cholesterol to a "mature" plasma VLDL particle (Fig. 5). This transformation is due to a transfer of esterified cholesterol to VLDL and the evidence for such a process as well as its regulation has been provided by studies from several laboratories. At first there were only apparently unrelated pieces of evidence, as for example the observation by Nichols and Smith (1965) that plasma VLDL can be further enriched in cholesterol ester upon incubation at 37°. Subsequently, it became apparent that the incorporation of cholesterol ester into VLDL is not a result of a direct action of LCAT on VLDL, but is due to a transfer of cholesterol ester from HDL, the preferred substrate of LCAT (Akanuma and Glomset 1968). More recently a cholesterol ester exchange protein in the d > 1.21 fraction of rabbit plasma has been described (Zilversmit et al. 1975). The evidence for net transfer of esterified cholesterol from HDL to VLDL in human plasma and the identification of apolipoprotein D as the transfer protein came from studies of Chajek and Fielding (1978). A possible role of HDL phospholipid phosphate groups in the interaction between HDL and the cholesterol ester transfer protein was suggested by Pattnaik and Zilversmit (1979). Results reported by Barter and Lally (1979) helped also to explain the riddle why no exchange of cholesterol ester has been observed in previous studies using rat plasma (Roheim et al. 1963), as the latter apparently does not contain the transfer protein. Finally studies in humans (Nestel et al. 1979) indicate that indeed transfer of labeled cholesterol ester from injected HDL to plasma VLDL occurs also in vivo. The scheme presented in Fig. 5 is an attempt to summarize in a graphic form the transfer of esterified cholesterol from HDL to VLDL in human plasma. The process begins with formation of esterified cholesterol by the LCAT reaction, the preferred substrate of which is the "nascent" HDL (Glomset 1979). The latter may be derived from hepatic secretion (Hamilton et al. 1976) or lipolysis of VLDL and chylomicrons (Eisenberg 1979). The formation of esterified cholesterol by the LCAT reaction is coupled to the transfer of the reaction product to VLDL by the transfer protein.

Stage 3
TRANSFER OF ESTERIFIED CHOLESTEROL (EC)

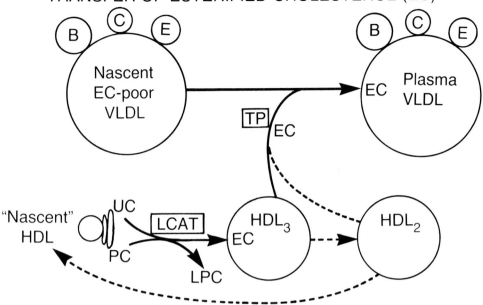

FIG. 5. Transfer of esterified cholesterol into VLDL. "Nascent" HDL is a fraction of HDL which consists of spherical particles < 60 Å and of discs and is the preferred substrate of lecithin cholesterol acyl transferase (LCAT). The HDL_3 particle contains newly formed cholesterol ester (EC) which is transported to VLDL by a transport protein (TP). The broken lines indicate pathways which have not yet been well characterized.

Attachment of the VLDL particle to the endothelial cell surface and hydrolysis of the triglyceride core. This phase of VLDL metabolism bears many similarities to and some differences from the events described for chylomicrons. The sequence of events is represented in Fig. 6 and it appears that in analogy to chylomicrons, hydrolysis of VLDL triglyceride is linked to the attachment of the particle to the endothelial cell surface. The finding of receptors for LDL and remnants of VLDL on cultured human endothelial cells (Stein et al. 1978) could suggest that these receptors might play a role in the attachment of the lipoproteins at the site of lipolytic activity. However, while in chylomicrons the ratio of apolipoprotein E : B is ∿3.0, it is only 0.35 in VLDL. Hence, one might assume that if surface receptors for apo B or apo E influence VLDL attachment, apoprotein B would play a more prominent role in the case of VLDL than in the case of chylomicrons. One might consider the possibility that since the affinity of apo E for cellular receptor is ∿20 times higher than of apo B (Innerarity and Mahley 1978) a less tight binding of the VLDL to the plasma membrane might promote a more rapid detachment and help to explain why delipidation of VLDL is a multistep process. Evidence for sequential delipidation of VLDL is indirect and based on kinetic analyses of turnover data (Eisenberg et al. 1973) and on isolation of subfractions of VLDL by rate zonal ultracentrifugation (Patsch et al. 1978). The main events occuring during delipidation are hydrolysis of triglyceride by lipoprotein lipase and delivery of FFA to peripheral tissues and a concomitant reduction in VLDL surface. The latter process has been studied extensively both in model systems in vitro (Eisenberg and Rachmilewitz 1975; Glangeaud et al. 1977; Eisenberg and Schurr 1976; Eisenberg 1978a) and in the perfused rat heart (Chajek and Eisenberg 1978). The surface components consist

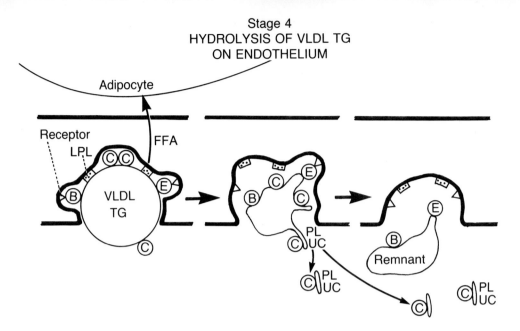

FIG. 6. Attachment of VLDL to endothelium and hydrolysis of triglyceride. Owing to the higher ratio of apo B : E in VLDL apo B might take part in the attachment of the lipoprotein to the cell surface. As in the case of chylomicrons during hydrolysis of TG there is a loss of unesterified cholesterol, phospholipid and apoprotein C.

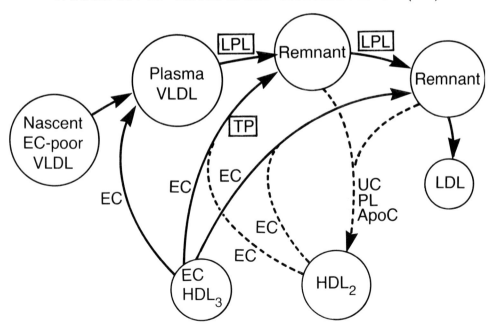

FIG. 7. Transfer of esterified cholesterol to VLDL and remnants formed during VLDL hydrolysis. The final step of lipolysis results in the formation of LDL.

mainly of phospholipids, unesterified cholesterol and apolipoprotein C which are transferred to a HDL density range and in negatively stained preparations appear in the form of stacked discs. It seems important to point out that as delipidation is a stepwise process which in the human takes 4-6 h, it is accompanied by a continuous transfer of esterified cholesterol from HDL to the various remnant particles being formed during the lipolytic process (Fig. 7). The remnant particle thus formed has retained all of its apolipoprotein B, has still about 20% of its original triglyceride load and has lost about half of its apolipoprotein E and more than 90% of apolipoprotein C (Eisenberg 1978b).

We shall now consider some quantitative aspects of the above-described transfer of cholesterol ester. The rate of the LCAT reaction was determined in vivo after injection of labeled mevalonic acid (Barter 1974) and the mean value obtained was 4724 μmoles/day. This rate, measured in males in post-absorptive state, agreed well with the rate determined in vitro. An equivalent number of phosphatidylcholine molecules must be available for the LCAT reaction to produce the cholesterol ester. It is quite apparent that the phosphatidylcholine which could be derived from daily catabolism of HDL (8.2 mg protein day/kg b.w., Blum et al. 1977) could amount to not more than 344 μmoles in a 70 kg man. Therefore additional sources of phosphatidylcholine have to be invoked. The potential donors of phosphatidylcholine are the chylomicrons or VLDL, which were shown to lose their surface phospholipid during lipolysis. One can calculate that secretion of 100 g triglyceride in the form of chylomicrons would introduce about 5.0 g of lecithin into the circulation (Green et al. 1979). Hydrolysis of 90% of the chylomicron-TG would be accompanied by a loss of 75% of the phospholipid (Redgrave and Small 1979) and this amount could account for all the phosphatidylcholine required for the LCAT reaction. Since the rate of the LCAT reaction is similar, also during carbohydrate consumption (Barter 1974), one might calculate whether hepatic VLDL secretion could supply enough substrate in the absence of fat consumption. It has been shown (Wolfe and Ahuja 1977) that individuals infused with a carbohydrate load can secrete up to 80 g of VLDL triglyceride/day. If the liver secreted 30 g triglyceride per day, which would be accompanied by 4 g phosphatidylcholine, and if 70% of the VLDL triglyceride is hydrolyzed (Eisenberg and Rachmilewitz 1975) then about 4500 μmoles of phosphatidylcholine would be provided for the LCAT reaction. Thus, it seems that the results obtained with the various experimental models in which a net transfer of phospholipid from VLDL to HDL was shown to occur during triglyceride hydrolysis (Eisenberg 1979) are in good agreement with reactions occurring in vivo.

Remnant removal and formation of LDL. The fate of the remnant particles formed during lipolysis of VLDL differs in the rat from that in the human. In the former the VLDL remnants are cleared rapidly from the circulation and following surface binding they are taken up by hepatocytes (Stein et al. 1974). There the protein and lipid moieties undergo intralysosomal hydrolysis (Stein et al. 1977). One may speculate that perhaps during the remodeling of the VLDL surface certain sites might become exposed on the apoprotein E which facilitate the binding of the remnant particle to the hepatocyte surface. Whether this is connected to the extensive loss of apoprotein C remains to be established. In the human the remnant particle is further metabolized to LDL and the two possible enzymes responsible for the additional hydrolysis of triglyceride are hepatic triglyceride hydrolase or lipoprotein lipase. Some support for the role of the latter enzyme may be seen in a recent study (Deckelbaum et al. 1979) in which LDL particles had been produced in vitro by exposing VLDL to milk lipoprotein lipase. Thus in the human the delipidation of VLDL terminates in the formation of LDL and the clearance of the latter provides the main exit route of cholesterol ester from the circulation. However, as has been discussed in the previous section, about 5000 μmoles of esterified cholesterol are formed by the LCAT reaction in the circulation per day, of which more than 90% are transferred to VLDL (Nestel et al. 1979). The fractional catabolic rate of LDL could account for the removal of about 50% of the cholesterol ester formed (Schaefer et al. 1978). Not more than 7% could be cleared as part of HDL catabolism (Blum et al. 1977). Therefore about 30-40% of the cholesterol ester formed by the LCAT reaction would require an additional clearing pathway. This removal of cholesterol ester would have to take place at a stage prior to the formation of LDL. This postulate is based on the premise that one VLDL particle results in the formation of one LDL particle with full conservation of apolipoprotein B (Eisenberg 1978b) and on the finding that the ratio of esterified cholesterol to apo B decreases from about 3 in VLDL to about 2 in LDL (Havel and Goldstein 1979; Schaefer et al. 1978). So far no direct evidence has been provided for such a pathway, apart for the finding that chylomicron cholesterol ester may be cleared by heart capillaries (Fielding 1978). One of the possibilities is that at the stage when a remnant particle is transformed into LDL it loses its apolipoprotein E and the latter carries with it the surplus cholesterol ester to be removed by extrahepatic tissues or by the liver (Glomset, personal communication).

As this review will not deal with the metabolism of LDL or HDL (subjects to be covered by others) it seems appropriate to close by posing the question why is the half life of chylomicrons in the circulation much shorter (minutes) than that of VLDL (hours). Three factors might influence the rate of clearance of these lipoproteins: 1) the number of particles needed to carry the same load of triglyceride; 2) The apo E : apo B ratio; 3) The differences in the remnant formed. As seen in Table 2 about 27 times more VLDL particles are formed for each unit mass of TG than chylomicron particles. If binding to sites of hydrolysis is saturable, then processing of VLDL-TG would be slower than of chylomicron TG. The different apo E : apo B ratio in the two lipoprotein species might play also a role in the tighter binding of chylomicrons to the hydrolytic site. Such a binding might reduce the number of delipidation steps and hence favor a more rapid hydrolysis. Indeed, a more rapid hydrolysis of chylomicron than of VLDL TG by lipoprotein lipase was observed (Fielding et al. 1977). In addition the clearance of the remnants formed from hydrolysis of VLDL and chylomicrons could be affected by their different diameter, surface and apo E : B ratio, which in all instances are greater in the chylomicron remnants than in VLDL remnants. Hence, if the apo E determines hepatic removal then chylomicron remnants would be preferred to VLDL remnants.

Table 2. Differences between VLDL and chylomicrons which might affect rates of clearance from circulation.

	VLDL	Chylomicron
Diameter, Å	∿500	∿1500
Particles needed to carry unit mass of TG	∿ 27	1
Apo E : Apo B	∿0.35	∿3.0

Acknowledgement

Some of the concepts presented in this series were elaborated during long
and fruitful discussions with Dr. John Glomset of the University of
Washington, Seattle, to whom most sincere thanks are extended.

References

Akanuma Y, Glomset JA (1968) In vitro incorporation of cholesterol-^{14}C into
    very low density lipoprotein cholesteryl esters. J Lipid Res 9: 620-626
Barter PJ (1974) Production of plasma esterified cholesterol in lean, normo-
    triglyceridemic humans. J Lipid Res 15: 234-242
Barter PJ, Lally JI (1979) In vitro exchanges of esterified cholesterol
    between serum lipoprotein fractions: Studies of humans and rabbits.
    Metabolism 28: 230-236
Blum CB, Levy RI, Eisenberg S, Hall M III, Goebel RH, Berman M (1977) High
    density lipoprotein metabolism in man. J Clin Invest 60: 795-807
Chajek T, Eisenberg S (1978) Very low density lipoprotein. Metabolism of
    phospholipids, cholesterol and apolipoprotein C in the isolated perfused
    rat heart. J Clin Invest 61: 1654-1665
Chajek T, Fielding CJ (1978) Isolation and characterization of a human serum
    cholesteryl ester transfer protein. Proc Natl Acad Sci USA 75: 3445-3449
Chajek T, Stein O, Stein Y (1978) Lipoprotein lipase of cultured mesenchymal
    rat heart cells: II. Hydrolysis of labeled very low density lipoprotein
    triacylglycerol by membrane supported enzyme. Biochim Biophys Acta
    52: 466-474
Davis RA, Engelhorn SC, Pangburn SH, Weinstein DB, Steinberg D (1979) Very
    low density lipoprotein synthesis and secretion by cultured rat hepato-
    cytes. J Biol Chem 254: 2010-2016
Deckelbaum RJ, Eisenberg S, Fainaru M, Barenholz Y, Olivecrona T (1979) In
    vitro production of human plasma very low density lipoprotein-like
    particles. A model for very low density lipoprotein catabolism. J Biol
    Chem 254: 6079-6087
Eisenberg S (1978a) Effect of temperature and plasma on the exchange of apo-
    lipoproteins and phospholipids between rat plasma very low and high den-
    sity lipoproteins. J Lipid Res 19: 292-236
Eisenberg S (1978b) Structure-function relationship in lipoprotein metabol-
    ism. In: Peeters H (ed) Proceedings of 25th Colloquium, Protides of
    the Biological Fluids. Pergamon Press, Oxford, pp 135-142
Eisenberg S (1979) Very-low-density lipoprotein metabolism. In: Eisenberg S
    (ed) Lipoprotein Metabolism (Progress in Biochemical Pharmacology). Kar-
    ger, Basel, Vol 15, pp 139-165
Eisenberg S, Bilheimer DW, Levy RI, Lindgren FT (1973) On the metabolic
    conversion of human plasma very low density lipoprotein to low density
    lipoprotein. Biochim Biophys Acta 326: 361-377
Eisenberg S, Rachmilewitz D (1975) The interaction of rat plasma very low
    density lipoprotein with lipoprotein lipase rich (post-heparin) plasma.
    J Lipid Res 16: 451-461
Eisenberg S, Schurr D (1976) Phospholipid removal during degradation of rat
    plasma very low density lipoprotein in vitro. J Lipid Res 17: 578-587
Felker TE, Fainaru M, Hamilton RL, Havel RJ (1977) Secretion of the arginine-
    rich and A-I apolipoproteins by the isolated perfused rat liver. J Lipid
    Res 18: 465-473
Fielding CJ, Higgins JM (1974) Lipoprotein lipase: Comparative properties of
    the membrane-supported and solubilized enzyme species. Biochemistry
    13: 4324-4330
Fielding CJ (1978) Metabolism of cholesterol-rich chylomicrons. Mechanism of
    binding and uptake of cholesteryl ester by the vascular bed of the per-
    fused rat heart. J Clin Invest 62: 141-151

Fielding PE, Shore VG, Fielding CJ (1977) Lipoprotein lipase. Isolation and characterization of a second enzyme species from postheparin plasma. Biochemistry 16: 1896-1900

Glangeaud MC, Eisenberg S, Olivecrona T (1977) Very low density lipoprotein. Dissociation of apolipoprotein C during lipoprotein lipase induced lipolysis. Biochim Biophys Acta 486: 23-35

Glomset JA (1979) Lecithin:cholesterol acyltransferase. An exercise in comparative biology. In: Eisenberg S (ed) Lipoprotein Metabolism (Progress in Biochemical Pharmacology). Karger, Basel, Vol 15, pp 41-66

Green PHR, Glickman RM, Saudek CD, Blum CB, Tall AR (1979) Human intestinal lipoproteins. Studies in chyluric subjects. J Clin Invest 64: 233-242

Hamilton RL (1972) Synthesis and secretion of plasma lipoproteins. In: Holmes WL, Paoletti R, Kritchevsky D (eds) Advances in Experimental Medicine and Biology: Pharmacological Control of Lipid Metabolism. Plenum, New York, Vol 26, pp 7-24

Hamilton RL, Williams MC, Fielding CJ, Havel RJ (1976) Discoidal bilayer structure of nascent high density lipoproteins from perfused rat liver. J Clin Invest 58: 667-680

Havel RJ, Goldstein J (1979) In Duncan's Diseases of Metabolism, 8th edition Saunders & Co, Phila. In press

Imaizumi K, Fainaru M, Havel RJ (1978a) Composition of proteins of mesenteric lymph chylomicrons in the rat and alterations produced upon exposure of chylomicrons to blood serum and serum proteins. J Lipid Res 19: 712-722

Imaizumi K, Havel RJ, Fainaru M, Vigne JL (1978b) Origin and transport of the A-I and arginine-rich apolipoproteins in mesenteric lymph of rats. J Lipid Res 19: 1038-1046

Innerarity TL, Mahley RW (1978) Enhanced binding of cultured human fibroblasts of apo-E-containing lipoproteins as compared with low density lipoproteins. Biochemistry 17: 1440-1447

Mahley RW, Bennett BD, Morre J, Gray ME, Thistlethwaite W, LeQuire VS (1971) Lipoproteins associated with Golgi apparatus isolated from epithelial cells of rat small intestine. Lab Invest 25: 435-444

Marsh JB (1976) Apoproteins of the lipoproteins in a nonrecirculating perfusate of rat liver. J Lipid Res 17: 85-90

Minari O, Zilversmit DB (1963) Behavior of dog lymph chylomicron lipid constituents during incubation with serum. J Lipid Res 4: 424-436

Mjøs OD, Faergeman O, Hamilton RL, Havel RJ (1975) Characterization of remnants produced during the metabolism of triglyceride-rich lipoproteins of blood plasma and intestinal lymph in the rat. J Clin Invest 56: 603-615

Nestel PJ, Reardon M, Billington T (1979) In vivo transfer of cholesteryl esters from high density lipoproteins to very low density lipoproteins in man. Biochim Biophys Acta 573: 403-407

Nichols AV, Smith L (1965) Effect of very low density lipoproteins on lipid transfer in incubated serum. J Lipid Res 6: 206-210

Pattnaik NM, Zilversmit DB (1979) Interaction of cholesteryl ester exchange protein with human plasma lipoproteins and phospholipid vesicles. J Biol Chem 254: 2782-2786

Patsch W, Patsch JR, Kostner GM, Sailer S, Braunsteiner H (1978) Isolation of subfractions of human very low density lipoproteins by zonal ultracentrifugation. J Biol Chem 253: 4911-4915

Rachmilewitz D, Albers JJ, Saunders DR, Fainaru M (1978) Apoprotein synthesis by human duodenojejunal mucosa. Gastroenterology 75: 677-682

Rachmilewitz D, Fainaru M (1979) Apolipoprotein A-I synthesis and secretion by cultured human intestinal mucosa. Metabolism. 28: 739-743

Redgrave TG, Small DM (1979) Quantitation of the transfer of surface phospholipid of chylomicrons to the high density lipoprotein fraction during the catabolism of chylomicrons in the rat. J Clin Invest 64: 162-171

Redgrave TG (1970) Formation of cholesteryl ester-rich particulate lipid during metabolism of chylomicrons. J Clin Invest 49: 465-471

Roheim PS, Haft DE, Gidez LI, White A, Eder HA (1963) Plasma lipoprotein metabolism in perfused rat liver. II. Transfer of free and esterified cholesterol into the plasma. J Clin Invest 42: 1277-1285

Schaefer EJ, Eisenberg S, Levy RI (1978) Lipoprotein apoprotein metabolism. J Lipid Res 19: 667-687

Schoefl GI, French JE (1968) Vascular permeability to particulate fat: morphological observations on vessels of lactating mammary gland and of lung. Proc Roy Soc (Biol) 169: 153-169

Stein O, Stein Y (1967) Lipid synthesis, intracellular transport, storage, and secretion. I. Electron microscopic radioautographic study of liver after injection of tritiated palmitate or glycerol in fasted and ethanol treated rats. J Cell Biol 33: 319-339

Stein O, Stein Y, Fidge A, Goodman DS (1969) The metabolism of chylomicron cholesteryl ester in rat liver. A combined radioautographic-electron microscopic and biochemical study. J Cell Biol 43: 410-431

Stein O, Rachmilewitz D, Sanger L, Eisenberg S, Stein Y (1974) Metabolism of iodinated very low density lipoprotein in the rat. Autoradiographic localization in the liver. Biochim Biophys Acta 360: 205-216

Stein O, Sanger L, Stein Y (1974) Colchicine-induced inhibition of lipoprotein and protein secretion into the serum and lack of interference with secretion of biliary phospholipids and cholesterol by rat liver in vivo. J Cell Biol 62: 90-103

Stein Y, Ebin V, Bar-On H, Stein O (1977) Chloroquine induced interference with degradation of serum lipoproteins in rat liver, studied in vivo and in vitro. Biochim Biophys Acta 486: 286-297

Stein Y, Friedman G, Stein O (1978) Intralysosomal accretion of cholesterol ester in vascular cells in culture and its translocation into the cytoplasma. In: Paoletti R, Gotto AM (eds) Atherosclerosis Reviews. Raven Press, New York, Vol 3, pp 97-108

Strauss EW (1968) Morphological aspects of triglyceride absorption. In: Code CF (ed) Handbook of Physiology, Alimentary Canal. American Physiological Socity, Washington DC, Vol 3, pp 1377-1406

Windmueller HG, Herbert PN, Levy RI (1973) Biosynthesis of lymph and plasma lipoprotein apoproteins by isolated perfused rat liver and intestine. J Lipid Res 14: 215-223

Wolfe BM, Ahuja SP (1977) Effects of intravenously administered fructose and glucose on splanchnic secretion of plasma triglycerides in hypertriglyceridemic men. Metabolism 26: 963-978

Wu AL, Windmueller HG (1979) Relative contributions by liver and intestine to individual plasma apolipoproteins in the rat. J Biol Chem 254: 7316-7322

Zilversmit DB, Hughes LB, Balmer J (1975) Stimulation of cholesterol ester exchange by lipoprotein-free rabbit plasma. Biochim Biophys Acta 409: 393-398

Possible Mechanisms of Lipid Storage in Tangier Disease

G. Assmann[1] and H.-E. Schaefer[2]

Tangier disease is a rare hereditary disorder characterized by the virtual absence of normal high density lipoproteins (HDL) from plasma and widespread tissue accumulation of cholesteryl esters, mostly cholesteryl oleate(Assmann 1979; Herbert et al. 1978a). Prominent clinical features include enlarged, orange-yellow tonsils, splenomegaly and, frequently, peripheral neuropathy; early atherosclerosis is not a manifestation of the disease. Histological and ultrastructural observations have provided evidence that the intracellular lipid storage is mainly confined to macrophages (tissue histiocytes), Schwann cells of peripheral nerves and myenteric plexus, nonvascular smooth muscle cells of the intestine, nevus cells and, occasionally, mast cells and fibroblasts. Endothelial cells and smooth muscle cells of large and small arteries are not affected by lipid storage. The tissue macrophage is the site of most of the lipid deposition, and the conversion of histiocytic cells to foam cells is the predominant abnormality in affected tissues. The foam cells contain sudanophilic, cytoplasmic lipid droplets and, upon occasion, crystalline material ; on examination at room temperature in plane polarized light, the storage material is birefringent and partially exhibits a maltese cross pattern. At body temperature a large proportion of the cholesteryl ester droplets within foam cells are in the smectic liquid crystalline state (Katz et al. 1977). Two major mechanisms may account for the intracellular accumulation of cholesteryl esters in various tissues: phagocytosis ofabnormal lipoproteins and/or ineffective removal of cholesterol from cells. These two mechanisms are discussed in the light of present biochemical and morphological evidence.

Phagocytosis of abnormal lipoproteins

Delayed clearance of chylomicrons from plasma is an immediate consequence of HDL deficiency (Assmann 1978) and results in fasting chylomicronemia and the formation of abnormal products of chylomicron catabolism in Tangier patients. On diets high in fat, large (68-nm) flattened, translucent particles (Herbert et al. 1978b) and lamellar bilayered structures (Assmann et al. 1980) can be visualized by electron microscopy in Tangier plasma. These abnormal lipoproteins are thought to derive from chylomicrons since they disappear when fat is removed from the diet. Normally, chylomicron surface remnants are either transferred to HDL during lipolysis or converted into spherical HDL by in-

---

[1] Supported by a Thyssen fellowship,Deutsche Forschungsgemeinschaft und Institut für Arterioskleroseforschung an der Universität Münster.

[2] Supported by Minister für Wissenschaft und Forschung des Landes Nordrhein-Westfalen, GFR.

teracting with lecithin-cholesterol acyltransferase (Tall and
Small 1978). Due to the intrinsic defect in Tangier disease
these mechanisms are inoperative and, as a consequence, abnormal
products of chylomicron catabolism accumulate.

Ultrastructural data are consistent with the concept that such
abnormal products of chylomicron catabolism are components of
the lipid deposits in various cells, particularly histiocytes.
In the spleen, gray-appearing lipid droplets that fuse with lysosomal granules can be visualized by electron microscopy (Fig.1a).
For the following reasons these particles seemingly represent
phagocytized chylomicrons: a) their size is compatible with that
of chylomicrons, and b) their content reacts osmiophilic, indicative of the presence of polyunsaturated fatty acids. By contrast,
cholesteryl oleate as a product of cellular cholesterol reesterification has a low binding capacity of OsO_4 and is extracted
by solvents applied in the procedure of tissue embedding. In
dermal biopsies we have occasionally traced extracellular foamy
material of fused particles ranging from 500 to 3000 Å in size
(Fig. 2). This material can be observed in intimate contact with
lipid-storing nevus cells or within the adventitia of small
subepidermal blood vessels; it most likely represents chylomicrons
or chylomicron remnants. Non-phagocytizing cells such as intestinal smooth muscle cells, nevus cells and Schwann cells may inter-
nalize lipoproteins by endocytotic vesicles. Because of the small
size of such vesicles and the presence of a surrounding basement
membrane, only particles smaller than chylomicrons can be metabolized. However, lipoproteins smaller than 500 Å are scarcely
resolved in tissues because of the relative thickness of thin
sections. Taking these limitations into account, the hidden uptake of abnormal lipoproteins (e.g. postprandial, discoidal
lipoproteins, Tangier A-II particles) even by non-phagocytotic
cells seems reasonable.

Ineffective removal of cholesterol from cells

The lipid-storing histiocytes in Tangier patients occur in
abundance a) in tissues which are engaged in the breakdown of
cells under physiological condition (spleen pulp, bone marrow)
and b) at sites of chronic inflammatory processes (tonsils,
rectal mucosa, inflamed stroma of a cervical ectopia)(Assmann
and Schaefer 1978; Ferrans and Fredrickson 1975). It is likely,
therefore, that at least to a certain degree the histiocytic
lipid content originates on the basis of the obligate intake of
cholesterol in the form of cell debris and membranes, which is
not compensated for by an effective cholesterol removal mechanism. Macrophages differ from most other cells in the body in
that they do not biosynthesize cholesterol and totally depend
upon cholesterol influx and efflux to maintain a cellular
equilibrium. Non-effective efflux could render macrophages most
vulnerable to cholesterol and cholesteryl ester storage. On the
basis of our observations in Tangier tissues one could speculate
that those cells which have the ability to control their cholesterol uptake (e.g. through regulation of LDL receptor sites)
may be in part protected from cholesteryl ester accumulation;
on the other hand macrophages take up cholesterol from various
sources in a random fashion and may, therefore, critically depend upon an effective removal mechanism. It is not clear,
however, whether this removal mechanism specifically resides
with HDL, HDL precursors or other plasma proteins.

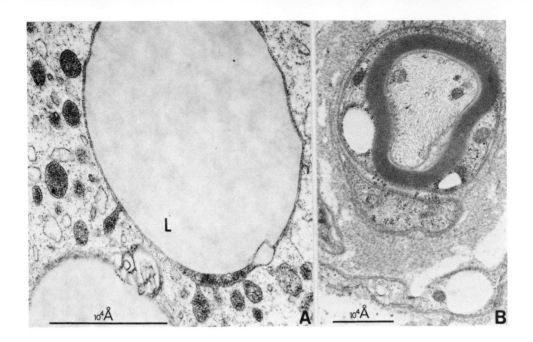

FIG. 1a, left: Tangier disease. Cytoplasm of a lienal macrophage containing lipoprotein-derived osmiophilic lipid (L) surrounded by dense lysosomal
bodies (x 40,000).
FIG. 1b, right: Dermal Schwann cell with a myelinated axon containing membraneless-lipid droplets (x 20,000).

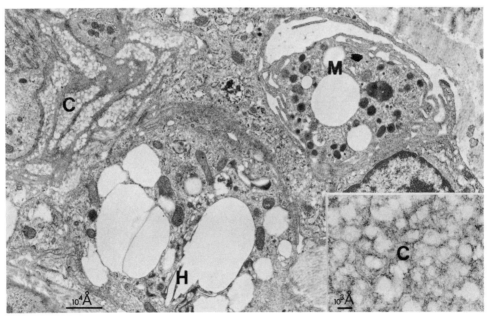

FIG. 2. Dermal lipid-storage in Tangier disease. Histiocyte (H) with electron-lucent lipid droplets; membrane-bound vacuoles in part combined with
crystalline residual bodies. Part of a tissue mast cell (M) containing
membraneless-lipid droplets. Extracellular foamy deposits of chylomicrons
(C), discoidal remnants, see inset. (x 12,000, inset x 50,000).

Recently, we have demonstrated the occurrence of lamellar bilayer structures in postprandial Tangier plasma (Assmann et al. 1980). These folds of lipid-apoprotein bilayers, absent from fasting serum, derive from the surface of chylomicrons during in vivo lipolysis and account for a significant proportion of the cholesterol uptake capacity from human fibroblasts (tissue culture) contained in postprandial Tangier serum. We propose that such HDL precursors (discoidal structures originating from the chylomicron surface or direct tissue synthesis) may be critically involved in cholesterol-uptake from peripheral cells (Fig. 3). In Tangier disease, cholesterol of peripheral cells (e.g. smooth muscle cells of the artery) may be scavanged into macrophages instead of becoming HDL cholesterol (Fig. 3). This hypothesis is consistent with the absence of lipid-storage in smooth muscle cells of large and small arteries and the accumulation of cholesteryl oleate in macrophages.

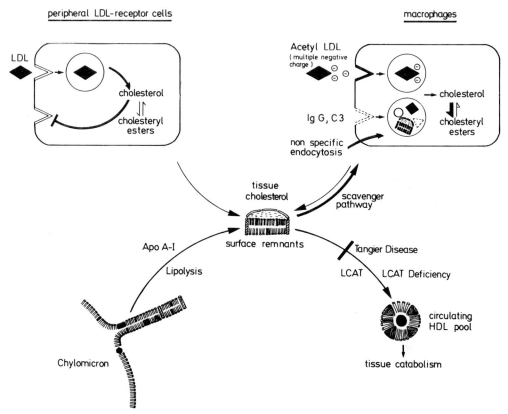

Fig. 3: Hypothetical pathway of cholesterol from peripheral LDL-receptor cells (e.g. smooth muscle cells of the artery) to macrophages in Tangier disease.

There is no direct morphological evidence for hampered removal of lipoproteins from macrophages and other cells in Tangier disease. The major amount of lipid stored is in the form of droplets unbound by membranes (Fig.1b). Contrary to phagocytized chylomicrons (Fig.1a) these droplets are electron-lucent because of the predominance of cholesteryl oleate. These cytoplasmic lipid droplets likely represent a storage form of re-esterified cholesterol, suggestive of a disturbed cholesterol efflux. It cannot be excluded, however, that a nonlysosomal cholesteryl esterase is impaired in lipid-storing cells in Tangier disease. Undoubtedly, the further elucidation of the biochemical defect in Tangier disease has implications for our understanding of the role of HDL in atherogenesis and tissue cholesterol metabolism.

References

Assmann G (1978) The metabolic role of high density lipoproteins: perspectives from Tangier disease. In: Gotto AM, Miller NE, Oliver MF (eds) High density lipoproteins and atherosclerosis. Elsevier, North Holland Biomedical Press, pp 77-89

Assmann G (1979) Tangier disease and the possible role of HDL in atherosclerosis. In: Paoletti R, Gotto AM, Jr (eds) Atherosclerosis Reviews, Volume 7. Raven Press, New York, in press

Assmann G, Schaefer H-E (1978) High density lipoprotein deficiency and lipid deposition in Tangier disease. In: Carlson LA, Paoletti R, Sirtori CR, Weber G (eds) International Conference on Atherosclerosis. Raven Press, New York,pp 97-101

Assmann G, Schmitz G, Schaefer H-E (1980) Tangier disease. A biochemical explanation for the absence of early atherosclerosis. Europ J Clin Invest, in press

Ferrans VJ, Fredrickson DS (1975) The pathology of Tangier disease. A light and electron microscopic study. Am J Pathol 78: 101-158

Herbert PN, Gotto AM, Fredrickson DS (1978a) Familial lipoprotein deficiency (Abetalipoproteinemia, Hypobetalipoproteinemia, and Tangier Disease) In: Stanbury JB, Wyngaarden JB, Fredrickson DS (eds) The Metabolic Basis of Interited Disease. Mc Graw-Hill, New York, pp 544-588

Herbert PN, Forte T, Heinen RJ, Fredrickson DS (1978b) Tangier disease. One explanation of lipid storage. N Engl J Med 299: 519-521

Katz SS, Small DM, Brook JG, Lees RS (1977) The storage lipids in Tangier disease. A physical chemical study. J Clin Invest 59: 1045-1054

Tall AR, Small DM (1978) Plasma high-density lipoproteins. N Engl J Med 299: 1232-1236

Introduction to Deficiencies of Apolipoproteins CII and EIII With Some Associated Clinical Findings[1]

J.A. Little, D. Cox, W.C. Breckenridge, and V.M. McGuire

Type III hyperlipoproteinemia (HLP) was characterized by Fredrickson et al. (1967) as having β migrating lipoproteins with a density less than 1.006. They referred to a prior description by Gofman et al. (1954) of patients with adult onset tuberous xanthomata, premature ischemic vascular disease, decreased Sf 0-12 and increased 12-400 lipoproteins, as probably having Type III. They suspected that it was "likely to be secondary to the presence of an abnormal lipoprotein" and from family studies that "several mutant alleles" might determine Type III HLP. A number of discoveries by several groups have further characterized the disorder: an increase in the cholesterol/glyceride ratio in β-VLDL; the precipitation of abnormal VLDL by heparin manganese; the increased concentration of arginine rich apolipoprotein (apo E) in VLDL and its description as a dysbetalipoproteinemia due to an accumulation of remnants from chylomicron and VLDL catabolism.

Finally, Utermann et al. (1975,1979) demonstrated genetic polymorphism of apo E determined by two autosomal codominant alleles, one of which results in a deficiency of the isoprotein EIII. The homozygotes for EIII deficiency have dysbetalipoproteinemia, but only individuals carrying a gene or genes for other types of HLP develop elevated total lipid levels and Type III HLP. This fulfills the prophecy of Fredrickson et al. (1967) that Type III HLP may be polygenic. The heterozygotes for EIII deficiency have a mild form of dyslipoproteinemia.

Type I HLP or hyperchylomicronemia was originally attributed to a deficiency of lipoprotein lipase (LPL) (Havel & Gordon 1960; Fredrickson et al. 1963); thus the current name, familial LPL deficiency. LaRosa et al. (1970) showed that apolipoprotein CII activated LPL.

In 1976 we investigated a man with chylomicronemia, pancreatitis, pancreatic calcification and apparently absent post heparin lipolytic activity (Breckenridge et al. 1978). A blood transfusion for anemia resulted in a dramatic fall in plasma triglyceride concentration from 1750 to 196 mg% in two days, suggesting that the transfused blood supplied a factor that lowered plasma lipoprotein levels. Dr. Breckenridge noted the absence of apolipoprotein CII in the polyacrylamide gel electrophoresis of the patients' VLDL soluble apoproteins and attributed the disease to apo CII deficiency. Intravenous infusion of an apo C preparation from human VLDL lowered the patients' plasma triglycerides in a manner similar to whole plasma or blood.

The VLDL isolated by zonal ultracentrifugation from 2.5 1 of fresh human plasma was partially delipidated with aqueous ether and sterilized by filtration and was pyrogen free. The "apo VLDL" product contained apoCII as determined by polyacrylamide gel electrophoresis and activation of guinea pig post heparin plasma. The "apo VLDL" was infused intravenously over a 7-hour period. Figure 1 shows the fall in the patient's plasma triglyceride from 948 to 216 mg%, an equivalent decrease in chylomicrons and only a questionable increase in LDL

---

[1] Supported in part by a contract from National Institutes of Health (NIH-NHLBI 1-HV2-2917-L) and by the Ontario Heart Foundation.

and HDL lipids. The effect of the infusion lasted 3 or more days. One-half and 24-hours after the infusion the patients' plasma stimulated lipolytic activity of guinea pig post heparin plasma whereas before there was no such stimulation. The diet was kept constant.

A report on a portion of his very large family (Cox et al. 1978) reveals that apo CII deficiency is inherited as an autosomal recessive trait, the homozygotes having no detectable apo CII and a lipoprotein pattern similar to LPL deficiency. The heterozygotes, despite having about half the normal concentration of apo CII relative to CIII in their VLDL and half the ability of normal plasma to activate lipoprotein lipase, generally have no gross elevation of lipids.

We now report the findings in more relatives. Table 1 shows the 14 homozygotes. Apo CII deficiency, compared with the 32 cases of LPL deficiency of Fredrickson and Levy (1972), has an early age of detection (14 vs 10 Yr.) and high prevalence of pancreatitis (64 vs 38%, not age adjusted), but has no xanthomata (0 vs 47%) and no hepatomegaly (0 vs 75%) (a liver biopsy of the proband was normal). Also there is no premature ischemic vascular disease and corneal arcus. In this symposium Breckenridge et al. describe the plasma lipids and lipoproteins in detail. Why homozygous CII deficiency has no xanthomata or gross infiltration of lipid into tissues despite triglyceride levels up to 5000 or more is a matter for speculation. Anemia, as defined by a hemoglobin concentration less than 14 g% for men and 12 g% for women, was present in 8 homozygotes. Table 2 compares the values of 11 sex matched homo- and heterozygote relatives living in the same environment. The homozygotes have significantly lower Hb levels. Dietary records did not indicate that a nutritional deficiency might be responsible. Some of their blood smears have increased polychromasia of red cells. The proband had a sudden drop in Hb level, suggesting hemolysis. Possibly the chronic hypertriglyceridemia destabilizes the red cell membrane. Anemia is not mentioned in previous reviews of LPL deficiency. The male CII deficient homozygote just reported by Yamamura et al. (1979) had a hemoglobin of 13.6 g%. Neither of their two homozygotes had pancreatitis, xanthomata or hepatosplenomegaly. Zieve (1958) reported hemolysis in association with lipemia, alcoholic cirrhosis and jaundice.

In our family, 23 obligate heterozygotes for apo CII deficiency are now identified (Table 3). By comparing their plasma lipid and lipoprotein concentrations with age/sex specific percentiles from the Toronto Lipid Research Clinic Population Study (Jones et al. 1979) it is evident that they have significantly low HDL-cholesterol and high total triglyceride and VLDL-cholesterol levels. Their diets conformed with the norm for the population. Breckenridge et al report the actual values elsewhere in this symposium. Total plasma cholesterol and LDL-cholesterol levels are normal. As controls, the plasma lipids of the unrelated spouses in this family were examined by the same method and show no deviation from normal. The clinical histories and findings in heterozygotes do not suggest premature ischemic vascular disease despite their tendency for decreased HDL and increased VLDL levels. One heterozygote had marked chylomicronemia on one examination and definitely elevated plasma triglycerides without chylomicronemia on a second test. A questionnaire indicated good health but detailed medical examination was not possible. It is possible that heterozygotes, with relatively reduced amounts of circulating apo CII, may maintain normal or nearly normal levels of triglyceride-rich lipoproteins except when their metabolism is stressed by dietary excesses or causes for secondary HLP.

In conclusion the findings of Utermann et al. and Breckenridge et al. provide a better understanding of lipoprotein metabolism and a refinement of the classification of HLP into more specific phenotypes and genotypes. The gene frequency in the population is high for EIII deficiency and probably is low for

Table 1. Homozygotes for apo CII Deficiency
(8 males & 6 females, ages 16–64 years)[a,b]

N	Findings
14	chylomicronemia
9[a]	pancreatitis
	1 diabetes & malabsorption
	1 pseudocyst
2	peptic ulcer
3	splenomegaly
0	hepatomegaly
0	xanthomata
1	corneal arcus, age 62
8	anemia
3	hypertension (age 39,41,63 Yr.)
2	CHD (age 59 & 62)
2	cataracts (age 59 & 62)
2	peripheral pain at rest
3	chronic rashes
1	ecchymoses
2	obese

[a] In addition to these, one sib of a homozygote died of acute pancreatitis prior to this study and presumably was a homozygote.
[b] Mean age of onset: symptoms at 10 years, detection of lipemia at 14 years.

Table 2. Hemoglobin (G%) in apo CII deficiency.

Sex	Homozygotes			Heterozygotes			p
	N	M	S.D.	N	M	S.D.	
M	6	12.05 ± 2.7		6	$15.1 \pm .63$		<.025
F	5	$11.7 \pm .65$		5	$14.2 \pm .82$		<.001

Table 3. Obligate Heterozygotes for apo CII Deficiency
(13 males & 10 females, ages 11–78 years).

N	Findings
19[a]	Total TG >50th percentile[b]
18[a]	HDL–chol <50th percentile[b] (8 <5th percentile)
19[a]	VLDL–chol >50th percentile[b]
1	Chylomicronemia transiently (TG 2160 & 326 mg%)
1	Diabetes, hypertension & ischemic vasc. dis., age 62
1	Cataracts, age 62
1	Duodenal ulcer

[a] Significantly different than the expected number above or below the 50th percentile, p <.001.
[b] Age and sex specific from the LRC Population Study.

CII deficiency since only two families are reported to date. Both EIII and CII deficiency are recessive traits. The homozygote for EIII deficiency sometimes has Type III HLP depending on the presence of other genes for HLP. The CII deficient homozygote always has severe chylomicronemia. Type III HLP has an excess while apo CII deficiency has a scarcity of chylomicron and VLDL remnants. Type III HLP has distinctive xanthomata and premature atherosclerosis whereas apo CII deficiency so far has neither complication, suggesting that apoprotein composition and the physicochemical properties of lipoprotein particles influence their uptake atopically by tissues. The heterozygotes for both deficiencies have dyslipoproteinemias intermediary between the normal and homozygote and we do not yet know if they are at increased or decreased risk for future disease complications.

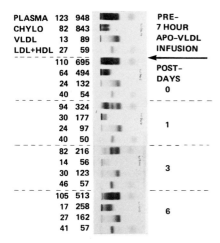

FIG. 1. The effect of an intravenous infusion of apoproteins from normal VLDL into a patient with apo CII deficiency. The plasma lipoproteins are separated by ultracentrifugation and by agarose gel electrophoresis. (C=cholesterol, TG= triglyceride.)

REFERENCES

Breckenridge WC, Little JA, Steiner G, Chow A and Poapst M (1978) Hypertriglyceridemia associated with deficiency of apolipoprotein CII. N Engl J Med 298:1265-1273

Cox DW, Breckenridge WC and Little JA (1978) Inheritance of apolipoprotein CII deficiency with hypertriglyceridemia and pancreatitis. N Engl J Med 299:1421-1424

Fredrickson DS, Levy RI, Lees RS (1967) Fat transport in lipoproteins – an integrated approach to mechanisms and disorders. N Engl J Med 276:32-44, 94-108, 148-156, 215-226, 273-281

Fredrickson DS and Levy RI (1972) Familial hyperlipoproteinemia. In: The Metabolic Basis of Inherited Disease. Stanbury, Wyngaarden and Fredrickson. 3rd ed p545. New York: McGraw-Hill

Gofman JW, deLalla O, Glazier F, Freeman NK, Lindgren FT, Nichols AV, Strishower EH and Tamplin AR (1954) The serum lipoprotein transport system in health, metabolic disorders, atherosclerosis and coronary artery disease. Plasma 2:413-486

Havel RJ and Gordon RS Jr (1960) Idiopathic hyperlipemia: metabolic studies in an affected family. J Clin Invest: 39:1777-1790

Jones GJL, Hewitt D, Godin GJ, Breckenridge WC, Bird J, Mishkel MA, Steiner G and Little JA (1979) Plasma lipoprotein levels and the prevalence of hyperlipoproteinemia in a Canadian population. Can Med Assoc J, In Press

LaRosa JC, Levy RI, Herbert P, Lux SE and Fredrickson DS (1970) Specific apoprotein activator for lipoprotein lipase. Biochem Biophys Res Commun 41:57

Utermann G, Jaeschke M and Menzel J (1975) Familial hyperlipoproteinemia type III: Deficiency of a specific apolipoprotein (Apo E-III) in the very low density lipoproteins. FEBS Lett 56:352-355

Utermann G, Vogelberg KH, Steinmetz A, Schoenborn W, Pruin N, Jaeschke M, Hees M and Canzler H (1979) Polymorphism of apolipoprotein E. Clin Genet 15:37-62, 63-72

Yamamura T, Sudo H, Ishikawa K and Yamamoto A (1979) Familial Type I hyperlipoproteinemia caused by apolipoprotein C-II deficiency. Atherosclerosis 34:53-65

Zieve L (1958) Jaundice, hyperlipemia and hemolytic anemia: A heretofore unrecognized syndrome associated with alcoholic fatty liver and cirrhosis. Ann Int Med 48:471-496

Apolipoprotein CII Deficiency[1]

W.C. Breckenridge, D. Cox, and J.A. Little

Introduction

The importance of lipoprotein lipase in the catabolism of chylomicrons has been recognized since the discovery of a deficiency of this enzyme in familial Type I hyperlipoproteinemia. Although apolipoprotein CII (apo CII) was demonstrated to be important in the activation of lipoprotein lipase in vitro a definitive role for apo CII for catabolism in vivo of triglyceride rich lipoproteins was clearly established with the report of a patient lacking this apoprotein (Breckenridge et al. 1978). The patient had an apparent deficiency of post heparin lipoprotein lipase which was obviated upon addition of apo CII. Furthermore , the patient's plasma triglycerides could be reduced by infusions of plasma or apo VLDL from normal subjects. As a result of family studies of the proband we reported (Cox et al. 1978) that apo CII deficiency appeared to be inherited as an autosomal recessive trait. This report describes the results of our continuing study of a rather large pedigree containing 14 homozygous subjects and 23 obligate heterozygotes identified at present.

Methods

The methods for estimation of plasma lipids and lipoproteins and the assay of activation of lipoprotein lipase and double immunodiffusion against anti apo CII have been reported elsewhere (Cox et al. 1978). Apolipoproteins were delipidized with ethanol ether 3:1, solublized in Tris (0.001M) urea (8M) containing dithiothreitol and analyzed by isoelectric focusing in urea acrylamide gels (9 cm) with a pH gradient of 3-7. The gels were stained overnight according to the method of Reisner et al.(1975). The optical density of dye uptake of each apoprotein band was proportional to the amount of protein applied up to 100 ug of apoprotein. All results are expressed as a ratio of apo CII/apo CIII. Apo CIII includes optical density due to apo CIII 0,1 and 2.

Results

Apoprotein profiles obtained by isoelectric focusing are shown in Figure 1 for lipoprotein fractions. The method gives good resolution of apo $CIII_2$, apo $CIII_1$, apo CII and apo $CIII_0$. Apo AII is resolved from $CIII_0$. Apo AI isomorphs are also resolved from the apo E isomorphs but it is important to use dithiothreitol to prevent band spreading of apo E. All homozygotes studied to date lacked detectable apo CII by isoelectric focusing in the chylomicron or VLDL fraction. The homozygotes have a normal compliment of apo E_1, 2 and 3 isomorphs as well as some minor bands migrating in the region of apo AI. Both apo AI and AII appear to be increased slightly in the homozygotes.

[1] Supported in part by a contract from National Institutes of Health (NIH-NHLBI 1-HV2-2917-L) and by the Ontario Heart Foundation.

The obligate heterozygotes have a reduction in apo CII relative to apo CIII peptides. None of the heterozygotes or homozygotes, examined to date have significant amounts of the apo CII isomorph reported by Kane et al. (1979) although a minor band between apo $CIII_1$ and apo $CIII_2$ corresponding to this species can be seen in normal subjects. Apo CII/CIII ratios for a group of normal Toronto subjects ranged from 0.22-0.35 (Table I). The mean ratio for obligate heterozygotes was 0.16 with a range of 0.03-0.27. Fifteen out of 18 obligate heterozygotes fell below the minimum value of 0.22 noted for healthy subjects. However in one branch of the family we have detected 3 obligate heterozygotes who have apo CII/CIII ratios well within the normal range.

The activation of skim milk lipoprotein lipase increased linearly with up to 0.6 ml of normal plasma (Figure 2). Homozygous plasma gave no significant release over the blank value and there was no activation with increasing concentrations of plasma. Plasma of heterozygotes usually gave an activation of about 50% of the normal pool although there was considerable variation among individual heterozygotes. The activity, under these assay conditions, appeared to be a reflection only of apo CII and not due to an inhibition by apo CIII since the release of fatty acids increased in a linear fashion but at about 50% of the value of the normal plasma. The activation assay gave a mean value of 25 for normals (Table I) while obligate heterozygotes had a mean value of 16 with a range from 10-31. Of the twenty-three obligate heterozygotes studied, 18 had activation values of 20 or less.

Thus the estimates of apo CII indicated that values of less than 0.20 for apo CII/CIII or 20 for activation are indicative of the heterozygous subjects. Of the 18 homozygotes tested by both methods, 14 gave values below these limits for both assays, 2 subjects had normal values and 2 subjects had values below normal for 1 assay but normal by the second assay. The combination of the two assays gives a relatively good predication of the heterozygote but suggests that a few heterozygotes overlap with the normal range.

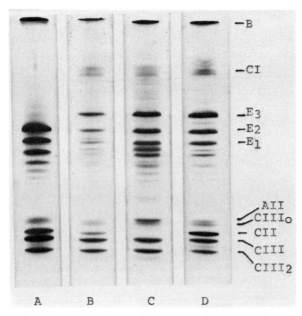

FIG. 1. Isoelectric focusing of urea soluble apoproteins of VLDL, A, Type III Hyperlipoproteinemia; B, Obligate Heterozygote apo CII deficiency; C, Homozygous apo CII deficiency; D, Normal.

The lipid and lipoprotein distributions for homozygous subjects are shown in Table II. The homozygotes had normal or elevated cholesterol levels depending on triglyceride concentrations. Triglyceride concentrations ranged from about 500 to 5000 mg/100 ml and were quite volatile for any individual. There were extensive accumulations of cholesterol in the chylomicron fractions and VLDL. The content of cholesterol in the LDL and HDL was extremely low, but total lipid analyses of these lipoproteins revealed that triglycerides account for 34% of LDL and 15% of HDL. The increase in triglyceride was primarily associated with a reduction of cholesterol ester in the lipoprotein. Estimates of total lipid mass indicated both lipoprotein fractions were reduced by 50-75% compared to normal values. The lipid and lipoprotein concentrations for heterozygotes are not grossly abnormal. The lipid composition of VLDL and LDL from heterozygous subjects showed no major differences compared to normal subjects. HDL cholesterol ranged from a low of 21 mg/100 ml to a high of 61 mg/100 ml. In heterozygous subjects who had HDL cholesterol levels less than 45 mg/100 ml the reduction in HDL cholesterol was primarily restricted to the HDL_2 fraction while the homozygote had a considerable reduction of HDL_2 and HDL_3.

Thus all homozygotes show severe alterations in lipoprotein composition consistant with the observations in the original proband. It is clear that apolipoprotein CII is essential for normal catabolism of triglyceride rich lipo-

Table 1. Estimation of Apolipoprotein CII in Obligate Heterozygotes for Apolipoprotein CII Deficiency.

Assay		Heterozygotes	Normal Spouses	Normal
Apo CII/Apo CIII Ratio	M	0.16 (18)	0.35 (15)	0.27 (25)
	R	0.03-0.27	0.21-0.64	0.22-0.35
LPL Activation Units	M	16 (23)	33 (15)	25 (55)
	R	10-31	19-48	18-45

Results are means (M) and range (R). Values in parentheses are number of subjects.

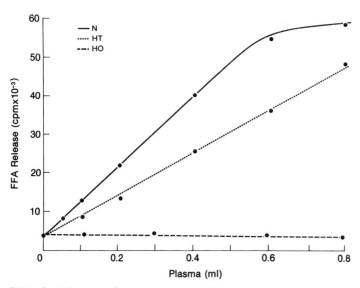

FIG. 2 Release of fatty acids with increasing amounts of plasma in lipase assay. N, normal plasma; HT and HO, heterozygote and homozygote for apo CII deficiency.

Table 2. Lipids and Lipoproteins in Homozygotes and Obligate Heterozygotes for Apo CII Deficiency.

Homozygotes	N		Plasma[a]		Lipoprotein Cholesterol[a]			
			C	TG	Chylo	VLDL	LDL	HDL
				mg/100 ml				
Homozygotes Males	8	M	307	2731	168	105	21	12
		R	176–530	1760–5270	94–310	30–188	12–28	4–26
Females	6	M	213	1640	88	101	26	14
		R	108–370	555–2250	69–144	41–252	15–44	7–18
Heterozygotes								
Males	13	M	159	112		22	97	42
		R	105–211	52–326[b]		8–59	62–155	25–61
Females	10	M	182	128		20	102	40
		R	144–293	67–298		9–31	89–139	21–61

[a] mg/100 ml.
[b] One subject tested twice had values of 326 and 2160 mg/100 ml.

proteins. The lack of apo CII results in extensive reductions in LDL and HDL which are believed to be remnants of the lipolytic process. The data on heterozygotes suggest that relatively low proportions of apo CII in plasma are sufficient to maintain fasting plasma levels in or near the normal range. However it is possible that the rate of catabolism of VLDL may be slightly decreased in these subjects. As shown by Little et al. in this symposium, plasma triglycerides and VLDL cholesterol are increased and HDL cholesterol decreased compared with an age/sex matched population. Fat tolerance or VLDL turnover studies in heterozygous subjects may help elucidate whether lower relative levels of apo CII influence VLDL clearance and possibly HDL levels. Other studies (Ballantyne 1976) have suggested that a low ratio of apo CII/apo CIII might be an important mechanism of Type V hyperlipoproteinemia. However the studies of obligate heterozygotes as well as our original studies of plasma infusion in the proband suggest that a low ratio of apo CII/apo CIII would not be the sole reason for severe hypertriglyceridemia.

In view of the number of homozygous subjects that we have found that the report of a second pedigree in Japan (Yamamura et al. 1979) apo CII deficiency should be considered in subjects with severe hypertriglyceridemia and pancreatitis. Most heterozygotes can be identified quite effectively by the measurement of apo CII/CIII ratios and the lipoprotein lipase activation assay but there is some overlap with normal values for a few heterozygotes. However the data from the entire pedigree indicates that apo CII deficiency is transmitted as an autosomal recessive trait.

References

Breckenridge WC, Little JA, Steiner G, Chow A and Poapst M (1978) Hypertriglyceridemia associated with a deficiency of apolipoprotein CII. N Engl J Med 298:1265-1273

Carlson LA, Ballantyne D (1976) Changing relative proportions of apolipoprotein CII and CIII of very low density lipoproteins in hypertriglyceridemia. Atherosclerosis 23:563-568

Cox DW, Breckenridge WC, Little JA (1978) Inheritance of apolipoprotein CII deficiency with hypertriglyceridemia and pancreatitis. N Engl J Med 299:1420-1424

Havel RT, Kotite L and Kane PJ (1979) Isoelectric heterogeneity of the cofactor protein for lipoprotein lipase in human blood plasma. Biochem Med 21:121-128

Reisner AH, Nemes P and Bucholtz C (1975) The use of Coomassie Brilliant Blue G-250 perchloric acid solution for staining in electrophoresis and isoelectric focusing on polyacrylamide gels. Anal Biochem 64:509-516

Yamamura T, Sudo H, Ishikawa K, Yamamoto A (1979) Familial Type I hyperlipo-proteinemia caused by apolipoprotein CII deficiency. Atherosclerosis 34:53-65

Tangier Disease

H.B. Brewer, Jr., E.J. Schaefer, L.A. Zech, and T.J. Bronzert

Tangier disease is a rare hereditary disease characterized by hypocholesterolemia and normal to elevated plasma triglycerides. The cardinal
feature of the plasma lipoproteins of patients with Tangier disease is a
marked deficiency of high density lipoproteins (HDL), and a reduction in
low density lipoproteins (LDL) (Fredrickson et al. 1961). The plasma
concentration of apoA-I and apoA-II in Tangier disease is decreased to
1 to 2% and 5 to 7 percent of normal respectively (Assmann et al 1977;
Schaefer et al 1978a).

The clinical features of patients homozygous for Tangier disease include
enlarged orange tonsils, corneal infiltrates, hepatosplenomegaly, lympha-
denopathy, and intermittent peripheral neuropathy. Histological examini-
nation of tissues from several organs has revealed intracellular cholesterol ester deposits particularly in macrophages, nonvascular smooth
muscle cells and Schwann cells (Ferrans and Fredrickson 1975).

Metabolic Studies in Homozygous Patients with Tangier Disease

Our initial studies to delineate the metabolism of HDL in Tangier disease
were conducted in eight normal subjects, two homozygotes and two oligate
heterozygous patients utilizing normal ^{125}I-HDL. Normal ^{125}I-HDL was catabolized at a rapid rate in heterozygotes and extraordinarily rapidly in
homozygous patients (Schaefer et al. 1976, 1978a). These studies were
extended by analysis of the kinetics of normal ^{125}I-apoA-I and ^{131}I-apoA-
II metabolism in 14 normal subjects and three homozygous patients. A
very rapid catabolism of apoA-I and apoA-II was observed in Tangier
patients similar to results obtained with radiolabeled HDL (Table I)
(Schaefer et al. 1978a). In addition, the catabolism of apoA-I was significantly faster than apoA-II (Table I). These studies were interpreted
to indicate that the catabolism of HDL, apoA-I, and apoA-II isolated from
normal individuals was very rapid in patients with Tangier disease
(Schaefer et al. 1976, 1978a). Similar conclusions were drawn from
studies on ^{125}I-HDL metabolism during an HDL infusion by Assmann et al.
1978. The assessment of fractional catabolic rates of apoA-I and apoA-II
in these studies is, however, difficult since the patients were not in
steady state during the HDL infusion.

Determination of the synthesis rates of apoA-I and apoA-II in our patients
with Tangier disease revealed a mild reduction, indicating that these
patients did not have a primary defect in synthesis of either apoA-I or
apoA-II (Table I).

Additional studies were then undertaken to elucidate the major site(s) of
synthesis and metabolic fate of human lipoprotein particles containing
apoA-I and apoA-II. Utilizing the immunoperoxidase technique, apoA-I and
apoA-II were shown to be synthesized in normal as well as Tangier intestine (Schwartz et al. 1978). Similarly apoA-I was reported to be present
in the intestine of Tangier patients by the immunofluorescence technique
(Glickman et al. 1978). Analysis of intestinal lipoproteins revealed that
apoA-I and apoA-II were constitutive apolipoproteins of chylomicrons and

HDL; the daily transport of apoA–I and apoA–II in thoracic duct lymph was 26 mg/kg–hr and 3.7 mg/kg–hr respectively (Anderson et al. 1979). Studies employing ^{125}I–apoA–I and ^{131}I–apoA–II associated with nascent chylomicrons demonstrated that the A–I and A–II apolipoproteins were rapidly transferred to HDL in normal subjects (Schaefer et al. 1978b). These combined results suggested that the intestine was a major site of synthesis of human apoA–I and apoA–II, and that the A–I and A–II apolipoproteins associated with intestinal triglyceride rich lipoproteins can serve as precursors for apoA–I and apoA–II within HDL.

The fate of normal ^{125}I–apoA–I and ^{131}I–apoA–II associated in vitro with Tangier chylomicrons was studied in two normal subjects and two Tangier homozygotes. In normal individuals apoA–I and apoA–II were rapidly transferred to HDL, while no significant apoA–I and apoA–II mass or radioactivity was isolated within HDL in Tangier patients (Schaefer and Brewer 1978). These studies provided the evidence for our concept that the normal conversion of apoA–I and apoA–II on chylomicrons to native HDL does not occur in patients with Tangier disease.

Molecular Defect in Patients with Tangier Disease

The molecular defect responsible for the plasma lipoprotein abnormalities and increased catabolism of apoA–I and apoA–II in Tangier disease remains elusive. Of fundamental importance is the differentiation of primary vs secondary manifestations of the disease. This is of particular importance with respect to the changes observed in the plasma lipoproteins. Electron microscopic examination of the plasma lipoproteins reveals large pleomorphic particles which increase in concentration during dietary hyperlipidemia (Herbert et al. 1978). These particles represent, at least in part, intestinal lipoproteins. As outlined above, we found no significant conversion of chylomicron proteins or lipid constituents into native HDL particles in Tangier disease. The uptake of chylomicrons and/or chylomicron remnants including large vesiculated particles as well as surface components in the form of discs or fragmentary surface constituents into the reticuloendothelial system is consistent with the experimental and clinical findings in Tangier patients.

Whether the abnormal morphology of the plasma lipoproteins and the enhanced catabolism of apoA–I and apoA–II are secondary manifestations of the molecular defect in Tangier disease or are due to a defect in the structure of synthesized lipoprotein particle(s) or a specific apolipoprotein remains to be elucidated. Particular attention has focused on the possibility that the defect in Tangier disease is due to a structural defect in apoA–I. The evidence to support a structural defect in apoA–I is inconclusive. The electrophoretic charge, molecular weight, amino acid composition, and immunological properties of apoA–I from Tangier patients appears virtually identical to apoA–I from control subjects (Lux et al. 1972; Utermann and Beisiegel 1979). The plasma distribution of radiolabeled apoA–I injected into Tangier patients was identical to that of Tangier apoA–I (Schaefer et al. 1978a). The enhanced catabolism of apoA–I was observed in Tangier patients following an HDL infusion which increased the HDL concentration to near normal levels. Kinetic analysis of ^{125}I–apoA–I and ^{131}I–apoA–II during the HDL infusion revealed a rapid catabolism and a decrease in specific activity of both apoA–I and apoA–II within plasma and HDL (Fig. 1). These results would suggest that de novo synthesized apoA–I and apoA–II can become associated with apoA–I and apoA–II containing lipoprotein particles and decrease the specific activity of radiolabeled normal apoA–I and apoA–II. These data are at variance with the results reported by Assmann et al. 1978 who observed no decrease in the specific activity of apoA–I during HDL infusion and emphasized the importance of a probable structural defect of apoA–I. The reason for the difference in these re-

Table 1. Synthesis rates and residence time of apoA–I and apoA–II in normal and homozygous Tangier patients.

	Synthesis Rates[a,b]		Residence Time[a]	
	apoA–I	apoA–II	apoA–I	apoA–II
Normal (N=14)	11.5±2.4	2.1±0.3	4.46±1.04	4.97±1.06
Tangier Homozygotes (N=3)	3.7±0.1	1.3±0.4	0.23±0.06	0.09±0.17

[a]mean values.
[b]mg/kg/day.

sults is as yet unexplained and may represent heterogeneity in the molecular defect in Tangier patients or differences in methodology. Further studies will be required to definitively establish the molecular defect(s) in patients with Tangier disease.

Premature Atherosclerosis and Tangier Disease

The recent recognition that HDL–cholesterol is a negative risk factor for the development of premature cardiovascular disease is of particular interest with respect to patients with Tangier disease. We have recently reviewed our own clinical experience and the published cases of Tangier disease (Schaefer et al. 1979). No homozygous patients below the age of 40 have been reported with vascular disease. Of patients over 40 years of age 6 of 9 homozygotes had evidence of vascular disease. The number of Tangier patients is small and definitive conclusions regarding vascular disease are therefore difficult to make. With the present data it would appear that Tangier patients may have some increase in premature vascular disease, however it is clear that these patients do not experience the strikingly premature vascular disease seen in patients with homozygous familial hypercholesterolemia.

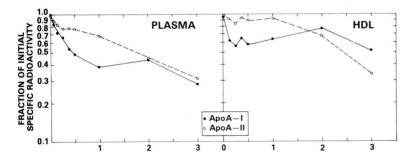

FIG. 1. Plasma decay of injected normal ^{125}I–apoA–I and ^{131}I–apoA–II in a homozygous patient with Tangier disease.

References

Anderson DW, Bronzert TJ, Schaefer EJ, Niblack GD, Zech LA, Forte T, Brewer HB Jr (1979) Evidence for recirculation of apolipoproteins A-I and A-II between plasma and human thoracic duct lymph. Clin Res 27: 362A

Assmann G, Smootz E, Adler K, Capurso A, Oette K (1977) The lipoprotein abnormality in Tangier disease, quantitation of A apoproteins. J Clin Invest 59: 565-575

Assmann G, Capurso A, Smootz E, Wellner U (1978) Apoprotein A metabolism in Tangier disease. Atherosclerosis 30: 321-332

Ferrans VJ, Fredrickson DS (1975) The pathology of Tangier disease: a light and electron microscopic study. Am J Pathol 78: 101-158

Fredrickson DS, Altrocchi PH, Avioli LV, Goodman DS, Goodman HC (1961) Tangier disease. Ann Int Med 55: 707-714

Glickman RM, Green PHR, Lee RS, Tall A (1978) Apolipoprotein A-I synthesis in normal intestinal mucosa and in Tangier mucosa. N Eng J Med 299: 1424-1427

Herbert PN, Gotto AM Jr, Fredrickson DS (1978) Familial lipoprotein deficiency (abetalipoproteinemia, hypobetalipoproteinemia and Tangier disease). In: Stanbury JB, Wyngaarden JB, Fredrickson DS (eds) The metabolic basis of inherited disease. 4th edn. McGraw-Hill, New York, pp 544-588

Lux SE, Levy RI, Gotto AM Jr, Fredrickson DS (1972) Studies on the protein defect in Tangier disease: isolation and characterization of an abnormal high density lipoprotein. J Clin Invest 51: 2505-2519

Schaefer EJ, Blum CB, Levy RI, Goebel RH, Brewer HB Jr, Berman M (1976) High density lipoprotein metabolism in Tangier disease. Circulation 54: 27-II

Schaefer EJ, Blum CB, Levy RI, Jenkins LL, Alaupovic P, Foster D, Brewer, HB Jr (1978a) Metabolism of high density lipoprotein apolipoproteins in Tangier disease. N Engl J Med 299: 905-910

Schaefer, EJ, Brewer, HB Jr (1978) Tangier disease: a defect in the conversion of chylomicrons to high density lipoproteins. Clin Res 26: 532A

Schaefer EJ, Jenkins LL, Brewer, HB Jr (1978b) Human chylomicron apolipoprotein metabolism. Biochem Biophys Res Commun 80: 405-412

Schaefer EJ, Zech LA, Schwartz DE, Brewer HB Jr (1979) Clinical features and coronary artery disease prevalence in familial high density lipoprotein deficiency (Tangier disease). Ann Int Med (in press).

Schwartz DE, Liotta L, Schaefer EJ, Brewer HB Jr (1978) Localization of apolipoproteins A-I, A-II, and B in normal, Tangier, and abetalipoproteinemia intestinal mucosa. Circulation 58: II-90

Utermann G, Beisiegel U (1979) Charge-shift electrophoresis of apolipoproteins from normal humans and patients with Tangier disease. FEBS Lett 97: 245-248

Abetalipoproteinemia and Hypobetalipoproteinemia: Questions Still Exceed Insights[1]

Peter N. Herbert, Robert J. Heinen, Linda L. Bausserman, Karen M. Lynch, L. Omar Henderson, and Thomas A. Musliner

The absence from plasma of all lipoproteins ordinarily containing apolipo-protein B (apoB) is the only unique characteristic of abetalipoproteinemia. The typical clinical features of this disease including acanthocytic defor-mation of the erythrocyte, fat malabsorption, retinitis pigmentosa, and spino-cerebellar and posterior column degeneration occur alone or in combination in a variety of other syndromes. This natural biochemical ablation experi-ment has yielded many insights relevant to normal plasma lipid transport. Nevertheless, much of our knowledge of abetalipoproteinemia is still largely descriptive. Data available for almost three decades still await integra-tion and interpretation. Only selected areas of ignorance and apparent enlightenment are briefly considered here.

Genetics

At least two distinct genetic abnormalities are characterized by the absence of apo-B (Herbert and Fredrickson 1976). The classical form of the disease has a typical autosomal recessive pattern of inheritance in which no signal abnormality has been detected in obligate heterozygotes. It is tempting to postulate that a structural mutation in one apoB gene may be without biologi-cal consequence in the presence of a normal allele. Obviously any post-tran-scriptional mechanism for which full compensation is possible could be simi-larly invoked. The fact that no "cross-reacting material" has been identified in abetalipoproteinemic plasma cannot be extrapolated to the conclusion that the mutant gene elaborates no product. The intracellular assembly of very low density lipoproteins (VLDL) and chylomicrons involves a series of biosynthetic and transport processes. Many of these are not well defined and the secretion of a mutant apoB could be blocked at one of several steps. The absence of apoB immunofluorescence in intestinal biopsies in abetalipoproteinemia simi-larly cannot be construed as evidence that no translation of a mutant apoB occurs. Antisera to apoB predictably do not react nearly as well (if at all) with apoB used as immunogen while immunoprecipitation with low density lipo-proteins (LDL) is readily demonstrated.

Recently a second form of "abetalipoproteinemia" due to familial homozygous hypobetalipoproteinemia has been described (Cottrill et al. 1974; Biemer and McCammon 1975). Obligate heterozygotes have had reduced plasma levels of LDL and, since male-to-male transmission has been documented, inheritance through a dominant autosomal gene seems probable. Here again the product of the mu-tant gene is unknown and, moreover, the degree of genetic heterogeneity en-compassed by "familial hypobetalipoproteinemia" is uncertain. Levy et al. (1970) and Sigurdsson and co-workers (1977) have studied two kindred with a familial form of hypobetalipoproteinemia and shown that apoB synthetic rates were reduced while catabolic rates were normal. These metabolic studies, however, were not performed in first degree relatives of patients with abeta-

---

[1]Supported in part by The Miriam Hospital Cardiology Research and Education Fund

lipoproteinemia secondary to homozygous hypobetalipoproteinemia. Thus the assumption that VLDL synthesis in the latter subjects is low remains unproved. The prevalence of familial hypobetalipoproteinemia is not known. Only three families with affected homozygotes have been described (Table 1).

Table 1. Plasma cholesterol levels in homozygotes and obligate heterozygotes with hypobetalipoproteinemia.

	Cottrill et al.(1974)	Biemer et al.(1975) (mg/100 ml)	Kindred "R"
Heterozygotes	78–99	100	70,84
Homozygotes	22,13	31	19

The highest cholesterol level documented in these "obligate" heterozygotes, 100 mg/100 ml, is well below the five-percentile fiducial limit in most populations. Unless most homozygotic hypobetalipoproteinemics have eluded detection, we must conclude that the gene for hypobetalipoproteinemia is very rare even among hypocholesterolemics.

Lipids, Lipoprotein, and the Acanthocyte

Comparison of the plasma lipids in abetalipoproteinemia and Tangier disease (Table 2) is informative because these states provide an opportunity to separately view the chylomicron-VLDL-LDL and the high density lipoprotein (HDL) systems uncomplicated by their usual extensive interactions. Comparable

Table 2. Plasma lipids in abetalipoproteinemia (ABL), Tangier disease, (TD) and normals (N).

	ABL	TD (range, mg/100 ml)	N
Cholesterol	18–96	25–101	∿100–250
Triglyceride	0–36	72–362	∿ 40–200
Phospholipid	24–105	40–150	∿150–250
Phosphatidylcholine/sphingomyelin	1.5	5.5	3.3

degrees of hypocholesterolemia are seen in both disorders. Triglyceride elevations are not uncommon in Tangier disease while only very small amounts of triglyceride are present in abetalipoproteinemic plasma. The plasma phospholipid derangements in these two disorders are particularly noteworthy (Table 2). Plasma concentrations of phosphatidylcholine are normally threefold greater than levels of sphingomyelin. Sphingomyelin constitutes about 26% of the phospholipid in normal LDL whereas it comprises only 14% in normal HDL. In Tangier disease, however, the absolute and relative amounts of plasma sphingomyelin are greatly reduced. Blumenfeld and co-workers (1979) have recently provided a plausible explanation for this observation. They showed that the sphingomyelin of cultured smooth muscle cells was much more exchangeable than phosphatidylcholine (86% vs. 21%) and the sphingomyelin was selectively transferred to HDL. The in vivo changes in phosphatidylcholine and sphingomyelin in Tangier disease and abetalipoproteinemia (Table 2) suggest, therefore, that HDL are the principal acceptors of tissue sphingomyelin and, moreover, that the sphingomyelin of HDL may be the origin of much of that phospholipid species eventually transported in LDL.

Absolute and relative amounts of phosphatidylcholine are diminished in abetalipoproteinemic plasma and, together with the proportional increase in sphingomyelin, this likely accounts for the sphingomyelin enrichment of erythrocytes in this disorder. We have reviewed evidence that the acanthocyte is formed after release into the circulation and that the membrane deformity is not a primary abnormality (Herbert and Fredrickson 1976). Cooper and co-workers (1977), moreover, have demonstrated that the sphingomyelin enrichment of the acanthocytes greatly reduces the fluidity of its plasma membrane and probably contributes to its "remodeling" during circulation. Thus alteration of the plasma phosphatidylcholine:sphingomyelin ratio probably causes the discocyte to acanthocyte transformation. This hypothesis is buttressed by the normal morphology of erythrocytes in Tangier disease even when plasma cholesterol concentrations are less than 20 mg/100 ml.

Apolipoproteins

All of the apolipoproteins in abetalipoproteinemic plasma are secreted as HDL or at least transported in this lipoprotein fraction. ApoB is the only well characterized apolipoprotein known to be absent. The monosialylated apoprotein C-III, apoC-III-1, has not been isolated from abetalipoproteinemic plasma (Herbert and Fredrickson 1976) and it has been postulated that this polymorph is secreted with VLDL. We have similarly found no evidence for the presence of apoC-III-1 in abetalipoproteinemia, but a protein of the same mobility has been repeatedly identified in the apoHDL of two subjects with homozygous hypobetalipoproteinemia (Fig. 1).

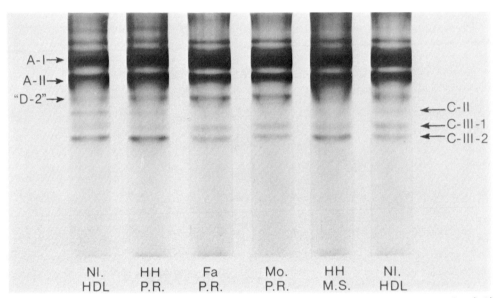

FIG. 1. Polyacrylamide gel electropherograms of apoHDL from two normals (N1), two subjects with homozygous hypobetalipoproteinemia (HH), and two obligate heterozygotes with hypobetalipoproteinemia (Fa, father; Mo, mother). An anionic (pH=9.4) system containing urea was employed.

The significance of this finding is unclear but one might speculate that traces of VLDL are elaborated in the latter disorder and sensitive immunoassays should certainly be applied in a search for apoB in the plasma of affected subjects.

HDL cholesterol concentrations are usually quite low in both abetalipoproteinemia and homozygous hypobetalipoproteinemia. We have quantified plasma apoA-1 and apoA-II in four patients with abetalipoproteinemia and one with homozygous hypobetalipoproteinemia. Mean apoA-I levels were 51 mg/100 mg (range 38-74 mg/100 ml), approximately half normal. ApoA-II concentrations were 60-70 percent of normal ($\overline{X}$=22 mg/100 ml; range 18-29 mg/100 ml). This disproportionate reduction in apoA-I levels has not previously been noted, and may relate to reduced intestinal contribution to the apoA-I plasma pool. Conversely, augmented HDL-catabolism in the absence of the lower density lipoproteins has not been excluded.

One additional feature of abetalipoproteinemic apoHDL, recently recognized, is the prominence of the E-A-II apoprotein (Fig. 2).

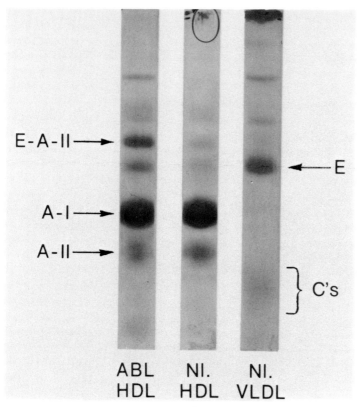

FIG. 2. SDS polyacrylamide (7½% monomer) gel electropherograms of apoHDL and apoVLDL from a normal (N1) and apoHDL from a patient with abetalipoproteinemia (ABL).

It is not known if this "mixed-disulfide" is a "pro-apolipoprotein" or is formed by reaction of the apoA-II disulfide dimer with the single cysteine in apoE (Weisgraber and Mahley 1978). The prominence of this apoprotein complex in abetalipoproteinemic HDL may result from the absence of VLDL in which apoE is a major constituent. ApoE enrichment of HDL may therefore favor production of the mixed disulfide, apoE-A-II.

Organ Dysfunction

The retinitis pigmentosa, and spinocerebellar and posterior column degeneration in abetalipoproteinemia are the most devastating complications in this syndrome. Even brief consideration of this disorder would be irrelevant if the readers attention was not called to the possible role for vitamin E in the management of these patients (Muller et al. 1977; H. Kayden, personal communication; Herbert et al. 1978). The possibility that a unique degree of vitamin E deficiency causes the profound morbidity in this disorder may prove to be the single most important lesson derived from studies of these disorders.

References

Blumenfeld OO, Schwartz E, Adamany AM (1979) Efflux of phospholipids from cultured aortic smooth muscle cells. J Biol Chem 254: 7183-7190

Biemer JJ, McCammon RE (1975) The genetic relationship of abetalipoproteinemia and hypobetalipoproteinemia: a report of the occurence of both diseases within the same family. J Lab Clin Med 85: 556-565

Cooper RA, Durocher JR, Leslie MH (1977) Decreased fluidity of red cell membrane lipids in abetalipoproteinemia. J Clin Invest 60: 115-121

Cottrill C, Glueck CJ, Leuba V, Millett F, Puppione D, Brown WV (1974) Familial homozygous hypobetalipoproteinemia. Metabolism 23: 779-791

Herbert PN, Fredrickson DS (1976) The hypobetalipoproteinemias. In: Schettler G, Greten H, Schlierf G, Seidel D (eds) Handbuch der Inneren Medizin, VII/4: Fettstoffwechsel. Springer-Verlag, Heidelberg

Herbert PN, Gotto AM, Fredrickson DS (1978) Familial lipoprotein deficiency (abetalipoproteinemia, hypobetalipoproteinemia and Tangier disease). In: Stanbury JB, Wyngaarden JB, and Fredrickson DS (eds) The Metabolic Basis of Inherited Disease. McGraw-Hill, New York

Levy RI, Langer T, Gotto AM, Fredrickson DS (1970) Familial hypobetalipoproteinemia, a defect in lipoprotein synthesis. Clin Res 18: 539

Muller DPR, Lloyd JK, Bird AC (1977) Long term management of abetalipoproteinemia. Possible role for vitamin E. Arch Dis Childh 52: 209-214

Sigurdsson G, Nicoll A, Lewis B (1977) Turnover of apolipoprotein-B in two subjects with familial hypobetalipoproteinemia. Metabolism 26: 25-31

Weisgraber KH, Mahley RW (1978) Apoprotein (E-A-II) complex of human plasma lipoproteins. J Biol Chem 253: 6281-6288

688

Polymorphism of Apolipoprotein E

Gerd Utermann

Plasma cholesterol levels are under multifactorial control. Environmental as well as genetic factors contribute to the considerable variance of cholesterol concentrations within and in between populations. Individual genes responsible for the normal variance of cholesterol in plasma have however not yet been identified. Conceptually such gene loci should be polymorphic and certain combinations of these genes may lead to polygenic familial hypercholesterolemia. On the other hand conditions are known where one rare mutant gene drastically affects the concentration of plasma lipids. Carriers of those genes have a monogenic familial dyslipoproteinemia. Among those are familial hypercholesterolemia, abetalipoproteinemia, Tangier disease, familial LCAT-deficiency and familial hyperchylomicronemia. Hence rare mutant genes, polymorphic gene loci and environmental factors have to be considered as determinants of plasma lipid levels. This makes the plasma lipoprotein system an excellent model to study the interaction of genes and environment in producing a multifactorial disease. Mutations resulting in familial dyslipoproteinemia may afflict: 1. the synthesis, assembly and secretion of lipoproteins, 2. the structure of apolipoproteins, 3. enzymes involved in the interconversion and intravasal catabolism of lipoproteins (lipase, LCAT) and 4. recognition, uptake and degradation of lipoproteins by cells. The same gene loci afflicted in familial dyslipoproteinemia also have to be considered responsible for normal genetic variance of plasma lipid and lipoprotein levels.

We have focused our attention on the search for possible genetic polymorphism of apolipoproteins. Methods recently developed in our laboratory that combine specific precipitation of lipoproteins (Burstein et al., 1970) with lipid extraction and subsequent electrofocusing of urea soluble apolipoproteins allow routine screening for charge variants of human apolipoproteins A-I, A-II, C-II, C-III and E (Utermann et al. 1977a,c 1978; Utermann unpublished). Application of these methods has lead to the discovery of a complex genetic system of apolipoprotein E. The genes controling this system have a significant effect on plasma lipoprotein concentrations.

Genetics of the Apo E-System

Apolipoprotein E is a major component of human VLDL. Isoelectric focusing of apo-VLDL yields five different Apo E-phenotypes (FIG. 1). These are controlled by two codominant alleles Apo E^n and Apo E^d at the Apo E-N/D locus (phenotypes Apo E-N, -ND and -D) and by two alleles the dominant Apo $E4^+$ and the recessive Apo E^O at the Apo E4 locus (phenotypes Apo E4 (+), Apo E4 (-); Utermann et al. 1977a,c, 1979a,b). Analysis of the frequency distribution of Apo E-phenotypes in blood donors demonstrated a highly significant association between both systems (X^2_{df1}=6.15; p∿o.o1).

The Apo E4 (+) phenotype is about twice as frequent in phenotype Apo E-N than in phenotype Apo E-ND (Table 1). The phenotypic combination Apo E-D/E4 (+) was not observed among the blood donors and also not in our total published material that includes 23 non-related Apo E-D subjects (p<0.0001). The association between both systems may be explained assuming very close linkage of the two Apo E-loci and a linkage disequilibrium of Δ=0.0147. The observed frequencies are in good agreement with those expected from Hardy-Weinberg's law (X^2_{df2}=0.43; p~0.8; Utermann et al. 1979b). The segregation of Apo E-phenotypes in 72 matings with a total of 167 offsprings is consistent with the close linkage of both loci. Apo E^n and Apo $E4^+$ cosegregate in all informative matings. The data may be explained by a formal genetic model where three haplotypes (Apo $E^n/E4^+$ (0.1452), Apo $E^n/E4^0$ (0.7660), and Apo $E^d/E4^0$ (0.0888)) determine the five different Apo E-phenotypes. The data may alternatively be explained by a second model where also the fourth hypothetical haplotype Apo $E^d/E4^+$ exists but where the gene Apo $E4^+$ is not expressed while in coupling with Apo E^d. A control function of the Apo E-N/D locus over the Apo E4 locus in the sense of an operator/promoter has to be anticipated in the four haplotype models. On the basis of present data the two models can not be distinguished by formal genetic criteria. However the four haplotype model seems more atractive in view of the quantitative character of the Apo E-N/D polymorphism and of biochemical results. These show that apolipoproteins E from phenotypes Apo E-N and Apo E-D differ in M_r according to their mobility in SDS-PAGE (FIG. 1) and that this reflects a difference in size of Apo E-II and Apo E-III, that are the major Apo E polymorphic forms of the two phenotypes, respectively. Hence the Apo E-N/D-locus may control structural genes involved in the posttranslational modification of Apo E (Utermann et al. 1979b,d).

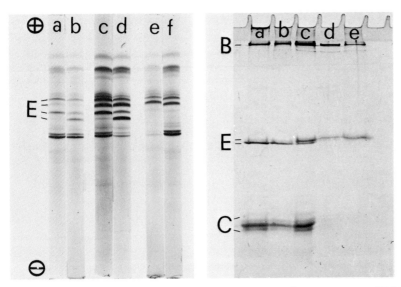

FIG. 1. left: Analytical electrofocusing of apo-VLDL (heparin/Mg-precipitate) from phenotypes Apo E-N/E4- (a), Apo E-N/E4+ (b), Apo E-ND/E4- (c), Apo E-ND/E4+ (d) and Apo E-D/E4- (e,f). pH-gradient from 3.5-1o. right: SDS-PAGE of apo-VLDL from phenotypes Apo E-N (a,b), Apo E-ND (c) and Apo E-D (d,e).

Table 1: Frequency of Apo E4-variant in Apo E-N/D-phenotypes

	Total	Apo E4 (+)	Apo E4 (-)
Apo E-N	574 (8o.1%)	173 (3o.1%)	4o1 (69.9%)
Apo E-ND	134 (18.7%)	22 (16.4%)	112 (83.6%)
Apo E-D	9 (1.2%)	0 (0 %)	9 (100 %)

Apo E-Polymorphism and Plasma Lipoproteins

The genes Apo E^n and Apo E^d have a significant effect on the concentration of plasma lipids and on the distribution of cholesterol among lipoprotein fractions (Utermann et al. 1979c). All
individuals of the homozygous phenotype Apo E-D exhibit a characteristic dyslipoproteinemia. LDL concentration is low and many
Apo E-D subjects have hypobetalipoproteinemia (Utermann et al.
1977c, 1979c; Weidman et al. 1979).VLDL usually is elevated,
rich in cholesterol and contains a subfraction of beta-mobility
(beta-VLDL). This typical lipoprotein distribution has been designated primary dysbetalipoproteinemia and corresponds to the
lipoprotein pattern seen in hyperlipoproteinemia type III (Utermann et al. 1977c, 1979a). However most of the Apo E-D subjects
detected in population based studies had remarkably low total
plasma cholesterol and not at all hypercholesterolemia. A systematic comparison of the phenotypic groups Apo E-N, -ND and -D revealed that cholesterol concentrations differ significantly between the three phenotypes. Mean cholesterol at age 4o years was
lowest in phenotype Apo E-D (161$\pm$51 mg/1ooml), intermediate in
phenotype Apo E-ND (186$\pm$32 mg/1ooml) and highest in phenotype
Apo E-N (2o4$\pm$41 mg/1ooml). In contrast, plasma triglyceride, VLDL-triglyceride and VLDL-cholesterol were highest in phenotype Apo E-D
(Utermann et al. 1979c). The hypocholesterolemic effect of the
gene Apo E^d was confirmed by a study of subjects with primary
hypocholesterolemia (plasma cholesterol on repeated determinations <13omg/1ooml, no evidence for secondary hypocholesterolemia). From the hypocholesterolemic subjects 1o% were of phenotype Apo E-D compared to 1% in the general population (Utermann
et al. unpublished). These data show that the alleles Apo E^n and
Apo E^d determine three overlapping distributions of cholesterol
in the population. This is the first example of a polymorphic
gene locus in man with a significant effect on the normal variance of plasma lipid levels. Moreover phenotype Apo E-D characte-
rises the most frequent monogenic (autosomal recessive) dyslipoproteinemia in man.

Apo E-Phenotypes and Myocardial Infarction

The significant effect of the Apo E-genes on plasma cholesterol
levels implies a major role of this gene locus in the development
of human atherosclerosis. The frequency distribution of Apo E-
phenotypes was determined in 328 individuals with myocardial infarction and compared to that in 49o blood donors (table 2). The
frequency of Apo E-D individuals was not significantly different
in both groups. This indicates that phenotype Apo E-D per se
(that is primary dysbetalipoproteinemia without hyperlipoproteinemia) is not a risk factor for atherosclerosis. The frequency

691

Table 2: Frequencies of Apo E-Phenotypes

Blood donors	observed	expected[a]	x^2/p
Apo E-N/4+	119 (24.3%)	119.3	
Apo E-N/4-	289 (59.o%)	287.5	x^2_{df2}=o.43
Apo E-ND/4+	13 (2.7%)	12.6	
Apo E-ND/4-	64 (13.1%)	66.6	p < o.8
Apo E-D/4-	5 (1.o%)	3.9	
Total	49o (1oo %)	49o.o	

Myocardial Infarction			
Apo E-N/4+	65 (19.8%)	79.9	
Apo E-N/4-	22o (67.1%)	192.5	x^2_{df4}=9.95
Apo E-ND/4+	5 (1.5%)	8.5	
Apo E-ND/4-	36 (11.o%)	44.6	p < o.o5
Apo E-D/4-	2 (o.6%)	2.6	
Total	328 (1oo %)	328.o	

[a]Expected numbers were calculated in blood donors assuming Hardy-Weinberg's equilibrium. Expected numbers in the patients with myocardial infarction were calculated from the gene frequencies determined in blood donors.

of Apo E-phenotypes in patients with myocardial infarction was significantly different from those expected from the gene frequencies determined in blood donors. Interpretation of this result however is difficult and more extensive studies obviously are necessary.

Hyperlipoproteinemia Type III

All individuals (N=42) studied so far in our laboratory that had hyperlipoproteinemia type III according to conventional contemporary definitions are of phenotype Apo E-D (Utermann et al. 1975, 1977b, 1979a). This observation has been confirmed by others (Pagnan et al. 1977, Warnick et al. 1979, Weidman et al. 1979). The frequency of phenotype Apo E-D (1:1oo) however is an order of magnitude higher than that of hyperlipoproteinemia type III (1:1ooo - 1:5ooo). Moreover most Apo E-D individuals have no hyperlipoproteinemia but all have dysbetalipoproteinemia. Hence presence of the Apo E-D phenotype seems a necessary but not sufficient condition for the development of clinical hyperlipoproteinemia type III. Comparative studies of 19 kindreds ascertained by a proband of phenotype Apo E-D support this concept. Non-type III forms of familial hyperlipidemia segregated in kindreds of grossly hyperlipidemic but not of normolipidemic Apo E-D probands (Utermann et al.1979a). Hyperlipidemia and Apo E-phenotypes segregated independently in the hyperlipidemia kindreds. We therefore concluded that hyperlipoproteinemia type III results from the coexistence of the homozygous genotype Apo E^d/E^d and "hyperlipidemia genes" in one individual. Since "hyperlipidemia genes" may be either those for the dominant forms of hyperlipidemia (Goldstein et al. 1973) or may be different kinds of sets of genes resulting in polygenic hyperlipidemia there will be several kinds of genotypic combinations that all share the basic Apo E^d/E^d genotype. Familial hyperlipoproteinemia type III than is caused by mutation at at least two non allelic gene loci and is dimeric in some and polygenic in other individuals. Moreover exogenous factors may interfere and aggravate the hyperlipidemia in individuals with a polygenic disposition. This model predicts that there will be considerable phenotypic variation in hyperlipoproteinemia type III.

None of the individuals with simple dysbetalipoproteinemia seen in this study had signs of atherosclerotic vascular disease. It therefore seems that normolipidemic Apo E-D subjects have no increased risk to develop premature atherosclerosis but that the coexisting "hyperlipidemia genes" convert a benign variant of lipoprotein metabolism into a severe disorder.

References

Burstein M, Scholnick HR, Morfin R (197o) Rapid method for the isolation of lipoproteins from human serum by precipitation with polyanions. J Lipid Res 11: 583-595

Goldstein JL, Schrott HG, Hazzard WR, Bierman EL, Motulsky AG, (1973) Hyperlipidemia in coronary heart disease. II. Genetics analysis of lipid levels in 176 families and delineation of a new inherited disorder, combined hyperlipidemia. J Clin Invest 52: 1544-1568

Pagnan A, Havel RJ, Kane JP, Kotite L (1977) Characterisation of human very low density lipoproteins containing two electrophoretic populations: double pre-beta lipoproteinemia and primary dysbetalipoproteinemia. J Lipid Res 18: 613-622

Utermann G, Jaeschke M, Menzel J (1975) Familial hyperlipoproteinemia type III: Deficiency of a specific apolipoprotein (Apo E-III) in the very low density lipoproteins. F E B S Letters 56: 352-355

Utermann G, Beisiegel U, Hees M, Mühlfellner G, Pruin N, Steinmetz A (1977a) A further genetic polymorphism of apolipoprotein E from human very low density lipoproteins. Protides of the Biological Fluids XXV, ed. Peeters H, Pergamon, Oxford-New York, pp 277-284

Utermann G, Canzler H, Hees M, Jaeschke M, Mühlfellner G, Schoenborn W, Vogelberg KH (1977b) Studies on the metabolic defects in Broad-ß disease (hyperlipoproteinemia type III). Clin Genet 12: 139-154

Utermann G, Hees M, Steinmetz A (1977c) Polymorphism of apolipoprotein E and occurence of dysbetalipoproteinemia in man. Nature 269: 6o4-6o7

Utermann G, Albrecht G, Steinmetz A (1978) Polymorphism of apolipoprotein E. I. Methodological aspects and diagnosis of hyperlipoproteinemia type III without ultracentrifugation. Clin Genet 14: 351-358

Utermann G, Canzler H, Hees M, Jaeschke M, Pruin N, Schoenborn, W, Steinmetz A, Vogelberg KH (1979a) Polymorphism of apolipoprotein E. II. Genetics of hyperlipoproteinemia type III. Clin Genet 15: 37-62

Utermann G, Langenbeck U, Beisiegel U, Weber W (1979b) Genetics of the Apo E-system in man. Am J Hum Genet in press

Utermann G, Pruin N, Steinmetz A (1979c) Polymorphism of apolipoprotein E. III. Effect of a single polymorphic gene locus on plasma lipid levels in man. Clin Genet 15: 63-72

Utermann G, Weber W, Beisiegel U (1979d) Different mobility in SDS-polyacrylamide-gel-electrophoresis of apolipoprotein E

from phenotypes Apo E-N and Apo E-D. F E B S Letters lol:
21-26

Warnick GR, Mayfield C, Albers JJ, Hazzard RW (1979) Gel Isoelectric focusing method for specific diagnosis of familial
hyperlipoproteinemia type III. Clin Chem 25: 279-284

Weidman WS, Suarez B, Falko JM, Witzum JL, Kolar J, Raben M,
Schoenfeld G (1979) Type III hyperlipoproteinemia: Development of a VLDL Apo E gel, isoelectric focusing technique and
application in family studies. J Lab Clin Med 13: 549-569

Renin Sodium Profiling and Vasoconstriction Volume Analysis of Hypertensive Patients. A New Era for Diagnosis and Treatment

John H. Laragh

A series of studies in humans and in animal models have led us to formulate an all-encompassing hypothesis for exposing and analyzing the mechanisms in all forms of human hypertension. The hypothesis, the vasoconstriction-volume hypothesis, proposes that blood pressure is always ultimately determined by the interplay of two factors: first, the size of the container between the aortic valves and the capillaries, and secondly the amount of liquid filling this container. Thus, whatever the myriad of inputs that may affect arterial pressure, ultimately they must be expressed by affecting one of these two final determinants (Figure 1).

This hypothesis is useful because it can be applied for a quantitative analysis of pressor mechanisms in all patients. By using one of three pharmacological probes that block any dynamic reaction of the renin system it becomes possible to evaluate the volume factor (determined by the state of sodium balance) either by controlling sodium balance or by manipulating it with natriuretic-diuretic drugs, in the presence of a maintained renin blockade.

The drugs that block the renin system and produce parallel effects or lack of effects are (1) beta blockers all of which lower renin secretion, (2) the angiotensin II receptor antagonists (e.g. saralasin), and (3) the converting enzyme inhibitors that block angiotensin II formation (e.g. Teprotide and Captopril). Our parallel research in humans and in animals using these three probes provides the proof of the active long-term participation of the renin system in most forms of high blood pressure and also for its active participation in the regulation of normal pressure. Moreover, unilateral renovascular hypertension in humans is similarly renin-dependent. It exhibits a high plasma renin-sodium profile, responds to anti-renin drugs and is surgically curable. In contrast, the hypertension of patients with bilateral kidney disease resembles the one-kidney volume dependent animal model. These latter patients are characterized by low total GFR, impaired sodium excretion and normal or low plasma renin values. They are correctible by volume depletion, using diuretics or ultrafiltration hemodialysis.

Using renin-sodium profiling, it can be shown that, contrary to the traditional view, essential hypertension is not homogeneous but can be physiologically differentiated into 3 subgroups of low, "normal" or high renin. Our companion research shows that these different renin patterns have pathophysiologic relevance. Thus, using the depressor responses to the anti-renin system drugs, it can be shown that angiotensin II actually actively participates in maintaining the hypertension of most essential hypertension, the high and "normal" renin types. Patients within the renin subgroups also exhibit correspondingly different and predicted hemodynamic and rheologic abnormalities. Moreover, our attendant epidemiologic studies have correlated these differences in physiology with differences in clinical course and prognosis. Thus, low renin patients live longer and suffer less heart attack and strokes than those who have varying degrees of renin vasoconstriction.

According to their renin profiles, all clinical forms of hypertension can be placed in a spectrum that ranges between the predominance of arterial vasoconstriction or a predominant excess of one component relative to the other

(Figure 2). Malignant hypertension and primary aldosteronism are the polar
extremes of this spectrum. These two are due largely to excess vasoconstriction or excess volume respectively. In most patients, this vasoconstriction-
volume pathophysiologic imbalance can be revealed easily by renin-sodium
profiling and verified by the clinical response to anti-renin or to volume-
reducing drugs.

The new level of understanding created by these findings has practical application for more modern treatment strategies. In practice, a baseline renin-
sodium profile test together with determination of plasma potassium levels
becomes the basic first step in screening all patients for surgically curable
renovascular or adrenocortical hypertensions. Then, for the former, a mathematical analysis of renal vein renin values is the definitive test, whereas
for the latter a urinary aldosterone sodium profile plus an appropriate
plasma aldosterone measurement establishes the diagnosis. For the remaining
majority of patients not surgically curable but with so-called essential
hypertension, renin profiling defines their heterogeneity by revealing the
degree of participation of vasoconstriction and volume factors sustaining
the high blood pressure. For most patients, this analysis steers and hastens
simpler, more specific, predictable treatments by guiding the use of either
anti-renin or anti-volume agents as the first drug. In particular, the renin
profile picks out those who should be started with an anti-renin drug first
as opposed to a diuretic.

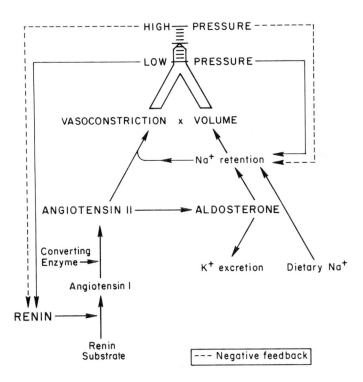

FIG. 1. Renin-angiotensin-aldosterone system. Renin secreted in response to reduced arterial pressure or renal
tubular sodium acts to release angiotensin II. Angiotensin
II raises pressure and stimulates aldosterone secretion,
leading to sodium and water retention. These pressure and
volume effects turn off more renin release. From Laragh
JH, et al., JAMA 241: 151-156, 1979.

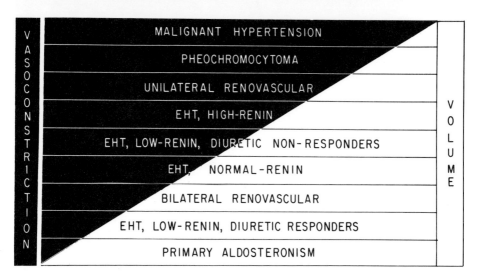

FIG. 2. Vasoconstriction-volume spectrum in hypertension. Abbreviation EHT
indicates essential hypertension. From Laragh JH, et al., JAMA 241:
151-156, 1979.

This approach thus separates out at the beginning major fractions of patients
in whom one drug instead of two will be effective for the long-term because
in them the drug selected works to contain the particular abnormal physiology
identified. In low-renin patients the test suggests a physiologic setup with
overfilling, which can be maintained on a diuretic alone for the longer term.
In contrast, diuretic drugs are less effective, and may be contraindicated,
in most patients with high or normal renin values. These drugs produce
hypovolemia, hemoconcentration, high renin and low K+ levels, all influences not theoretically attractive for long-term maintenance. Only for a
small remaining group of refractory patients is the older traditional trial
and error therapy with superimposition of other less palatable agents necessary. Moreover, besides its diagnostic and therapeutic and prognostic values,
this new analytical method also serves to expose those exceptional patients
with still undefined pressor mechanisms for more research into their causation and treatment.

Meanwhile, for major fractions, this new construction offers long-term control with one drug instead of two with the attraction of lesion specific
treatment. Fewer drugs adds up to lower cost, less disturbance of physical
and mental function. This means better compliance and long term results.

Summary

Recent research shows that the renin-angiotensin-aldosterone axis either
maintains or causes some or all of the high blood pressure of most patients
and demonstrates anew that renin-sodium profiling defines this involvement.
Performed with a serum potassium measurement, this now reliable test is useful for primary screening and then, in conjunction with renal vein renin
studies or an aldosterone profile, for the final diagnosis or exclusion of
surgically curable renovascular or adrenocortical hypertensions. For the
remaining majority who have essential hypertension, renin profiling exposes
the relative participation of either vasoconstriction or volume factors,
thereby guiding simpler, more specific and predictably effective anti-renin
or anti-volume treatments. Renin profiling identifies those who should be
started with a beta blocker as opposed to a diuretic while not infrequently

also providing baseline information about severity and prognosis in individual patients.

References

Ames RP, Borkowski AJ, Sicinski AM, Laragh JH (1965) Prolonged infusions of angiotensin II and norepinephrine and blood pressure, electrolyte balance, aldosterone and cortisol secretion in normal man and in cirrhosis with ascites. J Clin Invest 44: 1171–1186

Bühler FR, Laragh JH, Baer L, Vaughan ED Jr, Brunner HR (1972) Propranolol inhibition of renin secretion. A specific approach to diagnosis and treatment of renin-dependent hypertensive disease. N Engl J Med 287: 1209–1214

Brunner HR, Kirshman JD, Sealey JE, Laragh JH (1971) Hypertension of renal origin: Evidence for two different mechanisms. Science 174: 1344–1346

Brunner HR, Laragh JH, Baer L, Newton MA, Goodwin FT, Krakoff LR, Bard RH, Bühler FR (1972) Essential hypertension: Renin and aldosterone, heart attack and stroke. N Engl J Med 286: 441–449

Case DB, Wallace JM, Keim HJ, Weber MA, Sealey JE, Laragh JH (1977) Possible role of renin in hypertension as suggested by renin-sodium profiling and inhibition of converting enzyme. N Engl J Med 296: 641–646

Laragh JH, Ulick S, Januszewicz V, Deming QB, Kelly WG, Lieberman S (1960) Aldosterone secretion and primary and malignant hypertension. J Clin Invest 39: 1091–1106

Laragh JH, Angers M, Kelly WG, Lieberman S (1960) Hypotensive agents and pressor substances. The effect of epinephrine, norepinephrine, angiotensin II and others on the secretory rate of aldosterone in man. JAMA 174: 234–240

Laragh JH (1960) The role of aldosterone in man: Evidence for regulation of electrolyte balance and arterial pressure by renal-adrenal system which may be involved in malignant hypertension. JAMA 174: 293–295

Laragh JH, Sealey JE, Ledingham JGG, Newton MA (1967) Oral contraceptives. Renin, aldosterone and high blood pressure. JAMA 201: 918–922

Laragh JH (1973) Vasoconstriction-volume analysis for understanding and treatment of hypertension: The use of renin and aldosterone profiles. Am J Med 55: 261–274

Laragh JH, Sealey JE, Bühler FR, Vaughan ED Jr, Brunner HR, Gavras H, Baer L (1975) The renin axis for vasoconstriction volume analysis for understanding and treating renovascular and renal hypertension. Am J Med 58: 4–13

Laragh JH, Sealey JE (1977) Renin-sodium profiling: Why, how and when in clinical practice. Cardiovasc Med 2: 1053–1075

Laragh JH (1978) Renin as a predictor of hypertensive complicatons: Discussion. Ann NY Acad Sci 304: 165–177

Laragh JH, Letcher RL, Pickering TG (1979) Renin profiling for diagnosis and treatment of hypertension. JAMA 241: 151–156

Sealey JE, Bühler FR, Laragh JH, Vaughan ED Jr (1973) The physiology of renin secretion in essential hypertension: Estimation of renin secretion rate and renal plasma flow from peripheral and renal vein renin levels. Am J Med 55: 391–401

Sealey JE, Laragh JH (1974) A proposed cybernetic system for sodium and potassium homeostasis: Coordination of aldosterone and intrarenal physical factors. Kidney Int 6: 281–290

Sealey JE, Laragh JH (1977) How to do a plasma renin assay. Cardiovasc Med 2: 1079–1092

Vaughan ED Jr, Laragh JH, Gavras I, Bühler FR, Gavras H, Brunner HR, Baer L (1973) Volume factor in low and normal renin essential hypertension: Treatment with either spironolactone or chlorthalidone. Am J Cardiol 32: 523–532

Aortic Endothelial Changes During the Development and Reversal of Experimental Hypertension[1]

Aram V. Chobanian, Margaret Forney Prescott, and Christian C. Haudenschild

Relatively little is known of the role of the arterial endothelium in the development of hypertensive vascular disease. A variety of endothelial changes have been reported in experimental hypertensive models including focal increases in endothelial cell replication (Schwartz and Benditt 1977), changes in shape of the cells and their nuclei (Haudenschild et al. 1980), constriction of the cells (Gabbiani et al. 1975), decrease in their surface coating (Grodan et al. 1976), and increased permeability to certain tracers (Wiener et al. 1969). The current study has been designed to examine quantitatively the morphologic alterations in the aortic endothelium occurring during the development and correction of hypertension.

Methods

Uninephrectomized male Wistar-Kyoto rats (6-10 in each experimental group) were made hypertensive with deoxycorticosterone and salt (DOC/salt) as previously described (Brecher et al. 1978). Two control groups were used: untreated animals and uninephrectomized rats receiving 1% saline. Correction of hypertension was achieved by withdrawal of the DOC treatment and maintenance of the animals on a low sodium diet. Blood pressures were measured weekly using the tail cuff technique (Brecher et al. 1975).

For preparation of tissue, anesthetized rats were perfused through the left ventricle with cacodylate buffered 2.5% glutaraldehyde fixative at a pressure maintained 30 mmHg below the systolic pressure measured individually prior to fixation. Post-fixation of rings of the thoracic aorta was done with 1% OsO_4 which for selected studies contained 0.3% ruthenium red (Luft 1971). The tissues were dehydrated through graded alcohols, stained en bloc with uranyl acetate, embedded in epon, cut with diamond knives, stained with uranyl acetate and lead citrate, and examined with a Philips EM 300 transmission electron microscope. Scanning electron micrographs (SEM) were taken on a Jeol JSM-35 microscope after dehydration, critical point drying and gold sputtering. Measurements of endothelial cell number and of the circumferential length of the internal elastic lamina were performed on toluidine-blue stained thick epoxy sections using a manual image analyzer (MOP III, Zeiss Inc.).

Results

A characteristic change in early hypertension consisted of endothelial cell bulging and rounding with infolding of the nuclei (Figure 1). The junctional complexes remained intact. While endothelial cells in control rats were closely apposed to the internal lamina, the attachment of endothelium in hypertensive rats was limited to a few cytoplasmic extensions usually exhibiting a semi-desmosome. SEM demonstrated that areas of endothelial bulging in the hypertensive animals were numerous, though focal in nature (Figure 2). Pairs of endothelial cells were present with a villous surface suggesting mitoses.

---

[1] Supported by Hypertension SCOR Grant (HL 18318) from the USPHS

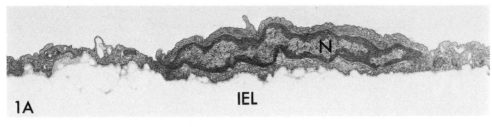

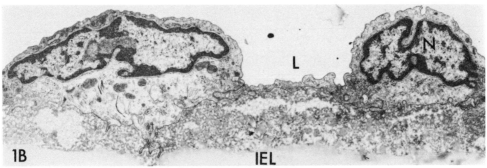

FIG. 1A and B. Electron micrographs of endothelium of thoracic aorta. The control (1A) shows a flat endothelial cell tightly adherent to the internal elastic lamina (IEL). The nucleus (N) has smooth contours. In the aorta of a hypertensive rat (1B), the endothelial cells bulge toward the lumen (L) and show folded nuclei (N). Amorphous extracellular material accumulates between the endothelial cells and the internal elastic lamina (IEL). Mag: (A) and (B) 15,000X.

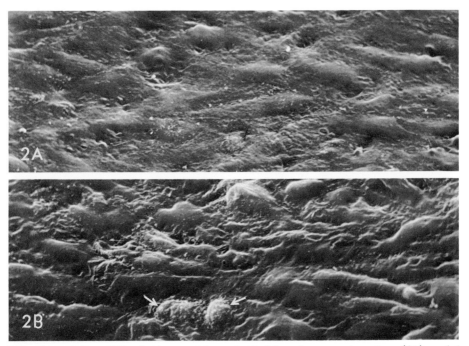

FIG. 2A and B. SEM of the aortic endothelium in normotensive (2A) and hypertensive rats (2B). In contrast to the flat smooth intimal surface seen in the control, the hypertensive endothelium shows increased cellularity and bulging of the cells toward the lumen. Arrows point to adjacent cells with villous surfaces. Mag: (A) and (B) 1300X.

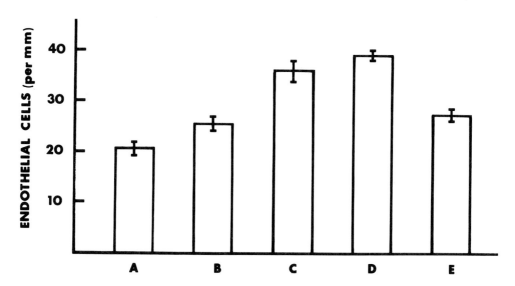

FIG. 3. Effects of hypertension on endothelial cell number in thoracic aorta
of rats. A = untreated controls, BP 132 ± 4 (mean ± S.E.); B = uninephrectomized controls, BP 139 ± 6; C = DOC/salt, 1-2 weeks treatment, BP 151 ± 4;
D = DOC/salt, 4 weeks treatment, BP 201 ± 4; E = DOC/salt 7 weeks followed
by withdrawal for 11 weeks, BP 137 ± 4.

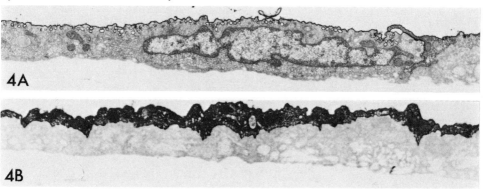

FIG. 4A and B. The flat aortic endothelial cell of a control animal (4A)
shows ruthenium red staining of the luminal cell surface and the luminal
pinocytotic vesicles. In a hypertensive animal (4B), ruthenium red staining
often is not limited to the endothelial cell surface but stains the entire
endothelial cytoplasm. MAG: (A) 13,000X, (B) 11,000X.

Quantitative analysis of the entire cross-sectional intimal circumference
showed a significant increase in the number of endothelial cell nuclei per
mm circumference, beginning as early as 1-2 weeks after the onset of hypertension (Figure 3). After 4 weeks of hypertension the number of endothelial
cells increased to 39 cells per mm as opposed to 20.7 in controls. However,
following reduction of blood pressure to control levels, the number of endothelial cells decreased to 27.6 cells per mm circumference.

Ruthenium red stained primarily the luminal glycoprotein coat (glycocalyx) of
control aortae, while cytoplasmic staining was common and often intense in
hypertensive rats (Figure 4). The thickened subendothelial space in hypertensive animals did not stain positively with ruthenium red unless there was
a discontinuity of the endothelial cell layer.

Discussion and Conclusions

These studies have demonstrated major alterations in the number and structure of aortic endothelial cells even after very brief periods of hypertension. The observed changes may reflect in part a proliferative response of the endothelium to the hypertension and would support the study of Schwartz and Benditt (1977) demonstrating focal increases in endothelial cell replication in aortas of rats with renovascular hypertension. The cause of the endothelial changes are uncertain although an increase in cell turnover in response to cell injury or a change in cell function somehow related to the hypertension may be important. The observed changes in cell number did not merely reflect an increase in luminal surface as a result of distention of the vessel since the measurements were related to the unit length of circumference of the vessel. Actual crowding and changes in shape of the cells were present.

The increased cytoplasmic staining of endothelial cells with ruthenium red in the hypertensive aorta is of interest and has not been reported previously. The significance of these observations is unclear but the findings support the concept that changes in the integrity or function of the arterial endothelium may be induced by hypertension. Whether the changed staining properties reflect the frequently hypothesized non-denuding endothelial damage has yet to be clarified.

Correction of hypertension produced return of the endothelial cell number toward control levels. Thus, some vascular changes induced by hypertension appear to regress with normalization of blood pressure, in accordance with our prior biochemical findings (Brecher et al. 1978). However, other hypertensive vascular alterations remain, such as increases in connective tissue protein content (Wolinsky 1971), subendothelial accumulation of both cellular and intra-cellular elements (Haudenschild et al. 1980), and changes in the activity of certain enzymes (Brecher et al. 1978; Chobanian et al. 1979).

References

Brecher P, Chan CT, Franzblau C, Faris B, Chobanian AV (1978) Effects of hypertension and its reversal on aortic metabolism in the rat. Circ Res 43:561

Chobanian AV, Brecher PI, Haudenschild C, Franzblau C, Kramsch D (1979) Studies on arterial metabolism and morphology in spontaneous and DOC-induced hypertension. In: Onesti G, Klimt CR (eds) Hypertension: Determinants, Complications, and Intervention. Grune and Stratton, New York pp 157-167

Gabbiani G, Badonnel M, Rona G (1975) Cytoplasmic contractile apparatus in aortic endothelial cells of hypertensive rats. Lab Invest 32:227.

Grodan P, Hüttner I, Rona G, Peters H, Laks M (1976) Surface acid mucopolysaccharides (AMPS): A marker of increased permeability in acute hypertension in the rat. Circulation 54:Suppl 2-137

Haudenschild CC, Prescott MF, Chobanian AV (1980) Effects of hypertension and its reversal on aortic intimal lesions of the rat. Hypertension (in press)

Luft JH (1971) Ruthenium red and violet. I. Chemistry, purification, methods of use for electron microscopy and mechanism of action. Anat Rec 171:347

Wiener J, Lattes RG, Meltzer AB, Spiro D (1969) The cellular pathology of experimental hypertension: IV. Evidence for increased vascular permeability. Am J Path 54:187

Wolinsky H (1971) Effects of hypertension and its reversal on the thoracic aorta of male and female rats. Circ Res 28:622

Atherosclerosis and Its Risk Factors in Japan

Y. Goto

It is known that the general characteristics of atherosclerotic disease in Japan are somewhat different from those of Western countries. Numerous studies intend to explain these characteristics from the standpoint of risk factors by the epidemiological studies. It is my purpose here to review some of Japanese studies.

Atherosclerotic Disease in Japan

The ranking of the causes of death in Japan is characteristically different from that of other countries. Cerebrovascular disease (CVD) including cerebral bleeding and infarction ranks as the highest cause of death in the last 25 years and comprises about one fourth of the total death in 1975. Cardiac disease, which is the leading cause of death in Western countries, accounts for 14% of all deaths in Japan and ranks after malignancy.

Cerebral bleeding and infarction accounts for 37% and 39% of the total cerebrovascular death, respectively. When the mortality rate is compared in several countries after adjusted for the age distribution of Japan in 1965, Japanese mortality of CVD is extremely higher than those of others (Figure 1).

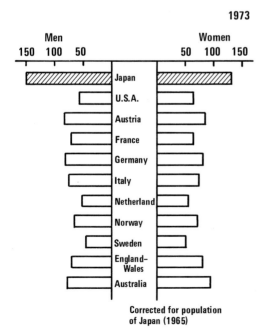

FIG. 1. Corrected mortality of cerebro-vascular diseases (per 100,000 population).

703

When the mortality rate is compared for different regions in Japan, it is higher in the northern part and lower in the southern part of the main island in this country. The mortality rate of CVD has increased until 1965 and then reached a plateau and began decreasing in 1970. While cerebral bleeding has decreased markedly after 1960 in every age group, cerebral infarction has increased slightly, but it is confined only in the age group of over 70.

The mortality rate of ischemic heart disease is around 300 per 100,000 of population in North America or Northern European Countries, whereas it is only 39 per 100,000 in Japan (Figure 2). The mortality rate of ischemic heart disease has increased gradually in the last twenty years in Japan. Dietary analysis has revealed that the increase of ischemic heart disease coincides with the increase of dietary intake of fat in the last twenty years, therefore, the relationship between the two factors cannot be over-emphasized, since the annual increment in ischemic heart disease is due to the increase in the population of the age group over 60 which dies often of heart disease, while the mortality rate in younger persons is decreasing rather than increasing.

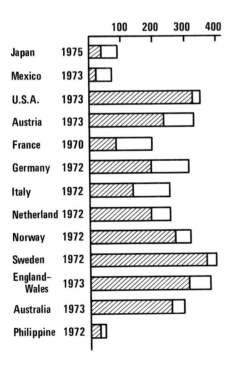

FIG. 2. Mortality of cardiac disease and ischemic heart disease (per 100,000 population).

There is no doubt that hypertension is one of the major risk factors for the development of atherosclerotic diseases. In particular for cerebral bleeding, hypertension seems to have the strongest influence. The number of patients are listed in Table 1, who developed atherosclerotic diseases during eight years follow up of 320 healthy rural population of over 40 years of age in our prevention trial study. Also the number of patients who possess each risk factor at the time of entry is listed.

Table 1. Total number of patients who developed atherosclerotic disease and number of patients who possessed each risk factor at the time of entry during eight year follow-up of 320 healthy rural persons over age 40.

	myocardial infarction	cerebral infarction	cerebral bleeding	at entry
number of patient	2	12	5	320
age (66 years)	1	8	3	79
cholesterol (220mg/dl)	1	9	3	183
triglyceride (140mg/dl)	0	4	1	111
B.P. systolic (160 mmHg)	0	5	4	87
B.P. diastolic (95 mmHg)	1	3	3	86
obesty (10%)	1	3	2	85
smoking	1	3	0	39

The data on the prevalence rate of hypertension in Japan can be obtained from the national survey which was done for 12,000 adults who had been randomly chosen from every part of Japan. The percentage of hypertension among Japanese over 30 years of age, categorized as 160mmHg of systolic pressure and 95 mmHg of diastolic pressure, is 25.2% for males, 21.5% for females and 23.1% for total. The percentage of hypertension in each age group is 7% in 30-39 years, 16% in 40-49 years, 30% in 50-59 years, 42% in 60-69 years and 54% in over 70 years of age in 1971. These Japanese values, when compared with those of Western countries, are not considered to be particularly high.

It is also known that there is a regional difference of the mortality rate from cerebrovascular disease in Japan. One of the factors for this regional difference is considered as diet. People in the northern area have such high salt intake as more than 25 a day and also less intake of animal proteins. The incidence of hypertension also roughly coincides with that of cerebrovascular disease in each district with some exception.

For the development of hypertension it seems necessary for several environmental factors such as diet, climate and others to act at the same time on the genetic factors which penetrate each individual.

The medical circumstance for a hypertensive population in Japan is generally favorable. Actually, increasing numbers of hypertensive patients are receiving medical treatment. Also the national project to reduce the incidence of stroke has reduced mortality rate from cerebral bleeding which can be observed in an annual decrease for the entire population.

It is interesting that the use of some hypotensive drugs have some relation to plasma lipid, (especially high-density lipoprotein (HDL) cholesterol concentration). Our data on the effect of hypotensive drugs on the concentration of plasma HDL cholesterol revealed that patients receiving B-blocker had higher (not significant) HDL cholesterol, and those receiving a mixture of resespine, hydralazine and thiazide had lower HDL cholesterol concentration than untreated control patients. It may suggest some relationship between hypotensive drugs and HDL cholesterol metabolism, which will need further investigation.

Controlled Therapeutic Trial in Mild Hypertension—Initial Results

Richard Lovell and the Australian Blood Pressure Study Management Committee[1]

This study aimed to answer the question whether antihypertensive treatment benefited symptomless persons with mild hypertension. It was a single blind prospective controlled trial in men and women aged 30 to 69 years, who, at population screening, had diastolic blood pressure (V) (DBP) from 95 to 109mmHg, and systolic blood pressure (SBP) under 200mmHg.

Design of the Trial

A trial population large enough to demonstrate a 30% reduction in mortality over 5 years was sought. It was required that the hypothesis that there was no benefit from treatment should be rejected at the 5% level of signifificance. Eventually 103,647 subjects were screened giving a trial population of 3,943.

Subjects qualified to enter the trial if the mean of their DBP measured twice at each of two screening visits averaged 95 to 109mmHg with SBP under 200mmHg. If no exclusion factors were found at a clinic visit, they were randomly assigned to active or placebo treatment groups. At this visit, if the DBP was 95mmHg or more, they started taking their tablets (active or placebo) and attended for follow-up. If the DBP was under 95mmHg, tablets were withheld, the subjects were seen 4-monthly and if their DBP later rose to 95mmHg or more, tablets were started according to the regimen to which they were originally assigned.

If having started tablets, a subject sustained a DBP of 110mmHg or more, definitive antihypertensive medication was started, such subjects continued under observation and trial end-points occurring in them were counted against their original randomized group. There were 185 such subjects, all but 2 in the placebo group. The study was thus a comparison between two regimens. In the active regimen, antihypertensive drugs were given from entry (or when the DBP later rose to 95mmHg or more), doses being aimed to keep the DBP under 95mmHg. In the placebo regimen, placebo tablets were given from entry (or when the DBP later rose to 95mmHg or more) except that if the DBP rose to 110mmHg or more, antihypertensive medication was given.

The first order drug used was chlorothiazide; second order drugs added were methyldopa, propranolol or pindilol and supplementary ones were hydrallazine and clonidine. There were corresponding placebos for each.

Trial end-points (TEP) defined by the protocol were: death from all causes; cerebrovascular accident; transient ischaemic attack with neurological deficit; myocardial infarction (WHO categories 1 & 2); other evidence of ischaemic heart disease (defined); congestive cardiac failure; dissecting aneurysm of aorta; retinal haemorrhages, exudates and papilloedema; hypertensive encephalopathy; onset of renal failure (defined).

A sequential analysis of the numbers of TEP occurring in the active and placebo treatment groups was reported throughout the study to an Ethics

---

[1]See Appendix.

Committee, the Management Committee being unaware of the results. In October, 1978, the Management Committee was advised by the Ethics Committee that there were certain trends in the occurrence of TEP that were differentiating the groups but that the difference was not sufficient to pose an ethical problem. It was also advised that, because of the number and pattern of premature withdrawals and the rate at which TEP were occurring, it had become unlikely that prolonging the trial would add greatly to the results. The Management Committee determined that the trial should continue but that a comparison of TEP rates for the entire population and for sub-groups according to entry characteristics such as age, sex and BP, and corresponding survival analyses by the Cox (1972) method, should be undertaken, using results as at 26 October, 1978. Analyses were done by the "intention to treat" approach taking account of outcome whether or not subjects adhered to their regimen and by the "on treatment" approach taking account of outcome only while subjects adhered to their regimen. The Management Committee considered these findings in March, 1979, and in view of the results and having regard for the distribution of additional TEP reported since October, 1978, it decided that 5 March, 1979, should be the final censoring date. The decision to stop the trial was thus made as a result of a single comprehensive analysis. This paper reports the results on the 3323 subjects started on tablets and analysed by the "on treatment" approach as at 26 October, 1978, when the average follow-up period was 3 years and 8 months.

Results

Subjects in the active and placebo groups were well matched for relevant characteristics at entry (Table 1). The status of the trial population at the October, 1978, censoring date is shown in Table 2. Overall 25.2% (786 + 53) of subjects had prematurely stopped their regimens and the status of 7.0% was unknown. Entry characteristics of those prematurely stopping did not differ significantly between the groups. TEP in 186 subjects were available for this analysis.

The TEP are shown in Table 3. For all subjects, in the active treatment group the rates of total fatal, total non-fatal and of total TEP were significantly less than in the placebo group. The rates of BP-related deaths and non-fatal cerebrovascular events were also significantly less. The non-fatal

Table 1. Entry Characteristics

| | Numbers | |
	Active (n 1663)	Placebo (n 1660)
Age (Years)		
30- 49	758	723
50- 69	905	937
Sex		
Male	1050	1057
Female	613	603
Entry DBP (mmHg)		
90- 99	625	600
100-109	769	789
110+	269	271
Cigarettes		
No	1252	1216
Yes	411	444
Serum Cholesterol (mg%)		
< 220	670	729
220+	993	931

Table 2. Status of Subjects at 26 October, 1978.

	Numbers	%
Subjects with no TEP		
Continuing Regimen	2065	
Prematurely stopped	786	
Sub-total	2851	85.8
Subjects with TEP		
While on regimen	186	
After stopping	53	
Sub-total	239	7.2
Lost to follow-up	233	7.0
Total at entry	3323	100.0

Table 3. Trial End-Points at 26 October, 1978, by Entry DBP.

| | Numbers (rates per 1000 person-years exposure) | | | | | |
| | All entry DBP | | DBP <100mmHg | | DBP 100+mmHg | |
	Active (1663)	Placebo (1660)	Active (625)	Placebo (600)	Active (1038)	Placebo (1060)
Fatal						
BP-related	4	10	2	2	2	8
	(0.81)	(2.12)*	(1.10)	(1.16)	(0.64)	(2.67)*
Not BP-related	4	7	2	3	2	4
	(0.81)	(1.49)	(1.10)	(1.75)	(0.64)	(1.34)
Total fatal	8	17	4	5	4	12
	(1.61)	(3.61)*	(2.19)	(2.91)	(1.28)	(4.01)*
Non-fatal						
Ischaemic heart disease	58	66	23	24	35	42
	(11.71)	(14.01)	(12.62)	(13.97)	(11.17)	(14.03)
Cerebrovascular	8	17	2	3	6	14
	(1.61)	(3.61)*	(1.10)	(1.75)	(1.92)	(4.68)*
Other	5	7	1	2	4	5
	(1.01)	(1.41)	(0.55)	(1.10)	(1.28)	(1.60)
Total non-fatal	71	90	26	29	45	61
	(14.33)	(19.10)*	(14.26)	(16.88)	(14.37)	(20.38)*
Total TEP	79	107	30	34	49	73
	(15.94)	(22.71)**	(16.46)	(19.79)	(15.64)	(24.38)**

* p < 0.05   ** p < 0.01

TEP were mostly ischaemic heart disease (IHD) events. Differences between groups were contributed to by subjects of both sexes and of all age groups.

When TEP rates were related to different levels of entry BP, differences between active and placebo rates increased with entry DBP and 100mmHg was the lowest level above which significant differences existed and below which they did not. (Table 3). In those with entry DBP 100+mmHg, the fatal TEP rate in the active group was one-third of that in the placebo group and the total TEP rate was two-thirds.

The estimate of numbers of subjects needed in the trial was based on the aim to test overall benefit of treatment, not to establish differences in respect of individual TEP. Nevertheless major clinical categories of TEP have been compared. Table 4 shows, for subjects with entry DBP 100+mmHg, significantly lower rates in the active compared with the placebo group for myocardial infarction and all cerebrovascular events, the reduction in both cases being by about one-half. Rates for other IHD events did not differ significantly.

Table 4. Trial end-points at 26 October, 1978 by entry DBP.

	Numbers (rates per 1000 person-years exposure)							
	DBP <100mmHg				DBP 100+mmHg			
	Numbers		Rates		Numbers		Rates	
	Active	Placebo	Active	Placebo	Active	Placebo	Active	Placebo
Myocardial infarction	10	6	5.49	3.49	8	17	2.55	5.68*
Other ischaemic heart disease	15	19	8.23	11.06	27	30	8.62	10.02
Cerebrovascular events	2	3	1.10	1.75	8	17	2.55	5.68*

* $p < 0.05$

To estimate changes in BP, for each subject the DBP at entry was compared
with the average of all their DBP recorded after starting tablets. In both
active and placebo groups, mean DBP while on tablets was less than entry
DBP, the higher the entry level the greater was the fall, and for each entry
class of DBP the fall was greater in the active group (ranging from 8.9 to
26.1 mmHg) than in the placebo group (ranging from 4.9 to 20.0 mmHg). The
difference between the groups in average DBP after entry ranged from 4.1 mmHg
for those with entry DBP 95 to 99mmHg, to over 7mmHg for those with entry DBP
110mmHg or more.

Discussion

Bias can be introduced into controlled trials when subjects prematurely stop
their randomized regimen, particularly if prognostic characteristics of those
stopping in active and placebo groups differ. There was no significant difference in such characteristics between the groups in the 25% of subjects who
stopped prematurely. Bias from premature stopping may affect "intention to
treat" and "on treatment" analysis differently. Comparably favourable effects
were seen with both types of analysis.

The observed reduction in cerebrovascular events accords with findings in
the Veterans Administration (VA) trial (1970). In that trial, cases of
myocardial infarction (and sudden death) numbered 13 in the control and 11
in the treated group compared with 23 and 18 in our trial. The VA trial did
not report myocardial infarction separately in those with entry DBP 100+mmHg
who had lower rates in our active treatment group.

The proportion of subjects on beta adrenergic blocking drugs was no less among
those experiencing IHD TEP than among those having other TEP. Thus an action
other than an antihypertensive one, of these drugs, appears not to have influenced the results.

Conclusion

Treatment of mild hypertension in symptomless persons aged 30 – 69 was beneficial. Reduction of TEP rates was greater in those with higher than in
those with lower entry DBP. In people with entry DBP 100+mmHg, as defined,
treatment led to 9 fewer hypertension-associated events, including 3 fewer
deaths, per year per 1000 persons treated.

Appendix

The Australian Blood Pressure Study Management Committee:
R. Reader (Chairman), G.E. Bauer, A.E. Doyle, K.W. Edmondson, S. Hunyor,
T.H. Hurley, P.I. Korner, P.W. Leighton, R.R.H. Lovell, M.G. McCall,

J.M. McPhie, M.J. Rand, H.M. Whyte; Study Centre Directors, J.A. Abernethy, J. Baker, M. Bullen, R. Edwards, G. Francis, M. Lamb, M. Stewart; Statistician, G. Santow; Computer Programmers, W. Clapton and H. Knight.

References

Cox DR (1972) Regression models and life tables. Jl R Statist Soc B 34: 187-220

Veterans Administration Co-operative Study Group on Antihypertensive Agents (1970). Effects of treatment on morbidity in hypertension. JAMA 213:1143-1152

Clinical and Pathogenic Relevance of Erythrocyte Cation Fluxes Measurement in Human Hypertension

Ricardo P. Garay, Jean-Luc Elghozi, Georges Dagher, and Philippe Meyer

In a recent investigation studying net Na^+ and K^+ fluxes in erythrocytes of essential hypertensives, we reported a decreased net Na^+ efflux in accelerated cases, while moderate hypertensives had an increase in net K^+ influx. Therefore in all essential hypertensives, the ratio of Na^+/K^+ net fluxes was reduced. These observations led us to propose that erythrocyte flux measurements could be used as a simple laboratory test for the diagnosis of essential hypertension (Garay and Meyer 1979).

In an effort to confirm the validity and reproducibility of this test as a routine screening procedure in clinical practice, we further investigated essential hypertensives, hypertension of renal and adrenal origin and normotensives with and without hypertension among their first degree relatives.

Methods

Net Na^+ and K^+ fluxes were measured in Na^+-loaded, K^+-depleted erythrocytes according to a previous described method (Garay and Meyer 1979; Garay et al. 1979).

Patients. Essential hypertension (42 cases), secondary hypertension (9 renal, 12 renovascular, 2 phaeochromocytoma) were defined according to criteria previously reported (Garay et al. 1979). Hypertension was considered to be benign when mean arterial blood pressure ranged between 95–120 mmHg. None of the secondary hypertensives had any known familial history of hypertension.

Results

The present clinical investigation confirms the preliminary report. As shown in Figure 1, all essential hypertensives have a reduced erythrocyte ratio of Na^+/K^+ net fluxes as compared to normotensive controls. All cases with secondary hypertension had a normal erythrocyte net flux ratio.

As previously reported (Garay et al. 1979) a reduced ratio was also observed in 13 out of 21 normotensives born of hypertensives. Those individuals with a reduced ratio were grouped as ⊕ normotensives.

Erythrocytes of normotensive controls and secondary normotensives showed in the presence of ouabain a net Na^+ efflux against the gradient, while ⊕ normotensives and essential hypertensives had a net Na^+ influx. Furthermore Na^+-K^+-pump fluxes in erythrocytes of ⊕ normotensives and moderate hypertensives showed a 30% increase.

712

Discussion

The clearcut difference observed in the ratios of Na^+/K^+ net fluxes of essential hypertensives on the one hand and normotensive controls and secondary hypertensives on the other hand, added to the simplicity and reproducibility of the previously described erythrocyte flux measurements, highly support the use of this test in the clinical investigation of essential hypertension. A detailed clinical application of this test is discussed in a previous communication (Garay et al. 1979).

The presence of a decreased erythrocyte net flux ratio in essential hypertensives, its absence in secondary hypertensives and in human devoid of familial history of hypertension suggest that the erythrocyte membrane defect is closely related to hypertension. The observed reduced flux ratios in some children of essential hypertensives indicate that the erythrocyte membrane abnormality accompanies the genetic transmission of hypertension.

Flux measurements in presence of ouabain indicate that erythrocytes of ⊕ normotensives and all essential hypertensives lack a Na^+ extrusion mechanism different from the Na^+- K^+-pump. Preliminary studies indicate that in normotensive controls net Na^+ outflux in presence of ouabain is a function of the K^+

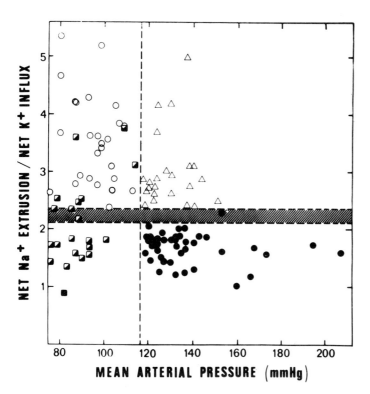

FIG. 1. Individual values of the erythrocyte test for the different studied groups as a function of mean arterial pressure. 0 = normotensive control; ◪ = normotensive born of one hypertensive parent; ■ = normotensive born of both hypertensive parents; Δ = secondary hypertensive; 0 = essential hypertensive.

gradient across the erythrocyte membrane (unpublished results). Therefore, it seems likely that in essential hypertension a functional defect in a Na^+-K^+ cotransport system is responsible for the reduced ratio of Na^+/K^+ net fluxes. Furthermore the increase in net K^+ influx observed in ⊕ normotensives and moderate hypertensives is consequent to an increase in the turnover rate of cation translocation by the Na^+-K^+-pump, as ouabain binding failed to reveal an increase in pump site number. This appears to be a compensatory mechanism preventing cell Na^+ retention before or in early stages of hypertension.

The alteration in cell Na^+ extrusion observed in essential hypertensives and in ⊕ normotensives suggests that this inherited functional defect might be of pathogenic importance if present in excitable cells with high surface/volume ratio, as the resulting increase in intracellular Na^+ concentration could lead to an increase in intracellular Ca^{++} (Blaustein 1977). Other investigators (Wessels, Junge-Hülsing,Losse 1966); Edmondson 1975; Postnov et al. 1976; Araoye et al. 1978) have already described altered permeability in hypertensive rats and human blood cells. The relationship between these abnormalities and the present observations deserves further investigation.

References

Araoye MA, Khatri I, Yao L, Freis ED (1978) Leukocyte intracellular cations in hypertension: Effect of antihypertensive drugs. Am Heart J 96:731-758
Blaustein MP (1977) Sodium ions, calcium ions, blood pressure regulation and hypertension: A reassessment and hypothesis. Am J Physiol 232:c165-c173
Edmondson R, Thomas R, Hilton P, Jones N (1975) Abnormal leucocyte composition and sodium transport in essential hypertension. Lancet 1:1003-1005
Garay RP, Elghozi JL, Dagher G, Meyer P (1979) Laboratory distinction between essential and secondary hypertension by measurement of erythrocyte cation fluxes. N Engl J Med, in press
Garay RP, Meyer P (1979) A new test showing abnormal net Na^+ and K^+ fluxes in erythrocyte of essential hypertensive patients. Lancet 1:349-353
Postnov Y, Orlov S, Gulak P, Shevchenko A (1976) Altered permeability of the erythrocyte membrane for sodium and potassium ions in spontaneous hypertensive rats. Pflügers Arch 365:257-263
Wessels Von F, Junge-Hülsing, Losse H (1961) Untersuchungen zur natriumpermeabilität der erythrozyten bei hypertonikern. Zeitschrift für Kreislaufforschung Band 56, Heft 4, 374-380

Estimated Rates of Progression and Regression of Human Femoral and Coronary Atherosclerosis in 45-Year-Old Men

David H. Blankenhorn

During studies of atherosclerotic lesion induction, the experimental questions frequently asked are: What sort of lesions have formed? How extensive are these lesions? How rapidly did lesions form? All of this information can be obtained by sacrificing test and control animals at intervals during a lesion induction regimen. Regression studies are relatively new to atherosclerosis research; the majority have been conducted in animals by extension of procedures previously developed to study lesion production. Regression studies randomly select a sample of animals with induced lesions for assignment to a regression regimen and ask very similar experimental questions. The most important difference between progression and regression studies is the expected direction of lesion change. These obvious similarities suggest the merit of interpreting lesion regression studies in light of what is already known about lesion production. It is generally expected that lesions will improve after an atherogenic stimulus is removed at about the same rate at which they previously were formed.

Recently it has been possible to extend studies of lesion regression to man by obtaining serial angiograms in selected volunteer subjects. Angiograms were first used to assign patients to one of three classes -- progression, no change, and regression (Ost et al. 1967; DePalma et al. 1970; Barndt et al. 1977). Later, instrumental measurement of films was used to quantitate lesion change and estimate lesion change rates (Blankenhorn et al. 1978). This approach allows each patient's risk factor level between angiograms to be analyzed in relation to this individual's lesion change -- a more powerful procedure than comparing risk factor levels against a three-way classification.

At this time, reports of humans showing lesion regression are confined to small studies which do not fulfill requirements of a controlled clinical trial (Barndt et al. 1977; Thompson et al. 1978; Ost and Stenson 1967; DePalma et al. 1970). A basic element of the controlled clinical trial is the assignment of subjects at random to test or control groups. This is difficult to do when studies involve angiography but one such study is now in progress (Buchwald et al. 1979). Selective arterial angiography is the only procedure which has provided images with sufficient resolution to detect lesion regression so far, but there is good reason to expect that non-invasive ultrasound procedures will soon have this capability also. This will greatly broaden the scope and number of regression studies possible in man. It should facilitate controlled clinical trials of lesion stabilization and regression.

In planning clinical trials, the number of subjects and study length is greatly influenced by the magnitude of expected difference between test and control groups. A fundamental aspect of these considerations is what is to be expected from the control group and it is reasonable to project this from what is now known about lesion progression. This rationale is similar to comparison of progression and regression rates in animal studies.

This paper presents two estimates of what may be expected for atherosclerosis change rates in human control subjects. One estimate has been obtained from autopsy data. The other has been obtained from measurement of lesion change in a small number of humans when risk factor levels were not greatly altered.

Autopsy data provides biased information about the population at large, but this bias is minimized if a large proportion of all who die are autopsied. Five European communities with very high autopsy rates were selected for a recent cooperative pathologic study supported by the World Health Organization (WHO) -- Malmo, Prague, Ryazan, Yalta and Talin. Table 1 presents age- and sex-specific data from the five communities. The percent of intimal surface covered by all types of atheroma increased an average of 1.42 percent per year in the aorta of men age 45. In the coronary arteries of 45-year-old men this increase was 1.40 percent per year. Rates of increase were lower in women of the same age; 0.75 percent per year in the aorta, and 0.94 percent per year in the coronary artery.

The angiographic estimate obtained from measurement of femoral lesions was in men with previous myocardial infarction of average age 46 at the time of the first angiogram. They were enrolled in a program for weight loss and exercise which achieved an average lowering of serum cholesterol of 4.7 percent as compared to their level on entry into the study. The average serum total cholesterol on entry was 234 mg. percent; between angiograms it was 223 mg. percent. This amount of change was similar to the 5.6 serum cholesterol reduction in the intervention group of the MRFIT (Christakis et al. 1979), but appears not to have been sufficient to stop lesion progression. Table 2 shows average levels for computer estimated atherosclerosis in three femoral segments at each of the three angiograms (Brooks et al. 1979). The scale for computer estimated atherosclerosis is 1 - 128, and so the change observed is equivalent to 1.94 percent per year.

Some indication of what we might hope for if risk reduction achieved effects on atherosclerosis equal to spontaneous differences occurring in Europeans is available from the WHO autopsy data. Men who died of coronary disease were compared with an age-matched low atherosclerosis group. The low atherosclerosis group died of trauma and were known to be free of hypertension and diabetes. Table 3 compares the extent of raised coronary lesions in men of these two groups. There were no deaths from coronary lesions before age 30, and therefore no data for coronary involvement at this age. If we assume from data for the population at large (Table 1) that 4.3 percent of the coronary surface was covered at 22.5 years, the rate of change from 22.5 to 45 years would be $(53-4.3)/22.5 = 2.16$ percent per year. In the low atheroscle-

Table 1. Percent of vessel surface area covered by all types of atherosclerotic lesions. Pooled data: five European communities; deaths.

| Age | Males | | Females | |
	Abdominal Aorta	Coronary[a]	Abdominal Aorta	Coronary[a]
15 - 19	14	3.2	20	1.8
20 - 24	17	4.3	28	5.1
25 - 29	22	7.6	31	6.1
30 - 34	25	13.0	35	7.3
35 - 39	30	19.0	34	11.0
40 - 44	36	26.0	37	12.0
45 - 49	43	34.0	42	17.0
50 - 54	50	40.0	46	26.0
55 - 59	59	46.0	53	30.0
60 - 64	65	48.0	60	37.0
65 - 69	70	52.0	66	44.0

[a]Average value: left anterior descending, circumflex and right.

rosis group this change rate was (17.0-2.6)/22.5 = .64 percent per year. Reduction of the accelerated atherosclerosis seen in men dying at 45 of coronary disease to the rate of a low atherosclerosis group is therefore a 1.52 percent change per year. In a separate communication (Blankenhorn and Brooks, in press) we argue that ischemic heart disease rate data from the two control groups in the Cooperative Clinical Trial in Primary Prevention and Ischemic Heart Disease using Clofibrate (Oliver et al. 1978) suggest that a spontaneous 27 percent difference in serum cholesterol level may be associated with the 2.7 percent difference in the rate of growth of stenotic coronary lesions. It is not known whether any therapy can consistently produce rate changes of this magnitude in human atherosclerosis although a 27 percent reduction in serum cholesterol level can be achieved by a variety of therapies. Lesion regression rates equal to or exceeding 2.7 percent per year were observed in several of the hyperlipoproteinemic patients reported by Barndt et al. (1977). In this report, the group of patients showing regression had maintained an average reduction of serum cholesterol of 25 percent as compared with pre-angiographic levels.

Table 2. Computer estimated atherosclerosis in three femoral segments on three occasions in 27 men.

Time of Measurement	Segment			
	Lower	Middle	Upper	Averages
First Angiogram	42.5	50.0	45.2	45.9
Second Angiogram[a]	44.6	51.4	46.8	47.6
Third Angiogram[b]	49.0	56.2	50.5	51.9

[a]15 months, on the average, after the first angiogram.
[b]14 months, on the average, after the second angiogram.

Table 3. Average percentage of coronary surface area covered by raised lesions in two groups of patients: coronary heart disease and low atherosclerosis.

Age	Males	
	Coronary Heart Disease	Low Atherosclerosis
20 - 29	--	2.6
30 - 39	43.0	8.8
40 - 49	53.0	17.0
50 - 59	58.0	30.0
60 - 69	62.0	32.0
70 - 79	64.0	42.0

References

Barndt R, Blankenhorn DH, Crawford DW, Brooks SH (1977) Regression and progression of early femoral atherosclerosis in treated hyperlipoproteinemic patients. Ann Intern Med 86: 139–146

Blankenhorn DH, Brooks SH, Selzer RH, Barndt R (1978) The rate of atherosclerosis change during treatment of hyperlipoproteinemia. Circ Vol 57: 2

Brooks SH, Blankenhorn DH, Chin HP, Sanmarco ME, Hanashiro PK, Selzer RH, Selvester RH (in press) Design of human atherosclerosis studies by serial angiography. J Chronic Dis Vol II

Buchwald H, McMullen JB, Varco RL, Tuna N, Amplatz K, Matts JP, Long JM, Moore RB, and the POSCH Group/University of Minnesota Hospitals, Minneapolis (1979) Graded exercise testing and arteriography in POSCH clinical trial. Circ Vol 59 & 60, Suppl II (abstract)

Christakis G, Wilcox M (1979) Serum cholesterol changes in 6,000 MRFIT participants after 2 years of intervention. Proc of the Amer Heart Assoc Coun on Epid and Cardio Dis, pp 446

DePalma RG, Hubay, CA, Insull W, Robinson AV, Hartman PH (1970) Progression and regression of experimental atherosclerosis. Surg Gynec Obstet, Vol 131: 633–647

Oliver MF, Heady JA, Morris JN, et al (1978) A co-operative trial in the primary prevention of ischemic heart disease using clofibrate. Brit Heart J Vol 40: 1069–1118

Ost CR, Stenson S (1967) Regression of peripheral atherosclerosis during therapy with high doses of nicotinic acid. Scand J Clin Lab Invest, Suppl 99, Vol 19: 241–245

Thompson G, Kilpatrick D, Oakley C, Steiner R, Myant N (1978) Reversal of cholesterol accumulation in familial hypercholesterolemia by long-term plasma exchange. Circ, Suppl II, Vol 57 & 58 (abstract)

Community Pathology of Atherosclerosis and Coronary Heart Disease in New Orleans: Relationship of Risk Factors to Atherosclerotic Lesions[1,2]

J.P. Strong, W.D. Johnson, M.C. Oalmann, R.E. Tracy, W.P. Newman, III, W.A. Rock, G.T. Malcom, M.G. Kokatnur, and V. Toca

Introduction

Epidemiological studies of living populations have identified personal attributes associated with increased risk of developing cardiovascular diseases such as coronary heart disease (CHD) and cerebral vascular disease. The clinical end-points for CHD (myocardial infarction or sudden death due to coronary disease) are presumably due to a combination of factors including the amount and distribution of coronary atherosclerosis, the size and workload of the heart, mechanisms related to the occlusive episode, the sequelae such as cardiac arrhythmias. It is important to establish whether the risk factors for clinically overt CHD are related to the development of atherosclerosis per se. Relationships between recognized CHD risk factors and the extent of atherosclerosis as measured at autopsy have been reported; however, much of the information concerning the risk factors was gathered from routine autopsy protocols, and carefully collected antecedent information on the risk factors was not available (Strong and Eggen 1970; Strong 1977). Recently, several studies have used standardized methods for evaluating atherosclerosis at autopsy to investigate its relationship to antecedent risk factors measured during life (Garcia-Palmieri et al. 1977; Hatano and Matsuzaki. 1977; Solberg et al. 1977; Stemmermann et al. 1977; Sternby 1977). An alternative approach involves the community-wide study of deceased persons in settings where a high percentage of autopsies are performed together with detailed standardized protocols for evaluating atherosclerotic lesions. This report presents results concerning the association of autopsy derived risk factor variables with (1) disease categories and (2) quantitative assessment of coronary and aortic atherosclerosis. Selected findings have been reported by Strong (1979), Newman et al. (1979), and Johnson et al. (1979).

Materials and Methods

This report pertains to an autopsy sample of all black and white men 25-44 years of age who resided and died in Orleans Parish, Louisiana, U.S.A., between 1968 and 1972. Of 1,008 eligible subjects, 778 were autopsied. Specimens were obtained according to our protocol for 579 (57.4% of all deaths). Methods used to obtain and evaluate the hearts and arteries have been described by Guzman et al. (1968), Rock et al. (1972) and Oalmann et al. (1979). The summary measure of atherosclerosis, raised atherosclerotic lesions, is the sum of fibrous plaques, complicated lesions, and calcified lesions. Weight and length of the body, length of the trunk, weight of the heart, and other data were obtained at autopsy. Thickness of the panniculus adiposus was measured at a point halfway between the xiphoid process and the umbilicus. Postmortem serum cholesterol levels were determined on blood samples taken from

---

[1]Supported by U.S.P.H.S. grant HL- 08974, N.H.L.B.I.
[2]Originally delivered at the Workshop on Epidemiology of Atherosclerotic Lesions (see pp. 52-70).

the inferior vena cava and analyzed by the method of Abell et al. (1952). Total lipid content of liver samples was determined gravimetrically after extraction by the Folch method. Coded histologic samples of renal tissue were examined to quantitate the arterial and arteriolar changes associated with hypertension (Tracy 1970). The triglyceride fatty acids distribution in adipose tissue taken from the perirenal area and buttock was determined (Kokatnur et al. 1979). Five pathologists independently evaluated hearts, coronary arteries and aortas, resolved disagreements by consensus, and assigned a cause of death for each man after review of all pertinent information.

Results

Four broad disease categories were considered in the analysis of data: 40 men died from CHD; 52 died with Related disease (e.g., stroke, hypertension, diabetes, or chronic renal disease); 7 were classified as Uncertain whether CHD was cause of death; and 480 died from all other conditions, including trauma (the Basal group). In each age-race subgroup, the CHD group is most extensively involved with lesions, the Related group intermediate, and the Basal group least involved (Fig. 1).

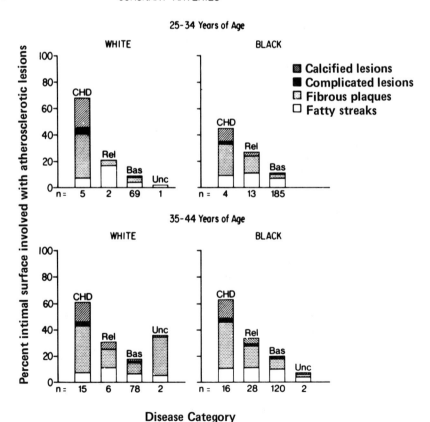

FIG. 1. Mean percent of intimal surface of coronary arteries involved, four types of lesions, by age, race, and broad disease category.

Lesions are not significantly different among the CHD subgroups. Lesions in the Basal group show the expected increase with age (more extensive lesions in the 35-44 year-old age group) for both races. The extent of lesions is approximately the same for blacks and whites in the Basal group. The extent of lesions in the abdominal aorta (not shown here) follows the same general pattern as in the coronary arteries.

Table 1. Summary of comparisons of means for selected risk factor variables in the CHD group versus the Basal group.

Variable	Result of Comparison
Postmortem cholesterol	CHD > Basal except young blacks
Heart Weight	CHD > Basal
Heart Weight/Body Length	CHD > Basal
Renal Hypertensive Index	CHD > Basal
Thickness of Panniculus Adiposus	CHD > Basal except young whites
Body Weight	CHD > Basal except young whites
Body Length	CHD < Basal except older whites
Trunk Length	Inconsistent differences
Body Weight/Body Length	CHD > Basal except young subjects
Ponderal Index	CHD < Basal except young whites
Liver Lipid	CHD < Basal except older subjects
Adipose Tissue Fatty Acids	
Myristic (14:0)	CHD < Basal
Palmitic (16:0)	Inconsistent differences
Palmitoleic (16:1)	CHD < Basal
Stearic (18:0)	Inconsistent differences
Oleic (18:1)	CHD < Basal
Lineoleic (18:2)	CHD > Basal

Mean serum cholesterol levels are greater in the CHD group for 3 of the 4 age-race subgroups (Text Table 1 and Appendix Table 1). Means for three postmortem indices of blood pressure and hypertension are greater in the CHD group. Body length is less in the CHD group except for older whites. Measures of obesity consistently indicate more obesity in the CHD group in older blacks and whites; less consistent trends exist in the younger groups. Liver lipid concentrations are less in the young CHD groups and more in the older CHD groups than in their Basal counterparts. Although not shown because of space limitations, means for myristic, palmitoleic, and oleic acids are consistently lower, whereas linoleic acid is consistently higher in the CHD group. Age and raised lesions in the abdominal aorta and coronary arteries are significantly intercorrelated in blacks and whites for the Total sample and the Basal group (Appendix Tables 2 and 3). Postmortem serum cholesterol is significantly correlated with aortic raised lesions and coronary raised lesions in the whites (Total sample) and with coronary raised lesions in the whites (Basal group). Heart weight, heart weight/body length, and renal hypertensive index are significantly correlated with either aortic raised lesions, coronary raised lesions or both for blacks and whites in the Total sample and the Basal group. Measures of obesity (body weight/body length, thickness of panniculus, and ponderal index) are significantly correlated with coronary raised lesions, but not aortic raised lesions in both races for the Total sample and for the Basal group (one exception). Body length is not significantly correlated with lesions; however, trunk length is significantly correlated with coronary raised lesions in whites in the Total sample and in both races in the Basal group. Liver lipid concentration is significantly correlated with aortic raised lesions in two subgroups. Significant correlations for the many fatty acids are difficult to summarize and will be the subject of a separate report.

Stepwise multiple regression analyses (backward elimination) were performed to show the significant contributions of age and the autopsy derived risk factors to the variability in coronary and aortic raised lesions. Separate regression equations were determined for the Total sample and the Basal group for each race using raised lesions in the abdominal aorta and coronary arteries as dependent variables. The percentage of total variability in raised lesions accounted for ranges from 17.4 (abdominal aorta, black men, Basal group) to 53.9 (abdominal aorta, white men, Total sample). The subset of variables making significant contributions varies from subgroup to subgroup. Age is a predominant variable, and this variable alone accounts for a significant portion of the variability in raised lesions (both aorta and coronary arteries) in all subgroups. Postmortem cholesterol and renal hypertensive index are also important variables in most subgroups. The contributions of the remaining variables are not consistent for the various subgroups. Nevertheless, other variables make significant contributions independently of age. Some of the variables with significant simple correlation coefficients do not make significant independent contributions (possibly due to co-relationships with age or other variables); and some of the variables which are not significantly correlated with lesions in the initial analyses do make a significant contribution in these multiple regression analyses.

Discussion

We had direct or indirect "markers" of three of the known or suspected risk factors for CHD--serum cholesterol levels, blood pressure levels, and obesity. In addition, we used adipose tissue fatty acids as potential indices of dietary and metabolic markers and lipid content of liver samples as a potential index of fatty liver and alcoholism. Our results provide only crude estimates of the associations between risk factors and raised lesions. The effects of measurement errors were reduced by replicating measurements where practical, but we were necessarily restricted to single determinations for most of the risk factors. Despite these limitations, our study shows statistically significant relationships between many risk factors and raised lesions, independently of age. The particular subset of risk factors that are statistically significant varies with race, disease category, and arterial segment; explanations for this finding are being sought. A large amount of variability remains unexplained. Measurement errors undoubtedly account for some of the remainder. Unfortunately, we do not have smoking histories, but previous reports suggest that this important risk factor may independently account for a sizable amount of variability in raised lesions (Strong et al. 1969; Strong and Richards 1976). Although it is not reasonable to expect a total explanation of the variability in lesions, arterial "susceptibility" remains an area of interest in atherosclerosis research.

Acknowledgments

The authors wish to thank Mrs. Rhea Dupeire and Mrs. Mary Engelhardt for their assistance in preparing and typing the manuscript.

References

Abell LL, Levy BB, Brodie BB, Kendall FE (1952) A simplified method for the estimation of total cholesterol in serum and demonstration of its specificity. J Biol Chem 195: 357-366

Garcia-Palmieri MR, Castillo MI, Oalmann MC, Sorlie PD, Costas R Jr (1977)
    The relation of antemortem factors to atherosclerosis at necropsy.
    In: Schettler GY, Goto Y, Hata Y, Klose G (eds) Atherosclerosis IV,
    Springer-Verlag, New York pp 108-113

Guzman MA, McMahan CA, McGill HC Jr, Strong JP, Tejada C, Restrepo C, Eggen DA,
    Robertson WB, Solberg LA (1968) Selected methodologic aspects of the
    International Atherosclerosis Project. Lab Invest 18: 479-497

Hatano S, Matsuzaki T (1977) Atherosclerosis in relation to personal attri-
    butes of a Japanese population in homes for the aged. In: Schettler G,
    Goto Y, Hata Y, Klose G (eds) Atherosclerosis IV, Springer-Verlag, New
    York, pp 116-123

Johnson WD, Oalmann MC, Strong JP, Newman WP III, Tracy RE, Rock WA Jr (1979)
    Implications of pathologic findings for prevention of sudden death in
    premature coronary heart disease. In: Proceedings of the Florence
    International Meeting on Myocardial Infarction. Florence, Italy, in
    press

Kokatnur MG, Oalmann MC, Johnson WD, Malcom GT, Strong JP (1979) Fatty acid
    composition of human adipose tissue from two anatomical sites in a
    biracial community. Am J Clin Nutr 32, in press

Newman WP III, Strong JP, Johnson WD, Oalmann MC, Tracy RE, Rock WA Jr (1979)
    Community pathology of atherosclerosis and coronary heart disease in
    New Orleans: Pathogenic factors and racial comparisons. In: Proceedings
    of the Florence International Meeting on Myocardial Infarction. Florence,
    Italy, in press

Oalmann MC, Strong JP, Johnson WD, Newman WP III, Rock WA Jr, Tracy RE (1979)
    Community pathology of atherosclerosis, coronary heart disease, and
    sudden death: Study methods. In: Proceedings of the Florence Inter-
    national Meeting on Myocardial Infarction. Florence, Italy, in press

Rock WA Jr, Oalmann MC, Stary HC, Tracy RE, McMurry MT, Palmer RW, Welsh RA,
    Strong JP (1972) A standardized method for evaluating myocardial and
    coronary artery lesions. In: Wissler RW, Geer JC (eds) The Pathogenesis
    of Atherosclerosis. Williams & Wilkins, Baltimore, p 247

Solberg LA, Hjermann I, Helgeland A, Holme I, Leren PA, Strong JP (1977)
    Association between risk factors and atherosclerotic lesions based on
    autopsy findings in the Oslo study: A preliminary report. In: Schettler
    G, Goto Y, Hata Y, Klose G (eds) Atherosclerosis IV, Springer-Verlag,
    New York, pp 98-102

Stemmermann GN, Rhoads GG, Blackwelder WC (1977) Atherosclerosis and its
    risk factors in the Hawaiian Japanese. In: Schettler G, Goto Y, Hata Y,
    Klose G (eds) Atherosclerosis IV, Springer-Verlag, New York, pp 113-116

Sternby NH (1977) Atherosclerosis and risk factors. In: Schettler GY, Goto Y,
    Hata Y, Klose G (eds) Atherosclerosis IV, Springer-Verlag, New York,
    pp 102-104

Strong JP (1979) Myocardial infarction in patients with patent coronary bed--
    A pathologist's viewpoint. In: Proceedings of the Florence International
    Meeting on Myocardial Infarction. Florence, Italy (in print)

Strong JP (1977) An introduction to the epidemiology of atherosclerosis. In:
    Schettler GY, Goto Y, Hata Y, Klose G (eds) Atherosclerosis IV, Springer-
    Verlag, New York, pp 92-98

Strong JP, Eggen DA (1970) Risk factors and atherosclerotic lesions. Athero-
    sclerosis: Proceedings of the Second International Symposium. Jones RJ
    (ed) Springer-Verlag, New York, pp 355-364

Strong JP, Richards ML (1976) Cigarette smoking and atherosclerosis in
    autopsied men. Atherosclerosis 23: 451-476

Strong JP, Richards ML, McGill HC Jr, Eggen DA, McMurry MT (1969) On the
    association of cigarette smoking with coronary and aortic atherosclerosis.
    J Atheroscl Res 10: 303-317

Tracy RE (1970) Quantitative measures of the severity of hypertensive nephro-
    sclerosis. Am J Epidemiol 91:25-31

Appendix Table 1. Summary data for coronary heart disease risk factors by age, race and cause of death.

Cause of Death

RISK FACTOR	AGE	RACE	CHD			RELATED			BASAL		
			n	MEAN	S.E.	n	MEAN	S.E.	n	MEAN	S.E.
Postmortem Cholesterol mg/dl	25-34	Black	2	173	34.3	12	176	20.7	140	175	6.3
		White	5	283	46.5	2	219	97.0	51	192	10.1
	35-44	Black	10	212	24.4	20	163	12.3	96	170	8.2
		White	10	276	34.0	3	304	29.0	55	182	11.9
Heart Weight gm	25-34	Black	4	426	63.5	13	512	45.4	194	369	6.0
		White	5	435	65.3	2	550	200.0	70	364	11.4
	35-44	Black	16	442	29.9	29	479	23.6	127	373	6.7
		White	15	495	37.8	7	442	48.9	83	387	9.0
Heart Weight/Body Length	25-34	Black	4	2.5	0.4	13	2.9	0.3	187	2.1	0.03
		White	3	2.6	0.6	2	3.2	1.3	68	2.1	0.06
	35-44	Black	13	2.5	0.1	26	2.8	0.1	113	2.1	0.04
		White	14	2.9	0.2	6	2.6	0.3	80	2.3	0.05
Renal Hypertension Index	25-34	Black	4	0.88	0.31	12	1.37	0.27	189	0.38	0.03
		White	5	0.48	0.14	1	1.53	-	67	0.34	0.03
	35-44	Black	15	0.88	0.17	27	1.77	0.17	118	0.83	0.05
		White	13	0.89	0.13	6	1.32	0.17	80	0.65	0.04
Thickness Panniculus Adiposus mm	25-34	Black	3	16.7	3.3	13	16.8	3.6	190	14.8	0.7
		White	4	10.8	1.5	2	15.0	0.0	69	20.1	1.5
	35-44	Black	15	21.3	3.4	25	17.7	3.0	116	14.4	0.9
		White	14	25.4	3.8	6	27.5	4.2	80	20.1	1.5

Appendix Table 1. (continued)

Body Weight kg	25–34	Black	3	77.0	4.7	13	72.4	5.1	189	74.9	1.1
		White	4	70.3	2.8	2	71.5	3.5	68	77.5	1.8
	35–44	Black	15	74.7	4.1	25	67.4	3.2	113	71.8	1.6
		White	14	87.6	5.9	6	82.2	12.9	80	75.5	2.1
Body Length (Height) cm	25–34	Black	4	170	3.8	13	174	1.5	188	175	0.6
		White	3	170	2.3	2	177	7.0	68	176	0.8
	35–44	Black	13	172	2.1	26	171	1.9	113	174	0.6
		White	14	175	2.4	6	173	2.6	80	172	1.1
Trunk Length cm	25–34	Black	3	52.7	1.76	13	53.2	0.8	188	52.5	0.22
		White	4	53.3	0.6	2	51.5	1.5	68	53.1	0.31
	35–44	Black	15	51.4	0.7	23	53.0	0.6	115	53.0	0.34
		White	13	55.9	1.9	5	54.8	1.4	79	54.1	0.44
Body Weight/Body Length	25–34	Black	3	0.44	0.02	13	0.42	0.03	187	0.43	0.01
		White	3	0.40	0.01	2	0.41	0.04	67	0.44	0.01
	35–44	Black	13	0.44	0.03	25	0.39	0.02	112	0.41	0.01
		White	14	0.50	0.03	6	0.47	0.07	80	0.44	0.01
Ponderal Index	25–34	Black	3	41.1	0.80	13	42.9	0.98	187	42.4	0.21
		White	3	42.1	0.42	2	43.3	2.41	67	42.2	0.32
	35–44	Black	13	41.5	0.79	25	43.2	0.69	112	42.9	0.31
		White	14	40.4	0.63	6	41.5	1.79	80	41.8	0.41
Liver Lipid mg/100 g	25–34	Black	4	53.3	5.5	13	59.6	11.0	190	63.8	3.1
		White	5	46.3	2.8	2	45.5	3.0	66	65.3	5.5
	35–44	Black	15	80.4	13.1	26	61.0	5.2	117	77.7	5.6
		White	13	115.0	26.8	5	109.0	39.3	76	94.4	8.5

Appendix Table 2. Total sample: Correlations coefficients.

Variables	Black			White		
	Raised Lesions		Heart Weight	Raised Lesions		Heart Weight
	Abd. Aorta	Coronary Arteries		Abd. Aorta	Coronary Arteries	
Raised Lesions in Abdominal Aorta	--	0.53**	0.21**	--	0.52**	0.13
Raised Lesions in Coronary Arteries	0.53**	--	0.32**	0.52**	--	0.41**
Age	0.39**	0.38**	0.13*	0.58**	0.33**	0.18*
Postmortem Cholesterol	0.00	0.11	0.04	0.26**	0.36**	0.17
Heart Weight	0.21**	0.32**	--	0.13	0.41**	--
Heart Weight/Body Length	0.19**	0.30**	0.98**	0.13	0.41**	0.98**
Renal Hypertension Index	0.36**	0.35**	0.43**	0.46**	0.26**	0.28**
Thickness Panniculus Adiposus	0.06	0.24**	0.39**	0.02	0.18*	0.37**
Body Weight	-0.05	0.17**	0.40**	-0.02	0.22**	0.53**
Body Length	0.00	-0.07	0.16**	-0.12	-0.01	0.15*
Trunk Length	0.07	0.07	0.28**	0.22**	0.24**	0.34**
Body Weight/Body Length	-0.05	0.20**	0.38**	0.00	0.21**	0.51**
Ponderal Index	0.05	-0.20**	-0.27**	-0.02	-0.23**	-0.39**
Liver Lipid	0.07	0.01	-0.03	0.19*	0.13	0.08

Appendix Table 2. (continued)
Adipose Tissue Fatty Acids:

Myristic (14:0)						
Perirenal	-0.03	-0.12*	-0.04	-0.09	-0.14	-0.28**
Buttock	-0.04	-0.16**	-0.11*	-0.03	-0.12	-0.24**
Palmitic (16:0)						
Perirenal	-0.05	-0.04	0.03	-0.08	0.02	0.06
Buttock	-0.05	-0.03	0.05	-0.10	0.02	0.00
Palmitoleic (16:1)						
Perirenal	0.08	-0.05	-0.11*	0.16*	-0.05	-0.09
Buttock	0.05	-0.03	-0.07	0.15	0.01	-0.01
Stearic (18:0)						
Perirenal	-0.07	-0.07	-0.02	-0.15	-0.05	-0.10
Buttock	0.00	-0.07	-0.08	-0.07	-0.08	-0.08
Oleic (18:1)						
Perirenal	0.12*	0.03	-0.05	0.10	-0.04	0.04
Buttock	0.08	0.01	-0.04	-0.05	-0.13	0.01
Linoleic (18:2)						
Perirenal	-0.06	0.11*	0.08	-0.08	0.12	0.07
Buttock	-0.06	0.13*	0.09	0.01	0.18*	0.07

*Significant at 0.05 level.   **Significant at 0.01 level.

Appendix Table 3. Basal group: Correlation coefficients.

Variable	Black			White		
	Raised Lesions			Raised Lesions		
	Abd. Aorta	Coronary Arteries	Heart Weight	Abd. Aorta	Coronary Arteries	Heart Weight
Raised Lesions in Abdominal Aorta	--	0.30**	0.16**	--	0.40**	-0.04
Raised Lesions in Coronary Arteries	0.30**	--	0.25**	0.40**	--	0.27**
Age	0.32**	0.30**	0.05	0.57**	0.36**	0.15
Postmortem Cholesterol	0.00	0.12	0.09	0.13	0.20*	0.03
Heart Weight	0.16**	0.25**	--	-0.04	0.27**	--
Heart Weight/Body Length	0.13*	0.15*	0.97**	-0.03	0.26**	0.97**
Renal Hypertension Index	0.40**	0.31**	0.24**	0.39**	0.13	0.10
Thickness Panniculus Adiposus	0.02	0.07	0.39**	-0.10	0.20*	0.40**
Body Weight	-0.04	0.22**	0.53**	-0.18*	0.22**	0.53**
Body Length	0.00	0.01	0.21**	-0.16	0.01	0.13
Trunk Length	0.07	0.19**	0.29**	0.13	0.19*	0.27**
Body Weight/Body Length	-0.04	0.22**	0.50**	-0.14	0.20*	0.51**
Ponderal Index	0.05	-0.18**	-0.38**	0.08	-0.21*	-0.36**
Liver Lipid	0.14*	0.02	-0.04	0.15	0.11	0.03

Appendix Table 3. (Continued)
Adipose Tissue Fatty Acids:

Myristic (14:0)						
Perirenal	-0.02	-0.09	0.02	-0.07	-0.11	-0.21*
Buttock	0.01	-0.08	-0.06	0.09	0.01	-0.19*
Palmitic (16:0)						
Perirenal	-0.01	-0.02	0.08	-0.17	0.04	0.11
Buttock	-0.03	-0.01	0.14*	-0.18*	0.01	0.00
Palmitoleic (16:1)						
Perirenal	0.14*	0.00	-0.06	0.28**	0.13	-0.01
Buttock	0.12*	0.08	-0.04	0.18*	0.14	-0.01
Stearic (18:0)						
Perirenal	-0.13*	-0.12*	-0.04	-0.15	-0.20*	-0.18*
Buttock	-0.06	-0.10	-0.10	-0.02	-0.16	-0.06
Oleic (18:1)						
Perirenal	0.14*	0.13*	-0.04	0.13	0.06	0.08
Buttock	0.10	0.08	-0.04	0.02	-0.04	0.08
Linoleic (18:2)						
Perirenal	-0.13*	-0.01	0.00	-0.15	-0.03	-0.02
Buttock	-0.11	-0.02	0.02	-0.06	0.01	-0.02

*Significant at 0.05 level. ** Significant at 0.01 level.

Regression Sequences After Experimental Atherosclerosis[1]

Mark L. Armstrong, Marjorie B. Megan, and Emory D. Warner

Basic Elements of Regression Studies

All regression studies conform to a general model of intervention (Fig. 1).
As new experimental settings are used to explore the limits of regressive
change, some interventions will doubtless have only minimal or no favorable effects, and the possibility of lesion worsening is always present.
In this presentation, however, we are not concerned with factors that might
tend to override all regressive effects. Our focus is on the sequences of
change that may occur in studies in which regression has been unequivocally
established.

The single defining criterion for lesion regression is a decrease in lesion
size. For this reason morphometric evaluation has been a primary consideration in classifying regression studies as positive or negative. The changes
in lesion composition have also been duly noted, in part to gain some understanding of the regressibility of lesion components (Armstrong and Megan
1972, Kokatnur et al. 1975). The method of lesion induction clearly influences both lesion composition and the possibility of regression. The
neointima following simple balloon-injury has a less complex composition
than the hypercholesterolemic intima, and its relatively rapid regression
has been well documented (Baumgartner and Studer 1977). In arterial lesions
induced by hypercholesterolemia, the only lesion-forming model we will discuss, the amount and type of lipid seem to affect subsequent lesion behavior during intervention regimens.

Regression in Terms of Depletable Pools

The most obvious change in lesion composition during regression is loss of
lipid, mainly cholesterol and its esters (Armstrong and Megan 1972, Kokatnur et al. 1975). A significant amount of lipid is not lost from large
fatty streaks and fibrofatty plaques. A lost/retained ratio has been operationally defined in terms of pools of cholesterol bound or unbound to
arterial matrix (Wagner and Clarkson 1973). The possibility of lipid depletion has also been related to its physical state in the arterial lesions
(Small 1977). Are there depletable lesion components other than the lipid
constituents? We have argued elsewhere that a reduction in total proteoglycans might be anticipated in regression (Armstrong 1978), but the evidence to date stops short of proof. There is loss of cellularity that might
be regarded as depletion. Changes in the fibrous matrix of the lesion are
best regarded as remodeling although the amount of collagen determined biochemically is sometimes decreased in long-term regression (Armstrong and
Megan 1975).

Depletability may not always correlate with change in lesion size. This
is illustrated by the early finding that coronary lesion size was not per-
ceptibly diminished at 5 months regression but that visible lipid had

[1]This work was supported by grants USPHS HL-14230 (Arteriosclerosis Specialized Center of Research) and HL-14388.

diminished (Maruffo and Portman 1968). Strictly speaking, regression had not occurred although a principal feature of regression was evident. Since lesion size defines regression and is the physical expression of the change in all "pools", whether depleted, increased or unchanged, we have used size as the endpoint in examining two questions. The first question is: do changes in regression vary among arterial beds apart from the type of lipid deposition? In Figure 2 are shown the regression slopes for aorta and coronary artery. The data are from a study in which rhesus monkeys were given an atherogenic diet for 28 months and a regression diet for 24 months. The relative resistance of the aorta to regression has been noted by numerous investigators. Is this an intrinsically different response? Much of the lipid in the coronary arteries and in the thoracic aorta was intracellular, and there was more extracellular "bound" lipid in the abdominal aorta. If we look at the comparative regression of the two aortic segments (Fig. 3), the thoracic segment behaves like the coronary arteries and regression is much less in the abdominal segment. Among the determinants of regressive changes, the general type of lesion lipid present at the start of regression has major importance. The second question is, what are the effects of successive time intervals of regression on changes in lesion size?

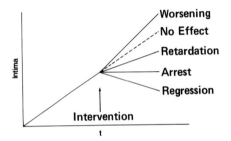

Figure 1. A general model of intervention, in which decrease in lesion size (regression) is shown as the most favorable of five outcomes of an intervention trial.

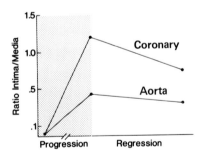

Figure 2. Coronary versus aortic regression. Details in text. Intima/media ratios are shown to facilitate comparison; medial size in each bed did not differ significantly between progression and regression, providing a relatively constant point of reference.

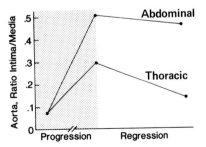

Figure 3. Regression of abdominal and thoracic segments of aorta.

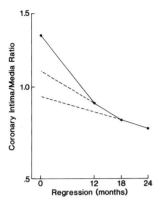

Figure 4. Coronary regression at 12, 18, and 24 months. The broken lines extending to the onset of regression represent sequential regression slopes following the rapid regression noted during the first year.

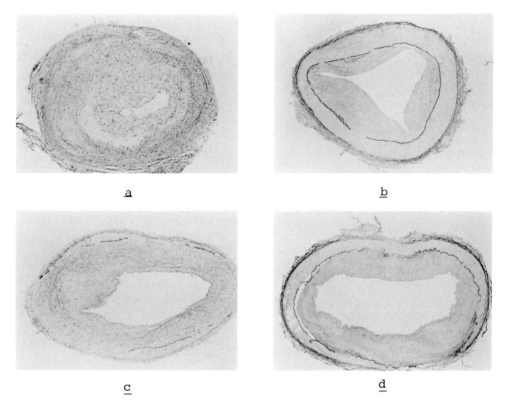

Figure 5. Coronary atherosclerosis and sequential regression. <u>a.</u> Reference atherosclerosis. Small lumen with moderate concentric fibrosis, underlying lipid (mainly intracellular) and pocks of necrosis. <u>b.</u> Regression, 12 months. Larger lumen with loss of intimal mass. Reduction of intracellular lipid is subtotal. <u>c.</u> Regression, 18 months. There is further reduction of cellularity and of intimal intracellular lipid. <u>d.</u> Regression, 24 months. Lumen is large. Intima has a prominent fibrous matrix and little intracellular lipid is visible.

Regression As a Series of Rates

The data in Figures 2 and 3 show regression effects between reference atherosclerosis and regression at 24 months. In Fig. 4 are shown interim values
for regression in coronary arteries at 12 and 18 months, yielding three sequences of size change. If the regression effect is construed in terms of
lipid loss, the three sequences might be considered to represent lipid sequentially mobilized. There is an inverse relation between the amount of
visible lipid and the time of regression, but the lipid "pools" are an obvious artefact of the number of observation periods. With less constraint
we may think of the intimal changes as depicting rate changes in regression.
The first regression interval at 12 months regression shows the greatest
decrease in intimal size. This is the period of greatest foam cell loss
(Fig. 5B versus A). The more dramatic changes in regression of experimental atherosclerosis come from this effect. The intima decreased about
30% during the first year of regression. The second sequence at 18 months
shows a further reduction in lesion size of 18% at an annual rate. The
morphologic data show less lipid in cells and probably less extracellular
lipid. The third regression sequence at 24 months shows a further reduction
in lesion size at an annual rate of 13% with even less visible lipid.

Summary

The possibility of lesion regression may be considered in terms of depletable lesion constituents. Lesion mass may be decreased by the loss of
mobilizable cholesterol and by the reduction of cell numbers. Regression
of experimental lesions is nonlinear, and may be regarded in terms of sequentially decreasing rates with continuing mass changes and lipid depletion during observation periods up to 2 years.

References

Armstrong ML, Megan MB (1972) Lipid depletion in atheromatous coronary ar-
    teries in rhesus monkeys after regression diets. Circ Res 30:675-680
Armstrong ML, Megan MB (1975) Arterial fibrous proteins in cynomolgus mon-
    keys after atherogenic and regression diet. Circ Res 36:256-261
Armstrong ML (1978) Connective tissue in regression. In: Paoletti R, Gotto
    AM Jr (eds) Atherosclerosis Reviews. Raven Press, New York, pp 147-168
Baumgartner HR, Studer A (1977) Platelet factors and the proliferation of
    vascular smooth muscle cells. In: Schettler G, Goto Y, Hata Y, Klose G
    (eds) Atherosclerosis IV. Springer-Verlag, Berlin, pp 609-612
Kokatnur MG, Malcom GT, Eggen DA, Strong JP (1975) Depletion of aortic free
    and ester cholesterol by dietary means in rhesus monkeys with fatty
    streaks. Atherosclerosis 21: 195-203
Maruffo C, Portman OW (1968) Nutritional control of coronary artery athero-
    sclerosis in the squirrel monkey. J Atheroscler Res 8:237-247
Small DM (1977) Cellular mechanisms for lipid deposition in atherosclerosis.
    N Engl J Med 297:873-877, 924-929
Wagner WD, Clarkson TB (1973) Slowly miscible cholesterol pools in regress-
    ing atherosclerotic aortas. Proc Soc Exp Biol Med 143:804-809

Changes in Atherosclerotic Lesions Following Surgical Cholesterol Reduction

Henry Buchwald, Richard D. Rucker, Richard B. Moore, and Richard L. Varco

Surgical procedures specifically employed to lower the plasma cholesterol concentration include partial ileal bypass, portacaval shunt, and various biliary drainage operations. These operations have all been used clinically and in the animal laboratory to assess changes in atherosclerotic plaque lesions induced by marked cholesterol reduction. Interesting and promising data have been derived from these studies.

White New Zealand rabbits placed on a 2% cholesterol diet (by weight) predictably developed severe atherosclerotic plaque lesions, including those in the coronary arteries resulting in a 50% myocardial infarction rate (Buchwald 1965a). Using this model, it was demonstrated that rabbits subjected to partial ileal bypass and then placed on the 2% atherogenic diet showed no elevation of the cholesterol concentration; indeed, they averaged circulating cholesterol values below that of the control group on ordinary diet. Furthermore, they developed no plaque lesions (Buchwald 1965b). Another group of animals was placed and maintained on the 2% cholesterol diet, but at either 2 or 4 months underwent a partial ileal bypass. In these animals, the blood cholesterol concentration was drastically lowered from average values in the 600-1000 mg% range to levels below 100 mg%. Concurrently, atherosclerotic plaques evolved from an acute proliferative process to a healing, flatter, fibrotic lesion, with 34% less total aortic cholesterol content per residue weight (Buchwald 1965b). We essentially duplicated these findings in a study of infant rabbits (Buchwald et al. 1972).

Okuboye and associates (1968) confirmed these results in the rabbit and extended the time of observation from 4 to 8 months after cholesterol reduction. They were thereby able to demonstrate, by gross plaque grading, evidence of plaque regression.

Using the white Carneau pigeon, an avian species with naturally occurring atherosclerosis, Gomes et al. (1971) showed that partial ileal bypass decreased the severity of aortic atherosclerosis, without interfering with growth or weight in both young and old birds. In pigeons initiated on an atherogenic diet at 6 months, and continued thereon for 28 months, the mean aortic plaque area was 10.1 mm in the controls and 4.2 mm in the bypass group. After 27 months on diet, in 6 year old pigeons, the mean aortic plaque area in the controls was 22.1 mm, whereas in the bypassed birds it was only 14.3 mm.

In the hypercholesterolemic canine model, partial ileal bypass, or biliary diversion procedures, have been shown to prevent atherosclerosis: Scott et al. (1966) utilized a 40% partial ileal bypass in the dog with demonstrable prevention; DePalma (1970) and Morgan (1972), using biliary diversion to the distal small intestine, also showed protective effects against experimentally-induced atherosclerosis; similar findings were reported by Wilk et al. (1976) by diverting the bile into the urinary bladder. In addition to demonstrating atherosclerosis prevention, DePalma's study gave evidence for regression of plaque lesions after marked cholesterol reduction.

Finally, with respect to animal data and surgically-induced atherosclerotic plaque changes, both DePalma (1972) and the group of Younger and Scott (1976) have published on prevention of lesion formation in the Rhesus monkey protected by biliary diversion or a partial ileal bypass.

Clinical Studies

There have been approximately 50 portacaval shunt procedures performed in the world to-date (personal communication, Starzl 1979), of which 17 are reported in the literature (see review elsewhere in this Symposium). Improvement in symptomatology, peripheral xanthomata, and in one case the aortic pressure gradient, have been reported in 8 of these patients.

We have reported clinical angina pectoris and xanthomata improvement in partial ileal bypass patients (Buchwald et al 1974) and this has been confirmed by other authors (Swan and McGowan 1968; Sodal et al. 1970; Miettinen et al. 1970; Fritz and Walker 1966; and DePalma 1978).

In a biochemical study, we (Moore et al. 1969, 1970) have calculated the total, freely miscible, and less freely miscible exchangeable cholesterol pools in hypercholesterolemic subjects before, and one year after, partial ileal bypass. At one year, there is an approximately 1/3 reduction in the total exchangeable cholesterol pools, with a relatively greater reduction in each patient in the slowly miscible pool than in the more freely miscible pool. This would suggest a loss of cholesterol from tissues other than the blood, liver, and intestinal mucosa.

The hardest human data of atherosclerosis arrest, and possible regression, comes from arteriographic studies of partial ileal bypass patients (Baltaxe et al. 1969; Knight et al. 1972). Of 22 carefully documented sequential arteriograms, at an average of 36.5 months between studies, plaque progression was read in five (22.7%), no change in 12 (54.5%), questionable angiographic improvement in 2 (9.1%), and fairly definitive evidence of angiographic improvement in 3 (13.6%). The rate of progression in other arteriographic studies in the literture, following patients with no marked cholesterol reduction, has been twice that reported in our series (Gensini and Kelly 1972; Bemis et al. 1973; Bruschke et al. 1973; Mark et al. 1973; Kimbiris et al. 1974; Rosch et al. 1976).

In the current National Heart, Lung, and Blood Institute sponsored secondary intervention trial, designated as POSCH — Program on Surgical Control of the Hyperlipidemias — each of the 1,000 study patients to be recruited (500 controls and 500 partial ileal bypass patients) will be followed by three sets of sequential coronary arteriograms, over a course of 5 years. These angiographic assessments of the disease process will not only be analyzed visually but by the computer technique of Blankenhorn and associates (1977). This study will be a definitive test of the lipid-atherosclerosis hypothesis and a prospective, controlled evaluation of the capacity of the atheroscler- otically diseased human artery to respond to marked total cholesterol and LDL-cholesterol reductions by plaque retardation, stabilization, or regression.

References

Baltaxe H, Amplatz K, Varco RL, Buchwald H (1969) Coronary arteriography in hypercholesterolemic patients. Am J Roentg 105:784-790

Bemis CE, Gorlin R, Kemp HG, Herman MV (1973) Progression of coronary artery disease: A clinical arteriographic study. Circulation 47:455-463

Blankenhorn DH (1977) Angiographic evidence of atherosclerosis regression in man. In Schettler G, Goto Y, Hata Y, Klose G (eds) Atherosclerosis IV. Springer-Verlag, Berlin, pp414-423

Bruschke AVG, Proudfit WL, Sones FJ Jr (1973) Progress study of 590 consecutive nonsurgical cases of coronary disease followed 5-9 years: II. Ventriculographic and other correlations. Circulation 47:1154-1163

Buchwald H (1965a) Myocardial infarction in rabbits induced solely by a hypercholesterolemic diet. J Atheroscler Res 5:407-419

Buchwald H (1965b) The effect of ileal bypass on atherosclerosis and hypercholesterolemia in the rabbit. Surgery 58:22-36

Buchwald H, Moore RB, Bertish J, Varco RL (1972) Effect of ileal bypass on cholesterol levels, atherosclerosis, and growth in the infant rabbit. Ann Surg 175:311-319

Buchwald H, Moore RB, Varco RL (1974) Surgical treatment of hyperlipidemias: Part I - Apologia; Part II - The laboratory experience; Part III - Clinical status of the partial ileal bypass operation. Circulation 49(I):1

DePalma RG, Clowes AW (1978) Interventions in atherosclerosis: A review for surgeons. Surgery 84:175-189

DePalma RG, Hubay CA, Insull W Jr, Robinson AV, Hartman PH (1970) Progression and regression of experimental atherosclerosis. Surg Gyn & Ob 131:633-647

DePalma RG, Insull W Jr, Bellon EM, Roth TW, Robinson AV (1972) Animal models for the study of progression and regression of atherosclerosis. Surgery 72:268-278

Fritz SH, Walker WJ (1966) Ileal bypass in the control of intractable hypercholesterolemia. Am J Surg 32:691-694

Gensini GG, Kelly AE (1972) Incidence and progression of coronary artery disease. Arch Intern Med 129:814-827

Gomes MM, Kottke BA, Bernatz P, Titus JL (1971) Effect of ileal bypass on aortic atherosclerosis of white Carneau pigeons. Surgery 70:353-358

Kimbiris D, Lavine P, VanDenBroek H, Najmi M, Likoff W (1974) Devolutionary pattern of coronary atherosclerosis in patients with angina pectoris. Am J Card 33:7-11

Knight L, Scheibel R, Amplatz K, Varco RL, Buchwald H (1972) Radiographic appraisal of the Minnesota partial ileal bypass study. Surg Forum 23:141

Mark RJ, Lansdown EL, Mymin D, Jackson D (1973) Second look at coronary angiography. J Am Med Assoc 225:979-981

Miettinen TA, Lempinen M (1970) Ileal bypass operation in familial hypercholesterolemia. Scan J Clin Lab Inv 112:55

Moore RB, Frantz ID Jr, Buchwald H (1969) Changes in cholesterol pool size,
turnover rate, and fecal bile acid and sterol excretion after partial
ileal bypass in hypercholesterolemic patients. Surgery 65:98–108

Moore RB, Frantz ID Jr, Varco RL, Buchwald H (1970) Cholesterol dynamics
after partial ileal bypass. In Jones RJ (ed) Proceedings Second International Symposium on Atherosclerosis. Springer-Verlag, New York pp295–
305

Morgan CV Jr, Lanier VC, Finch WT, Younger RK, Scott HW Jr (1972) Protective
effects of bile diversion to the distal fourth of small intestine against
experimental hypercholesterolemia and atherosclerosis in dogs. Am Surgeon
38:10–12

Okuboye JA, Ferguson CC, Wyatt JP (1968) The effect of ileal bypass on dietary-
induced atherosclerosis in the rabbit. Can J Surg 11:69–77

Rosch J, Antonovic R, Trenouth RS, Rahimtoola SH, Dim DN, Dotter CT (1976) The
natural history of coronary artery stenosis. Radiology 119:513–520

Scott HW Jr, Stephenson SE Jr, Younger R, Carlisle RB, Turney SW (1966) Prevention of experimental atherosclerosis by ileal bypass: Twenty-percent
cholesterol diet and I^{131} induced hyperthyroidism in dogs. Ann Surg
163:795–807

Sodal G, Gjertsen KT, Schrumpf A (1970) Surgical treatment of hypercholesterolemia. Acta Chir Scandinav 136:671–674

Swan DM, McGowan JM (1968) Ileal bypass in hypercholesterolemia associated
with heart disease. Am J Surg 116:22–27

Wilk PJ, Karipineni RC, Pertsemlidis D, Danese CA (1976) Prevention of induced atherosclerosis by diversion of bile or blockade of intestinal
lymphatics in dogs. Ann Surg 183:409–414

Younger RK, Curtis JJ, Butts WH, Scott HW Jr (1976) Protective effects of
ileal bypass versus administration of clofibrate on experimental hypercholesterolemia and atherosclerosis in monkeys. So Med J 69:1141–1142

Approaches to the Study of Atherosclerosis Regression in Rhesus Monkeys: Interpretation of Morphometric Measurements of Coronary Arteries[1]

Thomas B. Clarkson, M. Gene Bond, Carol A. Marzetta, and Bill C. Bullock

Introduction

During the past decade there has been considerable interest in whether and to what extent atherosclerotic lesions can be made to regress. There is increasing evidence that regression of atherosclerotic lesions can occur in human beings; although, there is generally a lack of definitive experimental data on the subject. Particular problems in the study of human atherosclerosis regression concern difficulties in determining the sequence of morphologic changes under control conditions.

Because of these difficulties in studying atherosclerosis regression in human beings there has been a strong interest in using nonhuman primate models of man for making these determinations. Since 1970 there have been numerous reports concerning the potential for regression of atherosclerotic lesions of nonhuman primates fed atherogenic diets (Armstrong et al. 1970; Tucker et al. 1971; Armstrong and Megan 1972; Jones et al. 1973; Armstrong and Megan 1974; Eggen et al. 1974; Stary 1974; Armstrong and Megan 1975; Kokatnur et al. 1975; Radhakrishnamurthy et al. 1975; Vesselinovitch et al. 1976). In all but one of these studies (which used Macaca fascicularis) rhesus monkeys were used as the primate model. Except in our own experiments pressure fixation of coronary arteries has not been utilized and rhesus monkeys of varying ages and at varying stages of body growth have been the experimental subjects. In this report we shall focus attention on the problems encountered in a long-term experiment in which the monkeys increased in body size and on some morphometric problems imposed by variations in tissue preparation. Also, in this report we shall cite examples of the types of morphometric measurements that can be made using digitizers and approaches to the interpretation of these data.

Experimental Material

The data on coronary arteries presented in this report were derived from a large, long-term experiment on atherosclerosis regression in rhesus monkeys done at the Arteriosclerosis Research Center of the Bowman Gray School of Medicine at Wake Forest University since 1971. The details of the design of the experiment have been reported elsewhere (Clarkson et al. 1979).

The purpose of the experiment was to determine the potential therapeutic benefit of plasma cholesterol concentrations of about 300 vs 200 mg/dl among rhesus monkeys with diet-induced atherosclerosis. The animals in this experiment were fed an atherogenic diet containing 40% of calories from lard and 1 mg/Cal of cholesterol for 19 months. At the end of this 19 month induction period the animals were divided into three groups (Groups A, B, and C) on the basis of total plasma cholesterol concentrations during

[1] Supported by a grant from the National Heart, Lung and Blood Institute (SCOR-HL 14164).

the induction period. Group A animals were killed at the end of the atherosclerosis induction period for baseline observations on the extent and
severity of atherosclerosis. Group B was fed diets with varying amounts of
cholesterol to maintain total plasma cholesterol concentrations between
280 and 320 mg/dl which we intended to be comparable to human beings with
modest hyperlipidemia. Group C was also fed diets with varying amounts of
cholesterol but in this case to maintain total plasma cholesterol concentrations between 180 and 220 mg/dl, which we intended to be comparable to
human beings who had modest hyperlipoproteinemia previously but had reduced
their plasma cholesterol concentrations by approximately 100 mg/dl using
diet and/or drugs. The regression period was either for 24 or 48 months.
The groups that were maintained on a regression regimen for 24 months are
designated as the B_1 and C_1 groups while those that were extended for 48
months are designated as the B_2 and C_2 groups.

At the time of necropsy, the coronary arteries from all of the animals were
flushed briefly with normal saline and perfused at 100 mmHg pressure with
either fresh 10% neutral buffered formalin or with barium sulfate-gelatin-
formalin mass (Schlesinger 1957). After the gelatin mass had solidified
the hearts were removed and fixed in 10% neutral buffered formalin. Perfusion and fixation of the coronary arteries at a standard pressure almost
always provided consistent distention of these arteries for histopathologic
and morphometric evaluation.

To study the extent and severity of coronary artery atherosclerosis among
these animals, 15 tissue blocks (each 3 mm in length) were cut perpendicularly to the long axis of the arteries. Five of these were serial blocks
from the left circumflex, five from the left anterior descending and five
from the right coronary artery. The tissue blocks were dehydrated through
increasing concentrations of ethanol and embedded in paraffin. Two 5 µ
sections were cut from each block and stained with either hematoxylin and
eosin or Verhoeff Van Gieson stains.

We have used two digitizers in making measurements of the characteristics
of coronary artery atherosclerosis. One of us (Dr. Bond) developed and
used a system consisting of a   pressure activated sonic digitizer interfaced with a programmable Hewlett-Packard computer. Data storage was on
flexible discs. The second digitzer was a Zeiss MOP III Image Analyzer.
Although we have made measurements of 20 arterial characteristics, we shall
report here on four of these: (1) the area within the internal elastic
lamina, (2) the area within the coronary artery lumens, (3) the cross
sectional area intimal lesions, and (4) the maximum thickness of intimal
lesions.

Interpretational Considerations

Growth of arteries during the experimental period

There is considerable variation among nonhuman primates concerning the
relationship between body weight at the time of puberty and body weight
when fully grown. Rhesus monkeys (Macaca mulatta) and cynomolgus macaques
(Macaca fascicularis) represent two of the most discordant species in this
regard in the genus Macaca. Male rhesus monkey, for example, reach puberty
between 3.0 and 4.0 years of age at which time they weigh about 4 kg. Full
body size is reached at about 10 years of age when the animals weigh 12 to
16 kg (a 300-400% increase). In contrast, male cynomolgus macaques also
reach puberty at about the same age as rhesus monkeys and weigh about 3 kg;
however, these animals reach full body size at between 7 and 8 years of age
when the body weight is about 5 kg (a 170% increase).

740

The experiment described in this communication extended for 67 months and during that time there was considerable increase in the size of the animals. This increase in body weight was associated with a corresponding increase in heart weight and coronary artery size. Data on these relationships are shown in Figure 1. During the course of this 67 month experiment, heart weights increased from about 25 gm to about 55 gm. Coronary artery size, as determined by the area within the elastic lamina, increased from about 1 to 2 mm^2. An illustration of this growth in coronary arteries is depicted in Figure 2. Figure 2a is a section of a coronary artery from a rhesus monkey 5 years of age (4.6 kg), while 2b is a coronary artery from a rhesus monkey 10 years of age (10.1 kg).

Differences in coronary artery size can markedly affect the interpretation of change in lumen stenosis if such data are used to imply changes in the area occupied by intimal lesions. For example, in a situation in which there are no changes in the areas of intimal lesions, but there are increases in the size of the arteries, one would find a decrease in lumen stenosis.

In Figure 3 we illustrate the effect of coronary artery size on lumen stenosis. Figures 3a and b are examples of sections of coronary arteries with comparable intimal lesions expressed as intimal area (0.51 mm^2 and 0.51 mm^2). Because the section illustrated in 3a is taken from a smaller coronary artery (area within the internal elastic lamina is 0.77 mm^2) than the artery illustrated in Figure 3b (area within the internal elastic lamina is 2.10 mm^2) the calculated lumen stenosis is 69% for Figure 3 a and 24% for 3b.

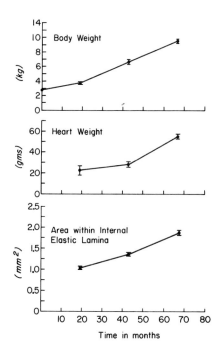

FIG. 1. The relationships between body weight gain, heart weight and coronary artery size (expressed as area within the internal elastic lamina) in a long-term experiment on rhesus monkeys.

While there are merits to both expressions it seems important to regression experiments to use measurements of change in plaque size as the determinant of changes in atherosclerotic lesions as opposed to possible improvement in "atherosclerotic heart disease". As regards the later, measurements of lumen stenosis and lumen area are particularly relevant.

In experiments in which animals grow or experiments on physical activity, increases in coronary artery lumens are due in large part to increases in coronary artery size. Using a single expression of atherosclerotic extensiveness such as lumen stenosis, it is not possible to disassociate the increase in lumen area due to growth or physical activity from that due to atherosclerosis regression. However, by determining the area within the internal elastic lamina and the area of the intimal lesions of coronary arteries fixed under uniform pressure, such a disassociation can be made.

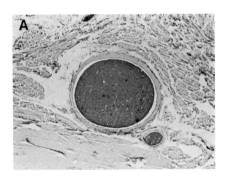 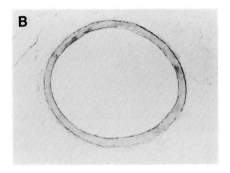

FIG. 2a and b. Photomicrographs of histologic sections taken from the same anatomic location of the left anterior descending coronary artery of rhesus monkeys of different ages. Fig. 2a was taken from a rhesus monkey 5 years of age that weighed 4.6 kgs. Fig. 2b is a section of coronary artery from a rhesus monkey 10 years of age that weighed 10.1 kgs. Both sections are stained with Verhoeff Van Gieson, 40X.

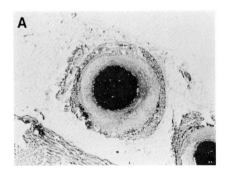 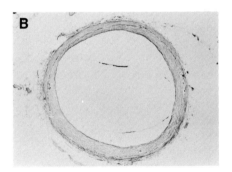

FIG. 3a and b. Photomicrographs of sections of coronary arteries from two rhesus monkeys with comparable intimal lesions expressed as intimal area (the intimal area of both sections was calculated to be 0.51 mm^2). Because the section illustrated in Fig. 3a was from a smaller artery than the artery illustrated in 3b, the calculated lumen stenosis is 69% for Fig. 3a and 24% for Fig. 3b although intimal areas were determined to be identical. Verhoeff Van Gieson, 40X.

Compression artifacts

Although the arteries in our study were perfused and fixed under pressure we did observe microscopic sections in which the contour of the artery was irregular rather than circular. Artifacts may be produced at several stages of tissue preparation. Some artifacts are caused by isolated difficulties in perfusion, embedding, dehydration, cutting and mounting the sections. The angle of tissue sectioning with the long axis of the artery may also present a problem. In this study the major difficulty appeared to be artifactual reduction of the lumen area when integration was used to make the measurement. This was simply corrected by using internal elastic lamina as the circumference of a circle and calculating internal elastic lamina area. An example of the effect of this correction is shown in Figure 4. Figure 4a is a photomicrograph of a section of a coronary artery that has maintained its shape through all stages of processing. Figure 4b depicts a section of an artery that has an irregular shape due to tissue processing. Correction of the area within the internal elastic lamina is important in regression studies for two reasons. First, if internal elastic lamina areas are used as measures of artery growth the growth of compressed arteries would be underestimated. Second, if there are experimental reasons for calculating lumen stenosis the values obtained from compressed arteries would be overstated. The magnitude of the compression effect can be seen in comparing internal elastic lamina area and percent lumen stenosis of the artery illustrated in Figure 4b before and after mathematical correction of the artifact. Before correction, the internal elastic lamina area determined by the integration method would be 1.05 mm^2 and lumen stenosis 16%; after correction using the length of the internal elastic lamina as the circumference of a circle, the internal elastic lamina area was 1.38 mm^2 and lumen stenosis 12%. We also corrected the lumen area estimate in arteries with this type of artifact by subtracting the intimal area as determined by integration from the area enclosed within the corrected internal elastic lamina. This mathematical model is based on the assumption that the intimal area remains constant. Using the example shown in Figure 4b, the calculated lumen area changes from 0.88 to 1.21 mm^2.

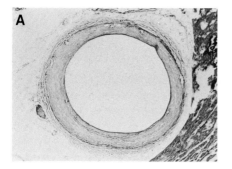 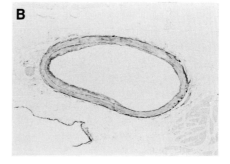

FIG. 4a and b. Photomicrographs of sections of coronary arteries from two rhesus monkeys. Fig. 4a is a photomicrograph of a section of a coronary artery that has maintained its shape through all stages of processing. Fig. 4b depicts a section of the coronary artery that has an irregular shape due to tissue processing. Both sections are stained with Verhoeff Van Gieson, 40X.

Table 1. Coronary artery measurements of rhesus monkeys fed an atherogenic diet for 19 months (Group A) and groups fed an atherogenic diet for 19 months followed by diets that maintained plasma cholesterol concentrations at about 300 (B_1/B_2 Groups) vs 200 (C_1/C_2 Groups) mg/dl for 24 or 48 Months[a]

Group	Area Within Internal Elastic Lamina (mm^2)	Area Within Coronary Artery Lumen (mm^2)	Area Occupied By Intimal Lesion (mm^2)	Maximum Thickness Of Intimal Lesion (mm)
A	1.080 $\pm$0.097	0.778 $\pm$0.066	0.301 $\pm$0.065	0.234 $\pm$0.037
B_1	1.306 $\pm$0.158	0.865 $\pm$0.104	0.441 $\pm$0.080	0.315 $\pm$0.034
C_1	1.347 $\pm$0.156	1.086 $\pm$0.118	0.262 $\pm$0.078	0.174 $\pm$0.028
B_2	1.803 $\pm$0.124	1.513 $\pm$0.092	0.289 $\pm$0.067	0.161 $\pm$0.023
C_2	1.802 $\pm$0.094	1.595 $\pm$0.069	0.207 $\pm$0.046	0.127 $\pm$0.018

[a] Data are expressed as composites of left anterior descending, left circumflex and right coronary arteries, means for the groups followed by the standard error of the mean.

Observations and Interpretations

Based on our experience in using morphometric methods to evaluate coronary artery atherosclerosis in a long-term regression study, the critical measurements are the area within the internal elastic lamina, the area within the coronary artery lumens, the area occupied by the intimal lesions, and the maximum thickness of the intimal lesions. We have summarized our observations concerning these measurements made on the rhesus monkeys from one portion of our lesion regression study in Table 1.

Of primary concern in this experiment is the interpretation of the changes from baseline in the area occupied by the intimal lesions and the increases from baseline in the area within the coronary artery lumens. In Table 2 we have summarized the changes from baseline in intimal area (amount of atherosclerotic plaque). After 24 months of maintaining plasma cholesterol concentrations at 300 vs 200 mg/dl there were marked differences in the change from baseline between the two groups (B_1 vs C_1). The animals maintained at about 300 mg/dl for 24 months increased the amount of intimal plaque. In contrast, those maintained at about 200 mg/dl plasma cholesterol decreased the amount of intimal plaque. As can be seen from the data in Table 2 the contrast in intimal area change was an increase of 32% from baseline in the higher plasma cholesterol concentration group and a decrease of 13% at the

Table 2. Change (Δ) in intimal area (plaque) of atherosclerotic coronary arteries of rhesus monkeys maintained at 300 (B_1/B_2 Groups) vs 200 (C_1/C_2 Groups) mg/dl total plasma cholesterol concentration

Group	Months of Regression	Δ in Intimal Area (mm^2)	% Change from Baseline[a] in Intimal Area
B_1	24	+ 0.14	+ 32 %
C_1	24	− 0.04	− 13 %
B_2	48	− 0.01	− 4%
C_2	48	− 0.10	− 31%

[a] Basline refers to the intimal area of the group of animals fed the the atherogenic diet for 19 months.

lower plasma cholesterol concentration. Similarly, after 48 months the groups at the higher plasma cholesterol concentrations were essentially unchanged from baseline while those at 200 mg/dl had a decrease of 31% in amount of intimal plaque.

The primary value of having made measurements of the area within the internal elastic lamina was to provide information on the changing size of the coronary arteries. As we have indicated there was considerable growth of the monkeys during the course of this 67 month experiment. With this increase in body size there was a corresponding increase in heart weight and of coronary artery size. The area within the internal elastic lamina increased from baseline of about 1.08 mm^2 to 1.80 mm^2 in the final groups. Similarly, after 67 months the coronary artery lumen changes were from a baseline of about 0.78 mm^2 to 1.60 mm^2. It was of particular interest to us to utilize our collected morphometric measurements to determine if we could partition the amount of increase in lumen area that was due to growth of the coronary arteries and that due to change in intimal lesions. This can be done by dividing the change in internal elastic lamina area by the change in lumen area to determine the contribution of growth and likewise by dividing the change in intimal area by the change in lumen area to determine the amount of increase in lumen area due to plaque regression. By knowing the increase in internal elastic lamina area for the groups, the change in area occupied by intimal lesion and the change in coronary artery lumen size, it was possible for us to make such a determination. These observations are summarized in Figure 5. Two points of particular interest are seen in these data. First, the growth of coronary arteries makes a very significant contribution of the increase in coronary artery lumen area. Second, among those animals maintained at the higher plasma cholesterol concentrations, essentially none of the increase in lumen area was due to reduction in the area of the atherosclerotic lesions. In contrast, 11 to 13% of the increase in lumen area of animals maintained at the lower plasma cholesterol concentrations can be explained on the basis of a decrease in intimal area.

Of particular concern to cardiologists has been whether it is possible to obtain any notion, based on nonhuman primate studies of atherosclerosis regression, about rates of regression with decreases in plasma cholesterol concentration of about 100 mg/dl. We examined our data to determine the rates of change per month among our atherosclerotic rhesus monkeys maintained at 300 vs 200 mg/dl plasma cholesterol concentrations. These observations are summarized in Table 3. There is little or no regression in amount of coronary artery intimal plaque at 300 mg/dl while at 200 mg/dl the mass of coronary plaques decreases at a rate between 0.65 and 0.54% per month. These data would suggest that the differential between 300 and 200 mg/dl plasma cholesterol concentration might be expected to induce a decrease in mass of coronary artery plaque of about 25 to 30% in four years.

Conclusions

We have presented data to indicate the usefulness and in some cases the necessity of using morphometric measurements to evaluate atherosclerotic coronary arteries. Apparent from this experiment is that investigators must be aware of interpretational problems resulting from such things as changing sizes of coronary arteries as a result of growth and compression artifacts. We have also focused attention on the usefulness of intimal area rather than "lumen stenosis" as a descriptor of changes in amount of coronary artery atherosclerosis per se, particularly, if the coronary arteries are changing in size as a result of growth or physical activity. In contrast, lumen stenosis and lumen areas are useful descriptors if one is investigating atherosclerotic heart disease as distinct from coronary artery lesions.

Our observations on the effect of maintaining atherosclerotic rhesus monkeys at plasma cholesterol concentrations of 300 vs 200 mg/dl would suggest that the differential of 100 mg/dl results in decreases in the mass of coronary artery plaques of about 30% in four years.

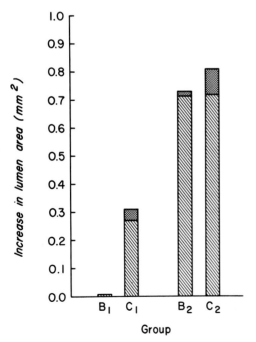

FIG. 5. Proportion of increase from baseline in lumen areas of rhesus monkeys fed regression diets (B_1/B_2 at 300 mg/dl and C_1/C_2 at 200 mg/dl plasma cholesterol concentrations) that is due to artery growth is indicated as ▨ , the proportion due to decreased intimal area is indicated as ▨

Table 3. Calculated rates of change in atherosclerotic plaques expressed as intimal area (IA) of coronary arteries of rhesus monkeys maintained at 300 (B_1/B_2 Groups) vs 200 (C_1/C_2 Groups) mg/dl total plasma cholesterol concentration

Group	Δ in IA/Month		% Δ in IA/Month	
	24 Mos.	48 Mos.	24 Mos.	48 Mos.
$B_1 + B_2$ (300 mg/dl)	+ 5.8 μ^2	-0.20 μ^2	+1.33%	-0.08%
$C_1 + C_2$ (200 mg/dl)	- 1.7 μ^2	-2.10 μ^2	-0.54%	-0.65%

References

Armstrong ML, Warner ED and Connor WE (1970) Regression of coronary atheromatosis in rhesus monkeys. Circ Res 27: 59-67

Armstrong ML and Megan MB (1972) Lipid depletion in atheromatous coronary arteries in rhesus monkeys after regression diets. Circ Res 30: 675-680

Armstrong ML and Megan MB (1974) Responses to two macaque species to atherogenic diet and its withdrawal. In: Schettler G and Weizel A (eds) Atherosclerosis: Proceedings of the Third International Symposium. Springer-Verlag, Berlin, pp. 336-338

Armstrong ML and Megan MB (1975) Arterial fibrous proteins in cynomolgus monkeys after atherogenic and regression diets. Circ Res 36: 256-261

Clarkson TB, Lehner NDM, Wagner WD, St. Clair RW, Bond MG and Bullock BC (1979) A study of atherosclerosis regression in Macaca mulatta. I. Design of experiment and lesion induction. Exp Mol Path 30: 360-385

Eggen DA, Strong JP, Newman WP III, Catsulis C, Malcom GT, and Kokatnur MG (1974) Regression of diet-induced fatty streaks in rhesus monkeys. Lab Invest 31: 294-301

Jones R, Vesselinovitch D, Hughes R, and Wissler RW (1973) Ultrastructure of advanced atherosclerosis and its reversal in rhesus monkey. Fed Proc 32: 158

Kokatnur MG, Malcom GT, Eggen DA and Strong JP (1975) Depletion of aortic free and ester cholesterol by dietary means in rhesus monkeys with fatty streaks. Atherosclerosis 21: 195-203

Radhakrishnamurthy B, Eggen DA, Kokatnur M, Jirge S, Strong JP, and Berenson GS (1975) Composition of connective tissue in aortas from rhesus monkeys during regression of diet induced fatty streaks. Lab Invest 33: 136-140

Schlesinger MJ (1957) New radiopaque mass for vascular injection. Lab Invest 6: 1-11

Stary HC (1974) Cell proliferation and ultrastructural changes in regressing atherosclerotic lesions after reduction of serum cholesterol. In: Schettler G and Weizel A (eds) Atherosclerosis: Proceedings of the Third International Symposium. Springer-Verlag, Berlin, pp 187-190

Tucker CF, Catsulis C, Strong JP and Eggen DA (1971) Regression of early cholesterol-induced aortic lesions in rhesus monkeys. Am J Pathol 65: 493-514

Vesselinovitch D, Wissler RW, Hughes R, and Borensztajn J (1976) Reversal of advanced atherosclerosis in rhesus monkeys. Part 1. Light microscopic studies. Atherosclerosis 23: 155-176

Regression of Advanced Atherosclerotic Lesions in Swine[1]

A.S. Daoud, J. Jarmolych, J.M. Augustyn, and K.E. Fritz

Introduction

At the 4th International Symposium on Atherosclerosis we reported that relatively advanced atherosclerotic lesions can be produced in the abdominal
aortas of swine by a combination of mechanical injury and high cholesterol
(HC) diet in a short period of time (4 months). We also reported that such
lesions rapidly regressed within 14 months after withdrawal of the dietary
stimulus. The features of regression were a decrease in the size of the
lesion, virtual disappearance of necrosis and sudanophilia, a decrease in
DNA concentration and rate of DNA synthesis and a depletion of lipids, namely
cholesteryl esters and phospholipids. While calcification had persisted, the
size of calcific foci appeared, by visual inspection, to be smaller than
those in the reference group (Daoud et al. 1976; Fritz et al. 1976). Although
these rapidly produced, advanced lesions showed an appreciable amount of necrosis and calcification, their cholesterol content was low as compared to
that of human atherosclerosis, as reported by Smith (1965), Scott et al. (1966),
Smith et al. (1967) and Chobanian and Manzur (1970). Hence it is possible
that the rapidity of regression in our experiment was due to the short period
of induction, the low cholesterol concentration of the lesions, or both. More
advanced atherosclerosis, with higher cholesterol concentration in the lesions,
can be produced by injury and 6 months of the HC diet feeding (Scott et al.
unpublished data). This report describes serial assessment of features of regression in advanced, complicated atherosclerotic lesions with a high cholesterol content. In addition, these data will be discussed in light of the
above experiment.

Material and Methods

The abdominal aortas of 28 male Yorkshire swine, weighing 6-15 kg each, were
abraded with an inflated balloon. Sixteen swine were fed a high fat, high
cholesterol diet for 6 months and the remaining 12 were maintained on hog
mash to serve as controls. At the end of 6 months, 4 HC diet fed animals
(reference group) and 3 controls were killed. The remaining 12 HC swine
were transferred to the hog mash diet and divided into 3 groups of 4. One
group was killed at 6 weeks, another at 5 months and the third at 14 months.
At each time 3 mash swine were killed as controls. Due to the death of one
animal of the 14 mos regression group at 10 months of regression and of another just prior to sacrifice, the morphologic data of this group are derived
from 3 animals and the chemical data from only two.

The techniques of inducing injury, the mode of sacrificing the animals and
the morphologic and biochemical procedures were the same as reported pre-

---

[1] The authors' personal research was supported by the Medical Service of the
Veterans Administration and by Grant #210038 NIHL

749

viously (Daoud et al. 1976; Fritz et al. 1976). Quantitative analysis of calcium was done according to the Manual of the Perkin-Elmer atomic absorbence spectrometer. Use of the word "significant" implies statistical significance at a confidence level of 0.05 or less, determined by analysis of variance, paired "t" or unpaired "t" tests as appropriate.

Results

By six weeks of regression, the serum cholesterol levels had returned virtually to control levels. The aortas of all control groups were, in general, smooth, and, on microscopic examination, showed focal, varying but slight degrees of intimal thickening. No necrosis or calcification was observed. The cells were almost exclusively smooth muscle cells.

Grossly, some of the lesions from the reference group were flat and yellow in color, but the majority were raised, many with calcification. Histologically, the flat lesions were composed chiefly of foam cells. The raised lesions were a mixture of foam cells and spindle cells. Most revealed necrotic centers and fibrous caps. In many, necrosis was extensive and involved over 1/3 of the atheroma. Calcification was often present in varying amounts in the raised lesion.

After six weeks on the regression diet, the gross and histologic appearance of the lesions was similar to that of the lesions of the reference group. However, there appeared to be more calcification and somewhat fewer foam cells in the 6 wks regression lesions.

After 5 months on the regression diet, no yellow flat lesions were observed. Microscopic examination of the raised lesions disclosed a marked decrease in the number of foam cells. These were chiefly present at the base of the lesion. The extent of necrosis was greatly diminished and consisted mainly of minute foci around the dense calcium deposits which were rather abundant. The center of most lesions was composed of loose connective tissue which was slightly cellular. The lesions were commonly covered at the luminal surface by a thick, dense fibrous cap.

After 14 months on the regression diet, the lesions were, in general, composed of dense fibrous tissue surrounding dense and abundant calcium deposits. Only occasional small foci of necrosis and minute accumulation of foam cells were observed. Around areas of calcification, cholesterol crystals and some giant cells were noted. The quantitative data are presented in Tables 1 and 2. It should be noted that these are derived from lesion "pools" which include flat and raised lesions for the reference and 6 wks regression tissue and only raised lesions from the 5 and 14 mos regression animals, since in the latter all flat lesions had disappeared. We have reported higher values of all of the biochemical features studied, except DNA concentration, in the raised lesions (Fritz et al. unpublished data). Hence, were complete data for raised lesions alone available in the reference and 6 wks regression groups, the decrease in values reported in the latter periods would have been accentuated.

Table 1 shows a significant decrease in sudanophilia of the aortas of 5 and 14 month regression animals from those of the reference and 6 wks regression animals. Necrosis was also significantly less extensive in the former groups. In contrast, there was no decrease in the ratio of mean thickest lesion thickness to mean medial thickness during the course of the experiment.

Table 1. Morphological data.

	Reference			6 Wks Regression			5 Mos Regression			14 Mos Regression		
	#[a]	Mean	SEM[b]	#	Mean	SEM	#	Mean	SEM	#	Mean	SEM
% intimal sudanophilia	4	43	5.8	4	51	13.6	4	9[c]	0.9	3	14[c]	2.9
Ratio: lesion/ media	4	1.27	0.07	4	1.27	0.4	4	0.88	0.35	3	1.22	0.33
% lesion necrosis	4	27	4.2	4	29	6.9	4	8[c]	2.7	3	4[c]	2.2

[a] # = number of animals.
[b] SEM = standard error of the mean.
[c] Sig. reference and 6 wk regression.

Table 2 shows that, at 5 months regression, mean total cholesterol concentration was significantly lower than the mean concentration of the lesions of the reference group. More importantly, a major contribution to this decrease in total cholesterol was the decrease in esterified cholesterol, which was no longer the predominant form as it was at 6 weeks. Mean calcium concentration of the 5 mos regression lesions was significantly elevated over the mean values of either the reference or 6 wks regression lesions.

After 14 months on the regression diet, the cholesterol component of the lesions had undergone no further depletion from the 5 mos regression values. However, rates of both DNA and protein synthesis and phospholipid concentration had decreased significantly; in fact, except for phospholipid, had reached control levels which were 190 dpm ^{3}H-thymidine and 1282 dpm ^{14}C-leucine/µg DNA, respectively.

Table 2. Biochemical data.

	Reference			6 Wks Regression			5 Mos Regression			14 Mos Regression		
	#[a]	Mean	SEM[b]	#	Mean	SEM	#	Mean	SEM	#	Mean	SEM
DNA conc. (µg/ mg dry wt)	6	4.3	0.2	8	4.7	0.2	9	2.7[c,d]	0.2	4	2.4[c,d]	0.6
DNA synthesis (dpm ^{3}H-thy-midine/µg DNA)	6	713	312	8	2974	1580	10	1108	224	4	290[e]	59
Protein Synth. (dpm ^{14}C-leu-cine/µg DNA)	6	1444	613	8	2434	888	10	2554	529	4	1255[e]	228
Calcium conc. (µg/mg dry wt)	5	9.4	2.8	7	55.5	17.3	5	87.3[c]	20.0	4	129.0[c]	46.4
Cholesterol (µg/mg dry wt)												
Total	4	107.8	31.8	4	63.5	21.6	10	53.0[c]	5.8	2	55.8	22.6
Free	4	33.6	11.3	4	13.4[f]	3.7	10	27.0	3.3	2	28.3	13.2
Esterified	4	74.5	23.5	4	50.0[f]	18.5	10	26.1[c]	2.7	2	27.6[c]	9.5
Phospholipids (nmoles P/mg dry wt)	3	70.7	13.2	4	68.2	15.7	5	99.5	4.2	2	72.9[e]	2.8
Triglycerides (µg/mg dry wt)	3	10.0	3.8	4	7.0	1.2	5	14.4	2.3	2	8.1	3.3

[a] # = number of determination.
[b] SEM = ± standard error of the mean.
[c] Sig. different from reference value.
[d] Sig. different from 6 wks regression value.
[e] Sig. different from 5 mos regression value.
[f] Cholesteryl esters sig. > free cholesterol in 6 wks regression animals.

Discussion and Conclusions

In comparing this study with our previous work it appears that there are differences in the rate and features of regression between lesions. Grossly, in the previous experiment, there was a remodeling of the intimal surface which had become smooth by 14 months after withdrawal of the HC diet. After the same interval, the aortas in the present study showed only minimal evidence of remodeling and flattening of the lesion. Sudanophilia decreased in both groups but to a greater extent in the former.

Histologically, both lesions showed a decrease in the number of foam cells and in necrosis, this being more marked, however, in the former experiment. The size of the atheromata was significantly decreased in the former but not in the latter.

Biochemically, after 14 months on a regression regimen, total cholesterol, cholesteryl esters, phospholipids, DNA concentration and DNA synthesis had returned to control levels in the first work; while in the present study only DNA and total protein synthesis had returned to control levels.

Although we are dealing with a small number of animals in this experiment, still the serial studies indicate that foam cells and necrosis decrease rapidly while the decrease in rates of DNA and total protein synthesis occurs later. Calcification continues to increase throughout the experiment.

In conclusion, the current study shows that the various types of atherosclerotic lesions regress at different rates and the features of regression do not change simultaneously, nor do these changes follow a linear pattern. Taken together, the two studies indicate that the length of the induction period, the lipid concentration in the lesions and their severity may be important factors in the determination of the rate of regression.

Acknowledgements

The expert technical assistance of Elsie Collier, William Raab, John Safarik and Terry Tedeschi is gratefully acknowledged.

References

Chobanian AV and Manzur F, (1972) Metabolism of lipid in the human fatty streak lesion. J Lipid Res 13: 201

Daoud AS, Jarmolych J, Augustyn JM, Fritz KE, Singh JK and Lee KT, (1976) Regression of advanced swine atherosclerosis. Arch Pathol Lab Med 100: 372

Fritz KE, Augustyn JM, Jarmolych J, Daoud AS and Lee KT, (1976) Regression of advanced swine atherosclerosis. Chemical studies. Arch Pathol Lab Med 100:380

Scott RF, Daoud AS, Wortman B, Morrison ES and Jarmolych J, (1966) Proliferation and necrosis in coronary and cerebral arteries. J Atheroscler Res 6:499

Smith EB, (1965) The influence of age and atherosclerosis on the chemistry of aortic intima. Part 1. The lipids. J of Atheroscler Res 5:224

Smith EB, Evans PH and Downman MD, (1967) Lipid in the aortic intima. The correlation of morphologic and chemical characteristics. J Atheroscler Res 7:171

Differences in the Degradation-Rate of Intracellular Lipid Droplets in the Intimal Smooth Muscle Cells and Macrophages of Regressing Atherosclerotic Lesions of Primates[1]

Herbert Chr. Stary, Jack P. Strong, and Douglas A. Eggen

Introduction

Cells overloaded with lipid droplets are one of the main characteristics of lesions associated with hypercholesterolemia. Accumulation and degradation of droplet inclusions are accompanied by characteristic ultrastructural changes within the cells. We have investigated the stages in droplet degradation while studying regressing atherosclerotic lesions in groups of monkeys killed at short intervals after lowering high serum cholesterol levels by diet. This paper reports on differences in the rate whereby the two main cell types of lesions, smooth muscle cells and macrophages, degrade droplets. We have already reported that the labeling index of cells decreased in the aortic lesions of these animals after we lowered the serum cholesterol (Stary 1974), and that cell death was the cause of the disappearance of macrophage foam cells (Stary 1977).

Methods

We previously described the design of the experiments on which these observations are based (Eggen et al. 1974; Strong et al. 1976; Stary et al. 1977). Briefly, 53 male rhesus monkeys were given the same high-cholesterol diet (commercial monkey diet supplemented with butter, beef tallow, cholesterol) for 12 weeks. At the end of that period, the animals were divided into groups, and one group was killed. The high-cholesterol diet was then changed to low-cholesterol (commercial monkey diet), and the remaining groups were killed after 2,3,4,8,12,16,24,32,40,64, and 128 weeks. In addition, we studied 11 control monkeys that received only low-cholesterol food for various periods. From each animal, tissues for electron microscopy were taken from the proximal left coronary artery, the thoracic, and the abdominal segments of the aorta, fixed in buffered osmium tetroxide, and embedded in Maraglas. Fine sections were stained with lead citrate and uranyl acetate.

Results and Discussion

Normocholesterolemic Phase. Control animals had mean serum cholesterol levels in the range of 110-165 mg/dl. The intima of many coronary artery and aortic segments consisted of one or more layers of smooth muscle cells (SMC). Intimal SMC were of three phenotypes. The main phenotype was rich in thick filaments (myofilaments) and resembled medial SMC; the second was rich in rough endo-

[1]Supported by N.I.H., Program Project Grant HL-08974.

plasmic reticulum (ER) and poor in myofilaments; and a third was poor in myofilaments and poor in rough ER. Macrophages were rare and always isolated.

Hypercholesterolemic Phase. Monkeys on the high-cholesterol diet had mean serum cholesterol levels in the range of 230–640 mg/dl over that 12-week period. Some hypercholesterolemia persisted for 4–8 weeks after return to low-cholesterol food. At the end of this phase, individual monkeys had coronary artery and aortic lesions. Within lesions, intimal SMC of all three phenotypes contained lipid inclusions. Lesions also contained numerous macrophages without and with inclusions. The inclusions were of five varieties: 1. Lipid droplets without a limiting membrane, the periphery merging imperceptibly with the cell cytoplasm. 2. Droplets peppered at their periphery with dark granules and vesicles (precursors of secondary lysosomes; small vesicles formed by the Golgi complex and by certain portions of the smooth ER carry hydrolytic enzymes (Novikoff 1973); fusion of vesicles with droplets represents generation of secondary lysosomes). 3. Droplets surrounded completely by double-contoured membranes (secondary lysosomes). 4. Pleomorphic bulbous inclusions made of finely laminated arrays of membranes but containing within them one or more small droplets (late stages of secondary lysosomes). 5. Pleomorphic or oval inclusions consisting entirely of irregular arrays of membranes (post-lysosomes; telolysosomes; residual bodies). Although any of the five could be in a cell, the hypercholesterolemic phase was characterized by the dominance of inclusions of the first and second variety (Fig. 1, Ib and IIb). Golgi complexes and small vesicles were increased in cells with inclusions, more so in macrophage foam cells.

Early Phase of Lesion Regression. A striking acceleration of intracellular lipid degradation became generally apparent about 12 weeks after low serum cholesterol levels were reestablished. Morphological evidence of degradation consisted of a decrease in the percentage of droplets without a limiting membrane and an increase in those having various degrees of membrane. A striking difference emerged between SMC and macrophages in the proportion of inclusions without and with membrane. Although more SMC droplets now had a peripheral membrane, most were not membrane-bound. Instead they had more granules and vesicles at their periphery (Fig. 1, Ic). The inclusions of macrophage foam cells, on the other hand, were membrane-bound. Most were the late stages of secondary lysosomes and many were post-lysosomes (Fig. 1, IIc). Shrinkage of droplets into late stage secondary lysosomes and post-lysosomes caused macrophage foam cells to decrease in size, reassuming an appearance morphologically closer to that of conventional macrophages. The size of SMC had not changed much from the hypercholesterolemic phase. Golgi and small vesicles were increased in both SMC and in macrophage foam cells.

Late Phase of Lesion Regression. The main characteristic of this phase, which generally began about 32 weeks after low serum cholesterol levels were reestablished, was an almost complete absence of macrophages with and without inclusions. Extracellular lipid and cell debris from dead cells, and inclusions in SMC persisted. Most inclusions of SMC were now late-stage secondary lysosomes and post-lysosomes (Fig. 1, Id). Decrease of secondary lysosomes and increase of post-lysosomes continued as this phase progressed. During the final stages of the late phase, the SMC of residual lesions contained mainly post-lysosomes, smaller in number and in size than the original lipid droplets. The Golgi complex also was small. Post-lysosomes probably have very low enzyme activity or lack activity (de Duve and Wattiaux 1966). Between the end of the first and the end of the second year after diet change, the number of post-lysosomes decreased little. Nevertheless, a far smaller

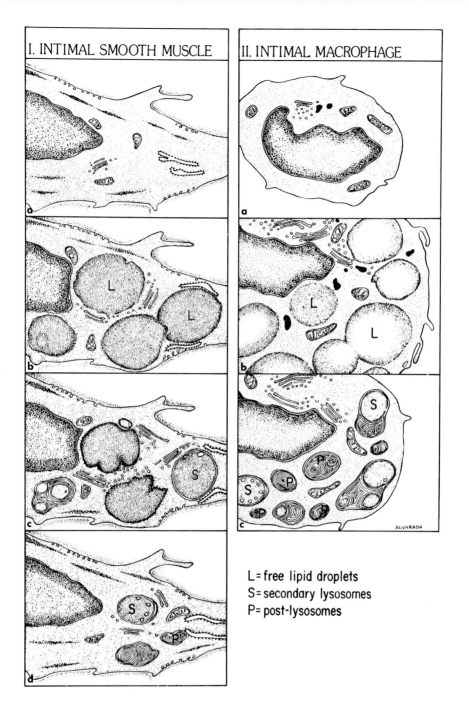

I. INTIMAL SMOOTH MUSCLE   II. INTIMAL MACROPHAGE

L= free lipid droplets
S= secondary lysosomes
P= post-lysosomes

FIG. 1, Ia–d, and IIa–c. Main steps in degradation of cytoplasmic lipid inclusions. I Intimal smooth muscle cells. a Normocholesterolemia: inclusions absent or infrequent. b Hypercholesterolemia: free lipid droplets without membranes. c Early regression: droplets with peripheral vesicles and granules. d Late regression: membrane-bound secondary and post-lysosomes. II Intimal macrophages. Hypercholesterolemia: a without inclusions and b with free droplets lacking membranes. c Early regression: membrane-bound secondary and post-lysosomes.

number of intimal SMC contained post-lysosomes than had contained droplets in the hypercholesterolemic phase. We have evidence that several non-lysosomal pathways can play a role in the removal of residuals from cells. First, dilution of residuals may occur when SMC divide, although SMC proliferation is low in regression (Stary 1974). Second, extrusion of residual bodies in toto from SMC can occur. In other cell types this process has been described as defecation (Ericsson et al. 1965). Third, we discovered that residual body-containing cytoplasmic projections of SMC frequently are trapped between elastic lamellae and severed from the main body of the cells. Separated cell processes die, adding residual inclusions and cell debris to the interstitial space.

Conclusions

High serum cholesterol levels induced in rhesus monkeys with a high cholesterol diet caused intimal SMC and macrophages to accumulate lipid droplets that were largely free, that is, without a limiting membrane. Cellular lysosomal mechanisms apparently were grossly insufficient to handle the excessive influx of lipid. Our experiments showed that this inadequacy was relative and temporary, as digestion and reduction of lipid droplets became morphologically apparent when we drastically reduced high serum cholesterol levels for at least 12 weeks. Both intimal SMC and macrophage foam cells then converted free lipid droplets to secondary lysosomes and post-lysosomes, but the rate of conversion was more rapid in macrophage foam cells. The morphological sequence of intracellular events was similar in both cell types. Although macrophages catabolized lipid inclusions rapidly, they did not survive long in the lesions and died while containing residual inclusions. We do not know whether or not macrophages could rid themselves of residuals if they continued to live beyond the 6-8 month life span they reached under our experimental conditions. We do know that many SMC can eventually rid themselves of residuals, although in some residuals persist for as long as 2 years.

References

de Duve C, Wattiaux R (1966) Functions of lysosomes. Ann Rev Physiol 28:435-492

Eggen DA, Strong JP, Newman WP, et al (1974) Regression of diet-induced fatty streaks in rhesus monkeys. Lab Investigation 31:294-301

Ericsson JLE, Trump BF, Weibel J (1965) Electron microscopic studies of the proximal tubule of the rat kidney. Lab. Investigation 14:1341-1365

Novikoff AB (1973) Lysosomes: A personal account. In: Hers HG, van Hoof F (eds) Lysosomes and storage diseases. Academic Press, New York, pp 1-41

Stary HC (1974) Cell proliferation and ultrastructural changes in regressing atherosclerotic lesions after reduction of serum cholesterol. In: Schettler G, Weizel A (eds) Atherosclerosis III. Springer-Verlag, Berlin, pp. 187-190

Stary HC (1977) Arterial cell injury and cell death in hypercholesterolemia and after reduction of high serum cholesterol levels. Progr Biochem Pharmacol 13:241-247

Stary HC, Eggen DA, Strong JP (1977) The mechanism of atherosclerosis regression. In: Schettler G et al (eds) Atherosclerosis IV. Springer-Verlag, Berlin, pp. 394-404

Strong JP, Eggen DA, Stary HC (1976) Reversibility of fatty streaks in rhesus monkeys. Primates in Medicine 9:300-320

Quantitating Rhesus Monkey Atherosclerosis Progression and Regression with Time[1]

R.W. Wissler, D. Vesselinovitch, T.J. Schaffner, and S. Glagov

Introduction

Numerous studies from several laboratories have demonstrated that advanced atherosclerotic lesions of the aorta and coronary arteries can be observed to undergo substantial regression when the serum lipids are reduced to "basal levels"[2] or below (Armstrong et al. 1970; Vesselinovitch et al. 1976; Daoud et al. 1976).

The space-occupying components of the advanced plaque which seem to be most consistantly reduced in size and/or number are the necrotic "lipid-rich" core, the extra-cellular lipid in the fibrous cap or other parts of the periphery of the plaque, the intracellular lipid, the cellularity of the lesion (Wissler 1978), and in some lesions the quantity of fiber proteins when collagen and elastin are determined and expressed as units per anatomical segment (Armstrong 1976).

There are also indications that visible and stainable calcium deposits decrease in size and number (Daoud et al. 1976; Vesselinovitch et al. 1979) and that damaged endothelium is replaced or healed (Weber et al. 1977; Jones and Wissler 1978).

While most of these results have been reported in arteries of rhesus monkeys or swine there are also indications that substantial lesion regression can be observed in arteries of individuals who have been treated with lipo-protein-cholesterol lowering regimens and who have responded with sizable, sustained reductions (Blankenhorn 1977; Barndt et al. 1977; Buchwald et al. 1978.

Although several of these studies have promising implications for the treatment of progressive human atherosclerosis, there has been very little quantitation of the morphological changes that occur in these lesions and few attempts to relate these changes to the duration of therapy have been reported.

This report will outline an approach to this type of morphometric study of regression, as well as progression, with time that is now being conducted in our laboratory. This approach is designed to yield data that will permit the calculation of the rates of progression and regression of specific components of plaques. It will also reveal overall plaque size, lumen narrowing and/or intimal thickness (as related to nearby normal media) in predetermined standard sites of the arterial tree.

[1] Supported by USPHS Grants HL 15062-08 and HL 17648-05, by the Block Fund at the University of Chicago and by the Heart Research Foundation, Inc.
[2] The levels usually observed for that species when it is fed a low fat, low cholesterol ration for most of its life span.

The Evolution of the Study

Although the need to quantitate atherosclerotic plaque components in human and experimental atherosclerosis has been recognized for some time, the methods available to accomplish the task have been laborious and time consuming and therefore not widely applied. The chemical methods also yield valuable data, but it is difficult at times to relate the results to the morphologic aspects of the lesions that are often most meaningful in respect to the threat of clinical consequences. Nevertheless, we have recently reported the results of rather revealing studies of the quantitative changes in lesion components during regression using chemical methods as well as the time-honored point-counting approach (Vesselinovitch et al. 1976, 1979).

With considerable help and encouragement from other members of the Atherosclerosis SCOR network, in particular Dr. Gene Bond of the Bowman-Gray SCOR (MG Bond, unpublished work 1979) we have developed a plan of study along with the hardware and software needed to make relatively swift and reproducible measurements possible.

In general, the same experimental design is now being used in all of our SCOR studies of progression and regression of atherosclerosis in rhesus and cynomolgus monkeys. Its essential features are shown in Figure 1. It includes autopsy and examination of lesion progression (12 months) and regression (12 months) at 4 month intervals in animals subjected to an extremely potent atherogenic ration and then treated with a previously demonstrated effective regimen to lower serum lipids and to produce regression of advanced plaques (Vesselinovitch et al. 1976, 1979).

The lesions found in standard histological samples taken from the aorta and coronary arteries and prepared for study by uniformly applied methods of fixation, embedding, sectioning and staining, that have been reported earlier (Vesselinovitch et al. 1974, 1979), are then subjected to morphometric analysis using an unusually versatile and reliable computer linked to microprojection and digitizer system. This was designed and assembled by us after careful consultation and planning with colleagues

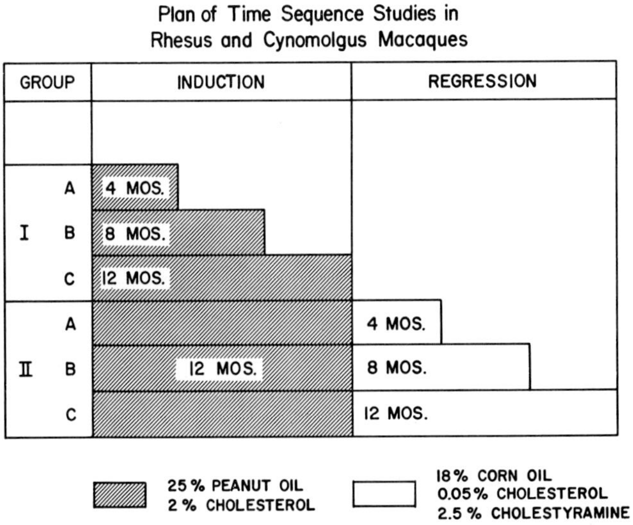

FIG. 1. Plan of time sequence studies in rhesus and cynomolgus macaques.

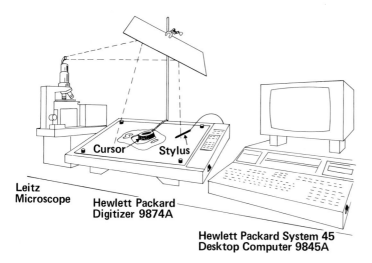

FIG. 2. Apparatus for performing morphometric analysis:
Computer linked to microprojection and digitizer system.

in the SCOR system and on our campus (Figure 2). The software which is
necessary to make maximum use of this apparatus has been largely developed
by Professor Seymour Glagov with the help of experienced systems engineers
on our campus.

The arteries, lesions and measurements taken on coronary arteries are
displayed as a visual image with numbers or letters identifying each
measured point. The program that has been developed gives the following
measurements: area of lesion, area of media, width of media at thickest
point, percentage of lumen still open, percentage of media involved in
lesion, % of wall that is necrotic lesion, % of total lesion made up of
fibrous capsule, maximum lesion thickness, maximum media thickness at its
most normal point, minimum media thickness at its narrowest dimension.

The data (exact measurements) derived from utilizing the program developed
for our standard aortic samples make it possible to express the lesion
size as a percent of the total section, the measurements of the fibrous
cap, the necrotic center and areas of calcification as percentages of the
total lesion and to measure lesion thickness and total wall thickness at
their most severe point, as well as the media and wall thickness at their
most normal-looking segment. We anticipate utilizing this system for a
reasonable separation of intracellular and extracellular lipid as well as
for enumeration of lesion cell types.

Current Status of Studies

At the time of the Vth International Symposium on Atherosclerosis, three
separate experiments are underway to ascertain the rates of progression
and regression in atheromatous lesion components in the aortas and
coronary arteries of adult male rhesus and cynomolgus monkeys by utilizing
this approach. Furthermore, the methodology has been used to quantitate
the coronary artery lesions in the experimental comparison of the response
(progression and regression at one year) in three species of monkeys that
Dr. Vesselinovitch and I have studied and reported at another workshop of
this symposium (Vesselinovitch and Wissler 1979). It is evident that the

system permits relatively speedy, easy and reproducible measurements which can be duplicated within very small limits by two independent observers.

We trust that long before the next International Symposium on Atherosclerosis we will be able to reach the goal that the chairman of this workshop and some of us participating in it have had for many years. We hope to learn much more about the rate at which various visible components of the plaques develop and regress under various types of experimental conditions.

Summary

1. Although valuable quantitative post mortem data regarding the progression and regression of atherosclerosis can be obtained by chemical and point-counting techniques, the methods are cumbersome and not always very helpful in predicting "clinical" effects.

2. An experimental plan now being used is presented. It makes it possible to evaluate the rates of progression and regression of atherosclerosis in macaque studies. This involves time interval autopsies of representative groups as well as standard sampling and tissue preparation approaches.

3. A computer linked-microprojection-digitizer approach to measuring lesion components at these intervals is described.

4. This morphometric system has been successfully utilized in a comparison of development and regression of coronary artery disease in 3 species of monkeys.

5. It yields data about the lesion components in a readily usable form and provides a hard copy of the artery section, the areas measured and the results of calculations made.

6. This approach should furnish valuable data regarding the rate of progression and regression of various components of the atherosclerotic plaque in animal model studies.

Acknowledgements

The authors are grateful for the excellent assistance they have received in preparing this manuscript from Barbara Ann Baxter, Lauren Brown and other members of the SCOR - Atherosclerosis staff.

References

Armstrong ML (1976) Regression of atherosclerosis. In: Paoletti R, Gotto AM Jr (eds) Atherosclerosis Reviews. Raven Press, New York, pp 137-182
Armstrong ML, Warner ED Connor WE (1970) Regression of coronary atheromatosis in rhesus monkeys. Circ Res 27:59-67
Barndt R Jr, Blankenhorn DH, Crawford DW, Brooks SH (1977) Regression and progression of early femoral atherosclerosis in treated hyperlipoproteinemia. Ann Int Med 86:139-146
Blankenhorn DH (1977) Studies of regression/progression of atherosclerosis in man. In: Manning GW, Haust MD (eds) Atherosclerosis: Metabolic, Morphologic, and Clinical Aspects (Adv Exp Med Biol, Vol 82). Plenum Press, New York, pp 453-458

Buchwald H, Amplatz K, Knight L, Guzman I, Varco RL (1978) Arteriography changes after partial ileal bypass. In: Hauss WH, Wissler RW, Lehmann R (eds) International Symposium: State of Prevention and Therapy in Human Arteriosclerosis and in Animal Models. Westdeutscher Verlag, Opladen, Germany, pp 469-482

Daoud AS, Jarmolych J, Augustyn JM, Fritz KE, Singh JK, Lee KT (1976) Regression of advanced atherosclerosis in swine. Arch Path Lab Med 100:372-379

Jones RM, Wissler RW (1978) Surface features of experimental atherosclerosis plaques in rhesus monkeys with and without treatment. Scanning Electron Microscopy AMF O'Hare, IL, Vol II, pp 975-982

Vesselinovitch D, Wissler RW (1980) Reversal of atherosclerosis: Comparison of non-human primate models. This volume

Vesselinovitch D, Getz GS, Hughes RH, Wissler RW (1974) Atherosclerosis in the rhesus monkey fed three food fats. Atherosclerosis 20:303-321

Vesselinovitch D, Wissler RW, Hughes R, Borensztajn J (1976) Reversal of advanced atherosclerosis in rhesus monkeys. I. Gross and light microscopic studies. Atherosclerosis 23:155-176

Vesselinovitch D, Wissler RW, Schaffner TJ (1979a) Quantitation of lesions during progression and regression of atherosclerosis in rhesus monkeys. In: Cardiovascular Disease in Nutrition, Symposium of American College of Nutrition. Spectrum Publications, New York, in press

Vesselinovitch D, Wissler RW, Schaffner TJ, Borensztajn J (1979b) The effect of various diets on atherogenesis in rhesus monkeys. Atherosclerosis, in press

Weber G, Fabbrini P, Resi L, Jones RM, Vesselinovitch D, Wissler RW (1977) Regression of arteriosclerotic lesions in rhesus monkey aortas after regression diet: Scanning and transmission electron microscope observations of the endothelium. Atherosclerosis 26:535-547

Wissler RW (1978) Current status of regression studies. In: Paoletti R, Gotto AM Jr (eds) Atherosclerosis Reviews. Raven Press, New York, pp 213-229

Prostacyclin and Atherosclerosis—A Hypothesis[1]

Ryszard J. Gryglewski

Properties of Prostacyclin

In 1976 we discovered (Bunting et al. 1976; Gryglewski et al. 1976; Moncada et al. 1976a,b) that prostaglandin (PG) endoperoxides are transformed by arterial microsomes to an unstable substance with anti-aggregatory and vasodilator properties. This new lipid factor was called PGX, and when it was later synthesized its name was changed to prostacyclin (PGI_2) (Johnson et al. 1976). Prostacyclin spontaneously decomposes to a biologically inactive prostaglandin. In extravasated blood at 37°C the half life of prostacyclin is 3 min (Dusting et al. 1978).

Prostacyclin is the most potent endogenous inhibitor of platelet aggregation so far discovered. Its anti-aggregatory activity is at least 15 times greater than that of PGD_2 and 40 times more than that of PGE_1 (Gryglewski et al. 1976; Moncada et al. 1976b). The anti-aggregatory activity of prostacyclin is due to stimulation of adenylate cyclase (Gorman et al. 1977) and thus increasing platelet cAMP. Recently, it has been shown (Dembińska-Kieć et al. 1979a) that prostacyclin increases cAMP levels also in vascular tissue provided that its phosphodiesterase is inhibited. Prostacyclin prevents thrombus formation in animals (Gryglewski et al. 1978c) and disperses circulating platelet aggregates in man (Gryglewski et al. 1978e; Szczeklik et al. 1978). Vasodilator activity of prostacyclin shows up in man as a profound erythema located on the face, neck, palms and feet, as well as a decrease in diastolic blood pressure (Szczeklik et al. 1978).

Regulation of Prostacyclin Release

Prostacyclin is the major metabolite of arachidonic acid in vascular walls, especially in vascular endothelium (Moncada et al. 1977; Weksler et al. 1978). The vast area of pulmonary endothelium seems to be a rich source of prostacyclin, so much that it is continuously secreted into the arterial blood (Gryglewski et al. 1978b,d; Moncada et al. 1978). Prostacyclin is also generated by perfused heart (De Dekere et al. 1977; Dembińska-Kieć et al. 1977) and by kidney (Silberbauer et al. 1979).

In anesthetized animals hyperventilation, air embolism, platelet embolism and serotonin stimulate the release of prostacyclin from lungs, while other sources of endogenous prostacyclin are activated by angiotensin II and bradykinin (Gryglewski et al. 1979).

Prostacyclin synthetase is inhibited by 15-hydroperoxyarachidonic acid (Gry-

---

[1]The author's and Dr. A. Szczeklik's personal research in 1979 was supported by a grant from the Upjohn Company, Kalamazoo, Michigan, USA.

glewski et al. 1976) and by other lipid peroxides (Salmon et al. 1978).

Biosynthesis of Prostacyclin in Experimental Atherosclerosis

At the early stage of experimental atherosclerosis in rabbits (one month of
the atherogenic diet) there occurs a severe depression (by 6C-90%) in generation of prostacyclin by heart, aorta, mesenteric arteries (Gryglewski et
al. 1978a), lungs and kidney (Dembińska et al. 1979b), whereas the metabolism
of arachidonic acid in platelet remains unchanged. At this early stage of
the disease hyperlipidemia does not yet induce atheromatic plaques. An increase in thromboxane synthesizing capacity of platelets appears later when
anatomical lesions of arteries are visible (Żmuda et al. 1977). At the same
time a slight tendency to recovery of prostacyclin biosynthesis in arteries
is observed (Dembińska et al. 1977; Gryglewski et al. 1978a). Also in human
atheromatic plaques the generation of prostacyclin hardly occurs (Angelo et
al. 1978). This generalized suppression of the prostacyclin generating system in atherosclerosis is associated with an increased susceptibility of
platelet adenylate cyclase and endothelial adenylate cyclase to the stimulatory action of exogenous prostacyclin (Dembińska-Kieć et al. 1979c). The
hypersensitivity of "the second messenger system" in atherosclerosis may be
a consequence of prostacyclin deficiency, just as has been observed many
times in other biological systems deprived of a primary physiological mediator.

Hypothesis

We postulate that atherosclerosis is a disease resulting from deficiency of
prostacyclin. This hormonal defect is the result of intoxication of prostacyclin synthetase with lipid peroxides or with corresponding free radicals
which are likely to be generated during hyperlipidemia. Deficiency of prostacyclin leads to a decrease in cAMP levels both in platelets and in arterial
walls, thus increasing platelet aggregability and endothelial permeability
(Numano 1977). Arterial endothelium, when deprived of its capacity to synthesize prostacyclin (Angelo et al. 1978; Gryglewski et al. 1978a), becomes
a surface prone to platelet adhesion and aggregation. Aggregating platelets
are activated not only by lack of "prostacyclin resistance" at the endothelial surface, but also by low concentrations of circulating prostacyclin and
by diversion of arachidonic acid metabolism from prostacyclin to pro-aggregatory metabolites. Activated platelets adhere and aggregate on the endothelial cells and release harmful substances that cause endothelial damage,
mural inflammatory response, migration of myocytes and formation of atheromatic plaque (Ross and Harker 1976). The aggressive behavior of platelets
in atherosclerosis (Harker et al. 1976) is facilitated by low levels of cAMP
in arterial walls (Numano et al. 1976). Both phenomena are growing from the
same stem, i.e., an injury to an enzymatic system which synthesizes prostacyclin.

Should the above reasoning be correct, then the substitution therapy with
prostacyclin should alleviate the symptoms of atherosclerosis in man.

Indeed, we have shown (Szczeklik et al. 1979) that intra-arterial infusion of prostacyclin (5-10 ng/kg/min for 72 hrs) into patients suffering from advanced arteriosclerosis obliterans of lower extremities results in a dramatic alleviation of pain, regression of focal necrosis and healing of ischemic ulcers. Although the prostacyclin therapy does not remove atheromatic obstructions to big arteries as evidenced by angiograms, there is a significant increase in capillary blood flow through the affected leg as shown by the xenon clearance technique. The treatment of advanced obstructive vascular diseases with various vasodilators was totally unsuccessful (Coffman 1979). We believe that the substitution prostacyclin therapy opens a new era in the treatment of atherosclerosis. We assume that in our patients prostacyclin cleared still functioning small arteries from platelet aggregates and offered the time necessary for recovery of the damaged endothelial prostacyclin synthetase. The disease was not cured but its progress was inhibited. The only other drug effective in the treatment of advanced arteriosclerosis obliterans is PGE_1 (Olsson and Jogestrand 1978). I believe that this therapeutical efficacy of PGE_1 can be explained by its biological similarity to PGI_2, as pointed out by Dr. B. Whittle (personal communication): "What E can do I can do better." The successful therapy of advanced arteriosclerosis obliterans with prostacyclin supports our concept that atherosclerosis is a disease resulting from deficiency of prostacyclin.

Conclusions

The above laboratory and clinical data encourage the following lines of research: protection against atherosclerosis by antioxidants, substitution therapy with prostacyclin or its stable analogs and stimulation of endogenous generation of prostacyclin by peptides.

References

Angelo V, Myśliwiec M, Donati MB, Gaetano G (1978) Defective fibrynolytic and prostacyclin-like activity in human atheromatous plaques. Thrombos Haemostas 39:535-536

Bunting S, Gryglewski R, Moncada S, Vane JR (1976) Arterial walls generate from prostaglandin endoperoxides a substance (prostaglandin X) which relaxes strips of mesenteric and coeliac arteries and inhibits platelet aggregation. Prostaglandins 12:897-913

Coffman JD (1979) Drug Therapy: Vasodilator drugs in peripheral vascular diseases. N Engl J Med 300:713-721

De Dekere EAM, Nugteren DH, Ten Hoor F (1977) Prostacyclin is the major metabolite released from the isolated perfused rabbit and rat heart. Nature 268:160-163

Dembińska-Kieć A, Gryglewska T, Żmuda A, Gryglewski RJ (1977) The generation of prostacyclin by arteries and by the coronary vascular bed is reduced in experimental atherosclerosis in rabbits. Prostaglandins 14:1025-1035

Dembińska-Kieć A, Rücker W, Schönhofer PS (1979a) Effects of dipyridamole in experimental atherosclerosis: Action of PGI_2, platelet aggregation and atherosclerotic plaque formation. Atherosclerosis, in press

Dembińska-Kieć A, Rücker W, Schönhofer PS (1979b) Atherosclerosis decreases prostacyclin synthesis in rabbit lungs and kidneys. Prostaglandins, in press

Dembińska-Kieć A, Rücker W, Schönhofer PS (1979c) Effects of dipyridamole in vivo on ATP and c-AMP content in platelets and arterial walls and on atherosclerotic plaque formation. Naunyn-Schmiedeberg's Arch Pharmacol, in press

Dusting GJ, Moncada S, Vane JR (1978) Recirculation of prostacyclin (PGI$_2$) in the dog. Br J Pharmacol 63:315-320

Gorman RR, Bunting S, Miller OV (1977) Modulation of human platelet adenylate cyclase by prostacyclin (PGX). Prostaglandins 13:377-388

Gryglewski RJ, Bunting S, Moncada S, Flower RJ, Vane JR (1976) Arterial walls are protected against deposition of platelet thrombi by a substance (prostaglandin X) which they make from prostaglandin endoperoxides. Prostaglandins 12:685-713

Gryglewski RJ, Dembińska-Kieć A, Chytkowski A, Gryglewska T (1978a) Prostacyclin and thromboxane A$_2$ biosynthesis capacities of heart, arteries and platelets at various stages of experimental atherosclerosis in rabbits. Atherosclerosis 31: 385-394

Gryglewski RJ, Korbut R, Ocetkiewicz A (1978b) Generation of prostacyclin by lungs in vivo and its release into the arterial circulation. Nature 273:765-767

Gryglewski RJ, Korbut R, Ocetkiewicz A (1978c) De-aggregatory action of prostacyclin in vivo and its enhancement by theophylline. Prostaglandins 15:637-644

Gryglewski RJ, Korbut R, Ocetkiewicz A, Splawiński J, Wojtaszek B, Świes J (1978d) Lungs as a generator of prostacyclin - hypothesis on physiological significance. Naunyn Schmiede-berg's Arch Pharmacol 304:45-50

Gryglewski RJ, Korbut R, Splawiński J (1979) Endogenous mechanisms which regulate prostacyclin release. Haemostasis, in press

Gryglewski RJ, Szczeklik A, Niżankowski R (1978e) Antiplatelet action of intravenous infusion of prostacyclin in man. Thromb Res 13:153-163

Harker LA, Ross R, Glomset J (1976) Role of the platelet in atherogenesis. Ann NY Acad Sci 275:321-329

Johnson RA, Morton DR, Kinner JH, Gorman RR, McGuire JC, Sun FF, Whittaker N, Bunting S, Salmon J, Moncada S, Vane JR (1976) The chemical structure of prostaglandin X (prostacyclin). Prostaglandins 12:915-928

Moncada S, Gryglewski R, Bunting S, Vane JR (1976a) An enzyme isolated from arteries transforms prostaglandin endoperoxides to an unstable substance that inhibits platelet aggregation. Nature 263:663-665

Moncada S, Gryglewski RJ, Bunting S, Vane JR (1976b) A lipid peroxide inhibits the enzyme in blood vessel microsomes that generates from prostaglandin endoperoxides the substance (prostaglandin X) which prevents platelet aggregation. Prostaglandins 12:715-733

Moncada S, Herman AG, Hihhs EA, Vane JR (1977) Differential formation of prostacyclin (PGX or PGI$_2$) by layers of the arterial wall. An explanation for anti-thrombotic properties of vascular endothelium. Thromb Res 11:323-344

Moncada S, Korbut R, Bunting S, Vane JR (1978) Prostacyclin is a circulating hormone. Nature 273:767-768

Numano F (1977) Progression and regression of atherosclerosis. Asian Med J 20:625-644

Numano F, Maezawa H, Shimamoto T, Adachi K (1976) Changes of cyclic AMP and cyclic AMP phosphodiesterase in the progression and regression of experimental atherosclerosis. Ann NY Acad Sci 275:311-320

Olsson AG, Jogestrand T (1978) Effects of prostaglandin E$_1$ in peripheral artery disease. In: Carlson LA, Paoletti R, Sirtori CR, Weber G (eds) Atherosclerosis. Raven Press, New York, pp 403-411

Ross R, Harker L (1976) Hyperlipidemia and atherosclerosis. Science 193: 1094-1100

Salmon JA, Smith DR, Flower RJ, Moncada S, Vane JR (1978) Some characteristics of the prostacyclin synthesising enzyme in porcine aorta. Biochim Biophys Acta 523:250-262

Silberbauer K, Sinzinger H, Winter M (1979) Prostacyclin activity in rat kidney stimulated by angiotensin II. Br J Exp Path 60:38-44

Modulation by Prostaglandins of Vascular Reactivity to Adrenergic Stimuli[1]

Kafait U. Malik and Alberto Nasjletti

The response of peripheral vascular beds to adrenergic nerve stimulation depends upon numerous factors including the intrinsic vascular tone, the density and distribution of sympathetic innervation, the sensitivity and heterogeneity of adrenergic receptors, the characteristics of the neurotransmitter-receptor coupling, the relative magnitude of alpha and beta receptor mediated responses, and the level of activity of vasoactive hormones with capacity to modify events at pre and post-junctional sites (Bevan, 1979; Malik, 1978a). Research efforts over the past two decades have prompted recognition of the potential role of several vasoactive hormones, e.g., prostaglandins, angiotensins, kinins, histamine, and serotonin in influencing the events at the adrenergic neuroeffector junction. A relationship between prostaglandins and vascular reactivity to adrenergic stimuli was first suggested by the observations that 1) prostaglandins of the E series reduced the vascular responses and release of norepinephrine evoked by sympathetic nerve stimulation (Hedqvist and Brundin, 1969; Hedqvist, 1970) and 2) stimulation of adrenergic nerves increased the release of prostaglandins from the spleen (Davies et al, 1968; Gilmore et al, 1968). These findings led to the proposition that PGE functions as a modulator of the activity of the adrenergic nervous system. In examining the evidence that prostaglandins modulate vascular reactivity to adrenergic stimuli we shall discuss 1) the effect of norepinephrine on the biosynthesis and release of prostaglandins, 2) effects of arachidonic acid metabolites on the vascular responses to adrenergic stimuli, and 3) effects of alterations in prostaglandin biosynthesis on adrenergically-induced vasoconstriction.

Effect of Norepinephrine on the Biosynthesis and Release of Prostaglandins

Arachidonic acid is released from tissue phospholipids by a lipase, presumably phospholipase A_2, and is converted by a microsomal cyclo-oxygenase to an endoperoxide precursor of prostaglandins and thrombaxane A_2 (Moncada and Vane, 1979). Prostaglandins are not stored in tissues; their release in response to sympathetic nerve stimulation and administered norepinephrine denotes increased biosynthesis rather than secretion from any preformed store. Adrenergic nerve stimulation or exogenous norepinephrine stimulate the synthesis and release of prostaglandins from post-junctional sites (Hedqvist, 1973; Junstad and Wennmalm, 1973); however, prostaglandin release from prejunctional sites cannot be excluded (Greenberg, 1978). The range of products of arachidonic acid metabolism released by adrenergic stimuli from different tissues has not yet been fully established. Both stimulation of sympathetic nerves or infusion of norepinephrine releases from the spleen of several species products which have the chemical, chromatographic and biological characteristics of PGE_2 and $PGF_{2\alpha}$ (Davies et al, 1968; Gilmore et al, 1968; Ferreira et al, 1973: Malik, 1978b; Hidaka and Malik, 1979).

---

[1] The authors' personal research cited is supported by the Grants HL-19134 and HL-18574 from the United States Public Service Health Service. K.U. Malik and A. Nasjletti are recipients of USPHS Research Career Development Awards 1K04-HL-00142 and 5KO-HL-099163, respectively.

PGE$_2$ has also been identified as the major arachidonic acid metabolite released from the kidney in response to sympathetic nerve stimulation and
exogenous norepinephrine (Dunham and Zimmerman, 1970; McGiff et al, 1972;
Davis and Horton, 1972). In contrast, PGI$_2$ is the principal prostaglandin
released from the heart (Wennmalm, 1978; Khan and Malik, 1979). PGI$_2$ is
also the major product of arachidonic acid metabolism in several blood vessels (Moncada et al, 1977). From these observations we infer that the prod-
uct(s) of arachidonic acid metabolism released by adrenergic stimuli differ
among tissues.

Effect of Arachidonic Acid Metabolites on the Vascular Responses to
Adrenergic Stimuli

There is ample evidence that the end products of prostaglandin endoperoxide
metabolism produced by a tissue during adrenergic receptor stimulation are
capable of modifying vascular reactivity. For example, PGE$_2$ and/or PGI$_2$
reduce vascular responses to sympathetic nerve stimulation and to exogenous
norepinephrine in the spleen of different species (Hedqvist, 1970; Malik
and McGiff, 1976; Malik, 1978a), dog, rabbit and cat kidneys (Lonigro et al,
1973; Malik and McGiff, 1975; Hedqvist, 1979), rabbit mesenteric arteries
(Malik et al, 1976; Armstrong et al, 1979), rabbit portal vein (Greenberg,
1974) and ear artery (De La Lande, 1975). Attenuation by PGI$_2$ and PGE$_2$ of
norepinephrine-induced vasoconstriction denotes a postjunctional effect.
However, PGE$_2$ also acts at prejunctional sites to reduce the release of norepinephrine evoked by sympathetic nerve stimulation (Hedqvist, 1977). The
effects of PGI$_2$ at prejunctional sites are variable: the output of neurotransmitter evoked by stimulation of adrenergic fibers was increased by PGI$_2$
in the canine blood vessels (Herman et al, 1979), reduced in the pulmonary
artery (Weitzell et al, 1978) and rat heart (Khan and Malik, 1978) and unaffected in the rabbit kidney (Hedqvist, 1979).

The work of Malik and McGiff (1975) indicate a major species difference in
the postjunctional effects of PGE$_2$. They found that PGE$_2$ which inhibited
vascular responses to adrenergic stimuli in the rabbit kidney caused augmentation of the adrenergically-induced vasoconstriction in the rat kidney.
Similar results were obtained with PGI$_2$ (Malik and Nasjletti, 1980; Malik,
unpublished work). The potentiating effect of PGE$_2$ on the vasoconstrictor
responses to adrenergic stimuli was also observed in the rat mesenteric
arteries (Malik et al, 1976). Prostaglandin F$_{2\alpha}$,which is also released by
adrenergic stimuli, acts prejunctionally to inhibit release of the neurotransmitter and postjunctionally to increase vascular reactivity to adrenergic stimuli (Endo et al, 1977; Kadowitz et al, 1971; Malik and McGiff,
1975; Malik, 1978a). Therefore, stimulation of prostaglandin synthesis in
tissues may result in the formation of products, having distinct and often
opposing actions on neuroeffector events. A corollary of this conclusion
is that prostaglandins synthesized in tissues innervated by adrenergic nerves
may contribute to the modulation of vascular responses to adrenergic stimuli.

Effect of Alterations in Prostaglandin Biosynthesis on
Adrenergically-Induced Vasoconstriction

Evidence that endogenous prostaglandins influence vascular reactivity to
adrenergic stimuli derives largely from experiments on the effect of prostaglandin synthesis inhibitors on adrenergically-induced vasoconstriction.

Inhibition of prostaglandin synthesis with indomethacin augments adrenergically-induced vasoconstriction in the isolated perfused spleen, kidney and mesenteric arteries of rabbit (Malik, 1978a; Malik and McGiff, 1975; Malik et al, 1976). Similar observations have been made in the cat spleen (Ferreira et al, 1973), the dog cutaneous vasculature (Zimmerman et al, 1973), the rabbit ear artery (Jackson and Hall, 1973), the rabbit portal vein (Greenberg, 1974), the human omental blood vessels (Stjärne and Brundin, 1976) and the fetal and neonatal lamb mesenteric arteries (Yabek and Avner, 1979). Furthermore, inhibition of prostaglandin synthesis increased the release of the adrenergic transmitter evoked by sympathetic nerve stimulation (Hedqvist, 1977; Stjärne and Brundin, 1976). Collectively, these observations on the effect of prostaglandin synthesis inhibition suggest that one or more products of prostaglandin endoperoxide metabolism may function as inhibitors of pre and postjunctional events. However, this may not apply to all tissues. First, neither indomethacin nor meclofenamate increased norepinephrine release by sympathetic nerve stimulation in the cat spleen (Dubocovich and Langer, 1975; Hoszowska and Panczenko, 1974). Similarly these agents produced variable effects on the adrenergically-induced renal vasoconstriction in this species (Chapnick et al, 1977). Second, indomethacin reduced the vasoconstrictor responses to adrenergic nerve stimulation and to exogenous norepinephrine in the isolated perfused kidney and mesenteric arteries of rat (Malik and McGiff, 1975; Malik et al, 1976).

Further support for the proposition that endogenous prostaglandins modulate the reactivity of blood vessels to adrenergic stimuli, derives from the demonstration in several tissues that stimulation of prostaglandin synthesis modifies events at the adrenergic neuroeffector junction. For example, stimulation of prostaglandin synthesis by infusion of arachidonic acid reduces vascular reactivity to adrenergic stimuli in the dog paw (Ryan and Zimmerman, 1974), and in the isolated perfused kidney, spleen and mesenteric arteries of the rabbit (Malik and McGiff, 1975; Malik et al, 1976; Malik 1978b). Similarly, stimulation of prostaglandin synthesis by bradykinin inhibits the vasoconstriction evoked by sympathetic nerve stimulation and by injected norepinephrine in the rabbit pulmonary artery (Starke et al, 1977) and kidney (Malik and Nasjletti, 1977a)(Figure). Furthermore, arachidonic acid and bradykinin were found to reduce the release of the neurotransmitter evoked by sympathetic nerve stimulation in the rabbit kidney (Frame and Hedqvist, 1975) and pulmonary artery (Starke et al, 1977) respectively; these effects were blocked by the cyclo-oxygenase inhibitor indomethacin suggesting mediation by a prostaglandin. From the preceeding observations on the effects of altered prostaglandin biosynthesis on the events at the adrenergic neuroeffector junction one may infer that one or more products of arachidonic acid metabolism, probably PGE_2 or PGI_2, reduces vascular reactivity to adrenergic stimuli. However, this conclusion cannot be applied to all tissues and species. This is inferred from the observations of Malik and McGiff (1975) and Malik et al (1976) that in the isolated kidney and mesenteric arteries of the rat, stimulation of prostaglandin biosynthesis by arachidonic acid potentiates adrenergically-induced vasoconstriction. This difference between the renal and mesenteric vasculature of rat and rabbit could be due to differences in prostaglandin receptors or in the events resulting from the interaction of prostaglandins with the receptors at the neuroeffector junction.

The overall conclusion emerging from this presentation is that arachidonic acid metabolites, particularly PGE_2 and PGI_2, could function as modulators of vascular reactivity to adrenergic stimuli. However, a possible involvement of other products of cycloxygenase ($PGF_{2\alpha}$, PGD_2, thromboxanes A_2 and B_2) and lipoxygenase activity cannot be excluded.

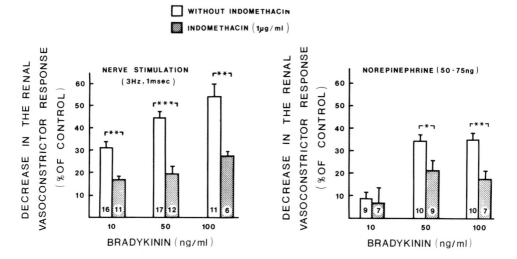

WITHOUT INDOMETHACIN

INDOMETHACIN (1μg/ml)

FIGURE 1. Percent decrease produced by bradykinin of the renal vasoconstrictor response to sympathetic nerve stimulation (3Hz, 1 msec duration for 22 sec) and to injected norepinephrine (50-75 ng) in the absence and presence of indomethacin. Bars represent SEM and numbers at the bottom of the columns indicate group size. *P<0.05; **P<0.01; ***P<0.001 (Significance of difference between decreases produced by bradykinin in the absence and presence of indomethacin, of renal vasoconstriction evoked by nerve stimulation and by injected norepinephrine).

References

Armstrong TM, Thirsk G, Biol. MI, and Salmon JA (1979) Effects of prostacyclin (PGI$_2$), 6-oxo-PGF$_{1\alpha}$ and PGE$_2$ on sympathetic nerve function in mesenteric arteries and veins of the rabbit in vitro. Hypertension 1: 309-315

Bevan JA (1979) Some bases of differences in vascular responses to sympathetic activity. Variation on a theme. Circ Res 45: 161-171

Chapnick BM, Paustian PM, Feigen LP, Joiner PD, Hyman AL, and Kadowitz PJ (1977) Influence of inhibitors of prostaglandin synthesis on renal vascular resistance and on renal vascular responses to vasopressor and vasodilator agents in the cat. Circ Res 40: 348-354

Davies BN, Horton EW, and Withrington PG (1968) The occurrence of prostaglandin E$_2$ in splenic venous blood of the dog following splenic nerve stimulation. Brit J Pharmacol Chemother 32: 127-135

Davis HA, and Horton EW (1972) Output of prostaglandins from the rabbit kidney: Its increase on renal nerve stimulation and its inhibition by indomethacin. Brit J Pharmacol 46: 658-675

De La Lande IS, Hall RC, Kennedy JA, and Higgins GD (1975) Prostaglandins, antipyretic analgesics and adrenergic stimuli on the isolated artery. Europ J Pharmacol 30: 319-327

Dubocovich ML, and Langer SZ (1975) Evidence against a physiological role of prostaglandins in the regulation of noradrenaline release in the cat spleen. J Physiol (London) 251: 737-762

Dunham EW and Zimmerman BG (1970) Release of prostaglandin-like material from dog kidney during nerve stimulation. Am J Physiol 219: 1279-1285

Endo T, Starke K, Bangerter A, and Taube HD (1977) Presynaptic receptor systems on the noradrenergic neurons of the rabbit pulmonary artery. Naunyn-Schmiedeberg's Arch Pharmacol 296:229-247

Ferreira SH, Moncada S, and Vane JR (1973) Some effects of inhibiting endogenous prostaglandin formation on the responses of the cat spleen. Brit J Pharmacol 47: 48-58

Frame MH, and Hedqvist P (1975) Evidence for prostaglandin mediated prejunctional control of renal sympathetic transmitter release and vascular tone. Brit J Pharmacol 54: 189-196

Gilmore N, Vane JR, and Wyllie JH (1968) Prostaglandins released by the spleen. Nature 218: 1135-1140

Greenberg R (1974) The effects of indomethacin and eicosa-5,8,11,14- tetraynoic acid on the response of the rabbit portal vein to electrical stimulation. Brit J Pharmacol 52: 61-68

Greenberg R (1978) The neuronal origin of prostaglandin released from the rabbit portal vein in response to electrical stimulation. Brit J Pharmacol 63: 79-85

Hedqvist P (1970) Control by prostaglandin E_2 of sympathetic neurotransmission in the spleen. Life Scis 9: 269-278

Hedqvist P (1973) Autonomic neurotransmission. In: Ramwell PW (ed.) The Prostaglandins. Plenum Press, New York, pp. 101-131

Hedqvist P (1977) Basic mechanisms of prostaglandin action on autonomic neurotransmission. Ann Rev Pharmacol Toxicol 17: 259-279

Hedqvist P (1979) Actions of prostacyclin (PGI_2) on adrenergic neuroeffector transmission in the rabbit kidney. Prostaglandins 17: 249-258

Hedqvist P and Brundin J (1969) Inhibition by prostaglandin E_1 of noradrenaline release and of effector response to nerve stimulation in the cat spleen. Life Scis 8: 389-395

Hidaka T and Malik KU (1978) Prostaglandin E_2 is the major product formed from arachidonic acid by sympathetic nerve stimulation (SNS), administered norepinephrine (NE) and bradykinin (BK) from isolated perfused rabbit spleen. Fed Proc 38, 751

Herman AG, Verbeuren TJ, Moncada S, and Vanhourre PM (1978) Effect of Prostacyclin on myogenic activity and adrenergic neuroeffector interaction in canine isolated veins. Prostaglandins 16: 911-921

Hoszowska A and Panczenko B (1974) Effects of inhibition of prostaglandin biosynthesis on noradrenaline release from isolated perfused spleen of the cat. Pol J Pharmacol Pharm 26: 137-142

Jackson HR, and Hall RC (1973) The effect of aspirin on the response to the rabbit ear artery. Europ J Pharmacol 21: 107-110

Junstad M and Wennmalm A (1973) On the release of prostaglandin E_2 from the rabbit heart following infusion of noradrenaline. Acta Physiol Scand 87: 573-574

Kadowitz PJ, Sweet CS, and Brody MJ (1971) Differential effects of prostaglandins E_1, E_2, $F_{1\alpha}$ and $F_{2\alpha}$ on adrenergic vasoconstriction in the dog hind paw. J Pharmacol Exp Therap 177: 641-649

Khan MT and Malik KU (1978) Inhibitory effect of prostaglandins (PG)I_2 and E_2 on the release of ^{3}H-norepinephrine (^{3}H-NE) evoked by potassium or electrical stimulation of the isolated rat heart. The Pharmacologist 20, 185

Khan MT and Malik KU (In Press) Sympathetic nerve stimulation of the isolated rat heart: Release of a prostaglandin (PG)I_2-like substance and the inhibitory effect of PGI_2 on the output of $[^3H]$-norepinephrine. In: Samuelsson B, Paoletti R (eds) Advances in Prostaglandins and thromboxane Research. Raven Press, New York, vol. 6-7

Lonigro AJ, Terragno NA, Malik KU, and McGiff JC (1973) Differential inhibition by prostaglandins of the renal action of pressor stimuli. Prostaglandins 3: 595-606

Malik KU (1978a) Prostaglandins - modulation of adrenergic nervous system. Fed. Proc. 37: 203-207

Malik KU (1978b) Prostaglandin-mediated inhibition of the vasoconstrictor responses of the isolated perfused rat splenic vasculature to adrenergic stimuli, Cir Res 43: 225-233

Malik KU and McGiff JC (1975) Modulation by prostaglandins of adrenergic transmission in the isolated perfused rabbit and rat kidney. Cir Res 36: 599-609

Malik KU and McGiff JC (1976) Modulation of adrenergic transmission by prostaglandins (PG) in the isolated splenic vasculature of rabbit and rat. Fed Proc 35, 297

Malik KU, Ryan P, and McGiff JC (1976) Modification by prostaglandins E_1 and E_2, indomethacin, and arachidonic acid of the vasoconstrictor responses of the isolated perfused rabbit and rat mesenteric arteries to adrenergic stimuli. Circ Res 39: 163-168

Malik KU and Nasjletti A (1979, In Press) Attenuation by bradykinin of adrenergically induced vasoconstriction in the isolated perfused kidney of the rabbit. Relationship to prostaglandin synthesis. Brit J Pharmacol

Malik KU and Nasjletti A (1980) Effect of bradykinin at the vascular neuroeffector junction. In: Bevan JA, Godfraind Th, Maxwell RA and Vanhoutte PM (eds) Vascular Neuroeffector Mechanisms. Raven Press, New York, pp 76-82

McGiff JC, Crowshaw K, Terragno NA, Malik KU, Lonigro AJ (1972) Differential effect of noradrenaline and renal nerve stimulation on vascular resistance in the dog kidney and the release of a prostaglandin E-like substance. Clin Sci 42: 223-233

Moncada S and Vane JR (1979) Arachidonic acid metabolites and the interaction between platelets and blood vessel walls. New England J Med 300: 1142-1147

Moncada S, Higgs EA, and Vane JR (1977) Human arterial and venous tissues generate prostacyclin (prostaglandin X), a potent inhibitor of platelet aggregation. The Lancet 1: 18-20

Ryan MJ and Zimmerman BG (1974) Effect of prostaglandin precursors, dihomo-γ-linolenic acid and arachidonic acid on the vasoconstrictor response to norepinephrine in the dog paw. Prostaglandins 6: 179-192

Starke K, Peskar BA, Schumacher KA and Taube HD (1977) Bradykinin and postganglionic sympathetic transimssion. Naunyn-Schmeideberg's Arch Pharmacol 299: 23-32

Stjärne L and Brundin J (1976) Additive stimulating effects of inhibitor of prostaglandin synthesis and of β-adrenoceptor agonist on sympathetic neuroeffector function in human omental blood vessels. Acta Physiol Scand 97: 267-269

Weitzell R, Steppeler A, and Starke K (1978) Effects of prostaglandin E_2, prostaglandin I_2 and 6-keto-prostaglandin $F_{1\alpha}$ on adrenergic neurotransmission in the pulmonary artery of the rabbit. Europ J Pharmacol 52: 137-141

Wennmalm Å (1978) Prostaglandin-mediated inhibition of noradrenaline release: III. Separation of prostaglandins released from stimulated hearts and analysis of their neurosecretion inhibitory capacity. Prostaglandins 15: 113-120

Yabek SM and Avner BP (1979) Effects of prostaglandin E_1 and indomethacin on fetal and neonatal lamb mesenteric artery responses to norepinephrine. Prostaglandins 17: 227-233

Zimmerman BG, Ryan MJ, Gomer S, and Kraft E (1973) Effect of prostaglandin synthesis inhibitors indomethacin and eicosa-5,8,11,14- tetraynoic acid on adrenergic responses in dog cutaneous vasculature. J Pharmacol Exp Therap 187: 315-323

Prostaglandins, Thrombin Receptors and Platelet Aggregation in Normal and Hypercholesterolemic Subjects

Rodolfo Paoletti and Elena Tremoli

The recent discovery of many new arachidonic acid metabolites active in the process of platelet aggregation, and their modification in experimental and human hypercholesterolemia has prompted us to investigate the action of inhibitors of platelet aggregation in hypercholesterolemic subjects in relation to the effect on arachidonic acid release and metabolism.

Patients with type II hypercholesterolemia are known to be at increased risk of atherosclerosis and thrombosis (Fredrickson et al. 1968; Miettinen 1974). In these patients platelet hypersensitivity, as documented by a number of abnormal functional tests in vitro, has been reported by several authors (Murphy and Mustard, 1971; Nørdoy and Rødset 1971; Carvalho et al. 1974). Carvalho et al. (1974) demonstrated that platelets in type IIA were a mean 140-fold sensitive than normal to epinephrine and released increased amounts of nucleotides in response to ADP, epinephrine and collagen.

More recently an enhanced biosynthesis of arachidonic acid products, i.e. Malondialdehyde (Tremoli et al. 1979) and Thromboxane B_2 (Tremoli et al. 1979) has been documented in type IIA patients.

These findings indicate an altered lipid peroxidation and an increased formation of arachidonic acid metabolites, with powerful aggregating effect, in hypercholesterolemia. Drugs affecting platelet function and prostaglandin biosynthesis in platelets are potentially useful in this pathological condition.

Indobufen. Indobufen is a new compound which has been demonstrated to be effective on platelet aggregation (Tamassia et al. 1979). The effects of repeated oral administrations (200 mg, twice a day) of Indobufen on platelets from type IIA patients has been studied. Responses to epinephrine and arachidonic acid sodium salt (AASS) are significantly enhanced in platelets from patients, when compared with controls. MDA production induced by serial concentrations of thrombin (range 2,5-25 U NIH/ml platelet rich plasma) is also increased. Indobufen administration significantly inhibits platelet aggregation, although the overcoming concentrations of both aggregating agents are significantly lower in patients than in controls (Fig. 1). MDA production is completely inhibited by Indobufen in both groups.

Metformin, platelet aggregation in experimental hyperlipidemia. Metformin has been shown to inhibit the onset of cholesterol atheromatosis

772

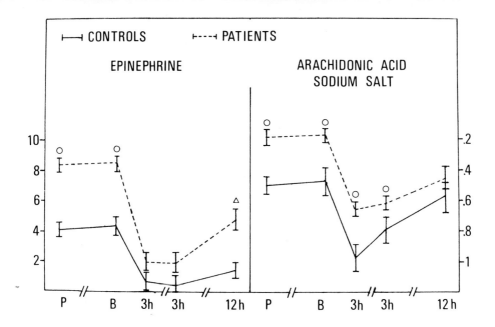

Fig. 1. Effect of repeated administrations of Indobufen or a corresponding placebo (P) on platelet aggregation induced by threshold concentration of Epinephrine and AASS to type IIA patients (n=8) and controls (n=8).

in rabbits without significantly reducing plasma cholesterol levels (Sirtori et al. 1977). Aggregation in platelets from rabbits fed for 1 month diet with a 2% cholesterol supplementation (HC) and with or without the addition of 0.5% Metformin (HC + MET) has been investigated. Platelets from normal and HC + MET rabbits showed a similar response to aggregation induced by threshold concentrations of arachidonic acid sodium salt (AASS) and collagen, in contrast platelets from HC rabbits required significantly lower concentrations of collagen and AASS to aggregate (Fig. 2).

Thrombin inhibitors and platelet aggregation. Thrombin induces platelet aggregation and secretion at concentrations which are generated in human blood physiologically and are present in many pathological conditions (Packam et al. 1977; Shuman and Levine 1978). The mechanism by which thrombin stimulates the platelet release reaction has yet to be clarified. However Majerus et al. (1976) indicate that the first step is the binding of thrombin to a specific receptor on platelet surface. GYKI 14,451, a synthetic tripeptide (Boc-D-Phe-Pro-Arg-H) synthetized at the Hungarian Institute of Drug Research and known for its anticoagulant activity has been studied in vitro on platelet aggregation induced by thrombin and other aggregating agents. This molecule shows a powerful activity in inhibiting thrombin induced aggregation at very low concentrations (2,5-5 microg/ml PRP) (Fig. 3) in human platelet rich plasma as well in washed

773

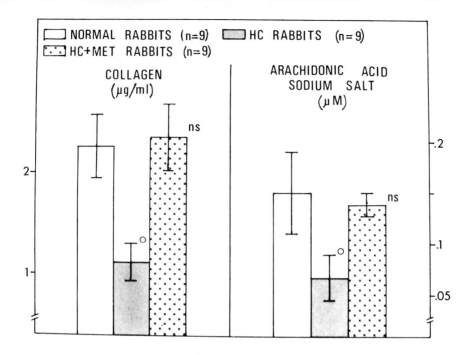

Fig. 2. Response to aggregation of platelets from normal, hypercholesterolemic (HC) and hypercholesterolemic + metformin (HC + MET) rabbits, p < 0.001.

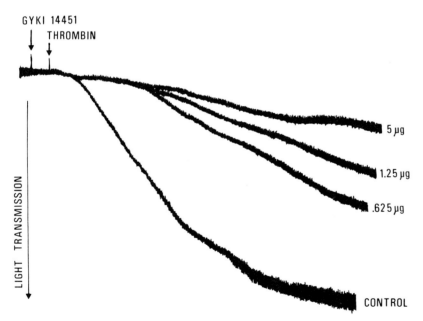

Fig. 3. Effect of different concentrations of GYKI 14,451 on aggregation
of washed platelets induced by thrombin (0.5 U NIH/ml PRP).

platelets, in the absence of Antithrombin III. Preliminary studies suggest a specific effect of this new compound as a thrombin antagonist; the anti-aggregating activity appears to be selective for thrombin: ADP and collagen induced aggregation are inhibited by much higher concentrations of the drug (160-200 microg /ml PRP). Further investigations are now under way in order to correlate the antiaggregating effect of GYKI 14,451 and that of arachidonic acid cascade products.

REFERENCES

Carvalho A, Colman RW and Lees RS (1974) Platelet function in hyperlipoproteinemia. New Engl J Med 290:434-438

Fredrickson DS, Levy RI and Lees RS (1967) Fat transport in lipoproteins. An integrated approach to mechanisms and disorders. New Engl J Med 276:32, 94, 148, 215, 273

Majerus PW, Tollefsen DM and Shuman MA (1976) The interaction of platelets with thrombin. In JL Gordon (ed) North-Holland, Amsterdam, 241-260.

Miettinen TA (1974) Hyperlipoproteinemia-relation to platelet lipids, platelet function and tendency to thrombosis. Thromb Res 4 suppl 1:41-47

Murphy EA, Mustard JF (1971) Coagulation tests and platelet economy in atherosclerotic and control subjects. Circulation 25:114-125

Nørdoy A and Rødset JM (1971) Platelet function and platelet phospholipids in patients with hyperbetalipoproteinemia: effect of nicotinic acid and clofibrate. Acta Med Scand 189:385-389

Packam MA, Guccione MA, Greenberg JP, Kinlough-Rathbone RL and Mustard JF (1977) Release of ^{14}C serotonin during initial platelet changes induced by thrombin, collagen or A23187. Blood 50:915-926

Sirtori CR, Catapano A, Ghiselli GC, Innocenti AL and Rodriguez J (1977) Metformin: an antiatherosclerotic agent modifying low density lipoproteins in rabbits. Atheroscler 26:78-89

Shuman MA, Levine SP (1978) Thrombin generation and secretion of platelet factor 4 during blood clotting. J Clin Invest 61:1102-1106

Tamassia W, Corvi GC, Fuccella LM, Moro E, Tosolini G and Tremoli E (1979) Indobufen (K3920) a new inhibitor of platelet aggregation: effect of food on bioavailability, pharmacokinetic and pharmacodynamic study during repeated oral administrations to man. Europ J clin Pharmacol 15:329-333

Tremoli E, Maderna P, Sirtori M and Sirtori CR (1979) Platelet aggregation and Malondialdehyde formation in type IIA hypercholesterolemic patients. Haemostasis 8:47-53

Tremoli E, Folco GC, Agradi E and Galli C (1979) Platelet thromboxanes and serum cholesterol. Lancet i:107-108

Prostaglandins, Thromboxanes and Leukotrienes[1]

Bengt Samuelsson

The hemostatic defense mechanism involves adhesion of circulating platelets to subendothelial structures. Platelets activated by this process release ADP, serotonin, various factors and enzymes and oxygenated products of arachidonic acid (Weiss 1975). A platelet aggregate is formed by the action of thromboxane A_2 and ADP. The same sequence of events seems to contribute to the development of the thrombus in human pathology. It has also been demonstrated that platelets generate products of arachidonic acid which stimulate leukocyte chemotaxis. This chapter deals with our current knowledge of the role of prostaglandins, thromboxanes and a more recently discovered group of compounds, leukotrienes, in these reactions.

In the course of studies on the mechanism of the transformation of polyunsaturated fatty acids into prostaglandins it was discovered that endoperoxide structures are involved (Samuelsson 1965 and 1972). Subsequently two unstable derivatives, PGG_2 and PGH_2 were isolated and found to act as intermediates in prostaglandin biosynthesis (Hamberg and Samuelsson 1973; Hamberg et al. 1974b; Nugteren and Hazelhof 1973) (FIG 1). Of particular interest, however, was the finding that the endoperoxides had biological effects which were not mediated by the prostaglandins known at that time (Hamberg et al. 1975). These effects included stimulation of respiratory and vascular smooth muscle and aggregation of human platelets. The endoperoxides caused release of ADP and serotonin and since aggregating agents as thrombin, gave release of endoperoxides it seemed reasonable to assume that the endoperoxides were the mediators in the reactions leading to the release reaction and aggregation (Malmsten et al. 1975). However, more detailed quantitative studies revealed that a very active and unstable ($t_{1/2}$ = 30 sec) aggregating factor was formed from arachidonic acid and the endoperoxides (Hamberg and Samuelsson 1974; Hamberg et al. 1974a). This was identified as a bicyclic oxane-oxetane structure and was named thromboxane A_2 (TXA_2) (Hamberg et al. 1974a; Samuelsson 1976) (FIG 2).

In collagen induced aggregation the initial event is the liberation of arachidonic acid from complex lipids. This reaction was earlier proposed to involve stimulation of phospholipase A_2 (Bills et al. 1977), however, more recent studies indicate that phosphatidyl inositol, after the actions of phospholipase C and diglyceride lipase, provide the main part of the free arachidonic acid (Bell et al. 1979). Oxygenation and further transformation yield the endoperoxide, PGH_2, which is isomerized to TXA_2. Studies with thromboxane synthetase inhibitors indicate that the conversion of PGH_2 to TXA_2 is essential (Gorman et al. 1977; Gryglewski et al. 1977). The aggregating activity of TXA_2 is mainly mediated by the ADP released (Claesson and Malmsten 1977). ADP stimulates further release of arachidonic acid and therefore constitutes a positive feed-back regulator. Thrombin can also cause ADP release by a cyclo-oxygenase independent mechanism (Malmsten et al. 1975). These reactions have been studied in various platelet disorders as summa-

---

[1] This work was supported by grants from the Swedish Medical Research Council (proj. no 03X-217).

776

MECHANISM OF PG BIOSYNTHESIS.

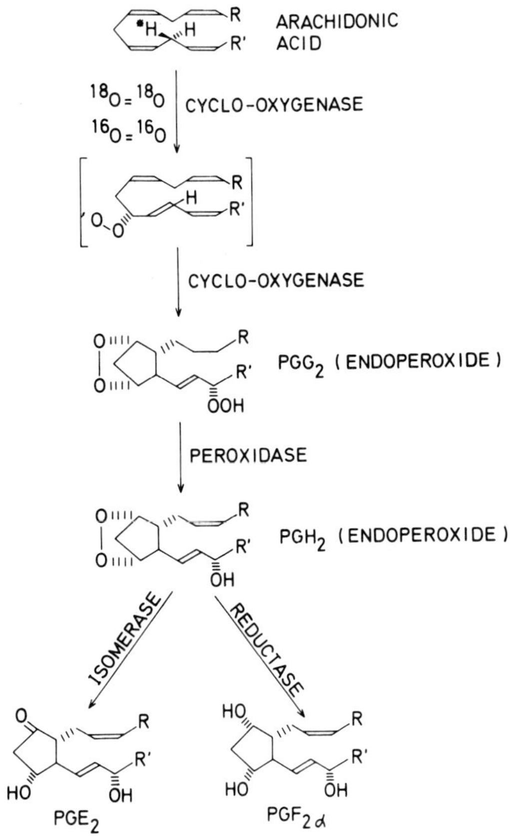

FIG. 1. Mechanism of prostaglandin
         biosynthesis.

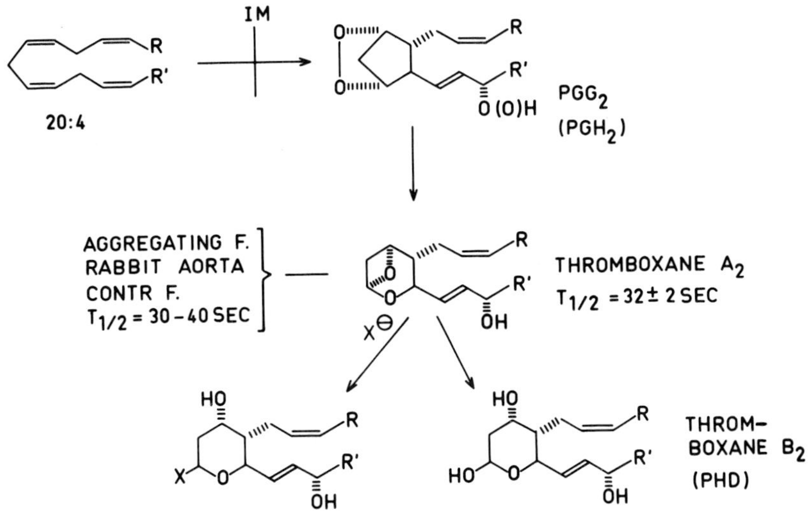

FIG. 2. Formation of thromboxanes.

rized in FIG 3 (Malmsten et al. 1975; Granström et al. 1976).

Thromboxane A_2 is a very potent vasoconstrictor, an effect which is of interest both in the hemostatic process and in pathological conditions. Radioimmunological methods have been developed for assay of TXA_2 and its stable hydrolysis product TXB_2 (Granström et al. 1976a, 1976b; Granström and Kindahl 1978). In the blood albumin exerts a protecting effect on TXA_2 against hydrolysis (Folco et al. 1977). However, it also reacts with the molecule to form TXA_2-albumin conjugates (Maclouf et al. 1980). The physiological significance of these reactions are unknown.

Following the isolation of the endoperoxides and the discovery of thromboxane A_2, it was found that arterial tissue converts the endoperoxide into a product with opposite effects (Moncada et al. 1976). Structural work demonstrated that it was an enol ether derivative (Johnson et al. 1976) (FIG 4). This vasodilator and antiaggregating compound was named PGI_2 or prostacyclin. It was proposed that PGI_2 synthesis by the vessel wall prevents deposition and aggregation of platelets through stimulation of platelet adenylate cyclase. The original proposal that platelets provide the endoperoxide for PGI_2 synthesis by the vessel wall has not been generally accepted (Bunting et al. 1976; Hornstra et al. 1979). Another endoperoxide derived product, PGD_2, the formation of which is facilitated by albumin, also stimulates formation of cAMP in platelets. These platelet and vessel wall reactions, which are of considerable interest in antithrombotic therapy are summarized in FIG 5. The main focus is now on the development of specific thromboxane synthetase inhibitors. Several structures with such activity have been described e.g. endoperoxide analogs, imidazole derivatives, pyridine derivatives and other compounds (Gorman et al. 1977; Gryglewski et al. 1977; Fitzpatrick et al. 1979; Diczfalusy and Hammarström 1977; Needleman et al. 1977; Moncada et al. 1977). Also, thromboxane antagonists (FIG 6) have recently become available for experimental work (Nicolaou et al. 1979; Fitzpatrick et al. 1978). Knowledge about the prostacyclin formation in the vessel wall has made antithrombotic therapy with aspirin type drugs less attractive. However, the longer duration of action of aspirin on platelets compared with endothelial cells has encouraged therapeutic trials with less frequent and low doses of aspirin.

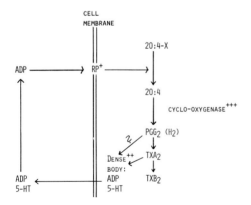

+)   MISSING OR REDUCED IN GLANZMANN'S THROMBASTHENIA
++) REDUCED IN HERMANSKY-PUDLAK SYNDROME
+++) MISSING IN PLATELET CYCLO-OXYGENASE DEFICIENCY

FIG. 3. Interrelationship between arachidonic acid derived products and ADP.

An alternative antithrombotic therapy is suggested by studies of the effects of products from eicosapentaenoic acid. Thus, thromoxane A₃, which is derived from this acid was found to be a vasoconstrictor but not an aggregating agent (Raz et al. 1977). However, the prostacyclin, PGI₃, derived from the same precursor acid has properties similar to those of PGI₂ (Johnson et al. 1978). Greenland eskimos, who have a very low incidence of myocardial infarction have been found to have a considerable increase in the amount of eicosapentaenoic acid in the lipids (Dyerberg et al. 1978). It therefore seems of interest to study the effects of dietary regimens in more detail in the search for new antithrombotic methods.

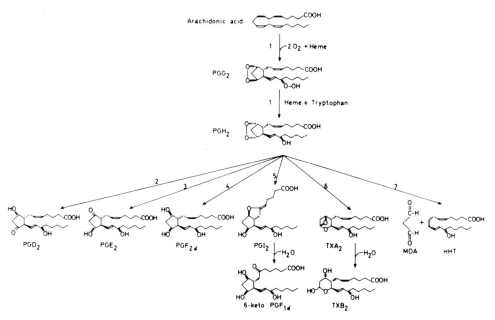

FIG. 4. Transformations of arachidonic acid.

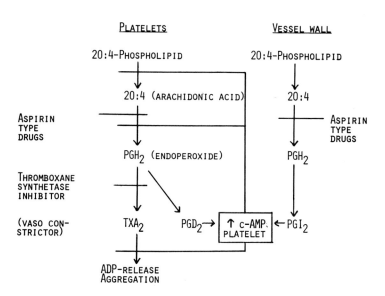

FIG. 5. Reactions in platelets and vessel wall.

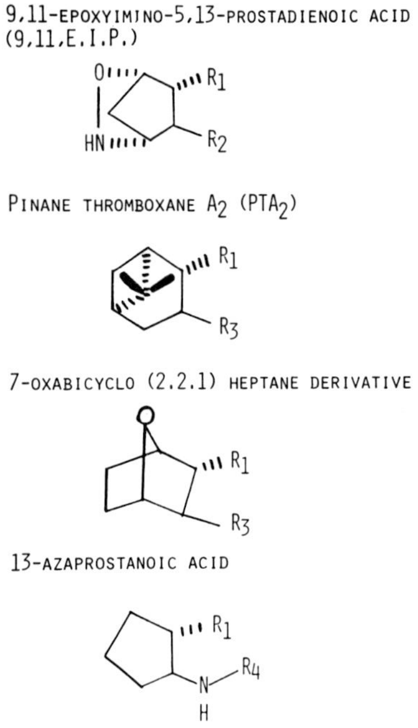

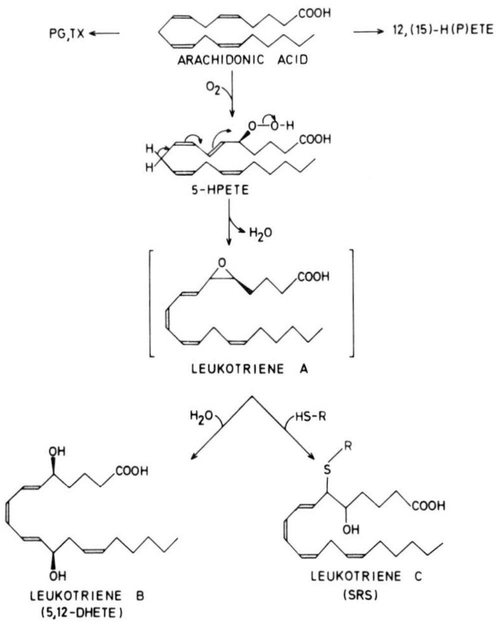

9,11-EPOXYIMINO-5,13-PROSTADIENOIC ACID
(9,11,E.I.P.)

PINANE THROMBOXANE A$_2$ (PTA$_2$)

7-OXABICYCLO (2.2.1) HEPTANE DERIVATIVE

13-AZAPROSTANOIC ACID

PG,TX ← ARACHIDONIC ACID → 12,(15)-H(P)ETE

5-HPETE

LEUKOTRIENE A

LEUKOTRIENE B
(5,12-DHETE)

LEUKOTRIENE C
(SRS)

FIG. 6. Thromboxane A$_2$ antagonists.   FIG. 7. Formation of leukotrienes.

The transformations of arachidonic acid in platelets also include a lipoxy-genase catalyzed reaction forming 12-hydroperoxy-eicosatetraenoic acid (12-HPETE) which is reduced to 12-hydroxy-eicosatetraenoic acid (12-HETE) (Hamberg and Samuelsson 1974). The physiological significance of this path-way is essentially unknown, however, the platelet product 12-HETE has chemo-tactic activity toward leukocytes (Turner et al. 1975; Goetzl et al. 1977). It is of interest in this context that leukocytes synthesize arachidonic acid derived products with pronounced biological activities.

Thus, arachidonic acid is oxygenated in leukocytes at C-5 to give 5-hydro-peroxy-eicosatetraenoic acid (5-HPETE) which is converted into an unstable epoxide intermediate with a conjugated triene (leukotriene A) (Borgeat et al. 1976; Borgeat and Samuelsson 1979a, 1979b, 1979c, 1979d) (FIG 7). Leuko-triene A can be hydrolyzed enzymatically to 5,12-dihydroxy-eicosatetraenoic acid (leukotriene B). A mast cell tumor forms leukotriene C which is a 5-hydroxy-eicosatetraenoic acid derivative with a cystein containing substi-tuent at C-6 (Murphy et al. 1979; Samuelsson et al. 1979). Leukotriene C has biological effects which are similar to those of SRS (Slow Reacting Substance), a substance also formed in leukocytes.

SRS is a very strong stimulant of bronchial smooth muscle, however, it has also been shown to be a vasodilator and to increase capillary permeability (Strandberg and Uvnäs 1971). It is an important mediator in immediate hyper-sensitivity reactions as asthma. Additional studies are required to eluci-date the role of leukotrienes and other lipoxygenase products in the inter-relationship between platelets, leukocytes and the vessel wall.

References

Bell RL, Kennerly DA, Stanford N, Majerus PW (1979) Diglyceride lipase: A pathway for arachidonate release from human platelets. Proc Natl Acad Sci USA 76:3238-3241

Bills, TK, Smith JB, Silver MJ (1977) Selective release of arachidonic acid from the phospholipids of human platelets in response to thrombin. J Clin Invest 60:1-6

Borgeat P, Hamberg M, Samuelsson B (1976) Transformation of arachidonic acid and homo-γ-linonelic acid by rabbit polymorphonuclear leucocytes. J Biol Chem 251:7816-7820, Correction: (1977) 252:8772

Borgeat P, Samuelsson B (1979a) Transformation of arachidonic acid by rabbit polymorphonuclear leukocytes: Formation of a novel dihydroxy-eicosatetraenoic acid. J Biol Chem 254:2643-2646

Borgeat P, Samuelsson B (1979b) Metabolism of arachidonic acid in polymorphonuclear leukocytes: Structural analysis of novel hydroxylated compounds. J Biol Chem 254:7865-7869

Borgeat P, Samuelsson B (1979c) Arachidonic acid metabolism in polymorphonuclear leucocytes: Effects of the ionophore A23187. Proc Natl Acad Sci USA 76:2148-2152

Borgeat P, Samuelsson B (1979d) Arachidonic acid metabolism in polymorphonuclear leukocytes: Unstable intermediate in formation of dihydroxy acids. Proc Natl Acad Sci USA 76:3213-3217

Bunting S, Gryglewski R, Moncada S, Vane JR (1976) Arterial walls generate from prostaglandin endoperoxides a substance (Prostaglandin X) which relazed strips of mesenteric and coeliac arteries and inhibits platelet aggregation. Prostaglandins 12:897-913

Claesson HE, Malmsten C (1977) On the interrelationship of prostaglandin endoperoxide G_2 and cyclic nucleotides in platelet function. Eur J Biochem 76:277-284

Diczfalusy U, Hammarström S (1977) Inhibitors of thromboxane synthase in human platelets. FEBS Lett 82:107-110

Dyerberg J, Bang HO, Stoffersen E, Moncada S, Vane JR (1978) Eicosapentaenoic acid and prevention of thrombosis and atherosclerosis? Lancet 8081:117

Fitzpatrick FA, Bundy GL, Gorman R, Honohan T (1978) 9,11-Epoxy-iminoprosta-5,13-dienoic acid is a thromboxane A_2 antagonist in human platelets. Nature (Lond) 275:764-766

Fitzpatrick F, Gorman R, Bundy G, Honohan T, McGuire J, Sun F (1979) 9,11-Iminoepoxyprosta-5,13-dienoic acid is a selective thromboxane A_2 synthetase inhibitor. Biochim Biophys Acta 573:238

Folco GC, Granström E, Kindahl H (1977) Albumin stabilizes thromboxane A_2. FEBS Lett 82:321-324

Goetzl EJ, Woods JM, Gorman RR (1977) Stimulation of human eosinophil and neutrophil polymorphonuclear leukocyte chemotaxis and random migration by 12-L-hydroxy-5,8,10,14-eicosatetraenoic acid (HETE). J Clin Invest 59:179-183

Gorman RR, Bundy G, Peterson D, Sun F, Miller O, Fitzpatrick F (1977) Inhibition of human platelet thromboxane synthetase by 9,11-azoprosta-5,13-dienoic acid. Proc Natl Acad Sci USA 74:4007-4011

Granström E, Kindahl H, Samuelsson B (1976a) Radioimmunoassay for thromboxane B_2. Anal Lett 9:611-627

Granström E, Kindahl H, Samuelsson B (1976b) A method for measuring the unstable thromboxane A_2: Radioimmunoassay of the derived mono-O-methyl-thromboxane B_2. Prostaglandins 12:929-941

Granström E, Kindahl H (1978) Radioimmunoassay of prostaglandins and thromboxanes. In: Frölich JC (ed) Advances in Prostaglandin and Thromboxane Research, vol 5 pp 119-210. Raven Press, New York

Gryglewski R, Zmuda A, Korbut R, Kreicioch E, Bieron K (1977) Selective inhibition of thromboxane A_2 biosynthesis in blood platelets. Nature 267:627-628

Hamberg M, Samuelsson B (1973) Detection and isolation of an endoperoxide intermediate in prostaglandin biosynthesis. Proc Natl Acad Sci USA 70:899-903

Hamberg M, Samuelsson B (1974) Prostaglandin endoperoxides. Novel transformations of arachidonic acid in human platelets. Proc Natl Acad Sci USA 71:3400-3404

Hamberg M, Svensson J, Samuelsson B (1974a) Prostaglandin endoperoxides. A new concept concerning the mode of action and release of prostaglandins. Proc Natl Acad Sci USA 71:3824-3828

Hamberg M, Svensson J, Wakabayashi T, Samuelsson B (1974b) Isolation and structure of two prostaglandin endoperoxides that cause platelet aggregation. Proc Natl Acad Sci USA 71:345-349

Hamberg M, Hedqvist P, Strandberg K, Svensson J, Samuelsson B (1975) Prostaglandin endoperoxides. IV. Effects on smooth muscle. Life Sci 16:451-462

Hornstra G, Haddeman E, Don JA (1979) Blood platelets do not provide endoperoxides for vascular prostacyclin production. Nature 279:66

Johnson RA, Lincoln FH, Nidy EG, Schneider WD, Thompson JL, Axen U (1978) Synthesis and characterization of prostacyclin, 6-keto-prostaglandin $F_{1\alpha}$, prostaglandin I_1, and prostaglandin I_3. J Am Chem Soc 100:7690-7705

Johnson RA, Morton DR, Kinner JH, Gorman RR, McGuire JC, Sun FF, Whittaker N, Bunting S, Salmon J, Moncada S, Vane JR (1976) The chemical structure of prostaglandin X (Prostacyclin). Prostaglandins 12: 915-928

Maclouf J, Kindahl H, Granström E, Samuelsson B (1980) Thromboxane A_2 and prostaglandin H_2 form covalently linked derivaties with human serum albumin. In: Samuelsson B, Ramwell P, Paoletti R (eds) Advances in Prostaglandin and Thromboxane Research, vol 6 pp xx-xx. Raven Press, New York

Malmsten C, Hamberg M, Svensson J, Samuelsson B (1975) Physiological roles of an endoperoxide in human platelets: Hemostatic defect due to platelet cyclo-oxygenase deficiency. Proc Natl Acad Sci USA 72:1446-1450

Moncada S, Bunting S, Mullane K, Thorogood P, Vane JR, Raz A, Needleman P (1977) Imidazole: A selective inhibitor of thromboxane synthetase. Prostaglandins 13:611-618

Moncada S, Gryglewski RJ, Bunting S, Vane JR (1976) An enzyme isolated from arteries transforms prostaglandin endoperoxides to an unstable substance that inhibits platelet aggregation. Nature 263:663-665

Murphy RC, Hammarström S, Samuelsson B (1979) Leukotriene C: A slow reacting substance (SRS) from murine mastocytoma cells. Proc Natl Acad Sci USA 76:4275-4279

Needleman P, Raz A, Ferendelli JA, Minkes M (1977) Application of imidazole as a selective inhibitor of thromboxane synthetase in human platelets. Proc Natl Acad Sci USA 74:1716-1720

Nicolaou KC, Magolda RL, Smith JB, Aharony D, Smith EF, Lefer AM (1979) Synthesis and biological properties of pinane-thromboxane A_2, a selective inhibitor of coronary artery constriction, platelet aggregation, and thromboxane formation. Proc Natl Acad Sci USA 76:2566-2570

Nugteren DH, Hazelhof E (1973) Isolation and properties of intermediates in prostaglandin biosynthesis. Biochim Biophys Acta 326:448-461

Raz A, Minkes MS, Needleman P (1977) Endoperoxides and thromboxanes. Structural determinant for platelet aggregation and vasoconstriction. Biochim Biophys Acta 488:305-311

Samuelsson B (1965) On the incorporation of oxygen in the conversion of 8,11,14-eicosatrienoic acid to prostaglandin E_1. J Am Chem Soc 87:3011-3113

Samuelsson B (1972) Biosynthesis of prostaglandins. Fed Proc 31:1442-1450

Samuelsson B (1976) Introduction: New trends in prostaglandin research. In: Samuelsson B, Paoletti R (eds) Advances in Prostaglandin and Thromboxane Research, vol 1 pp1-6. Raven Press, New York

Samuelsson B, Borgeat P, Hammarström S (1979) Introduction of a nomenclature: Leukotrienes. Prostaglandins 17:785-787

Strandberg K, Uvnäs B (1971) Purification and properties of the slow reacting substance formed in the cat paw perfused with compound 48/80. Acta physiol scand 82:358-374

Turner SR, Tainer JA, Lynn WS (1975) Biogenesis of chemotactic molecules by the arachidonate lipoxygenase system of platelets. Nature 257:680-681

Weiss HJ (1975) Platelet physiology and abnormalites of platelet function. N Engl J Med 293:580-588

Role of Hormones Associated with Atherogenesis in Modulating Cellular Metabolism of Lipoproteins

Edwin L. Bierman

It should be apparent from the information presented by the participants in this workshop that the cellular metabolism of lipoproteins is a finely regulated process. There appears to be tissue specificity for binding, uptake, and degradation of certain classes of lipoproteins, particularly LDL, VLDL and chylomicron remnants, and perhaps subclasses of HDL. Newer in vivo techniques such as the one described by Dr. Steinberg, will help to unravel the role of metabolism of lipoproteins by particular tissues and cells in overall lipoprotein transport.

We are now beginning to understand the role of non-receptor mediated pathways for lipoprotein degradation that collectively comprise the "scavenger pathway". The role of macrophages in this process, as described by Dr. Fogelman, is undoubtedly important, perhaps as it may relate to the removal and degradation of lipoproteins that have been "altered" by prolonged retention in the circulation resulting from a transport defect in one or another form of hyperlipidemia.

Delivery of lipoprotein cholesterol to cells appears to be a key component of normal cell physiology. We know that endogenous synthesis of cholesterol is linked to cholesterol flux into and out of the cell. Cholesterol esterification and hydrolysis are important regulatory components of intracellular cholesterol homeostasis. Understanding how regulation at these steps can be altered, particularly in cells that may accumulate abnormal quantities of esterified cholesterol, such as arterial smooth muscle cells appears to be critical. Dr. Stein has provided us with many new insights into the factors that control cellular accumulation and depletion of cholesterol and other lipids.

How cellular cholesterol is transported out of cells is obviously of key interest in any attempt to understand and promote reversal of atherosclerotic lesions. Dr. Rothblat's observations point to the complexity of the process, which clearly involves apoproteins, apoprotein-lipid complexes, transport proteins, and enzymes such as LCAT.

Superimposed on all of these processes regulating the cellular metabolism of lipoproteins is the influence of hormonal factors, some of which (insulin, thyroid hormone, glucocorticoids, gonadal steroids) have been implicated in atherogenesis. Recent work in our laboratory, using cultured human skin fibroblasts as a model, has shown that insulin in physiological concentrations (100 uU/ml) stimulates LDL receptor activity (LDL binding and degradation), presumably involving a mechanism leading to an increased number of LDL receptors (Chait et al. 1978, 1979a). Coupled with insulin-induced stimulation of endogenous cellular cholesterol synthesis, this effect of insulin provides a mechanism whereby cells theoretically could increase its supply of cholesterol during times of additional need, i.e., during active proliferation.

Furthermore, the role of insulin in modulating cell LDL receptor activity could be relevant to in vivo LDL (and perhaps VLDL) degradation. Several recent well-controlled studies in which lipoproteins have been quantified in diabetics (Bennion and Grundy; Howard et al.; Paisey et al.) have shown increased LDL levels in the insulin deficient state. Preliminary (unpublished) observations in our laboratory indicate that provision of excess insulin (with glucose) to non-diabetics will accelerate the catabolism of intravenously administered ^{125}I-labeled LDL and lower plasma LDL cholesterol levels.

Thus both insulin excess (as in the non-insulin dependent adult diabetic and in treatment of the insulin-dependent diabetic) and insulin deficiency can be implicated in atherogenesis by effects on cellular metabolism of lipoproteins. Insulin excess would promote arterial smooth muscle cell LDL uptake, cholesterol synthesis, and cell proliferation. Insulin deficiency would promote decreased LDL and VLDL degradation by peripheral cells via the receptor mediated pathway leading to hyperlipidemia. As shown by Wolinsky (1978) in streptozotocin-induced diabetic rats, insulin lack is also associated with decreased activity of lysosomal enzymes, which would impair the degradation of LDL and cholesterol esters by arterial cells.

Thyroid hormone also stimulates LDL receptor activity (Chait et al. 1979b). L-triiodothyronine in physiological concentrations (10^{-10}M in serum-free medium) appears to increase the number of LDL receptors of cultured human skin fibroblasts which leads to enhanced LDL degradation. This effect may be additive to that of insulin. Thus thyroid hormone may play an important independent regulatory role in cellular cholesterol metabolism. This effect on the LDL receptor presumably in part may explain the known impaired catabolism of LDL in vivo in the thyroid deficient state.

In contrast, as reported elsewhere in this symposium by Dr. Henze, hydrocortisone in physiological concentrations (15 mg/ml in serum-free medium) profoundly reduces LDL receptor activity by decreasing receptor number. Hydrocortisone also appears to decrease endogenous cholesterol synthesis. Thus the regulatory role of corticosteroid hormones on cellular metabolism of lipoproteins appears to counter that of insulin.

Thus far we have been unable to show any effect of gonadal steroids (estrogens, progestagens, androgens) on LDL receptor activity in cultured fibroblasts. However, since these hormones appear to influence lipoprotein transport in vivo, it is possible that metabolic products of these agents could play a regulatory role on lipid metabolism at the cellular level. Certainly a specific role for estrogen in modulating the binding, uptake, and degradation of VLDL and chylomicron remnants in the hepatocyte remains a distinct possibility.

Thus some of the key hormones that have been associated with atherogenesis have been shown to influence the cellular metabolism of lipoproteins by directly regulating LDL receptor activity. Further studies are necessary to elucidate the in vivo consequences of this regulation.

References

Bennion LJ, Grundy SM (1977) Effects of diabetes mellitus on cholesterol metabolism in man. N Engl J Med 296: 1365-1571
Chait A, Bierman EL, Albers JJ (1978) Regulatory role of insulin in the degradation of low density lipoprotein by cultured human skin fibroblasts. Biochim Biophys Acta 529: 292-299
Chait A, Bierman EL, Albers JJ (1979a) Low density lipoprotein receptor activity in cultured human skin fibroblasts: mechanism of insulin-induced stimulation. J Clin Invest, in press
Chait A, Bierman EL, Albers JJ (1979b) Regulatory role of triiodothyronine in the degradation of low density lipoprotein by cultured human skin fibroblasts. J Clin Endocrinol Metab 48: 887-889

Howard BV, Savage PJ, Bennion LJ, Bennett PH (1978) Lipoprotein composition in diabetes mellitus. Atherosclerosis 30: 153–162

Paisey R, Elkeles RS, Hambley J, Magill P (1978) The effects of chlorpropamide and insulin on serum lipids, lipoproteins and fractional triglyceride removal. Diabetologia 15: 81–85

Wolinsky H, Goldfischer S, Capron L, Capron F, Coltoff-Schiller B, Kasak L (1978) Hydrolase activities in the rat aorta. I. Effects of diabetes mellitus. Circ Res 42: 821–831

Platelet Production of Pathological LDL[1]

Alan M. Fogelman,[2] Ishaiahu Shechter,[3] Janet Seager, Martha Hokom, John S. Child, and Peter A. Edwards[4]

There is increasing evidence that the foam cells found in the atherosclerotic reaction are macrophages which are derived from blood borne monocytes and/or smooth muscle cells which have taken on many of the properties of macrophages (Gerrity and Naito 1978; Schaffner et al.1979; Fowler and Haley 1979). The hallmark of these cells is their high cholesteryl ester content (≥50% of the total cholesterol content). Our objective has been to define the conditions and mechanisms leading to cholesteryl ester accumulation within these cells. We began our work by asking if the conversion of blood monocytes into macrophages was associated with an increase in the cholesteryl ester content of the cells. In order to test this question we prepared pure monocytes (Fogelman et al, 1979) and cultured the cells using a modification of the method of Johnson, Mei and Cohn (1977). By cytochemical, morphological, ultrastructural and functional criteria the monocytes were converted into macrophages. However, the cholesteryl ester content did not increase appreciably (from approximately 0.5 to 0.8 μg per mg cell protein, or approximately 1.5% of the total cellular cholesterol content after 14 days of culture). There was no increase in the cholesteryl ester content of the cells when the concentration of serum was varied from 10% to 50%. Nor was there an increase in cellular cholesteryl esters when the cells were incubated in 50% serum that was taken after a meal containing 250 gm of saturated fat and 2.5 gm of cholesterol.

It is a widely held notion that the relative amounts of LDL and HDL are prime determinants of the intracellular cholesterol concentration and hence predictors of susceptibility to atherosclerosis. We tested this notion by supplementing the incubation medium with LDL so that the LDL/HDL ratio was increased from 1.7:1 to 10.2:1 and the concentration of LDL-cholesterol was increased to 2,470 μg/ml, more than twice that which the cells had been exposed to in vivo as monocytes. After periods of incubation ranging from 3 to 15 days the maximum cholesteryl ester concentration observed was 3.8 μg per mg cell protein or 3.5% of the total cholesterol content. Freshly isolated monocytes incubated in Teflon FEP containers (a surface to which the cells could not adhere) were seen to take up and degrade ^{125}I-LDL by a saturable, high affinity process with maximum velocity at 25 to 50 μg ^{125}I-LDL/ml and a slower, nonsaturable process which was apparent at higher concentrations. After the cells were cultured for 7 days in 30% autologous serum containing 180 μg LDL protein/ml, LDL uptake via the receptor was increased by more than an order of

[1]This work was supported in part by U.S.P.H.S. Grants HL 20807, HL 22474 and HL 19063.
[2]Dr. Fogelman is the recipient of a U.S.P.H.S. Research Career Development Award (HL 00426).
[3]Dr. Schechter participated in this work as a co-principal investigator while on leave from Tel Aviv University, Israel.
[4]Dr. Edwards is an Established Investigator of the American Heart Association.

787

magnitude. At a concentration of 186 µg of ^{125}I–LDL/ml the cells degraded approximately 5 µg ^{125}I–LDL/mg cell protein in 4 hours and approximately three-fourths of this could be accounted for by high affinity degradation. At this rate the cells would have degraded 30 µg of LDL protein/mg cell protein in 24 hours. Had the cells retained the cholesterol liberated from this LDL their cholesterol content would have doubled each 24 hours. However, such an increase was not observed and there was no accumulation of cholesteryl esters under these conditions. In parallel experiments it was seen that the ^{125}I–LDL was not degraded in the medium outside the cells by enzymes that may have been released from the cells. We concluded, therefore, that monocyte-macrophages have a very active LDL receptor pathway (Goldstein and Brown 1977), but that the vast majority of the cholesterol liberated from the LDL taken up by this pathway is not retained within the cell and therefore is incapable of causing cholesteryl ester accumulation. On reviewing the literature we found that these cells were not unique in this regard. Cultured arterial smooth muscle cells have been shown to take up and degrade ^{125}I–LDL by the LDL receptor pathway but they did not accumulate cholesteryl esters when incubated with high concentrations of normal LDL. However, the cells did accumulate cholesteryl esters when incubated with LDL from hypercholesterolemic animals (St. Clair and Leight 1978). In the monkey these hyperlipidemic LDL molecules were found to be larger than normal LDL molecules (St. Clair and Leight 1978). In order to test whether particle size might be an important determinant of cholesteryl ester accumulation we set out to chemically produce an enlarged molecular weight LDL. In searching for a suitable method we considered the possibility that glutaraldehyde might form a Schiff's base with the ε-amino group of lysines located on two different LDL molecules and thus serve to cross link LDL and form a high molecular weight polymer. When glutaraldehyde was added to ^{125}I–LDL and the lipoproteins analyzed by gel filtration chromatography on Sepharose 4–B it was seen that the resulting lipoproteins had a molecular weight of at least 10 million daltons. (It should be noted that before analysis or incubation these lipoprotein preparations and all other lipoprotein preparations were first filtered through a 0.45 µ filter in order to remove denatured lipoproteins.) On electrophoresis the glutaraldehyde treated LDL showed an intensely staining band at the origin and a band which ran ahead of native LDL. In between these two bands there was a trail of stain consistent with particles of differing molecular weights and/or charge. Glutaraldehyde–^{125}I–LDL was degraded by the two processes described above for native–^{125}I–LDL but the glutaraldehyde–^{125}I–LDL was degraded at least five times faster than the native–^{125}I–LDL. After 3 days incubation with the glutaraldehyde treated–LDL the cholesteryl ester content of the cells increased to approximately 28 µg of esterified cholesterol per mg protein compared to 0.9 µg of esterified cholesterol per mg protein in cells incubated with the same concentration of native–LDL (500 µg/ml.) We concluded that modification of the size and/or charge of native–LDL was required in order to produce cholesteryl ester accumulation. We reasoned that altered LDL produced at the site of the atherosclerotic lesion would be taken up by the monocyte–macrophages and smooth muscle cells with macrophage properties that are present at such sites. However, LDL that was altered at a site distant from the atherosclerotic reaction would probably be cleared from the circulation by the reticuloendothelial cells of the liver. In considering mechanisms by which LDL could be altered at the site of the atherosclerotic reaction we remembered the important role attributed to blood platelets in causing the proliferation of smooth muscle cells (Ross and Glomset 1976). Furthermore, it is known that in the metabolism of arachidonic acid by platelets there is one mole of malondialdehyde produced for every mole of thromboxane A_2 (Smith et al. 1976; Samuelsson et al. 1978). Since thromboxane A_2 and malondialdehyde are produced by the platelets only at sites at which platelets aggregate and release, this mechanism seemed ideally suited to explain the focal nature of the atherosclerotic process. Moreover, malondialdehyde has a structure similar to glutaraldehyde, and Chio and Tappel

(1969) demonstrated that malondialdehyde produced intra and intermolecular cross linking of ribonuclease A due to the formation of Schiff's bases between malondialdehyde and the ε-amino groups of the protein.

In order to test this hypothesis we prepared malondialdehyde from malondialdehyde bis(dimethyl acetal) and reacted it with LDL. Upon reisolation the LDL was found in a single band with an electrophoretic mobility more negative than native-LDL. Malondialdehyde-^{125}I-LDL was seen to be taken up and degraded by two processes: a high affinity, saturable process with maximum velocity at 10 μg protein/ml and a slower, nonsaturable process. The degradation of 25 μg/ml of malondialdehyde-^{125}I-LDL was readily inhibited by increasing concentrations of non-radioactive malondialdehyde-LDL but was not inhibited by increasing concentrations of non-radioactive acetyl-LDL or native-LDL (up to 1600 μg/ml). We interpreted these data to indicate that the malondialdehyde-^{125}I-LDL was being taken up by a receptor distinctly different from that responsible for the uptake of either acetyl-LDL or native-LDL. After three days of incubation with malondialdehyde-LDL the cholesteryl ester content of the cells increased to approximately 17 μg of esterified cholesterol per mg protein compared to 1.0 μg of esterified cholesterol per mg protein in cells incubated with the same concentration of native-LDL (500 μg/ml).

Encouraged by these results we caused human blood platelets to aggregate and release in the presence of native-^{125}I-LDL. Upon reisolation the platelet-^{125}I-LDL was analyzed. In contrast to the glutaraldehyde-^{125}I-LDL, very little of the platelet-^{125}I-LDL was found to have a high molecular weight. However, on electrophoresis the platelet-^{125}I-LDL was found to have an electrophoretic mobility intermediate between native-^{125}I-LDL and acetyl-^{125}I-LDL. After three days of incubation with the platelet-LDL the cholesteryl ester content of the cells increased to approximately 9 μg per mg cell protein compared to approximately 2 μg per mg cell protein in cells incubated with the same concentration of control-LDL (native-LDL that was treated identically to the platelet-LDL except that platelets were omitted from the reaction mixture). Evidence that malondialdehyde released from the platelets reacted with the LDL was obtained from experiments in which platelets were caused to aggregate and release in the presence of native-LDL. Subsequently, the LDL was reisolated and precipitated with heparin-manganese. The precipitate was washed and then exposed to acid conditions in order to hydrolyze the Schiff's base bonds. The malondialdehyde released was then measured spectrophotometrically: 1.74 ± 0.21 nanomoles of malondialdehyde per mg of LDL protein were recovered from the LDL which had been exposed to the platelets, while there was no detectable malondialdehyde recovered from control-LDL.

We conclude from these experiments that the widely held notion that the relative amounts of LDL and HDL outside the cell primarily determine the cholesterol concentration within the cell is not true. When native-LDL was added to the cells in high concentrations for prolonged periods during which HDL concentrations were low, the cells did not accumulate cholesteryl esters. They degraded native-LDL at a rate that should have liberated an amount of cholesterol sufficient to double the cellular cholesterol content every 24 hours. Such an increase was not observed. However, when LDL was polymerized by glutaraldehyde or its charge modified by malondialdehyde or by the action of human platelets, the resultant molecules readily caused the cells to accumulate cholesteryl esters. Moreover, the malondialdehyde-LDL was taken up by a receptor distinctly different from that which takes up acetyl-LDL and native-LDL. Based on these experiments we propose that modification of native-LDL is a prerequisite to the accumulation of cholesteryl esters within the macrophages and smooth muscle cells of the atherosclerotic reaction. We further hypothesize that the modification of LDL in vivo that leads to cholesteryl ester accumulation in the cells of the arterial wall is mediated by the action of blood platelets. The vast majority of persons with atherosclerosis have "normal" levels of LDL. Our hypothesis provides an explanation

for the accumulation of cholesteryl esters within the cells of the atherosclerotic reaction of these individuals. Their "normal" LDL levels provide
sufficient substrate for the production of pathological LDL by platelets.
Since malondialdehyde-LDL is taken up by a receptor different from the native-
LDL receptor, this hypothesis may also provide an explanation for the accumulation of cholesteryl esters within the cells of the atherosclerotic reaction
of receptor negative homozygous familial hypercholesterolemics.

References

Chio KS, Tappel AL (1969) Inactivation of ribonuclease and other enzymes by
    peroxidizing lipids and malonaldehyde. Biochem 8:2827-2832
Fogelman AM, Seager J, Hokom M, Edwards PA (1979) Separation of and chole-
    sterol synthesis by human lymphocytes and monocytes. J Lipid Res 20:
    379-388
Fowler S, Haley NJ (1979) Investigation of macrophage-like properties of
    rabbit aortic foam cells. Fed Proc 38:1076
Gerrity RG, Naito HK, Richardson M, Schwartz CJ (1979) Dietary induced athero-
    genesis in swine. Am J Path 95:775-792
Goldstein JL, Brown MS (1977) The low-density lipoprotein pathway and its
    relation to atherosclerosis. Ann Rev Biochem 46:897-930
Johnson WD Jr, Mei B, Cohn ZA (1977) The separation, long term cultivation,
    and maturation of the human monocyte. J Exp Med 146:1613-1626
Ross R, Glomset JA (1976) The pathogenesis of atherosclerosis. N Engl J Med
    295:420-425
St. Clair RW, Leight MA (1978) Differential effects of isolated lipoproteins
    from normal and hypercholesterolemic rhesus monkeys on cholesterol ester-
    ification and accumulation in arterial smooth muscle cells in culture.
    Biochim Biophys Acta 530:279-291
Samuelsson B, Goldyne M, Granstrom E, Hamberg M, Hammarstrom S, Malmsten C
    (1978) Prostaglandins and thromboxanes. Ann Rev Biochem 47:997-1029
Schaffner T, Vesselinovitch D, Wissler RW (1979) Macrophages in experimental
    and human atheromatous lesions, immunomorphologic identification. Fed
    Proc 38:1076
Smith JB, Ingerman CM, Silver MJ (1976) Malondialdehyde formation as an indi-
    cator of prostaglandin production by human platelets. J Lab Clin Med 88:
    167-172

Modulation of Cellular Cholesterol Metabolism by LCAT Treated Lipoproteins

George Rothblat, Fabrizio Bellini, and Eva Ray[1]

Introduction

Lecithin cholesterol acyl transferase (LCAT) plays a major role in regulating
the lipid composition of serum lipoproteins (Glomset 1972). It has been proposed that LCAT could also function to regulate cellular cholesterol metabolism by influencing the lipid composition of the lipoproteins that serve to
deliver and remove cholesterol from cells (Glomset 1968). In the present investigation we have studied the effect of LCAT modification of serum lipid
composition on cholesterol content and synthesis in primary hepatocytes and
hepatoma cells. In addition, we have obtained information on the mechanism
by which changes in lipoprotein lipid composition influence cellular cholesterol metabolism.

Results

Figure 1 shows the results obtained when primary rabbit hepatocytes were
incubated 24 hours in medium supplemented with different concentrations of
normal rabbit serum. As the concentration of rabbit serum was increased,there
was an increase in HMG Co-A reductase activity in the cells. Fig.1 also illustrates that an inverse correlation was observed between the serum concentration and cellular sterol content. Cells grown in 50% serum contained approximately 30% less cholesterol than did cells maintained in sterol-free
medium. Results obtained with monolayers of Fu5AH rat hepatoma cells also
demonstrated that growth of the cells in elevated concentrations of rabbit
serum resulted in a decrease in cellular cholesterol content and an elevation
in sterol synthesis. To determine if this phenomenon was linked to serum
LCAT activity, normal rabbit serum was incubated for 24 hours at 37° after
which the serum was heated or treated with N-ethyl-maleimide (NEM) to inactivate LCAT. The result of this incubation was a large increase in the
serum EC/FC ratio because the serum FC concentration was markedly reduced
with a concomitant rise in serum EC concentration. As a control, an aliquot
of the same serum was inactivated prior to the 24 hour preincubation period,
thus, this serum maintained an EC/FC within the normal range. Table 1 shows
the reductase activity and cholesterol content of Fu5AH hepatoma cells incubated for 18 hours in both unmodified and LCAT modified serum. The cells
maintained in the modified serum had a response pattern similar to that
previously observed with fresh rabbit serum. That is, the reductase activity
was stimulated at high serum concentrations and cellular cholesterol content
was reduced. However, cells maintained in unmodified serum had reductase
activities below that observed in DLP controls. In addition, these cells
exhibited an elevation in cholesterol content when compared to the control
cells grown in sterol-free medium. Rabbit serum was not unique in its ability
to stimulate cellular sterol synthesis when present at elevated concentrations;
rat and human serum produced similar effects. There was, however, considerable
variation among individual serum samples, as illustrated in Fig.2 which shows

[1] This work was supported in part by U.S.P.H.S. Grant number HL-22633 and
American Cancer Society Grant number IN-125.

the relative HMG Co-A reductase activities in Fu5AH cells following exposure to samples of human sera taken from normolipemic individuals and preincubated 18 hours before LCAT was inactivated by the addition of NEM. The reductase activity in the cells could be correlated with the magnitude of the LCAT modification (r = 0.8).

An experiment was conducted quantitating the release of labeled cholesterol from hepatoma cells exposed to fresh rabbit serum containing active LCAT. Increasing serum concentration resulted in greater loss of labeled cellular cholesterol which appeared in the culture medium. Exposure of prelabeled cells for 6 h to medium supplemented with 50% serum resulted in the efflux of 60% of the labeled cellular cholesterol. The increase in efflux observed with increasing serum concentration was accompanied by a reduction in cellular cholesterol content. After 6 hours incubation in 50% serum, approximately 30% of the FC that had been removed from the cells had been converted to EC via the action of LCAT.

Table 2 presents the results of an experiment designed to study the effect of LCAT modification of lipoprotein composition on cellular cholesterol flux. Monolayers of hepatoma cells prelabeled with ^{3}H-cholesterol were incubated for two hours in medium supplemented with either DLP, LCAT-modified HDL, or HDL which had undergone no modification because LCAT had been inhibited by the addition of NEM. The HDL was added to the culture medium together with the non-lipoprotein fraction of the serum. Incubation in DLP produced no significant changes in cellular cholesterol composition or specific activity

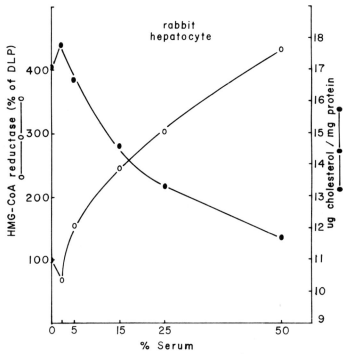

FIG.1. Influence of increasing concentrations of normal rabbit serum on HMG-CoA reductase activity and total cholesterol content of primary rabbit hepatocytes. Monolayers (60 mm dishes) of rabbit hepatocytes which had been plated for 18 h were refed with DLP supplemented medium for 24 h prior to refeeding with medium containing fresh, normal rabbit serum. Zero % serum samples were refed with DLP. Cells were incubated for 18 h. Points are the averages of three determinations.

during the two hour incubation period. Exposure of the cells to the modified HDL resulted in a 40% reduction of cellular FC content and efflux of 57% of the radiolabeled FC. The rate of cholesterol movement from cells to medium followed first order kinetics with a half time of cholesterol movement of 125 min. Assuming a linear change in cellular cholesterol specific activity during the two hour incubation, it can be calculated that the efflux averaged 0.08 ug/min/mg cell protein. When prelabeled cells were incubated with HDL which had not been modified by LCAT there was no significant change in FC content although 70% of the labeled FC appeared in the culture medium with its release following first order kinetics. The half time of release in this case was 72 minutes with a calculated efflux of 0.14 ug/min/mg cell protein. The specific activity of the FC remaining in the cells at the end of the incubation period was reduced by only 25% in cells exposed to the modified HDL, whereas control HDL produced a 65% reduction in specific activity. These results demonstrate that although extensive release of cellular cholesterol occurred with both lipoproteins, the influx of cholesterol was markedly reduced in cells exposed to the modified HDL. The reductase activity of the cells exposed to control and modified lipoproteins for 6 h are also shown in Table 2.

Discussion

The physiological significance of the action of LCAT on serum lipoproteins remains a topic of considerable controversy. One of the many roles which has been proposed for LCAT is in the removal of cellular cholesterol. In such a model, FC is released from peripheral cells onto HDL and is converted to EC by LCAT, thus, maintaining lipoprotein lipid composition and structure (Glomset 1968). This model can be further extended to predict that depletion in lipoprotein FC by the action of LCAT could result in the production of lipoproteins that stimulate efflux of cellular FC. If such a model were correct, exposure of tissue culture cells to lipoproteins which had been depleted in FC would result in enhanced cellular cholesterol efflux, which in turn would produce reduced cellular cholesterol content and elevated cholesterol synthesis. The results obtained from the present study using cultured liver cells demonstrated that exposure of such cells to LCAT-modified whole serum or serum HDL results in a reduction in cellular cholesterol content and stimulation in cholesterol synthesis; however, the mechanism by which LCAT produces these cellular responses does not appear to be

Table 1. Effect of LCAT modification of serum lipids on cholesterol content and synthesis in Fu5AH hepatoma cells.

Serum[a]	HMG-CoA Reductase (% of DLP) Serum Concentration		Cellular Cholesterol (ug/mg protein) Serum Concentration	
	5%	50%	5%	50%
Control Rabbit Serum	18	20	19.2	21.4
LCAT Modified Rabbit Serum	70	520	17.2	12.5

[a] Monolayers were incubated 24 hr. in DLP medium prior to refeeding with serum. Incubation time on serum was 18 hr. Control serum was heated(60° for 30 min) to inactivate LCAT prior to an 18 h preincubation at 37°. The EC/FC of this serum remained at 1.5. The LCAT modified serum was preincubated 18 h at 37° after which LCAT was inactivated by heating. The EC/FC of this serum rose to 6.6.

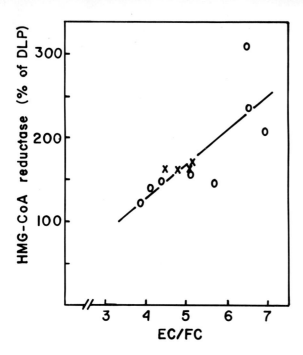

FIG. 2. Effect of individual samples of human serum on HMG-CoA reductase activity in Fu5AH cells. Serum obtained from normolipemic adults was preincubated 24 h at 37° after which LCAT was inactivated by the addition of NEM. Each sample was added to culture medium at a final concentration of 25%. Ru5AH cells were incubated in this medium for 4 h. HMG-CoA reductase activity, expressed relative to DLP grown controls, is plotted against the EC/FC ratio of the sera. 0---0 = female donor, X---X = male donor.

Table 2. Cholesterol flux in hepatoma cells exposed to control and LCAT modified HDL.

Medium Supplements	Cell Content (ug/mg protein)		^{3}H-cholesterol (cpm/mg protein)		FC Specific Activity (cpm x 10^{-3}/ug)	HMG-CoA Reductase [d] (% DLP control)
	FC	EC	FC	EC		
DLP(0 time)	12.9	0.6	101.9	5.2	7.9	--
DLP [a]	13.1	0.6	100.4	4.1	7.7	100
HDL (LCAT) modified) [b]	7.6	1.9	44.2	2.3	5.8	338
HDL (unmodified) [c]	12.3	1.8	32.0	2.5	2.6	50

[a] Delipidized serum protein at 5 mg/ml. Incubation time 2 h.
[b] Human serum protein d>1.063 preincubated 18 h at 37° prior to inactivation of LCAT by addition of NEM. Serum proteins added to culture medium at a concentration equivalent to 25% serum. Free cholesterol=1.7 ug/ml; cholesterol ester=138.6 ug/ml.Incubation time 2 h.
[c] Human serum proteins d>1.063 inactivated with NEM prior to preincubation. Serum proteins added to culture medium at a concentration equivalent to 25% serum. Free cholesterol=30.2 ug/ml; cholesterol ester=114.2 ug/ml. Incubation time 2 h.
[d] Reductase activity in cells after 6 hr incubation.

linked to a stimulation of cholesterol efflux, but rather, to a reduced uptake of cholesterol by cells exposed to serum in which the FC has been depleted by LCAT. That the increase in cellular HMG Co-A reductase activity
can be directly correlated to the EC/FC ratio achieved after LCAT modification of serum (Fig.2) lends support to a model in which the concentration of
FC in the serum lipoprotein plays a direct role in the regulation of cellular cholesterol metabolism. Previous studies using the Fu5AH hepatoma cells
demonstrated that increasing the FC to phospholipid molar ratio of HDL stimulated the net uptake of cholesterol by the cells and that this influx occurred, to large extent, without lipoprotein internalization (Rothblat 1978).
If increasing the FC/PL stimulates influx, it is probable that reducing this
ratio would decrease FC uptake by the cultured cells. If in the present experiments a reduction in the transfer of FC was the primary change provoked
by LCAT modification then surface transfer would have to be considered as a
quantitatively significant mechanism for supplying cholesterol to the cultured cells used in this study. Whether other cell types, such as smooth
muscle cells and fibroblasts would be as sensitive to the action of LCAT
remains to be investigated. It is probable that the ability of LCAT to modulate cellular cholesterol metabolism will be most obvious under conditions
where the physical/chemical transfer of cholesterol is the primary mechanism
for supplying cellular cholesterol.

References

Glomset JA (1972) In: Nelson GJ (ed) Blood Lipids and Lipoproteins: Quanti-
    tation, Composition and Metabolism. Wiley-Interscience, New York,
    pp 754-787
Glomset JA (1968) J Lipid Res 9:155-167
Rothblat GH, Arbogast LY, Ray EK (1978) J Lipid Res 19:350-358

Deposition and Hydrolysis of Cytoplasmic Triglyceride and Cholesterol Ester in Aortic Smooth Muscle Cells in Culture[1]

O. Stein, G.A. Coetzee, and Y. Stein

Introduction

Cellular cholesterol ester is localized in two main compartments, one intralysosomal, the other cytoplasmic (Fig. 1). The intralysosomal compartment is derived from the uptake of cholesterol ester containing lipoproteins and can be expanded either by increased uptake or by impairment of degradation. The extralysosomal compartment can be localized to cytoplasmic lipid droplets in cells which store normally esterified cholesterol, i.e., the adrenals. In human and in experimental atheroma, cholesterol ester accumulates apparently in both the intralysosomal and the cytoplasmic pools. Our previous studies have dealt mainly with the modulation of the intralysosomal pool (Stein et al. 1976; Stein et al. 1977; Stein et al. 1978) and the present investigation is concerned with the regulation of the cytoplasmic pool. In most instances, cytoplasmic cholesterol ester is found in close association with cytoplasmic triglyceride. Even though the enzymes active in the synthesis of both triglyceride and cholesterol ester are located in the endoplasmic reticulum, different enzyme systems are involved in the synthesis of these compounds. Neutral cholesterol ester hydrolase activity has been demonstrated in homogenates of cultured smooth muscle cells (Riddle et al. 1977). However, the exact localization, or the identity or nonidentity of triglyceride and cholesterol ester hydrolase has not been established. Studies in adipose tissue and in adrenal (Khoo et al. 1977; Pittman and Steinberg 1977) have shown a similarity between the enzymes acting on the two substrates and these neutral hydrolases have been shown to be hormone sensitive.

Selective perturbation of the cytoplasmic compartment

To study the degradation of cytoplasmic triglyceride and cholesterol ester in cultured aortic smooth muscle cells it was important to perturb and label selectively the cytoplasmic compartment only.

The triglyceride pool. Enrichment in cellular triglyceride was achieved with the help of a medium containing free fatty acid and in the presence of enhanced triglyceride synthesis. The addition of labeled glycerol resulted in a channeling of the label into triglyceride. To learn about the rate of hydrolysis of the cytoplasmic triglyceride the cells which had been labeled with ^{3}H glycerol were postincubated in the presence of chase glycerol. The appearance of the labeled glycerol in the medium and the disappearance of labeled triglyceride from the cells were compared in the presence or absence of Isuprel, or dibutyryl cyclic AMP and the results are shown in Fig. 2. Under the experimental conditions of multiple media changes and addition of

[1] This investigation was supported in part by a grant from the United States-Israel Binational Science Foundation and from the Delegation a la Recherche Scientifique et Technique of the French Government. Dr. G.A. Coetzee was a fellowship holder from the South African Medical Research Council. Dr. O. Stein and Dr. Y. Stein are Established Investigators of the Ministry of Health.

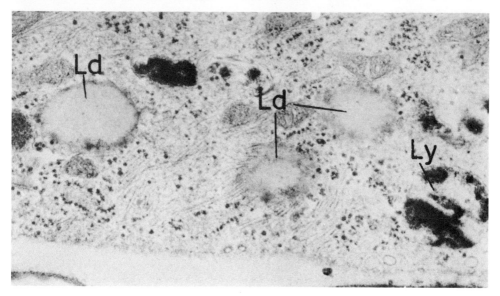

FIG. 1.   Electron micrograph of a section of cultured human skin fibroblasts demonstrating lipid deposition in the lysosomal (Ly) and cytoplasmic (Ld) compartments.   x 70,000.

TURNOVER OF ^{3}H-GLYCEROL LABELED TG IN BOVINE SMC

● Control   ○ dbcAMP   △ Isuprel

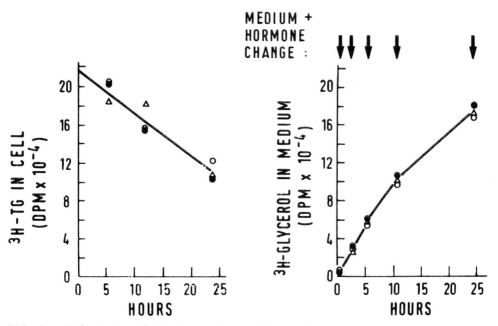

FIG. 2.   Hydrolysis of labeled triglyceride and release of labeled glycerol into medium.

the hormone or cyclic nucleotide at time intervals indicated by arrows the appearance of the label in the medium and loss of label from cellular triglyceride were not affected by the presence of Isuprel or dbc AMP. The smooth muscle cells derived from bovine aorta had a higher triglyceride content than the rat or rabbit aortic cells and a slower triglyceride loss following exposure to medium without added fatty acids. In order to determine whether indeed the catabolism of the triglyceride is due to the activity of a cytoplasmic rather than lysosomal hydrolases, the disappearance of labeled triglyceride was studied in the presence of high concentrations of chloroquine, and no changes in the rate of triglyceride hydrolysis were seen.

The cholesterol ester pool. A selective increase and labeling of the cytoplasmic cholesterol ester pool was made possible by using a medium enriched in unesterified cholesterol (Shinitzky 1978). It appears that when the ratio of free to esterified cholesterol in the medium is increased from 0.5 to 2.0 activation of acyl cholesterol transferase occurs. The events are depicted schematically in Fig. 3. This activation resulted in a 5-10 fold enhancement of incorporation of labeled free cholesterol into cholesterol ester, which could be used as a selective marker of the cytoplasmic cholesterol ester. At the same time there was a slight increase in cellular cholesterol ester content.

Intracellular hydrolysis of the labeled cholesterol ester was observed upon transfer of the cells to a medium containing the d > 1.25 fraction of serum (Fig. 4). The label appearing in the medium was in the form of free cholesterol. In analogy to the findings with the labeled triglyceride, addition of Isuprel or dbc AMP did not enhance cholesterol ester hydrolysis. In the presence of chloroquine there was no inhibition of the degradation of labeled cholesterol ester, and the residence time was even shortened apparently due to inhibition of cholesterol reesterification.

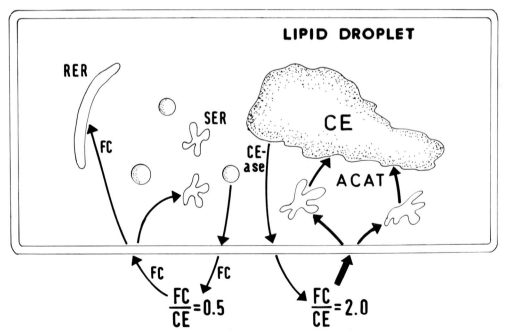

FIG. 3. Effect of increase in free cholesterol (FC) to esterified cholesterol (CE) in culture medium on deposition of cholesterol ester in cultured cells.

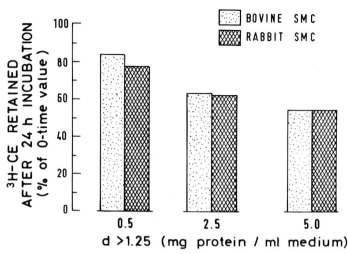

EFFECT OF PROTEIN CONCENTRATION OF d > 1.25
ON THE LOSS OF ^{3}H-CE

FIG. 4. Effect of d > 1.25 fraction of serum on loss of ^{3}H-cholesterol ester from cultured smooth muscle cells.

Conclusions

The possible role of cytoplasmic triglyceride and cholesterol ester hydrolases lies in the potential reversal of lesions in which the accumulated lipid is mainly intracellular. Some evidence for the regression of such lesions in experimental animals has been well documented. It would be most important to determine whether the rate of cholesterol ester hydrolysis can be further stimulated by agents such as prostaglandins or potent acceptors of free cholesterol and studies to be reported indicate that apoprotein phospholipid complexes might be active in this direction.

References

Khoo JC, Sperry PJ, Gill GN, Steinberg D (1977) Activation of hormone-sensitive lipase and phosphorylase kinase by purified cyclic GMP-dependent protein kinase. Proc Natl Acad Sci USA 74: 4843-4847

Pittman RC, Steinberg D (1977) Activatable cholesterol esterase and triacylglycerol lipase activities of rat adrenal and their relationship. Biochim Biophys Acta 487: 431-444

Riddle MC, Fujimoto W, Ross R (1977) Two cholesterol ester hydrolases. Distribution in rat tissues and in cultured human fibroblasts and monkey arterial smooth muscle cells. Biochim Biophys Acta 488: 359-369

Shinitzky M (1978) An efficient method for modulation of cholesterol level in cell membranes. FEBS Letters 85: 317-320

Stein O, Vanderhoek J, Friedman G, Stein Y (1976) Deposition and mobilization of cholesterol ester in cultured human skin fibroblasts. Biochim Biophys Acta 450: 367-378

Stein O, Vanderhoek J, Stein Y (1977) Cholesterol ester accumulation in cultured aortic smooth muscle cells. Atherosclerosis 26: 465-482

Stein Y, Friedman G, Stein O (1978) Intralysosomal accretion of cholesterol ester in vascular cells in culture and its translocation into the cytoplasma. In: Paoletti R, Gotto AM (eds) Atherosclerosis Reviews. Raven Press, New York, Vol 3, pp 97-108

The Role of the Liver in LDL Catabolism

Daniel Steinberg, Ray C. Pittman, Alan D. Attie, Thomas E. Carew, Sharon Pangburn, and
David Weinstein

In 1974 we showed that after total hepatectomy both pigs and dogs degrade
injected ^{125}I-LDL at a rate equal to or actually greater than the rate in
the intact animal (Sniderman et al. 1974). Those results established for
the first time the large potential capacity of extrahepatic tissues to degrade LDL in vivo. However, no final quantitative conclusions could be reached
regarding the relative roles of liver and extrahepatic tissues in the intact
animal because of the possible perturbations accompanying hepatectomy. The
very fact that fractional catabolic rate increased after hepatectomy indicated
that some acute change induced by the procedure must influence extrahepatic
LDL metabolism. A hypothesis that might explain the phenomenon was advanced
(Steinberg et al. 1974) but others are possible and the basis for the paradoxical finding remains undefined. Nor did those studies provide any independent assessment of the relative contribution of different extrahepatic
tissues to overall LDL degradation.

We have now devised a novel approach to the latter problem (Pittman and
Steinberg, 1978; Pittman, et al. 1979a,b). The method capitalizes on the
fact that sucrose is degraded very slowly if at all by lysosomal hydrolases
(i.e. mammalian lysosomes contain little if any sucrose) and the fact that
intact sucrose crosses the lysosomal membrane very slowly. These properties
of sucrose have made it a useful molecule for quantifying pinocytosis in
cultured cells (Cohn and Ehrenreich 1969). One simply incubates cells in
the presence of ^{14}C-sucrose, washes them and determines the ^{14}C accumulating.
Over periods up to 24 hours the leakage back to the medium is minor.

The rationale of the method is schematized in Fig. 1. ^{14}C-sucrose, activated
with cyanuric chloride, is coupled covalently to amino groups of the LDL
apoprotein. Each LDL molecule taken up by endocytosis thus carries ^{14}C-
sucrose with it into the lysosome. There the apoprotein is rapidly degraded
and the free amino acids escape rapidly to appear in the culture medium or
in the plasma. The sucrose derivative, however, (and probably a short peptide in the vicinity of its attachment to the protein), cannot escape and
the ^{14}C-sucrose accumulates. Knowing the specific activity of the $[^{14}$C-
sucrose]LDL, one can calculate the total number of LDL molecules degraded
over any given experimental period by simply measuring the total ^{14}C-sucrose
accumulated in low-molecular weight degradation products. These underlying
assumptions have been validated in cell culture studies and in in vivo studies
(Pittman et al. 1979a,b). Briefly stated, when $[^{14}$C-sucrose]LDL is incubated
with human skin fibroblasts, ^{14}C accumulates intracellularly in an amount
equivalent to the amount of LDL degraded (simultaneously determined using
^{125}I-LDL and measuring accumulation of TCA-soluble ^{125}I in the medium). Leakage of ^{14}C back to the medium was less than 10% in 24 h. Asialofetuin, a
protein known to be very rapidly and selectively removed by the liver (Ashwell and Morell 1974), was labeled with ^{14}C-sucrose and injected into rats.
At 1 h 88% of the ^{14}C was found in the liver and about 10% in the sum of
extrahepatic tissues. At 24 h the ^{14}C in extrahepatic tissues had not changed;
the ^{14}C in liver had decreased by about 25% but the loss was accounted for by
biliary excretion. These data suggest that there was no appreciable redistribution, i.e. that the ^{14}C-sucrose degradation products were effectively
trapped.

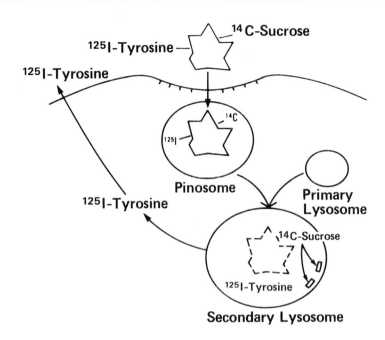

FIG. 1. Schematic representation of the rationale for the use of ^{14}C-sucrose covalently bonded to protein to quantify lysosomal protein degradation in a cumulative manner.

Swine LDL was tagged with ^{14}C-sucrose and injected intravenously into normal, conscious swine via an indwelling catheter. Analysis of the plasma decay curves showed that the fractional catabolic rates of the [^{14}C-sucrose]LDL were the same as those observed using ^{125}I-LDL. Recipients were killed at 24 or 48 h and tissues surveyed for ^{14}C-sucrose degradation products after precipitation of intact LDL. Organ contents of ^{14}C were related to the amount of LDL irreversibly catabolized (calculated from the plasma decay curve).

As shown in Fig. 2, the liver accounted for 39% of LDL catabolized over 24 h. Results at 48 h were similar. In 2 cases, parenchymal cells were separated from nonparenchymal cells. Over 90% of the ^{14}C was recovered in parenchymal cells. About 35% of LDL catabolized was accounted for by the sum of ^{14}C degradation products recovered in the extrahepatic tissues examined. Interestingly adipose tissue was a major site of LDL catabolism, consonant with the high rate of LDL degradation reported for isolated human adipocytes (Angel et al. 1979). The value for intestine may be high due to binding or uptake of ^{14}C excreted in bile. Every tissue examined contained ^{14}C, i.e evidently all tissues participate in LDL degradation to some extent.

In Fig. 3 the data are expressed in terms of the activity of each tissue in LDL degradation per gram wet weight, assigning liver a value of 100. The adrenal was the most active user of LDL per unit tissue weight, the only tissue more active than liver. Assuming LDL cholesterol is taken up in proportion to LDL protein we could calculate daily delivery of cholesterol to the adrenal in LDL. The value was 1.4 mg/d, enough to provide precursor for maximal steroidogenesis (Dvorak 1972). These results are consonant with those of Kovanen et al. (1979) showing that the plasma membrane isolated from bovine adrenal has the highest density of specific LDL receptors of any tissue membranes examined. The relatively high activity of spleen and lymph nodes suggests some preferential uptake in reticuloendothelial cells. Adipose tissue

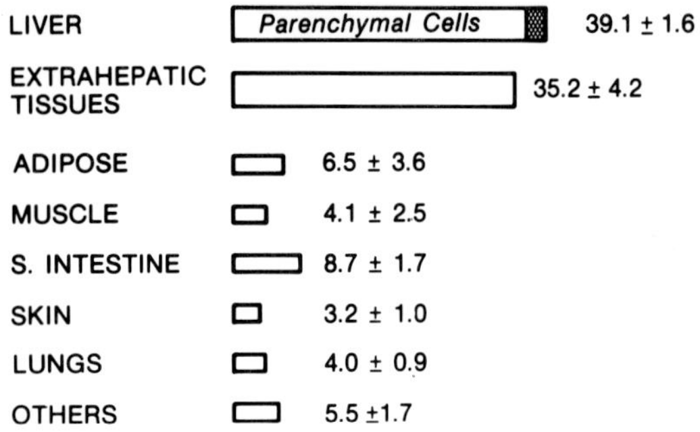

LIVER
Parenchymal Cells
39.1 ± 1.6
EXTRAHEPATIC TISSUES
35.2 ± 4.2
ADIPOSE
6.5 ± 3.6
MUSCLE
4.1 ± 2.5
S. INTESTINE
8.7 ± 1.7
SKIN
3.2 ± 1.0
LUNGS
4.0 ± 0.9
OTHERS
5.5 ±1.7

FIG. 2. Recoveries in major organs of ^{14}C-sucrose degradation products from [^{14}C-sucrose]LDL injected intravenously into pigs 24 h before sacrifice (mean and standard error for three studies). Recoveries expressed as a percentage of the total amount of labeled LDL irreversibly catabolized over 24 h (calculated from plasma decay curve).

is low in the ranking using total wet weight as denominator. However, if one neglects stored fat and expresses results per mg cell protein, adipose tissue is actually one of the most active tissues.

Knowing that liver is a major site of LDL degradation _in vivo_ we wanted to know if liver cells had a high affinity LDL receptor. Studies in cultured rat hepatocytes using human LDL showed little evidence for a specific receptor (Pangburn SH, Weinstein DB, Steinberg D, unpublished results). Recently we have been able to prepare from the liver of young pigs cells that adhere to cell culture dishes and proliferate in an arginine-free medium. Further characterization as parenchymal cells is in progress. Binding of homologous LDL to these cells as a function of concentration is biphasic as is also degradation as a function of concentration. Addition of excess unlabeled native LDL reduced degradation of ^{125}I-LDL by over 80% but prior reductive methylation of the unlabeled LDL markedly reduced its effectiveness as a competitor. Weisgraber et al. (1978) have shown that such methylation blocks lysine amino groups essential for binding of LDL to its receptor on human skin fibroblasts. Bachorik et al. (1978) have described specific binding of procine LDL to a plasma membrane fraction from procine liver although the specific cell type yielding the plasma membranes responsible for the specific binding was not determined. Thus pig liver appears to have a receptor analogous to the fibroblast receptor. Regulation of this receptor could play an important role in LDL homeostasis since almost one-half of the LDL degraded is degraded in the liver. For example, depletion of hepatic

0
100
200
ADRENAL
LIVER
SPLEEN
SKIN
LYMPH NODES
PANCREAS
AORTA
SMALL INTESTINE
LUNGS
KIDNEY
ADIPOSE TISSUE
LARGE INTESTINE, BRAIN, HEART, MUSCLE

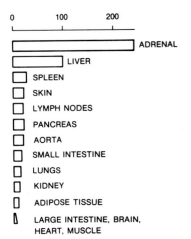

FIG. 3. Relative _in vivo_ activities of pig tissues in uptake of LDL per unit wet weight calculated from ^{14}C-sucrose degradation products recovered 24 h after intravenous injection of [^{14}C-sucrose]LDL.

cholesterol induced by diet or drugs may induce the hepatic receptor as it does in peripheral cells. This could lead to increased catabolism of LDL and reduction in LDL levels. We have previously suggested that an hepatic receptor may also play a role in regulation of lipoprotein secretion (Steinberg 1979). The absence of the hepatic receptor in homozygous familial hypercholesterolemia could then account for unrestrained production and the increased LDL production seen in such patients (Soutar et al. 1977).

References

Angel, A, D'Costa, MA, Yuen, R (1979) Low density lipoprotein binding, internalization, and degradation in human adipose cells. Canad J Biochem 57: 578–587

Ashwell, G, Morell, AG (1974) The role of surface carbohydrates in the hepatic recognition and transport of circulating glycoproteins. Avd Enzymol 41: 99–128

Bachorik, PS, Kwiterovich, PO, Cooke, JC (1978) Isolation of a porcine liver plasma membrane fraction that specifically binds low density lipoproteins. Biochem 17: 5287–5299

Cohn, ZA, Ehrenreich, BA (1969) The uptake, storage and intracellular hydrolysis of carbohydrates by macrophages. J exp Med 129: 201–225

Dvorak, M (1972) Adrenocortical functions in foetal, neonatal and young pigs. J Endocrinol 54: 473–481

Kovanen, PT, Basu, SK, Coldstein, JL, Brown, MS (1979) Low density lipoprotein receptors in bovine adrenal cortex. II. Low density lipoprotein binding to membranes prepared from fresh tissue. Endocrinology 104: 610–616

Pittman, RC, Steinberg, D (1978) A new approach for assessing cumulative lysosomal degradation of proteins or other macromolecules. Biochem Biophys Res Commun 81: 1254–1259

Pittman, RC, Green SR, Attie, AD, Steinberg, D (1979a) Radiolabeled sucrose covalently linked to protein: A device for quantifying degradation of plasma proteins catabolized by lysosomal mechanisms. J Biol Chem 254: 6876–6879

Pittman, RC, Attie, AD, Carew, TE, Steinberg, D (1979b) Tissue sites of degradation of low density lipoprotein: Application of a new general method for determining the fate of plasma proteins. Proc Nat Acad Sci 76: 5345–5349

Sniderman, AD, Carew, TE, Chandler, JG, Steinberg, D (1974) Paradoxical increase in rate of catabolism of low-density lipoproteins after hepatectomy. Science 183: 526–528

Soutar, AK, Myant, NB, Thompson, GR (1977) Simultaneous measurement of apolipoprotein B turnover in very-low- and low-density lipoproteins in familial hypercholesterolaemia. Atherosclerosis 28: 247–256

Steinberg, D (1979) Origin, turnover and fate of plasma low-density lipoprotein. Prog BiochemPharmacol 15: 166–199

Steinberg, D, Carew, TE, Chandler, JG, Sniderman, AD (1974) The role of the liver in metabolism of plasma lipoproteins. In: Lundquist, Tygstrup (eds) Munksgaard, Copenhagen (Regulation of Hepatic Metabolism, pp 144–156)

Steinberg, D, Pittman, RC, Attie, AD, Carew, TE (1979) Tissue sites of low density lipoprotein degradation determined by a novel tracer technique. Clin Res 27: 518A

Weisgraber, KH, Innerarity, TL, Mahley, RW (1978) Role of the lysine residues of plasma lipoproteins in high affinity binding to cell surface receptors in human fibroblasts. J Biol Chem 253: 9053–9062

Standardization of Apolipoprotein Immunoassays by an Isotope Dilution Method[1]

Philip Weech, Walter J. McConathy, Petar Alaupovic, and James Fesmire

Plasma lipoproteins consist of a mixture of lipid-protein particles differing in hydrated density, size and chemical composition (Nichols, 1967). The recognized existence of at least nine well-characterized apolipoproteins and their distribution throughout the entire density spectrum are further indications of the complex nature of this macromolecular system (Osborne and Brewer, 1977; Olofsson et al. 1978). As distinct constituents, the apolipoproteins represent suitable markers for the identification and differentiation of lipoprotein particles. To assess the physiological role of apolipoproteins in lipid transport processes and to evaluate the potential use of apolipoprotein profiles in clinical practice, various immunochemical procedures have been developed for the quantitative determination of almost all known plasma apolipoproteins (Alaupovic et al. 1978; Albers 1978). Although all three immunoassays, i.e., radioimmunoassay, radial immunodiffusion and electroimmunoassay, display a high degree of specificity, sensitivity and precision, the standardization of individual assays and the assessment of accuracy remain unsolved problems. To establish a standard for accuracy, we have applied a simple isotope dilution method to determine the A-II content in HDL_3. This method also furnishes a standard for electroimmunoassay, not as a delipidized polypeptide but as a lipoprotein.

The A-II polypeptide was isolated by chromatography of a totally delipidized HDL_3 (d 1.12 – 1.23 g/ml) on a column (200 x 2.5 cm) of Sephadex G-75 equilibrated with 2 M acetic acid. The totally delipidized HDL_3 was applied in 2 M acetic acid containing 2 M ultrapure urea and eluted by 2 M acetic acid. After concentration with polyethylene glycol (MW = 20,000) and rechromatography on the Sephadex G-75 column, the A-II peak was concentrated again, dialyzed against 6 M Gu·HCl, pH 7.2, and chromatographed in a column (100 x 2.5 cm) of Sephadex G-100 equilibrated with 6 M Gu·HCl, pH 7.2. The A-II polypeptide was characterized by polyacrylamide gel electrophoresis in the presence and absence of sodium dodecyl sulfate, double diffusion analyses with monospecific antisera to all known apolipoproteins and by amino acid analysis. An aliquot of this preparation (1.01 mg) was labeled with 0.5 mCi ^{125}I by the procedure described by Weech et al. (1978). This labeled A-II preparation was diluted with 10.6 mg of unlabeled A-II and dissolved in phosphate buffer. An aliquot of this solution was added to a sample of HDL_3 isolated from 200 ml plasma. This mixture was dialyzed against distilled water, lyophilized and delipidized by the procedure described by Olofsson et al. (1978). The A-II polypeptide was reisolated from this delipidized HDL_3 preparation by the same procedure as described above. The composition and concentration of A-II was determined by amino acid analysis and the radioactivity in the same A-II solution was measured in a Beckman Gamma 310 scintillation spectrometer with a NaI crystal. Data for ^{125}I counts were corrected to disintegrations per minute (dpm) using efficiencies determined individually for each sample by the method described by Horrocks (1975). The ^{125}I dpm were corrected for isotope decay back to a reference time.

[1] This study was supported in part by Grant HL-23181 from the U.S. Public Health Service.

The amount of A-II polypeptide in the aliquot of HDL_3 was calculated using the following relation:

$$Mu = \frac{Ao}{SA_r} - Mo$$

where, Mu is the unknown mass (mg) of A-II in the HDL_3 aliquot
Mo is the mass (mg) of labeled A-II added to the HDL_3 aliquot
Ao is the activity (in dpm) of ^{125}I-A-II added to the HDL_3 aliquot
SA_r is the specific activity (in dpm/mg protein) of reisolated A-II polypeptide.

As an example, the following experimental values were obtained:

$$Mu = \frac{1.850 \cdot 10^8}{3.555 \cdot 10^6} - 2.170$$

Therefore, 49.9 mg of A-II polypeptide were present in the original aliquot of HDL_3.

By amino acid analysis this HDL_3 aliquot contained 135 mg of protein, containing 16.3 μmoles of histidine. Since histidine is missing from A-II, we estimated the amount of protein in the HDL_3 that could be accounted for by A-I polypeptide. Based on the presence of 5 moles of histidine residues per mole of A-I, a sample of 135 mg of delipidized HDL_3 could have contained 92.4 mg of A-I. Since there are small amounts of other polypeptides containing histidine in HDL_3, this figure represents the maximum content of A-I and will be in error proportionally to the content of other polypeptides. Nevertheless, it predicts that the maximum amount of A-I is the difference between the total protein in this HDL_3 preparation and the measured content of A-II. Thus, the amino acid analysis of HDL_3 appears to offer a rapid way to estimate the maximum A-I content of HDL_3 which can then be used as a standard for calibrating immunoassays.

Using a pool of HDL_3 as a standard with A-I content calculated in this manner, Table 1 summarizes the values for levels of A-I and A-II polypeptides in the plasma of normolipidemic subjects. The conditions for electroimmunoassays were those described by Curry et al.(1976). The data demonstrated a significant ($p < 0.05$) age-related increase of both A-I and A-II considering both men and women together. This same effect was also evident when the sexes were considered separately, though the differences in A-II levels were less significant. A sex-difference in A-I level was evident between men and women in the young age group. There were no significant differences between men and women in the older age group.

The accuracy with which we determined the content of A-II in an HDL_3 sample depended on at least five factors

1. The accuracy of protein determinations by amino acid analysis
2. The accuracy of radioactivity determinations
3. The identical behavior of the labeled and unlabeled compound during fractionation
4. The ability to isolate and reisolate the polypeptide in an adequately pure form
5. The acceptability of that polypeptide as a 'true and unique' compound

The action of the first two factors is simple and obvious. A basic assumption with this method is that the third factor holds true. The action of the latter two factors would be to generate a discrepancy between the protein determination and the amount of A-II. If the isolated or reisolated poly-

Table 1. Concentration of apolipoproteins A-I and A-II in plasma of normolipidemic men and women[*]

Age		A-I			A-II	
	n	Men	n	Women	Men	Women
< 39	11	114 + 15	16	125 + 13	53 + 7.9	58 + 8.4
> 40	15	136 + 31	14	151 + 29	64 + 20.2	63 + 8.8

[*]Mean (mg/dl) + S.D.

peptide contains an impurity then the estimate of A-II in HDL3 will be excessive. If the A-II preparation was in fact a mixture then the result of the determination will reflect the total of that mixture only so long as each component of the mixture can be recovered to the same extent during isolation. The use of the radioactive label permitted us to observe the behavior of the labeled polypeptide, and comparison with the mass of protein during isolation allowed us to verify that they both had the properties of A-II, a necessary criterion for this method.

The results indicate that the molar ratio of A-I:A-II in this HDL3 is close to 1. It seems that this method is equally applicable to A-II in plasma. Since methods exist for the isolation of other well-characterized apolipoproteins then the method should be applicable to them also.

Acknowledgments

We thank Mrs. R. Ballou and Mr. T. Gross for valuable technical assistance and Mrs. M. Farmer for typing the manuscript.

References

Alaupovic P, Curry MD, McConathy WJ (1978) Quantitative determination of human plasma apolipoproteins by electroimmunoassays. In: Carlson LA, Paoletti R, Sirtori CR, Weber G (eds) International Conference on Atherosclerosis. Raven Press, New York, pp 109–115
Albers JJ (1978) An introduction to lipoprotein immunoassays. Test of the Month 4, No. 2
Curry MD, Alaupovic P, Suenram CA (1976) Determination of apolipoprotein A and its constitutive A-I and A-II polypeptides by separate electroimmunoassays. Clin Chem 22: 315–322
Horrocks DL (1975) Standardizing ^{125}I source and determining ^{125}I counting efficiencies of well-type gamma counting systems. Clin Chem 21: 370–375
Nichols AV (1967) Human serum lipoproteins and their relationships. In: Lawrence TH, Gofman JW (eds) Advances in biological and medical physics. Vol 11, Academic Press, New York, pp 109–158
Olofsson SO, McConathy WJ, Alaupovic P (1978) Isolation and partial characterization of a new acidic apolipoprotein (apolipoprotein F) from high density lipoproteins of human plasma. Biochemistry 17: 1032–1036
Osborne JC, Brewer HB, Jr (1977) The plasma lipoproteins. Adv. Protein Chem. 31: 253–337
Weech PK, McTaggart F, Mills GL (1978) Comparison of guinea-pig serum lipoproteins after iodination by two different methods. Biochem J 169: 687–695

Rate-Nephelometry of A-I and Electrophoresis[1]

N. Weinstock, M. Bartholomé, and D. Seidel

Concentrations of A-I, HDL-C and α-lipoproteins have recently been determined and correlated as risk-factors for coronary heart disease. In order to evaluate and appraise the measurement of these compounds for epidemiological studies or general clinical use, the method applied must fulfill certain criteria. The method should be easy to perform, fast, not too laborious and should allow wide use in general clinical laboratories. The method must also fulfill basic criteria of quality control for a clinical chemical analysis, especially with respect to precision and accuracy.

Previous studies from our laboratory have shown that these criteria are fulfilled in principle by the quantitative lipoprotein electrophoresis on agarose, using a polyanion precipitation technique to visualize the bands. An important advantage of this method is not only the measurement of the individual lipoprotein bands, but also that of the relative concentration ratios with high precisions (Wieland and Seidel 1978).

As to A-I, in recent years several methods have been introduced to measure this apoprotein, most of which are based on an immunological reaction of a specific anti-A-I serum with this major apoprotein of the high-density-class or α-lipoprotein band. As noted in other presentations in this workshop as well as in previous publications, the widely used methods are in principle based either on electroimmunoassay, radioimmunoassay or radial immunodiffusion techniques. Since nephelometric measurement of proteins in body fluids has recently become attractive in general clinical chemistry, we utilized the Beckman rate-nephelometric system for apoA-I quantification. General advantages of the nephelometry are that it does not involve radioactivity and is fast (to perform); moreover, because rate-nephelometry utilizes the kinetic of the antibody:antigen reaction, it is far less influenced by background turbidity of the sample and works faster than any other nephelometric system. In rate-nephelometry the change of the forward scattered light (predominantly MIE-scattering) is measured.

Method

The experimental conditions of our method may be summarized as follows: We are using the Immunochemistry-System by Beckman. A 0.02 M phosphate buffer, pH 7.1, containing 4 g polyethyleneglycol per liter is used as reaction solution. To 100 ml of this buffer 12 ml of antiserum are added, and the mixture is incubated for at least 12 hours at room temperature before use. Thereafter the mixture is centrifuged for 15 to 20 min at 3000 RPM, filtered and degassed. Such a preparation may be kept at $4°C$ in a refrigerator for as long as 3 weeks without alteration.

[1] Supported by Deutsche Forschungsgemeinschaft, SFB 89.

807

In general serum samples are diluted 1:36 with 0.9% sodiumchloride and "delipidized" using Tween 20^R in a final concentration of 1% (v/v). For the reaction, 42 µl of the diluted serum are added to 600 µl of the antiserum buffer solution (∿ 65 µml antiserum per sample). The measurement taked place in a special glass cell under constant stirring at a wavelength in the range 400-500 nm. The time for measurement is usually less than 1 min per sample. The signals obtained by the system are plotted on a two-channel recorder as light scattering and as a curve of the first derivative of the light scattering signal expressed as rate units. The immunoprecipitin reaction of the system shows the typical behavior in both the antibody excess and antigen excess ranges. Under the conditions of our assay no antigen excess test is required because we are working far below the point of equivalence (Fig. 1). The maximum of this change, "the peak rate," is a measure of the antigen concentration under conditions of excess antibody. Using a polymer-reaction-enhancer, this maximum may be reached within one minute. Within the normal range of A-I concentrations the rate unit curves approximate straight lines for both "delipidized" and whole serum samples. It is of interest to note that the correlation between treated samples and whole serum samples are highly constant as long as normal serum samples are used. Standardization of apoprotein concentration from rate units is estimated and based on the following criteria and assumptions.

The experimental mean value of A-I rate units are determined on samples taken from 500 blood donors (aged 18 to 40 years). The mean values of A-I concentrations expressed in mg/dl are taken from previously published work (approximately 120 mg/dl) (Fainaru et al. 1975; Kostner et al. 1979; Reman et al. 1978; Schonfeld et al. 1974). The correlation between milligrams per deciliter and rate units follows a mathematical approach for the overall reaction kinetics of the rate nephelometric system which depends on the antigen and the antibody, as well as on factors specific to the system.

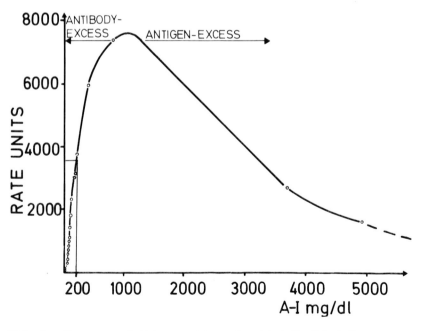

FIG. 1.   Immunoprecipitin reaction of anti-A-I with A-I as measured by rate nephelometry (rate units versus A-I concentration).

As the normal range for our A-I method shows a reaction curve close to linear, this mathematical approach of the overall reaction can be simplified to a linear equation. Conversion from rate units into mg/dl A-I can therefore be calculated according to equation 5 of Table 1.

As to the question of precision of the method we established a coefficient of variance of 1.44% within one series of 20 samples. The day-to-day precision is also remarkably good in both lyophilized and deep frozen (-80° C) serum samples, with a coefficient of variance of 1.75% for lyophilized sera and of 3.65% for deep frozen (-80° C) sera.

Since it was thought that parts of the antigen side of A-I may be covered by lipids or may be inaccessible to the antibody in the intact lipoprotein particle, the influence of delipidation and temperature incubation was studied on both whole serum and on isolated lipoproteins. While for whole serum, temperatures up to 37°C and incubation up to 14 hours have no significant influence, the A-I accessibility to the antibody shows a slight increase for isolated HDL by incubation at temperatures as low as 25°C for a period of 14 hours. Incubation at 56°C revealed for isolated HDL a preliminary increase followed by a decrease probably due to denaturation after 14 hours, and for whole serum a significant and constant increase during the incubation time of 14 hours. Delipidation with both butanol-di-isopropyl ether and Tween 20R causes an increase of the signals close to 250% compared with the untreated whole serum. It is interesting, however, and important to note that a change of this magnitude holds only for normal sera and may be different or even zero in different pathological states. This phenomenon is currently under investigation in our laboratory. Estimation of the distribution of A-I in plasma fractions revealed that only 1-3% of A-I are found within the density class d < 1.063 g/ml while 85-87% are concentrated in the HDL fractions; up to 12% can be

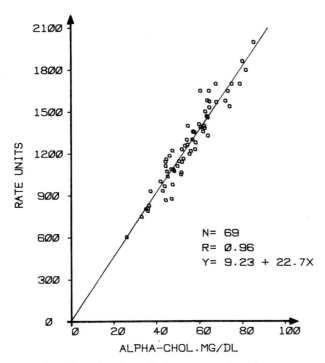

FIG. 2. Correlation of A-I concentration versus alpha-cholesterol.

Table 1. Standardization of the rate nephelometric method for the determination of A-I.

---

1) Experimental mean value for the A-I concentration (RU) of 500 female blood donors aged 18-40 years.

$$\bar{X}_{RU} = 1280 \text{ RU}$$

2) Mean value for the A-I concentration (mg/dl) taken from the published work of other authors.

$$\bar{X}_{A-I} = 120 \text{ mg/dl}$$

3) Mathematical approach for the overall reaction kinetic.

$$RU_{A-I} = \frac{K \cdot U \cdot (A-I)^2 \cdot (1-\frac{1}{s} \cdot A-I)}{1 + (U-\frac{1}{s}) \cdot A-I}$$

4) Mathematical approach valid for values in normal range.

$$RU_{A-I} = m \cdot A-I + b$$

5) The concentration of A-I in mg/dl can be calculated from the measured RU by using the rearranged equation 4). b and m are calculated from 1) and 2).

$$A-I = \frac{RU_{A-I} - b}{m}$$

$$m = 16.64 \qquad b = -718.6$$

---

found in the 1.21 g/ml bottom fraction after ultracentrifugation of whole plasma. Precipitation by polyanions revealed 15-25% in the lipoprotein free fraction.

Comparison of the quantitative serum lipoprotein electrophoresis with rate-nephelometry revealed an excellent correlation of A-I versus α-cholesterol concentration of $r = 0.96$ (Fig. 2). These findings indicate a very constant composition of normal α-lipoproteins for both A-I and cholesterol.

In conclusion the presented rate-nephelometric method for A-I determination has proved to fulfill critical criteria necessary for clinical chemical methods. It is easy to handle, timesaving, and is characterized by high sensitivity and excellent precision. The correlation between A-I determined by rate-nephelometry and α-cholesterol determined by quantitative lipoprotein electrophoresis is excellent ($r = 0.96$). We therefore can recommend rate-nephelometry as an additional tool to measure A-I concentration in whole serum. Its clinical value will have to be established in future studies.

References

Fainaru M, Glangeaud MC, Eisenberg S (1975) Radioimmunoassay of human high density lipoprotein apoprotein A-I. Biochim Biophys Acta 386:432
Kostner GM, Avogaro P, Bon GB, Cazzolato G, Quinci GB (1979) Determination of high-density lipoproteins: Screening methods compared. Clin Chem 25: 939
Reman FC, Vermond A (1978) The quantitative determination of apolipoprotein A-I (apo-1p-Gln I) in human serum by radial immunodiffusion assay (RID). Clin Chim Acta 87:387
Schonfeld G, Pfleger B (1974) The structure of human high density lipoprotein and the levels of apolipoprotein A-I in plasma as determined by radioimmunoassay. J Clin Invest 54:236
Wieland H, Seidel D (1978) Advances in the analysis of plasma lipoproteins. Innere Medizin 5:290

Methodological Considerations in Apolipoprotein Immunoassay[1]

J.J. Albers,[2] M.C. Cheung, and C.-H. Floren

The radial immunodiffusion technique has been used for quantification of immunoglobulins and various plasma proteins (Fahey and McKelvey 1965; Storiko 1968). In our laboratory, we have used it to quantitate various apoproteins, including A-I, A-II, and B, and the Lp(a) lipoprotein (Albers et al. 1975, 1976; Albers and Hazzard 1974; Cheung and Albers 1977).

Quantification by radial immunodiffusion has been reported to be very precise by Mancini et al. (1965), but the application of this method for the determination of apoproteins and lipoproteins is not without difficulties. The present discussion will focus on the difficulties one encounters in apoprotein radial immunodiffusion assays. Some of these difficulties apply also to the other two immunochemical techniqes already discussed, namely, radioimmunoassay and electroimmunoassay.

The principle of radial immunodiffusion assay is simple. When an antigen is allowed to diffuse freely and radially from a well into an agar gel medium homogeneously impregnated with antibody, an immune complex in the form of a precipitate is formed around the well. At equilibrium, the surface area of the precipitation ring is directly proportional to the initial concentration of the antigen. To be able to apply this technique successfully as a quantification method, one has to meet certain basic requirements:

1. The antibody used must be specific for the given antigen so that multiple rings of precipitation will not form.

2. The antigen must be in a soluble state to be able to migrate freely into the agar gel.

3. The concentration of the antigen should be greater than 1 µg/ml, for two reasons. First, the concentration of the antigen must be higher than the antibody in the agar gel for the antigen to diffuse into the gel. Secondly, the sensitivity of the method depends on the visibility of the precipitate at equilibrium. When the concentrations of antigen and antibody are too low, the precipitation ring becomes so faint that one cannot visualize it without further treatment of the agar gel. Under the usual conditions, the lower limit of sensitivity of the technique is approximately 10 µg/ml. However, by intensifying the precipitation rings with various agents such as tannic acid (Simmons 1971), DL-DOPA (DL- 3, 4 dihydroxyphenylalanine) (Sieber and Becker 1974), ethanol (Wieja and Smith 1976), or a second anti-

[1]Supported in part by Contract HV-12157, Lipid Metabolism Branch, National Heart, Lung, and Blood Institute, National Institutes of Health.
[2]J.J. Albers is an Established Investigator of the American Heart Association.

body directed against the immunoglobulin used (Darcy 1972) one can increase the sensitivity of the radial immunodiffusion assay approximately tenfold to 1 μg/ml.

4. The accuracy of radial immunodiffusion assay relies on the comparability of the precipitation rings formed between standard antigen and antibody with those formed between test antigen and the same antibody at a fixed antibody concentration. The diameter of the precipitation ring varies not only with the antigen concentration but also with the molecular size of the migrating antigen. Hence, it is essential that the test and standard antigens are of similar size if monodisperse, or of similar size distribution if polydisperse.

5. Furthermore, the test and standard antigens should have similar immunoreactivity per unit of protein antigen.

Requirements 1–3 can be easily met in the development of lipoprotein or apoprotein immunoassays; but because of a number of unique physicochemical properties of lipoproteins, requirements 4 and 5 sometimes create difficulties. Some of these properties are as follows:

1. Lipoprotein polydispersity and immunochemical heterogeneity. Most of the apoproteins, such as the B, C, D, and E apoproteins, are common to different lipoprotein classes, which differ not only in size and hydrated density but also in lipid and protein composition. Hence, the immunoreactivity of a given apoprotein in intact lipoproteins may vary with the particular lipoprotein species.

2. Masking of antigen determinants by lipid. Apoproteins have a strong affinity for lipids, particularly phospholipids, because of their ability to form amphipathic helices. The presence of lipids may sometimes mask the antigenic sites or change the conformation of the apoprotein, so that partial or total loss of reactivity toward its specific antisera results. This loss poses special problems in quantifying apoproteins in whole plasma or lipoprotein fractions because the accuracy of immunoassays is based on the assumption that test and standard antigens have similar immunoreactivity per unit of protein antigen. Since standard antigens are usually purified apoproteins, it is often necessary to dissociate the lipid from the protein prior to measurement. Dissociation has been achieved in various laboratories by the use of sodium decylsulfate (Fainaru et al. 1976), tetramethylurea (Albers et al. 1976; Cheung & Albers 1977), heating (Karlin et al. 1976), or prior extraction of lipids with organic solvents (Schonfeld & Pfleger 1974).

3. Self-association and aggregation of apoproteins. Most purified apoproteins self-associate or aggregate in aqueous solution. This condition may alter the availability of immunochemical determinants and subsequently change the amount of immunoreactivity per unit weight. Aggregation and self-association also change the molecular size and form of the apoprotein; and these changes may create further problems, the extent of which depends on the nature of the immunoassay. In radial immunodiffusion assay molecular size and form affect the diffusion coefficient; thus aggregation and self-association could affect the ring size of the precipitate and error would result in the assay.

4. Instability of isolated lipoproteins and apoproteins. Purified lipoproteins and apoproteins are generally unstable. By this, we mean their immunoreactivity changes with sample storage time. To circum-

vent this effect, one either has to prepare fresh standard periodically or set up a secondary standard such as plasma or serum pools
in which lipoprotein or apoprotein concentration has been determined
by multiple analyses with freshly prepared standards.

5. <u>Multivalence of apoproteins</u>. Specific antisera have been produced
   against most of the known apoproteins. They are considered
   "specific" only insofar as they react against only one kind of apoprotein. However, since apoproteins are polypeptides of some 60–250
   amino acids, sometimes containing carbohydrate residues, they are
   likely to contain multiple antigenic determinants (Schonfeld et al.
   1977, 1977). Hence, immunization with purified apoprotein can lead
   to production of mixed antibody populations, each with different affinity and specificity toward different antigenic determinants.
   Therefore, measurement of apoprotein in plasma or plasma fraction
   with apoprotein specific antisera could vary with the nature and
   composition of antibody populations in the antisera.

6. <u>Polymorphic forms of apoproteins</u>. Polymorphs of apoproteins have
   been identified for apolipoproteins A-I, C-II, C-III, and E by the
   isoelectricfocusing method. It has yet to be determined whether
   these various forms of a given apoprotein have the same immunoreactivity or molecular form. The distribution of these isoforms can
   vary significantly among individuals. Differences in immunoreactivity among isoforms could lead to systematic errors in immunochemical measurements of these apoproteins.

Of the three immunoassay techniques discussed, i.e., radioimmunoassay,
electroimmunoassay, and radial immunodiffusion assay, electroimmunoassay
can be performed most rapidly. Radioimmunoassay is more time-consuming
but is the most sensitive of the three. Radial immunodiffusion is the
least sensitive but is simple to perform. Since the plasma concentrations
of lipoproteins and apoproteins are well within the sensitivity limit of
radial immunodiffusion assay, this technique is suitable for mass screening work in this field. When applied to various lipoprotein classes or
fractions, it proves to be an excellent tool in the study of lipoprotein
structure and composition. We have used radial immunodiffusion assays of
apo A-I, A-II, and B to evaluate precipitation methods for high-density
lipoprotein cholesterol determination (Warnick et al. 1979) and to study
the plasma levels in a selected population (Cheung and Albers 1977). We
have quantitated apo A-I and A-II levels in various physiological or
diseased states such as pregnancy (Cheung et al. 1977), juvenile and
adult onset diabetes mellitus (Eckel et al. 1979), myocardial infarction
(Albers et al. 1978), and abnormal coronary arteries (Tan et al. 1978).
We have also looked at the effects of drugs (Cheung et al. 1980), hormones (Albers et al. 1976; Cheung and Albers 1977), exercise (Krauss et
al. 1977) and diet (Applebaum-Bowden 1979), on the composition and
content of high-density lipoprotein apoproteins. We have also used the
assays to study the compositions of various HDL subfractions obtained by
CsCl gradient centrifugation (Cheung and Albers 1979).

After discussing how the properties of apoproteins and their antibodies
can affect immunochemical determinations, we feel it appropriate to conclude with an example to illustrate these problems.

Since apo B is insoluble in the absence of lipid and B-containing lipoproteins vary widely in size and hydrated density, radial immunodiffusion
assay of apo B provides only a reasonable estimate of apo B in plasma or
serum. Recognizing this limit, we have developed a double-antibody radioimmunoassay procedure for apo B (Albers et al. 1975). Since radio-

813

immunoassay involves competition of labeled and unlabeled antigens for a common antibody, the procedure does not require that the test and standard antigens be structurally identical (as long as they are immunologically identical to the reacting antibody). However, since apo B is a multivalent antigen associated with lipoproteins containing from 65 to over 99% lipid, the problem of masking of antigenic site(s) by lipid has not yet been circumvented. This is illustrated in Table 1.

Table 1. Changes in apo B immunoreactivity as a function of triglyceride hydrolysis of chylomicrons.

Fraction	% triglyceride hydrolysis	Ratio of apo B immunoreactivity, Anti-B(1)/ Anti-B(2)
1	34	1.25
2	52	1.48
3	61	1.72
4	70	1.81

The apo B radioimmnoassay was applied to chylomicron remnant fractions. Each fraction differed significantly in apo B immunoreactivity as determined by two different antisera (1 and 2) to apo B. As the triglyceride hydrolysis increased from 30 to 70%, the difference in immunoreactivity between the two antibodies increased from 25 to 81%. This implies that for apo B in chylomicron remnant fractions, the specificity of antibody and the degree of masking of antigenic determinants by lipid are of major importance in the apo B quantification. It is therefore important that any immunoassay should be validated with respect to various lipoprotein classes or fractions before it be applied for quantification of apoproteins of that certain class (fraction).

References

Albers JJ, Hazzard WR (1974) Immunochemical quantification of human plasma Lp(a) lipoprotein. Lipids 9: 15–26
Albers JJ, Cabana VG, Hazzard WR (1975) Immunoassay of human plasma apolipoprotein B. Metabolism 25: 1339–1351
Albers JJ, Wahl PW, Cabana VG, Hazzard WR, Hoover JJ (1976) Quantitation of apolipoprotein A-I of human plasma high density lipoprotein. Metabolism 25: 633–644
Albers JJ, Cheung MC, Hazzard WR (1978) High-density lipoproteins in myocardial infarction survivors. Metabolism 27: 479–485
Applebaum-Bowden D, Hazzard WR, Cain J, Cheung MC, Kushwaha RS, Albers JJ (1979)Short-term egg yolk feeding in humans. Atherosclerosis 33: 385–396
Cheung MC, Albers JJ (1977) The measurement of apolipoprotein A-I and A-II levels in men and women by immunoasay. J Clin Invest 60: 43–50
Cheung MC, Chapman M, Albers JJ, Knopp RH (1977) High density lipoprotein composition in the hypertriglyceridemia of pregnancy. Abstract of the 31st annual meeting of the council on Atherosclerosis, American Society for the study of Atherosclerosis, American Heart Assoc., November 28–30, 1977, p 7
Cheung MC, Albers JJ (1979) Distribution of cholesterol and apolipoprotein A-I and A-II in human high density lipoprotein subfractions separated by CsCl equilibrium gradient centrifugation: evidence for HDL subpopulations with differing A-I/A-II molar ratios. J Lipid Res 20: 200–207

Cheung MC, Albers JJ, Wahl PW, Hazzard WR (1980) High density lipoproteins during hypolipidemic therapy: a comparative study of four
drugs. Atherosclerosis, in press

Darcy DA (1972) A general method of increasing the sensitivity of
immune diffusion. Its application to CEA. Clin Chim Acta 38: 329-337

Eckel RH, Albers JJ, Cheung MC, Wahl PW, Bierman EL (1979) Antiatherogenic high density lipoprotein composition in juvenile onset
diabetes mellitus. Clin Res 27: 44A

Fahey JL, McKelvey EM (1964) Quantitative determination of serum immunoglobulins in antibody-agar plates. J Immunology 94: 84-90

Fainaru M, Havel J, Felker TE (1976) Radioimmunoassay of apolipoprotein A-I of rat serum. Biochim Biophys Acta 446: 56-58

Karlin JB, Juhn DJ, Starr JI, Scanu AM, Rubenstein AH (1976) Measurement of human high density lipoprotein apolipoprotein A-I in serum by
radio-immunoassay. J Lipid Res 17: 30-37

Krauss RM, Lindgren FT, Wood PD, Cheung MC (1977) Differential increases in plasma high density lipoprotein subfractions and apolipoproteins (apo-Lp) in runners. Circulation part II, 56:III-4

Mancini G, Carbonara AO, Heremans JF (1965) Immunochemical quantitation of antigens by single radial immunodiffusion. Immunochemistry
2: 235-254

Schonfeld G, Pfleger B (1974) The structure of human high density
lipoprotein and the levels of apolipoprotein A-I in plasma as determined by radioimmunoassay. J Clin Invest 54: 236-246

Schonfeld G, Chen J-S, Roy RG (1977) Antigenic properties of apoproteins A-I and A-II in intact high density lipoprotein. J Biol Chem
252: 6651-6654

Schonfeld G, Chen J-S, Roy RG (1977) Use of antibody specificity to
study the surface disposition of apoprotein A-I on human high density
lipoproteins. J Biol Chem 252: 6655-6659

Sieber A, Becker W (1974) Quantitative determination of IgE by single
radial immunodiffusion. A comparison of three different methods for
intensification of precipitates. Clin Chim Acta 50: 153-155

Simmons P (1971) Quantitation of plasma proteins in low concentrations using RID. Clin Chim Acta 35: 53-57

Storiko K (1968) Normal values for 23 different human plasma proteins
determined by single radial immunodiffusion. Blut 16: 200-208

Tan MH, Albers JJ, Cheung MC (1978) Serum apo A-I and HDL-Cholesterol
levels in patients with abnormal coronary arteries. Clin Res 26:
282A

Warnick GR, Cheung MC, Albers JJ (1979) Comparison of current methods
for high-density lipoprotein cholesterol quantitation. Clin Chem 25:
596-604

Wieja JG, Smith CJ (1976) Enhanced visibility of precipitin disks in
radial immunodiffusion measurements. Anal Biochem 74: 636-637

Plasma Levels of Some Apolipoproteins in Human Atherosclerosis

Pietro Avogaro, Gabriele Bittolo Bon, Giuseppe Cazzolato, Giobatta Quinci, and Fabio Belussi

The major emphasis in the study of the biochemical abnormalities of atherosclerosis have been put on the lipid counterpart of lipoproteins since 30
years (Jones et al. 1951; Barr et al. 1951). The study of the protein moiety
of lipoproteins has been hampered by technical difficulties which do not
appear completely overcome even now.

This paper refers data obtained in a group of 328 survivors of myocardial
infarction (MI), all males with a mean age 52.1 ± 10.6; all of them had
suffered the acute infarction at least six months previously. As controls
330 males were randomly selected from a population freely participating to
an Health Survey Program; all were males aged 53.3 ± 13.8. The criteria of
selection for both survivors and controls have been published elsewhere (Avogaro et al. 1979). In all the subjects the following analyses have been performed: cholesterol, triglycerides, HDL-C, apolipoproteins A_I and B. In 55
survivors and in 80 controls the pattern of analyses has also included:
VLDL-C, VLDL-TG, LDL-C, apo-A_{II}, apo-D and apo-Lp(a).

In our laboratory quantification of the various apolipoprotein has been performed through electroimmunoassay according to Curry et al. (1976); for the
determination of apo-Lp(a) the procedure outlined by Kostner (1976) has been
followed. The isolation of the various lipoprotein classes has been
accomplished according to the method of Havel et al. (1955).

According to the criteria followed for selection, survivors showed cholesterol and triglycerides plasma levels not significantly different from
controls (Tables 1, 2). Despite this, survivors had significantly lower
values of HDL-C, apo-A_I, ratio TC/apo-B and ratio apo-A_I/ apo-B than
controls and significantly higher levels of apo-B (Table 1). The same
behaviour was present even when all the subjects were divided according to
the various phenotypes, although some differences did not prove to be significant, i.e. for HDL-C in type IIB and IV and for apo-A_I in type IV (Table 1).
In the subgroups in which more analyses have been performed, significantly
higher amounts of LDL-C have been recorded while no significant variations
have been observed in chemical components of VLDL (Table 2). In the same
subgroups, survivors displayed more apo-B and less apo-A_I than controls
while no significant variations in plasma levels of apo-A_{II} and apo-D have
been stressed (Tab. 3). Mean plasma levels of apo-Lp(a) did not show significant variations between survivors and controls. Apo-Lp(a) negative were a
5.5 percentage in survivors and 13.8 in controls; a 18.2 percentage of survivors showed values higher than 50 mg/dl while only 11.3% of controls had
values above this level (not shown).

Previous researches have stressed reduced levels of apo-A (Berg et al. 1976) and apo-A$_I$ (Albers et al. 1976; Avogaro et al. 1978) and increased levels of apo-Lp(a) (Albers et al. 1977) and apo-B (Avogaro et al. 1978, 1979). When survivors and controls having similar values of plasma lipids were matched significantly lower plasma levels of apo-A$_I$ and significantly higher plasma levels of apo-B have been found out in survivors (Avogaro et al. 1978, 1979). These findings are confirmed by the present experience which has considered a much larger numeber of patients. When the subjects have been clustered according to their phenotypes, apoproteins still kept a relevant role; this

Table 1. Concentrations of lipids and apolipoproteins in survivors of myocardial infarction (MI) and in a control population (C). Subjects have also been considered according to their lipidic phenotype; normal (NL); type IIA, type IIB and IV. Mean values (mg/dl) plus values of one standard deviation are given.

	TC	TG	HDL-C	A-I	B	TC/B	A-I/B
C	234	139	52	124	124	1.96	1.08
(330)	46	69	11	19	29	.20	.28
MI	245	138	46++	106++	157++	1.58++	0.72++
(328)	48	70	9	18	34	.23	.15
C-NL	209	108	53	124	106	2.00	1.21
(210)	30	28	10	19	18	.29	.25
MI-NL	214	109	46++	105++	134++	1.61++	0.80++
(183)	33	27	10	20	29	.21	.27
C-IIA	308	119	58	137	159	1.96	0.88
(60)	32	26	11	16	27	.25	.21
MI-IIA	295	119	50+	110++	192++	1.55++	0.59++
(91)	28	27	10	15	27	.21	.20
C-IIB	298	241	42	113	168	1.76	0.69
(30)	28	41	8	12	13	.25	.14
MI-IIB	300	252	41	102+	197++	1.53++	0.53++
(28)	32	47	7	13	21	.28	.15
C-IV	204	297	41	109	118	1.88	0.96
(30)	26	47	9	16	18	.26	.18
MI-IV	222	285	39	103	151++	1.48++	0.78++
(26)	28	94	8	14	24	.28	.19

[a] TC = total cholesterol, TG = triglycerides; HDL = high density lipoproteins; A$_I$ = apo-A$_I$; B = apo-B
[b] Significant differences are given for subjects of the same group:
+ P < 0.05   ++ P < 0.01

Table 2. Concentrations of lipids and lipoproteins in survivors of myocardial infarction (MI) and in a control population (C). Mean values (mg/dl) plus values of one standard deviation are given.

	TC	TG	VLDL–C	VLDL–TG	LDL–C	HDL–C
C (80)	225.6	156.8	27.7	85.9	148.5	48.1
	50.4	72.2	20.3	43.2	45.5	12.7
MI (55)	243.3	178.4	29.6	95.2	173.3[++]	40.4[+]
	54.2	88.9	23.8	50.3	48.5	11.2

+ P < 0.05   ++ P < 0.01

Table 3. Concentrations of apolipoproteins in survivors of myocardial infarction (MI) and in a control population (C). Mean values (mg/dl) plus values of one standard deviation are given.

	Apo–B	Apo–A$_I$	Apo–A$_{II}$	Apo–D	Apo–Lp(a)
C (80)	126.3	117.8	33.8	14.8	23.8
	34.5	18.8	7.9	4.2	18.5
MI (55)	167.5[++]	101.3[++]	31.2	12.9	30.2
	40.3	17.2	9.9	4.5	20.2

+ P < 0.01

is expecially true for apo–B. In our hands the determination of plasma levels of apo–A$_{II}$ and apo–D has proved to be without any value as discriminators between the two populations. The quantitative determination of apo–Lp(a) confirm the data of Albers et al. (1977) about a tendency in survivors to higher values of this apolipoprotein than in controls. These studies support previous views about a major role played by proteins both as a biochemical marker of lipoproteins (Alaupovic 1971) and as discriminators between atherosclerotic subjects and normal population (Avogaro et al. 1979).

REFERENCES

Alaupovic P (1971) Apolipoproteins and lipoproteins. Atherosclerosis 13: 141–146

Albers JJ, Adolphson JL, Hazzard WR (1977) Radioimmunoassay of human plasma Lp(a) lipoprotein. J Lipid Res 18: 331–338

Albers JJ, Wahl PW, Cabana GV, Hazzard WR, Hoover JJ (1976) Quantitation of apolipoprotein A$_I$ of human plasma high density lipoprotein. Metabolism 25: 633–644

Avogaro P, Bittolo Bon G, Cazzolato G, Quinci GB, Belussi F (1978) Plasma levels of apolipoprotein A$_I$ and apolipoprotein B in Human Atherosclerosis. Artery 4: 385–394

Avogaro P, Bittolo Bon G, Cazzolato G, Quinci GB (1979) Are apolipoproteins better discriminators than lipids for atherosclerosis? Lancet i: 901-903

Barr DP, Russ EM, Eder HA (1951) Protein-lipid relationship in human plasma: II. In atherosclerosis and related conditions. Amer J Med 11: 480-484

Berg K, Borresen AL, Dahlen G (1976) Serum high density lipoprotein and atherosclerotic heart disease. Lancet i: 499-501

Havel RJ, Eder HA, Bragdon JH (1955) The distribution and chemical composition of ultracentrifugally separated lipoproteins in human serum. J Clin Invest 34: 1345-1353

Jones HB, Gofman JW, Lindgren F, Lyon Tp, Graham D, Strisower B (1951) Lipoproteins in Atherosclerosis. Am J Med 11: 358-380

Kostner GM (1976) Lp(a) Lipoproteins and the genetic polymorphism of Lipoprotein B. In: Day CE, Levy RS (eds.)Low Density Lipoproteins. Plenum Press, New York pp. 229-265

Quantitation of C Apolipoprotein Metabolism in Human Subjects

Noel H. Fidge, Paul J. Nestel, and Murray W. Huff

Considerable progress has been made recently in understanding the structure
and function of the C group of apolipoproteins which in human plasma are
mainly associated with triglyceride rich lipoproteins (chylomicrons and
very low density lipoproteins) and high density lipoproteins. C apoproteins
are peptides of low molecular weight (ca 8-10,000) which can be separated on
the basis of differences in charge into three major subgroups, namely CI,
CII and CIII apoproteins, the latter existing in polymorphic forms e.g.
CIII-0, CIII-1, CIII-2 etc. due to variation in the content of carbohydrate
attached to a common primary polypeptide chain (Morrisett et al. 1975).
The sequence of all C proteins have now been determined; CII apoprotein
has been identified as a powerful activator of lipoprotein lipase while the
CI (Lee et al. 1976) and CIII (Brown et al. 1972) apoproteins may be
involved both in the activation and inhibition of lipolytic systems.
Several laboratories have studied the metabolism of the C proteins and have
demonstrated that C apoproteins exchange freely among the plasma lipoproteins (Eisenberg and Levy 1975). We have recently been concerned with
attempts to quantitate the metabolism of individual C proteins and this
report describes the development of methods which have enabled us to use a
kinetic approach to the measurement of production rates, pool sizes and
clearance of C proteins in human subjects.

Methodology

The following is a summary of our methodological approach: (1) Administration of radioactively labeled C proteins (pulse) within VLDL followed by
blood sampling at multiple time points; (2) separation of individual C
proteins of VLDL and HDL by a system providing rapid and accurate estimates
of specific radioactivity (SA); (3) use of compartmental analysis to
describe C protein metabolism.

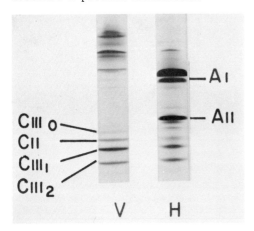

FIG. 1. Isoelectric focusing (pH 4-6) of VLDL (V) and HDL (H) apoproteins
on polyacrylamide gels in 6M urea illustrating resolution of C apoproteins
of both lipoproteins.

The separation of C proteins for SA measurement was achieved by isoelectric focusing (IEF) of the soluble (isopropranol) fraction of VLDL and HDL on 7.5% polyacrylamide gels in 6 M urea (using carrier ampholytes) with a pH gradient of 4-6 (Fig. 1).

After focusing, the gels were stained with an extract of Coomassie Blue (Malik and Berrie 1972) and the separated bands quantitated by densitometric scanning of each gel, run in duplicate. Purified C apoproteins (CII, CIII-1 and CIII-2) were prepared by either preparative IEF on a flat bed electrophoresis system (Pharmacia) or by ion exchange chromatography using DEAE-Sephacel (Pharmacia). Each protein was identified by electrophoretic mobility and amino acid composition and CII by its cofactor action for lipoprotein lipase. Standard curves were obtained for each C apoprotein of which the mass was determined by gravimetric analysis and the mass of unknown samples was obtained by reference of integrated peaks to appropriate standard curves. Linear responses were obtained in the 5-40 ug range and CII had a chromogenicity 1.3 fold higher than CIII. CI was not appreciably labeled with ^{125}I and not quantitated further. To determine counts, bands were excised and radioassayed for ^{125}I content. The injected dose for each C apoprotein was determined by isoelectric focusing the isopropranol soluble fraction of the injected VLDL.

The SA data was plotted against time and conformed to a biexponential curve (Fig. 2) permitting the use of an appropriate two-pool model for calculating kinetic parameters (Gurpide et al. 1964) providing estimates of production rates (PR), mass of C protein (MI) and total fractional removal rates (-KAA) in the more rapidly exchanging pool.

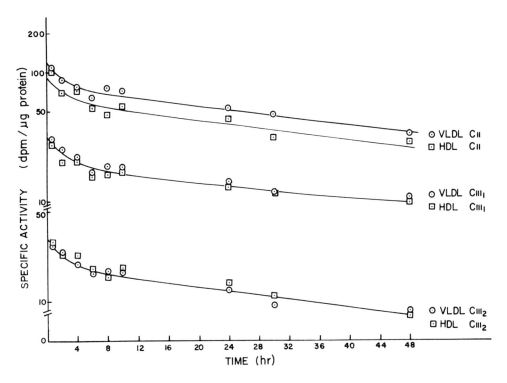

FIG. 2. Specific radioactivities of CII, CIII-1 and CIII-2 in VLDL and HDL after injecting ^{125}I-labeled VLDL into a normal subject.

The data in Table 1 shows that mass of CII was directly related to the
plasma triglyceride concentration and also with VLDL triglyceride concentration (not shown). This is illustrated in Fig. 3A which also suggests
that the proportional relationship between CII mass and triglyceride concentration is apparent at low triglyceride levels only. Of further interest
is the suggestion that the removal rate (-KAA) rather than synthesis rate
influences CII pool size as shown in Fig. 3B and Table 1. Production rates
of CII apoprotein for normal and hypertriglyceridemic subjects were very
similar, being approximately 1 mg/kg/day.

Table 1. Pool size, production and removal rates of C apoproteins

Subject	Lipoprotein Phenotype	Plasma triglyceride mg/100 ml	Mass mg		Pool 1 kinetics Fractional Removal hr^{-1}		Production mg/kg/d	
			CII	CIII-1	CII	CIII-1	CII	CIII-1
1	Normal	100	104	277	0.30	0.23	1.1	2.5
2	Hyper-cholesterolemia	177	134	843	0.13	0.15	1.2	6.5
3	Normal (obese)	176	159	469	0.24	0.19	1.1	3.2
4	Normal (obese)	195	170	753	0.24	0.16	1.6	6.0
5	Combined hyper-lipoproteinemia	298	210	659	0.11	0.12	1.2	3.2
6	Type 5	1030	288	456	0.09	0.07	1.0	1.5
7	Type 5	1105	233	1225	0.09	0.15	0.7	3.7

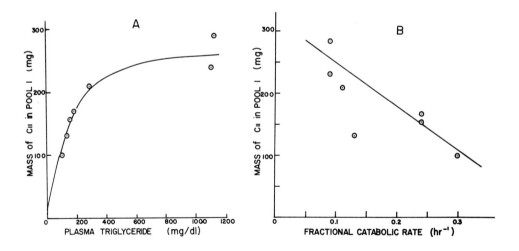

FIG. 3a and b.   A. Relationship between mass of CII apoprotein in pool 1
and plasma TG concentration and B. relationship between CII mass and
fractional catabolic rate.

822

This suggests that the production of this important cofactor protein does not increase in proportion to increased triglyceride transport. Both VLDL triglyceride and VLDL B apoprotein production tend to increase in hyper-triglyceridemic subjects. The finding that CII removal rates fall with raised triglyceride levels may be related to the increased residence time in plasma of VLDL particles, observed in studies of VLDL triglyceride and VLDL B kinetics (Nestel, Reardon and Fidge, 1979).

In several normal subjects, the SA of HDL-C proteins was also determined following injection of ^{125}I labeled VLDL. The data (Fig. 1) shows identical CIII-1 and CIII-2 SA and very close SA of CII in VLDL and HDL, suggesting that a rapid exchange of both CII and CIII proteins occurs between VLDL and HDL leading to similar clearance rates. The $T\frac{1}{2}$ of the slow exponential of CII and CIII proteins were similar in normal subjects (approximately 25-35 hr) and although higher (55-90 hr), were also similar in hypertriglycerid-emic subjects.

These kinetic studies have thus allowed estimates of pool sizes, production and removal rates of C proteins. Immunoassays recently developed to quant-itate C proteins (Kashyap et al. 1977) only measure plasma pool sizes but are of a similar order of magnitude to the mass of C apoproteins, determined kinetically, in pool 1. This suggests that the dimensions of pool 1 are similar to those of plasma.

References

Brown WV, Baginsky ML (1972) Inhibition of lipoprotein lipase by an apoprotein of human very low density lipoprotein. Biochem Biophys Res Comm 46: 375-382

Eisenberg S, Levy RI (1975) Lipoprotein metabolism. Adv Lipid Res 13: 1-89

Gurpide E, Mann J, Sandberg E (1964) Determination of kinetic parameters in a two pool system by administration of one or more tracers. Biochemistry 3: 1250-1255

Kashyap ML, Srivastava LS, Chen CY, Perisutti G, Campbell M, Lutmer RF, Glueck CJ (1977) Radioimmunoassay of human apolipoprotein CII. A study in normal and hypertriglyceridemic subjects. J Clin Invest 60: 171-180

Lee DM, Ganesan D, Bass HB (1976) Studies of the hydrolysis of triacyl-glycerols in chylomicrons, very low- and low-density lipoproteins by C-1 activated lipoprotein lipase from post-heparin plasma of normal human subjects. FEBS Lett 64: 163-168

Malik N, Berrie A, (1972) New stain fixative for proteins separated by gel isoelectric focusing based on Coomassie brilliant blue. Anal Biochem 49: 713-716

Morrisett JD, Jackson RL, Gotto AM (1975) Lipoproteins: Structure and function. Ann Rev Biochem 44: 183-207

Nestel PJ, Reardon MF, Fidge NH (1979) Very low density lipoprotein B-apoprotein kinetics in human subjects. Circ Res 45: 35-40

Quantitation of Apolipoproteins C-II and C-III in Plasma

Gustav Schonfeld

Introduction

Apolipoproteins have been assigned a variety of important physiologic roles in lipoprotein metabolism. ApoC-II is a potent stimulator of lipo-protein lipase (LPL), and ApoC-III, a glycoprotein which contains from 0 to 3 or more moles of sialic acid residues per mole of protein (ApoC-III$_0$, ApoC-III$_1$, etc.), inhibits ApoC-II-stimulated LPL activity <u>in vitro</u> (Havel et al. 1973). The essential role of ApoC-II <u>in vivo</u> has been established in a patient with gross hypertriglyceridemia who had normal levels of post-heparin plasma LPL, but no detectable levels of ApoC-II in his plasma VLDL. The hypertriglyceridemia was corrected only by intravenous infusions containing ApoC-II. Several other homozygotes with ApoC-II deficiency and hypertriglyceridemia have been identified (Breckenridge et al. 1978; Cox et al. 1978). The specific role of ApoC-III as a modulator of LPL activity <u>in vivo</u> is not nearly so secure, because in addition to ApoC-III there are several apoproteins which can inhibit ApoC-II activated LPL activity. In this paper, we report on the development of double antibody radioimmuno-assays for ApoC-II and ApoC-III and on the levels of ApoC-II and ApoC-III in whole plasmas and in lipoproteins of subjects with various forms of hyper-lipidemia.

Methods

<u>Clinical Procedures.</u> Subjects with hyperlipidemia were Caucasian patients of the Washington University Lipid Research Center. Hyperlipidemia was defined by values in the upper 5th percentile for the appropriate age and sex. Subjects with Type III hyperlipidemia, in addition to having the appropriate lipid levels and VLDL-Chol:VLDL-TG ratios [< 0.42], had grossly diminished or absent ApoE-III bands. Type V subjects had fasting chylo-micronemia. Secondary causes of hyperlipidemia were ruled out by appro-priate clinical procedures. None of the subjects were taking medication. Normal controls (both TG and Chol levels < 90th percentile) were self-referred Caucasian volunteers and people who were identified during the various population screens. All venous bloods were drawn into EDTA tubes (1 mg/ml) after 12-14 hours of fasting from untreated subjects who were eating ad lib diets.

<u>Lipoprotein Lipid and Apoprotein Analyses.</u> Total plasma and lipoprotein triglyceride (TG) and cholesterol (Chol) levels were determined by Auto-analyzer II according to Lipid Research Clinic procedures [Lipid Research Clinics Manual of Laboratory Operations 1974]. Apoproteins were measured in whole plasma and in d< 1.006 supernates and infranates. In selected cases, density distributions of apoproteins were assessed in greater detail. For this purpose, plasmas were divided into several aliquots and any given aliquot was ultracentrifuged only once at one of the following densities: d 1.006, d 1.063, and d 1.21. Apoproteins were measured on

both the supernates and infranates of these centrifugations and density distributions were obtained by appropriate subtractions.

Radioimmunoassays. ApoC-II and ApoC-III were isolated from VLDL of hypertriglyceridemic subjects by column chromatography, first on Sephadex G200 and then on DEAE cellulose (Brown et al. 1969). Apoproteins C-II and C-III$_1$ which yielded single bands on polyacrylamide disc gel electrophoresis and on isoelectric focusing (IEF) and which had appropriate amino acid compositions (Jackson et al. 1977; Brewer et al. 1974) were used as immunizing antigens in rabbits, as ^{125}I-labelled tracers in assays, and as assay standards. Second antibodies consisting of antirabbit IgG were produced in goats.

Iodinations were with lactoperoxidase and H_2O_2 and ^{125}I-ApoC-II and ^{125}I-ApoC-III were purified by column chromatography. 80-90% of ^{125}I-ApoC-II and ^{125}I-ApoC-III$_1$ were precipitated by 10% TCA, and equal proportions were bound by appropriate antisera. But anti ApoC-II antisera bound only 5-8% of ^{125}I-ApoC-III, and anti ApoC-III antisera bound only 2-6% ^{125}I-ApoC-II. The assay test tubes contained antiserum, ^{125}I-ApoC-II or ^{125}I-ApoC-III, plasma or lipoprotein sample, non-immune rabbit serum and sufficient assay buffer to raise the total volume to 500 µl. The above mixtures were incubated at 4°C for 42 hr., then goat antirabbit IgG was added and incubations were continued for another 16 hrs. Immune precipitates were harvested by centrifugation and counted. Assays were calculated on a programmable calculator using the logit transformation of B/B_0.

Statistical Analysis. Data were entered into the SAS statistical analysis and data management system (Nie et al. 1970) for subsequent display and analysis. Group means, standard deviations, and non-paired t-tests were calculated on data which had been subjects to logarithmic transformation, because of the well known log normal distribution of lipid values in populations. For the same reasons Spearman rather than Pearson correlations were computed.

Results and Discussion

Specificity and Precision. The addition of ApoC-II to the system containing anti ApoC-II and ^{125}I-ApoC-II produced typical radioimmunoassay displacement curves, with slopes and intercepts on logit plots of -3.10 ± 0.50 and +2.63 ± 0.33 (mean ± 1 S.D., n=18 curves). Similarly, ApoC-III also produced usable displacement curves in the appropriate system with slopes and intercepts of -3.00 ± 0.31 and 2.08 ± 0.31, respectively (n=25). ApoC-III$_1$ and ApoC-III$_2$ yielded superimposable curves, thus, the assay measured both ApoC-III$_1$ and ApoC-III$_2$. Further to assess the specificity of the ApoC-III assay, a VLDL preparation was subjected to digestion by neuraminidase and analyzed by IEF. Following digestion, >80% of the sialylated forms of ApoC-III were converted to ApoC-III$_0$. Yet upon reassay, the apparent ApoC-III contents of the VLDL preparations were unaltered. Therefore, the assay was able to detect all of the subspecies of ApoC-III. ApoC-III$_1$ was used routinely as the standard. The addition of ApoC-II to the ApoC-III assay or of ApoC-III$_1$ to the ApoC-II assay resulted in <1% displacement of counts. ApoA-I, ApoA-II, and ApoE displaced no counts in either assay even in at doses of 2000 ng. Normal LDL (1.025-1.050) appeared to contain <1% of either ApoC-II or ApoC-III. Thus, each assay was specific for its respective apoprotein.
Coefficients of variation for triplicate points in standard curves ranged 3-5%. Intra- and interassay coefficients of variation for plasma samples

were 6 and 11% for ApoC-II and 9 and 13% for ApoC-III. (Frozen plasma pool assayed at 2 doses in duplicate over ∿1 year in 25–30 assays.)

Parallelism. The addition of increasing doses of VLDL, HDL or of whole normal or hyperlipidemic plasma to the assays produced displacement curves which paralleled those produced by either the ApoC-II or ApoC-III standards, i.e. the calculated slopes of the lipoprotein and plasma samples were within the mean ± 1 S.D. of the slopes of the logit plots.

Accuracy. On column chromatography of 10 VLDL preparations, ApoC-II and ApoC-III represented 12.5% ± 2.5 and 40% ± 7.9 of VLDL protein, respectively. In VLDL preparations taken from three subjects with Type IV hyperlipidemia, the percent contribution of ApoC-II to VLDL protein ranged from 12–17, 7–9, and 3–5% for the S_f 100–400, S_f 60–100, and S_f 20–60 VLDL fractions, respectively. In similar VLDL subfractions prepared from the plasma of a Type III patients, the percent contributions of ApoC-II were 2, 4, and 7% and the contributions of ApoC-III were 11, 19, and 22%. Delipidations of lipoproteins had no effect on the results, and, in recovery experiments, 95–99% of the ApoC-II and ApoC-III added to plasma were detected. Thus, the assays appeared to be accurate.

Levels of ApoC-II and ApoC-III in Plasma. Levels of ApoC-II and ApoC-III were measured in 171 fasting plasmas (Table 1). There were no differences in apoprotein levels due to sex. Levels of both apoproteins were high in the hypertriglyceridemias. Levels of both ApoC-II and ApoC-III were strongly correlated with the concentrations of total TG, VLDL-TG, and VLDL-Chol (r_s 0.88 to 0.92, p<0.001). But levels of VLDL-ApoC-II and VLDL-ApoC-III did not rise at the same rate as did VLDL-TG. The proportion of total ApoC-II (or ApoC-III) in VLDL were also strongly correlated with the proportion of total TG in VLDL [VLDL-ApoC-II or C-III/Total ApoC-II or C-III vs VLDL-TG/Total TG, r_s +0.77 and +0.83, p<0.001].

These correlations agree with the fact that about 40% of ApoC-II and 35% of ApoC-III were in the d 1.006 fractions of normal subjects, but this rose to 80+% in the hypertriglyceridemias (Fig. 1). The d 1.006–1.063 range contained 15% or less of ApoC-II and ApoC-III in normals and in subjects with Types II, IV, and V hyperlipidemia, but it contained about 25% of these apoproteins in Type III hyperlipidemia. The d 1.063–1.21 fractions contained about 30 and 40% of ApoC-II and ApoC-III, but this fell to 10–20% in the

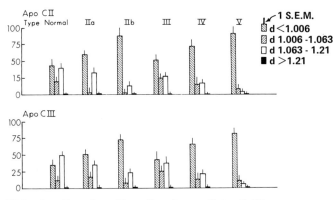

FIG. 1. Density distributions of ApoC-II and ApoC-III in plasmas of normal subjects and patients with hyperlipidemia. Each category contains plasma of 3–5 subjects. Results are means ± 1 SEM of percent of total.

Table 1. Plasma levels of apoC-II and apoC-III in hyperlipidemia.

Phenotype	n	Total Plasma		n	VLDL ApoC/Plasma ApoC Ratios	
		ApoC-II	ApoC-III		ApoC-II	ApoC-III
		mg/dl			mass ratio	
Normal	(93)	3.9 ±1.4	15.4 ± 6.2	(12)	0.45 ±0.15	0.35 ±0.13
IIA	(19)	5.2* ±1.7	18.0* ± 6.6	(8)	0.49 ±0.17	0.35 ±0.14
IIB	(14)	7.8* ±2.7	20.6* ± 6.1	(9)	0.64 ±0.19±	0.46* ±0.11
III	(17)	9.1* ±3.3	33.4* ±10.8	(8)	0.60 ±0.24	0.51 ±0.29
IV	(17)	9.6* ±3.0	33.3* ±12.8	(9)	0.71* ±0.21	0.63* ±0.14
V	(11)	13.2* ±5.0	51.7* ±29.9	(6)	0.91* ±0.20	0.75* ±0.15

Results are means ± 1 S.D.. ( ) = number of subjects; * = p<0.01;
** = p<0.05 by non-paired t-test (hyperlipidemics vs normal). Ratios
were calculated using individual results. The results are means
(± 1 S.D.) of the individual ratios.

hypertriglyceridemias. The d>1.21 fractions contained <5% of total ApoC-II
and ApoC-III. Note that the density distribution of ApoC-II and ApoC-III
were not identical. These assays should be useful in further studies of
lipoprotein metabolism.

Acknowledgements

The contributions of P. K. George, M.D., Joyce Miller, Ph.D.,
Joseph Witztum, M.D., Mary Ann Dillingham, P.A.-C., William E. Giese,
P.A.-C., Janet B. Kolar, P.A.-C., Ingming Jeng, Ph.D., Pat Reilly,
Barbara Pfleger, and Robert Roy are gratefully acknowledged. We
appreciate the secretarial assistance of Lillian Beal and the help of
Dr. Ralph Bradshaw with the amino acid analyses.

References

Breckenridge WC, Little JA, Steiner G, Chow A, Poapst M (1978) Hypertri-
    glyceridemia associated with deficiency of apolipoprotein C-II. N Engl
    J Med 298: 1265-1273
Brewer Jr HB, Shulman R, Herbert P, Ronan R, Wehrly K (1974) The complete
    amino acid sequence of alanine apolipoprotein (ApoC-III), an apolipo-
    protein from human plasma very low density lipoproteins. J Biol Chem
    249: 4975-4984
Brown WV, Levy RI, Fredrickson DS (1969) Studies of the proteins in human
    plasma very low density lipoproteins. J Biol Chem 244:5687-5694
Cox DW, Breckenridge WC, Little JA (1978) Inheritance of apolipoprotein C-II
    deficiency with hypertriglyceridemia and pancreatitis. N Engl J Med
    299: 1421-1424

Havel RJ, Fielding CJ, Olivecrona T, Shore VG, Fielding PE, Egelrud R
(1973) Cofactor activity of protein components of human very low
density lipoproteins in the hydrolysis of triglycerides by lipoprotein lipase from different sources. Biochemistry 12: 1828–1833
Jackson RL, Baker HN, Gilliam EB, Gotto Jr AM (1977) Primary structure of
very low density apolipoprotein C-II of human plasma. Proc Natl Acad
Sci USA 74: 1942–1945
Lipid Research Clinics Program Manual of Laboratory Operation, Lipid and
Lipoprotein Analysis (DHEW Publication No. NIH 75-628) Vol. 1, 1974
Nie NH, Hull CH, Jenkins JG, Steinbrenner K, Bent DH (1970) Statistical
package for the social sciences, 2nd edn. McGraw Hill, St. Louis, Mo.

Addendum to B.M. Rifkind, J. LaRosa, and G. Heiss, "Prevalence of
Hyperlipoproteinemia in Selected North American Populations," (pp. 264-267)

Acknowledgements

This work was supported by National Heart, Lung and Blood Institute
contracts numbered: NO1-HV1-2156-L, NO1-HV1-2160-L, NO1-HV2-2914-L,
YO1-HV3-0010-L, NO1-HV2-2913-L, NO1-HV1-2158-L, NO1-HV1-2161-L,
NO1-HV2-2915-L, NO1-HV2-2932-L, NO1-HV2-2917-L, NO1-HV1-2157-L
NO1-HV1-2243-L, NO1-HV1-2159-L, NO1-HV3-2961-L, and NO1-HV6-2941-L.

References

Fredrickson DS, Levy RI (1972) Familial hyperlipoproteinemia. In: Stanbury
    JB, Wyngaarden JB, Fredrickson DS (eds) The Metabolic Basis of Inherited
    Diseases (3rd edition). McGraw Hill, New York, pp 545-614
Fredrickson DS, Levy RI, Lees RS (1967) Fat transport in lipoproteins: An
    integrated approach to mechanisms and disorders. N Engl J Med 276:32-44,
    94-103, 148-156, 215-226, 273-281
Gibson TC, Whorton EB (1973) The prevalence of hyperlipidemia in a natural
    community. J Chronic Dis 26:227-236
Gustafson A, Elmfeldt D, Wilhemson L, Tibblin G (1972) Serum lipids and
    lipoproteins in men after myocardial infarction compared with represen-
    tative population sample. Circulation 46:709-716
Heiss G, Tamir I, Davis CE, Tyroler HA, Rifkind BM, Schonfeld G, Jacobs D,
    Frantz, ID Jr, (1980) Lipoprotein cholesterol distributions in selected
    North American populations: The Lipid Research Clinics Program Preva-
    lence Study. Circulation (in press)
Manual of Laboratory Operations, Lipid Research Clinics Program, Vol 1,
    Lipid and Lipoprotein Analysis (1974) National Heart, Lung and Blood
    Institute, National Institutes of Health, Bethesda, Maryland. DHEW
    Publication No. (NIH)75-628
Nikkila EA, Aro A (1973) Family study of serum lipids and lipoprotein in
    coronary heart disease. Lancet 1:954-959
The Lipid Research Clinics Program Epidemiology Committee (1979) Plasma
    lipid distributions in selected North American populations: The Lipid
    Research Clinics Program Prevalence Study. Circulation 60:427-439
Wallace RB, Hoover J, Barrett-Connor E, Rifkind BM, Hunninghake, DB, Mack-
    enthun A, Heiss G (1979) Altered plasma lipid and lipoprotein levels
    associated with oral contraceptive and oestrogen use. Lancet 2:111-115

Appendix

Collaborators in the Lipid Research Clinic Program are: Lipid-Lipoprotein
Working Group - C.E. Davis, M. Feinleib, W. Hazzard, G. Heiss, D. Jacobs,
P. Kwiterovich, I. Tamir, H.A. Tyroler; LRC Epidemiology Committee - H.A.
Tyroler, Chairman, P. Anderson, E. Barrett-Connor, M. Brockway, G. Chase,
B. Christensen, M. Criqui, M. Davies, A. Deev, I. de Groot, M. Feinleib, M.
Fisher, I. Glasunov, G. Godin, S.T. Halfon, R. Harris, W. Haskell, G.
Heiss, D. Hewitt, J. Hill, J. Hoover, D. Jacobs, K. Kelly, J.A. Little, A.
Mackenthun, I. Mebane, J. Medalie, R. Mowery, J. Morrison, J.B. O'Sullivan,
B. Rifkind, C. Rubenstein, W.J. Schull, D. Shestov, I. Tamir, H. Taylor, P.

Van Natta, R. Wallace, O.D. Williams, A. Zadoja; <u>LRC Directors Committee</u>
F. Abboud, E. Bierman, R. Bradford, V. Brown, W. Connor, G. Cooper, J.
Farquhar, I. Frantz, C. Glueck, E. Gerasimova, A.M. Gotto, Jr., V.
Grambsch, J. Grizzle, W. Hazzard, F. Ibbott, W. Insull, A. Klimov, R.
Knopp, P. Kwiterovitch, J. LaRosa, J.A. Little, F. Mattson, M. Mishkel, B.
Rifkind, G. Schonfeld, R. Shank, T. Sheffield, Y. Stein, D. Steinberg, G.
Steiner.

INDEX

Apolipoprotein *(cont.)*
  hyperlipidemia and phenotypic expression of, 260–263
  immunoassay of
    methodological considerations in, 811–814
    standardization of, by isotope method, 804–806
  from LDL
    associating system in, 176–179
    electrophoresis of soluble, 177–179
    immunoelectrophoresis of fractions of, 179
    molecular weights of components of, 178
    size of, 176
  and lipids, transfer of, 658–659
  in lymph and plasma, 654–656
  spatial arrangement of, 174
Apoprotein, *see also* Apolipoprotein
  chylomicron composition and, 655
  hypolipidemic drugs and, 90–92
  infusion of, in apo-CII deficiency, 674
  levels of, in children, 287–288
    determinants of, 289–290
  origin and synthesis of, 144–145
  secretion of, from human intestine, 160–162
Arachidonic acid
  metabolites of, and vascular responses, 767, 768
  products of, ADP and, 776, 778
  transformations, 778, 779
Arterial injury and atherogenesis, 330–332
Arterial LPL and atherogenesis, 601
Artery growth during experimental period, 740–742, 744–745
Artery lesions and diet, 372
Artery wall
  atherogenetic factors of, 98–101
  and atherosclerotic lesions, 520–523
  elastic element in, 136–139
  progressive atherosclerosis and, 407–411
  transport of macromolecules across, 525–528
  unique reactivity of, 94–96
Aspirin, PGI2 and TXA2, 430–431
Atherogenesis
  arterial endothelium in, 103–109
  chylomicrons and, 600–602
  immunologic arterial injury and, 330–332
  intimal-endothelial injury and, 410
  SMC in, 99–100
Atherosclerotic lesions
  changes in, following surgical cholesterol reduction, 735–738
  epidemiology of, 52
  morphology of, 126–127
  raised, 57–61, 717
  regression of advanced, 749–752
Atherosclerosis
  autoimmune mechanisms in, 348–350
  childhood, smoking and, 278–281
  clinical significance of, 6–7
  diet treatment of, 305–306
  epidemiology of coronary, 54–56
  in Japan, 703–704

patterns of, 3–5
PGI2 deficiency and, 763–764
rates of progression of, 5–6
regression sequences after experimental, 731–734
smoking and various risk factors and, 67–70
study of regression of, 739–747
Atherosclerosis-diet-lipid relationship, 220–233
Attitude as mechanism of progress, 28
Authority and mechanisms of progress, 30

Barrier
  endothelial, 121–122, 133–134, 404, 551
  permeability, in arterial wall, 133–135
Bezafibrate and hyperlipidemia, 86, 87
Biliary lipid composition and hypolipidemic diets, 320–322
Binding, determinants responsible for, 644–645
Biologic mechanisms and CV disease, 274–275
Blood and artery, permeability and interaction of, 121–124
Blood-compatible container, endothelium as, 417–419
Blood pressure
  CHD death and, 54–56
  in children, 513–514
  coronary atherosclerosis and, 57–61
  coronary risk factors and, 297, 299–301
  diets and, 363
  after vasectomy, 326, 328
Body weight and dietary fat and hyperlipidemia, CHD and, 307–310
Bradykinin, PG synthesis and, 768, 769
Bran, 312
Butter consumption, 206–207

C-HDL, *see* HDL cholesterol
CAD, *see* Coronary artery disease
600-Calorie diet and bile lipids, 321
Cancer and viral hepatitis and immunoregulatory lipoproteins, 340–343
Cardiac catheterization, 12
Cardiological results of plasma exchange, 460–461
Cardiovascular disease, 272–276
  death rates for, 44
  mechanisms of, 272–276
  portacaval shunt and, 451
  risk factors, 359–363
    population characteristics and, 273–276
  tobacco and immunologic injury and, 337–338
Cardiovascular surgery, progress in, 26–34
  animal experiments, 29–30
  attitude and, 28
  authority and, 30
  clinical utilization of new operative techniques, 32–33
  necessity of, 27–28
  publication and, 29
  serendipity, 28
  spilling over of ideas, 31
  World War II and, 32
Carotid artery reendothelialization, 106

Cytoplasmic TG, deposition and hydrolysis of, in SMC, 796−799

Death, smoking and, 68
Death rates
 for cardiovascular disease, 44
 for ischemic heart disease, 230
Deendothelialization (DEE), 104−107
Demographic factors, C-HDL levels and, 488−492
Diet
 artery lesions and, 372
 atherosclerosis and, 351−352, 355−356
  reversal of, 369−373
  treatment of, 305−306
 blood pressure and, 363
 CA disease prevention and, 199−207
 CH disease and, 233, 307−310
  body weight and, 307−310
  fatty acids and, 235−241
  prevention of, 209−218
 CH disease death and, 63−65
 cholesterol and, 206−207, 215, 230
 disease and, 219
 fat in, 307−310
  analysis of, in United Kingdom, 239
 fatty acids in, 237−238
 fiber in, *see* Fiber, dietary
 hyperlipidemia and, 86, 88, 307−310, 365−368
 LDL cholesterol and, in FH, 79−80
 lipoprotein changes and, 356−357
Diet-lipid-atherosclerosis relationship, 220−233
Dietary change
 body weight and serum lipids and, 308
 eggs and, 206−207
 milk and cream and, 206−207
 plasma LPL and, 316−319
 vegetable fats and oils and, 206−207
Dietary goals, U.S., 1977, 236
DMPC (dimyristoyl phosphatidylcholine) hydrolysis, 182
DNA, specific activity of, 568
DPE-chylomicrons, LPL and, 180, 181
DPE-VLDL fluorescence, LPL and, 180, 181
Dimyristoyl phosphatidylcholine (DMPC) hydrolysis, 182
Drugs
 FH and, 78−81
 HDL metabolism and, 591−594
 hyperlipidemia and, 71−72, 86−89
 hypolipidemic, 90
 Type II hyperlipoproteinemia and, 74−77

E-A (ethanolamine-agarose) and lipoproteins, 467
EC (esterified cholesterol), *see* Cholesteryl esters
Education, humanistic, 517
Egg consumption, 206−207
Elastins
 biosynthesis of, 136−137
 degradation of, 137−138

lipids and, 138
Electrophoresis, rate-nephelometry of A-I and, 807−810
Endocytosis recycling via coated pits, 283−285
Endothelial biology, 415−421
Endothelial cells, 112−118
 undulating pattern of, 113, 117
Endothelial dysfunction
 and pathogenesis of atherosclerosis, 415−421
 and response-to-injury hypothesis, 421
Endothelial injury hypothesis of atherogenesis, 563
Endothelial permeability barrier, 121−122, 133−134, 404, 554
 selective, 416−417
Endothelium, 98
 alterations of, in arteriosclerosis, 557−560
 aortic, 113, 118
  changes in, 699−702
 arterial, in atherogenesis, 103−109
 as blood-compatible container, 417−419
 blue area, showing short junctions, 112, 114
 chylomicron attachment to, 655, 656−657
 in experimental atherosclerosis, 563−565
 functions of, 415−419
 hydrolysis of VLDL-TG on, 660
 injury to, 99, 419−420
 intimal thickening and, 563−565
 passage of cells through intact, 99
 passage of soluble material through intact, 98−99
 PGI₂ formation by, 141−142
 repair of, 419−420
 selective permeability of, 416−417
 synthetic-metabolic-secretory activities of, 417
 turnover rate of, 551
 ultrastructure of arterial, 112−118
 vascular, 415
 white area elongated, 112, 114
Environmental agents causing natural selection, CH disease and, 326−327
Environmental factors
 in atherosclerosis, 57, 324−328
 and C-HDL, 492
 in lipid regulation, 230−231
Enzymatic regulation of LP catabolism, 631−639
Enzyme activation in apolipoprotein, 624−625
Epidemiological data on CH disease incidence, 229−232
Epidemiology
 of atherosclerotic lesions, 52
 of coronary atherosclerosis, 54−56
 and HDL, 495−498
Erythrocyte cation fluxes measurement in hypertension, 712−714
Erythrocyte-hemodynamics hypothesis for arterial thrombosis, 554
Estrogen
 CH disease mortality and, 498
 CH disease risk and, 498
Ethanolamine-agarose (E-A), lipoprotein and, 467